Abdominal Imaging

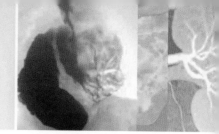

Abdominal Imaging

Dushyant V. Sahani, MD

Associate Professor of Radiology, Harvard Medical School
Assistant Radiologist, Abdominal Imaging & Intervention
Director, CT Imaging Services
Massachusetts General Hospital
Boston, MA

Anthony E. Samir, MD

Clinical Instructor of Radiology, Harvard Medical School
Assistant Radiologist, Abdominal Imaging & Intervention
Associate Director, Ultrasound Imaging Services
Massachusetts General Hospital
Boston, MA

SAUNDERS

ELSEVIER

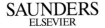

3251 Riverport Lane
Maryland Heights, Missouri 63043

Notice

Knowledge and best practice in this field are constantly changing. As new research and experience broaden our knowledge, changes in practice, treatment and drug therapy may become necessary or appropriate. Readers are advised to check the most current information provided (i) on procedures featured or (ii) by the manufacturer of each product to be administered, to verify the recommended dose or formula, the method and duration of administration, and contraindications. It is the responsibility of the practitioner, relying on their own experience and knowledge of the patient, to make diagnoses, to determine dosages and the best treatment for each individual patient, and to take all appropriate safety precautions. To the fullest extent of the law, neither the publisher nor the editors assumes any liability for any injury and/or damage to persons or property arising out of or related to any use of the material contained in this book.

The Publisher

Library of Congress Cataloging-in-Publication Data
Abdominal imaging / [edited by] Dushyant V. Sahani, Anthony E. Samir.—1st ed.
     p. ; cm.—(Expert radiology series)
   Includes bibliographical references and index.
   ISBN 978-1-4160-5449-8 (alk. paper)
   1. Abdomen—Imaging.   I. Sahani, Dushyant V.   II. Samir, Anthony E.   III. Series: Expert radiology
series.
   [DNLM: 1. Digestive System Diseases—diagnosis.   2. Abdomen—physiopathology.   3. Abdomen—
radionuclide imaging.   4. Diagnostic Imaging—methods. WI 141 A1353 2010]
   RC944.A172   2010
   617.5'507572—dc22
                                                                              2010002582

Acquisitions Editor: Rebecca Gaertner
Developmental Editor: Roxanne Halpine
Publishing Services Managers: Tina Rebane, Jeff Patterson
Project Managers: Norm Stellander, Megan Isenberg
Design Direction: Steve Stave
Illustration Manager: Ceil Nuyianes
Marketing Manager: Radha Mawrie

Working together to grow
libraries in developing countries

www.elsevier.com | www.bookaid.org | www.sabre.org

ELSEVIER   BOOK AID International   Sabre Foundation

Printed in China

Last digit is the print number: 9   8   7   6   5   4   3   2   1

With great fondness I dedicate this book to mentors, colleagues, and students for their contributions in my personal and professional life that made me worthy of editing this book, and to my family for their unconditional love, encouragement, and unwavering support.
Dushyant V. Sahani

I dedicate this book to my wife, Susan, whose love and support make everything possible; to my son, Noah, whose loving smile brings me the purest joy; and to my parents, Charlotte and Moshe, who sacrificed much so that I could achieve something meaningful.
Anthony E. Samir

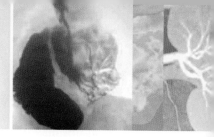

Contributors

Abhishek Rajendra Agarwal, MD, DNB
Research Scholar, Abdominal Imaging, Department of
Radiology, Emory University School of Medicine,
Atlanta, Georgia
Normal Anatomy and Variants of the Colon

Diego A. Aguirre, MD
Assistant Professor of Radiology, El Bosque University;
Chairman, Department of Medical Imaging,
Fundación Santa Fe de Bogotá, University Hospital,
Bogotá, Columbia
*Normal Anatomy of the Abdominal Wall, Non-neoplastic Conditions
of the Abdominal Wall, Neoplastic Conditions of the Abdominal
Wall, Abdominal Wall Hernias*

Pritish Aher, MBBS, DMRD
Consultant Radiologist, Pune, Maharashtra, India
*Fluoroscopic Study of the Abdomen and Fluoroscopic
Contrast Media*

Stephan W. Anderson, MD
Assistant Professor, Department of Radiology, Director
of Body CT, Boston University Medical Center,
Boston, Massachusetts
*Acute Appendicitis, Hollow Viscus Perforation, Acute Gastrointestinal
Bleeding*

Ashwin Asrani, MD, MBBS
Clincal Fellow in Radiology, Harvard Medical School;
Clinical Assistant in Radiology, Massachusetts
General Hospital, Boston, Massachusetts
*Imaging of the Penis, Erectile Dysfunction, Penile Trauma and
Miscellaneous Penile Lesions, Imaging of the Scrotum, Benign
Testicular Lesions, Malignant Testicular Lesions*

Arpan K. Banerjee, MBBS (LOND), FRCP, FRCR, FBIR
Hon Senior Clinical Lecturer, Birmingham Medical
School; Consultant Radiologist, Heart of England
Foundation NHS Trust, Birmingham, England,
United Kingdom; Past President Radiology Section
2005-2007, Royal Society of Medicine, London,
England, United Kingdom
Peritonitis and Peritoneal Abscess

William Bennett, MD
Associate Professor of Radiology, Ohio State University,
College of Medicine; Attending Radiologist, Ohio
State Medicial Center, Columbus, Ohio
Small Bowel Obstruction

Senta Berggruen, MD
Assistant Professor of Radiology, Feinberg School of
Medicine, Northwestern University, Chicago, Illinois
Conventional Imaging of the Small Bowel

Michael Blake, MB, BCh, BSc, MRCPI, FRCR, FFR (RCSI)
Assistant Professor of Radiology, Harvard Medical
School; Assistant Radiologist, Massachusetts
General Hospital, Boston, Massachusetts
*PET/CT Technique and Instrumentation, Pearls and Pitfalls in
PET and PET/CT Interpretation, PET and PET/CT Clinical
Applications, Imaging of Adrenal Glands, Enlarged Adrenal
Glands, Adrenal Masses*

Giuseppe Brancatelli, MD
Associate Professor of Radiology, Department of
Radiology, University of Palermo, Palermo, Sicily,
Italy
Benign Focal Lesions, Malignant Focal Lesions

Wenli Cai, PhD
Assistant Professor of Radiology, Harvard Medical
School; Assistant Computer Scientist, Massachusetts
General Hospital, Boston, Massachusetts
*Principles of 3D Postprocessing, Advanced Applications in
Postprocessing*

Vito Cantisani, MD, PhD
Professor of Radiology, Instructor in Radiology,
Department of Radiological Sciences, University
Sapienza of Rome, Rome, Italy
Plain Radiography of the Abdomen

Giovanni Carbognin, MD
Department of Radiology, University Hospital, Verona,
Italy
Imaging of the Pancreas

Onofrio Catalano, MD
Clinical Fellow, Harvard Medical School; Clinical Fellow, Department of Radiology, Massachusetts General Hospital, Boston, Massachusetts
Hepatic Variants, Pancreas—Normal Variants, Solid Pancreatic Masses, Cystic Lesions of the Pancreas

Michael Chew, MBBS, BA
Fellow in Abdominal and Interventional Imaging, Massachusetts General Hospital, Boston, Massachusetts
Dilated Bile Ducts

Aqeel Ahmad Chowdhry, MD
Staff Radiologist, Department of Radiology, Cleveland Clinic—South Pointe Hospital, Cleveland, Ohio
Neoplastic Conditions of the Mesentery and Omentum

Garry Choy, MD, MS, MSc
Clinical Fellow, Department of Radiology, Harvard Medical School; Clinical Fellow, Massachusetts General Hospital, Boston, Massachusetts
Principles of MRI Physics, MRI Instrumentation and Safety, MRI Pulse Sequences, MRI Artifacts, Contrast Media and Contrast-Enhanced MRI, MR Angiography, Advanced MRI Applications

Rivka R. Colen, MD
Radiology Resident, Massachusetts General Hospital, Boston, Massachusetts
Gastric Function Imaging Techniques, Clinical Applications of Gastric Function Imaging, Imaging of the Scrotum, Benign Testicular Lesions

Carmel Cronin, MD, MB, BCh, MRCPI, FFR (RCSI)
Radiology Fellow, Department of Abdominal Imaging and Interventional Radiology, Massachusetts General Hospital, Boston, Massachusetts
Imaging of the Prostate and Seminal Vesicles, Benign Prostate Hypertrophy, Benign Focal Prostate Lesions, Malignant Focal Prostate Lesions, Seminal Vesicle Lesions

Abraham H. Dachman, MD, FACR
Professor of Radiology, Director of Fellowship Programs, The University of Chicago Medical Center, Chicago, Illinois
Benign Neoplasms and Wall Thickening of the Small Bowel

Ugo D'Ambrosio, MD
Resident, Department of Radiological Sciences, University Sapienza of Rome, Rome, Italy
Plain Radiography of the Abdomen

Hemali Desai, MD
Research Fellow, Massachusetts General Hospital, Boston, Massachusetts; Resident, Beth Israel Medical Center, Newark, New Jersey
Imaging of Chronic Pancreatitis

Mirko D'Onofrio, MD
Assistant Professor of Radiology, G.B. Rossi University Hospital, University of Verona, Verona, Italy
Imaging of the Pancreas

Silvana C. Faria, MD, PhD
Assistant Professor, MD Anderson Cancer Center, Houston, Texas
Fatty Liver Disease, Hepatic Storage Disorders, Hepatitis, Cholestatic Hepatic Disorders

Todd Fibus, MD
Assistant Professor, Department of Radiology, VA Medical Center, Emory University School of Medicine, Atlanta, Georgia
Conventional Imaging of Colon and Rectum

Efrén J. Flores, MD
Harvard Medical School, Department of Radiology, Massachusetts General Hospital, Boston, Massachusetts
Imaging of the Postoperative Bowel

Mark Frank, MD
Associate Professor of Radiology, Indiana University School of Medicine, Indianapolis, Indiana
Anatomy of Peritoneum and Retroperitoneum, Non-neoplastic Conditions of the Peritoneum

Anna Galluzzo, MD, FRCR
Research Fellow, Division of Abdominal Imaging and Intervention, Massachusetts General Hospital, Boston, Massachusetts; Department of Radiology, University of Palermo Policlinico, Palermo, Italy
Ultrasonography of the Liver

Karthik Ganesan, DNB
Radiologist, Liver Imaging Group, Department of Radiology, University of California San Diego, San Diego, California; Consultant Radiologist, Piramal Diagnostics and Jankharia Imaging, Mumbai, India
Hepatic Iron Overload

Alpa G. Garg, MD
Clinical Assistant, Massachusetts General Hospital, Boston, Massachusetts
Benign Bladder Lesions

Arunas E. Gasparaitis, MD
Assistant Professor, Department of Radiology, University of Chicago; Director of Fluoroscopic Services, University of Chicago Medical Center, Chicago, Illinois
Benign Neoplasms and Wall Thickening of the Small Bowel, Malignant Neoplasms and Wall Thickening of the Small Bowel

Michael S. Gee, MD, PhD
Instructor in Radiology, Harvard Medical School; Assistant Radiologist, Divisions of Pediatric Radiology and Abdominal Imaging and Intervention, Massachusetts General Hospital, Boston, Massachusetts
Small Bowel Anomalies and Variants

Sukanya Ghosh, MBBS, MRCP, FRCR
St. Bartholomew and the Royal London Hospital, London, England, United Kingdom
Conventional Imaging of the Stomach and Duodenum, CT of the Stomach and Duodenum, Anatomic Variants of the Stomach and Duodenum

Thomas Grant, DO
Professor of Radiology, Feinberg School of Medicine, Northwestern University; Attending Radiologist, Northwestern Memorial Hospital, Chicago, Illinois
Ultrasound Imaging of the Small Bowel

Rossella Graziani, MD
Radiologist, University Hospital, University of Verona, Verona, Italy
Imaging of the Pancreas

Kavita Gulati, MD
Radiology, Brigham and Women's Hospital, Boston, Massachusetts
Imaging Techniques for the Gallbladder and Bile Ducts, Gallbladder and Bile Ducts—Variants and Anomalies

Arti Gupta, MD, DABR
Assistant Professor of Radiology, University of Kansas School of Medicine; Radiologist, Wesley Medical Center, Wichita, Kansas
Nuclear Medicine Techniques for the Small Bowel

Peter F. Hahn, MD, PhD
Associate Professor of Radiology, Harvard Medical School; Radiologist, Massachusetts General Hospital, Boston, Massachusetts
Dilated Bile Ducts

Nancy A. Hammond, MD
Assistant Professor of Radiology, Feinberg School of Medicine, Northwestern University; Staff Radiologist, Body Imaging, Northwestern Memorial Hospital, Chicago, Illinois
MRI of the Small Bowel

Robert Hanna, MD
Radiologist (Physician), Department of Radiology, University of California San Diego, San Diego, California
Cirrhosis, Hepatic Iron Overload

Peter A. Harri, MD
Resident Physician, Department of Radiology, Emory University School of Medicine, Atlanta, Georgia
Normal Anatomy and Variants of the Colon

Gordon J. Harris, PhD
Associate Professor of Radiology, Harvard Medical School; Director of 3D Imaging Service, Department of Radiology, Massachusetts General Hospital, Boston, Massachusetts
Principles of 3D Postprocessing, Advanced Applications of Postprocessing, CT of Liver

Donald Hawes, MD
Associate Professor of Radiology, Indiana University School of Medicine, Indianapolis, Indiana
Anatomy of Peritoneum and Retroperitoneum, Non-neoplastic Conditions of the Peritoneum

Miguel Hernandez Pampaloni, MD, PhD
Assistant Professor of Radiology, Chief, Nuclear Medicine, University of California San Francisco, San Francisco, California
Nuclear Imaging of the Liver

Mai-Lan Ho, MD
Clinical Fellow in Radiology, Harvard Medical School; Resident—Scholar's Track, Department of Radiology, Beth Israel Deaconess Medical Center, Boston, Massachusetts
Tumors of Gallbladder, Intrahepatic Bile Duct Tumors, Extrahepatic Bile Duct Tumors

Nagaraj-Setty Holalkere, MD, DNB
Instructor, Department of Radiology, Boston Medical Center, Boston, Massachusetts
Imaging of Adrenal Glands, Enlarged Adrenal Glands, Adrenal Masses

Kedar Jambhekar, MD, DNB
Assistant Professor, Department of Radiology, University of Arkansas for Medical Sciences, Little Rock, Arkansas
Diffuse Renal Parenchymal Diseases, Renal Parenchymal Infections, Renal Vascular Diseases, Miscellaneous Diffuse Renal Diseases

Bijal Jankharia, MBBS, DMRE, DMRD, DNB
Teacher and Consultant, Piramal Diagnostics, Jankharia Imaging, Mumbai, Maharashtra, India
Doppler Ultrasound Imaging

Saurabh Jha, MBBS, MRCS
Assistant Professor of Radiology, University of Pennsylvania, Philadelphia, Pennsylvania
Nuclear Imaging of the Liver

Akash Joshi, MD, DABR
Assistant Professor of Radiology, University of Kansas School of Medicine; Radiologist, Wesley Medical Center, Wichita, Kansas
Nuclear Medicine Techniques for the Small Bowel

Sanjeeva P. Kalva, MD, MB, BS

Assistant Professor, Department of Radiology, Harvard Medical School; Associate Director of Clinical Affairs, Division of Vascular Imaging & Intervention, Department of Radiology, Massachusetts General Hospital, Boston, Massachusetts

Acute Small Bowel Ischemia, Chronic Small Bowel Ischemia

Avinash Kambadakone R., MBBS, MD, DNB, FRCR

Clinical Fellow in Abdominal Imaging and Intervention, Massachusetts General Hospital, Boston, Massachusetts

Recent Advances, CT Protocols for Abdomen and Pelvis, Diffuse Gallbladder Wall Thickening, Focal Gallbladder Wall Thickening, Lymph Node Imaging Techniques, Clincal Role of Lymph Node Imaging

David P. Katz, MD

Assistant Professor, Department of Radiology, Baylor College of Medicine, Houston, Texas

Conventional Imaging of the Kidneys and Urinary Tract, Cystic Renal Lesions

Keerthana Kesavarapu, BS

Department of Biology, Georgia Institute of Technology, Atlanta, Georgia

Conventional Imaging of the Colon and Rectum

Danny Kim, MD

Assistant Professor, Department of Radiology, New York University Langone Medical Center, New York, New York

MRI of Liver: From Sequences to Protocol

Kyoung Won Kim, MD

Assistant Professor, Department of Radiology, University of Ulsan College of Medicine; Asan Medical Center, Seoul, Korea

Focal Splenic Lesions, Diffuse Splenic Lesions

Min Ju Kim, MD

Department of Radiology, National Cancer Center, Goyang-si, Gyeonggi-do, Korea

Focal Splenic Lesions, Diffuse Splenic Lesions

Marie R. Koch, MD

Resident, Radiology, Brigham and Women's Hospital, Boston, Massachusetts

Small Bowel Obstruction

Kirti Kulkarni, MD

Assistant Professor, Department of Radiology, University of Chicago, Chicago, Illinois

Malignant Neoplasms and Wall Thickening of the Small Bowel

Naveen M. Kulkarni, MD, DNB

Fellow, Abdominal Imaging and Interventional Radiology, Massachusetts General Hospital, Boston, Massachusetts

Fluoroscopic Study of the Abdomen and Fluoroscopic Contrast Media, Instrumentation and Radiation Safety, Colonic Vascular Lesions, Imaging of Chronic Pancreatitis

A. Nick Kurup, MD

Instructor, Department of Radiology, Mayo Clinic College of Medicine, Rochester, Minnesota

CT of the Kidneys and Urinary Tract, Malignant Focal Renal Lesions

Somesh Lala, MBBS, DMRD, DNB

Teacher, Consultant Radiologist, and Sonologist, Piramal Diagnostics; Consultant Radiologist and Sonologist, Midtown Diagnostics, Jankharia Imaging, Mumbai, Maharashtra, India

Doppler Ultrasound Imaging

Chandana G. Lall, MD

Associate Professor of Clinical Radiology, Indiana University School of Medicine, Indianapolis, Indiana

Peritoneal Fluid Collections

Dipti K. Lenhart, MD

Department of Radiology, Massachusetts General Hospital, Boston, Massachusetts

Colon Cancer and Screening Strategies

Bob Liu, PhD

Instructor in Radiology, Harvard Medical School; Director of Radiological Physics, Department of Radiology, Massachusetts General Hospital, Boston, Massachusetts

Instrumentation and Radiation Safety

Xiaozhou Ma, MD

Research Fellow, Harvard Medical School; Fellow, 3D Imaging, Massachusetts General Hospital, Boston, Massachusetts

Harmonic Imaging, Four-Dimensional Ultrasound Imaging, Contrast Media and Contrast-Enhanced Ultrasound Evaluation

Michael Macari, MD

Vice Chair of Operations, Section Chief of Abdominal Imaging, New York University Langone School of Medicine, New York, New York

Inflammatory and Infectious Colonic Lesions

Riccardo Manfredi, MD

Associate Professor, Department of Diagnostic Imaging, University of Verona, Verona, Italy

Imaging of the Pancreas

Andrea Marcantonio, MD

Resident, Department of Radiological Sciences, University Sapienza of Rome, Rome, Italy

Plain Radiography of the Abdomen

Daniele Marin, MD
Department of Radiology, Duke University Medical Center, Durham, North Carolina; Department of Radiology, University of Rome Sapienza, Rome, Italy
Benign Focal Lesions, Malignant Focal Lesions

Jaime Martinez, MD
Associated Radiologist, Body Imaging Section, Fundación Santa Fe de Bogotá University Hospital, Bogotá, Columbia
Normal Anatomy of the Abdominal Wall, Abdominal Wall Hernias

Deepa Masrani, MD
Clinical Assistant Professor, Women's Imaging, Upstate Medical University, State University of New York, Syracuse, New York
Imaging of the Penis, Erectile Dysfunction

Sameer M. Mazhar, MD
Fellow, Division of Gastroenterology, University of California San Diego, San Diego, California
Fatty Liver Disease, Cirrhosis, Hepatic Iron Overload, Hepatic Storage Disorders, Hepatitis, Hepatic Veno-occlusive Diseases, Cholestatic Hepatic Disorders

Vishakha Mazumdar, MBBS
Fellow, Radiology, Piramal Diagnostics, Jankharia Imaging, Mumbai, Maharashtra, India
Doppler Ultrasound Imaging

Jennifer McDowell, MM
Ultrasound and 3D Ultrasound Technical Manager, Massachusetts General Hospital, Boston, Massachusetts
Ultrasound Physics and Instrumentation: A Condensed View, Abdominal Ultrasound Imaging

Pardeep Mittal, MD
Assistant Professor, Department of Radiology, Emory University School of Medicine, Atlanta, Georgia
Conventional Imaging of Colon and Rectum, CT of the Colon and Rectum, Normal Anatomy and Variants of the Colon

Michael Moore, MB, BCh, FFR (RCSI)
Radiologist, Abdominal Imaging, Massachusetts General Hospital, Boston, Massachusetts; Consultant Radiologist, Mercy University Hospital, Cork, Ireland
PET/CT Technique and Instrumentation, Pearls and Pitfalls in PET and PET/CT Interpretation, PET and PET/CT Clinical Applications

Giovanni Morana, MD
Director, Radiological Department, General Hospital, Treviso, Italy
Gallbladder and Bile Duct Functional Imaging

Ajaykumar Morani, MBBS, MD
Clinical Lecturer I, Body Imaging, Department of Radiology, University of Michigan, Ann Arbor, Michigan
Imaging of the Penis, Erectile Dysfunction, Penile Trauma and Miscellaneous Penile Lesions, Imaging of the Scrotum, Benign Testicular Lesions, Malignant Testicular Lesions

Massimiliano Motton, MD
Department of Radiology, G.B. Rossi Hospital Verona, Verona, Italy
Imaging of the Pancreas

Ozden Narin, MD
Research Fellow, Department of Radiology, Massachusetts General Hospital, Boston, Massachusetts
Colonic Vascular Lesions

Vamsidhar R. Narra, MD
Associate Professor of Radiology, Co-Chief, Body MRI, Washington University School of Medicine; Chief, Abdominal Imaging, Chief of Radiology, Barnes-Jewish West County Hospital, St. Louis, Missouri
Tumors of the Gallbladder, Intrahepatic Bile Duct Tumors, Extra-hepatic Bile Duct Tumors

Paul Nikolaidis, MD
Associate Professor of Radiology, Feinberg School of Medicine, Northwestern University; Staff Radiologist, Body Imaging, Northwestern Memorial Hospital, Chicago, Illinois
MRI of the Small Bowel

Aytekin Oto, MD
Associate Professor of Radiology, Chief of Abdominal Imaging; Chief, Body MRI, Department of Radiology, University of Chicago, Chicago, Illinois
Benign Neoplasms and Wall Thickening of the Small Bowel, Malignant Neoplasms and Wall Thickening of the Small Bowel

Tarun Pandey, MD, DNB, FRCR
Assistant Professor of Radiology, University of Arkansas for Medical Sciences, Little Rock, Arkansas
Diffuse Renal Parenchymal Diseases, Renal Parenchymal Infections, Renal Vascular Diseases, Miscellaneous Diffuse Renal Diseases

Ralph C. Panek, MD
Staff Radiologist, Department of Radiology, St. Elizabeth's Hospital, Brighton, Massachusetts
Malignant Bladder Lesions

Heather M. Patton, MD
Assistant Clinical Professor of Medicine, Division of Gastroenterology, University of California San Diego, San Diego, California
Fatty Liver Disease, Hepatic Iron Overload

Rocio Perez Johnston, MD
Research Fellow, Abdominal Imaging, Massachusetts General Hospital, Boston, Massachusetts
Ultrasonography of the Liver

Rodolfo F. Perini, MD
Fellow, Medical Oncology and Nuclear Medicine, Hospital of the University of Pennsylvania, Philadelphia, Pennsylvania
Nuclear Imaging of the Kidneys and Urinary Tract

Christine M. Peterson, MD
Assistant Professor of Radiology, Body Imaging Section, Penn State Hershey Radiology, Hershey, Pennsylvania
Tumors of the Gallbladder, Intrahepatic Bile Duct Tumors, Extrahepatic Bile Duct Tumors

Michael R. Peterson, MD, PhD
Assistant Clinical Professor, Pathology, University of California San Diego, San Diego, California
Cirrhosis, Hepatic Iron Overload, Hepatic Storage Disorders, Hepatitis, Hepatic Veno-occlusive Diseases, Cholestatic Hepatic Disorders

Giuseppe Petralia, MD
Radiologist, Division of Radiology, European Institute of Oncology, Milan, Italy
Gallbladder and Bile Duct Functional Imaging

Niall Power, MRCPI, FRCR
Consultant Radiologist, Radiology Department, Royal London Hospital, London, England, United Kingdom
Conventional Imaging of the Stomach and Duodenum, CT of the Stomach and Duodenum, Anatomic Variants of the Stomach and Duodenum

Anand M. Prabhakar, MD
Clinical Fellow in Abdominal Imaging, Harvard Medical School, Massachusetts General Hospital, Boston, Massachusetts
Malignant Mucosal Diseases of the Stomach, Gastric Stromal Tumors

Hima B. Prabhakar, MD
Staff Radiologist, South Texas Radiology Group, San Antonio, Texas
Benign Mucosal Diseases of the Stomach, Malignant Mucosal Diseases of the Stomach, Gastric Stromal Tumors, Gastric Outlet Obstruction, Abnormal Positions of the Stomach

Priya D. Prabhakar, MD, MPH
Clinical Assistant Professor of Radiology, Department of Radiology, Jefferson Medical College; Staff Radiologist, Department of Radiology, Albert Einstein Medical Center, Philadelphia, Pennsylvania
Gastric Outlet Obstruction, Abnormal Positions of the Stomach

Srinivasa R. Prasad, MD
Professor, Radiology Department, University of Texas Health Science Center at San Antonio, San Antonio, Texas
Imaging of the Urethra, Imaging of Disorders of the Female Urethra, Imaging of Disorders of the Male Urethra

Daniel A. Pryma, MD
Assistant Professor of Radiology, Modality Chief, Nuclear Medicine/Molecular Imaging, Department of Radiology, University of Pennsylvania, Philadelphia, Pennsylvania
Nuclear Imaging of the Liver, Nuclear Imaging of the Kidneys and Urinary Tract

Arumugam Rajesh, MBBS, FRCR
Consultant Radiologist, Honorary Senior Lecturer, University Hospitals of Leicester NHS Trust, Leicester, England, United Kingdom
Peritonitis and Peritoneal Abscess

Anuradha S. Rebello, MBBS
Instructor, Department of Radiology, Boston University, Boston, Massachusetts
Imaging of Acute Pancreatitis

Maryam Rezvani, MD
Assistant Professor, Department of Radiology, University of Utah, Salt Lake City, Utah
CT of the Small Bowel

Oscar M. Rivero, MD
Assistant Professor of Radiology, El Bosque University; Associate Radiologist, Department of Medical Imaging, Fundación Santa Fe de Bogotá University Hospital, Bogotá, Columbia
Normal Anatomy of the Abdominal Wall, Non-neoplastic Conditions of the Abdominal Wall, Neoplastic Conditions of the Abdominal Wall, Abdominal Wall Hernias

Johannes B. Roedl, MD
Department of Radiology, Harvard Medical School, Massachusetts General Hospital, Boston, Massachusetts
Gastric Function Imaging Techniques, Clinical Applications of Gastric Function Imaging

David A. Rosman, MD, MBA
Assistant Radiologist, Abdominal Imaging and Intervention, Department of Radiology, Massachusetts General Hospital, Boston, Massachusetts
Colon Cancer and Screening Strategies

Dushyant V. Sahani, MD
Associate Professor of Radiology, Harvard Medical School; Assistant Radiologist, Abdominal Imaging & Intervention; Director, CT Imaging Services, Massachusetts General Hospital, Boston, Massachusetts

Principles of 3D Postprocessing, Advanced Applications in Postprocessing, Colon Cancer and Screening Strategies, Imaging of the Postoperative Bowel, Ultrasonography of the Liver, CT of the Liver, Hepatic Variants, Pancreas—Normal Variants, Solid Pancreatic Masses, Cystic Lesions of the Pancreas, Imaging of Acute Pancreatitis, Imaging Techniques for the Gallbladder and Bile Ducts, Gallbladder and Bile Ducts—Variants and Anomalies, Diffuse Gallbladder Wall Thickening, Focal Gallbladder Wall Thickening, Lymph Node Imaging Techniques, Clincal Role of Lymph Node Imaging

Nisha I. Sainani, MD
Clinical Fellow, Abdominal Imaging and Interventional Radiology, Massachusetts General Hospital, Boston, Massachusetts

Miscellaneous Pancreatitis, Diffuse Pancreatic Disease

Anthony E. Samir, MD
Clinical Instructor of Radiology, Harvard Medical School; Assistant Radiologist, Abdominal Imaging & Intervention; Associate Director, Ultrasound Imaging Services, Massachusetts General Hospital, Boston, Massachusetts

Conventional Imaging of the Kidneys and Urinary Tract, CT of the Kidneys and Urinary Tract, MRI of the Kidneys and Urinary Tract, Benign Focal Renal Lesions, Malignant Focal Renal Lesions, Cystic Renal Lesions, Urinary Tract Obstruction, Benign Ureteral Strictures, Malignant Ureteral Strictures, Benign Bladder Lesions, Malignant Bladder Lesions

Kumaresan Sandrasegaran, MD
Associate Professor of Radiology, Indiana University School of Medicine, Indianapolis, Indiana

Principles of CT Physics, Recent Advances, CT Protocols for Abdomen and Pelvis, Anatomy of Peritoneum and Retroperitoneum, Peritoneal Fluid Collections, Peritonitis and Peritoneal Abscess, Non-neoplastic Conditions of the Peritoneum, Neoplastic Conditions of the Mesentery and Omentum

Cynthia S. Santillan, MD
Assistant Clinical Professor of Radiology, University of California San Diego, San Diego, California

Hepatic Veno-occlusive Diseases

Rupan Sanyal, MD
Clinical Associate, Staff Radiologist, Radiology HBG, Cleveland Clinic, Cleveland, Ohio

CT Contrast Media and Principles of Contrast Enhancement

Alissa Saunders, MD
Clinical Assistant, Massachusetts General Hospital, Boston, Massachusetts

Benign Ureteral Strictures, Malignant Ureteral Strictures

Richard T. Scuderi, MD, PhD
Fellow, Surgical Pathology, University of California San Diego, San Diego, California

Fatty Liver Disease

Melanie Seale, MBBS, FRANZCR
Radiologist, St. Vincent's Hospital Melbourne, University of Melbourne, Fitzroy, Victoria, Australia

Urinary Tract Obstruction

Sunit Sebastian, MD
Assistant Professor, Department of Radiology; Chief, Division of Body Imaging, University of Mississippi Medical Center, Jackson, Mississippi

Conventional Imaging of the Colon and Rectum, CT of the Colon and Rectum, CT Colonography, Normal Anatomy and Variants of the Colon

Hemendra Shah, MD, FACR
Professor of Radiology and Urology, University of Arkansas for Medical Sciences, Little Rock, Arkansas

Diffuse Renal Parenchymal Diseases, Renal Parenchymal Infections, Renal Vascular Diseases, Miscellaneous Diffuse Renal Diseases

Shetal N. Shah, MD
Visiting Associate Professor of Radiology, Cleveland Clinic Lerner School of Medicine at Case Western Reserve University; Co-Director, Center for PET and Molecular Imaging; Staff, Cleveland Clinic Imaging Institute, Cleveland, Ohio

CT Contrast Media and Principles of Contrast Enhancement, Neoplastic Conditions of the Mesentery and Omentum

Zarine K. Shah, MD, MBBS
Assistant Professor, Department of Radiology, Divison of Abdominal Imaging, Ohio State University Medical Center, Columbus, Ohio

Small Bowel Obstruction

Masoud Shiehmorteza, MD
Liver Imaging Group, Department of Radiology, University of California San Diego, San Diego, California

Hepatitis

Ajay Singh, MD
Assistant Professor of Radiology, Massachusetts General Hospital, Boston, Massachusetts

Pearls and Pitfalls in PET and PET/CT Interpretation

Anand Singh, MD, AFIH
Research Fellow, Harvard Medical School, Massachusetts General Hospital, Boston, Massachusetts

Principles of 3D Postprocessing, Advanced Applications in Postprocessing, CT of the Liver

Claude B. Sirlin, MD
Associate Professor, Liver Imaging Group, Department of Radiology, University of California San Diego, San Diego, California

Fatty Liver Disease, Cirrhosis, Hepatic Iron Overload, Hepatic Storage Disorders, Hepatitis, Hepatic Veno-occlusive Diseases, Cholestatic Hepatic Disorders

William Small, MD, PhD
Associate Professor, Department of Radiology; Director of Abdominal Imaging, Department of Radiology, Emory University School of Medicine, Emory University Hospital, Atlanta, Georgia

Conventional Imaging of the Colon and Rectum, CT of the Colon and Rectum, CT Colonography, Normal Anatomy and Variants of the Colon

Jorge A. Soto, MD
Professor of Radiology, Boston University School of Medicine; Vice Chairman, Department of Radiology, Boston Medical Center, Boston, Massachusetts

Ureteral and Kidney Stones, Acute Appendicitis, Hollow Viscus Perforation, Acute Gastrointestinal Bleeding

Lance L. Stein, MD
Center for Liver Disease and Transplantation, Columbia University New York Presbyterian Hospital, New York, New York

Hepatic Storage Disorders

Venkateswar R. Surabhi, MD
Assistant Professor, Department of Radiology, University of Texas Health Science Center at Houston, Houston, Texas

Imaging of the Urethra, Imaging of Disorders of the Female Urethra, Imaging of Disorders of the Male Urethra

Bachir Taouli, MD
Associate Professor of Radiology and Medicine, Director of Body MRI, Department of Radiology, Mount Sinai Medical School, New York, New York

MRI of Liver: From Sequences to Protocol

Marco Testoni, MD
Department of Radiology, G.B. Rossi Hospital Verona, Verona, Italy

Imaging of the Pancreas

Ashraf Thabet, MD
Clinical Fellow, Division of Abdominal Imaging and Intervention, Department of Radiology, Harvard Medical School, Massachusetts General Hospital, Boston, Massachusetts

Acute Small Bowel Ischemia, Chronic Small Bowel Ischemia

Ernesto Tomei, MD
Associate Professor, Department of Radiology, University Sapienza of Rome, Rome, Italy

Plain Radiography of the Abdomen

Michelle Udeshi, MD
Department of Radiology, Hospital of St. Raphael, New Haven, Connecticut; Griffin Hospital, Derby, Connecticut

MRI of the Kidneys and Urinary Tract, Benign Focal Renal Lesions

Raul N. Uppot, MD
Assistant Professor, Department of Radiology, Harvard Medical School; Interventional Radiologist, Massachusetts General Hospital, Boston, Massachusetts

Urinary Tract Anomalies and Variants

Sujit Vaidya, MD
Barts and the London NHS Trust, London, England, United Kingdom

Conventional Imaging of the Stomach and Duodenum, CT of the Stomach and Duodenum, Anatomic Variants of the Stomach and Duodenum

Sanjaya Viswamitra, MD
Assistant Professor, Department of Radiology, University of Arkansas for Medical Sciences, Little Rock, Arkansas

Diffuse Renal Parenchymal Diseases, Renal Parenchymal Infections, Renal Vascular Diseases, Miscellaneous Diffuse Renal Diseases

T. Gregory Walker, MD
Instructor of Radiology, Harvard Medical School; Associate Radiologist, Massachusetts General Hospital, Boston, Massachusetts

Acute Small Bowel Ischemia, Chronic Small Bowel Ischemia

Sjirk J. Westra, MD
Associate Professor of Radiology, Harvard Medical School; Associate Radiologist, Director, Pediatric Radiology Fellowship, Massachusetts General Hospital, Boston, Massachusetts

Small Bowel Anomalies and Variants

Vahid Yaghmai, MD, MS
Associate Professor of Radiology, Feinberg School of Medicine, Northwestern University; Medical Director of CT Imaging, Northwestern Memorial Hospital, Chicago, Illinois

CT of the Small Bowel, Nuclear Medicine Techniques for the Small Bowel

Takeshi Yokoo, MD, PhD
Department of Radiology, University of California San Diego, San Diego, California

Fatty Liver Disease

Hiroyuki Yoshida, PhD
Associate Professor, Harvard Medical School; Director, 3D Imaging Radiology, Massachusetts General Hospital, Boston, Massachusetts

Principles of 3D Postprocessing, Advanced Applications in Postprocessing, CT of the Liver

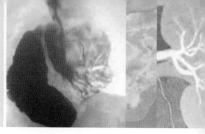

Preface

In 2006, when Elsevier approached us about *Abdominal Imaging,* we were initially doubtful. Our uncertainty arose from a simple question: *is there truly a need for another abdominal radiology text?* Several excellent comprehensive multi-volume reference texts are available, and there are a number of handbooks that provide busy Radiologists with quick access to images and abbreviated information at the interpretation station. Elsevier piqued our interest by explaining that the approach for *Abdominal Imaging* would be entirely new. Their market research had determined that the traditional problems faced by comprehensive texts—portability and quick access—could be solved by creating an accessible online knowledge platform. This platform, titled *Imaging Consult,* comprises a online radiology support tool that presents high yield content and numerous annotated images in an easy-to-use format specifically designed for rapid retrieval of clinically useful information. But electronic search and retrieval is not sufficient in isolation: the text must permit swift review, quick understanding, and a clear distillation of the key facts. The objective of *Abdominal Imaging* is to provide readers with the best of both worlds: a reference that is both comprehensive and that incorporates features more typically found in handbooks—short, readable sentences, key fact boxes, summary tables, abbreviated reference lists, listings of important review articles, and, above all, a highly integrated knowledge base that allows readers to rapidly access key content from any Internet-connected computer anywhere in the world.

To achieve this objective we assembled an international group of over 130 expert authors who contributed a total of 136 chapters. Each author created a chapter based on adherence to a template. This approach allows the reader to treat the text as a dynamic resource; instead of reading an entire chapter to find a pertinent fact, the reader can simply turn to the section of interest and rapidly access needed knowledge. We are well aware that useful Radiology texts should have many images for review, and we have taken care to richly illustrate the chapters with over 2,500 images of excellent quality. The chapters have also been supplemented with illustrative boxes titled Key Points, Classic Signs, and What the Referring Physician Needs to Know. These boxes provide tightly focused synopses so that a busy reader may glean the most crucial information in the precious few minutes that are available during a typical day at the reporting workstation. For those who wish to deepen their knowledge beyond the text, a list of key references and review articles has been provided in every chapter. In this way, we hope to facilitate self-study in the many potential areas of reader interest. The text also comes with access to *Imaging Consult* online, the searchable decision support tool that allows the reader to rapidly retrieve useful information and greatly facilitates the practical use of our two-volume "handbook."

Producing a text of this type is necessarily an undertaking that is the work of many people. There are several people whose contribution stands out. The numerous chapter authors whose work was so essential to this project: it is a testament to your dedication and knowledge that we were able to complete this mammoth task. We have also been privileged to work with superb editorial assistants. Dr. Melanie Seale's editorial contribution was simply outstanding: for many chapters Melanie read not only the chapter text, but also the source references. Melanie—thanks so much for everything. We couldn't have done this without you. Our efforts would not have been possible without the understanding and strong support of our families and colleagues. We have also been privileged to work with an indefatigable team at Elsevier. Roxanne Halpine demonstrated a remarkable combination of patience and perseverance. No matter how busy the editors and authors, Roxanne somehow managed to coax us all to complete our chapters. We would also like to thank Rebecca Gaertner, who managed the project, and Norm Stellander, our production manager. Elsevier has a great team, and we have been lucky to work with them.

Dear Reader: we'd like to share a small secret with you. Editing the 1,476 pages that make up *Abdominal Imaging* has been an arduous task. But it's also been fun. We've learned so much new about our own subspecialty that we did not know before we started that we believe that there will be something useful and fun in this text for every physician who interprets diagnostic images of the abdomen and pelvis.

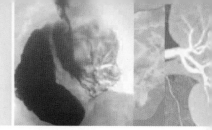

Contents

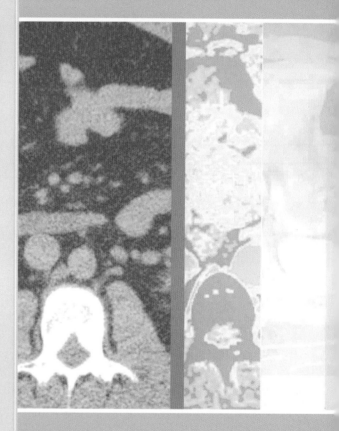

PART
ONE

Imaging
Techniques

Conventional Imaging of the Abdomen

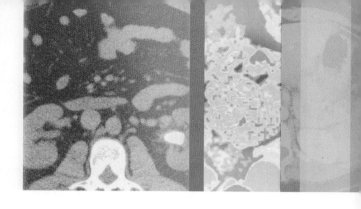

CHAPTER 1

Plain Radiography of the Abdomen

Ernesto Tomei, Vito Cantisani, Andrea Marcantonio, and Ugo D'Ambrosio

TECHNICAL ASPECTS

A plain abdominal radiograph must be read with a complete knowledge of the clinical situation. The patient's history and results of the physical examination and laboratory studies are always important to evaluate an acute abdomen, which may be caused by a number of different diseases. Obtaining plain films with the patient supine and erect and that include the diaphragm is the "classic" approach. Because chest abnormalities may produce an acute abdomen, a chest posteroanterior radiograph is sometimes ordered.

The standard abdominal radiograph is a supine projection: x-rays are passed from front to back (anteroposterior projection) in a patient lying on his or her back (Fig. 1-1). In some circumstances an abdominal radiograph taken with the patient erect is requested: its advantage over a supine film is the visualization of air/fluid levels. A decubitus film (with the patient lying on his or her side) is also of use in certain situations, especially to visualize fluid levels in the large bowel.

It is important, as with any imaging technique, that the technical details of an abdominal radiograph are assessed. The date the film was taken and the name, age, and sex of the patient are all worth noting. This ensures you are reviewing the correct film with the correct clinical information, and it also may aid your interpretation. Unless the order is specifically labeled, the film is taken with the patient supine. The best way to appreciate normality is to look at as many films as possible, with an awareness of anatomy in mind. Although an abdominal radiograph is a plain radiograph, it has a radiation dose equivalent to 50 posteroanterior chest radiographs or 6 months of standard background radiation.[1]

PROS AND CONS

There are many ways of getting images of the abdomen, including ultrasonography, CT, and MRI, but the plain abdominal radiograph is the technique that is most readily available in the emergency situation when a patient presents with acute abdominal pain.

Radiographs should never be requested without due consideration. They expend resources and expose the patient to ionizing radiation. They are an adjunct to a careful history and thorough physical examination.

The abdominal radiograph has the advantage of low cost. It is easy to perform and can be done on uncooperative patients, and, if correctly carried out and carefully interpreted,[2] it can still today be used with a dual purpose. It can be used to evaluate the catheter placement, identify ingested, inhaled, or introduced foreign bodies or free air in patients with a gastrointestinal perforation (conditions for which the examination is often diagnostic), or assess a condition of intestinal occlusion or an abdomen in the postoperative phase. It can also be of use in documenting the intestinal morphodynamics, the findings of which at the direct examination of the abdomen are dependent on both the etiology of the acute pathologic process and the time when the examination is performed with respect to the onset of the insult.[3] In addition, plain abdominal radiographs are an accessible, relatively inexpensive, convenient, and accurate method of detecting retained surgical needles. They can be used effectively to locate needles over 10 mm in length retained in the abdomen, with a sensitivity of 92% in this size range. In this scenario, plain abdominal radiographs should continue to be used after incorrect needle counts. It is also recommended that the requesting physician provide the radiologist the size of the lost needle. However, for missing needles of 10 mm or less in length, the utility of plain abdominal radiographs is more debatable.[4]

Conversely, criticisms of requests for abdominal films: http://www.patient.co.uk/showdoc/40001570/-ref1#ref1, often quote a low number of cases in which the diagnosis or management was changed by the radiographic findings. However, the diagnostic value is questionable, and very often there is no clear indication. In the majority of cases the results are negative or nonspecific. The reasons that abdominal radiography remains routinely requested are

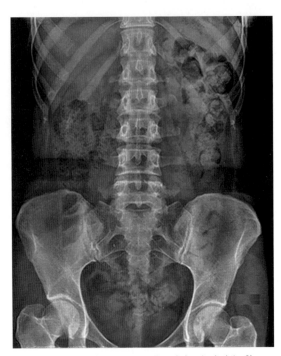

■ FIGURE 1-1 Normal anteroposterior abdominal plain film.

likely multifactorial. The modality has been available for decades and is found on many investigational algorithms for the assessment of abdominal emergency abnormalities. It is relatively inexpensive, is widely available, and exposes the patient to lower radiation doses than does abdominal CT. However, as reported in a recent article by Kellow and colleagues,[5] the results of abdominal radiography are neither sensitive nor specific. Flak and Rowley[6] have suggested that there are only two clinical entities in which sensitivity of abdominal radiography approaches 100%: free intraperitoneal air and, to a lesser extent, bowel obstruction. For the latter indication, a prospective trial conducted by Frager and associates[7] determined that clinical and radiographic evaluation was never precise enough to provide the exact location or cause of small bowel obstruction. Furthermore, Taourel and coworkers[8] demonstrated that not only is CT valuable in making a more accurate diagnosis but also that clinical treatment was correctly modified in 21% of patients because of the additional information provided by using CT. Therefore, abdominal radiography appears of limited value in the initial diagnosis of obstruction. For the indication of free air, the diagnosis is better made by evaluation of a chest radiograph obtained with the patient erect.[9] In addition, only a few physicians are aware of the relatively high radiation dose of an abdominal film, which is equal to 50 chest radiographs.[10]

CONTROVERSIES

In the 1950s gastrointestinal radiology consisted of plain abdominal films and single-contrast barium studies to assess gastrointestinal diseases.[11] Today the plain radiograph of the abdomen may be still the first step to evaluate acute abdominal diseases. However, with the advent of

CT, and to a lesser extent, ultrasonography, the importance of the plain abdominal film is decreasing. In past years plain radiography was also used to help diagnose abdominal pathologic processes such as stones in the kidney, gallbladder, or bladder. Plain radiography is now limited to emergency radiology in the acute abdomen. However, despite the undoubted advantages of the speed of examination, the multiplanar capabilities, and the objectivity of interpretation, CT subjects the patient to a higher dose of ionizing radiation,[12] which cannot be justified, particularly in groups of patients with a limited prevalence of pathologic processes, such as in emergency departments. The role of plain radiography of the abdomen in the diagnosis of acute abdomen needs to be reconsidered.[13] According to some authors, plain radiography should be performed only in patients for whom there are known advantages, such as those with suspected gastrointestinal perforation,[14] intestinal occlusion, ingestion of or the search for foreign bodies,[15] and in the assessment of the postoperative abdomen[16]; in these cases it is still the examination of choice, and only if it does not prove diagnostic should a CT examination be recommended.[17] In addition to these situations, however, there is another indication: the ability of plain radiography to assess the evolution of intestinal morphodynamism, that is, the variations in the motility, shape, and position of the small bowel in acute pathologic conditions.[18] Even though in the first instance assessing the etiology or the precise site of the obstruction is advisable, differentiating at least a mechanical ileus from a paralytic ileus,[19] and above all having an understanding of the seriousness and the extension of the cause and the time elapsed since its onset,[20] can prove to be clinically more useful. There are few comparisons of plain abdominal radiographs and CT scans in the literature. Siewert and associates[21] reported on 91 admitted patients with acute abdominal pain who eventually received CT because of continuing symptoms or failure to respond to therapy. In this series, treatment was changed after CT in 25 patients (27%), but the authors did not state the relative contribution of the plain abdominal radiographs to the pre-CT diagnosis. In particular, the percentage of patients who had abnormal plain abdominal radiographs was not described. A retrospective review of 23 patients with proven mesenteric infarction compared plain abdominal radiographs with CTs and showed that 6 patients (26%) had abnormal plain abdominal radiographs only, 8 patients (35%) had abnormal CTs only, and in only 1 patient (4%) were both tests abnormal.[22] Both studies were normal or nonspecific in 8 patients (35%). That 26% of patients had signs of an acute abdominal syndrome shown only on plain abdominal radiographs and not on CT is in sharp contradiction to our findings, in which the plain abdominal radiographs provided minimal additional information in 2 of 74 patients (3%) and at the cost of 33 (57%) potentially misleading false-negative results. There are several possible explanations. Mesenteric infarction may represent one of a series of specific syndromes that have either relatively low CT sensitivity, high plain abdominal radiograph sensitivity, or both. In the review just cited there were no patients diagnosed on plain abdominal radiographs, CT, or clinical course with this syndrome. Other possibilities include individual or institutional variations in radiologic interpretations or improvement in the interpretation of CTs for this and other syndromes over the past decade. The increased imaging capabilities of this newer technology would most likely make the test characteristics of the newer CT scanners even more favorable. Despite these limitations, for emergency department patients with acute abdominal, flank, or back pain, in whom a CT is likely to be obtained, a preliminary plain abdominal radiograph adds almost no additional information and is potentially misleading. Given the utilization of resources required for plain abdominal radiographs as well as the time delay to obtain them, some authors believe that patients in whom the clinical suspicion of significant intra-abdominal pathology is high should go directly to CT.[23]

NORMAL ANATOMY

As with any plain radiograph, only five main densities may be distinguished, four of which are natural: black for gas, white for calcified structures, gray representing a host of soft tissue, with a slightly darker gray for fat (because it absorbs slightly fewer x-rays). Metallic objects are seen as an intense bright white. The clarity of outlines of structures depends, therefore, on the differences between these densities. On the chest radiograph this is easily shown by the contrast between lung and ribs as black air against the white calcium-containing bones. These differences are much less apparent on the abdominal radiograph because most structures are of similar density, mainly soft tissue. A systematic approach to plain abdominal radiographs will help to avoid errors in interpretation. Interpretation of the abdominal radiograph depends on the assessment of the bowel gas pattern, solid organ outlines, a search for abnormal calcification, and a review of the skeleton. A search should be made for extraluminal gas. A bowel gas pattern distinguishing the colon from the small bowel may be difficult. The presence of solid feces and the distribution, caliber, and mucosal pattern of the bowel help in deciding whether a particular loop of bowel is stomach, small intestine, or colon. The presence of solid feces indicates the large bowel, which may also be recognized by the incomplete haustral band crossing the colonic gas shadow. Haustra are usually present in the ascending and transverse colon but may be absent from the splenic flexure and descending colon. The valvulae conniventes of the small bowel are closer together and cross the width of the bowel. The distal ileum when dilated can appear smooth, which makes differentiation more difficult. The small bowel when obstructed is generally centrally positioned with numerous loops of tighter curvature than the large bowel. Maximal small bowel caliber is 3.5 cm in the jejunum and 2.5 cm in the ileum. Maximal caliber of the transverse colon on plain films is taken to be 5.5 cm in diameter, and the maximal cecal diameter is 9 cm. Solid organs, the liver edge, renal outlines, and the splenic tip may all be demonstrated.

Intraluminal Gas

One should begin by looking at the amount and distribution of gas in the bowels (intraluminal gas). There is con-

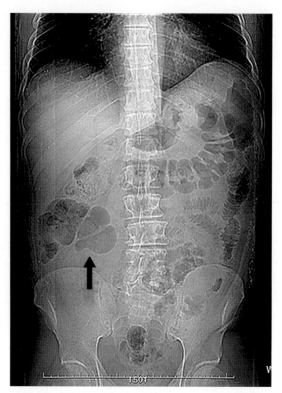

■ **FIGURE 1-2** Diverticulitis and peridiverticulitis. There is no evidence of bowel distention at the level of either the colon or the small bowel. It is possible to see a mild air dilation of the small bowel. The cecum seems to be medially moved (*arrow*).

siderable normal variation in distribution of bowel gas (Fig. 1-2). On the abdominal radiograph taken with the patient erect, the gastric gas bubble in the left upper quadrant of the film is a normal finding. Gas is also normally seen within the large bowel, most notably the transverse colon and rectum. Small and large bowel can also be distinguished, most easily when dilated, by their different mucosal markings. Small bowel has valvulae conniventes that transverse the full width of the bowel; large bowel has haustra that cross only part of the bowel wall. These features are important in the next part of this series, which considers abnormal intraluminal gas. Occasionally, fluid levels in the small bowel are a normal finding. Fecal matter in the bowel gives a "mottled" appearance. This is seen as a mixture of gray densities representing a gas/liquid/solid mixture.

Extraluminal Gas

Gas outside the bowel lumen is invariably abnormal (Fig. 1-3). The largest volume of gas one might see is likely to be under the right diaphragm: this occurs after a viscus has been perforated. This gas within the peritoneal cavity is termed *pneumoperitoneum*. Gas in the right upper quadrant within the biliary tree is a "normal" finding after sphincterotomy or biliary surgery, but it can indicate the presence of a fistula between the biliary tree and the gut. One must beware of gas in the portal vein, because this can look very similar to biliary air. Gas in the portal vein is always pathologic and frequently fatal. It occurs in ischemic states, such as toxic megacolon, and it may be

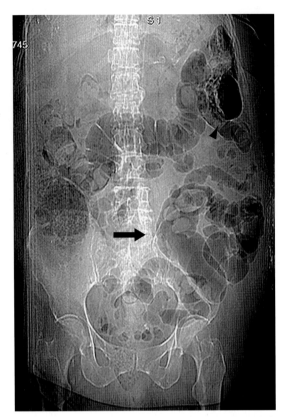

■ **FIGURE 1-3** Mesenteric ischemia and spleen infarction. Abdominal radiograph shows a colonic dilation (*arrow*) that is especially marked at distal segments. Furthermore, extracolonic air collections are visible at the spleen level (*arrowhead*) in the upper left quadrant. Bowel dilation is evident without the finding of bowel obstruction.

BOX 1-1   Areas to Search for Abnormal Extraluminal Gas

- Under the diaphragm
- In the biliary system
- Within the bowel wall

---

accompanied by gas within the bowel wall (intramural gas) (Box 1-1).

Calcification

Calcium is visible in a variety of structures, both normal and abnormal, and becomes more common with advancing age. Calcification should be identified and anatomically located. In some locations (e.g., vascular calcification) it is common and benign. Vascular calcification may be seen within the aorta, in the splenic artery in the left upper quadrant, or in the pelvis. Abdominal aortic aneurysms are usually below the second lumbar vertebra. Calcification can make them obvious and can give a rough indication of the internal diameter. Abdominal ultrasonography is required for accurate assessment and to determine the need for surgery or follow-up. Uterine fibroids can become calcified.

Calcified renal tract stones should be looked for around the renal outlines and down the line of the ureters. More

rarely, calcified gallstones are seen in the right upper quadrant or a calcified (porcelain) gallbladder is present. The pancreas lies at the level of the T9 to T12 vertebrae. Calcification occurs in chronic pancreatitis and may show the whole outline of the gland.

In the pelvic region, bladder calculi may occasionally be seen. Bladder stones are usually quite large and often multiple. Calcification of a bladder tumor may also occur. Schistosomiasis may produce calcification of the bladder wall.

Other causes of pelvic calcification include phleboliths, calcified fibroids, and, rarely, calcification in ovarian teratodermoids, which may also contain teeth and hair.

Soft Tissues and Bone

A review of the soft tissues entails evaluating the outlines of the major abdominal organs. Observing these structures is made easier by the "fatty" rim (properitoneal fat lines) surrounding them. In fact, the loss of these fat planes may indicate an ongoing pathologic process, such as peritonitis.

The liver is seen in the right upper quadrant and extends downward a variable distance. The tip of the right lobe may be seen extending below the right kidney; this is a normal variant called Riedel's lobe. The spleen may be visualized (especially in thin individuals) even when of normal size. It enlarges inferiorly and toward the left lower quadrant. It is often possible to identify both kidneys and the psoas shadows within the retroperitoneum. The kidneys are lateral to the midline in the region of the T12 to L2 vertebrae (*note:* a useful way to identify vertebrae is that the lowest one to give off a rib is T12 and thus can serve as a reference point).

Soft tissue masses or abscess can sometimes be identified on plain films. An abscess generally has a rather heterogeneous density due to the presence of gas and necrotic tissue. Mass lesions are of soft tissue density and will displace bowel gas shadows.

The assessment of bones entails evaluating the spine and pelvis for evidence of a bony pathologic process. Osteoarthritis frequently affects the vertebral bodies, as well as the femoral and the acetabular components of the hip joint. Paget's disease may also be identified, commonly along the iliopectineal lines of the pelvis. The bone survey should also include a check for fractures, especially subtle femoral neck fractures in elderly persons. The spine and pelvis are also common locations for metastatic deposits. In the spine this is classically seen as "the absent pedicle."

Artifacts

"Man-made" structures should be correctly identified. These may be iatrogenic (put there by health care professionals), accidental (put there by the patient or another person), or projectional (lying in front of or behind the abdomen but spuriously projected within it on the abdominal radiograph). Examples of iatrogenic structures would be surgical clips, an intrauterine contraceptive device, a renal or biliary stent, an endoluminal aortic stent, or an inferior vena cava filter. Accidental findings include bullets or an object in the rectum. Projectional findings include pajama buttons, coins in pockets, or body piercings.

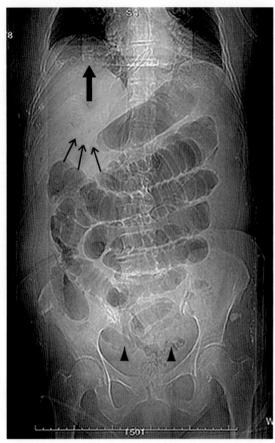

■ **FIGURE 1-4** Sigmoid carcinoma. Wide sickle-shaped free air is evident under the right hemidiaphragm (*large arrow*). A small, linear, free air collection is also shown along the lower margin of the liver (*small arrows*). Marked air distention of jejunum with a transitional area between dilated jejunum and normal ileum is visible (*arrowheads*).

PATHOLOGIC FINDINGS

Abdominal radiographs obtained with the patient erect are requested to look for fluid levels in obstruction or ileus. Air under the diaphragm may be seen in an erect film if the bowel has been perforated, although a chest radiograph is more usually done to look for that sign (Fig. 1-4). An abdominal radiograph is of no value in hematemesis. Avoiding obtaining erect films when unnecessary and avoiding plain films for hematemesis will reduce the level of radiation exposure.

Renal Colic

If a patient presents with loin pain, the possibility of renal colic is high; therefore, a kidney/ureter/bladder (KUB) view is requested. About 90% of renal stones are radiopaque. Uric acid stones especially may be missed. False-positive findings may occur from phleboliths, which are most common in the pelvic veins, and false-negative findings occur from small stones. On the right, calcification may represent gallstones but only a minority of gallstones are radiopaque. The presence of gallstones does not confirm biliary colic as the cause of pain because gallstones become more frequent with age and are often asymptomatic.

Intestinal Obstruction

Erect and supine films are used to confirm the diagnosis. Obstruction of the small bowel shows a ladder-like series of small bowel loops, but this also occurs with an obstruction of the proximal colon. Fluid levels in the bowel can be seen in upright views. Distended loops may be absent if obstruction is at the upper jejunum. Obstruction of the large bowel is more gradual in onset than small bowel obstruction. The colon is in the more peripheral part of the film, and distention may be very marked. Fluid levels will also be seen in paralytic ileus when bowel sounds will be reduced or absent rather than loud and tinkling as in obstruction. In an erect film a fluid level in the stomach is normal, as may be a level in the cecum. Multiple fluid levels and distention of the bowel are abnormal.

Perforation of the Intestine

If the bowel has been perforated and a significant amount of gas has been released, it will show as a translucency under the diaphragm on an erect film. Gas will also be found under the diaphragm for some time after laparotomy or laparoscopy.

Appendicitis

An appendicolith may be apparent in an inflamed appendix in 15% of cases, but as a diagnostic point in the management of appendicitis the plain radiograph is of very limited value, although it may be of value in infants.

Intussusception

Intussusception occurs in adults and children. A plain abdominal radiograph may show some characteristic gas patterns. A sensitivity and specificity of 90% adds to this rather difficult diagnosis, but ultrasonography is vastly superior.

Body Packers

An increasing problem occurs with people who swallow drugs, usually in condoms, to evade detection. There may be signs that the drugs are leaking, but the carrier is unwilling to disclose the fact for fear of a long prison term, even if his life is at risk. A plain abdominal radiograph will show 90% of cases, but there will be false-positive findings in 3%. Therefore, a positive result is likely to be true but a negative result does not exclude the clinical suspicion adequately and an ultrasound examination may be considered (Boxes 1-2 and 1-3).

PATHOPHYSIOLOGY
Small Bowel

The small bowel contains a small amount to no gas in normal subjects, so it is not visible on a plain film. The presence of gas more than normal should be seen with suspicion and interpreted in the proper clinical setting. Some clinical situations, such as indigestion or viral

BOX 1-2   Key to Densities in Abdominal Radiographs

- Black—gas
- White—calcified structures
- Gray—soft tissues
- Darker gray—fat
- Intense white—metallic objects

BOX 1-3   Radiographic Review Points

- Technical specifics of the radiograph
- Amount and distribution of gas
- Extraluminal gas
- Calcification
- Soft tissue outlines and bony structures
- Iatrogenic, accidental, and incidental objects

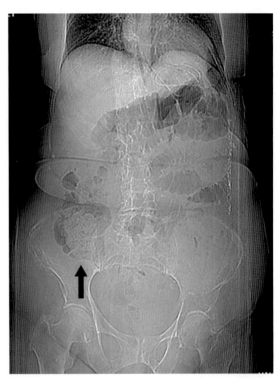

■ **FIGURE 1-5** Volvulus. Visible fecal material (*arrow*) is evident in the right colon, whereas the left and sigmoid colon are not represented. Moderate distention of bowel in the upper abdomen can be seen. In left lower quadrant a mass is suspected because of the lack of intestinal air.

enteritis, show an increase of intestinal gas, usually without air/fluid levels; these are self-limiting diseases, and usually they do not need diagnostic efforts.

Intestinal obstruction is a common radiographic finding in an emergency department. Distended intestinal loops with air/fluid levels with scarcely visible colonic gas are among the most commonly seen features of small bowel obstruction; the clinical history of the patient may be the key to the diagnosis in the case of suspected postoperative adhesions, Crohn's disease, or a known tumor. In some cases, however, depending on the gas and fluid distribution it is not impossible to have a near-normal plain film with a true obstruction. On the other hand, diffuse peritoneal metastasis may produce air/fluid levels without obstruction. The level of the intestinal obstruction may be, in some cases, understood; however, in prestenotic loops the fluid may be abundant and gas is not visible so that only proximal loops are distended by gas. Again, fluid-filled intestinal loops showing the cause of obstruction either of the bowel wall or extraintestinal are often easily seen at CT. The diagnosis of strangulation requires expertise because the intramural gas and a rigid loop are well-known features but not so commonly seen. It should be remembered that the shape of valvulae conniventes is generally preserved also in severe distention so that they can be used to differentiate small intestinal disease from colonic disease.

The adhesions are not directly seen, but a transition zone (dilatation of the bowel followed by a collapsed loop) without any other visible cause of obstruction may lead to the diagnosis in a patient with a history of surgery.

CT performed after a plain abdominal film can be obtained without oral contrast administration, but intravenous administration of a contrast agent usually cannot be avoided in these often severely ill patients.

A set of CT criteria that may help surgeons to decide if a patient needs surgery for small bowel obstruction has been implemented.[24] Although plain radiography can be used with good results by experienced surgeons, CT has been reported to have 100% sensitivity in complete obstruction.[25] Daneshmand and colleagues compared CT and plain radiography and found a sensitivity and specificity of 75% and 53% for plain film, respectively, and 92% and 71% for CT; they suggest that CT be used as the primary diagnostic tool for small bowel obstruction.[26] The approach to evaluate patients with small bowel obstruction is not generally accepted; however, CT is considered the preeminent imaging modality to evaluate these patients.[27] Last but not least, the accuracy of a plain film is influenced by the experience of the radiologist.[28]

Colon

Because of the presence of haustra, feces, and gas, understanding diseases of the colon is apparently easier than recognizing diseases of the small bowel on a plain radiograph. An obstruction of the sigmoid colon shows the transition from a dilated to a nondilated colon, and it is not difficult to recognize. On the other hand, an obstruction of the ascending colon may be similar, in some cases, to an obstruction of the last ileal loop. Colonic obstruction producing a severe cecal dilatation greater than 10 to 11 cm is an indication for immediate surgery, to avoid perforation. In elderly constipated patients a sigmoid volvulus is among the possible causes of obstruction; the dilated sigmoid that is seen as a "kidney bean" may also mimic an abdominal mass. Cecal volvulus, seen in younger patients, produces distention of the cecum (Fig. 1-5). In both cases CT can provide crucial information.

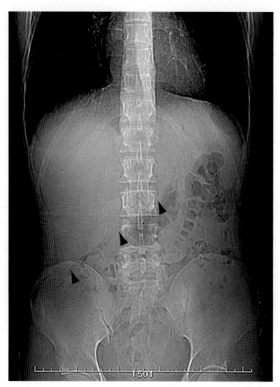

■ **FIGURE 1-6** Perisigmoid abscess. Note enlargement of the hepatic area (*arrowheads*). Small bowel and colon are within the normal range for size.

The loss of a haustral pattern is important to distinguish a patient with an obstruction of the distal colon from a patient with colitis, in which a haustral pattern is usually lost, even with mild disease. Small bowel distention, often with air/fluid levels, may be seen in a subgroup of patients with severe ulcerative colitis at higher risk of both toxic megacolon and multiple organ dysfunction syndrome. The poor response to therapy and the persistence of gastrointestinal distention are monitored with plain radiography, which is important to evaluate patients who need colectomy.[29]

Miscellaneous Findings

Free intraperitoneal or subphrenic air is commonly seen in postoperative patients, and the only thing to do is wait for its resorption. A deep intestinal or colonic biopsy can also produce, as a rare complication, free or subphrenic air collection. Perforation of a duodenal ulcer or perforation of a diverticulum of the colon are not as common causes of extraintestinal air collections.

Cholecystitis, pancreatitis, and other causes of acute abdomen in which a collection of air or fluid may be misleading should now be assessed by ultrasonography or CT. Fecaloma is easy to detect on a plain film; however, a digital exploration of the rectum is preferred to diagnose this lesion.

However, severe clinical situations such as perirectal or perisigmoid abscesses or a carcinoma infiltrating bowel wall without obstruction may have a completely normal appearance on a plain film (Fig. 1-6); these situations are easily seen on CT.

Distention of the colon, accompanied often by diffuse distention of the small bowel without mechanical obstruction, is the feature of paralytic or adynamic ileus. The intestinal distention may be limited to some part of the intestine so that it may be difficult to distinguish mechanical from paralytic ileus. The clinical situation of the patient may be enough, in some cases, to make the diagnosis. If the diagnosis is not clear, CT is mandatory.

Ischemic bowel disease produces many different abnormalities on a plain radiograph, ranging from intestinal distention to a gasless abdomen. "Thumbprinting" is a famous, but not so specific, feature of intestinal ischemia; a linear shadow of gas within the bowel wall is difficult to detect on a plain film; when visible, it indicates a poor prognosis.

Toxic megacolon may be a lethal complication of ulcerative colitis. A plain film shows a dilatation of the transverse colon greater than 6 to 8 cm with loss of haustra.

KEY POINTS

■ The history, physical examination, and laboratory findings are always important to evaluate an acute abdomen, which may be caused by a number of different diseases.

■ Plain radiography, because it is relatively inexpensive and convenient, should be performed as an initial imaging modality only in patients for whom there are known advantages, such as those with suspected gastrointestinal perforation, intestinal occlusion, and ingestion of, or in a search for, foreign bodies, and in the assessment of the postoperative abdomen to detect retained needles; in these cases it is still the examination of choice, and if it does not prove diagnostic, a CT examination is recommended. In addition, another indication is the ability of plain radiography to assess the evolution of intestinal morphodynamism, which is the variation in the motility, shape, and position of the small bowel in acute pathologic conditions.

■ The lack of positive findings at abdominal radiography is falsely reassuring in nontrauma emergency department patients.

■ Further imaging is often required to better characterize abnormalities identified at abdominal radiography.

SUGGESTED READINGS

Best evidence topic reports. Role of plain abdominal radiograph in the diagnosis of intussusception. Emerg Med J 2008; 25:106-107.

Brazaitis MP, Dachman AH. The radiologic evaluation of acute abdominal pain of intestinal origin: a clinical approach. Med Clin North Am 1993; 77:939-961.

Burkill G, Bell J, Healy J. Small bowel obstruction: the role of computed tomography in its diagnosis and management with reference to other imaging modalities. Eur Radiol 2001; 11:1405-1422.

Gupta H, Dupuy DE. Advances in imaging of the acute abdomen. Surg Clin North Am 1997; 77:1245-1263.

Hayes R. Abdominal pain: general imaging strategies. Eur Radiol 2004; 14(Suppl 4):L123-L137.

Kidmas AT, Ekedigwe JE, Sule AZ, Pam SD. A review of the radiological diagnosis of small bowel obstruction using various imaging modalities. Niger Postgrad Med J 2005; 12:33-36.

Reuchlin-Vroklage LM, Bierma-Zeinstra S, Benninga MA, Berger MY. Diagnostic value of abdominal radiography in constipated children: a systematic review. Arch Pediatr Adolesc Med 2005; 159:671-678.

Roszler MH. Plain film radiologic examination of the abdomen. Crit Care Clin 1994; 10:277-296.

REFERENCES

1. Levine MS. Plain film diagnosis of the acute abdomen. Emerg Med North Am 1985; 3(3).

2. Baker SR: The abdominal plain film: what will be its role in the future? Radiol Clin North Am 1993; 31:1335-1344.

3. Grassi R, Di Mizio R, Pinto A, et al. Semeiotica radiografica dell'addome acuto all'esame radiologico diretto: ileo riflesso spastico, ileo riflesso ipotonico, ileo meccanico ed ileo paralitico. Radiol Med 2004; 108:56-70.

4. Ponrartana S, Coakley FV, Yeh BM. Accuracy of plain abdominal radiographs in the detection of retained surgical needles in the peritoneal cavity. Ann Surg 2008; 247:8-12.

5. Kellow ZS, MacInnes M, Kurzencwyg D, et al. The role of abdominal radiography in the evaluation of the non-trauma emergency patient. Radiology 2008; 248:887-893.

6. Flak B, Rowley VA. Acute abdomen: plain film utilisation and analysis. Can Assoc Radiol J 1993; 44:423-428.

7. Frager DH, Baer JW, Rothpearl A, Bossart PA. Distinction between postoperative ileus and mechanical small-bowel obstruction: value of CT compared with clinical and other radiographic findings. AJR Am J Roentgenol 1995; 164:891-894.

8. Taourel P, Pradel J, Fabre JM, et al: Role of CT in the acute non-traumatic abdomen. Semin Ultrasound CT MR 1995; 16:151-164.

9. McCook TA, Ravin CE, Rice RP. Abdominal radiography in the emergency department: a prospective analysis. Ann Emerg Med 1982; 11:7-8.

10. Campbell JP, Gunn AA. Plain abdominal radiographs and acute abdominal pain. Br J Surg 1988; 75:554-556.

11. Goldberg HJ, Margulis AR. Gastrointestinal radiology in US: an overview of the past 50 years. Radiology 2000; 216:1-7.

12. Baker SR: Musings at the beginning of the hyper-CT era. Abdom Imaging 2003; 28:110-114.

13. Feyler S, Williamson V, King D: Plain abdominal radiographs in acute medical emergencies: an abused investigation? Postgrad Med J 2002; 78:94-96.

14. Grassi R, Pinto F, Rotondo A, et al: Contributo della radiologia tradizionale alla diagnosi di pneumoperitoneo. In Pinos A: Pneumoperitoneo. Napoli, Guido Gnocchi, 1996, pp 7-158.

15. Baker SR: Plain films and cross-sectional imaging for acute abdominal pain: unresolved issues. Semin US CT MRI 1999; 20:142-147.

16. Frassineti A: La Radiologia dell'Addome Acuto Postoperatorio. Padua, Piccin, 1982.

17. Wiest P, Roth P. Fundamentals of Emergency Radiology. Philadelphia, WB Saunders, 1996, pp 96-112.

18. Taourel P, Kessler N, Lesnik A, et al: Non-traumatic abdominal emergencies: imaging of acute intestinal obstruction. Eur Radiol 2002; 12:2151-2160.

19. Krestin GP, Choyke PL: Acute Abdomen: Diagnostic Imaging in the Clinical Context. Stuttgart, Georg Thieme, 1996, p 139.

20. Silen W: Cope's Early Diagnosis of the Acute Abdomen. New York, Oxford University Press, 2005, p 159.

21. Siewert B, Raptopoulos V, Mueller M, et al. Impact of CT on diagnosis and management of the acute abdomen in patients initially treated without surgery. AJR Am J Roentgenol 1997; 168:173-178.

22. Smerud MJ, Johnson CD, Stephens DH. Diagnosis of bowel infarction: a comparison of plain films and CT scans in 23 cases. AJR Am J Roentgenol 1990; 154:99-103.

23. Nagurney JT, Brown DF, Novelline DA, et al. Plain abdominal radiographs and CT scans. Am J Emerg Med 1999; 17:668-671.

24. Jones K, Mangram AJ, Lebron RA, et al. Can a computed tomography scoring system predict the need for surgery in small-bowel obstruction? Am J Surg 2007; 194:780-784.

25. Frager D, Medwid SW, Baer JW, et al. CT of small bowel obstruction: value in establishing the diagnosis and determining the degree and cause. AJR Am J Roentgenol 1994; 162:37-41.

26. Daneshmand S, Hedley CG, Stain SC. The utility and reliability of CT in the diagnosis of small bowel obstruction. Am Surg 1999; 65:922-926.

27. Ros PR, Huprich JE. ACR appropriateness criteria on suspected small bowel obstruction. J Am Coll Radiol 2006; 3:838-841.

28. Thompson WM, Kilani RK, Smith BB, et al. Accuracy of abdominal radiography in acute small-bowel obstruction: does reviewer experience matter? AJR Am J Roentgenol 2007; 188:233-238.

29. Latella G, Vernia P, Viscido A, et al. GI distension in severe ulcerative colitis. Am J Gastroenterol 2002; 5:1169-1175.

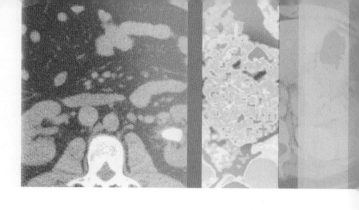

CHAPTER 2

Fluoroscopic Study of the Abdomen and Fluoroscopic Contrast Media

Naveen M. Kulkarni and Pritish Aher

Fluoroscopy is a type of imaging technique in which real-time movements of body organs and radiopaque contrast material are visualized. During a fluoroscopic examination the operator or radiologist controls the functions of radiography equipment and x-ray tubes for real-time imaging of the patient. In abdominal imaging, fluoroscopy has a role in the diagnosis of various clinical conditions with gastrointestinal studies, postoperative studies, genitourinary studies, and more.

TECHNICAL ASPECTS

Fluoroscopy

History

Early fluoroscopes had an x-ray tube and fluorescent screen made of barium platinocyanide. Gradually the screens were replaced by cadmium tungstate and then zinc-cadmium sulfide, which produced a yellow-green emission.[1]

Fluoroscopy has evolved from the early days of images on a fluoroscopic screen of a poor quality, a dark radiography room, and eye adaptation with red goggles to improved images with image intensifiers, video-recorders, and a variety of C-arm machines. Currently, it is available in many different configurations for use in various clinical applications. With technologic advancements in hardware design and image processing, fluoroscopy has gained substantially both qualitatively and quantitatively. The introduction of flat-panel detectors, high-quality image intensifiers with video-recording capabilities, state of the art C-arm design, and digital units has revolutionized the field of fluoroscopic imaging.[1,2] The superior spatial and contrast resolution combined with faster image reconstruction and reduced radiation along with a variety of

safe and effective contrast media has empowered fluoroscopy with advanced capabilities in the diagnostics and interventional realm. A variety of fluoroscopic units are now commercially available, and the components of basic fluoroscopic equipment are shown in Figure 2-1. The main uses of fluoroscopy are listed in Table 2-1.

Patient Preparation

It is important to have the patient empty his or her stomach to increase the sensitivity of the fluoroscopy examination, because food and food residue can mimic disease. Informed consent is required, and any medical history such as heart disease, asthma, allergy, thyrotoxicosis, and hypersensitivity to drugs should be elicited. Also important to consider: What medications (e.g., insulin) is the patient using? Is the patient pregnant or breast-feeding? Has there been a recent diagnosis of small bowel obstruction or perforation and, if so, what were the surgical details?

Patients scheduled for a double-contrast barium enema must adhere to a clear liquid diet for 24 hours before the procedure. Laxatives may be prescribed to ensure thorough bowel cleansing, and on the morning of the examination a bisacodyl suppository is given per rectum.

However, in the acute/emergency or postoperative setting, patient preparation is usually optional. Moreover, in this setting, iodinated contrast media are preferred over barium sulfate because the latter might interfere with a surgical procedure and any extraluminal collection of barium may create confusion with a diagnosis on subsequent examinations.[3-5] A medical history of severe hypersensitivity to iodinated contrast media or certain medications should be obtained if the procedure requires its use.

Fluoroscopic Examinations

Fluoroscopic examinations are of two types: single-contrast studies and double-contrast studies (Table 2-2). Single-contrast studies are performed either with barium or with iodinated contrast media.[6,7] For double-contrast media, air or carbon dioxide is used (Fig. 2-2).[8-10]

Gastrointestinal Fluoroscopic Procedures

● Swallowing study for pharynx (pharyngography)
● Esophagography
● Upper gastrointestinal series (UGI) for stomach and duodenum (barium meal)
● Small bowel series (SBS) for jejunal and ileal loops (barium meal follow-through and enteroclysis)
● Barium enema (BE) for colon, sigmoid colon, and rectum
● Stomal examinations, enema through ileostomy or colostomy for patency, recurrence of disease and leak
● Feeding tube studies
● Oral cholecystogram (OCG) and T-tube cholangiogram
● Hydrostatic reduction of pediatric abdominal emergencies such as intussusceptions and sigmoid volvulus

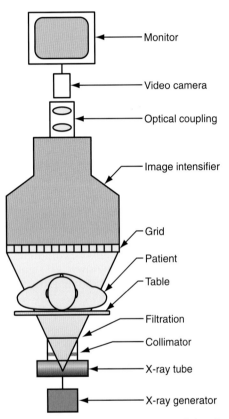

Monitor
Video camera
Optical coupling
Image intensifier
Grid
Patient
Table
Filtration
Collimator
X-ray tube
X-ray generator

■ **FIGURE 2-1** Schematic diagram of fluoroscopic imaging system.

TABLE 2-1 Main Uses of Fluoroscopy

Gastrointestinal imaging
Genitourinary imaging
Angiography
Other:
　Intraoperative
　Foreign-body removal
　Musculoskeletal

TABLE 2-2 Single-Contrast versus Double-Contrast Studies

Single-Contrast Studies	Double-Contrast Studies
Precise control of barium column	Thick barium coats lumen, and effervescent tablets are ingested to distend lumen with air.
Easier identification of filling defects	Produced see-through effect with better assessment of mucosal details
In suspected perforation, single contrast with water-soluble medium preferred.	Better distention and separation of the bowel loops
Can be used to evaluate mechanical problems (e.g., obstruction, fistula)	Better detection of small mucosal lesions, polyps, ulcers
Optimal for patients unable to swallow gas-forming tablets	

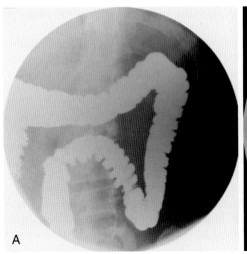

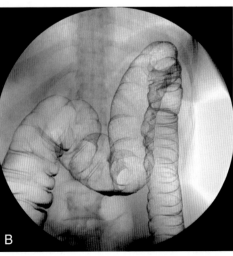

■ **FIGURE 2-2** Spot radiograph of the mid transverse colon obtained during single-contrast (**A**) and double-contrast (**B**) barium enema. The mucosal details are well seen on the double-contrast study.

Genitourinary Fluoroscopic Procedures

● Cystography for evaluation of urinary bladder and vesicoureteric reflux
● Voiding cystourethrography (VCUG) for visualization of urethra
● Retrograde urethrography (RUG) for anterior urethra
● Hysterosalpingogram for uterus and fallopian tubes

Interventional Procedures

● Placement of vascular catheter and stents
● Percutaneous biliary drainage procedures
● Urologic procedures—retrograde pyelography, percutaneous nephrostomies, and suprapubic cystotomies

Other Examinations

● Sinogram
● Fistulogram

FLUOROSCOPIC CONTRAST AGENTS

Fluoroscopic contrast agents are compounds that enable improved visualization of internal luminal structures, spaces, and tracts and also delineate tubes and catheters on fluoroscopy or radiography (Fig. 2-3).

Fluoroscopic contrast agents can be divided into two types: positive contrast and negative contrast. A positive contrast medium absorbs x-rays more strongly than the surrounding tissue or organ being examined and appears radiopaque. A negative contrast medium absorbs x-rays less strongly and hence appears radiolucent. Positive contrast media are barium and iodine compounds (Figs. 2-4 and 2-5). Negative contrast media can be obtained by air or carbon dioxide (Fig. 2-6).[11,12]

Barium

The higher the concentration of the barium sulfate suspension, the thinner are the layers that can be identified in the radiograph. The more viscous is the suspension, the better is the penetration into the finest folds and the more differentiated are the structures that become visible. Different barium preparations available for use are shown in Figure 2-7. Various barium suspensions used for the evaluation of different parts of gastrointestinal tract are depicted in Table 2-3.

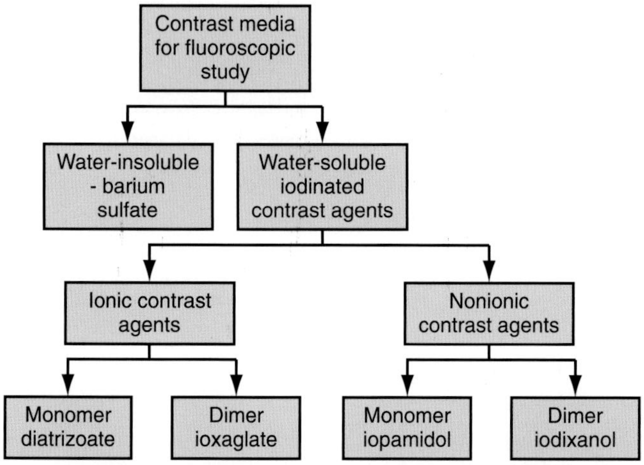

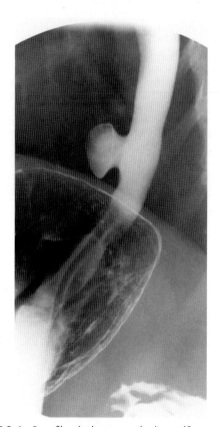

■ **FIGURE 2-4** Spot film single-contrast barium sulfate study of esophagus shows a pulsion diverticulum from the lower esophagus.

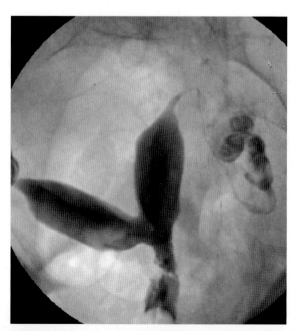

■ **FIGURE 2-5** Spot film from hysterosalpingography using iodinated contrast media shows a bicornuate uterus with free spill.

■ **FIGURE 2-3** Contrast media used in fluoroscopy.

Properties desirable for the conventional upper gastrointestinal and per-oral small bowel examinations include suspension stability, good coating ability for double-contrast views, and resistance to flocculation in the small intestine.[3,4] For dense, uniform coating in the esophagus, stomach, duodenum, and colon, it is also desirable that the barium suspension have the ability to delineate fine mucosal surface details with reasonable flow rate and resistance to flocculation.[3,4,9]

TABLE 2-3 Barium Formulations for Gastrointestinal Tract Radiography

Gastrointestinal Tract Study	Barium Formulations
Barium swallow	Single contrast: 50-100% w/v
	Double contrast: 250% w/v
Upper gastrointestinal tract (stomach and duodenum)	Single contrast: 35-80% w/v
	Double contrast: 250% w/v
Small bowel followthrough	40-60% w/v
Enteroclysis	50-95% w/v
Retrograde ileography	20-25% w/v
Barium enema	Single contrast: 12-25% w/v
	Double contrast: 60-120% w/v
	(80% commonly used)

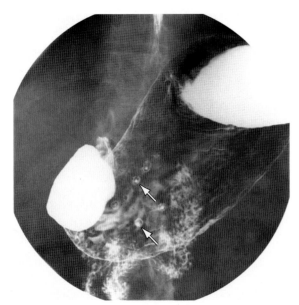

■ **FIGURE 2-6** Spot film of double-contrast barium study of stomach showing multiple aphthoid ulcers (*arrows*).

Water-Soluble Contrast Agents

Water-soluble contrast agents can be divided into ionic or nonionic agents or, depending on the osmolarity, as high- and low-osmolar agents (see Figs. 2-3 and 2-8). Ionic contrast media have higher osmolarity and more side effects. Nonionic contrast media have lower osmolarity and tend to have fewer side effects.[11,12] Water-soluble organic iodine compounds are used in certain circumstances where barium is contraindicated, for instance in suspected perforation of gut into the free peritoneal cavity, in postoperative cases to look for a leak, or when the risk of aspiration into the lung is high. Barium leakage into the peritoneal cavity can lead to formation of granuloma, and aspiration into the lung can leak to pneumonitis or pulmonary edema.[5,6]

In general to achieve good radiographic opacification of the gastrointestinal tract it is recommended that 60% or higher solutions of ionic contrast agents be used. Although ionic contrast agents stimulate intestinal peristalsis and result in more rapid visualization of distal small bowel loops as compared with barium preparations, this effect is quickly nullified by the dilution effect in the bowel secondary to hyperosmolarity of these agents.[11-13] Ideally, one of the nonionic contrast agents should be used when indicated for evaluation of gastrointestinal tract. Iodinated contrast agents such as diatrizoate meglumine preparations (Gastrografin and Hypaque) are commercially available for oral use (Fig. 2-9). For genitourinary fluoroscopic procedures, ionic contrast agents such as Renografin and Cystografin are preferred over nonionic contrast agents in most institutions owing to the lower cost.

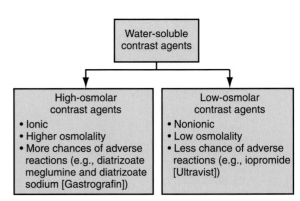

■ **FIGURE 2-8** Water-soluble contrast agents.

■ **FIGURE 2-7** Different barium sulfate preparations for gastrointestinal study.

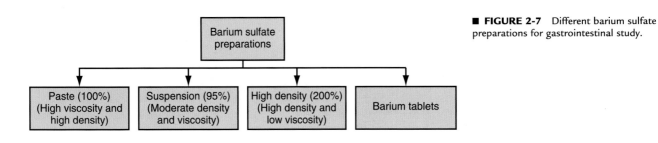

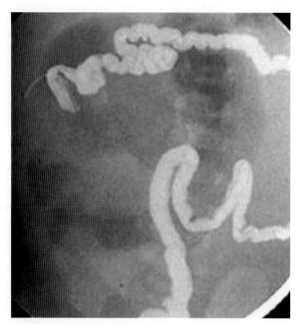

■ **FIGURE 2-9** Gastrografin enema performed in a neonate with intestinal obstruction shows microcolon.

Gastrografin

Gastrografin (diatrizoate meglumine and diatrizoate sodium) is a commercially available oral contrast medium for opacification of gastrointestinal tract. This preparation is particularly indicated when use of a more viscous agent such as barium sulfate, which is not water soluble, is not feasible or is potentially dangerous.

Oral Administration

Adult oral dosage usually ranges from 30 to 90 mL (11 to 33 g iodine), depending on the type of the examination and the size of the patient. For infants and children younger than 5 years of age, 30 mL (11 g iodine) is usually adequate; for children 5 to 10 years of age, the suggested dose is 60 mL (22 g iodine). These pediatric doses may be diluted 1:1, if desired, with water, carbonated beverage, milk, or mineral oil.

For very young (<10 kg) and debilitated children the dose should be diluted as 1 part Gastrografin in 3 parts water.

Enemas or Enterostomy Instillations

Gastrografin should be diluted when it is used for enemas and enterostomy instillations. When used as an enema, the suggested dilution for adults is 240 mL (88 g iodine) in 1000 mL of tap water. For children younger than 5 years of age, a 1:5 dilution in tap water is suggested; for children older than 5 years of age, 90 mL (33 g iodine) in 500 mL of tap water is a suitable dilution.

Oral Gastrografin Indications

Indications for oral use of Gastrografin include the following:

TABLE 2-4   Patient Factors in Gastrointestinal Fluoroscopy
Ability to Ingest Contrast   To get high-quality images, a relatively large volume of contrast agent needs to be ingested fairly quickly.
Mobility   Multiple positions are required for gastrointestinal examinations, particularly double-contrast examinations.   Limited mobility = fewer diagnostic images
Weight   Tables have weight limits.   Maximal radiographic technique is required, and exposure is often suboptimal.

- Cystic fibrosis and subacute intestinal obstruction, because risk of obstruction in the small bowel is greater with barium
- Intestinal perforation
- Suspected tracheoesophageal fistula and pyloric stenosis, to avoid barium aspiration
- Recent rectal biopsy, recent surgery, to visualize postoperative leak, or to visualize ileostomy or colostomy loops
- Infants and neonates with suspected intestinal obstruction, necrotizing enterocolitis, unexplained pneumoperitoneum, gasless abdomen, other bowel perforation, esophageal perforation, or postoperative anastomosis

For genitourinary evaluation the ionic contrast agents are preferred over the nonionic agents owing to the cost factor. However, in patients with a previous history of allergic reactions nonionic agents are preferred. The dose and dilution depend on the investigation and body part examined.

Equipment Factors

Equipment factors include the following:

- Source-to-image distance
- Fluoroscopic kilovolt peak
- Fluoroscopic milliampere
- Focal spot
- Field of view
- Grid use
- Fluoroscopic acquisition mode
- Dose rate selection
- Video frame rate

Patient Factors

Patient factors are listed in Table 2-4.

Side Effects

Barium

The side effects of barium include:

- Bloating
- Constipation (severe or continuing)
- Cramping (severe)

● Nausea or vomiting
● Stomach or lower abdominal pain
● Tightness in chest or troubled breathing
● Wheezing

Some people have reported sensitivity to the flavoring substance and exposure to latex (in gloves and tubes) used in barium contrast studies. Allergic reactions to barium sulfate suspensions are estimated to occur at a rate of less than 2 per million.

Iodinated Oral Contrast Media

The side effects of iodinated oral contrast media may vary from mild reactions such as itching or a rash to rare life-threatening reactions such as shock. These media should be used with caution in patients with known hypersensi-tivity to iodine, bronchial asthma, eczema, and thyroid disorders such as thyrotoxicosis. Also, patients with inflammatory bowel disease and those with conditions in which there is absorption of contrast media from a mucosal surface may have increased chances of a reaction.[14,15] With oral administration patients may experience nausea, vomiting, diarrhea, and stomach cramps.

PROS AND CONS

Fluoroscopic examinations may be affordable, but results depend on various factors, including the skill of the radiologist, quality of fluoroscopic equipment, and the patient's weight and compatibility. However, as compared with advanced modalities such as CT or MRI, fluoroscopy has limitations in cross-sectional imaging and radiologic tissue diagnosis.

SUGGESTED READINGS

Gelfand DW, Ott DJ, Chen YM. Optimizing single- and double-contrast colon examinations. Crit Rev Diagn Imaging 1987; 27:167-201.

Maglinte DD, Romano S, Lappas JC. Air (CO_2) double-contrast barium enteroclysis. Radiology 2009; 252:633-641.

Nolan DJ. Barium examination of the small intestine. Br J Hosp Med 1994; 6:136-141.

Op den Orth JO. Use of barium in evaluation of disorders of upper gastrointestinal tract: current status. Radiology 1989;173:601-608.

Rubesin SE, Maglinte DD. Double-contrast barium enema technique. Radiol Clin North Am 2003; 41:365-376.

Schueler BA. The AAPM/RSNA physics tutorial for residents: general overview of fluoroscopic imaging. RadioGraphics 2000; 20:1115-1126.

REFERENCES

1. Cowen AR, Davies AG, Sivananthan MU. The design and imaging characteristics of dynamic, solid-state, flat-panel x-ray image detectors for digital fluoroscopy and fluorography. Clin Radiol 2008; 63:1073-1085.

2. Schueler BA. The AAPM/RSNA physics tutorial for residents: general overview of fluoroscopic imaging. RadioGraphics 2000; 20:1115-1126.

3. Op den Orth JO. Use of barium in evaluation of disorders of upper gastrointestinal tract: current status. Radiology 1989; 173:601-608.

4. Nolan DJ. Barium examination of the small intestine. Br J Hosp Med 1994; 6:136-141.

5. Tanomkiat W, Galassi W. Barium sulfate as contrast medium for evaluation of postoperative anastomotic leaks. Acta Radiol 2000; 41:482-485.

6. Gottesman L, Zevon SJ, Brabbee GW, et al. The use of water soluble contrast enemas in the diagnosis of acute lower left quadrant peritonitis. Dis Colon Rectum 1984; 27:84-88.

7. Matsukawa H, Shiraga N, Tsugu T, et al. The use of water-soluble contrast enema without pretreatment for the diagnosis of colon disease. Nippon Shokakibyo Gakkai Zasshi 2007; 104:1344-1351.

8. Gelfand DW, Ott DJ, Chen YM. Optimizing single- and double-contrast colon examinations. Crit Rev Diagn Imaging 1987; 27:167-201.

9. Rubesin SE, Maglinte DD. Double-contrast barium enema technique. Radiol Clin North Am 2003; 41:365-376.

10. Jobling JC. Air versus carbon dioxide insufflation in double contrast barium enemas: the role of active gaseous drainage. Br J Radiol 1996; 69:89-89.

11. Ott DJ, Gelfand DW. Gastrointestinal contrast agents. Indications, uses, and risks. JAMA 1983; 249:2380-2384.

12. Rubin JD, Cohan RH. Iodinated radiographic contrast media: comparison of low-osmolar with conventional ionic agents [corrected]. Curr Opin Radiol 1991; 3:637-645.

13. Kory LA, Epstein BS. The oral use of iodinated water-soluble contrast agents for visualizing the proximal colon when barium enema examination reveals complete obstruction. Am J Roentgenol Radium Ther Nucl Med 1972; 115:355-359.

14. Ridley LJ. Allergic reactions to oral iodinated contrast agents: reactions to oral contrast. Australas Radiol 1998; 42:114-117.

15. Eisenberg RL, Hedgcock MW, Shanser JD, et al. Iodine absorption from the gastrointestinal tract during Hypaque-enema examination. Radiology 1979; 133:597-599.

Ultrasound

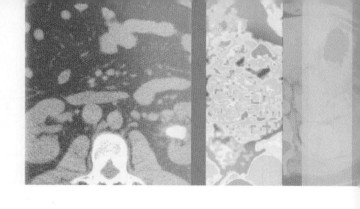

CHAPTER 3

Ultrasound Physics and Instrumentation: A Condensed View

Jennifer McDowell

TECHNICAL ASPECTS

Currently all diagnostic ultrasound systems rely on the ability of the sonographer to adjust certain parameters to demonstrate the most accurate image possible. Because of this user reliance, it is imperative to understand the physics of ultrasound.[1-3] There are several ways to adjust the displayed ultrasound image to obtain an accurate diagnosis. Understanding the knobology of the ultrasound system is important to optimize the image quality according to specific areas of interest and patient body habitus.

ULTRASOUND WAVES

Ultrasound travels at a rate of 1540 meters per second through soft tissue (Fig. 3-1). The density of the tissue being evaluated will affect the speed at which the sound waves travel. More dense tissue will cause the sound waves to slow, and less dense tissue will cause the ultrasound waves to increase in speed. Sound does not propagate well in gas because the molecules are far apart and therefore less dense.

TRANSDUCERS

A transducer is an instrument that converts one form of energy to another and acts as the receiver and processor of the returned sound waves. Ultrasound transducers are made of piezoelectric material that expands and contracts to generate the ultrasound pulses. Selecting the appropriate transducer is essential to optimally image the area in question. Ultrasound transducers have multi-frequency bandwidths that allow for a range of imaging options for each selected transducer. For example, a 3.5-MHz transducer will have a range of 2.5 to 4.0 MHz. This allows for better penetration using the 2.5 MHz on more dense tissue

and the 4.0 MHz on more easily penetrated tissue where better resolution is desired. The lower-frequency transducers will allow for more penetration into tissues, but there is a resolution compromise. When possible, a higher-frequency transducer should be used for maximum resolution.

Transducer Selection (Fig. 3-2)

Linear Sequential Array

The linear transducer is typically used for soft tissue imaging, such as for thyroid, scrotal, musculoskeletal, and vascular studies.

Curved Array

The curved array transducer has a bigger footprint, which allows for a larger structure to be evaluated. This transducer has a wider range of depths, giving better depth penetration and a larger field of view. It is typically used for general abdominal imaging and obstetric/gynecologic studies.

Matrix Array

Matrix array transducers consist of elements arranged in rows and columns usually totaling 2500 elements.[1] This allows four-dimensional viewing, which is live three-dimensional imaging.

Transducer Care

Each ultrasound transducer has crystals lined up under the damping material that actually come into contact with the gel and patient. It is very important to handle each

Speed of sound

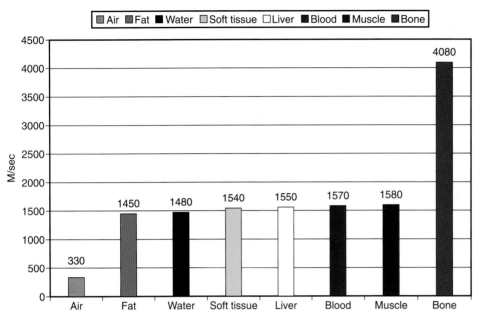

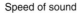

■ **FIGURE 3-1** Speed of sound as it travels through different tissues and structures within the body.

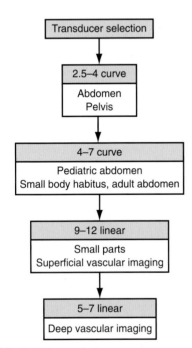

■ **FIGURE 3-2** Transducer selection.

transducer with care and finesse. If a transducer is dropped or mishandled and bumped, it can damage the crystals that send and receive the pulses. If there is a damaged crystal, there will be "drop out" and a portion of the image will not be present (Fig. 3-3).

KNOBOLOGY

● *Freeze:* causes the real-time image to stop and allows for permanent storage.
● *Overall gain:* increases the strength of sound and overall brightness of the entire area visualized on the ultrasound screen.

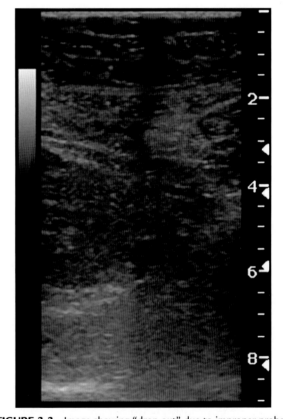

■ **FIGURE 3-3** Image showing "drop out" due to improper probe care and subsequent crystal damage.

● *Time gain compensation (TGC):* as ultrasound travels deeper into tissues, attenuation occurs. TGC allows the operator to adjust the strength of the beam in areas that would normally be weak due to the attenuated beam.
● *Depth:* the maximum depth is dependent on the transducer and area of interest. The ability to adjust the

imaging depth is important when attempting to evaluate deeper structures within the body.

- *Dual image:* the ultrasound screen can be split into two images; one side will be frozen and the other can be live. This is usually used to demonstrate images with and without calipers for measurements.
- *Focal zone:* focusing of the beam to specific areas of interest.
- *Color Doppler mode:* by activating this feature it allows the display of the blood flow to the area of interest. A color map appears that helps determine the direction of blood flow.
- *Power Doppler mode:* Power Doppler imaging is used to display a wide range of blood flow within a particular organ. It can display the amplitude of blood flow but not its direction.
- *Pulsed-wave Doppler mode:* by placing the pulsed-wave Doppler probe into a vessel it allows the operator to quantify the speed of blood flow to the particular organ that is being insonated.

IMAGING ARTIFACTS

Imaging artifacts can hinder a diagnosis by creating something that does not actually exist. However, ultrasound imaging artifacts can also help to aid in diagnosis.[1-3]

Propagation Artifact

When there is a great difference in density between two abutting tissues it will create a stronger return signal. This can create propagation artifacts within a seemingly normal anatomic structure.

Reverberation Artifact

This artifact occurs when the ultrasound signal is sent between two highly reflective tissues. This bouncing back and forth increases the speed of the ultrasound wave and creates linear lines or bands that do not actually exist within the structure being imaged (Fig. 3-4).

Comet Tail Artifact

This artifact can be referred to as a reverberation artifact. The differential criteria are that the linear lines or bands decrease in brightness the deeper they go into the body (Fig. 3-5).

Refraction Artifact

This is created by the ultrasound beam bending (Fig. 3-6) and has also been referred to as an edge shadow because this artifact has a tendency to appear along the edge of a curved structure.

Side Lobe Artifact

This artifact is a direct result of off-axis sound beams. This means that the ultrasound beam does not return parallel to the main beam axis. This artifact can make fluid appear

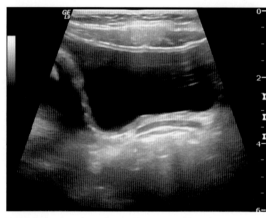

■ **FIGURE 3-4** Reverberation artifact seen within the urinary bladder.

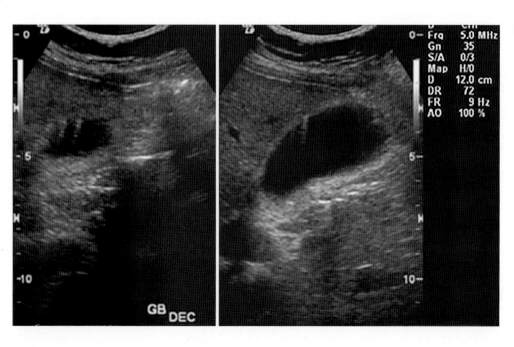

■ **FIGURE 3-5** Comet tail artifact demonstrating the linear bands decreasing in strength.

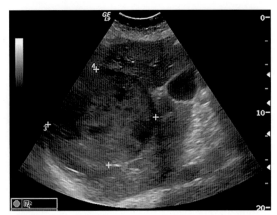

■ **FIGURE 3-6**   Edge shadow artifact showing a bending of the ultrasound beam.

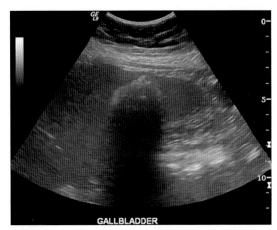

■ **FIGURE 3-7**   Shadowing artifact of the gallbladder wall.

more viscous or debris-filled and degrade lateral resolution.

Mirror Image Artifact

This artifact occurs most often when imaging the left upper abdomen. For example, it gives a false impression that the spleen is above the level of the diaphragm by creating a mirror image of the structure, the spleen, from below the diaphragm. This occurs because the diaphragm is a strong reflector of sound waves.

Shadowing Artifact

Shadowing occurs because of a loss of information. There is a dramatic decrease in the beam intensity owing to a strong reflector or attenuating structure, such as gallstones, renal calculi, or bone (Fig. 3-7).

Acoustic Enhancement

Increased acoustic enhancement occurs because sound travels quicker through less dense material, such as fluid-filled structures. This causes structures distal to the fluid-filled area to have more echoes than the adjacent areas that are not posterior to the structure. This artifact is used to advantage in many cases. Ultrasonography can better

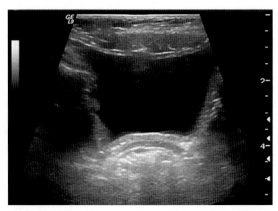

■ **FIGURE 3-8**   Image demonstrating posterior enhancement. There is an increase in the sound waves posterior to the fluid-filled object in comparison with other surrounding tissues.

evaluate structures when there is fluid above the area of interest. Most female and male bladders are filled to better visualize the anatomy that lies below (Fig. 3-8), which for the female patient is the uterus and ovaries and for the male patient is the prostate.

PROS AND CONS

Ultrasound studies are noninvasive, use no radiation, and have no known side effects. Ultrasonography is also fairly inexpensive and more portable in comparison with other imaging options such as MRI and CT. Ultrasonography is a user-dependent imaging modality that does take away the uniform structure that comes with a CT scan or an MR image. This can both benefit and hinder the interpretation of the images in diagnosing the questioned pathologic process. Obtaining a quality diagnostic ultrasound image can be difficult owing to anatomic barriers such as bowel gas in poorly prepped patients. Unlike other imaging modalities, ultrasonography does offer real-time evaluation of body parts and organs. This can be of great benefit when doing more invasive procedures that require a real-time view of needle placement. Current ultrasound technology not only allows for real-time needle placement in two dimensions but also allows for four-dimensional needle placement. This has been a recent and important advancement for complicated procedures that require four-dimensional real-time viewing.

CONTROVERSIES

Even though ultrasonography has no known side effects, it is still recommended that the ALARA (As Low As Reasonably Achievable) principle be practiced whenever possible. Prudent judgment should be used when scanning. Minimal exposure time is always optimum. Ultrasonography is a user-dependent modality that allows the operator more freedom when creating the images. This creates a less uniform study that can be somewhat unpredictable for the individual who has the responsibility of interpreting the acquired images. Having a skilled sonographer who is able to manipulate the ultrasound system to obtain the highest quality images is essential. This can aid the interpreting physician in attaining the correct diagnosis.

KEY POINTS

- Select the correct transducer for appropriate penetration of body part and resolution for optimal imaging.
- Understand the artifacts and recognize them when they appear in a seemingly normal structure.
- Adhere to the ALARA guidelines; image only as long as necessary to obtain an accurate diagnosis.
- Know the machine's knobology; this will help to optimize images and better evaluate the anatomy in question. This is especially important in patients with medical conditions that can complicate the examination.

SUGGESTED READINGS

Benacerraf B. Book review: Diagnostic Ultrasound Principles and Instruments, 7th ed. J Ultrasound Med 2006; 25:280.

Boote EJ. AAPM/RSNA physics tutorial for residents: topics in US, Doppler US techniques, concepts of blood flow detection and flow dynamics. RadioGraphics 2003; 23:1315-1327.

Hangiandreou NJ. B-mode US: basic concepts and new technology. RadioGraphics 2003; 23:1019-1033.

REFERENCES

1. Kremkau FW, Dripps RD, Eckenhoff JE, et al. Diagnostic Ultrasound Principles and Instruments, 7th ed. Philadelphia, Saunders, 2005.
2. Mittelstaedt CA. General Ultrasound. New York, Churchill Livingstone, 1992.
3. Rumack CM, Wilson SR, Charboneau WJ. Diagnostic Ultrasound, 3rd ed. St. Louis, Elsevier Mosby, 2005.

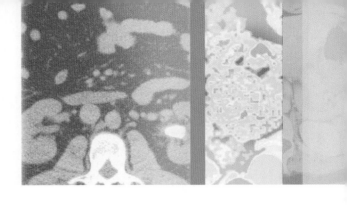

CHAPTER 4

Abdominal Ultrasound Imaging

Jennifer McDowell

TECHNICAL ASPECTS

Ultrasonography can be used for visualizing any solid structure within the abdomen. It can also be used to image the abdominal wall, certain types of bowel abnormalities, and soft tissue masses. The vasculature within these structures can be evaluated by initializing the color Doppler or power Doppler modes for low flow lesions. Ultrasonography is considered the gold standard for imaging the gallbladder and pathologic processes related to it. It is not the gold standard, nor is it recommended, for pathologic determinations involving the pancreas; instead, CT is considered to be the best means of evaluating pancreatic lesions.

PROS AND CONS

Ultrasonography is an inexpensive, portable, noninvasive imaging option. It has no known side effects. However, prudence should be used when utilizing this modality. Ultrasonography does have its limitations as far as what it can optimally image. Body habitus and dense tissues can create imaging obstacles for sonographers. These obstacles can make imaging difficult and sometimes impossible. Ultrasonography is a very user-dependent modality that can both hinder and aid in the diagnosis of pathologic processes within the body. The more experienced sonographer can optimize the images by adjusting the ultrasound machine settings and changing transducers. There are many manipulations of the ultrasound system that the sonographer can make to optimize an image. This variable creates a level of uncertainty when it comes to the interpretation of the actual images and any subsequent pathologic processes.

CONTROVERSIES

Ultrasonography is a user-dependent modality that allows the operator more freedom when creating representative images. This creates a less uniform study that can be somewhat unpredictable for the individual who has the responsibility of interpreting the acquired images. Having a skilled sonographer who is able to manipulate the ultrasound system is essential to help the interpreting physician visualize any pathologic process that may be present and obtain the correct diagnosis.

IMAGING OF SPECIFIC AREAS

Liver and Ducts

The liver occupies the majority of the right upper quadrant within the abdomen.[1-3] Its size generally makes it easy to find and image. Landmarks should be indicated to ensure it has been evaluated in its entirety. The left lobe of the liver can be visualized just below the xiphoid process in both sagittal and transverse planes. The right lobe of the liver sits under the ribs high in the right upper quadrant. However, there are many windows that can be used for complete organ visualization (Fig. 4-1). This can make it more challenging to image in comparison with the left lobe. There are also patient positioning options that should be explored (Fig. 4-2). The traditional window has been one that is anterior and medial to the rib cage (Fig. 4-3). Some of the scanning options for the liver include scanning subcostally (Fig. 4-4), intercostally, or with the patient upright, scanning while having the patient extend the abdomen or perform a Valsalva maneuver and scanning after rolling the patient into the left posterior oblique (LPO) position. If scanning is done subcostally, then the transducer must be angled in an extreme cephalic manner. Scanning the liver intercostally can be a challenge if using a large footprint probe (Fig. 4-5). The transducer typically used for abdominal scanning is curved and of 2 to 5 MHz. This transducer has a large footprint for a wider field of view and better resolution. It can be beneficial to switch to a smaller footprint sector probe to image both costally and subcostally (Fig. 4-6). Attempting to image through the ribs with a large footprint probe can be

Organ	Typical window	Alternate window
Liver	Anterior Coronal	Subcostal Intercostal
Gallbladder	Anterior Coronal	Subcostal Intercostal
Pancreas	Midline/subxiphoid	Sternal angling through the liver
Right kidney	Coronal	Intercostal Posterior
Left kidney	Coronal	Intercostal Posterior
Spleen	Coronal	Posterior
Aorta	Midline	Lt lateral medial to the kidney

■ **FIGURE 4-1** Alternate scanning windows.

Organ	Patient positioning options
Liver	LPO or left lateral decub Upright Standing
Gallbladder & Ducts	LPO or left lateral decub Upright Standing
Pancreas	Upright Standing
Right kidney	LPO or left lateral decub
Left kidney	RPO or right lateral decub Upright
Spleen	LPO
Pancreas	Upright Standing LPO
Aorta	RPO

■ **FIGURE 4-2** Alternate patient positioning options.

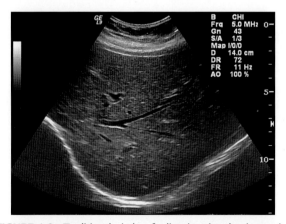

■ **FIGURE 4-3** Traditional window for liver imaging that is anterior and medial to the rib cage.

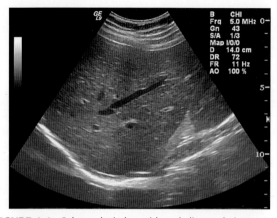

■ **FIGURE 4-4** Subcostal window with cephalic angulation.

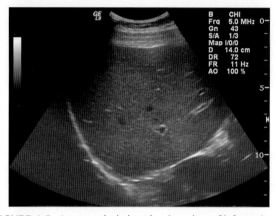

■ **FIGURE 4-5** Intercostal window showing a loss of information due to rib shadow.

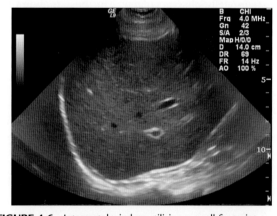

■ **FIGURE 4-6** Intercostal window utilizing a small footprint transducer to image between the ribs.

painful for the patient because of the costal nerves. Having the patient sit in the upright position and perform a Valsalva maneuver can essentially accomplish liver visualization more easily. Both maneuvers move the diaphragm down, thereby moving the liver into adequate visualization. Rolling the patient into an LPO position can move the liver out from under the ribs and closer to the midline. These techniques can be helpful when dealing with a patient with a partial liver transplant or a small cirrhotic liver.[1-3] All of these techniques can be used to better visualize the ductal system as well. The most commonly used alternative is rolling the patient into the LPO position. The power Doppler mode should be used to help differentiate the ductal system from the hepatic artery.

Gallbladder

When imaging the gallbladder it is imperative to visualize the neck of the organ for any obstructing stones. The neck of the gallbladder is also the most difficult image to obtain. If there is inadequate visualization, the patient should be rolled into the LPO or left lateral decubitus position. If these techniques do not help, then the patient can sit upright or stand while being scanned. The gallbladder should always be imaged with the patient rolled or standing in addition to the patient being supine. This is done to ensure that there are no stones hiding on the back wall of the gallbladder and that there is nothing within the neck of the gallbladder. When gallstones or sludge are present it is important to document that they move with the patient: a polyp or mass within the gallbladder will not move with patient manipulation. Additionally, hyperemia should be evaluated on all nonmobile pathologic processes within the gallbladder.[1-3]

Kidney and Spleen

Imaging the right kidney can be less complicated than imaging the left kidney. The liver can be used as a window for viewing the right kidney. Imaging the left kidney can prove to be a challenge because a normal-sized spleen does not allow for an optimal imaging window (Fig. 4-7). This can be especially difficult in patients with a barrel-shaped chest, those who are smaller than normal, or those with a surgically absent spleen. The best technique for visualization of the left kidney is having the patient perform a Valsalva maneuver while in the supine position. If the patient is not able to cooperate, then placing the patient into the right posterior oblique (RPO) position can bring the kidney into visualization. If the kidney is still not adequately visualized, the patient can be kept in the RPO position and scanned from the posterior aspect (Fig. 4-8). The best way to image for renal calculi is from the posterior aspect. It can be a very physically challenging task to visualize the entire kidney. It also may be necessary to image one portion of the kidney in one view and the remaining portion in another.

The Valsalva maneuver also should be used to image the spleen when necessary. If the spleen is atrophic, it also can be seen from the posterior aspect with the patient in the RPO position.

Pancreas

Ultrasound evaluation of the pancreas can be a challenge. Patients should be kept NPO for 6 to 8 hours to increase the probability of visualization. Because the pancreas is a retroperitoneal organ, and is seemingly smaller than other abdominal organs, it is common to have partial or no visualization in properly prepped patients. Imaging options in the instances that the pancreas is not fully visualized (Fig. 4-9) include imaging with the patient sitting upright, having the patient stand, rolling the patient onto either side, having the patient perform a Valsalva maneuver (Fig. 4-10), or filling the stomach to create a window for visualization. Having the patient drink two to three 8-ounce glasses of water can create a window to allow for full visualization. The patient can also be placed in the LPO position after drinking water to capitalize on the opportunity. Full evaluation of the other abdominal organs should be performed before having the patient

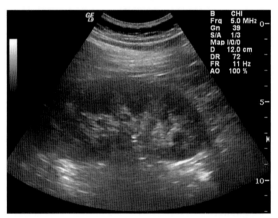

■ **FIGURE 4-8**   Posterior presentation showing the left kidney.

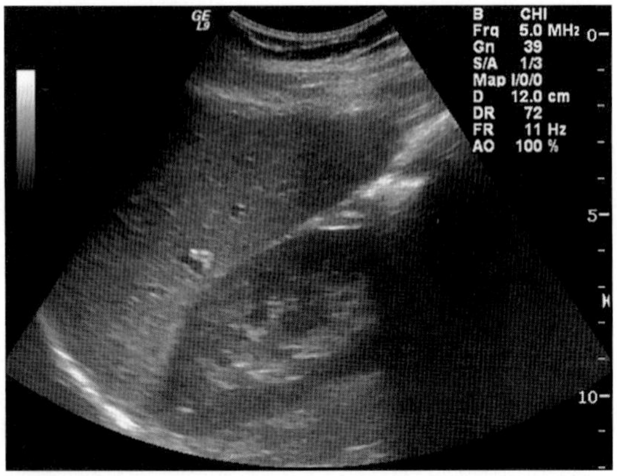

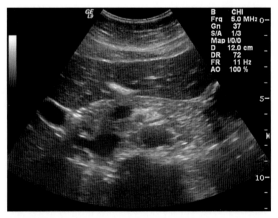

■ **FIGURE 4-7**   Typical coronal view of the left kidney.

■ **FIGURE 4-9**   Conventional midline view of the pancreas.

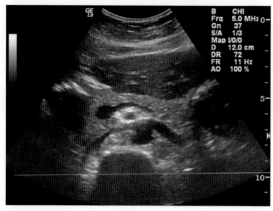

■ **FIGURE 4-10** Pancreas imaged with the patient performing a Valsalva maneuver.

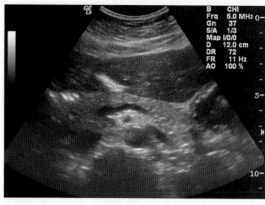

■ **FIGURE 4-12** Patient is performing a Valsalva maneuver, and the left lobe of the liver is being used as a window.

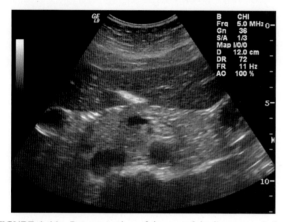

■ **FIGURE 4-11** Demonstration of the use of the liver as a window for pancreas evaluation.

drink water. An alternate window for pancreas visualization is going through the left lobe of the liver and angling the transducer caudad (Fig. 4-11). Having the patient perform a Valsalva maneuver and angling the transducer through the left lobe of the liver is another imaging option (Fig. 4-12).

Urinary Bladder

Adequate urinary bladder evaluation should be done while the bladder is distended. Polyps or bladder tumors are often not seen in an empty bladder. There is a higher risk of a reverberation artifact occurring when the bladder is full. Moving the transducer to the right or left of the urinary bladder and angling into the organ can decrease the probability of this artifact.

SUGGESTED READINGS

Baron RL, Tublin ME, et al. Imaging the spectrum of biliary tract disease. Radiol Clin North Am 2002; 40:vii, 1325-1354.

Boote EJ. AAPM/RSNA physics tutorial for residents: topics in US, Doppler US techniques, concepts of blood flow detection and flow dynamics. RadioGraphics 2003; 23:1315-1327.

Hangiandreou NJ. B-mode US: basic concepts and new technology. RadioGraphics 2003; 23:1019-1033.

Nienaber CA, von Kodolitsch Y, et al. The diagnosis of thoracic aortic dissection by noninvasive imaging procedures. N Engl Med J 1993; 328:1-9.

Wood BJ, Khan MA, McGovern F, et al. Imaging guided biopsy of renal masses: indications, accuracy and impact on clinical management. J Urol 1999; 161:1470-1474.

Zamir D, Jarchowsky J, et al: Inflammatory pseudotumor of the liver—a rare entity and a diagnostic challenge. Am J Gastroenterol 2004; 93:1538-1540.

REFERENCES

1. Rumack CM, Wilson SR, Charboneau WJ. Diagnostic Ultrasound, 3rd ed. St. Louis, Elsevier Mosby, 2005.
2. Mittelstaedt CA: General Ultrasound. New York, Churchill Livingstone, 1992.
3. Dogra V, Rubens DJ: Ultrasound Secrets. St. Louis, Elsevier, 2004.

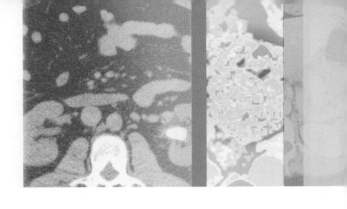

Harmonic Imaging

Xiaozhou Ma

TECHNICAL ASPECTS

Harmonics refers to the additional frequencies generated from the targeted tissue in the region of the ultrasound beam when a certain beam energy is reached. Harmonics is one of the acoustic phenomena, which are the integral (even) multiples of the fundamental frequency. *Fundamental frequency* is the original frequency of the acoustic beam emitted from the transducer. For instance, the fundamental frequency is 2 MHz and then its harmonic frequencies are 4 MHz, 6 MHz, 8 MHz, or more (Fig. 5-1).

Why Harmonic Imaging?

The large amounts of fat tissue, thickened skin layers (with or without scars), and the dehydrated status of patients are the predominant causes of ultrasound beam distortion and scattering. Grating lobes, slice thickness side lobes, and reverberation artifacts are the phenomena that frequently cause general image clutter.

Grating Lobes

Grating lobes are the secondary beams split off at angles to the main ultrasound beam, which are specific to nonlinear tissue, or nonlinear propagation (array transducers), that is caused by the regular, periodic spacing of the small array elements. When grating lobes are reflected from other structures surrounding the targeted area (e.g., fat), they cause off-axis artifacts and emulate unwanted effects on the ultrasound image as the echo returns to the transducer, resulting in "ghost images" blurring the main image.

Slice Thickness Side Lobes

Side lobes are unwanted parts of the ultrasound beam emitted off axis that produce image artifacts due to error in positioning of the returning echo.

Reverberation Artifacts

Reverberation artifacts are produced from the multiple reflections from a strong echo returning from a large acoustic interface: the detected echo does not run the shortest sound path because it bounces back and forth between the object and the transducer. In a reverberation artifact the sound wave is reflected back into the body usually from the transducer/skin interface, causing additional echoes parallel to the first.

How Harmonics Improve Imaging

The higher image quality is achieved by reducing the effects from grating lobes, slice thickness side lobes, and reverberation artifacts. The distorted and scattered energy from these artifacts is much weaker than the transmitted energy and therefore generates minimal energy of harmonics. As a result, a tissue harmonic image contains minimal noise and clutter produced in the back echoes.

The second harmonic (twice the fundamental frequency) is currently the frequency applied for harmonic imaging technically in ultrasonography. The third harmonic and even higher up to the fifth harmonic frequencies were recently analyzed and an improvement of signal-to-noise ratio in imaging in vitro was reported.[1,2]

EQUIPMENT

A broad transducer bandwidth is needed for harmonic imaging because the center frequency of the receiver must be set to twice the center frequency of the transmitted pulse.

PROCESS

Ultrasound equipment sends out a beam with a fundamental frequency and receives essentially the same frequency back as an echo. However, the sound wave becomes distorted when the tissue expands and compresses in response to the energy of the original wave. The reason for this is that the higher-pressure portions of the wave travel faster than the lower-pressure portions (see Fig. 5-1). When a certain energy level is reached, this distortion results in the generation of additional frequencies, which are the harmonics, that are two, three, or more times the fundamental emitted frequency. The echo containing the fundamental frequency and harmonic frequencies return to the transducer together.

Harmonic imaging is achieved by electronically filtering out the fundamental frequency and its grating lobes. The harmonic frequency can be isolated and can be used to create an alternative ultrasound image. Compared with the standard B-mode image, the harmonic image will typically show enhanced contrast by removing the noises.

TECHNICAL CHALLENGE

Tissue harmonic imaging provides a different view to the baseline ultrasound. The two imaging modes can therefore supplement each other to remove noise from images and provide a better basis for diagnosis. The challenge for the ultrasound system is to separate the clean harmonic signals from the fundamental signals. The simplest separation method is to lengthen the transmitted pulses. This technique will result in a clear separation of the fundamental and harmonic signals, and then a filter may be applied to remove the fundamental signals or the signals from grating lobes. Although this type of separation is easy to implement, using a lengthened transmit pulse will result in a narrower bandwidth harmonic signal and some degradation of image resolution.

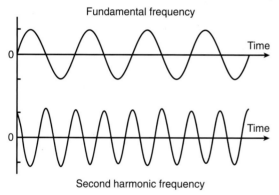

■ **FIGURE 5-1** Illustration of relationship between the fundamental frequency and the harmonic frequency.

Recently, a new technology called "pulse-inversion technique" has further improved the image quality with harmonic imaging (Fig. 5-2).[3]

CLINICAL APPLICATIONS

Because harmonics are generated within the targeted tissue itself, a certain distance from the transducer is required to build up the harmonic wave. Near-field imaging does not permit this. Conversely, the signal energy in the far field is decreasing. Therefore, harmonic imaging is most applicable when scanning structures in the middle field of the ultrasound beam. This technique is usually applied in the following situations.

"Technically Difficult" Patients

Patients with certain types of body composition, such as obesity, can be difficult to scan, and acoustic noise such as grating lobes can be easily generated. Therefore, the image quality can be improved with harmonic imaging (Fig. 5-3).

Cystic Structures

Cystic structures such as a large liver cyst, gallbladder, and urinary bladder have the round shape facing the ultrasound beam profile. Therefore, the phenomenon of grating lobes always exists in these kinds of situations. Harmonic imaging will increase the image conspicuity (Fig. 5-4).

Major Vascular Structures

Major vascular structures have a similar appearance as cystic structures, especially for deep-seated vessels, such as the inferior vena cava and abdominal aorta. The conspicuity of ultrasound images of the deep-seated vessels is easily affected by the anterior structures, causing grating lobes, slice thickness side lobes, and reverberation artifacts. Therefore, the harmonic imaging can improve conspicuity of these ultrasonic structures (Fig. 5-5).

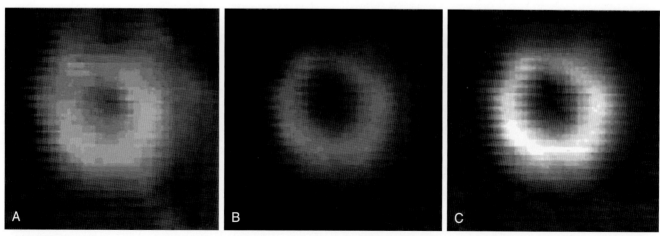

■ **FIGURE 5-2** Reconstructed images. **A,** Fundamental frequency image. Second harmonic image obtained before (**B**) and after (**C**) use of pulse-inversion technique. *(From Ma Q, Ma Y, Gong X, Xhang D. Improvement of tissue harmonic imaging using the pulse-inversion technique. Ultrasound Med Biol 2005; 31:889-894.)*

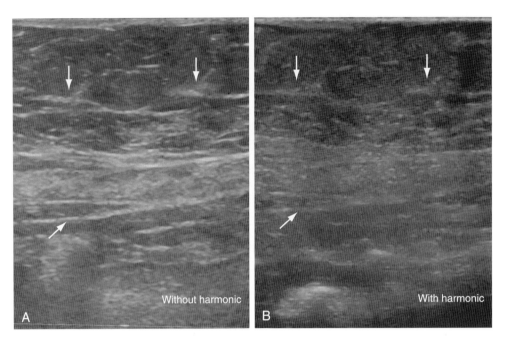

■ FIGURE 5-3 Comparison of normal thick superficial structures in ultrasound images: the microstructures such as the structure indicated by *arrows* appear blurred in the image without harmonic technique (**A**) and clear in the image using harmonic technique (**B**).

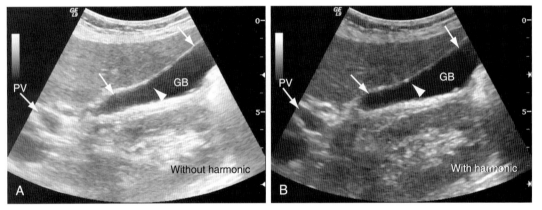

■ FIGURE 5-4 Comparison of images in the same location of the right upper quadrant without and with harmonic imaging. **A,** Image without harmonic imaging: the fundus and neck areas (GB, *arrows*) of gallbladder and intraportal venous area (PV, *arrow*) appear echogenic and cloudy. **B,** With harmonic technique, the figure shows a clear gallbladder and portal venous structure. In addition, the tiny calcification on the anterior wall of the gallbladder (*arrowhead*) is well shown on the harmonic image in **B** but invisible in the blurred image in **A**.

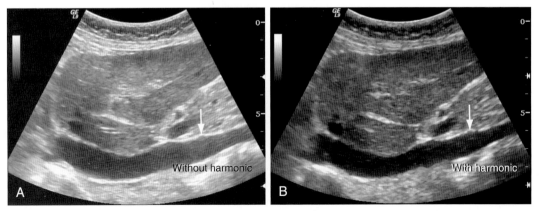

■ FIGURE 5-5 Comparison of image conspicuity without/with harmonic imaging in the sagittal plane of the left liver and the long axis of the inferior vena cava (IVC). The *arrow* points to the intra-IVC area, which is obviously cloudy and blurring in the nonharmonic image (**A**) compared with the harmonic image (**B**).

Contrast-Enhanced Ultrasonography

The harmonic echoes (usually the second harmonic) of the fundamental transmitted frequency are selectively detected and used for imaging; however, the higher harmonics may be created by nonlinear scattering, such as from gas microbubbles. Therefore, an improved detection of blood flow in small vessels can be achieved by selectively enhancing the Doppler signal from blood and at the same time suppressing the echoes from surrounding tissue when harmonic Doppler ultrasound imaging is used with microbubble contrast media.[4]

KEY POINT

■ Harmonic imaging technique fused in the gray-scale ultrasound image will improve the image conspicuity by decreasing grating lobes, slice thickness side lobes, and reverberation artifacts, especially in cystic structures.

SUGGESTED READINGS

Hykes D, Hedrick WR, Starchman D (eds). Ultrasound Physics and Instrumentation, 4th ed. Philadelphia, Mosby, 2005.

Kremkau FW. Ultrasound: Principles and Instruments, 6th ed. Philadelphia, WB Saunders, 2002.

Rumack CM, Wilson SR, Charboneau JW. Diagnostic Ultrasound, 3rd ed. St. Louis, Elsevier Mosby, 2005.

Wells PN. Ultrasound imaging. Phys Med Biol 2006; 51:R83-R98.

Zagebski J. Essentials of Ultrasound Physics. St. Louis, CV Mosby, 1996.

REFERENCES

1. Ma Q, Zhang D, Gong X, Ma Y. Phase-coded multi-pulse technique for ultrasonic high-order harmonic imaging of biological tissues in vitro. Phys Med Biol 2007; 52:1879-1892.

2. Ma Q, Gong X, Zhang D. Third order harmonic imaging for biological tissues using three phase-coded pulses. Ultrasonics 2006; 44(Suppl 1):e61-e65.

3. Ma Q, Ma Y, Gong X, Xhang D. Improvement of tissue harmonic imaging using the pulse-inversion technique. Ultrasound Med Biol 2005; 31:889-894.

4. Kim TK, Choi BI, Han JK, et al. Hepatic tumors: contrast agent–enhancement patterns with pulse-inversion harmonic US. Radiology 2000; 216:411-417.

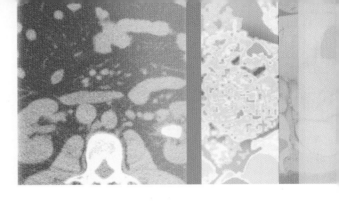

6

Doppler Ultrasound Imaging

Somesh Lala, Bijal Jankharia, and Vishakha Mazumdar

Doppler ultrasonography is a noninvasive technique that provides information about the condition of blood vessels and the flow direction. It also analyzes the flow velocity waveform and characterizes tissue to evaluate the vascularity of mass lesions. Color and pulsed-wave Doppler imaging are complementary and provide spatial orientation and a time velocity spectrum for quantification, respectively.[1] Sonographers who use this technique cultivate a combination of hand, eye, and ear coordination to achieve an accurate diagnosis.

TECHNICAL ASPECTS

Doppler examination requires not only a good quality machine with the appropriate probes but also a good person using the machine. This modality is highly operator dependent and requires a considerable amount of expertise. The following 5 "Ps" are important parameters to keep in mind:

- *Patient preparation:* Fasting for a Doppler examination of the abdomen is required and is particularly important for evaluation of the mesenteric, portal, and renal vessels. It is advisable not to chew gum or smoke before the examination.
- *Probes:* Commonly used probes are the (1) curvilinear-array probes (low frequency, 3-5 MHz), (2) phased-array probes (low frequency, 2 MHz), and (3) linear-array probes (high frequency, 4-10 MHz). Lower frequency produces greater tissue penetration, whereas the phased-array probes are useful in scanning through rib interspaces and in assessing the renal artery origins in obese patients.[2]
- *Person:* The sonographer should have a considerable amount of expertise to perform a Doppler examination. He or she should understand the normal anatomy, pathophysiology, and signature patterns of the various abdominal vessels and should optimize the machine to arrive at an appropriate diagnosis.
- *Picture quality (machine):* To obtain a good picture quality, the radiologist should consider the following operational parameters: (1) an appropriate anatomic window, (2) depth of field, (3) frame rate, (4) flow sensitivity with adjusted gain settings, (5) image vessel of interest at a Doppler angle of 30 to 60 degrees, and (6) low wall filter settings (if these are high, one can lose significant velocity information). The recorded color flow should occupy the full anteroposterior diameter or cross-sectional area of the vessel without color flow aliasing and noise in the surrounding tissues.
- *Positioning:* The various positions required for imaging every individual vessel are listed in Tables 6-1 to 6-5.

PROS AND CONS

Pros

- Doppler imaging is readily available and cost effective.
- It is portable and can be done by the bedside in sick or debilitated patients.
- It is noninvasive: no contrast agent is required, and it can be performed in patients with renal dysfunction.
- It can differentiate vascular and nonvascular structures (e.g., porta hepatis) (Fig. 6-1).
- It can provide information about the patency of blood vessels, direction of flow turbulence, phasicity, jet, impedance, and so on.
- It can provide quantification of stenosis and direct measurement of flow lumen reduction.
- It helps in tissue characterization of tumors.
- It is helpful in the preoperative and postoperative workup of liver and renal transplant patients and in the assessment of any complications.

Cons

- Doppler imaging is technically difficult to perform in obese patients and in those with overlying bowel gas or a distended abdomen, especially when desiring visualization of the mesenteric vessels or the portosplenic confluence, performing portosystemic collateral mapping, determining renal artery origin, evaluating a shunt anastomosis, and so on.

- Good spectral analysis cannot be achieved in patients who cannot hold their breath.
- The technique is operator dependent.
- Graft surveillance at the level of the distal abdominal aorta and iliac arteries is difficult.
- Abdominal aortic calcifications can be an obstacle in visualization of renal artery origin.

CONTROVERSIES

Doppler imaging may be controversial in certain situations:

1. In acute mesenteric ischemia, the patient is ill, is unable to hold his or her breath, and has a distended abdomen, which makes it virtually impossible to visualize the mesenteric vessels.
2. Nonvisualization of the origin of the renal artery occurs in obese patients or because of overlying bowel gas. Also, sometimes there is a kink or tortuosity in the vessel, which artifactually increases the peak systolic

TABLE 6-1 Positioning for Ultrasound Imaging of the Portal System

Vessel	Scanning View
Portal vein (PV), hepatic artery (HA), and right intrahepatic branches of these vessels	Right coronal oblique/anterolateral intercostal approach
Left intrahepatic portal vein and accompanying hepatic artery	Transverse and sagittal midline epigastric
Portal venous confluence	Sagittal midline (at level of epigastrium)
Anterior and posterior branches of right portal vein and proximal left portal vein	Transverse imaging centered at midclavicular line
Splenic artery and vein	Left coronal (right decubitus)

TABLE 6-2 Positioning for Ultrasound Imaging of the Hepatic Veins and Inferior Vena Cava

Vessel	Scanning View
Right hepatic vein	Right coronal (posterior and cephalad)
Middle hepatic vein	Right coronal (anterior and cephalad)
Left hepatic vein	Sagittal/transverse midline epigastric with cephalad angulation
Inferior vena cava	Sagittal midline, transverse epigastric (to trace downward up to the bifurcation)
Confluence of hepatic veins with inferior vena cava	Transverse subxiphoid approach

TABLE 6-3 Positioning for Ultrasound Imaging of the Mesenteric Vessels

Celiac axis and superior mesenteric artery	Sagittal midline (to see the origin of the two vessels along with the abdominal aorta) Transverse epigastric (for celiac axis bifurcation into hepatic and splenic arteries)
Superior mesenteric vein	Sagittal midline at same level of superior mesenteric artery
Inferior mesenteric artery	Sagittal midline (just above the aortic bifurcation and slightly oblique and left of the midline)
Inferior mesenteric vein	Sagittal midline (at same level of inferior mesenteric artery)

TABLE 6-4 Positioning for Ultrasound Imaging of the Great Vessels

Aorta lies to the left of inferior vena cava	Sagittal midline Transverse epigastric for axial view (trace downward up to the inferior vena cava/aorta bifurcation)

TABLE 6-5 Positioning for Ultrasound Imaging of the Renal Arteries

Right renal artery/vein	Right coronal (left decubitus)/right anterolateral transverse approach
Left renal artery/vein	Left coronal (right decubitus) from left posterolateral transverse/longitudinal approach
Renal artery origin	Transverse midline oblique (to locate origin of arteries on transverse aortic view just caudad to superior mesenteric artery)

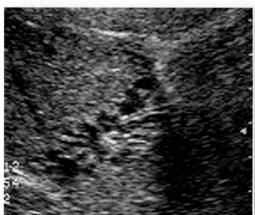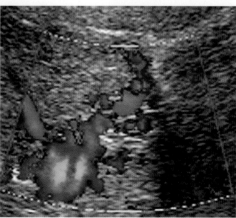

■ **FIGURE 6-1** Transverse Doppler imaging centered at midclavicular line reveals multiple collateral vessels in the porta hepatis that mimic dilated intrahepatic biliary radicles.

velocity and mimics a renal artery stenosis. There could be multiple renal arteries/accessory renal arteries in many patients that are often not picked up on Doppler imaging, and hence a stenosis can be missed.[3,4] In hemodynamically insignificant stenosis, renal Doppler imaging may be normal.

3. In the portal system due to a hyperdynamic circulation (e.g., congestive cardiac failure), the portal vein may be increased in caliber and a false-positive diagnosis of portal hypertension can be made. In the decompensated stage of portal hypertension the portal vein caliber may decrease owing to formation of portosystemic collateral vessels, and if one cannot visualize these vessels, a false-negative diagnosis of portal hypertension can be made.

Therefore, an alternate imaging modality needs to be considered and the clinician needs to be guided by the radiologist. However, because of its noninvasive nature Doppler imaging should always be the first line of investigation.

NORMAL ANATOMY

Portal System

The portal vein is formed by the union of the superior mesenteric and splenic veins behind the neck of the pancreas. It ends at the porta hepatis by dividing into right and left branches. After entering the liver, each branch divides along with the hepatic artery enclosed in Glisson's capsule to end ultimately in the hepatic sinusoids.[5,6]

At the porta hepatis, the common hepatic/common bile duct is normally anterior to the portal vein and hepatic artery (vein-artery-duct [VAD] from posterior to anterior).

The portal flow in normal individuals is hepatopetal (toward the liver) throughout the entire cardiac cycle. The normal caliber of the vein is 13 mm in quiet respiration and 16 mm in deep inspiration. It is commonly measured where the portal vein crosses the inferior vein cava. The mean flow velocity is 15 to 18 cm/s. Portal flow varies with cardiac activity and respiration, giving the waveform an undulating appearance (Fig. 6-2).

The superior mesenteric and splenic veins are two primary contributors of portal vein flow. The splenic vein lies posterior to the pancreas. The superior mesenteric vein extends caudad from the portosplenic confluence and parallels the course of the superior mesenteric artery (Fig. 6-3). The normal caliber of the superior mesenteric vein and splenic vein should be less than 10 mm.

Hepatic Veins

There are three major hepatic veins, which converge to the inferior vena cava at the level of the diaphragm. The right hepatic vein runs in a coronal plane between the anterior and posterior segments of the right hepatic lobe. The middle hepatic vein lies between the right and left hepatic lobes. The left hepatic vein runs between the medial and lateral segments of the left lobe. In most individuals the left hepatic and middle hepatic veins join to form a common trunk before entering the inferior vena cava. The caudate lobe has its own accessory venous drainage directly into the inferior vena cava. The inferior right hepatic vein is seen in 10% of cases.

Renal Arteries

The renal arteries arise from the aorta slightly below the origin of the superior mesenteric artery. The right renal artery arises from the anterolateral aspect of the aorta and then passes posterior to the inferior vena cava as it curves toward the renal hilum (Fig. 6-4). The left renal artery arises from the posterolateral aspect of the aorta and follows a posterolateral course to the left renal hilum.

The renal arteries are scanned from their origin at the level of the aorta up to the level of the cortex. Flow signals are obtained at the (1) origin, (2) mid segment, (3) hilum, (4) mid zone of kidney, and (5) cortical branches.[7]

Renal Veins

Renal veins are formed from tributaries that coalesce in the renal hilum. The left renal vein receives the adrenal vein from above and the left gonadal vein (ovarian or testicular) from below. The left renal vein passes posterior

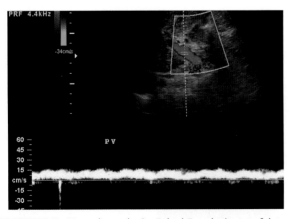

■ **FIGURE 6-2**　Normal portal vein. Pulsed Doppler image of the portal vein shows normal undulating signature pattern with phasic flow. Peak systolic velocity = 15 cm/s.

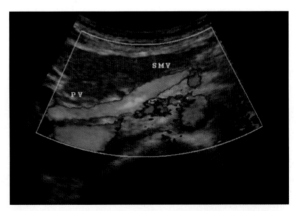

■ **FIGURE 6-3**　Superior mesenteric vein. Long-axis view shows a normal superior mesenteric vein (SMV) becoming confluent with the portal vein (PV).

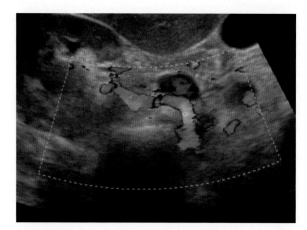

■ **FIGURE 6-4** Normal right renal artery. Right coronal oblique view with anterolateral transverse approach shows the course of the renal artery from the hilum to the origin.

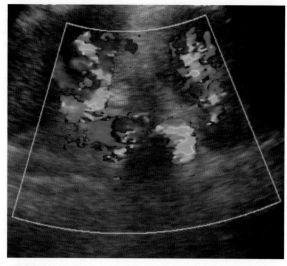

■ **FIGURE 6-6** Lienorenal collateral vessels. Transverse image of the left kidney shows tortuous collateral vessels between the splenic and renal hila.

to the superior mesenteric artery and anterior to the aorta to reach the left side of the inferior vena cava. The right renal vein, which is shorter than the left, extends directly into the inferior vena cava from the right renal hilum.

Abdominal Aorta

The aorta enters the abdomen through the aortic hiatus of the diaphragm immediately anterior to the 12th dorsal vertebra. It descends anterior and slightly to the left of the vertebral bodies. It is flanked on either side by the diaphragmatic crura. It bifurcates at the L4 level into the common iliac arteries, which are 5 cm long and run along with their respective veins. The main branches seen on ultrasonography include the celiac artery, paired renal arteries, superior mesenteric artery, common iliac artery, and inferior mesenteric artery (sometimes seen).

Inferior Vena Cava

The inferior vena cava is a large vein that returns blood from the lower limbs, pelvis, and abdomen to the right

atrium. It is formed by the paired common iliac veins on the anterior surface of the L5 vertebra and lies anteriorly and slightly to the right of the spine. The main branches are the renal, hepatic, and common iliac veins.

Abdominal Vessels

Portosystemic collateral vessels (Figs. 6-5 and 6-6) are explained in detail in Table 6-6.[5,6] The reader is referred to Table 6-7 for the normal appearance and signature pattern of abdominal vessels (Figs. 6-7 to 6-9).[8]

Celiac Artery

The celiac artery is also called the celiac trunk or axis. It is the most cephalad visceral branch of the abdominal aorta. It arises from the anterior aortic surface between the diaphragmatic crura and bifurcates 1 to 3 cm from its origin into the common hepatic and splenic arteries. It

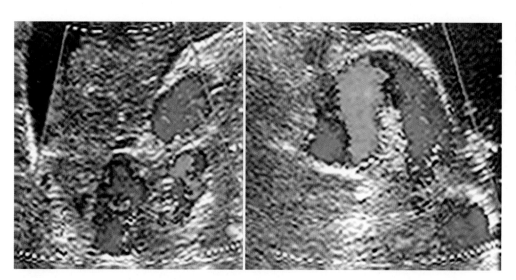

■ **FIGURE 6-5** Portosystemic collateral vessels. Long-axis view shows large, tortuous, left gastric vein collateral vessels along the inferior border of the left lobe of the liver.

TABLE 6-6 Portosystemic Collateral Vessels: Diagnostic Criteria

Site	Portosystemic	Appearance
Gastroesophageal junction. Normal coronary vein diameter < 6 mm	Between coronary/short gastric veins and systemic esophageal veins	Coronary veins > 7 mm are abnormal. Prominent cephalad-directed vessel arising from portal vein opposite superior mesenteric vein
Paraumblical vein (falciform ligament) Normal = 2 mm hepatopedal flow	Between left portal vein and systemic epigastric veins near umbilicus	Solitary vein originating from left portal vein courses inferiorly through falciform ligament and anterior abdominal wall to umbilicus, demonstrating hepatofugal flow
Gastroepiploic (see Fig. 6-5)	Between gastroepiploic and esophageal/paraesophageal veins	Cephalad directed vessel along the inferior border of the left lobe
Splenorenal and gastrorenal (splenic and renal hilum)	Between splenic, coronary, short gastric, and left adrenal or renal veins	Splenorenal (see Fig. 6-6). Tortuous, inferiorly directed vessels between spleen and upper pole of left kidney
Intestinal	Veins of ascending/descending colon, duodenum, pancreas, liver anastomosis with renal, phrenic and lumbar veins (systemic tributaries)	Collateral pathways identification on ultrasonography depends on the amount of air in the bowel at the time of study
Hemorrhoidal (perianal region)	Superior rectal vein anastomoses with systemic middle and inferior rectal veins	Rectal/pararectal varices can be detected with transvaginal or transrectal ultrasonography, cannot be visualized on transabdominal ultrasonography

TABLE 6-7 Normal Appearance and Signature Patterns of Abdominal Vessels

Vessel	Identification	Normal Signature Pattern
Portal vein: normal caliber = 13 mm (quiet respiration)	Anechoic structure, which runs in transverse plane and converges on the porta hepatis Surrounded by a sheath of echogenic fibrous tissue.	Undulating continuous waveform pattern with subtle phasic variation Hepatopetal flow (toward the liver)
Hepatic vein: normal caliber = 3 mm (measured 2 cm from inferior vena cava)	Longitudinally oriented sonolucent structures within liver parenchyma Best visualized with transverse subxiphoid approach to see the three main trunks with the inferior vena cava	Triphasic pulsatile waveform pattern with hepatofugal flow Naked margins
Hepatic artery[8]: normal velocity = 30-60 cm/s	Vascular structure anterior to portal vein	Low-resistance flow with spectral broadening
Inferior vena cava: normal caliber = 2.5 cm	Anechoic structure in the midline to the right of the aorta and anterior to the spine Upper part best visualized using liver as an acoustic window	Pulsatile flow near the heart: "sawtooth pattern" Phasic flow distally
Abdominal aorta: normal caliber = 2.3 cm (men), 1.9 cm (women)	Hypoechoic tubular pulsatile structure with echogenic walls best seen by longitudinal midline approach	High-resistance waveform pattern with a brief period of reversed flow (see Fig. 6-7)
Mesenteric vessels: normal caliber <10 mm	Superior mesenteric artery is surrounded by a triangular mantle of fat. It is to the right of superior mesenteric vein, which runs parallel to the superior mesenteric artery (see Figs. 6-8 and 6-9).	Superior mesenteric artery fasting view: high-resistance waveform pattern with sharp systolic peaks with absent late diastolic flow Postprandial shows low-resistance waveform pattern.
Celiac artery	Best visualized in transverse plane in which the "T"-shaped bifurcation of vessel into hepatic and splenic artery is characteristic	Low-resistance type of waveform
Renal artery and vein	Origin of artery is slightly caudad to superior mesenteric artery and best seen by transverse midline approach. Left renal vein is seen between superior mesenteric artery and aorta. Right renal vein can be traced from inferior vena cava.	Artery: low-resistance flow with broad systolic waveform and forward flow during diastole Vein: phasic with velocity varying with respiration and cardiac activity

also gives rise to the left gastric artery, which is not visualized on ultrasound imaging.

Splenic Artery

The splenic artery (left limb of "T" configuration) runs along the posterosuperior margin of the pancreatic body and tail. It gives rise to several pancreatic branches and the short gastric and left gastroepiploic arteries. None of

these branches can be seen on ultrasonography. The splenic artery terminates as a series of branches within the splenic hilum. The distal portion of the splenic artery is difficult to image because of tortuosity.

Hepatic Artery

The hepatic artery is the right limb of the celiac "T" configuration. It runs along the superior border of the

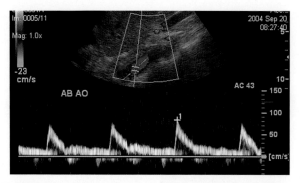

■ **FIGURE 6-7** Abdominal aorta. Long-axis view of the proximal abdominal aorta shows high-resistance flow with brief flow reversal. Doppler angle = 43 degrees.

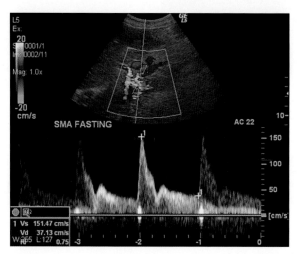

■ **FIGURE 6-8** Superior mesenteric artery. Long-axis view shows normal high-resistance waveform patterns of artery in fasting. Peak systolic velocity = 151 cm/s; resistive index = 0.75.

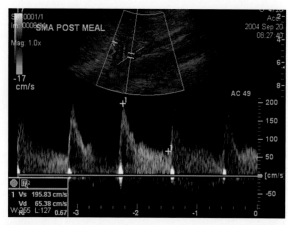

■ **FIGURE 6-9** Superior mesenteric artery. Postprandial Doppler image reveals low-resistance waveform pattern with increase in peak systolic velocity. Resistive index = 0.6.

IMAGING OF SPECIFIC CONDITIONS

Portal Hypertension

Common Causes

- Prehepatic: portal vein thrombosis (idiopathic, hypercoagulable states, pancreatitis), portal vein compression (tumor, trauma, lymphadenopathy)
- Intrahepatic: cirrhosis
- Post-hepatic: Budd-Chiari syndrome (idiopathic, hypercoagulable states, trauma, web, and tumor)

Pathophysiology

Portal hypertension is characterized by an increase in portal pressure, variously defined as hepatic venous pressure or direct portal vein pressure of more than 5 mm Hg greater than inferior vena cava pressure. Portosystemic collateral vessels form when the resistance to blood flow in the portal vein exceeds the resistance to flow in the small communicating channels between the portal and systemic circulation.[9-11] Hepatic vein thrombosis leads to elevated sinusoidal pressure, which causes delayed/reversal portal inflow and alteration in hepatic morphology. The combination of inferior vena cava and hepatic vein obstruction is the most common pattern of Budd-Chiari syndrome.[10]

Diagnostic Criteria

Gray Scale Imaging Findings

- Portal vein dilatation is greater than 13 mm.
- Superior mesenteric vein and splenic vein are greater than 10 mm.
- Lack of caliber variation in splanchnic veins is less than 20%.
- In thrombosis there may be partial visualization/failure to visualize the portal vein (chronic)/echogenic material within distended lumen (acute) (Figs. 6-10 and 6-11).

pancreatic head. Important tributaries are the gastroduodenal artery and the right gastric artery. Beyond the origin of the gastroduodenal artery, the common hepatic artery becomes the proper hepatic artery, which runs along with the portal vein to the porta hepatis and divides into the right and left hepatic arteries.

Superior Mesenteric Artery

The superior mesenteric artery arises from the anterior surface of the aorta immediately distal to the celiac artery. It consists of a short, anteriorly directed segment and a much longer, inferiorly directed segment that ends in the region of the ileocecal valve (see Figs. 6-8 and 6-9).

Inferior Mesenteric Artery

The inferior mesenteric artery arises from the anterior aspect of the aorta 3 to 4 cm proximal to the bifurcation. It runs downward and to the left and continues in the sigmoid mesocolon as the superior rectal artery.

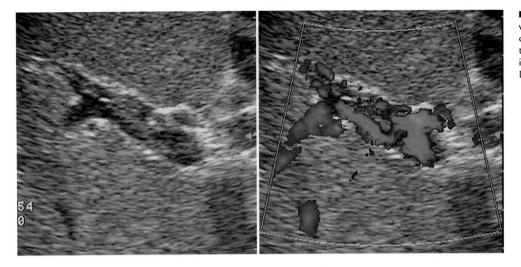

■ **FIGURE 6-10** Partial portal vein occlusion. Transverse imaging of the portal vein shows echogenic thrombus within the vein with incomplete filling on color flow Doppler imaging.

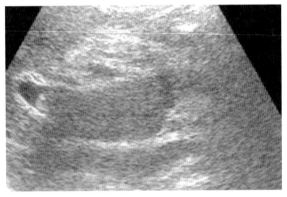

■ **FIGURE 6-11** Acute portal vein occlusion. Transverse image of the intrahepatic portal vein shows distended portal vein with thrombus within.

Doppler Imaging Findings

Portal Vein

- Thrombosis: absence of flow; malignant thrombus causes pulsatile flow, whereas bland thrombus does not (Fig. 6-12).

- Continuous monophasic flow is seen.
- Reduction in velocity is from 7 to 12 cm/s.
- Abnormal hepatofugal flow may be the only sign (Fig. 6-13).[12]
- Gallbladder varices may be associated with portal vein thrombosis (spontaneous portosystemic shunt) (Fig. 6-14).
- Chronic: echogenic/nonvisualized portal vein occurs with cavernoma formation (Fig. 6-15).[13]
- Aneurysmal dilatation of the portal vein occurs (Fig. 6-16).

Hepatic Artery

- The hepatic artery is dilated with increased resistance (renal resistive index > 0.78).

Hepatic Vein (Budd-Chiari Syndrome)

- Thrombus formation occurs (Fig. 6-17).
- The vein cannot be visualized.
- Stenosis/size reduction is noted as less than 3 mm (Fig. 6-18).
- Decreased/absent/reversed flow occurs in hepatic vein.

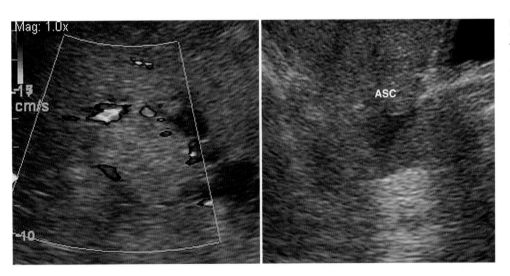

■ **FIGURE 6-12** Tumor thrombus from renal mass. Transverse image of the liver reveals echogenic material within the portal vein with peripheral flow along its walls. ASC, ascites.

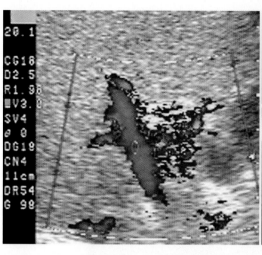
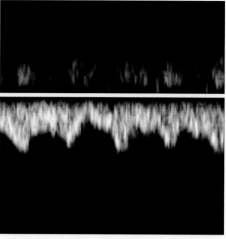

■ **FIGURE 6-13** Cirrhosis. Long-axis view of the liver shows hepatofugal flow (away from the liver) in the portal vein. Note that the signature pattern is below the baseline.

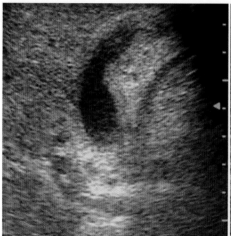
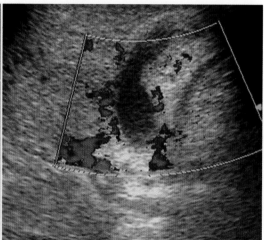

■ **FIGURE 6-14** Gallbladder varices. Transverse imaging of the liver shows hepatopetal collateral vessels involving the gallbladder wall.

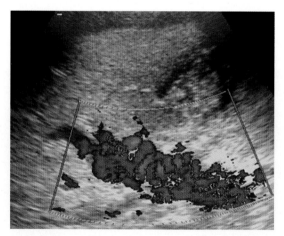

■ **FIGURE 6-15** Chronic portal vein thrombosis. Serpiginous tortuous collaterals along the porto-pancreatic axis suggestive of cavernoma formation.

● Communicating intrahepatic venous collateral vessels can be seen.

The reader is referred to Table 6-8 for the specifics of diagnostic imaging for portal hypertension.

Transjugular Intrahepatic Portosystemic Shunt (TIPS)

TIPS refers to portal decompression through a percutaneously established shunt between the hepatic and portal veins with an expandable metallic stent (Fig. 6-19).[14] It is done for esophageal/gastric variceal hemorrhage or refractory ascites in advanced liver disease with portal hypertension.

Doppler Imaging Findings

Post-TIPS spectral analysis should show a high-velocity turbulent flow (90 to 110 cm/s) and uniform flow at the portal and inferior vena cava end. Abnormal findings include generalized decrease in shunt velocity less than 60 cm/s, localized increase in shunt velocity, irregular filling defects, and absence of flow in the shunt.

Liver Transplantation

Doppler imaging plays an important role in assessing the vascular complications of liver transplants, which is the most frequent cause of graft loss. Most of the

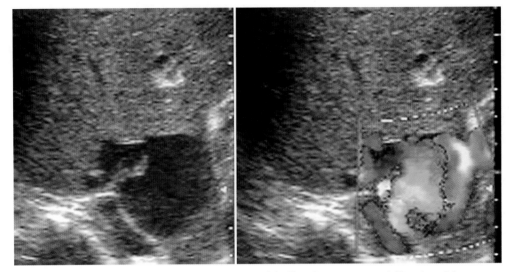

■ **FIGURE 6-16** Portal vein aneurysm. Long-axis view of the liver shows aneurysmal dilatation of the portal vein with "to and fro" flow within.

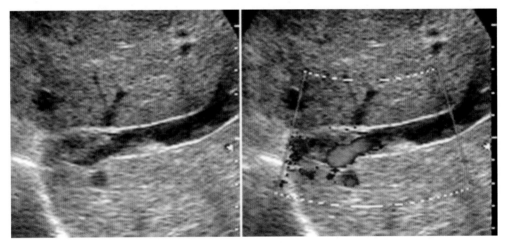

■ **FIGURE 6-17** Budd-Chiari syndrome. Right coronal oblique view shows echogenic thrombus partially obstructing the right hepatic vein.

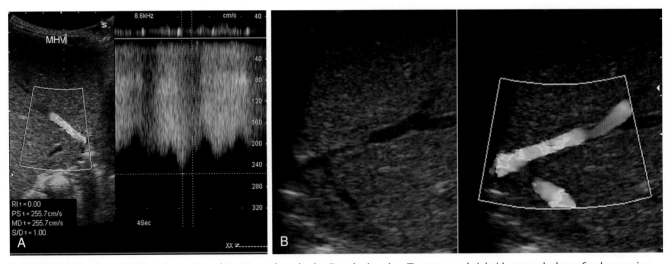

■ **FIGURE 6-18** Budd-Chiari syndrome. **A** and **B,** Gray scale and color Doppler imaging. Transverse subxiphoid approach shows focal narrowing and significant increase in peak systolic velocity in middle hepatic vein.

TABLE 6-8 Ultrasound Imaging of Portal Hypertension

	Prehepatic	Hepatic	Post-hepatic
Portal vein flow direction	Hepatopedal	Hepatofugal	Hepatofugal
Portal vein caliber (>13 mm)	Increased	Increased	Normal or increased
Liver texture/size	Normal	Altered	Altered
Caudate lobe hypertrophy	−	+	+
Hepatic wedge pressure	Normal	High	High
Secondary signs of portal hypertension (splenomegaly, ascites, portosystemic collateral vessels)	+	+	+

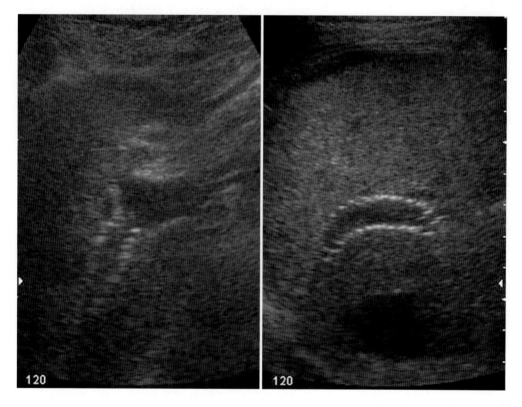

■ **FIGURE 6-19** Transjugular intrahepatic portosystemic shunt (TIPS). Right coronal view of liver shows a TIPS between the portal and hepatic veins.

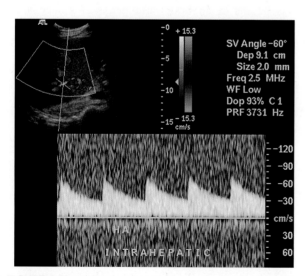

■ **FIGURE 6-20** Liver transplant. Post-transplant image of hepatic artery shows a normal low-resistance spectral waveform pattern with a renal resistive index of 0.57.

complications involve the inferior vena cava, portal vein, and hepatic artery (Fig. 6-20). The complications are commonly seen due to discrepancy in vessel caliber between the donor and the recipient, faulty surgical technique, and hypercoagulable states. The diagnostic criteria are listed in Table 6-9.

Mesenteric Ischemia

Mesenteric ischemia may be classified as occlusive or non-occlusive. Occlusion accounts for 75% of acute intestinal ischemia (Fig. 6-21). Mesenteric artery embolus/plaque due to rheumatic heart disease or atherosclerosis and venous occlusion due to infection or hypercoagulability states are the common causes (Fig. 6-22). Ischemia leads to breakdown of the mucosal barrier, which progressively leads to bowel infarction and eventual stricture formation. The diagnostic criteria are listed in Table 6-10.[15-18]

TABLE 6-9   Vascular Complications of Liver Transplant: Diagnostic Criteria

Complication	Diagnostic Criteria
Anastomotic narrowing of portal vein/inferior vena cava	Thinned-out portal vein with post-stenotic dilatation
Thrombus/stenosis in portal vein	Filling defect in portal vein
	Focal narrowing at anastomotic site with increase in velocity
Thrombus/stenosis in inferior vena cava	Focal increase in velocity at stenotic/anastomotic site
	Dilatation of inferior vena cava proximal to stenosis
	Damped waveform with absent periodicity in subanastomotic inferior vena cava
Hepatic artery stenosis	Increase in peak systolic velocity >200-300 cm/s and post-stenotic turbulence
	Intrahepatic tardus parvus distal to stenosis
Hepatic artery thrombosis	Absence of flow

TABLE 6-10   Ultrasound Imaging of Mesenteric Ischemia

Acute Ischemia	Chronic Ischemia
Gray scale findings: bowel wall thickening (normal, <2 mm)[15] *Doppler findings:* Arterial: Mesenteric artery not always well visualized, absence of arterial flow in the wall of the ischemic colon[16] Venous: Dilated vein with echogenic thrombus and no flow within (see Fig. 6-22)[17]	*Doppler findings:* stenosis (70% or more); superior mesenteric artery shows increase in peak systolic velocity > 275 cm/s and end-diastolic velocity > 45 cm/s with post-stenotic turbulence (see Fig. 6-21).[18] Celiac artery shows increase in peak systemic velocity > 200 cm/s and end-diastolic velocity > 55 cm/s. Low-resistance pattern in fasting is diagnostic of mesenteric ischemia.

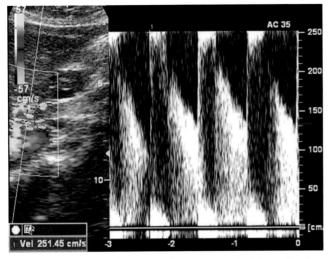

■ **FIGURE 6-21** Superior mesenteric artery stenosis. Atherosclerotic narrowing of the artery reveals significant increase in peak systolic velocity (251 cm/s) at its origin suggestive of moderate stenosis.

Renal Artery Stenosis

Atherosclerosis accounts for 75% of the causes of renal artery stenosis, whereas fibromuscular dysplasia accounts for 15%. Stenosis or occlusion of the artery causes ischemia, which triggers the renal-angiotensin mechanism and causes hypertension. Renal artery stenosis is hemodynamically significant when the luminal narrowing is 50% to 60% (Fig. 6-23). The diagnostic criteria are listed in Table 6-11.[19-23]

Renal Vein Thrombosis

The common causes of renal vein thrombosis in neonates are dehydration, and in adults they are low flow states, trauma, and tumor. The thrombotic process begins within the small intrarenal veins, reducing venous flow. In the acute stage, hemorrhagic renal infarction occurs from ruptured vessels and capillaries. Formation of collateral vessels begins at 24 hours and peaks at 2 weeks after onset of occlusion. The diagnostic criteria are listed in Table 6-12.

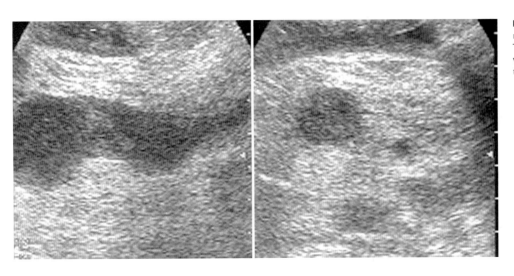

■ **FIGURE 6-22** Superior mesenteric vein thrombus. Transverse and long-axis epigastric views show distended vein with thrombus within.

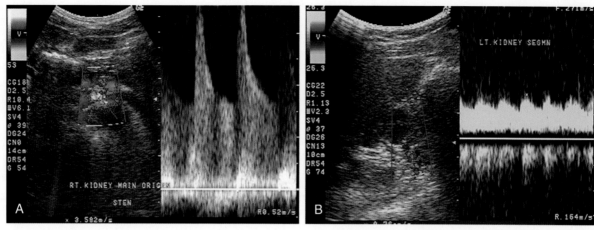

■ **FIGURE 6-23** Renal artery stenosis. **A** and **B**, Color Doppler image and spectral analysis at the level of right renal artery origin show significant increase in peak systolic velocity (251 cm/s) with poststenotic turbulence in the segmental artery.

TABLE 6-11 Ultrasound Imaging of Renal Artery Stenosis

Direct Signs	Indirect Signs
Peak systolic velocity > 180-200 cm/s with post-stenotic turbulence: significant stenosis (see Fig. 6-23).[20] Renal aortic ratio > 3.5 No flow detected: arterial occlusion	Dampened appearance: tardus parvus pulse Loss of early systolic peak Acceleration time > 80 ms (0.08 s) (see Fig. 6-23B).[21] In mild stenosis < 50% intrarenal Doppler is normal.[22] Difference in renal resistive index between normal and abnormal kidney[2]

TABLE 6-12 Ultrasound Imaging of Renal Vein Thrombosis

Gray Scale	Doppler
Enlarged kidney with focal or generalized areas of increased echogenicity Loss of corticomedullary differentiation Thrombus within distended renal vein/inferior vena cava	Main renal vein not traceable into inferior vena cava Steady, less-pulsatile venous flow as compared with contralateral renal vein Renal resistive index > 0.7 or reversed end-diastolic arterial flow

TABLE 6-13 Ultrasound Imaging of Medical Renal Disease

Gray Scale[25]	Doppler
Hyperechogenicity ± loss of corticomedullary differentiation Acute: enlarged/normal kidney Chronic: small shrunken kidney	Acute: increase in renal resistive index > 0.7. Chronic: increased renal resistive index ± absent end-diastolic or reversal of flow (see Fig. 6-24)

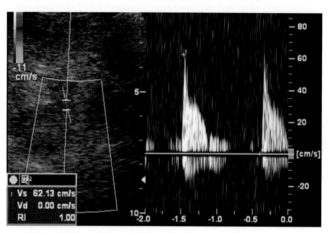

■ **FIGURE 6-24** Medical renal disease. Spectral analysis of renal artery at the hilum reveals high-resistance waveform pattern with absent end-diastolic flow. Resistive index = 1.00.

present in the renal artery with the renal resistive index not exceeding 0.7. Doppler imaging is also used to distinguish between obstructive and nonobstructive dilatation by measuring the renal resistive index of the arcuate arteries, in which the former shows an increase greater than 0.7 (Fig. 6-24).[24] The diagnostic criteria are listed in Table 6-13.[25]

Renal Transplantation

After renal transplantation, baseline ultrasound and Doppler imaging are mandatory 2 days after surgery. Doppler imaging plays an important role in assessing transplant-related complications. The normal renal resistive index in the parenchyma should not exceed 0.7 (Fig. 6-25).

Parenchymal Complications

● Acute tubular necrosis occurs due to prolonged ischemia leading to necrosis. On gray scale imaging there is increased cortical echogenicity. On Doppler imaging there is an increase in the renal resistive index to more

Medical Renal Disease

Flow resistance within the renal parenchyma may be increased by a variety of acute and chronic parenchymal disorders. Normally a large amount of diastolic flow is

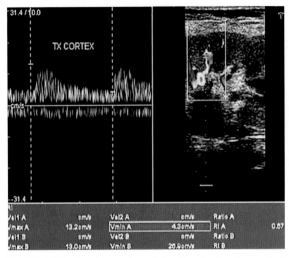

■ **FIGURE 6-25** Renal transplant. Color Doppler imaging at the level of the cortex using a high-frequency probe (7.5-10 MHz) shows normal low-resistance waveform pattern. Resistive index = 0.67.

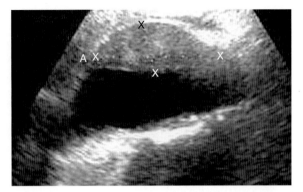

■ **FIGURE 6-26** Longitudinal midline color flow image shows a large abdominal aortic aneurysm with peripheral thrombus. A, aneurysm.

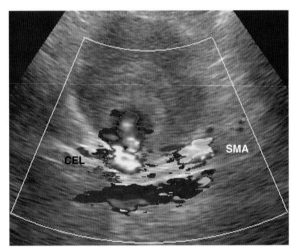

■ **FIGURE 6-27** Longitudinal color Doppler image shows a large thrombosed celiac artery (CEL) aneurysm. SMA, superior mesenteric artery.

than 0.7. Renal biopsy is required to confirm the diagnosis.

● Acute interstitial rejection occurs due to edema with lymphocytic infiltration. In vascular rejection there is proliferative endovasculitis and thrombosis.

● Diagnostic criteria: On gray scale imaging there is increased size and echogenicity of the graft with prominent pyramids. On color Doppler imaging a renal resistive index greater than 0.9 has a 100% positive predictive value.[9,26]

Vascular Complications

● Allograft renal artery stenosis occurs at the allograft artery origin (short segment), which is almost always due to a surgical complication. A later complication (long segment stenosis) commonly results from intimal hyperplasia or scarring. The findings are similar to those of renal artery stenosis.[27]

● Vascular occlusion (rare, arterial and venous) occurs due to rejection or faulty surgical technique. The findings are similar to those of renal arterial occlusion and renal vein thrombosis, respectively.

● Arteriovenous fistula occurs most commonly due to biopsy trauma. There is a high-velocity low-resistance flow in the feeding artery, a pulsatile "arterialized waveform" in the draining vein, and exaggerated focal color around the lesion called the "visible bruit."

● Pseudoaneurysm is commonly seen due to biopsy, mycotic infection, or anastomotic leakage. On gray scale imaging it could resemble a cyst. On Doppler imaging there is a to-and-fro waveform with high velocity jet within the neck of the aneurysm.

Aorta

Aneurysm

The common causes of aortic aneurysm are atherosclerosis, trauma, a congenital disorder, infection, and hyperten-

sion. The atheromatous plaque causes irregularity and structural defect of the wall by increased proteolysis. Progressive weakening of the media results in vessel dilatation and increased tension of the vessel wall, leading to aneurysm formation. Aortic aneurysms can be associated with visceral, iliac, and femoral aneurysms/stenosis (Figs. 6-26 to 6-28). On ultrasonography there is focal widening of the aorta more than 3 cm. Analysis of the aneurysm should include its dimension, shape, location, and extent and documentation of thrombus and involvement of any branches.

Aortic Dissection

The common causes of aortic dissection are hypertension, Marfan syndrome, Ehlers-Danlos syndrome, and valvular aortic stenosis. Usually, dissection begins in the thorax; less than 5% occur in the abdomen. There is separation of the intima and adventitia by circulating blood having gained access to the media of the aortic wall, splitting it into two. For an aortic dissection to occur a defect must exist in the intima.

On gray scale imaging there is a thin echogenic membrane (intimal flap) "fluttering" in the lumen. On color

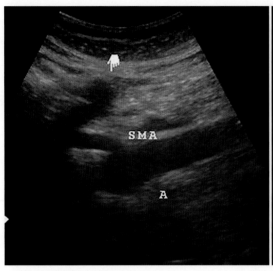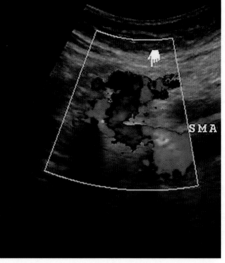

■ **FIGURE 6-28** Superior mesenteric artery aneurysm. Transverse midline imaging shows an aneurysm in the distal artery with turbulent flow within on color Doppler imaging.

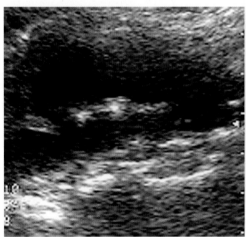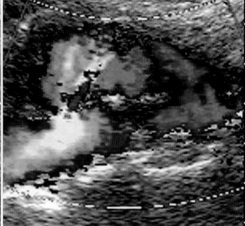

■ **FIGURE 6-29** Longitudinal midline gray scale and color Doppler imaging show an abdominal dissection with an intimal flap and flow within true and false lumens.

Doppler imaging there is blood flow in both true and false channels with higher velocity in the true lumen and retrograde flow being common in the false lumen (Fig. 6-29).

Inferior Vena Cava

The common causes of disorders of the inferior vena cava are neoplastic, idiopathic, thrombotic extension from femoroiliac veins and inferior vena cava filters, congenital webs, and extrinsic compression. Because of obstruction to the inferior vena cava, collateral vessels are established between it and the superior vena cava:

- Deep pathways: ascending lumbar veins to azygos and hemiazygos veins.
- Superficial pathway: external iliac to epigastric veins, internal mammary veins to subclavian veins
- Portal pathway: retrograde flow through internal iliac veins and hemorrhoidal veins into inferior mesenteric and splenic veins.

TABLE 6-14 Ultrasound Imaging of the Inferior Vena Cava

Gray Scale	Doppler
Distention of inferior vena cava	Absence of flow
	Loss of triphasic waveform pattern
Echogenic material within the lumen	Flow reversal in distal segment due to collateralization

The diagnostic criteria are listed in Table 6-14.[28]

SUMMARY

Although most abdominal vessels have a common origin, they have different signature patterns on Doppler ultrasound imaging. It is important to understand normal and abnormal flow patterns as well as know the importance and limitations of Doppler imaging to arrive at a definitive diagnosis.

KEY POINTS

- Doppler imaging is a very useful modality for evaluation of specific pathologic processes in the abdomen.
- It is particularly useful in portal hypertension, chronic mesenteric ischemia, and renal transplants.

- It has limitations in assessment of mild renal artery stenosis.
- There are technical limitations in the performance of the examination owing to respiratory variation, obesity, and poor patient preparation.

SUGGESTED READINGS

Al-Nakshabandi NA. Role of ultrasonography in portal hypertension. Saudi J Gastroenterol 2006; 12:111-117.

Al-Rohani M. Renovascular hypertension. Saudi J Kidney Dis Transplant 2003; 14:497-510.

Eapen CE, Mammen T, Moses V, Shyamkumar NK. Changing profile of Budd-Chiari syndrome in India. Indian J Gastroenterol 2007; 26:77-81.

Foley DW, Erickson SJ. Color Doppler flow imaging. AJR Am J Roentgenol 1991; 156:3-13.

Goldstein A. Overview of physics of US. RadioGraphics 1993; 13: 701-704.

Ponziak M, Zagzebski J, Scanlan KA. Spectral and color Doppler artifacts. RadioGraphics 1992; 12:35-44.

REFERENCES

1. Scoutt LM, Zawin ML, Taylor KJW. Doppler US: clinical applications. Radiology 1990; 174:309-319.

2. Taylor KJW, Burns PN, Woodcock JP, et al. Blood flow in deep abdominal and pelvic vessels: ultrasonic pulsed-Doppler analysis. Radiology 1985; 154:487-493.

3. Nchimi A, Biquet JF, Brisbois D, et al. Duplex ultrasound as first line screening test for patients suspected of renal artery stenosis: prospective evaluation in high-risk group. Eur Radiol 2003; 1413-1419.

4. Bude R, Rubbin JM. Detection of renal artery stenosis with Doppler sonography; it is more complicated than originally thought. Radiology 1995; 196:612-613.

5. Rumack CM, Wilson SR, Charboneau JW, Johnson JA. Diagnostic Ultrasound, 3rd ed. St. Louis, Mosby, 2004.

6. Zwiebel WJ. Introduction to Vascular Ultrasonography, 4th ed. Philadelphia, WB Saunders, 2000.

7. Taylor KJW, Burns PN, Woodcock JP, et al. Blood flow in deep abdominal and pelvic vessels: ultrasonic pulsed-Doppler analysis. Radiology 1985; 154:487-493.

8. Kruskal JB, Newman PA, Sammons L. Optimizing Doppler in color flow US: application to hepatic sonography. RadioGraphics 2004; 24:657-675.

9. Dänhert W. Radiology Review Manual, 6th ed. Philadelphia: Lippincott Williams & Wilkins, 2007.

10. Edward GG, Tessler FN, Gomes AS, et al. Color Doppler imaging of portosystemic shunts. AJR Am J Roentgenol 1990; 154:393-397.

11. Bolondi L, Gandolfi L, Arienti V, et al. Ultrasonography in the diagnosis of portal hypertension: diminished response of portal vessels to respiration. Radiology 1982; 142:167-172.

12. Wachsberg R, Bharamipur P, Sofocleous C. Hepatofugal flow in portal venous system: pathophysiology, imaging findings, and diagnostic pitfalls. RadioGraphics 2002; 22:123-140.

13. De Gaetano AM, Lafortune M, Patriquin H, et al. Cavernous transformation of the portal vein: pattern of intrahepatic and splanchnic collateral circulation detected with Doppler sonography. AJR Am J Roentgenol 1995; 165:1151-1155.

14. Liewer M, Hertzberg B, Heneghon J, et al. Transjugular intrahepatic portosystemic shunts (TIPS): effects of respiratory state and patient position on the measurement of Doppler velocities. AJR Am J Roentgenol 2000; 175:149-152.

15. Dietrich CF, Jedrzejezyk M, Ignee A. Sonographic assessment of splanchnic arteries and the bowel wall. Eur J Radiol 2007; 64: 202-212.

16. Danse EM, Van Beers BE, Jamart J, et al. Prognosis of ischemic colitis: comparison of color Doppler sonography with early clinical and laboratory findings. AJR Am J Roentgenol 2000; 175:1151-1154.

17. Amrapurkar DN, Patel ND, Jatania J. Primary mesenteric venous thrombosis: a study from western India. Indian J Gastroenterol 2007; 26:113-117.

18. Lim HK, Lee WJ, Kim SH. Splanchnic artery stenosis or occlusion: diagnosis at Doppler US. Radiology 1999; 211:405-410.

19. Soulez G, Oliva VL, Turpin S, et al. Imaging of renovascular hypertension: respective values of renal scintigraphy, renal Doppler US, and MR angiography. RadioGraphics 2000; 20:1355-1368.

20. House MK, Dowling RJ, King P, et al: Using Doppler sonography to reveal renal artery stenosis: an evaluation of optimal imaging parameters. AJR Am J Roentgenol 1999; 173:761-765.

21. Ripolles T, Aliaga R, Morote V, et al. Utility of intrarenal Doppler ultrasound in the diagnosis of renal artery stenosis. Eur J Radiol 2001; 40:54-63.

22. de Cobelli F, Venturini M, Vanzulli A, et al. Renal arterial stenosis: prospective comparison of color Doppler US and breath-hold, three-dimensional dynamic, gadolinium-enhanced MR angiography. Radiology 2000; 214:373-380.

23. Leiner T, De Haan MW, Nelemans PJ, et al. Contemporary imaging techniques for the diagnosis of renal artery stenosis. Eur Radiol 2005; 15:2219-2229.

24. Dwivedi US, Bishoyi SC, Shukla RC, et al. Renal resistive index: differentiation of obstructive from non-obstructive hydronephrosis. Indian J Urol 1998; 14:17-21.

25. Buturović-Ponikvar J, Visnar-Perovic A. Ultrasonography in chronic renal failure. Eur J Radiol 2003; 46:115-122.

26. Grant EG, Tessler FN, Perrella RR. Clinical Doppler imaging. AJR Am J Roentgenol 1989; 152:709-713.

27. Gottlieb RH, Lieberman JL, Pabico RC, et al. Diagnosis of renal artery stenosis in transplanted kidneys: value of Doppler waveform analysis of the intrarenal arteries. AJR Am J Roentgenol 1995; 165:1441-1446.

28. Rossi AR, Ponziak MA, Zarvan NP. Upper inferior vena caval anastomotic stenosis in liver transplant recipients: Doppler US diagnosis. Radiology 1993; 187:387-389.

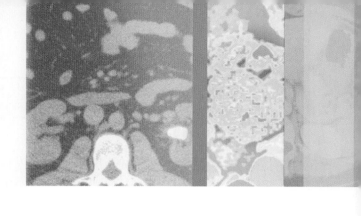

CHAPTER 7

Four-Dimensional Ultrasound Imaging

Xiaozhou Ma

TECHNICAL ASPECTS

Many technical improvements have been achieved because of the evolution of ultrasound equipment. With systematic ultrasound evaluation and follow-up, diagnoses can be made earlier and disease progression can be monitored.[1] The application of 3D volumetric ultrasonography has been reported to be more efficient than that of 2D imaging for radiologists to interpret in some cases, especially for fetuses,[2] with no additional side effects.[3,4] 4D ultrasound imaging provides an observation of moving organs or the fetus, and, recently, this technique is more often applied to studying the activities of the fetus.[2,5]

4D ultrasound imaging is the evolution of 3D imaging and is defined as real-time 3D ultrasound imaging. In other words, a "time axis" is added into the 3D imaging to make the 3D image animated or updated in real time, providing a "live show" in a 3D view of the target.[3,6]

A real 3D image (not a stretched 3D image) is the basis of 4D imaging because the 4D imaging process in an ultrasound system calculates the data of volumetric images (3D). However, the key point of a real 3D image is the regulated data of the z-axis adding to the conventional 2D image, because a constant continuous sweeping that is perpendicular to the 2D image is indeed needed. However, this kind of volumetric sweep is often very difficult for technologists to perform successfully. A specialized transducer, called a "4D transducer" or "volumetric transducer," standardizes the real 3D image (Fig. 7-1). The transducers for 4D application are usually mechanical transducers, whereas the phased-array transducers are commonly used in the modem equipment. Compared with the conventional ultrasound transducer, the 4D transducer is much thicker and provides enough space for the transducer crystals rocking inside. When scanning, the transducer crystals in the 4D transducer continuously rock, sending and receiving echoes. As the calculating speed of the ultrasound system is increased, 4D imaging can reach up to 40 volumes per second (Voluson 730, GE Healthcare) and make movement of the volume of interest real. 4D imaging is commonly applied for moving organs, such as in obstetric examinations.

The main types of 4D transducers include the following:

- Convex 4D transducer—mainly applied for imaging the abdomen and can be used for guidance in radiofrequency ablations.
- Endocavity 4D transducer—provides volume data for transvaginal scans, such as obstetric procedures and prostate imaging.
- Linear 4D transducer—used to image small parts of the anatomy, such as the testes, thyroid, and breasts.

All these 4D transducers might be applied for biopsy guidance depending on their availability.

During image acquisition, the 4D transducer is usually held steadily in place, facing and observing the region of interest. As in 3D imaging, there are usually four components that can be selectively involved in the 4D image display, including the longitudinal plane, transverse plane, coronal plane, and volume-rendered images. These planes are known as the x-axis, y-axis, and z-axis and are perpendicular (orthogonal, 90 degrees) to each other.

The acquisition plane is determined by the direction of the transducer, which determines the orientation of the other two perpendicular planes. However, an understanding of these multiplanar reconstructed planes and their orientation is necessary for manipulating 4D images.

The amount of information and the volume-rendered images are predetermined before the acquisition. The region of interest (ROI) or the volume of interest (VOI) allows the user to determine the area of the targets displayed in the 4D images. However, the ROI/VOI and the imaging frame (volumes per second) are inversely proportional, owing to the limitation of the current processing speed of U.S. systems. It is still imperative to choose a

	Description	Applications	Footprint	Bandwidth	FOV	Biopsy kit	Availability
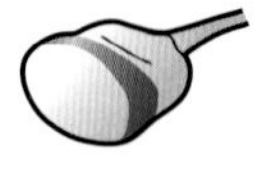 RAB2-5L H48621X	Micro4D convex is RealTime 4D transducer for general imaging and the technically difficult OB patient.	Abdomen, OB/GYN	53.2 x 40.6 mm	2.0 – 5.0 MHz	80° Volume 85° x 80°	Yes	Expert PRO
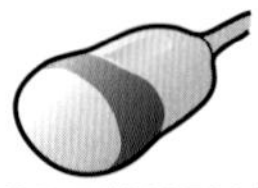 RAB2-5 H46701M	RealTime 4D transducer for general imaging and the technically difficult OB patient.	Abdomen, OB/GYN	65 x 55 mm	1.5 – 5.0 MHz	80° Volume 80° x 75°	Yes	Expert PRO PRO V
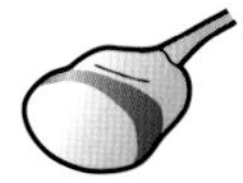 RAB4-8L H48621Z	Micro4D convex is a RealTime 4D transducer, great resolution, ideal for an OB practice.	OB/GYN, abdomen, pediatrics	53.2 x 40.6 mm	4.0 – 8.5 MHz	70° Volume 85° x 70°	Yes	Expert PRO
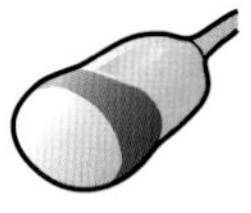 RAB4-8P H46701N	RealTime 4D convex transducer, higher frequency, great resolution, ideal for an OB practice.	OB/GYN, abdomen	65 x 55 mm	2.0 – 7.0 MHz	70° Volume 85° x 75°	Yes	Expert PRO PRO V
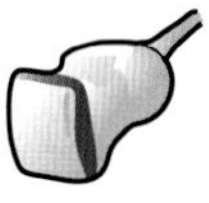 RSP6-16 H46701AB	RealTime 4D linear transducer. Excellent breast and small parts imaging.	Small parts, peripheral vascular, pediatrics, orthopedics	38.4 x 44.5 mm	5.6 – 18.4 MHz	37.4 mm Volume 37.4 mm x 29°	Yes	Expert PRO PRO V
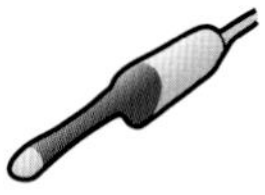 RIC5-9H H48651DA	Next generation RealTime 4D micro-convex endocavitary transducer. Ideal for GYN and first trimester scanning.	OB/GYN, urology	32 x 27 mm	3.7 – 9.3 MHz	146° Volume 146° x 90°	Yes	Expert PRO PRO V
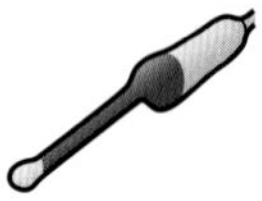 RRE6-10 H46701S	RealTime 4D side-fire micro-convex endocavitary transducer. Smaller footprint makes this ideal for urology applications.	Urology, GYN	32 x 35 mm	3.3 – 10.0 MHz	146° Volume 146°x135°	Yes	Expert
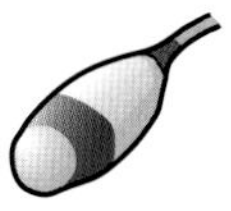 RNA5-9 H48651DB	Next generation RealTime 4D micro-convex transducer. Small footprint and hi-flex cabling well-suited for pediatrics.	Pediatrics, small parts, cardiac, abdomen, OB	32 x 29 mm	3.3 – 9.1 MHz	117° Volume 117° x 90°	Yes	Expert PRO

■ **FIGURE 7-1**   Illustration of different types of 3D/4D volumetric transducers and their corresponding features and appropriate applications. *(Courtesy of GE Healthcare.)*

large ROI/VOI that will reduce the imaging frame; otherwise, a smaller ROI/VOI (more specific area) will allow for better observation of the target's activity. Users need to be aware of this characteristic of 4D imaging and choose a suitable ROI/VOI, depending on the purpose of the examination.

Not all ultrasound equipment provides 3D/4D applications; the products of different vendors are listed in Table 7-1.

Different parameters and settings of the rendering methods will affect the presentation of the volume-rendered display. The four main types of rendering methods include opacity, maximum intensity projection (IP), minimum IP, and mean IP. The opacity mode demonstrates an object's surface anatomy by calculating the volume data. This mode can be used to show the surface anatomy, such as the fetal face, extremity, body surface, and polyp(s) in the gallbladder (Figs. 7-2 through 7-5) and can demonstrate the abnormalities by morphology changes, such as cleft lip. Maximum IP mode highlights the maximum hyperechoic signals in a volume-rendered image. This mode is helpful to present the hyperechoic structures such as fetal skeletal anatomy (Fig. 7-6) or stones in the gallbladder (Fig. 7-7) and urinary bladder. Minimum IP mode demonstrates the minimum values in the volume-rendered display. This mode is useful to highlight the hypoechoic structures such as hypoechoic lesions (cystic lesions) or large vascular structures (Fig. 7-8). Mean IP mode, also known as x-ray mode, shows the mean value in the volume-rendered display. This method enhances contrast resolution and is the mode used for biopsy guidance (Fig. 7-9; Table 7-2).

TABLE 7-1 Some Products and Vendors for 4D Ultrasound Applications	
Vendor	**Products**
GE	LOGIQ 9; VOLUSON 730
Medison	Voluson 530D; SonoAce 8000/9900
Philips	SONOS 7500
Siemens-Acuson	Aspen
Toshiba	Aplio; Xario

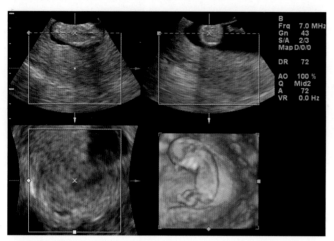

■ **FIGURE 7-2** Multiplanar 4D image of an early pregnancy. This image illustrates the typical layout in a 3D/4D display. The upper left, upper right, and lower left images are usually the transverse, sagittal, and coronal planes of the region of interest (ROI); the green cross (X) and line (----) represent the central point and line of the ROI of each plane, which can be adjusted by the operator. The lower right image is the reconstructed 3D/4D image corresponding to the ROIs selected in the prior three planes. *(Courtesy of LOGIQlibrary, GE Healthcare.)*

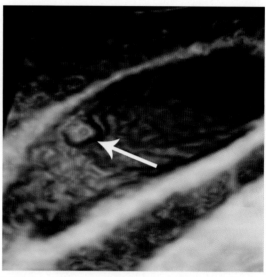

■ **FIGURE 7-4** Single reconstructed 3D image of the gallbladder. A polyp (*arrow*) in the anterior wall of the gallbladder neck is well shown using opacity mode. *(Courtesy of LOGIQlibrary, GE Healthcare.)*

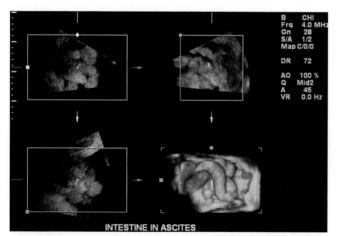

INTESTINE IN ASCITES

■ **FIGURE 7-3** Multiplanar 4D image of the intestines in a patient with ascites. The 3D reconstructed image at the lower right shows the intestine structure well using the opacity mode when a large amount of ascites is present. *(Courtesy of LOGIQlibrary, GE Healthcare.)*

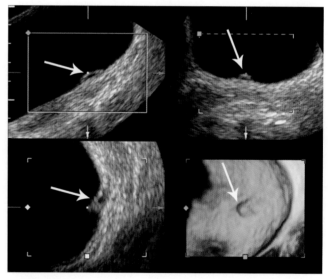

■ **FIGURE 7-5** Multiplanar 4D image of the urinary bladder. The normal left urine tract opening (*arrow*) in the bladder is well presented in the reconstructed 3D image at the lower right using opacity mode. *(Courtesy of LOGIQlibrary, GE Healthcare.)*

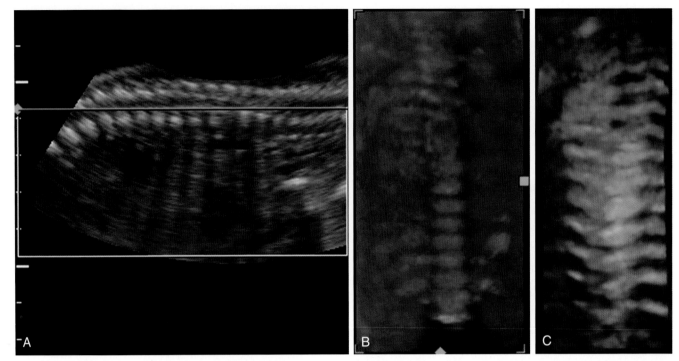

■ **FIGURE 7-6** The spine of a second-trimester fetus in 4D imaging using maximum IP mode. **A,** The green line in this image represents the central line of the ROI. **B,** Reconstructed image of the inside view of the fetus when supine. **C,** Reconstructed image of outside view of the fetus while supine. *(Courtesy of LOGIQlibrary, GE Healthcare.)*

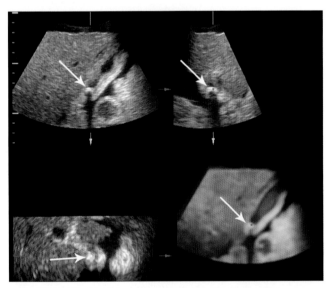

■ **FIGURE 7-7** Multiplanar 4D image of cholelithiasis with acute cholecystitis of the gallbladder. A hyperechoic focus (gallstone, *arrows*) is well represented in the sagittal plane (*upper left*), transverse plane (*upper right*), and coronal plane (*lower left*). The 3D reconstructed image at the *lower right* shows the gallstone using maximum IP mode. *(Courtesy of LOGIQlibrary, GE Healthcare.)*

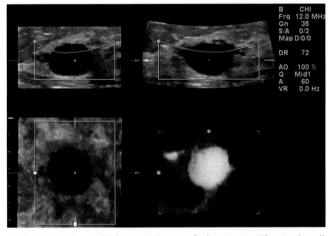

■ **FIGURE 7-8** Multiplanar 4D image of a breast cyst. The cyst is well shown in gray-scale images in different planes. The lower right 3D reconstructed image demonstrates the 3D view of the cyst and its adjacent structures (communications) using minimum IP mode. *(Courtesy of LOGIQlibrary, GE Healthcare.)*

PROS AND CONS

Benefits of 4D Ultrasound Imaging

- 4D imaging allows doctors to observe internal anatomy structures moving in real time and enables the investigation of the activities of internal anatomy, such as fetuses' activities.[3,6]

- 4D imaging provides volumetric data of an organ, fetus, or a lesion for further evaluation and comparison from the volume changes.
- The diagnostic confidence might be improved with the data from imaging in coronal planes.
- 4D applications are convenient for radiologists to analyze data after patient discharge; 3D "virtual rescan" enables the reviewer to easily display the 2D images in any desired orientation within the scanned volume and avoid the potential for rescans.

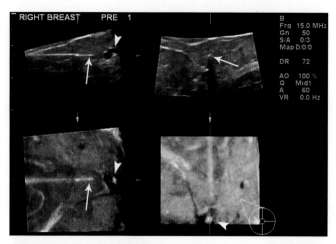

■ **FIGURE 7-9** Multiplanar 4D image of a percutaneous breast mass biopsy. The needle tip (*arrow*) is well shown in the sagittal, transverse, and coronal planes in the upper left/right and the lower left images, respectively. The 3D image at the lower right was processed using mean IP mode (x-ray mode). (*Courtesy of LOGIQlibrary, GE Healthcare.*)

- The 4D transducer results in less variation in the acquired image, and 3D images become standardized.
- Volumetric sweeps can image an entire organ within a few seconds and potentially reduce the examination time.
- During interventional procedures, the confidence of the needle placement increases owing to the confirmation of three planes simultaneously.
- Patients may benefit from 4D imaging because of reduced procedure time.
- The department's work flow is improved.

Limitations

- Large ROI/VOI results in slow frames on the screen.
- Although 3D/4D scanning has been reported safe,[3] increased awareness of safety issues should lead to the ALARA principle ("as low as reasonably achievable") in clinical practice, especially during obstetric 3D/4D.[7]

TABLE 7-2 Common Rendering Methods and Their Relevant Clinical Applications

Modes	Characteristics	Applications
Opacity mode	Blends volume data to demonstrate an objective's surface anatomy.	Fetal face
		Fetal extremities
		Obstetric anomalies (cleft lip)
		Inside surface of gallbladder
		Inside surface of urinary bladder
Maximum IP mode	Highlights the maximum intensity signals in a volume-rendered image, to emphasize the hyperechoic structures	Fetal skeletal anatomy
		Stones in the gallbladder/urinary bladder
Minimum IP mode	Demonstrates the minimum intensity in the volume-rendered image, to emphasize hypoechoic structures	Cystic lesions
		Major vessels or large vascular structures
Mean IP mode	Shows the mean value of the pixels in the volume-rendered image, to enhance contrast resolution.	Known as "X-ray" mode
		Organs with solid parenchyma
		Biopsy needles

IP, intensity projection.

KEY POINTS

- 4D ultrasound imaging is 3D ultrasound imaging plus time axis, hence real-time 3D imaging.

- 4D ultrasound imaging reduces the procedure time and improves the department work flow.

SUGGESTED READINGS

Avni FE, Cos T, Cassart M, et al. Evolution of fetal ultrasonography. Eur Radiol 2007; 17:419-431.

Rumack CM, Wilson SR, Charboneau JW. Diagnostic Ultrasound, 3rd ed. St. Louis, Elsevier Mosby, 2005.

Timor-Tritsch IE, Platt LD. Three-dimensional ultrasound experience in obstetrics. Curr Opin Obstet Gynecol 2002; 14:569-575.

Wells PN. Ultrasound imaging. Phys Med Biol 2006; 51:R83-R98.

REFERENCES

1. Avni FE, Cos T, Cassart M, et al. Evolution of fetal ultrasonography. Eur Radiol 2007; 17:419-431.
2. Benacerraf BR, Shipp TD, Bromley B. Three-dimensional US of the fetus: volume imaging. Radiology 2006; 238:988-996.
3. Sheiner E, Hackmon R, Shoham-Vardi I, et al. A comparison between acoustic output indices in 2D and 3D/4D ultrasound in obstetrics. Ultrasound Obstet Gynecol 2007; 29:326-328.
4. Xu HX, Zhang QP, Lu MD, Xiao XT. Comparison of two-dimensional and three-dimensional sonography in evaluating fetal malformations. J Clin Ultrasound 2002; 30:515-525.
5. Yigiter AB, Kavak ZN. Normal standards of fetal behavior assessed by four-dimensional sonography. J Matern Fetal Neonatal Med 2006; 19:707-721.
6. Timor-Tritsch IE, Platt LD. Three-dimensional ultrasound experience in obstetrics. Curr Opin Obstet Gynecol 2002; 14:569-575.
7. Nyborg WL. History of the American Institute of Ultrasound in Medicine's efforts to keep ultrasound safe. J Ultrasound Med 2003; 22:1293-1300.

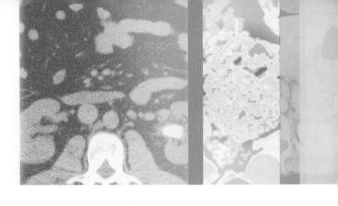

CHAPTER 8

Contrast Media and Contrast-Enhanced Ultrasound Evaluation

Xiaozhou Ma

TECHNICAL ASPECTS

Ultrasound contrast agents can be classified as microbubble-based or non–microbubble-based contrast agents. Microbubble-based contrast agents are exogenous substances that can be administered, either intravenously or into a cavity, to enhance ultrasonic backscattered signals, whereas non–microbubble-based ultrasound contrast agents are administered orally and employed for removing the interposing bowel gas, which impedes the imaging of anatomic structures.

Contrast-enhanced ultrasonography is the application of ultrasound contrast agents in conventional ultrasonography to enhance the image of anatomic structures, blood perfusion in organs, or blood flow in the cardiovascular system.

The contrast phenomenon of ultrasonic echo backscattered by air bubbles was first described by Gramiak and colleagues in 1968.[1] Subsequent to understanding the effects of air microbubbles, many investigations have been dedicated to developing contrast agents for clinical use.

Microbubble-based ultrasound contrast agents can be classified as targeted microbubbles and untargeted microbubbles. However, all the targeted microbubble contrast agents are in the laboratory stage of development and have not been approved for clinical use by the U.S. Food and Drug Administration (FDA).[2-5] Several untargeted microbubble contrast agents such as Definity (Bristol-Myers Squibb) and Optison (GE Healthcare) have been approved by the FDA and are marketed in the United States. A simethicone-coated cellulose suspension called SonoRx (ImaRx Pharmaceuticals, Tucson/Bracco, Princeton, NJ) has been introduced with the hope of improving the visualization of bowel and abdominal anatomy with reduction of gas artifacts.[6] Some major ultrasound contrast agents are listed in Table 8-1.

Physical Properties

When a microbubble goes into an ultrasound beam field it acts like a ball with high elasticity. It compresses, oscillates, and reflects the sound echo backward, but the reflected echo contains more energy than the echo from the adjacent tissue, which has less elasticity. As a consequence, a stronger energy is generated from the microbubbles at the second, third, or following harmonics (frequencies) compared with the energy generated from the adjacent tissue when using harmonic imaging. On the screen, the microbubbles appear brighter than other tissue (except bone).

The resistance of the microbubble-based ultrasound contrast agents is directly related to the gas nature, the shell composition, the fundamental ultrasound frequency, the pulse repetition frequency, and the acoustic power (mechanical index). The microbubbles are easily disrupted under a high mechanical index when performing contrast-enhanced ultrasonography. Therefore, the performance of real-time contrast-enhanced ultrasound imaging requires a low mechanical index, specific pulse sequences, and the use of harmonic imaging.[7,8]

The ideal microbubble-based ultrasound contrast agents should be smaller than red blood cells (<7 μm) with a narrow distribution of bubble sizes and an inactive nature with a biocompatible shell and should be stable enough during intravenous bolus injection and when passing through the left ventricle to provide enough time for imaging study. There should be a well-regulated reaction to the cycled acoustic energy of the ultrasound, persisting

TABLE 8-1 Characteristics of Some Major Ultrasound Contrast Agents

Type	Type of Shell	Agent (Code Name)	Size (Avg., Range)	Application	Availability	Characteristics (Advantage/ Disadvantage)
Carbon dioxide microbubbles	None	N/A	Variable	Focal liver lesion	N/A	Ready uptake for lung clearance, but low stability
Air-filled microbubbles with a shell	Galactose	Echovist (SH U454)	2 μm, 97% < 6 μm	Cardiac, vascular	Development stage	Small, but not sufficient to cross lungs
		Levovist (SH U508A)	2-3 μm, 99% < 7 μm	Most organs	Europe, Japan	Having a late hepatosplenic-specific parenchymal phase
	Albumin	Albunex (N/A)	3.8 ± 2.5 μm	Unknown	Withdrawn from market	Half-life < 1 min
		Quantison (AIP101)	Unknown (shell: 200-300 nm thick)	Myocardial perfusion	N/A	Mean uptake = 41.8 ± 10.4%, 1 hr after intravenous administration
		Myomap (AIP-201)	10 μm, 1.46-23.5 μm	Myocardial perfusion	Development stage	Viable microbubble sizes
	Cyanoacrylate	Sonavist (SH U563A)	2 μm	Wide	Development stage	Intact in blood pool for up to 10 min; taken up by Kupffer cells
Perfluorocarbon-filled microbubbles	Liquid perfluorocarbon emulsion	Perfluoro-chemical (N/A)	0.06-0.25 μm	Wide	N/A	Hours of half-life in blood, slower diffusion than air; applicable for radiography and CT; administered by inhaling, orally, and intravenously
	Phospholipid	BR 14 (BR14)	3 μm, 95% < 10 μm	Cardiac, organs	Preclinical stage	Persistent contrast enhancement of tissue perfusion
		Definity (DMP115, MRX115)	2.5 μm, 98% < 10 μm	Cardiac	FDA approval	
		Imavist/ Imagent (AFO150)	99.8% < 10 μm	Cardiac	FDA approval	Intravenous
		Sonazoid (NC100100)	3 μm		No	Relatively stable; exclusively internalized in Kupffer cells
	Albumin	Optison (FS069)	1.0-2.25 μm, 93% < 10 μm	Cardiac	FDA approval	To be captured and phagocytosed by activated neutrophils[28]
	Phase shift perfluorocarbon-filled microbubbles	EchoGen (QW3600)	3-8 μm	Cardiac	Withdrawn from market	Dodecafluoropentane liquid shift to a gas phase as temperature increased to body temperature
Sulfur hexafluoride-filled microbubbles		SonoVue (BR1)	3 μm, 90% < 8 μm	Wide	FDA approval	Stable; half-life = 6 min, 80% exhaled through lungs in 11 min[29]
Simethicone-coated cellulose suspension		SonoRx (N/A)	N/A	Bowel	FDA approval	Orally administered, reduces air artifacts, improves bowel visualization

N/A, not available.

within the blood pool, or the provision of a specific tissue distribution, such as with Levovist (Schering AG, Berlin, Germany), which may provide a late hepatosplenic-specific parenchymal phase. Levovist microbubbles can accumulate within the liver and the spleen up to 20 minutes after they disappear from the blood pool when the agent is administered intravenously.[9,10] This phenomenon might be mediated by the reticuloendothelial system or by being captured in the liver sinusoids, but the mechanism of the late selective uptake of the Levovist microbubble is not fully known.[11]

The stability of a microbubble-based ultrasound contrast agent is directly related to the gas component and the composition of the shell. The ideal gas should be inactive (dull), have a high vapor pressure, and be of low solubility. Heavy gases such as nitrogen, perfluorocarbon, and sulfur hexafluoride are filled into microbubble-based contrast agents owing to their low solubility and low diffusibility. An example of such an agent is SonoVue (Bracco Diagnostics, Inc., Milan, Italy), which is sulfur hexafluoride in a phospholipid shell. Lindner and associates demonstrated that the heavy gas dramatically improved the length of time that the microbubbles persist in the peripheral blood system.[12] SonoVue has a prolonged stability in the peripheral blood; the half-life of elimination was reported at about 6 minutes, which provides plenty of time for ultrasonography.

The microbubble is encapsulated in a shell. Currently, microbubble shells are built up with components with biocompatible features, such as albumin, galactose, lipid, or polymers.[12] An ideal shell may increase the mechanical elasticity of the microbubbles: the more elasticity of the shell material, the more acoustic energy it can withstand before bursting.[13] In addition, the selection of microbubble shells affects the persistency of the ultrasound contrast agents; a more hydrophilic component results in a shorter time available for contrast imaging.

Mechanical Index

Besides the nature of the microbubble itself, the value of the mechanical index directly affects the half-life of the ultrasound contrast agent. The mechanical index indicates the energy transmitted by the ultrasound transducer and the potential of nonthermal bioeffects. It is displayed on the screen edge of most modern ultrasound machines. Its value changes as it corresponds to the changes in operating mode or any control settings that affect acoustic output power.

The strength and flexibility of shells from different vendors differ. Therefore, there is not a specific mechanical index value that can predict the burst of microbubbles. In other words, there is no boundary between low and high mechanical indices relating to the stability or destruction of microbubbles and the power of energy is more about the possibility of the bubbles disrupting. A mechanical index of 1.0 is certainly considered to be high energy, whereas a mechanical index of 0.06 to 0.4 is usually considered to be low energy during contrast-enhanced ultrasonography.

Both high and low mechanical indices are employed during contrast-enhanced ultrasound scanning by two quite different theories. A high mechanical index is employed using larger pulse amplitudes (~1 MPa); the effective component is the difference in energy (echoes) released before and after the bubbles burst. A high mechanical index allows static, intermittent imaging. In addition, the sensitivity of ultrasound imaging is proportional to a higher mechanical index in conventional ultrasonography. However, this technique increases the rate of microbubble destruction and is not suitable when performing real-time imaging. On the contrary, a low mechanical index technique is employed using as little as the incident ultrasound energy to maximally slow down the destruction of microbubbles and prolong the effective scanning time. In addition, the low mechanical index technique reduces the magnitude of tissue harmonics and makes the best use of much greater nonlinearity of backscattering harmonic signals by microbubbles compared with the adjacent tissue. This technique allows dynamic, continuous acquisition, but using a low mechanical index

in imaging results in less sensitivity in viewing lesions and requires second-generation contrast media.

Applications of Microbubbles in Ultrasonography

Microbubble-based intravenous ultrasound contrast agents can be classified as untargeted or targeted. Targeted contrast agents are currently in various stages of development and not yet available for clinical use.[2-5]

Untargeted Ultrasound Contrast Agents

Untargeted microbubbles such as Definity, Optison, and Levovist are currently approved by the FDA for echocardiography in the United States and are available worldwide. The newer generation of ultrasound contrast agents such as SonoVue are available only in Asian and European countries.

With the newer-generation contrast media, microbubbles can survive long enough in the circulation so that all vascular phases can be covered for real-time imaging. In contrast-enhanced ultrasonography, the vascular phases can be divided into the arterial phase (15-35 seconds after the administration of contrast media), the portal venous phase (35-90 seconds), and the late (parenchymal or sinusoidal) phase (90-240 seconds).[14]

In abdominal applications, investigations of contrast-enhanced ultrasonography are predominantly performed on liver, kidney, pancreas, and spleen for screening of anatomic structures, lesion characterization, and blood volume and perfusion evaluation.

The different contrast media and contrast-specific technologies applied in the different investigations result in different hemodynamic characteristics of a lesion. However, the enhancement patterns are similar in benign or malignant lesions. The common enhancing patterns of focal lesions are well established in contrast-enhanced ultrasonography (Fig. 8-1).

Contrast-enhancing patterns in ultrasonography of focal liver lesions are variable in the arterial phase (Table 8-2). The typical patterns of liver lesions include (1) contrast absence (e.g., cyst, small hemangioma, or dysplastic/premalignant nodule); (2) diffuse hyperechoic enhancement (e.g., hepatocellular carcinoma [HCC], hypervascular metastasis or atypical columnar cell change, lymphoma, focal nodular hyperplasia) (Fig. 8-2); (3) heterogeneous enhancement (e.g., large HCC); (4) diffuse heterogeneous enhancement (e.g., HCC, lymphoma, metastasis); (5) rim-like enhancement (e.g., abscess, metastasis, cholangiocarcinoma); (6) peripheral nodular enhancement (e.g., cavernous hemangioma) (Fig. 8-3); (7) spoke-like enhancement (e.g., focal nodular hyperplasia); and (8) a stippled heterogeneous or "basket sign" (e.g., HCC). The enhancing patterns in portal or late phase are relatively less variable and less specific (see Fig. 8-1). However, malignant lesions usually present a rapid wash out, owing to arteriovenous shunts in the portal venous phase, and centripetal filling is not seen in malignancies.[15] The benign lesions usually present as an isoechoic homogeneous enhancing pattern; in addition, the residual central hypoechoic area is often a specific pattern for the diagnosis of focal nodular hyperplasia.[16]

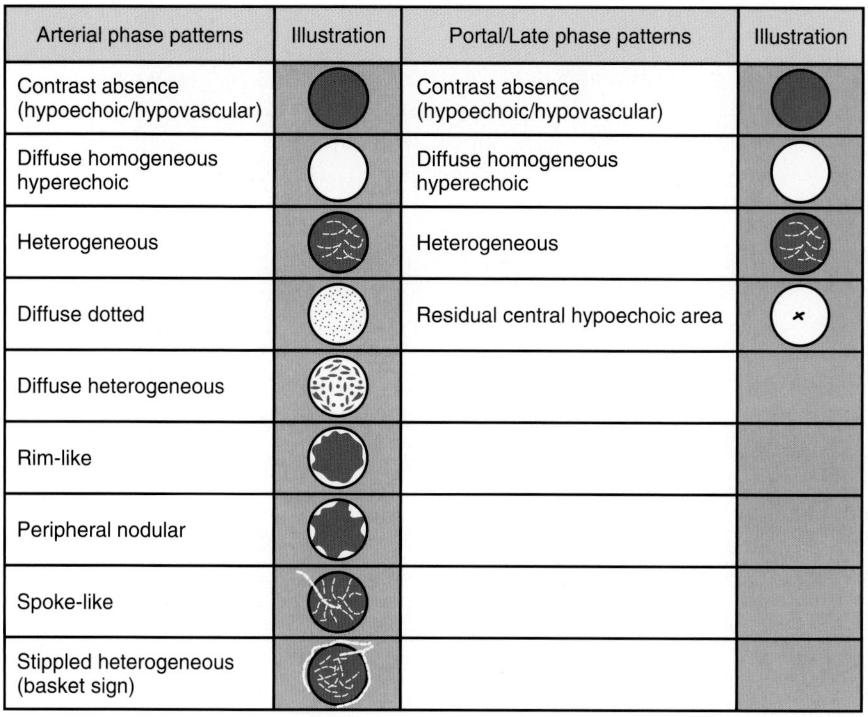

Arterial phase patterns	Illustration	Portal/Late phase patterns	Illustration
Contrast absence (hypoechoic/hypovascular)		Contrast absence (hypoechoic/hypovascular)	
Diffuse homogeneous hyperechoic		Diffuse homogeneous hyperechoic	
Heterogeneous		Heterogeneous	
Diffuse dotted		Residual central hypoechoic area	
Diffuse heterogeneous			
Rim-like			
Peripheral nodular			
Spoke-like			
Stippled heterogeneous (basket sign)			

■ **FIGURE 8-1** Illustrations of enhancing patterns of focal liver lesions in contrast-enhanced ultrasonography.

TABLE 8-2 Characterizations of Focal Liver Lesions of Gray-Scale Image and Enhancing Patterns

Focal Liver Lesions	Typical Gray Scale Features	Typical Enhancement Patterns Arterial Phase	Typical Enhancement Patterns Portal/Late Phase
Hemangioma			
Typical	Hyperechoic, sharp margin, often posterior enhancement	Progressively peripheral nodular	Slow fill in, iso- or hyperechoic
Atypical	Isoechoic, hypoechoic	No enhancement; or rapid fill in, hyperechoic	Iso- or heterogeneous
Focal nodular hyperplasia	Variable echogenicity (hyper- iso-, or hypo-echoic), central scar may be visible as hypoechoic area	Progressively spoke-like, centripetal, or diffuse hyperechoic	Diffuse iso- or hyper-echoic; residual central hypoechoic area (scar)
Hepatocellular adenoma	Variable echogenicity (hyper- iso-, or hypo-echoic), heterogeneous, halo sign (in large lesions), calcifications (rare)	Rapid fill in, diffuse homogeneous (small lesion), heterogeneous (large lesion)	Usually homogeneous; heterogeneous (large lesion)
Dysplastic and regenerative nodules	Predominantly hypo- to iso-echoic, may be hyperechoic, heterogeneous	Contrast absence or diffuse heterogeneous	Homogeneous
Focal hepatic steatosis	Geometric with sharp margin, usually hypoechoic, mimics a pseudo focal lesion	Progressively diffuse heterogeneous as adjacent liver parenchyma	Homogeneous as adjacent liver parenchyma
Abscess	Variable echogenicity: mature abscess, predominant hypoechoic, thick walled; immature abscess, iso-, hyper-, or hypo-echoic, infiltrating margins	Rapid fill in, rim-like	Rim-like, heterogeneous
Hepatocellular carcinoma			
Small	Predominantly hypoechoic, may be hyperechoic, rare for isoechoic	Rapid fill in, diffuse heterogeneous or homogeneous enhancement	Quick wash out during portal phase, hypo- or iso-echoic, contrast absence
Large	Variable echogenicity, heterogeneous with hypoechoic rim and irregular anechoic area (necrosis)	Rapid fill in, diffuse heterogeneous, or stippled heterogeneous	
Intrahepatic cholangiocarcinoma	Iso- to hypoechoic, heterogeneous and infiltrating margins, distal biliary dilation	Progressive fill in, heterogeneous and peripheral rim-like enhancement	Quick wash out similar to HCC, hypoechoic and heterogeneous
Lymphoma	Hypoechoic, heterogeneous, infiltrating margins	Progressively heterogeneous, or contrast absence	Contrast absence, or heterogeneous
Metastasis			
Hypovascular (predominant)	Variable, predominant hypoechoic, may anechoic (mimic a cyst)	Contrast absence	Contrast absence
Hypervascular	Variable, predominant hypoechoic, may isoechoic or hyperechoic, halo sign may present	Rim-like, homogeneous, or stippled heterogeneous	Usually quick wash out

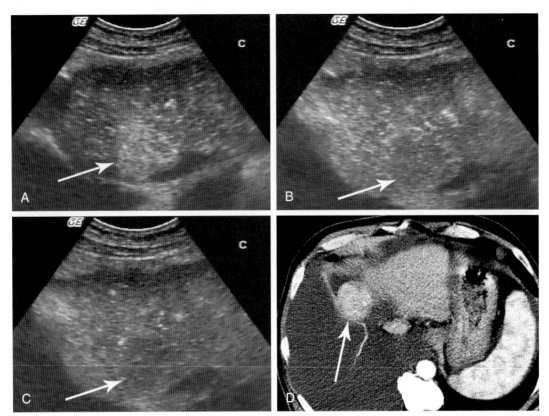

■ **FIGURE 8-2** Images from a 66-year-old man with cirrhosis show a hypoechoic mass (*arrows*) in the transverse plane of ultrasound and CT images. **A,** Image captured at 14 seconds after the administration of an ultrasound contrast agent represents the diffuse heterogeneous contrast enhancement in the early arterial phase. **B,** Image captured at 47 seconds represents the microbubble wash out quickly beginning in the portal venous phase. **C,** Image captured at 78 seconds demonstrates the full wash out of microbubbles in the hypoechoic mass. **D,** Corresponding contrast-enhanced CT image demonstrates the early arterial phase contrast enhancement. This lesion was histopathologically proven to be hepatocellular carcinoma.

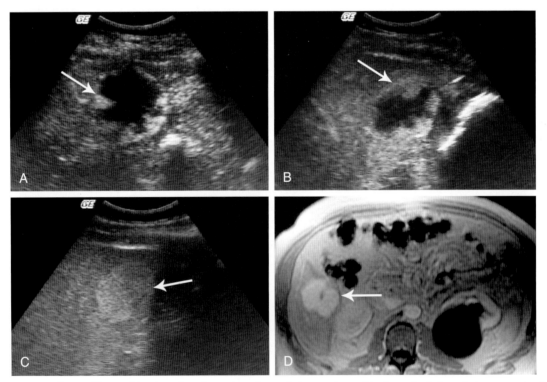

■ **FIGURE 8-3** Images from a 59-year-old male patient show a large hypoechoic mass (*arrows*) in the sagittal plane during contrast-enhanced ultrasonography that was incidentally discovered in segment 7 of the liver. **A,** Image captured at 23 seconds after the administration of an ultrasound contrast agent represents a typical peripheral nodular contrast enhancement pattern in the early arterial phase. **B,** Image captured at 47 seconds shows the microbubbles gradually centripetally filling in during the portal venous phase. **C,** Image captured at 161 seconds demonstrates the microbubbles to finally fill out the hypoechoic mass, which appears as homogeneous hyperechoic enhancement. The enhancing patterns demonstrate the lesion was a typical hemangioma. **D,** Corresponding contrast-enhanced MR image in the portal venous phase confirmed the lesion was a hemangioma.

The effectiveness of contrast-enhanced ultrasonography for diagnosing focal liver lesions has been studied by many investigators. The diagnostic sensitivity and specificity of hemangioma using contrast-enhanced ultrasonography were reported as up to 89% and 100%, respectively.[17] Peripheral nodular enhancement with centripetal filling is a specific indicator for a hemangioma. In the arterial phase, the peripheral nodular enhancement was found in 70% to 92% of hemangiomas, and rim-like and diffuse homogeneous enhancing patterns were revealed in 10% to 25% and 5% of hemangiomas, respectively.[15,18,19] Focal nodular hyperplasia usually has a spoke-like enhancing pattern in the arterial phase and is progressively diffuse in the lesion. The presence of a centripetal enhancing pattern has a high specificity of 100% but a lower sensitivity of only 67% for diagnosing focal nodular hyperplasia.[16]

The diagnostic sensitivity and specificity of HCC using contrast-enhanced ultrasonography were reported as up to 94% and 93%, respectively, and 91% to 96% of HCC vascularity could be demonstrated by contrast-enhanced ultrasonography.[17,20,21] In the arterial phase, homogeneous and heterogeneous contrast-enhancing patterns were found in 50% of HCCs, respectively.[15] In addition, a diffuse enhancing pattern on the early arterial phase followed by rapid wash out usually indicates HCC, and the presence of a stippled heterogeneous (basket sign) enhancing pattern had 92% sensitivity and 96% specificity of diagnosing a HCC in one study.[22] The sensitivity and specificity of contrast-enhanced ultrasonography in the diagnosis of cholangiocarcinoma have been reported as 90% and 95%, respectively.[22] A rim-like pattern is the predominant enhancing pattern in contrast-enhanced ultrasonography. The sensitivity and specificity of contrast-enhanced ultrasonography in the diagnosis of metastases have been reported as 77% and 93%, respectively.[17] Rim-like enhancing patterns in the arterial phase were found in 48% of metastases, and homogeneous and stippled enhancing patterns were found in 21% and 6%, respectively.[15]

Contrast-enhanced ultrasonography provides additional vasculature and blood perfusion information for lesion characterization compared with conventional and color Doppler ultrasound imaging.[23] However, the overlaps of the contrast enhancement patterns cause difficulties in differentiating some diseases, such as atypical HCC, small cholangiocarcinoma, lymphoma, cirrhotic nodule, and abscess. Although the early arterial phase enhancement is common in malignant liver lesions, the reported sensitivity and specificity of this enhancing feature were 67% and 60%, respectively.[16] Therefore, further study is needed in some cases.

The characterizations of contrast-enhanced ultrasonography for kidney, pancreas, and spleen are summarized in Tables 8-3, 8-4, and 8-5, respectively.

In addition to lesion characterization, contrast-enhanced ultrasonography can be employed for evaluating the degree of blood perfusion and blood volume in an organ or a region of interest to assess the organ functionally (Fig. 8-4). Also, the relative intensity of the microbubble echoes can provide a potential quantitative estimation for blood volume. The before and after evaluation of organ transplantation such as that of the liver and kidney benefits from blood perfusion and volume assessment using contrast-enhanced ultrasonography.

Owing to the capability of dynamic observation of lesion hemodynamics, contrast-enhanced ultrasonography has been reported as having improved localization of ultrasonically invisible hypervascular HCCs in percutaneous ultrasound-guided liver interventional procedures, liver biopsy, and interventional therapy.[24,25]

Targeted Ultrasound Contrast Agents

The targeted ultrasound contrast agent is the future of contrast-enhanced ultrasonography and currently not available.

Targeting Inflammations

The blood vessels in the inflammatory change area present some specific receptors such as vascular cell adhesion molecule-1 (VCAM-1), intercellular adhesion molecule-1 (ICAM-1), and E-selectin. When microbubbles with a specific ligand can bind these molecules, the early inflammatory change can be detected by contrast-enhanced ultrasonography, and, indeed, earlier treatment leads to a better prognosis of the disease. Patients with inflammatory diseases such as liver abscess, Crohn's disease, or myocardial infarction may benefit.

TABLE 8-3   Characterizations of Renal Lesions of Gray-Scale Image and Enhancing Patterns

Renal Lesions	Typical Gray-Scale Features	Typical Enhancement Patterns	
		Arterial Phase	Late Phase
Cyst	Anechoic, sharp margin	Contrast absence	Contrast absence
Angiomyolipoma			
Small	Hyperechoic, sharp margin	Homogeneous, dotted, or heterogeneous; iso-enhancing compared with adjacent parenchyma	Iso- to hypo-enhancement, progressive wash out
Large (>3 cm)	Mixed heterogeneous		
Oncocytoma	Hypoechoic with central scar	Homogeneous hypervascular enhancement	Progressive wash out
Renal cell carcinoma	Hypoechoic, 30% hyperechoic, anechoic rim	Homogeneous or heterogeneous hypervascular, quick wash in	Iso- to hyper-enhancement, progressive wash out
Cystic renal cell carcinoma	Thick-walled anechoic	Rim-like	Iso- to hyper-enhancement, progressive wash out
Metastasis	Variable	Contrast absence	Contrast absence

TABLE 8-4   Characterizations of Pancreatic Lesions of Gray-Scale Image and Enhancing Patterns

		Typical Enhancement Patterns	
Pancreatic Lesions	Typical Gray-Scale Features	Arterial Phase	Late Phase
Pancreatitis			
Acute	Enlarged, hypoechoic, peripheral anechoic, necrotic area	Heterogeneous, affected by inflammation portion	Heterogeneous
Chronic	Hyperechoic, heterogeneous, calcifications	Heterogeneous, depends on the degree of fibrosis	Heterogeneous
Pseudocyst	Thick-walled cystic mass	Contrast absence	Contrast absence
Serous cystic lesion	Anechoic, sharp margin	Contrast absence	Contrast absence
Mucinous cystic lesion	Dirty anechoic, sharp margin, septations	Enhancing may occur on septations	Heterogeneous
Adenocarcinoma	Hypoechoic, heterogeneous, ill-defined	Low-grade heterogeneous enhancement	Hypovascular
Intraductal papillary mucinous neoplasm	Heterogeneous mass	Peripheral nodular enhancement	Heterogeneous
Endocrine tumor			
Hypervascular	Iso- to hyperechoic, well-defined	Early arterial phase homogeneous enhancement	Quick wash out, contrast absence, hypo-enhancement
Hypovascular		Contrast absence	Contrast absence
Metastasis	Variable, depends on originals	Diffuse homogeneous, or contrast absence	Contrast absence

TABLE 8-5   Characterizations of Splenic Lesions of Gray-Scale Image and Enhancing Patterns

		Typical Enhancement Patterns	
Splenic Lesions	Typical Gray-Scale Features	Arterial Phase	Late Phase
Primary cyst	Anechoic, sharp margin	Contrast absence	Contrast absence
Hemangioma	Echogenic, calcifications	Variable due to different vascular supply	Iso-enhancement
Hamartoma	Hyperechoic homogeneous	Variable enhancement	Iso-enhancement
Lymphangioma	Cystic with septation/debris	Contrast absence	Contrast absence
Infarction	Anechoic, hypoechoic, wedge shaped	Contrast absence	Contrast absence
Abscess	Hypoechoic, ill-defined	Peripheral rim-like	Iso-enhancement
Lymphoma	Hypoechoic, infiltrated, cystic appearance, "target sign"	Irregular peripheral, heterogeneous	Heterogeneous
Metastasis	Variable, depends on originals	Irregular peripheral, heterogeneous	Heterogeneous

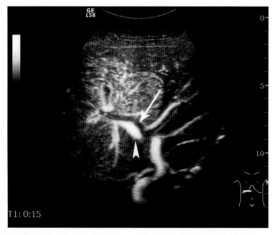

■ **FIGURE 8-4**   Contrast-enhanced image of the normal liver vasculature. Contrast-enhanced ultrasonography increases the conspicuity of intrahepatic vasculature (portal vein, *arrowhead*) and the intrahepatic biliary tree (right hepatic bile duct, *arrow*). *(Courtesy of LOGIQlibrary, GE Healthcare.)*

Targeting Cancers

Mainly because of angiogenesis, cancer cells also present some specific receptors, such as vascular endothelial growth factor (VEGF). When microbubbles with a ligand that can specifically bind a receptor such as VEGF are used, the early stage of cancers can be detected by contrast-enhanced ultrasonography, thus providing an alternative imaging study for noninvasive diagnosis of malignancy.

Lindner found microbubbles with monoclonal antibodies that were designed for binding endothelial markers of inflammations to enable contrast-enhanced ultrasonography for imaging inflammatory tissue[12]; however, current microbubble targeting strategies show low adhesion efficacy at physiologically high vessel shear stresses.[26] Effective contrast-enhanced ultrasonography requires microbubble binding at the targeting area that is more efficient and more stable.[27] Some research groups demonstrated dual-targeted microbubbles that have improved adhesion compared with single-targeted microbubbles,

TABLE 8-6 Common Advantages, Disadvantages, and Contraindications of Microbubble-Based Contrast-Enhanced Ultrasonography

Advantages	Disadvantages	Contraindications
Increased ability in distinguishing vasculature	Taken up quickly by immune system, liver, or spleen; usually not lasting long enough	Right-to-left, bidirectional, or transient right-to-left cardiac shunts
Increased ability in characterization of focal lesions	Impact sensitivity of ultrasound when using low mechanical index technique	Worsening or clinically unstable congestive heart failure
Evaluation of blood perfusion and blood volume for functional imaging	High mechanical index technique increases the image quality but increases the destruction rate of microbubbles.	Acute myocardial infarction or acute coronary syndromes
Targeting strategies for specific diagnosis and treatment, such as drug delivery	High mechanical index with microbubbles increases the acoustic cavitation and increases the potential risk of bioeffects.	Serious ventricular arrhythmias or high risk for arrhythmias due to prolongation of the QT interval
Real-time evaluation of hemodynamics	Unstable microbubbles may cause severe adverse reaction.	Respiratory failure, as manifested by signs or symptoms of carbon dioxide retention or hypoxemia
No radiation	Allergic reactions may occur in some patients owing to the coating material of the microbubbles.	Severe emphysema, pulmonary emboli, or other conditions that cause pulmonary hypertension due to compromised pulmonary arterial vasculature
		Hypersensitivity to coating materials

but this strategy is still ineffective for clinical use of targeted contrast-enhanced ultrasonography.[2,3,5]

PROS AND CONS

The common advantages, disadvantages, and contraindications of microbubble-based contrast-enhanced ultrasonography are summarized in Table 8-6.

KEY POINT

Contrast-enhanced ultrasonography increases the sensitivity and specificity of lesions by adding additional information about vasculature to the findings of the conventional ultrasound evaluation.

SUGGESTED READINGS

Hykes D, Hedrick WR, Starchman D (eds). Ultrasound Physics and Instrumentation, 4th ed. Philadelphia, Mosby, 2005.

Kremkau FW. Ultrasound: Principles and Instruments, 6th ed. Philadelphia, WB Saunders, 2002.

Rumack CM, Wilson SR, Charboneau JW. Diagnostic Ultrasound, 3rd ed. St. Louis, Elsevier Mosby, 2005.

Wells PN. Ultrasound imaging. Phys Med Biol 2006; 51:R83-R98.

Zagebski J. Essentials of Ultrasound Physics. St. Louis, Mosby, 1996.

REFERENCES

1. Gramiak R, Shah PM. Echocardiography of the aortic root. Invest Radiol 1968; 3:356-366.
2. Rychak JJ, Klibanov AL, Hossack JA. Acoustic radiation force enhances targeted delivery of ultrasound contrast microbubbles: in vitro verification. IEEE Trans Ultrason Ferroelectr Freq Control 2005; 52:421-433.
3. Omolola Eniola A, Hammer DA. In vitro characterization of leukocyte mimetic for targeting therapeutics to the endothelium using two receptors. Biomaterials 2005; 26:7136-7144.
4. Klibanov AL. Ligand-carrying gas-filled microbubbles: ultrasound contrast agents for targeted molecular imaging. Bioconjug Chem 2005; 16:9-17.
5. Weller GE, Villanueva FS, Tom EM, Wagner WR. Targeted ultrasound contrast agents: in vitro assessment of endothelial dysfunction and multi-targeting to ICAM-1 and sialyl Lewisx. Biotechnol Bioeng 2005; 92:780-788.
6. Lund PJ, Fritz TA, Unger EC, et al. Cellulose as a gastrointestinal US contrast agent. Radiology 1992; 185:783-788.
7. Meuwly JY, Correas JM, Bleuzen A, Tranquart F. [Detection modes of ultrasound contrast agents]. J Radiol 2003; 84:2013-2024.
8. Shen CC, Li PC. Pulse-inversion–based fundamental imaging for contrast detection. IEEE Trans Ultrason Ferroelectr Freq Control 2003; 50:1124-1133.
9. Kitamura H, Kawasaki S, Nakajima K, Ota H. Correlation between microbubble contrast-enhanced color Doppler sonography and immunostaining for Kupffer cells in assessing the histopathologic grade of hepatocellular carcinoma: preliminary results. J Clin Ultrasound 2002; 30:465-471.
10. Maruyama H, Matsutani S, Saisho H, et al. Different behaviors of microbubbles in the liver: time-related quantitative analysis of two ultrasound contrast agents, Levovist and Definity. Ultrasound Med Biol 2004; 30:1035-1040.
11. Kono Y, Steinbach GC, Peterson T, et al. Mechanism of parenchymal enhancement of the liver with a microbubble-based US contrast medium: an intravital microscopy study in rats. Radiology 2002; 224:253-257.
12. Lindner JR. Microbubbles in medical imaging: current applications and future directions. Nat Rev Drug Discov 2004; 3:527-532.
13. McCulloch M, Gresser C, Moos S, et al. Ultrasound contrast physics: a series on contrast echocardiography, article 3. J Am Soc Echocardiogr 2000; 13:959-967.
14. Solbiati L, Tonolini M, Cova L, Goldberg SN. The role of contrast-enhanced ultrasound in the detection of focal liver lesions. Eur Radiol 2001; 11(Suppl 3):E15-E26.
15. Kim TK, Choi BI, Han JK, et al. Hepatic tumors: contrast agent–enhancement patterns with pulse-inversion harmonic US. Radiology 2000; 216:411-417.

16. von Herbay A, Vogt C, Haussinger D. Pulse inversion sonography in the early phase of the sonographic contrast agent Levovist: differentiation between benign and malignant focal liver lesions. J Ultrasound Med 2002; 21:1191-1200.

17. Youk JH, Kim CS, Lee JM. Contrast-enhanced agent detection imaging: value in the characterization of focal hepatic lesions. J Ultrasound Med 2003; 22:897-910.

18. Kim JH, Kim TK, Kim BS, et al. Enhancement of hepatic hemangiomas with Levovist on coded harmonic angiographic ultrasonography. J Ultrasound Med 2002; 21:141-148.

19. Lee JY, Choi BI, Han JK, et al. Improved sonographic imaging of hepatic hemangioma with contrast-enhanced coded harmonic angiography: comparison with MR imaging. Ultrasound Med Biol 2002; 28:287-295.

20. Yamamoto K, Shiraki K, Deguchi M, et al. Diagnosis of hepatocellular carcinoma using digital subtraction imaging with the contrast agent Levovist: comparison with helical CT, digital subtraction angiography, and US angiography. Oncol Rep 2002; 9:789-792.

21. Honda T, Kumada T, Kiriyama S, et al. Comparison of contrast-enhanced harmonic ultrasonography and power Doppler ultrasonography for depicting vascularity of hepatocellular carcinoma identified by angiography-assisted CT. Hepatol Res 2003; 27:315-322.

22. Tanaka S, Ioka T, Oshikawa O, et al. Dynamic sonography of hepatic tumors. AJR Am J Roentgenol 2001; 177:799-805.

23. Migaleddu V, Virgilio G, Turilli D, et al. Characterization of focal liver lesions in real time using harmonic imaging with high mechanical index and contrast agent Levovist. AJR Am J Roentgenol 2004; 182:1505-1512.

24. Maruyama H, Kobayashi S, Yoshizumi H, et al. Application of percutaneous ultrasound-guided treatment for ultrasonically invisible hypervascular hepatocellular carcinoma using microbubble contrast agent. Clin Radiol 2007; 62:668-675.

25. Wu W, Chen MH, Yin SS, et al. The role of contrast-enhanced sonography of focal liver lesions before percutaneous biopsy. AJR Am J Roentgenol 2006; 187:752-761.

26. Takalkar AM, Klibanov AL, Rychak JJ, et al. Binding and detachment dynamics of microbubbles targeted to P-selectin under controlled shear flow. J Control Release 2004; 96:473-482.

27. Klibanov AL. Targeted delivery of gas-filled microspheres, contrast agents for ultrasound imaging. Adv Drug Deliv Rev 1999; 37:139-157.

28. Lindner JR, Dayton PA, Coggins MP, et al. Noninvasive imaging of inflammation by ultrasound detection of phagocytosed microbubbles. Circulation 2000; 102:531-538.

29. Gorce JM, Arditi M, Schneider M. Influence of bubble size distribution on the echogenicity of ultrasound contrast agents: a study of SonoVue. Invest Radiol 2000; 35:661-671.

Computed Tomography

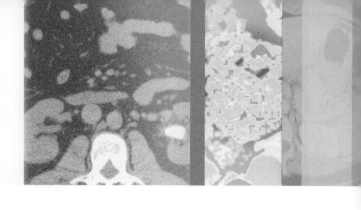

CHAPTER 9

Principles of CT Physics

Kumaresan Sandrasegaran

TECHNICAL ASPECTS

In the past decade CT has undergone tremendous technical advances. In 1992, the first dual-slice CT scanner (CT Twin, formerly Elscint Technologies, Haifa, Israel) was introduced. In 1998 the quad-slice CT scanners were introduced. In 2002, the 16-slice CT scanner became available. With these scanners it became possible to perform coronary CT angiography, multiphasic examinations, and virtual endoscopy studies. In 2004, 64-slice CT scanners were introduced. With 64-slice CT scanners it became possible to acquire submillimeter sections of large body regions, obtain high-quality coronary angiography in most patients, and perform perfusion studies. The development of CT technology is not only about an increase in the number of detector rows. Long-held concepts, based on single-slice CT scanners, have had to change. Newer features have been introduced as an adjunct to the superior capabilities of 64-slice CT scanners.

64-Slice CT Scanners

The detector configurations of the four main CT scanners are different (Table 9-1). In the 64-slice mode the beam coverage of GE (LightSpeed VCT, GE Medical Systems, Waukesha, WI) and Philips (Brilliance 64, Philips Medical Systems, Cleveland, OH) scanners is 40 mm, whereas the Toshiba 64-slice scanner (Aquilion 64, Toshiba Medical Systems, Tustin, CA) has a coverage of 32 mm. The Siemens 64-slice scanner (Somatom Sensation 64, Siemens Medical Solutions, Forchheim, Germany) has 32 inner detector rows that are 0.6 mm wide in the z-axis that are activated in the "64-slice mode." The beam coverage of this scanner is 19.2 mm. As per Table 9-1, apart from some unique features of the Siemens scanner, discussed later, there are no major differences between the scanners.

Flying Focal Spot Function

In the x-ray tube of the Siemens 64-slice CT scanner, the electron beam is deflected between two different focal spots, at a rate of almost 5000 times per second. The focal spot positions are such that the rapidly alternating x-ray beams are shifted by half a collimated slice width in the z-direction.[1] This means that that each detector element receives information almost simultaneously from two different projections (Fig. 9-1). This technique, also called the z-sharp function, allows 32 detector rows in the z-direction to acquire 64 overlapping 0.6-mm electronic channels of data per rotation.

The benefits of this arrangement include improved spatial resolution. Aliasing artifacts (windmill or splay artifacts) that occur due to inadequate sampling of data are also eliminated. The main disadvantage of this technique is the reduced z-axis coverage per gantry rotation.

Dual-Source CT Scanners

In 2005, a dual-source CT scanner (Somatom Definition, Siemens Medical Solutions) became available (Fig. 9-2). Potential advantages of this scanner include evaluation of coronary arteries without need for beta blockage,[2] lower radiation dose during cardiac examinations,[3] better image quality in obese patients, and the ability to perform dual-kilovoltage studies.[4] The main disadvantage is the additional cost of a second x-ray tube.

Reconstruction Algorithms

In single-slice CT scanners the x-ray beam is almost parallel. With multislice CT scanners the x-ray beam is cone shaped. As a result, newer reconstruction algorithms are required. The traditional two-dimensional filtered back-projection reconstructions, such as 180-degree linear interpolation reconstruction, assume that all of the rays used to reconstruct an image lie entirely within the axial plane of that image (Fig. 9-3A) and are unable to handle an x-ray beam that spans several detector rows in the z-axis (see Fig. 9-3B). Various reconstruction techniques have been proposed to deal with this cone beam problem in 16- and higher-slice scanners (4-slice CT scanners use traditional reconstruction algorithms). These cone beam

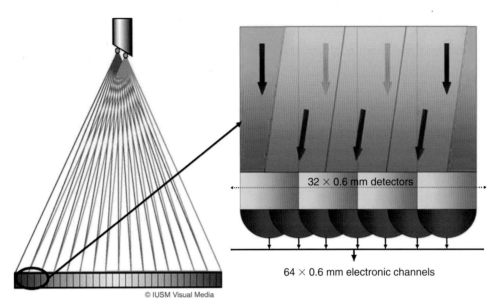

© IUSM Visual Media

32 × 0.6 mm detectors

64 × 0.6 mm electronic channels

■ **FIGURE 9-1** Simplified diagram of z-sharp technology. Line diagram shows that each detector receives, almost simultaneously, two separate x-ray beams originating from two different locations in the anode. Magnified inset shows that four detectors yield eight channels of electronic information. Extrapolating to the entire detector row, 32 detectors yield 64 channels of overlapping electronic information. (© *IUSM Visual Media. Reproduced with permission.*)

TABLE 9-1 Technical Aspects of 64-Slice CT Scanners

	GE LightSpeed VCT	**Philips Brilliance 64**	**Siemens Sensation 64**	**Toshiba Aquilion 64**
Detector configuration (inner rows)	64 × 0.625 mm	64 × 0.625 mm	32 × 0.6 mm	64 × 0.5 mm
Detector configuration (outer rows)	NA	NA	8 × 1.2 mm	NA
Z-axis detector length (64-slice mode) (mm)	40	40	19.2	32
Fastest gantry rotation (s)	0.35	0.40	0.33	0.40
Scan field of view (mm)	25, 50	25-50	50 (option to 70)	18, 24, 32, 40, 50
Coverage in 1 second with pitch of 1 in 64-slice mode (mm)	114.3	100	58.2	80
X-ray generator power (kW)	100	60	80	60
Anode heat capacity (MHU)	8	8	Equivalent to 30	8
Maximum mA at 120 kV	800	500	665	500
Matrix	512	512, 768, 1028	512	512
Automatic dose reduction	3D DOSE MODulation	DoseRight	CareDose 4D	SureExposure
Simultaneous ATCM in x-y and z-planes	Yes	Yes	Yes	Yes
Cone beam reconstruction algorithm	3D	3D	3D	3D
Automatic re-formation in multiple planes	Source axial images	Source axial images	Raw data	Source axial images
Simultaneous functions*	Yes	Yes	Yes	Yes
Speed of reconstruction†	22	14	2	2

NA, not applicable; ATCM, automatic tube current modulation; 3D, 3-dimensional algorithms that back-project each ray along its true path through the 3D volume and reconstruct each voxel independently based on multiple projections.
*Simultaneous scanning, reconstruction, archiving, and hardcopy filming.
†Time from start of scanning to appearance of 30th image in helical abdominal scan(s).
Modified from Lewis M, Keat N, Edyvean S. Report 06013: 32- to 64-Slice CT Scanner Comparison Report Version 14. London, ImPACT, 2006, pp 1-17.

reconstructions can be broadly classified into two-dimensional and three-dimensional types. Owing to complexity of calculations, reconstructions are not exact and use approximations (a potential source of artifacts).

Two-dimensional cone beam reconstruction uses a series of intermediate tilted image planes based on the trajectory of the gantry around the patient. The tilted image planes are used to create axial slices (Fig. 9-4): this technique is used on some 16-slice CT scanners. In contrast, all 64-slice scanners use three-dimensional cone beam reconstructions. These algorithms back-project each ray along its true path through the three-dimensional volume and reconstruct each voxel independently based on multiple projections.

Pitch, Noise, and Radiation Dose

In a single-slice scanner, the pitch of the helical scan refers to the ratio of the table movement per gantry rotation to the slice width. This definition is not entirely satisfactorily when applied to multislice CT scanners. Different slice widths may be created using the data acquired by a multislice CT scanner, resulting in different pitch for the same table movement speed. A better definition of pitch in multislice CT is the ratio of table movement to the total x-ray beam collimation. Using this definition, the lengths of volume scanned by 64-slice CT scanners, when a pitch of 1 is chosen, range from 58 to 114 mm (see Table 9-1).

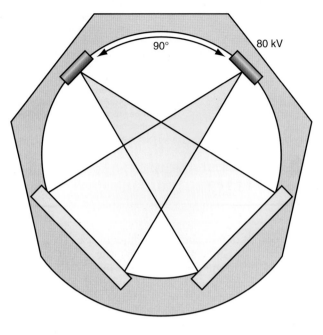

■ **FIGURE 9-2** Simplified diagram of dual-source CT scanner (Somatom Definition, Siemens Medical Solutions). The two x-ray tubes are in the same axial plane and are separated by 90 degrees. The gantry rotation is 330 ms, the same as Sensation 64 CT scanner (Siemens Medical Solutions). The temporal resolution in coronary CT angiography is the time taken to acquire 180 degrees of data. Each gantry has to rotate only 90 degrees to acquire this information from the two sets of detectors. Thus the temporal resolution of this scanner is only 83 ms (330/4), allowing assessment of coronary arteries with heart rates of 80 to 90 beats per minute. Note that the temporal resolution of catheter coronary angiography is about 20 ms.

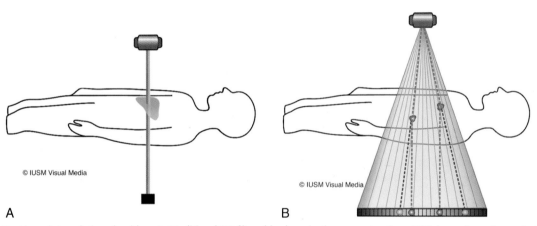

■ **FIGURE 9-3** Linear interpolation algorithm. **A,** Traditional 2D filtered back-projection reconstructions (180-degree linear interpolation) assume that all rays used to reconstruct an image lie entirely within plane. **B,** In 64-slice CT, the beam is not fan shaped but cone shaped. Linear interpolation algorithms may lead to incorrect positioning of lesions (as shown by *red dotted lines*). New reconstruction techniques are required.

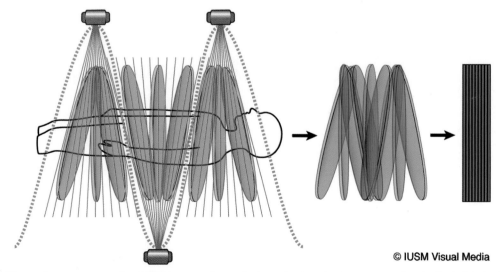

■ **FIGURE 9-4** 2D cone beam reconstruction. This reconstruction method uses back-projection to create slices in tilted planes, which are used to create overlapping projections, which are then filtered in the z-axis to make axial slices. (*© IUSM Visual Media. Reproduced with permission.*)

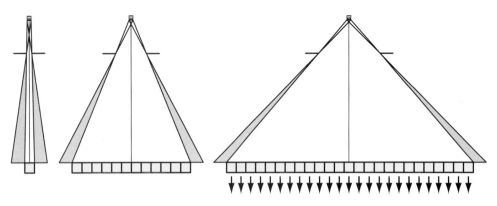

■ **FIGURE 9-5** Penumbra radiation. Diagrams show that as the beam becomes wider, the proportion of wasted penumbra radiation (shown as gray bands of radiation falling outside the active detectors) becomes smaller. The 64-slice CT scanners with wider, 40-mm beam collimation have lower penumbra radiation than those with narrower collimation.

In single-slice CT, the gantry always has to rotate through a specific angle, depending on the reconstruction algorithm used, to acquire the projection information needed to create an axial image. Thus, the number of photons that are used to produce an axial image (the principal determinant of image noise) depends on the tube current/time product and not on the pitch. However, as the pitch increases, the radiation dose reduces, because each part of the scanned volume spends less time in the x-ray beam.

The relationship between pitch, noise, and radiation dose is not the same with current multislice scanners.[5] In the noncardiac mode, as the pitch is increased, 64-slice scanners automatically increase the tube current to maintain a relatively constant noise level. With higher pitch, the larger focal spot may be automatically chosen. These secondary effects negate any reduction of radiation dose that is intuitively expected with an increase in pitch.[6] Therefore, changing the pitch per se, in current multislice CT scanners, does not result in alteration of the radiation dose. In addition, with multislice CT, pitch does not have a significant effect on the slice sensitivity profile. However, as the pitch is increased insufficient data may be collected for accurate reconstructions, leading to *windmill* or *splay artifacts* (see later).

On the other hand, in the cardiac mode of multislice CT, image reconstruction shows some similarities to single-slice CT. In this mode, the minimum data required to reconstruct an image are acquired over a rotation of 180 degrees plus the angle subtended by the x-ray beam in the x-y plane (known as the fan angle). Therefore, in the cardiac mode, noise is dependent on tube current and not on pitch. A major driving force in cardiac CT technology is the attempt to "freeze" the cardiac motion with the development of scanners with faster gantry rotation. With faster gantry rotation, the pitch has to be reduced to eliminate gaps in anatomic coverage in images reconstructed from consecutive heartbeats. This results in increased radiation dose to maintain the same noise.

Reducing Radiation Dose

CT examination is responsible for about 70% of the radiation dose received by the general population from imaging tests.[7] The use of multislice CT scanners has resulted in a rapid increase in radiation dose to the general population.

This increase is due to the more frequent use (sometimes with inadequate indication) of CT, the acquisition of thinner slices, and the performance of multiphasic examinations. However, when comparisons are made for scans using the same slice width, multislice CT scanners are more dose efficient than single-slice scanners. One reason is the reduction in the non–image-contributing penumbra radiation (Fig. 9-5). Modern scanners also employ techniques to reduce radiation dose. Automatic tube current modulation (ATCM) changes the tube current to produce an acceptable noise level for each slice. The tube current modulation may be in the radial (x-y) plane (Fig. 9-6A) or in the z-axis (see Fig. 9-6B). Although the modulation techniques work differently in each scanner, in general the mA is altered to maintain a selected noise level throughout the scanned volume. In some scanners, such as Sensation 64 (Siemens Medical Solutions) the tube current is constantly varied using dosimetry reading from prior gantry rotations. In others, the localizer image is used to calculate regions requiring higher and lower x-ray tube currents. It is possible on most 64-slice scanners to use simultaneously both radial and z-axis ATCM, leading to an overall reduction in dose of 40% to 60% compared with fixed mAs scanning. The use of ATCM has been shown to maintain image quality in assessment of structures with high inherent contrast differences, such as in chest CT and CT colonography.[8] However, there is a potential of ATCM to increase noise and adversely affect image quality in studies where the difference in tissue contrast is low.

Artifacts of Multislice Scanners

Artifacts due to beam hardening, photon starvation, and metallic implants occur less commonly in 40- and 64-channel scanners than they did in earlier CT generations. The use of beam-hardening reduction software, adaptive filtration, and ATCM reduces artifacts from dense bone such as in the shoulders and posterior cranial fossa. Adaptive filtration refers to software that smooths the attenuation differences at sites of highly variable attenuation, before reconstruction of source images. Several methods are now available to reduce artifacts from metallic implants, allowing diagnosis of prosthetic malfunction using CT. The use of thin-slice isotropic scanning technique almost completely eliminates stair-step artifacts seen on multiplanar reformatted images. Ring artifacts may be seen due to poorly functional or miscalibrated detector elements (Fig. 9-7).

The wide cone beam required for 40- and 64-slice scanning as well the obligatory reconstruction algorithms result in specific artifacts. These include cone beam, windmill, and zebra artifacts.

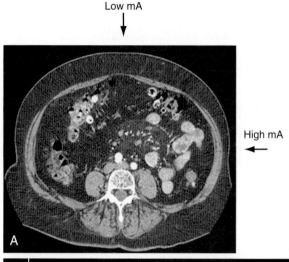

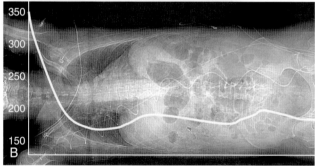

■ **FIGURE 9-6** Automatic tube current modulation (ATCM). **A,** Angular (x-y) ATCM is depicted as variation in tube current as the gantry rotates round the patient. **B,** Z-axis ATCM. Diagram shows that the tube current is constantly changed through the scan. It is high when scanning through the shoulders, low through the lungs, higher through the abdomen, and even higher through the pelvis. If extremities are scanned, the tube current reduces. The parameters used to alter the tube current vary for each vendor. In general, the tube current alters to maintain noise within a small range.

Cone Beam Artifact

Cone beam artifacts result from approximations in reconstruction algorithms that fail to exactly reconstruct a widely divergent x-ray beam. The artifact may manifest as geometric distortions or a glow around high-contrast objects such as bones (Fig. 9-8). They are more obvious on two-dimensional cone beam reconstruction algorithms compared with three-dimensional techniques. The widely divergent cone beam of 64-slice scanners would be expected to show worse cone beam artifact than narrower beams of 4- and 16-slice scanners. However, 64-slice scanners use three-dimensional reconstruction techniques that minimize this artifact.

Windmill Artifact

Windmill or splay artifacts occur as a result of inadequate sampling in the z-direction (Fig. 9-9). These artifacts are similar to aliasing artifacts seen in Doppler ultrasonography and are unrelated to the cone beam geometry. The appearance of artifacts is determined by the number of detector rows, the detector width, the helical pitch, and the reconstructed slice thickness. For example, splay is more prominent on thin-slice axial images where the slice thickness is approximately equal to the detector width, while they are minimized as the slice thickness is increased. Typically, splay artifact does not occur if the slice thickness is double that of the detector width. The number of vanes in the windmill artifact is proportional to the pitch; decreasing the pitch also reduces this artifact. Oversampling of z-axis data, as seen with the z-flying focus (Somatom Sensation 64, Siemens Medical Solutions) is less likely to cause this artifact.

Zebra Artifact

Weighting factors used in reconstruction algorithms are associated with inhomogeneity in noise, particularly away from the center of rotation.[9] The variation in noise between different axial slices becomes obvious on images oriented in the z-axis, including nonaxial reformatted images and maximum intensity projection images. The artifact appears as faint stripes of variable density and is termed the *zebra artifact* (Fig. 9-10). This artifact is reduced by ATCM

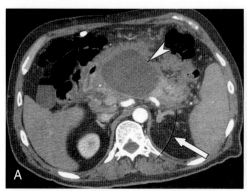

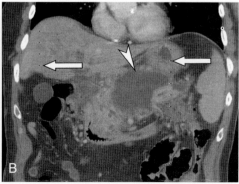

■ **FIGURE 9-7** Ring artifact. Axial (**A**) and coronal reformatted images (**B**) in a 67-year-old man with necrotic pancreatitis. Alternating black and white curves (**A**) or pixels (**B**) (*arrows*) are artifactual and due to malfunction of a detector element. Note large pseudocyst (*arrowheads*).

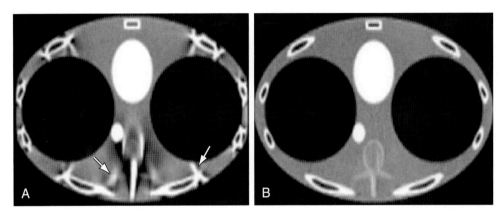

■ **FIGURE 9-8** Cone beam artifact. Reconstruction of an anthropomorphic phantom in 40-slice scanner, with standard (180-degree linear interpolation, **A**) and 3D Feldkamp-based (**B**) reconstructions. Note the glow around the "vertebra" and "ribs" (*arrows,* **A**) is eliminated by the use of algorithms that take into account the divergence of the x-ray beam in the z-axis.

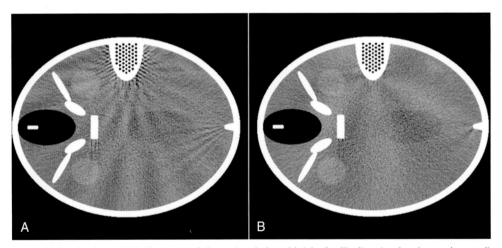

■ **FIGURE 9-9** Windmill (splay) artifact. Windmill pattern of alternating dark and bright fan-like lines is related to undersampling of data, similar in etiology to aliasing in Doppler sonography. **A,** Image of anthropomorphic head phantom performed using 16 × 1.5 mm configuration, 1.5 pitch, 2 mm slice width. **B,** Image performed using same parameters except for a 0.5 pitch. Splay artifact is less prominent with lower pitch due to better sampling in the z-axis. The artifact superficially resembles, but is unrelated in etiology to, beam-hardening artifacts.

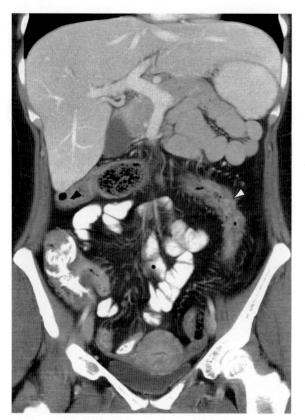

■ **FIGURE 9-10** Zebra artifact. Coronal reformatted images from a 64-slice CT scan show faintly visible lines best seen over the urinary bladder and gluteal and adductor muscles. These artifacts are due to variation in noise in axial source images that become obvious on images reformatted in the z-axis. Patient had active Crohn colitis, with thickened colon (*arrowhead*).

techniques that attempt to maintain a constant noise level at different axial locations. Adaptive filtration techniques also can be used to reduce variability of noise between different axial slices. Zebra artifact is not related to beam hardening or the effect of scatter radiation, which may cause a similar-appearing artifact on nonhelical scanners.

CONCLUSION

Knowledge of the technical and physics-related features of 64-slice CT scanners helps in pushing the limits of these versatile scanners, for example, to obtain good-quality images in an obese patient or to reduce the dose in a pediatric patient.

KEY POINTS

- Multislice CT requires new methods of reconstructions: the 2D and 3D cone beam reconstruction algorithms
- In the noncardiac mode, changing the pitch in current multislice CT scanners does not significantly change noise or radiation dose.

REFERENCES

1. Flohr TG, Stierstorfer K, Ulzheimer S, et al. Image reconstruction and image quality evaluation for a 64-slice CT scanner with z-flying focal spot. Med Phys 2005; 32:2536-2547.
2. Scheffel H, Alkadhi H, Plass A, et al. Accuracy of dual-source CT coronary angiography: first experience in a high pre-test probability population without heart rate control. Eur Radiol 2006; 16: 2739-2747.
3. Flohr TG, McCollough CH, Bruder H, et al. First performance evaluation of a dual-source CT (DSCT) system. Eur Radiol 2006; 16:256-268.
4. Johnson TR, Krauss B, Sedlmair M, et al. Material differentiation by dual energy CT: initial experience. Eur Radiol 2007; 17:1510-1517.
5. Mahesh M, Scatarige JC, Cooper J, Fishman EK. Dose and pitch relationship for a particular multislice CT scanner. AJR Am J Roentgenol 2001; 177:1273-1275.
6. Theocharopoulos N, Perisinakis K, Damilakis J, et al. Dosimetric characteristics of a 16-slice computed tomography scanner. Eur Radiol 2006; 16:2575-2585.
7. Mettler FA Jr, Wiest PW, Locken JA, Kelsey CA. CT scanning: patterns of use and dose. J Radiol Prot 2000; 20:353-359.
8. Graser A, Wintersperger BJ, Suess C, et al. Dose reduction and image quality in MDCT colonography using tube current modulation. AJR Am J Roentgenol 2006; 187:695-701.
9. Hsieh J. Investigation of an image artefact induced by projection noise inhomogeneity in multi-slice helical computed tomography. Phys Med Biol 2003; 48:341-356.

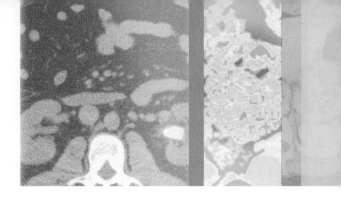

CHAPTER 10

Instrumentation and Radiation Safety

Bob Liu and Naveen M. Kulkarni

TECHNICAL ASPECTS

CT Instrumentation

The performance of CT, in terms of acquisition time, image quality, and radiation dose, has been improved significantly over the past 3 decades. For example, the scan time for a single 10-mm slice data acquisition was about 300 seconds in 1972.[1] Motion artifacts due to the long scanning time and the partial volume artifacts due to the thick-slice images were common. In contrast, the newest multidetector CT (MDCT) can complete a whole-body scan within a single breath-hold, producing hundreds of thin-slice images almost free from the motion and partial volume artifacts. Several breakthroughs in CT hardware and software developments have contributed to such tremendous advances. The first was the adoption of the slip ring technology in 1980s. This technology allows the x-ray source and the detector assembly to rotate continuously while the power and the data are exchanged between the rotating components and the fixed components. The second revolutionary development was the invention of the spiral scanning mode in the late 1980s. In this scanning mode, the patient table moves at a constant speed through the gantry opening while the x-ray source/detector assembly is rotating continuously. The projections of a volume, not just a slice, are obtained. Any axial slice within the volume can be reconstructed based on the projection data on both sides of the slice using various interpolation algorithms. The third major development wave was marked by the introduction of MDCT in 1998. At the time of this writing, one vendor has introduced a 320-row detector with a z-coverage as large as 16 cm. A complete heart can be scanned with just one rotation in 0.35 second.

The major components of a CT system are a gantry, a patient table, a control console, an image reconstruction computer, and a power distribution unit. Almost all new CT systems are third-generation scanners (i.e., the scanners with rotating x-ray sources and rotating detectors).

The typical configuration of a modern MDCT scanner is shown in Figure 10-1.

The gantry hosts the x-ray generator, the x-ray tube, the x-ray collimators, the x-ray filters, and the x-ray detector. Figure 10-2A shows the logical arrangement of these components, and Figure 10-2B is a photograph of the interior of a CT gantry. The x-ray generators are of high-frequency type with typical power between 60 and 100 kW and voltage between 80 and 140 kVp. The x-ray tubes for CT are usually equipped with two focal spots. The large one is used for applications requiring high x-ray photon flux. The small one is engaged when high spatial resolution is required. When prescribing scans on some CT models, users should be aware that a selection of high mA value may lead to the engagement of the large focal spot that may be undesirable for high spatial resolution applications. The multiple pre-patient collimators are used to define the desired x-ray beam dimension and to reduce unnecessary radiation dose to patients. The fixed post-patient collimators, positioned between the detector elements and aligned exactly in the direction of x-ray focal spot, are used to reduce the scatter radiation. The flat copper or alumina filter is used to remove the low-energy x-ray photons, which may contribute to patient dose significantly but not much for image formation. The bow-tie–shaped filters are used to compensate the tissue deficits at the periphery of patient contour such that signal dynamic range matches that of the detectors. These filters also reduce the patient dose in the periphery region significantly. The engagement of a specific bow-tie–shaped filter is usually triggered by the selection of a specific scan field of view. For example, the body filter will be placed in the x-ray beam path if the large scan field of view is selected. The x-ray detectors for modern CT are ceramics or scintillation crystal arrays usually arranged in multiple rows in the z-direction. Examples of multiple-row x-ray detectors are shown in Figure 10-3. Signals from several detector rows can be combined to produce slice thickness larger than the detector array pitch in the z-direction.

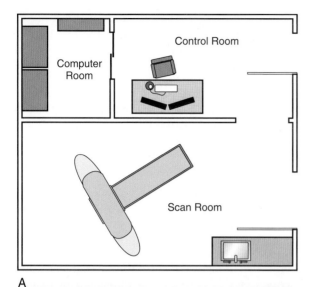

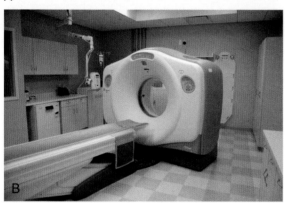

■ **FIGURE 10-1** **A,** Layout of the CT examination room and the operator's area. **B,** The CT gantry and the patient table.

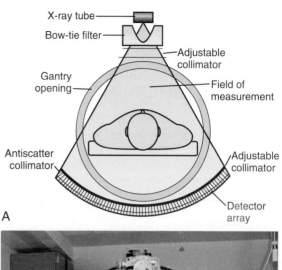

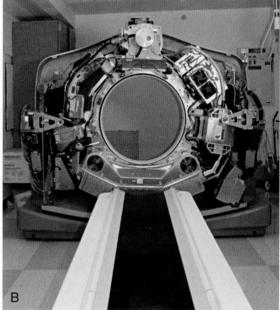

■ **FIGURE 10-2** **A,** Schematic representation of the scanning geometry and important components of the CT measuring system. **B,** View inside the CT gantry.

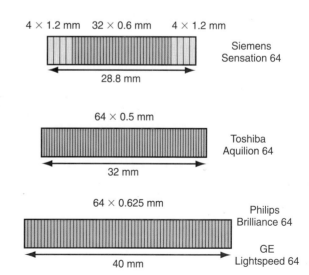

■ **FIGURE 10-3** Detector array designs for CT scanners that can yield 64 images per gantry rotation. (*From Cody DD, Mahesh M. AAPM/RSNA physics tutorial for residents: technologic advances in multidetector CT with a focus on cardiac imaging. RadioGraphics 2007; 27:1829-1837.*)

The patient table is used to move patients in and out of the gantry with high precision. Most vendors can accomplish a precision of ±0.25 mm in positioning with the maximum load, which is at least 450 lb. The table top is typically made of carbon fiber, which has low x-ray attenuation and high strength.

The system console is the main interface for the operator to interact with all components of the CT system. The console is used to input patient demographic information, to select scanning parameters, to initiate or stop scans, to display and review images, to print hard copy, and to communicate with the picture archiving and communications system (PACS), radiology information system, and other devices on the image network.

The image reconstruction computer performs preprocessing (data conditioning and calibration), image reconstruction, and postprocessing (e.g., artifacts reduction and image re-formation). This computer usually has multiple high-speed processors and very large memory. A parallel processing algorithm is implemented to maximize the performance. With reduced image matrix size and an advanced algorithm, 12-frame-per-second real-time images have been realized in CT fluoroscopy. In 2008, a reconstruction speed of 40 images per second was listed in one CT vendor's specification sheet.

The CT system can be operated in several different modes. Most common modes are scout scan mode, axial scan mode, and helical scan mode.

The scout scan mode is also called the topogram mode or preview mode. In this mode, the x-ray tube and the x-ray detector are parked at a fixed orientation (90 or 180 degrees). While the x-ray is on, the patient table moves at a constant speed through the gantry opening. The whole system is equivalent to a slot scanning digital radiography system. An anteroposterior or lateral digital radiograph is obtained. The purpose of the scout scan is to identify the area of interest and to define the scan range for an axial scan or a helical scan.

The axial scan mode is also called sequential scan mode. In this mode, the patient table is stationary when the x-ray beam is on. After one cross section is scanned, the table moves a certain distance and the next cross section is scanned. All CT systems were operated in this mode before the helical scan mode was introduced in late 1980s. The disadvantages of this mode are the long examination time and lack of flexibility of reconstruction from an arbitrary location. The axial mode is still available on all modern CT scanners and is used in several advanced applications such as CT perfusion and high-resolution chest imaging.

The helical scan mode is also called the spiral scan mode. This mode is used most often for modern CT scanners. While the x-ray tube/detector assembly is rotating, the patient table is moving at a constant speed through the gantry opening. The whole-body scan can be completed within one breath-hold, and the slice at any location can be reconstructed from the volume projection data.

Radiation Safety

As CT systems become more sophisticated and more user friendly, the categories of CT applications have expanded rapidly. As a result, the number of CT examinations has increased significantly over the past 20 years.[2] Compared with most x-ray imaging procedures, the patient dose from CT is much higher (Table 10-1). For example, the effective dose for a chest CT is about 200 times the effective dose for chest radiography and the effective dose for

an abdomen CT is more than 10 times the effective dose for abdominal radiography.[3] Although the number of CT examinations is about 12% of total radiology examinations, CT contributes about 45% of the collective dose from all medical examinations.[4]

Radiation risks from abdominal CT procedures can be classified into three categories: (1) malfunction of electric medical devices caused by high dose rate radiation, (2) deterministic bioeffects when the dose exceeds a threshold, and (3) stochastic bioeffects due to low-level radiation exposure.

High-dose CT may cause unintended "shocks" (i.e., stimuli) from neurostimulators, malfunctions of insulin infusion pumps, and transient changes in pacemaker output pulse rate. The U. S. Food and Drug Administration recently issued a public health notification on this problem and made the following recommendations[5]:

Before beginning a CT scan, the operator should use CT scout views to determine if implanted or externally worn electronic medical devices are present and if so, their location relative to the programmed scan range. For CT procedures in which the medical device is in or immediately adjacent to the programmed scan range, the operator should:

(a) Determine the device type;
(b) If practical, try to move external devices out of the scan range;
(c) Ask patients with neurostimulators to shut off the device temporarily while the scan is performed;
(d) Minimize x-ray exposure to the implanted or externally worn electronic medical device by using the lowest possible x-ray tube current consistent with obtaining the required image quality; and making sure that the x-ray beam does not dwell over the device for more than a few seconds.

For CT procedures that require scanning over the medical device continuously for more than a few seconds, as with CT perfusion or interventional examinations, attending staff should be ready to take emergency measures to treat adverse reactions if they occur.

The deterministic bioeffects of radiation will not occur unless a threshold dose is exceeded. For typical one-phase CT scan of abdomen and pelvis, the highest skin dose is under 80 mGy, which is much lower than the threshold for any deterministic effect. However, several special procedures may need attention. These include CT-guided interventional procedures, CT fluoroscopy, CT perfusion, CT biopsy, and so on. In these procedures, the same organ or skin area may be scanned multiple times in a short period and the accumulated skin dose can be more than 2 Gy, which is in the range of the warning level for deterministic skin effects. For instance, the same body section may be scanned up to 40 times in a CT biopsy procedure and the patient skin dose can be up to 3 Gy if improper technique is used.

An important safety issue with CT of the lower abdomen or pelvis of pregnant women is the radiation risk to fetus. Potential deterministic effects of the x-ray exposure include termination of viability, nonrecoverable growth retardation, small head size, malformation, and mental retardation. The probability of inducing the effect and the

TABLE 10-1 Estimated Effective Doses from Typical Abdominal Radiology Examinations	
Examination	Dose (mSv)
Abdominal radiograph (AP)	0.2-0.6
Abdominal series (KUB, upright, LLD)	0.6-1.8
Barium enema	5-7
Intravenous pyelogram	8-10*
Small bowel follow-through	4-7†
Abdomen CT	5-7
Pelvis CT	3-5
Abdomen and pelvis CT	8-12

*Four to five conventional tomograms and six to nine radiographs.
†Including fluoroscopy and spot views.
AP, anteroposterior; KUB, kidney/ureter/bladder; LLD, left lateral decubitus.

severity of radiation risks depend on gestation age and amount of radiation delivered. The most sensitive period for radiation-induced prenatal death is between 0 to 8 days after conception. Animal data suggest that radiation-induced prenatal death might occur at the dose of 50 to 100 mGy and higher if delivered before implantation. The critical period for inducing growth retardation occurs during organogenesis, which is between the second and seventh weeks after conception. The data from Japanese atomic bomb survivors suggested that the effect can occur if the fetus dose is more than 250 mGy. For the thresholds of other effects, the reader is referred elsewhere.[6] The fetal doses from abdomen or pelvis scans range from 6.7 to 56 mGy, with an average of 24.8 mGy.[7] It is obvious that high-dose interventional CT procedures should be avoided and multiple-phase CT scans should be used with great discretion for pregnant women. The volume CT dose index (CTDI$_{vol}$) displayed on the CT control console should not be used as an estimation of the fetus dose because, in general, it underestimates it.[6]

The stochastic effects may occur at any dose level and the probability of occurrence increases with the dose, according to the linear nonthreshold dose-response model. Stochastic effects include carcinogenesis and the induction of genetic mutations. The cancer induction is the primary risk resulting from CT examinations. The lifetime risk of fatal cancer is about 5% per Sievert for the general population.[8] Children are inherently more sensitive to radiation because they have more dividing cells and radiation acts on dividing cells. The lifetime mortality risk is significantly higher when the exposure is received just after birth.

The CT scanning protocols should be optimized in such a way that the quality of images is sufficient for diagnosis and the patient dose is kept as low as reasonably achievable (ALARA). To accomplish the optimization, operators must understand the basic relationship between the dose and image quality and the dependency of the dose on image acquisition parameters.

The quantity CTDI$_{vol}$ is often used to describe the patient dose. CTDI$_{vol}$ represents the average dose in a given scan volume. When a scan is prescribed, the system displays the CTDI$_{vol}$ in milligray on the console. However, the dose displayed is not the true dose for the specific patient under examination. Instead, it is the dose value when the patient is replaced with an acrylic phantom while the same image acquisition parameters are used. The body phantom is an acrylic cylinder with a diameter of 32 cm and a height of 15 cm. For neonates, the dose displayed may significantly underestimate the true patient dose.

The effective dose, E, is used to assess the radiation detriment from nonhomogeneous irradiation. The effective dose is a weighted sum of the doses to all exposed tissues.

$$E = \left[\sum \left(w_t \times H_t\right)\right],$$

where H$_t$ is the equivalent dose to a specific tissue and w$_t$ is the weight factor representing the relative radiosensitivity of that tissue. The unit of effective dose is the Sievert (Sv). The effective dose can be estimated by multiplying the dose-length-product (DLP) in a dose report with a conversion factor.[9] For a typical one-phase CT examination of the abdomen, the effective dose is about 6.5 mSv.

The patient dose depends on three group factors: equipment-related factors, patient-related factors, and application-related factors (Tables 10-2 and 10-3).

The factors in the first group include the x-ray beam filtration, the x-ray beam collimation, the system geometry, and the detector efficiency. Although users do not have control of most of these factors, it is important to understand that the z-axis dose efficiency is reduced when the total x-ray beam width becomes very small for MDCT owing to the need to keep the beam penumbra out of any detector row. Another dose-related issue with MDCT is over scan. To reconstruct a slice near the end of the prescribed range in the helical mode, the projection data on both sides of the slice are needed for proper interpolation. Therefore, the actual scan range is larger than the prescribed scan range. Some scanners require one additional rotation at each end of the prescribed scan range.

The dose is strongly dependent on patient size, as shown in Figure 10-4 and Table 10-4. If the same technique is used to scan an average adult and a newborn, the dose to the newborn is significantly higher.[10]

Image acquisition parameters such as kVp, mAs (the product of the tube current and the time in seconds per rotation), and pitch (the table travel per rotation divided by the total x-ray beam width) are selected by the operator. If all other conditions are fixed, the patient dose is proportional to the effective mAs, which is defined as the mAs (mA × seconds per rotation) divided by the helical pitch (Table 10-5). The dependency of the dose to kVp is more complicated. In general, the dose increases as a power function of kVp (CTDI$_{vol}$ ~ kVp^p) if all other parameters are fixed. The value of p is between 2 and 3 depending on the type of the scanner.[11]

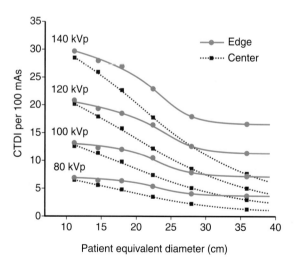

■ **FIGURE 10-4** Graph shows the CTDI per 100 mAs as a function of patient diameter for four tube voltages, given a 4 × 5-mm transverse acquisition (20-mm nominal collimation). The doses measured in the PMMA phantoms at the edge and at the center are shown. The lines (*solid lines* for edge data, *dotted lines* for center data) represent the computer-fit CTDIw values, which were used to interpolate dose values between patient thicknesses. (*From Boone JM, Geraghty EM, Seibert JA, Wootton-Gorges SL. Dose reduction in pediatric CT: a rational approach. Radiology 2003; 228:352-360.*)

TABLE 10-2   Principles of Scanning Factors

Tube Current (mA)	Determines photon fluence
	Most effective dose-reduction strategy
	50% reduction reduces radiation dose by half
	Decrease in mAs increases image noise
Tube Potential (kVp)	Determines x-ray beam energy
	Dose is approximately proportional to square of kVp
	Decreasing kVp increases attenuation of iodine
	Decrease in kVp significantly increases image noise. This needs a compensatory increase in mAs to maintain image quality
Gantry Rotation Time (seconds)	Faster gantry rotation reduces photon fluence (mAs)
	Increase in mA needed to maintain image noise
Pitch and Collimation (these are interlinked)	Ratio of table speed to beam collimation (mm)
	Dose is inversely proportional to pitch
	Higher pitch increases image noise (if mAs constant)
	Higher pitch can produce artifacts
	Wider collimation is more dose efficient
Scanning Length	Effective dose is proportional to length of scanned volume
	Scan coverage should be restricted to area of interest
	Minimize overlap scanning
	Minimize scan phases
Scanning Mode	Over-ranging contributes to extra dose
	Single helical scan volume is more dose efficient than multiple helical scan volumes to cover a large region

TABLE 10-3   Other Dose-Saving Factors

Low dose scout
Low dose smart prep
Patient positioning
Noise reduction
Improved dose efficiency of scanners
Over-range shielding

TABLE 10-6   Weight and Clinical Indication (Routine Abdomen and Pelvis MDCT) Adapted ATCM

Weight	Noise Index	Ref mAs
<61 kg	12.5	200
61-91 kg	15	220
>91 kg	18	250

TABLE 10-4   Practical Tips for CT of Obese Patients

kVp: 140
Automatic exposure control (AEC) with maximal current limit of 800 mA
Rotation time: 0.8-1.0 second
Noise reduction filters
Increase reconstruction thickness
Noise-reducing reconstruction algorithms

TABLE 10-5   Adjustable Parameters for Dose Radiation

Decrease in:	Increase in:
Tube current	Pitch (table speed)*
Tube potential	Beam collimation
Gantry rotation time*	
Scan length	
Overlap scanning	
Number of scan phases	

*Provided other scanning factors are kept constant.

Image quality is closely related to patient dose, and it is characterized by spatial resolution, contrast resolution, image noise, and other quantities. In practice, image noise has been widely used to judge the CT image quality because the detectability of low-contrast objects is strongly dependent on the contrast-to-noise ratio. The standard deviation of a region of interest in the image is usually used to represent the noise. For a given reconstruction kernel and slice thickness, the noise is inversely proportional to the square root of patient dose. To reduce the noise by a factor of 2, the dose must be increased by a factor of 4. In general, image quality is better when the patient dose is increased.

Many dose-reduction methods have been investigated and implemented over the past few years.[12] On the one hand, imaging professionals have adapted various weight-based or age-based scanning protocols that reduced the doses for pediatric or small-size patients significantly. On the other hand, CT equipment vendors have developed sophisticated automatic current modulation software to deliver just enough dose to accomplish a specified image quality (Table 10-6).

The principle of automatic tube current modulation (ATCM) is illustrated in Figure 10-5. The scout images are first obtained to assess the patient size and attenuation properties at each cross section along the z-direction. The current is modulated along the z-direction based on the information collected. The current may also change when the tube moves to different location in the scan plane. The tube current is generally lower when the x-ray tube is in the anteroposterior direction because the patient thickness is smaller in that direction. It must be pointed out that using the automatic current modulation does not guarantee the low patient dose. All current modulation software packages require users to specify the expected image quality. The expected image quality can be specified with an image noise or an image produced using a reference mAs. It is the user's responsibility to define the proper image quality for a specific imaging task. If the specified image noise is too low, the patient dose may be higher than the dose using a fixed technique (Fig. 10-6).

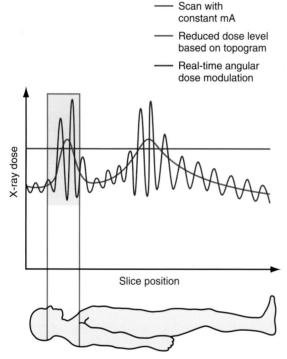

—— Scan with constant mA

—— Reduced dose level based on topogram

—— Real-time angular dose modulation

X-ray dose

Slice position

■ **FIGURE 10-5** Principle of automatic tube current modulation for a helical scan from shoulder to pelvis. Note the high tube current and strong modulation in shoulder and pelvis and lower tube current and low modulation in abdomen and thorax. (*Redrawn from Siemens SOMATOM Sensation 64 Application Guide.*)

Summary

Modern CT scanners can acquire whole-body volume images with isotropic resolution within a single breath-hold. The key enabling technologies are the slip ring, helical scanning mode, and multiple-row x-ray detector. The primary radiation risks from CT examinations are carcinogenesis and the induction of genetic mutations. The CT dose can be reduced significantly if the automatic current modulation feature is used properly.

PROS AND CONS

The major advantages of modern MDCT are fast image acquisition, large volume coverage in short time, less partial volume and motion artifacts, near-isotropic resolution, ability to retrospectively reconstruct images with different slice thickness, more efficient use of x-ray output, and contrast materials. However, widespread use of MDCT has increased the collective radiation dose significantly.

KEY POINTS

- Modern MDCT can acquire high-quality 3D images of the whole body within one breath-hold.
- Enabling technologies are the slip ring, helical scan mode, multiple-slice detector, and fast computer processors.
- The primary radiation risk from CT is the possible higher cancer rate.
- Patient skin dose in some CT interventional procedures may be in the range of the warning level for deterministic skin effects.
- High dose rate in some CT interventional procedures may cause malfunction of electric medical devices.
- Patient dose can be reduced significantly if automatic current modulation is configured properly.

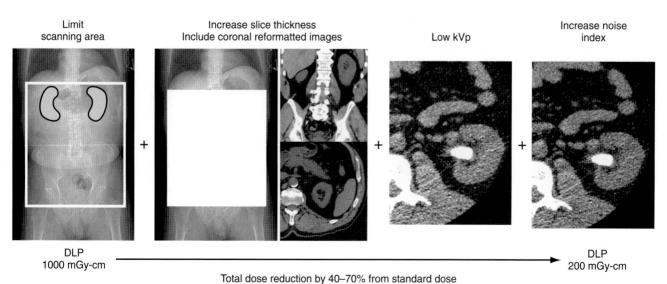

Limit scanning area

Increase slice thickness Include coronal reformatted images

Low kVp

Increase noise index

DLP 1000 mGy-cm

DLP 200 mGy-cm

Total dose reduction by 40–70% from standard dose

■ **FIGURE 10-6** Summary of strategies for dose reduction.

SUGGESTED READINGS

Hsieh J. Computed Tomography—Principles, Design, Artifacts, and Recent Advances. Bellingham, WA, SPIE Press, 2003.

Kalender W. Computed Tomography—Fundamentals, Systems Technology, Image Quality, Applications. Munich, Publicis MCD Verlag, 2006.

Rruening R, Kuettner A, Flohr T. Protocols for Multislice CT. Berlin, Springer-Verlag, 2006.

REFERENCES

1. Kalender WA. Computed Tomography, Fundamentals, System Technology, Image Quality, Application. Munich, Publicis MCD Verlag, 2000.
2. IMV 2006 CT Market Summary Report. Des Plains, IL, IMV Medical Information Division, 2006.
3. Lee CI, Haims AH, Monico EP, et al. Diagnostic CT scans: assessment of patient, physician, and radiologist awareness of radiation dose and possible risks. Radiology 2004; 231:393.
4. Mettler FA Jr. Magnitude of radiation uses and doses in the United States: NCRP scientific committee 6-2 analysis of medical exposures. Forty-third NCRP annual meeting program, 2007, pp 9-10.
5. FDA Preliminary Public Health Notification. Possible Malfunction of Electronic Medical Devices Caused by Computed Tomography (CT) Scanning. 2008. Available at http://www.fda.gov/MedicalDevices/Safety/AlertsandNotices/PublicHealthNotifications/ucm061994.htm.
6. Wagner LK, Lester RG, Saldana LR. Exposure of the Pregnant Patient to Diagnostic Radiations: A Guide to Medical Management, 2nd ed. Madison, WI, Medical Physics Publishing, 1997.
7. Goldberg-Stein S, Liu B, Hahn P, Lee S. Body CT in pregnancy: how to best minimize fetal radiation exposure. Presented before the RSNA annual meeting, Chicago, 2008.
8. National Council on Radiation Protection. Report 116, Limitation of Exposure to Ionizing Radiation. Bethesda, MD, 1993.
9. American Association of Physicists in Medicine. Report 96, The Measurement, Reporting, and Management of Radiation Dose in CT. College Park, MD, 2008.
10. Boone JM, Geraghty EM, Seibert JA, Wootton-Gorges SL. Dose reduction in pediatric CT: a rational approach. Radiology 2003; 228:352-360.
11. Nagal HD. Radiation Exposure in Computed Tomography. Hamburg, CTB Publications, 2002.
12. McCollough CH, Bruesewitz MR, Kofler JM Jr. CT dose reduction and dose management tools: overview of available options. RadioGraphics 2006; 26:503-512.

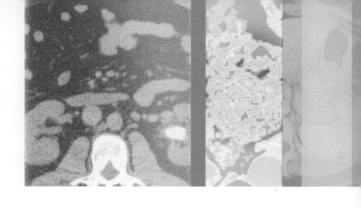

CHAPTER 11

Recent Advances

Avinash Kambadakone R. and Kumaresan Sandrasegaran

For almost 4 decades now, CT has made a remarkable impact on clinical practice, and the rapid advances in both CT technology and software have widened the clinical utility of CT of the abdomen and pelvis.[1] The benefits of multidetector CT (MDCT) over single-detector CT include increased temporal and spatial resolution, decreased image noise, and longer anatomic coverage. Better z-axis resolution and larger scan volumes result in improved multiplanar reconstruction in the coronal and sagittal planes. The reduced scanning time achieved by MDCT also helps to reduce respiratory and motion artifacts. The technologic advancements in MDCT technology have been paralleled by the development of sophisticated workstations with higher computational power, which not only allows rapid image processing but also permits complex navigation and quantification programs.

Perfusion CT is an exciting CT innovation that allows functional evaluation of tissue vascularity. This technique has many potential applications in abdominopelvic oncologic imaging.[2-4] Dual-energy CT, either using a single-source (single x-ray tube) or dual-source (dual x-ray tube), is another advance that shows promise for a broad spectrum of abdominal and pelvic applications.[5] Computer-aided detection is becoming more sophisticated and aids in diagnosis, particularly in CT colonography. Other developments include scanners with 256 or 320 detector rows, superior detector materials (gemstone detector technology), volume or helical shuttle mode techniques, and use of dose reduction iterative reconstruction algorithms.[6-8] In this chapter an overview is provided of the recent advances in CT with emphasis on clinical applications. Discussion of advances in postprocessing and software developments is beyond the scope of this chapter, and the reader is referred to Chapters 24 and 25.

TECHNICAL ASPECTS

Advances in X-Ray Tube

Several advances in the x-ray tube in the past few years have enabled CT to broaden its utility in the realm of cardiac imaging and in tissue material differentiation (Table 11-1). One of the best-known advancements has been the introduction of dual-source CT (Somatom Definition, Siemens Medical Solutions, Forchheim, Germany). Dual-source CT contains two sets of x-ray tube and detector arrays, which are arranged in a single gantry perpendicular (90 degrees) to each other in the x-y plane (Fig. 11-1A).[5,9,10] Dual-source CT has three main advantages over the single-source scanners, depending on the mode of scan acquisition. Operating the two tubes at different tube potentials allows dual-energy scanning and, thus, has applications in tissue differentiation. When the two x-ray tubes are used in unison at equal tube potentials, the resultant increased photon flux permits scanning larger patients with acceptable noise. The third, and most explored, capability of dual-source CT is the improved temporal resolution achieved by the use of two x-ray tubes. By using the two tubes at identical kVp levels, it is possible to acquire images using data from only 90 degrees of gantry rotation instead of the conventional 180 degrees of data required for the single-source CT. The resultant temporal resolution of only 83 ms is particularly advantageous in coronary artery imaging. It is possible to obtain diagnostic images at higher heart rates than previously possible and possibly obviate the need for β-adrenergic blockers.[9]

Dual-energy scanning, that is, simultaneous scanning using two different energies, can also be performed using single-source CT by rapid voltage and mA modulation (see Fig. 11-1B).[5] This technique may achieve dual-energy processing using projection data acquired in both axial and helical modes, unlike the image-based dual-energy processing of dual-source CT.[5] Theoretically, this permits accurate material decomposition and monochromatic CT image display, which should potentially facilitate more precise tissue characterization and also substantially decrease image artifacts.[5] Two disadvantages of single-source dual-energy scanning are the unequal noise levels that may result in the datasets owing to the rapid modulation of tube current and the fact that the use of the same filtration for the two energy beams may result in suboptimal spectral separation.[5]

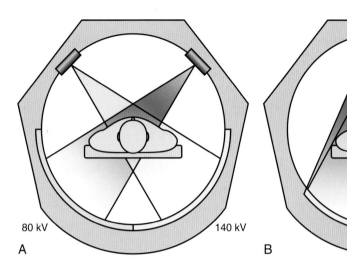

■ **FIGURE 11-1** Diagrammatic illustration of dual-source CT (**A**) with two x-ray tubes and detector assemblies and single-source dual-energy CT (**B**) with one x-ray tube and detector assembly. (*A redrawn from art provided courtesy of Christianne Leidecker, Siemens Medical Solutions; B modified from art provided courtesy of Mukta Joshi, GE Healthcare.*)

TABLE 11-1 Technical Details of Current CT Technology

	GE Discovery 750HD	Phillips Brilliance CT	Siemens Flash	Toshiba One
Rows (n × mm)	64 × 0.625	128 × 0.625 256 × 0.625	2 × 64 × 0.6	320 × 0.5
Width (cm)	4	8/16	3.8	16
Channels (n)	64	256/512	2 × 128	320
Tube power (kW)	100	120	2 × 100	72
Max current (mA)	800	950	2 × 850	600
Gantry rotation (ms)	350	270	280	350
Temporal resolution (ms)	175	135	75	175

From Rubin GD. Cardiac CT technologies: what is important. In Abdominal Radiology Course 2009. Maui, Hawaii, Society of Gastrointestinal Radiology, 2009.

Dual-Energy CT

Dual-energy computed tomography (DECT) is based on the same principles as dual-energy conventional radiography.[11] Owing to their differing electron configurations, the atoms of different elements absorb x-rays with different frequency signatures. This phenomenon can be used, with limitations, to identify the elemental makeup of compounds, including calcium density in bones and iron content,[12] to differentiate plaque from contrast-enhanced vessel lumen, to assess tissue fat, and to differentiate calcium and uric acid stones.[13-16] Although experiments in dual-energy CT have been performed for nearly 30 years, prior studies were restricted by the technologic limitations of the older generations of CT scanners. The ability of dual-energy CT to qualitatively and quantitatively assess calcium content has been used to assess urinary stones[17,18] and bone density more reliably than single-energy techniques.[19,20] The introduction of dual-source CT scanners has facilitated concurrent scanning with two different energy levels, avoiding even small misregistration artifacts.[13,16] The practical utility of DECT is likely to be enhanced by the introduction of rapid kV switching as another approach for dual-energy scanning.[5,13,16,21] A third approach also exists as an alternative for dual-energy scanning that involves a sandwich detector: the low-energy photons are absorbed in the top layers of the detector, while the higher energy photons are absorbed in the lower levels of the detector.[5]

Clinical Applications of Dual-Energy CT in the Abdomen

For most clinical applications, dual-energy scanning is performed at the tube potentials of 80 and 140 kVp, which allows for optimum tissue material differentiation because the quality of dual-energy postprocessing is inversely related to the overlap of the spectra, which is least at these two energies.

1. *Virtual unenhanced images:* Reconstruction of the 80 kVp and 140 kVp image datasets allows generation of "virtual unenhanced images" that may preclude the routine need for true unenhanced acquisitions.[5,10] As such, a dual-energy contrast-enhanced acquisition could yield both unenhanced and contrast-enhanced CT images and, thus, diminish radiation dose exposure to the patients.
2. *Determination of stone composition:* Dual-energy CT has been found to be a robust technique to determine the composition of urinary stones, particularly the differentiation of uric acid from non–uric acid stones, which has implications for treatment (Fig. 11-2).[17,18,22] Uric acid stones may be treated with urinary alkalinization as a first-line treatment, whereas non–uric acid stones are usually treated by lithotripsy or surgically.[17,18,22]
3. *Evaluation of renal masses:* Dual-energy scanning can be used to generate a color-coded image that shows

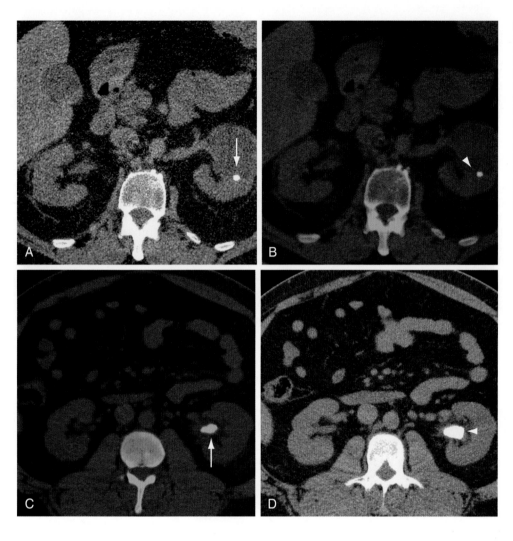

■ FIGURE 11-2 **A,** Axial unenhanced abdominal CT scan in a 43-year-old man shows a calculus in the left mid pole (*arrow*). **B,** Corresponding color-coded dual-energy postprocessed image shows the calculus coded as red (*arrowhead*) indicating a uric acid stone. **C,** Axial unenhanced abdominal CT scan in a 36-year-old man shows a large calculus in the left renal pelvis (*arrow*). **D,** Corresponding color-coded dual-energy image after postprocessing shows the calculus coded as blue (*arrowhead*), indicating a non–uric acid stone.

the distribution of iodine within a particular tissue. These iodine-based maps are sensitive for the detection of subtle enhancement and may be used to differentiate high-density benign cysts from solid renal masses.[5,10]

4. *CT angiography:* Dual-energy techniques may be used for rapid and accurate removal of bony structures and calcified plaques during postprocessing of CT angiographic images. Dual-energy CT angiography examination reduces radiation dose by 20% to 30%.[5]

5. Other applications include use of iodine maps for liver lesion characterization and classification of gallstones.[23]

Advances in Detector Technology

Since the introduction of four-slice CT scanner in 1998 there has been a series of advances in CT technology with the development of 8-, 16-, 32-, and 64-slice CT scanners. Currently, 64-slice CT scanners are the preferred MDCT technology. The detector widths in the currently available 64-slice CT scanners range from 2.8 to 4 cm and allow acquisition of slices, with widths ranging from 0.5 to 0.625 mm.[24] Reformatting of images in orthogonal planes is possible with isotropic resolution.[24] Current 64-slice CT scanners meet almost all of the expectations of radiolo-

gists and physicians for abdominal imaging. However, the craniocaudal coverage of the 64-slice scanners is limited to 3.2 to 4.0 cm, which restricts cine imaging over a wider coverage area.[6,7] Because the value of CT in the realm of functional imaging is gradually increasing, it is desirable to have a wider coverage area for cine imaging. This has led to the emergence of newer CT scanners with wider detector arrays with increasing numbers of rows.[6,7,24,25]

Wide-Area Detector

The latest entrants to the CT arena are scanners with a number of detectors in excess of 100 (128, 256, and 320), which eliminates the need for spiral scanning and has the potential to achieve a "single-shot" scan. The 128-slice scanner has a fluid metal-cooled x-ray tube and a 128-row detector array with coverage of 8 cm at 0.625 mm thickness (see Table 11-1).[24] Whereas the spiral scanning option with this CT allows a coverage of 8 cm, operating in the joggle mode (i.e., back and forth movements of the two table positions) helps expand the effective coverage for dynamic imaging.[24] The 256-slice CT scanner is able to achieve an isotropic resolution of less than 0.5 mm for a wide craniocaudal coverage in one rotation.[7] The 320-slice dynamic volume CT scanner has a gantry with an aperture of 70 cm and a 70-kW x-ray tube with detector width of 16 cm along the rotational axis of the gantry. The scanner has 320 rows of 0.5-mm-thick detector elements.[24] The wide detector coverage (16 cm) makes it possible to scan the entire heart without table motion and has the potential to allow dynamic imaging over a single heartbeat.[24] This scanner may also allow functional assessment of entire organs or large tumors.[24]

New Detector Materials

Another recent innovation in the CT detector systems has been the development of detectors with higher sensitivity to radiation and faster sampling rates. The novel gemstone detector is a garnet-based scintillator that has a fast primary speed (0.03 μs) and a short afterglow.[26] This detector material allows the use of rapid kV switching to acquire dual-energy data with almost simultaneous spatial and temporal registration.[24,26] As a result, the resolution is improved and artifacts due to beam hardening and metals are reduced.[24,26]

Sandwich Detectors

As previously discussed, dual-energy CT can be primarily accomplished (1) by scanning with two different energy spectra either from two sources operating at different voltages, (2) from a single source by rapid kV switching,

or (3) by analyzing the energy spectrum with a multilayered detector.[24] This third approach is not yet available in clinical practice. The design of this detector assembly consists of a first layer that predominantly receives photons with lower energy and a second, deeper layer that receives photons with higher energy.[24] The signal readout from both the detector layers can be used separately for spectral analysis.[24]

New Reconstruction Algorithms

There is increasing concern for the potentially harmful effects of machine-induced radiation.[27] Several approaches have been proposed to reduce radiation doses in CT examinations, such as the use of lower tube current or voltage.[28] An undesirable consequence of most of these techniques is the excessive image noise that can deteriorate image quality and diagnostic performance. A step ahead in this regard is the emerging use of new image reconstruction techniques, such as full or adaptive statistical iterative reconstruction (ASIR), which have the ability to eliminate image noise and also maintain lesion conspicuity in low-dose CT examinations. The algorithm typically used for reconstruction of CT data is filtered back-projection. Reconstructing CT data with a combined filtered back-projection and ASIR technique has been found to enable a reduction in radiation dose ranging from 20% to 80% for various abdominal applications (Fig. 11-3).

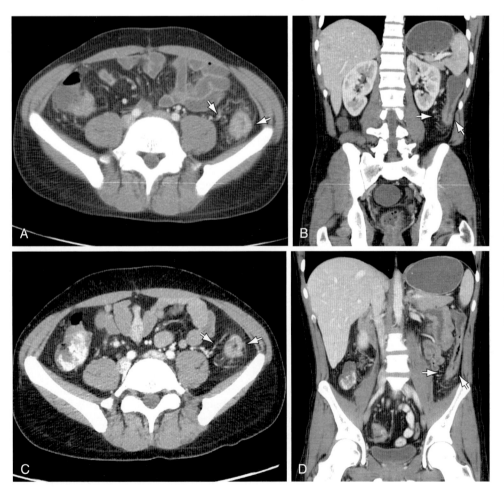

■ **FIGURE 11-3** Multiplanar CT images in a 22-year-old man (body weight: 56 kg) with Crohn's disease with multiple exacerbations. Axial (**A**) and coronal (**B**) contrast-enhanced CT images obtained during initial evaluation demonstrate wall thickening and enhancement with increased surrounding perienteric vascularity in the descending colon. Biopsy confirmed Crohn's disease. CT dose for this examination was 11.6 mSv. The patient underwent remission after therapy with corticosteroids. One year later, the patient presented with a relapse. Repeat axial (**C**) and coronal (**D**) contrast-enhanced CT scan images were obtained using the ASIR technique. The image quality and the depiction of enteric and extraenteric changes are comparable to the previous examination. The radiation dose for this CT study was 5.5 mSv (i.e., a radiation dose reduction of 53%).

Perfusion CT

CT perfusion imaging has been investigated as a functional tool to give information that is complementary or superior to anatomic information of conventional CT.[2-4] Perfusion CT measures the temporal changes in tissue density after intravenous injection of contrast medium bolus using a series of dynamically acquired images.[2] Perfusion imaging has attained significance in the field of oncology owing to the increasing use of targeted therapies such as antiangiogenic drugs targeting tumor vascularity, tumor ablation, and selective internal radiation with yttrium-90 particles. Because these therapies do not cause substantial change in tumor dimensions for several months, functional imaging techniques such as perfusion CT and MRI have shown promise in better assessing the tumor response long before changes in tumor dimension (Fig. 11-4).[2-4,29] The excellent spatial resolution of perfusion CT is an advantage compared with other functional imaging techniques such as positron emission tomography (PET). Another key advantage of perfusion CT is the linear relation between iodine concentration and tissue density changes, which makes quantification of tissue vascularity much simpler and straightforward.[2-4] Moreover, faster scanning times within a short breath-hold that are possible with current-generation MDCT scanners and easy availability of commercial software for perfusion analysis make it a desirable and practical technique for various abdominal applications.

In the realm of oncologic imaging, perfusion CT has been found to be effective to characterize tumor, detect occult tumor, and assess tumor response to therapy and also of use in prognostic evaluation.[4,29] Perfusion CT has also been found to be a useful tool for assessment of tissue perfusion in various nononcologic applications. However, there remain certain limitations. The total coverage area over which the perfusion analysis can be performed is limited to 2 to 4 cm depending on the CT technology. Patient movement during dynamic CT data acquisition may degrade image quality, resulting in inaccurate perfusion measurements. Another concern of repeat perfusion CTs is the risk of exposure to ionizing radiation, especially for nononcologic indications.

Technique

A limited noncontrast CT scan is performed initially for localization of the tumor or the organ in question. The dynamic CT acquisition is performed after intravenous administration of a contrast bolus of 40 to 70 mL at a rate ranging from 3.5 to 10 mL/s. The dynamic CT acquisition involves a first-pass phase (usually 45 to 60 s) followed by a delayed phase (usually 2 to 10 min) for optimal assessment of the tumor perfusion and permeability measurements. The dynamic CT data are then postprocessed with perfusion software to generate colored perfusion maps of blood flow, blood volume, mean transit time, and permeability. The quantitative perfusion parameters are then

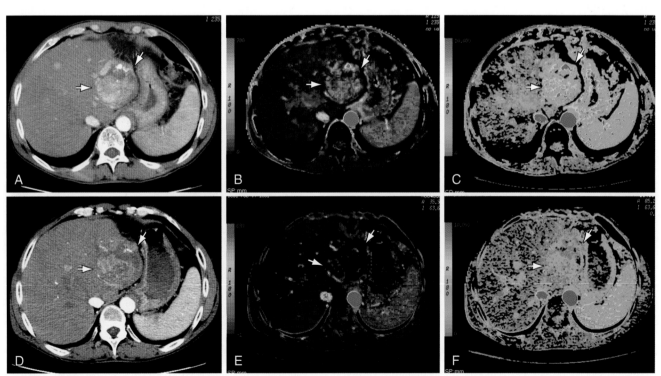

■ **FIGURE 11-4** CT perfusion images obtained before and after treatment with the antiangiogenic agent bevacizumab (Avastin) in a 56-year-old man with hepatocellular carcinoma. **A,** Axial contrast enhanced CT image in the dynamic phase shows the avidly enhancing rounded hepatocellular carcinoma (*arrows*) in the left lobe with corresponding colored perfusion maps demonstrating increased (**B**) blood flow (95 mL/100 g/min) and (**C**) increased blood volume (6.2 mL/100 g). After treatment with Avastin, axial contrast-enhanced CT image (**D**) shows reduced enhancement, with corresponding colored perfusion maps demonstrating (**E**) reduction in the blood flow (24 mL/100 g/min) and (**F**) reduced blood volume (1.64 mL/100 g).

obtained by drawing the region of interest around the tumor tissue. Perfusion software, the analytical methods employed for postprocessing, and the various quantitative perfusion parameters obtained vary from scanner to scanner and among commercial vendors.[2]

Abdominopelvic Applications of Perfusion CT

Liver Tumors

The detection of higher perfusion parameters in metastatic lesions using CT perfusion has been found to be a good prognostic indicator suggesting optimal response to treatment. In hepatocellular carcinoma, perfusion CT has benefits in differential diagnosis, evaluating tumor aggressiveness, and monitoring therapeutic effects.[2,30,31]

Pancreatic Tumors

On perfusion CT, substantially high blood perfusion was observed in hypervascular tumors such as insulinomas compared with background pancreatic parenchyma.[32]

Colorectal Cancer

The predominant application of perfusion CT in colorectal cancer is in the diagnosis and in assessing response to treatment.[2,33,34] Perfusion CT has been found to be able to distinguish colonic wall thickening due to diverticulitis from colorectal carcinoma based on the high perfusion values in the latter.[35]

Prostate Cancer

A potential application of perfusion CT is in the identification of tumor foci within the prostate, thus enabling targeted radiotherapy for the tumor foci with minimal radiation to the surrounding tissues.[36,37]

Lymphoma

The data on the utility of the perfusion CT in patients with lymphoma are limited because angiogenesis is not a predominant feature of lymphoma.[38]

Nononcologic Applications

Perfusion CT facilitates quantification of organ perfusion in liver, kidney, and pancreas in diverse applications such as renal functional assessment, renal transplant rejection, evaluation of the degree of hepatic fibrosis and cirrhosis, and determination of pancreatic ischemia and necrosis in acute severe pancreatitis.[2]

SUGGESTED READINGS

Fletcher JG, Takahashi N, Hartman R, et al. Dual-energy and dual-source CT: is there a role in the abdomen and pelvis? Radiol Clin North Am 2009; 47:41-57.

Geleijns J, Salvado Artells M, de Bruin PW, et al. Computed tomography dose assessment for a 160 mm wide, 320 detector row, cone beam CT scanner. Phys Med Biol 2009; 54:3141-3159.

Graser A, Johnson TR, Chandarana H, Macari M. Dual energy CT: preliminary observations and potential clinical applications in the abdomen. Eur Radiol 2009; 19:13-23.

Kambadakone AR, Sahani DV. Body perfusion CT: technique, clinical applications, and advances. Radiol Clin North Am 2009; 47: 161-178.

Mori S, Endo M, Obata T, et al. Clinical potentials of the prototype 256-detector row CT-scanner. Acad Radiol 2005; 12:148-154.

Mori S, Endo M, Obata T, et al. Properties of the prototype 256-row (cone beam) CT scanner. Eur Radiol 2006; 16:2100-2108.

Rogalla P, Kloeters C, Hein PA. CT technology overview: 64-slice and beyond. Radiol Clin North Am 2009; 47:1-11.

REFERENCES

1. Sahani DV, Yaghmai V. Advances in MDCT: preface. Radiol Clin North Am 2009; 47:xiii-xiv.
2. Kambadakone AR, Sahani DV. Body perfusion CT: technique, clinical applications, and advances. Radiol Clin North Am 2009; 47: 161-178.
3. Miles KA. Perfusion CT for the assessment of tumour vascularity: which protocol? Br J Radiol 2003; 76(Spec No 1):S36-S42.
4. Miles KA. Perfusion imaging with computed tomography: brain and beyond. Eur Radiol 2006; 16(Suppl 7):M37-M43.
5. Fletcher JG, Takahashi N, Hartman R, et al. Dual-energy and dual-source CT: is there a role in the abdomen and pelvis? Radiol Clin North Am 2009; 47:41-57.
6. Mori S, Endo M, Obata T, et al. Properties of the prototype 256-row (cone beam) CT scanner. Eur Radiol 2006; 16:2100-2108.
7. Mori S, Endo M, Obata T, et al. Clinical potentials of the prototype 256-detector row CT-scanner. Acad Radiol 2005; 12:148-154.
8. Hein PA, Romano VC, Lembcke A, et al. Initial experience with a chest pain protocol using 320-slice volume MDCT. Eur Radiol 2009; 19:1148-1155.
9. Achenbach S, Anders K, Kalender WA. Dual-source cardiac computed tomography: image quality and dose considerations. Eur Radiol 2008; 18:1188-1198.
10. Graser A, Johnson TR, Chandarana H, Macari M. Dual energy CT: preliminary observations and potential clinical applications in the abdomen. Eur Radiol 2009; 19:13-23.
11. Johnson TR, Krauss B, Sedlmair M, et al. Material differentiation by dual energy CT: initial experience. Eur Radiol 2007; 17:1510-1517.
12. Oelckers S, Graeff W. In situ measurement of iron overload in liver tissue by dual-energy methods. Phys Med Biol 1996; 41:1149-1165.
13. Flohr TG, McCollough CH, Bruder H, et al. First performance evaluation of a dual-source CT (DSCT) system. Eur Radiol 2006; 16: 256-268.
14. Raptopoulos V, Karellas A, Bernstein J, et al. Value of dual-energy CT in differentiating focal fatty infiltration of the liver from low-density masses. AJR Am J Roentgenol 1991; 157:721-725.
15. Ruzsics B, Lee H, Powers ER, et al. Images in cardiovascular medicine: myocardial ischemia diagnosed by dual-energy computed

tomography: correlation with single-photon emission computed tomography. Circulation 2008; 117:1244-1245.

16. Ruzsics B, Lee H, Zwerner PL, et al. Dual-energy CT of the heart for diagnosing coronary artery stenosis and myocardial ischemia—initial experience. Eur Radiol 2008; 18:2414-2424.

17. Graser A, Johnson TR, Bader M, et al. Dual energy CT characterization of urinary calculi: initial in vitro and clinical experience. Invest Radiol 2008; 43:112-119.

18. Primak AN, Fletcher JG, Vrtiska TJ, et al. Noninvasive differentiation of uric acid versus non-uric acid kidney stones using dual-energy CT. Acad Radiol 2007; 14:1441-1447.

19. Laan RF, van Erning LJ, Lemmens JA, et al. Single-versus dual-energy quantitative computed tomography for spinal densitometry in patients with rheumatoid arthritis. Br J Radiol 1992; 65:901-904.

20. Reinbold WD, Adler CP, Kalender WA, Lente R. Accuracy of vertebral mineral determination by dual-energy quantitative computed tomography. Skeletal Radiol 1991; 20:25-29.

21. Sosna J ST, Mifra A, Amin-Spector S, Libson E. Improved lesion conspicuity with single source dual energy MDCT. Presented before the Radiological Society of North America scientific assembly and annual meeting program. Oakbrook, IL, Radiological Society of North America, 2007, SSC14-09.

22. Matlaga BR, Kawamoto S, Fishman E. Dual source computed tomography: a novel technique to determine stone composition. Urology 2008; 72:1164-1168.

23. Voit H, Krauss B, Heinrich MC, et al. [Dual-source CT: in vitro characterization of gallstones using dual energy analysis]. Rofo 2009; 181:367-373.

24. Rogalla P, Kloeters C, Hein PA. CT technology overview: 64-slice and beyond. Radiol Clin North Am 2009; 47:1-11.

25. Geleijns J, Salvado Artells M, de Bruin PW, et al. Computed tomography dose assessment for a 160 mm wide, 320 detector row, cone beam CT scanner. Phys Med Biol 2009; 54:3141-3159.

26. Rubin GD. Cardiac CT technologies: what is important. In: Abdominal Radiology Course 2009. Maui, Hawaii: Society of Gastrointestinal Radiology, 2009.

27. Brenner DJ, Hall EJ. Computed tomography—an increasing source of radiation exposure. N Engl J Med 2007; 357:2277-2284.

28. Lee CH, Goo JM, Ye HJ, et al. Radiation dose modulation techniques in the multidetector CT era: from basics to practice. RadioGraphics 2008; 28:1451-1459.

29. Goh V, Padhani AR. Imaging tumor angiogenesis: functional assessment using MDCT or MRI? Abdom Imaging 2006; 31:194-199.

30. Sahani DV, Holalkere NS, Mueller PR, Zhu AX. Advanced hepatocellular carcinoma: CT perfusion of liver and tumor tissue—initial experience. Radiology 2007; 243:736-743.

31. Zhu AX, Holalkere NS, Muzikansky A, et al. Early antiangiogenic activity of bevacizumab evaluated by computed tomography perfusion scan in patients with advanced hepatocellular carcinoma. Oncologist 2008; 13:120-125.

32. Xue HD, Jin ZY, Liu W, et al. [Perfusion characteristics of normal pancreas and insulinoma on multi-slice spiral CT]. Zhongguo Yi Xue Ke Xue Yuan Xue Bao 2006; 28:68-70.

33. Bellomi M, Petralia G, Sonzogni A, et al. CT perfusion for the monitoring of neoadjuvant chemotherapy and radiation therapy in rectal carcinoma: initial experience. Radiology 2007; 244:486-493.

34. Sahani DV, Kalva SP, Hahn PF. Imaging of rectal cancer. Semin Radiat Oncol 2003; 13:389-402.

35. Goh V, Halligan S, Taylor SA, et al. Differentiation between diverticulitis and colorectal cancer: quantitative CT perfusion measurements versus morphologic criteria—initial experience. Radiology 2007; 242:456-462.

36. Henderson E, Milosevic MF, Haider MA, Yeung IW. Functional CT imaging of prostate cancer. Phys Med Biol 2003; 48:3085-3100.

37. Jeukens CR, van den Berg CA, Donker R, et al. Feasibility and measurement precision of 3D quantitative blood flow mapping of the prostate using dynamic contrast-enhanced multi-slice CT. Phys Med Biol 2006; 51:4329-4343.

38. Dugdale PE, Miles KA, Bunce I, et al. CT measurement of perfusion and permeability within lymphoma masses and its ability to assess grade, activity, and chemotherapeutic response. J Comput Assist Tomogr 1999; 23:540-547.

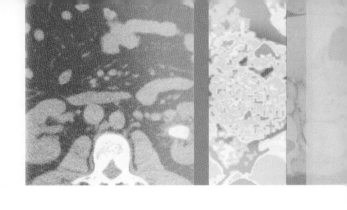

12

CT Contrast Media and Principles of Contrast Enhancement

Shetal N. Shah and Rupan Sanyal

All radiologic contrast media available for intravascular use depend on iodine for their radiopacity. Ideally, contrast media should be inert in every respect. But unlike other therapeutic medications, contrast media are used in larger quantities and participate in numerous physiologic and pharmacokinetic interactions after intravenous administration. Their interactions not only affect the tissue characteristics but also may have significant effects on patient health.

CONTRAST ENHANCEMENT PRINCIPLES

The principle of contrast enhancement is based on photoelectric interaction of the iodine atom with x-rays. The binding energy of the inner K shell electron of the iodine atom is called its K-edge and is equal to 33.2 KeV. The mean energy of diagnostic radiographs is close to this value. When diagnostic radiographs interact with iodine atoms in the body there is increased absorption of the x-rays by the iodine atoms compared with the surrounding soft tissues. The attenuation of the x-ray beam increases with the concentration of iodine in the tissue due to more K shell interactions. This is the fundamental basis of contrast enhancement. There is a linear relation between iodine concentration and attenuation. Every milligram of iodine in a milliliter of blood or cubic centimeter of tissue elevates the attenuation by 25 Hounsfield units (HU).[1]

TYPES OF CONTRAST MEDIA

All currently used CT contrast agents are based on the tri-iodinated benzene ring. Whereas the iodine atom is responsible for the radiopacity of contrast media, the organic carrier is responsible for its other properties, such as osmolality, tonicity, hydrophilicity, and viscosity. The organic carrier is responsible for most of the adverse effects and has received a lot of attention from researchers. Some patients react to small amounts of contrast media, but most of the adverse effects are mediated by the large osmotic load. Thus, over the past few decades researchers have focused on developing contrast media that minimize the osmotic load after contrast agent administration.

Contrast media are classified as ionic or nonionic and as monomers or dimers. Ionic contrast media dissolve in water to dissociate into an iodinated benzene ring containing an iodized carboxyl group and a cation. Nonionic contrast media are water soluble (hydrophilic) but do not dissociate in solution. Monomers have a single tri-iodinated benzene ring, whereas dimers have a double benzene ring containing six iodine atoms. Figure 12-1 shows the chemical structure of contrast media molecules.

The most commonly used classification of contrast media is by their osmolality, which is defined as the number of osmotically active particles per kilogram of solvent. This is determined by the size of the contrast media molecule and whether it dissociates in solution. Table 12-1 lists commonly used contrast media.

High Osmolar Contrast Media

Ionic monomers consisting of a cation (e.g., sodium, meglumine) and an anion (iodine-containing benzoic acid derivative) were developed in the 1950s. These molecules dissociate in solution to give three atoms of iodine for every two particles in solution (iodine atoms to particle in solution ratio of 3:2). The osmolality of these agents ranges from 1500 to 1800 mOsm/kg, whereas that of human plasma is 290 mOsm/kg; thus, they are named "high osmolar contrast media." Because of the higher

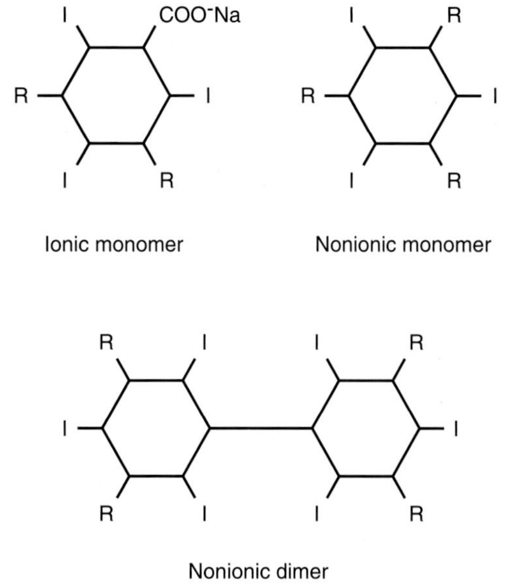

■ **FIGURE 12-1** Diagram showing the molecular structure of ionic monomer, nonionic monomer, and nonionic dimer contrast media molecules.

incidence of adverse reactions, these agents are infrequently used today.

Low Osmolar Contrast Media

Nonionic monomers are widely used today and have much better solubility and lower toxicity compared with ionic monomers.[2] Nonionic monomers consist of a benzoic acid derivative containing three iodine atoms per molecule but do not contain an ionizing carboxyl group (iodine atoms to particle in solution ratio of 3:1). These particles do not dissociate in solution. Their osmolality is 600 to 700 mOsm/kg (double that of human plasma). Other than eliminating ionicity and reducing osmolality, newer low osmolar contrast media also have an increased number of and more evenly distributed hydroxyl groups. This improves their hydrophilicity by restricting access to the lipophilic areas of the molecule, decreasing affinity for cell membrane and plasma proteins and improving tolerance.

Dimeric ionic contrast media contain six atoms of iodine per molecule. They dissociate in solution into an anion (six-iodine atom double-benzene ring) and a cation, yielding iodine atoms to particle in solution ratio of 6:2 or 3:1. The osmolality of ionic dimers is only slightly lower than that of nonionic monomers.

Isosmolar Contrast Media

Nonionic dimers have been more recently developed. These molecules consist of a double-benzene ring with six iodine atoms. Because they do not dissociate in solution, they have iodine atoms to particle in solution ratio of 6:1 and are isosmolar to plasma. The larger molecule size in isosmolar contrast media results in higher viscosity. Nonionic dimers have generally been shown to be less

TABLE 12-1 Classification of Contrast Media

Classification	Iodine per Particle Ratio	Osmolality (mOsm/kg)
High osmolar contrast media	3:2	1500-1800
Diatrizoate (Hypaque)		
Iothalamate (Conray)		
Nonionic monomer low osmolar contrast media	3:1	600-700
Iohexol (Omnipaque)		
Iomeprol (Iomeron)		
Iopamidol (Niopam)		
Iopromide (Ultravist)		
Ioversol (Optiray)		
Ioxilan (Oxilan)		
Iobitridol (Xenetix)		
Ionic dimer low osmolar contrast media	3:1	560
Ioxaglate (Hexabrix)		
Nonionic dimer isosmolar contrast media	6:1	300
Iodixanol (Visipaque)		
Iotrolan (Isovist)		

nephrotoxic compared with other compounds, but this is not established.[3]

PHARMACOKINETICS

All currently used iodinated contrast media have low lipid solubility. Contrast media molecules are not metabolized in the body and are excreted by glomerular filtration without tubular reabsorption. They have a half-life of 2 hours in patients with normal renal function, and 75% of the dose is excreted within 4 hours of administration.[2]

FACTORS AFFECTING ENHANCEMENT

There are a multitude of factors that determine the enhancement of a particular organ or tissue after contrast media administration. Broadly, these can be divided into organ-specific factors, patient-related factors, and injection-related factors.

Organ-Specific Factors

The enhancement patterns of organs vary mainly because of the differences in the vascular supply. Factors that affect enhancement include vascular anatomy, vascular resistance, and percentage of cardiac output received.

Liver

Seventy-five percent of the hepatic blood supply is from the portal venous system, while the remaining 25% is from the hepatic arterial circulation. This unique dual blood supply of the liver can be exploited to bring out the differences between normal parenchyma and pathologic lesions. The *hepatic arterial phase* occurs 20 to 30 seconds after the start of intravenous contrast injection (or 20- to 30-second delay). During this phase hepatic tumors that primarily derive blood supply from the hepatic artery "hypervascular tumors" enhance (Fig. 12-2). The normal hepatic parenchyma shows only minimal

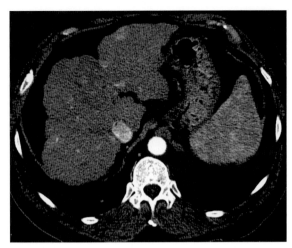

■ **FIGURE 12-2**   Axial image arterial-phase CT scan showing hyperenhancing hepatocellular carcinoma.

enhancement during this phase. The hepatic parenchyma enhances only after the contrast media pass through the splanchnic or splenic circulation and reach the portal vein. This phase is known as the *portal venous phase* (60- to 90-second delay). Hypovascular lesions are relatively hypoattenuating compared with the parenchyma during this phase.

After intravenous injection, the contrast media rapidly diffuse along the concentration gradient into the extravascular (interstitial) space. This redistribution occurs by passive diffusion along the concentration gradient until equilibrium is reached in the *equilibrium phase* (1.5- to 3-minute delay). Contrast media accumulate in the interstitial spaces of the tumor, reducing the attenuation difference with the hepatic parenchyma. The onset of equilibrium phase depends on injection duration. Because the attenuation difference between tumor and normal parenchyma is lost in equilibrium phase, hepatic imaging must be completed before the equilibrium phase.[1,4,5]

Pancreas

Although contrast dynamics for the pancreas is not as well defined as for the liver, the enhancement can be divided into arterial, parenchymal, and portal venous phases. The initial *arterial phase* (20- to 25-second delay) best opacifies the arterial tree and is followed by the *pancreatic phase* (40- to 45-second delay) when the parenchymal enhancement is maximum. The portal venous phase (60- to 70-second delay) opacifies the portal veins and is also useful for evaluating hepatic metastatic disease. Neuroendocrine tumors are hypervascular and are best seen on earlier phases,[6,7] whereas the peak tumor to parenchymal attenuation difference for hypovascular malignancies (e.g., adenocarcinoma) is best appreciated later during the parenchymal or portal venous phase.[8] Most practices use a biphasic pancreatic protocol, with some variation in the exact timing.

Kidneys

The kidney has unique enhancement characteristics because of the much greater vascularity of the renal cortex compared with the medulla, which results in a much greater enhancement of the renal cortex compared with the medulla during the *corticomedullary phase* (25- to 35-second delay). Small renal tumors can be obscured by this differential enhancement. A more homogeneous enhancement occurs during the *nephrographic phase* (90- to 110-second delay), which is primarily used to detect renal parenchymal tumors. A more delayed *excretory phase* (up to 8- to 10-minute delay) is used to opacify the collecting system and ureter and also in CT urography.[9]

Patient-Related Factors

In a healthy patient, the only significant factor that determines the amount of iodine required to achieve desired enhancement is body weight. Patient body weight is inversely related to hepatic enhancement, and the total iodine dose needs to increase with increasing body weight to achieve optimal enhancement. Certain comorbid conditions, such as cardiac failure, can alter circulation time and increase the time required to achieve maximal aortic and hepatic enhancement.

Injection-Related Factors

The total amount of iodine administered per second is obtained by multiplying the injection rate by the iodine concentration and is known as the iodine flux. Increasing iodine flux by either increasing the rate of injection or iodine concentration results in higher and earlier peak of aortic enhancement.

Test Bolus

A fixed delay before start of contrast injection is not advisable for dedicated hepatic or arterial studies. The injection of a small test bolus (15 to 20 mL) followed by nonincremental CT acquisition helps determine the transit time of contrast agent from site of injection to the reference vessel.

Contrast Medium Concentration

If the total iodine dose is administered using a contrast medium containing a higher concentration of iodine, then the total amount of contrast agent and injection duration can be decreased. When this is done, the intravascular iodine concentration increases and the peak aortic enhancement is higher and occurs earlier. The magnitude of enhancement in the hepatic arteries as well as any hypervascular lesion in the arterial phase is also increased. Although the peak hepatic enhancement occurs earlier with increasing contrast agent concentration, the magnitude of hepatic enhancement is unchanged because this depends on the total iodine dose. So, whereas 300 to 350 mg/mL is used for most adult patients for body imaging, a higher concentration (370 to 400 mg/mL) can be used when arteries or hypervascular lesions need to be evaluated. A lower concentration, 240 mg/mL, provides adequate contrast enhancement in thin patients.[1,4]

CONTRAST-INDUCED NEPHROPATHY

Contrast-induced nephropathy is defined as an increase of 25% or more, or an absolute increase of 0.5 mg/dL or more, in serum creatinine concentration from a baseline value at 48 to 72 hours after exposure to intravenous contrast media in absence of any other cause. In 80% of cases, the serum creatinine concentration begins to rise within 24 hours after contrast medium administration. The serum creatinine concentration typically peaks at 3 to 5 days and returns to baseline within 1 to 3 weeks.[10,11] Contrast-induced nephropathy varies from an asymptomatic nonoliguric transient form to severe oliguric acute renal failure requiring dialysis. The extensive use of contrast media in recent years has resulted in an increased incidence of iatrogenic renal function impairment. Contrast-induced nephropathy is now responsible for 11% of cases of hospital-acquired renal impairment. Coronary angiography and percutaneous coronary interventions are associated with higher rates and severity of contrast-induced nephropathy compared with intravenous contrast media used in radiologic procedures.

Risk Factors

It is important to identify risk factors for contrast-induced nephropathy in every patient so that appropriate measures can be taken before intravenous contrast agent administration.

Preexisting Renal Disease

Patients having preexisting renal disease with elevated creatinine concentrations are at highest risk of contrast-induced nephropathy. However, the serum creatinine concentration is not a good indicator of renal function to assess for the risk of contrast-induced nephropathy because it varies with age, muscle mass, physical activity, and gender. The estimated glomerular filtration rate provides a more accurate estimation of renal function. An estimated glomerular filtration rate of 60 mL/min/1.73m^2 is considered a cutoff for identifying patients at a high risk for contrast-induced nephropathy.[12,13]

Diabetes

Patients with diabetes often develop medical conditions that need radiologic evaluation and contrast agent administration. If these patients have concomitant diabetic nephropathy, a higher incidence of contrast-induced nephropathy has been noted. However, in the absence of an underlying renal disorder and any other risk factor, the rate of contrast-induced nephropathy in diabetics is comparable to that in the general population.[14]

Age

Older age is an independent risk factor for contrast-induced nephropathy. The reason is likely to be multifactorial, including age-related changes in the kidneys and other comorbidities.

Other Risk Factors

Congestive heart failure, anemia, dehydration, hypotension, myeloma, and recent use of nephrotoxic drugs all increase the risk of contrast-induced nephropathy. The presence of more than one risk factor may have an additive effect.[10]

Prevention

The pathophysiology of contrast-induced nephropathy is not clearly understood. Altered rheologic properties, renal vasoconstriction, certain paracrine factors, and direct toxic effects on renal epithelial cells all seem to play a role. It has been noted for many years that dehydration increases the risk of contrast-induced nephropathy, so hydrating a patient before contrast agent administration is a simple way to combat it. Volume supplementation increases renal blood flow, reduces renal vasoconstriction, reduces dwell time of contrast agent within the kidney, dilutes the agent, and avoids tubular obstruction.

Saline supplementation has now been established as an inexpensive and effective method of preventing contrast-induced nephropathy in high-risk patients. Intravenous volume supplementation is most effective when isotonic saline is started several hours before the procedure and continued several hours after. Sodium bicarbonate reduces free radical formation and can also be used for volume supplementation. However, it should be kept in mind that a high infusion rate or high total fluid volume may result in volume overload and trigger pulmonary edema in patients with predisposing cardiac conditions.[15] Pharmacologic agents such as *N*-acetylcysteine have been used to reduce nephrotoxicity through antioxidant and vasodilatory effects. However, there is no conclusive evidence to show that it provides consistent protection against contrast-induced nephropathy.[14]

Low osmolar contrast media have been shown to reduce the incidence of contrast-induced nephropathy in patients with impaired renal function compared with high osmolar contrast media. Whether the newer isosmolar agents have an advantage over low osmolar contrast media in reducing contrast-induced nephropathy is yet to be established.

ADVERSE EFFECTS OF CONTRAST MEDIA

Contrast media are one of the most widely prescribed drugs in clinical medicine and like any other medication can have adverse effects when introduced in the body. Adverse reactions to contrast media can be classified as general and organ specific, such as contrast-induced nephropathy, or as cardiovascular, pulmonary, and neurotoxic.

General Adverse Reactions

General adverse reactions can be divided into acute reactions, occurring within 1 hour of contrast agent administration, and delayed reactions occurring between 1 hour and 1 week of administration.

TABLE 12-2 Clinical Presentation of Acute General Reactions to Contrast Media

Mild	Moderate	Severe
Flushing	Severe vomiting	Severe manifestations of moderate symptoms
Nausea, vomiting	Extensive urticaria	
Pain	Moderate hypotension	
Headache	Laryngeal edema	
Mild urticaria	Bronchospasm	Pulmonary edema
Pruritus		Circulatory collapse
		Cardiac arrhythmia
		Convulsions
		Unconsciousness

TABLE 12-3 Predisposing Factors for General Adverse Reactions

Asthma
Prior adverse reaction to contrast media (excluding mild flushing and nausea)
Atopy
Cardiac disease
Preexisting renal disease
Dehydration
Anxiety
Infants and elderly
Hematologic and metabolic diseases (sickle cell disease, myelomatosis)

Acute Reactions

Acute reactions can be divided into mild, moderate, and severe. Table 12-2 lists the clinical presentation of each subtype. The incidence of general adverse reactions is lower with the use of low osmolar contrast media compared with high osmolar contrast media. Mild reactions are seen in 15% of patients given high osmolar contrast media compared with 3% given low osmolar contrast media, whereas very severe reactions are seen in 0.04% of patients given high osmolar contrast media compared with 0.004% given low osmolar contrast media. However, the incidence of fatal reactions (1 : 170,000) is the same for low osmolar contrast media and high osmolar contrast media.[2]

There are several predisposing factors to general contrast adverse reactions. These are listed in Table 12-3. The probability of a patient having a general adverse reaction is much higher in patients having these predisposing factors.[16]

Delayed Reactions

Delayed general adverse reactions occur between 1 hour and 7 days after contrast media administration. They are less common than acute reactions but occur when the patient is no longer under medical supervision. Delayed reactions usually are mild and consist of skin manifestations. However, rare cases of more serious delayed effects such as hypotension, dyspnea, and shock can occur. There have been reports of increased delayed reactions

with new isosmolar nonionic dimeric agents, resulting in withdrawal of Iotrolan for intravenous use.[17]

Pathophysiology of General Adverse Effects

There is no evidence to show that contrast media are allergic, because no antibodies have been consistently demonstrated. The pathogenesis of general adverse effects is not well understood and is likely multifactorial. Most adverse effects are either pseudoallergic or idiosyncratic. *Pseudoallergic reactions* are the same as allergic reactions but depend on nonspecific complement system activation and histamine release, mimicking type I allergic reactions. *Idiosyncratic reactions* are genetically determined, unpredictable reactions that are caused by metabolites and occur after administration of small amount of drugs.

Treatment

Mild contrast reactions usually require no treatment other than reassurance and restoration of the patient's confidence. Oral antihistamines can be offered for itching. Intravenous access must be retained in all cases and vital signs closely monitored. Moderate reactions are managed with intravenous or intramuscular antihistamines for urticaria and angioneurotic edema, fluids for hypotension, and salbutamol inhalation and oxygen for bronchospasm. Intravenous hydrocortisone and intravenous or subcutaneous epinephrine may need to be given for more severe bronchospasm. Management of more severe allergic reactions is described in Table 12-4.

Organ-Specific Adverse Effects

The hemodynamic, cardiovascular, neurologic, and subjective effects of contrast media can be explained by the osmolality, tonicity, and viscosity of these agents. After administration of intravascular contrast media there is a sudden increase in intravascular osmolality. This causes a shift of water into the vascular space. The contrast agent does not enter cell membranes, so intracellular water shifts out of red blood cells. This can cause red blood cell desiccation as well as influence cell membrane potential. Also, movement of water from the interstitium into the vascular compartment results in increased intravascular blood volume, increased cardiac output, and decreased peripheral vascular resistance. Peripheral vasodilation after contrast medium injection results in a feeling of warmth and discomfort. Systemic vasodilation leads to hypotension and decreased venous return, possibly leading to cardiac failure.

Contrast media can injure the endothelium, which along with complex effects on platelets and coagulation factors increases the risk of thrombosis. In the central nervous system, contrast media molecules cannot cross the blood-brain barrier. Pathologic increase in the permeability of the blood-brain barrier by infection or neoplasm exposes the brain tissue to the toxic effects of contrast media. All these effects are more common with high osmolar contrast media.

TABLE 12-4 Treatment of Severe General Adverse Reactions

Severe Bronchospasm
1. Provide oxygen by mask (6-10 L/min).
2. Provide salbutamol nebulization (5 mg in 2-mL saline).
3. Administer epinephrine injection if bronchospasm is progressive.

Laryngeal Edema
1. Provide oxygen by mask (6-10 L/min).
2. Administer epinephrine (1:1000) 0.5 mL IV injection with ECG monitoring.

Hypotension without Bradycardia
1. Elevate patient's legs.
2. Provide oxygen by mask (6-10 L/min).
3. Administer intravenous fluids (normal saline or lactated Ringer's).
4. If unresponsive, give dopamine, 2-5 µg/kg/min infusion, or epinephrine injection.

Vagal Reaction
1. Elevate patient's legs.
2. Provide oxygen by mask (6-10 L/min).
3. Administer intravenous fluids (normal saline or lactated Ringer's).
4. Inject atropine 0.6 mg IV; repeat if necessary at 3-5 minutes up to 3-5 mg total.

Anaphylactoid Generalized Reaction
1. Call for resuscitation team.
2. Ensure patent airways.
3. Elevate patient's legs.
4. Provide oxygen by mask (6-10 L/min).
5. Administer intravenous fluids (normal saline or lactated Ringer's).
6. Administer hydrocortisone, 500 mg intravenously.
7. Administer epinephrine (1:1000) 0.5 mL IV with ECG monitoring.

From Namasivayam S, Kalra MK, Torres WE, Small WC. Adverse reactions to intravenous iodinated contrast media: a primer for radiologists. Emerg Radiol 2006; 12:210-215.

Prevention

There is no prophylactic regimen that eliminates the risk of adverse reaction to contrast media. All patients who are considered to be at a high risk for contrast reaction should be considered for alternative forms of imaging. If administration of contrast media is necessary, low osmolar contrast media should be used because they significantly reduce the incidence of adverse effects compared with high osmolar contrast media. Oral corticosteroids are relatively safe when given for a brief period and are used for premedication. In our institution 50 mg of oral prednisone is given 13 hours before contrast media administration, followed by a second dose of 50 mg of oral prednisone along with 50 mg of oral diphenhydramine 1 hour before administration of the contrast agent. Because adverse reactions can occur even after premedication, prompt recognition and management are invaluable in preventing life-threatening outcomes.

KEY POINTS

- A molecule of contrast medium is composed of an iodine atom, which is responsible for radiopacity, and an organic carrier, which is responsible for its other properties and adverse effects.
- Contrast media are classified into high osmolar, low osmolar, and isosmolar agents.
- Knowledge of various phases of enhancement is critical in detecting and characterizing a pathologic process.
- Low osmolar contrast media have a lower incidence of adverse reactions.
- Contrast-induced nephropathy can be prevented by judicious hydration of at-risk patients with low estimated glomerular filtration rate.
- Patients at high risk of allergic reactions should be premedicated.

SUGGESTED READINGS

Morcos SK, Thomsen HS. Adverse reactions to iodinated contrast media. Eur Radiol 2001; 11:1267-1275.

Thomsen HS, Morcos SK, Barrett BJ. Contrast-induced nephropathy: the wheel has turned 360 degrees. Acta Radiol 2008; 49:646-657.

Weisbord SD. Iodinated contrast media and the kidney. Rev Cardiovasc Med 2008; 9(Suppl 1):S14-S23.

REFERENCES

1. Herman S. Computed tomography contrast enhancement principles and the use of high-concentration contrast media. J Comput Assist Tomogr 2004; 28(Suppl 1):S7-S11.
2. Morcos SK, Thomsen HS. Adverse reactions to iodinated contrast media. Eur Radiol 2001; 11:1267-1275.
3. Kuhn MJ, Chen N, Sahani DV, et al. The PREDICT study: a randomized double-blind comparison of contrast-induced nephropathy after low- or isoosmolar contrast agent exposure. AJR Am J Roentgenol 2008; 191:151-157.
4. Brink JA. Use of high concentration contrast media (HCCM): principles and rationale—body CT. Eur J Radiol 2003; 45 (Suppl 1):S53-S58.
5. Brink JA, Heiken JP, Forman HP, et al. Hepatic spiral CT: reduction of dose of intravenous contrast material. Radiology 1995; 197:83.
6. Fidler JL, Fletcher JG, Reading CC, et al. Preoperative detection of pancreatic insulinomas on multiphasic helical CT. AJR Am J Roentgenol 2003; 181:775-780.
7. Horton KM, Hruban RH, Yeo C, Fishman EK. Multi-detector row CT of pancreatic islet cell tumors. RadioGraphics 2006; 26: 453-464.
8. McNulty NJ, Francis IR, Platt JF, et al. Multidetector row helical CT of the pancreas: effect of contrast-enhanced multiphasic imaging on enhancement of the pancreas, peripancreatic vasculature, and pancreatic adenocarcinoma. Radiology 2001; 220:97-102.

9. Van Der Molen AJ, Cowan NC, Mueller-Lisse UG, et al. CT urography: definition, indications and techniques: a guideline for clinical practice. Eur Radiol 2008; 18:4-17.

10. Mehran R, Nikolsky E. Contrast-induced nephropathy: definition, epidemiology, and patients at risk. Kidney Int Suppl 2006; (100):S11-S15.

11. Katzberg RW, Barrett BJ. Risk of iodinated contrast material–induced nephropathy with intravenous administration. Radiology 2007; 243:622-628.

12. Swedko PJ, Clark HD, Paramsothy K, Akbari A. Serum creatinine is an inadequate screening test for renal failure in elderly patients. Arch Intern Med 2003; 163:356-360.

13. Baxmann AC, Ahmed MS, Marques NC, et al. Influence of muscle mass and physical activity on serum and urinary creatinine and serum cystatin C. Clin J Am Soc Nephrol 2008; 3:348-354.

14. Thomsen HS, Morcos SK, Barrett BJ. Contrast-induced nephropathy: the wheel has turned 360 degrees. Acta Radiol 2008; 49:646-657.

15. Mueller C. Prevention of contrast-induced nephropathy with volume supplementation. Kidney Int Suppl 2006; (100):S16-S19.

16. Namasivayam S, Kalra MK, Torres WE, Small WC. Adverse reactions to intravenous iodinated contrast media: a primer for radiologists. Emerg Radiol 2006; 12:210-215.

17. Idée JM, Pinès E, Prigent P, Corot C. Allergy-like reactions to iodinated contrast agents: a critical analysis. Fundam Clin Pharmacol 2005; 19:263-281.

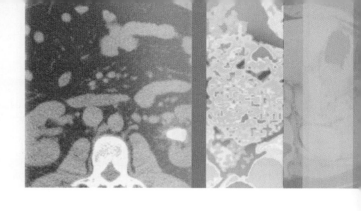

CHAPTER 13

CT Protocols for Abdomen and Pelvis

Kumaresan Sandrasegaran and Avinash Kambadakone R.

TECHNICAL ASPECTS

Computed tomography of the abdomen and pelvis is performed for the evaluation of a wide variety of clinical conditions. Specific protocols are designed to optimize imaging parameters and maximize diagnostic information while keeping the radiation dose to the minimum necessary. Appropriate scanning protocols are essential to tailor the CT examination to answer the particular clinical question. The scanning protocols comprise several key components, including the contrast agent used (oral, intravenous, or rectal), the number of intravenous contrast phases, and the technical parameters (tube voltage and current, pitch, rotation time). Nearly all abdominopelvic CT studies are postprocessed to yield 2D or 3D reformatted images. In this chapter, we discuss the requirements for an optimal CT examination.

Oral Contrast Media

Oral contrast agents are categorized as positive (denser than water), neutral, and negative (less dense than water). Neutral media, such as milk, are rarely used in North America and are not further discussed. Positive media include dilute barium (2% to 5%) and diluted ionic and nonionic iodinated media, such as diatrizoate meglumine sodium (Gastrografin) or iopamidol (Isovue). Some centers prefer nonionic contrast media for pediatric CT, mainly because of their taste. Neutral contrast media have an attenuation value of 10 to 30 Hounsfield units. These agents include water, water in combination with methylcellulose or locust bean gum, polyethylene glycol solutions, and a commercially available low-density (0.1%) barium sulfate suspension (VoLumen).[4,6] The advantages, limitations, and indications of positive and neutral oral contrast agents are listed and shown in Table 13-1 and Figures 13-1 and 13-2.[1-3]

Need for Oral Contrast Media

Several studies have looked at the use of oral contrast media in patients who present to an emergency department with acute abdomen[4-7] or blunt trauma[8-12] and found that using oral contrast media did not substantially improve the diagnostic performance. Because there are many disadvantages to the use of oral contrast media in these patients, including time delay, inability of patients to ingest large volumes of fluid, and potential need for emergency surgery, we do not use oral contrast agents in emergency department patients unless there is suspicion of postoperative bowel leak. Some studies have gone further and suggested that there may not be a need for oral contrast media in the vast majority of routine CT studies, such as those performed for cancer staging.[13] The traditional argument for use of oral contrast media was to delineate bowel from adenopathy or peritoneal masses.[14,15] However, current multidetector CT (MDCT) provides thin sections and multiplanar reformatted images, and the need for oral contrast media may be less than before, particularly if intravenous contrast media is also given. Nevertheless, in our practice, we use positive oral contrast media for routine cases, unless the patient has nausea or if the requesting physician does not want it used.

Intravenous Contrast Media

Screening Patients before Use

It is usual to screen for risks of intravenous contrast agents before CT. The two principal risks are allergic reactions and contrast-induced nephropathy. In our practice, those who have a history of mild (vomiting, mild itching) or moderate (symptomatic urticaria, vasovagal reaction, bronchospasm, transient hypotension or tachycardia)

TABLE 13-1   Salient Features of Oral Contrast Agents

Positive Oral Contrast	Neutral Oral Contrast
• Preferred agent in noncontrast (intravenous)-enhanced scans of abdomen • Best suited for the demonstration of fistulas, sinus tracts, and hollow viscus perforation • Used in most routine abdominopelvic CT studies	• Contrast agents of choice for CT enterography • Recommended for identifying subtle mucosal enhancement and abnormalities • Do not interfere with data manipulation during 3D imaging (CT angiography) • Gastrointestinal indications (e.g., Crohn's disease, unexplained abdominal pain, obscure bleeding and suspected mesenteric ischemia, duodenal lesions) • Nongastrointestinal indications: liver, pancreatic, or renal masses and CT urography

allergic reactions to intravenous contrast media are premedicated (Table 13-2). Low-osmolar intravenous contrast media are not believed to provoke hypertensive crisis in patients with pheochromocytoma, whether on or off α-adrenergic blocker therapy.[16-18] Similarly, those who are allergic to topical iodine or shellfish do not need to be premedicated.

Contrast-induced nephropathy is discussed in detail elsewhere in this book. In our practice, those with diabetes, myeloma, sickle cell anemia, cardiac failure, a personal or family history of renal disease, and renal surgery are screened. Inpatients and those with the just mentioned conditions have a serum creatinine (and estimated glomerular filtration rate [eGFR]) value checked before intravenous use of a contrast agent. Those with an eGFR of more than 60 mL/min/1.73 m² have the usual dose. Those with an eGFR of 30 to 60 mL/min/1.73 m² are given intravenous hydration and receive the standard or a

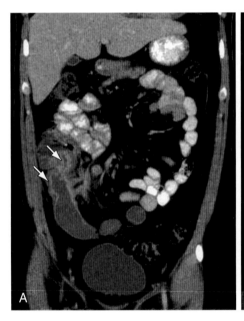
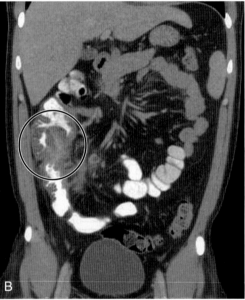

■ **FIGURE 13-1** A 22-year-old man presented with Crohn's disease. **A,** Postcontrast coronal CT images show excellent depiction of the mural enhancement (*arrows*) when the bowel lumen is distended with a neutral contrast agent. **B,** On a comparative image with use of a positive oral contrast agent the mural enhancement is less obvious (*circle*).

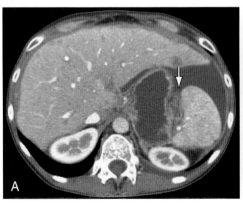
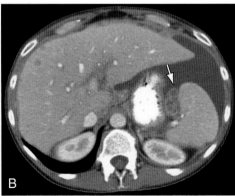

■ **FIGURE 13-2** MDCT images in a 60-year-old woman with ovarian carcinoma and peritoneal metastases. **A,** On an axial contrast CT image obtained with neutral oral contrast a nodular peritoneal metastasis (*arrow*) is seen in the perigastric region. **B,** This lesion (*arrow*) is more conspicuous on contrast-enhanced CT obtained with positive oral contrast. This set of images highlights the advantage of a positive oral contrast agent in demonstrating peritoneal disease compared with a neutral oral contrast agent.

reduced dose (depending on the clinical situation). Intravenous contrast media are not usually used in those patients with an eGFR of less than 30 mL/min/1.73 m^2. These general guidelines may be altered on discussion with the referring physician, depending on the indication for CT, a patient's comorbidities, and so on. Preventive measures for contrast-induced nephropathy, including the details of intravenous hydration, are discussed elsewhere.

Intravenous Contrast Media Protocols

CT without intravenous use of a contrast agent is obtained in patients for evaluation of urinary calculi and in the follow-up evaluation of an adrenal mass. In the absence of a history of severe allergy to intravenous media or other contraindications, such as grade 4 or 5 renal failure, it is usual to administer these agents for other indications for abdominopelvic CT. The phase(s) of CT image acquisition after contrast agent administration depends on the organ being scanned, the clinical indication, and the enhancement characteristics of different organs. Table 13-3 gives a brief overview of the enhancement timings of various organs after intravenous administration of a contrast agent.

Arterial phase scanning is performed for a limited number of indications (Table 13-4; Figs. 13-3 and 13-4). Routine abdominal and pelvic CT examinations are performed in the portal venous phase for a large variety of indications, including abdominal pain, staging of cancer, and postoperative complications (Fig. 13-5). Delayed scans are also helpful to clarify subtle bowel findings such as bowel leak or fistula.[19] The details of the contrast volume, concentration, injection rate, and the various phases of acquisition depend on the organ scanned (Figs. 13-6 and 13-7). Indications and details are discussed in the relevant chapters. A summary is given in Table 13-5. To obtain a high contrast during the short scanning time of MDCT, it is usual to use higher iodine concentration (>350 mg of I/mL) of intravenous media given at rates of more than 3 mL/s.

Timing of Bolus

The rapid scanning capability of MDCT (16 or more detector rows) has necessitated the precise timing of a concentrated bolus. In the past, fixed time intervals after intravenous injection of the contrast agent were commonly used. However, owing to variations in cardiac function, bolus tracking is now routinely used. Timing of an intravenous bolus of the contrast agent may be determined with a test bolus. However, our preference is bolus tracking with the intravenous injection of the entire dose.

TABLE 13-2 Premedication Protocols

Type of Prior Reaction	Drug and Dose	Times Given
Mild or moderate	Diphenhydramine (Benadryl), 25 or 50 mg intravenously or intramuscularly	Immediately before intravenous (IV) contrast media
Moderate	Prednisone, 50 mg orally	13, 7, and 1 hour before IV contrast media
Moderate	Alternate steroid regimen: methylprednisolone (Medrol), 32 mg orally	12 and 2 hours before IV contrast media

---

TABLE 13-4 List of Abdominal Indications for Arterial Phase Scanning

- Hepatocellular carcinoma
- Neuroendocrine tumors (islet cell tumors, carcinoid, pheochromocytoma)
- Melanoma
- Renal cell carcinoma
- Sarcoma
- Gastrointestinal stromal tumor
- Angiographic studies

TABLE 13-3 Contrast Delay Times of Various Organs after IV Injection of Contrast Media

Time after Start of IV Injection*	Phase	Structures Opacified and Indication for Phase
25-30 s	Arterial	Aorta and branches for CT angiogram or preoperative assessment of tumors, or in transplantation
40-50 s	Late arterial and pancreatic	Hypervascular liver tumors (see Table 13-4) Pancreas in severe acute pancreatitis or preoperative staging of cancer Bowel mucosa in CT enterography or obscure gastrointestinal bleeding
50-60 s	Corticomedullary	Renal cortex in characterization of cystic renal tumors (mural nodules enhancement), performed in precontrast and nephrographic phases
60-70 s	Portal or venous	Liver parenchyma (phase for routine single-contrast studies)
100-120 s	Nephrographic	Renal medulla (renal tumors)
5-10 min	Delayed/pyelographic	Collecting systems, ureters, and urinary bladder in CT urogram: different protocols possible Characterization of liver lesions suspected of being hemangioma or cholangiocarcinoma Characterization of adrenal mass (precontrast, venous phase, and delayed)

*These times are guidelines, and different centers may have slightly different timing of the phases. With slower rates of injection (<3 mL/s) the phases will be delayed by a few seconds.

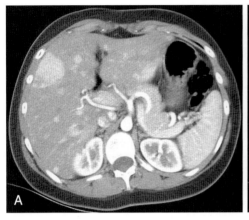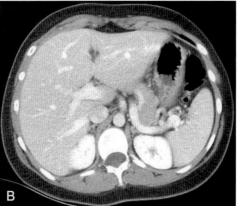

■ **FIGURE 13-3** MDCT axial images from the arterial (**A**) and portal venous (**B**) phases from a 69-year-old patient with terminal ileal carcinoid. On the arterial phase image, multiple hyperdense lesions are noted in the liver that turn isodense to liver on the portal phase and therefore are difficult to visualize. This case highlights the value of optimal phase imaging for detecting hypervascular tumors.

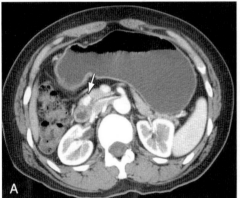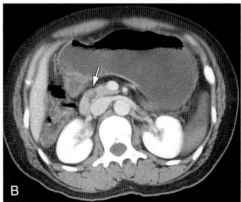

■ **FIGURE 13-4** MDCT of the pancreas of a 41-year-woman. **A,** Contrast-enhanced CT image through the pancreas acquired in the arterial phase demonstrates a hypervascular mass (*arrow*) in the uncinate process. **B,** On the portal venous phase, this lesion (*arrow*) turns iso-hypodense and is less conspicuous. The hypervascular mass was later surgically resected and was diagnosed as a pancreatic neuroendocrine tumor.

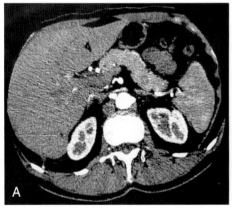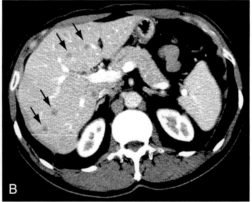

■ **FIGURE 13-5** Liver metastases on MDCT. **A,** Arterial phase image show subtle hypodense lesion in the liver without discernible tumors. **B,** However, on the portal venous phase, multiple small hypodense tumors are now obvious (*arrows*).

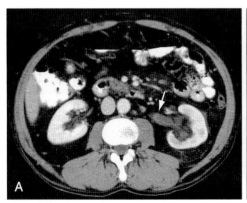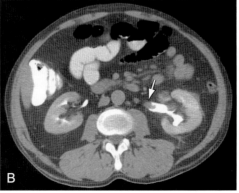

■ **FIGURE 13-6** MDCT of the kidney in a 56-year-old man presenting with hematuria. **A,** Contrast-enhanced CT image through the kidney acquired in the nephrographic phase shows mild dilatation of the pelvic calyceal system (*arrow*). **B,** In the pyelographic phase a soft tissue filling defect (*arrow*) is demonstrated in the renal pelvis that highlights the superiority of delayed images in depicting lesions of the urinary collecting system. Histopathology of the filling defect showed transitional cell carcinoma.

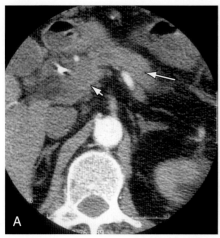
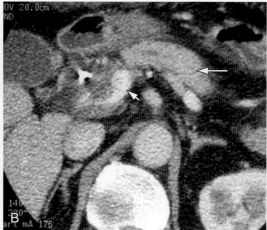

■ **FIGURE 13-7** CT angiography images from a patient with pancreatic adenocarcinoma. **A,** Arterial phase image demonstrates suboptimal enhancement of the superior mesenteric vein (*short arrow*) and poor conspicuity of the tumor in the pancreatic head because the pancreatic parenchyma is not yet enhancing (*long arrow*). **B,** On the corresponding pancreatic phase image, the parenchyma enhancement is now obvious (*long arrow*) with improved conspicuity of adenocarcinoma in the head of the pancreas that is also partially involving the superior mesenteric vein (*short arrow*).

Low-dose CT images are obtained every 0.5 second through a region of interest placed in the distal thoracic aorta at the diaphragmatic hiatus. When the density in the region of interest reaches a preset threshold, CT is started after an appropriate time delay. For instance, with dual-phase liver CT, we use an injection rate of 4 mL/s via a 20-gauge angiocatheter in the antecubital fossa vein. The preset density in the region of interest is 125 HU. Once this density is achieved, the scan is triggered after a delay of 18 seconds for the late arterial phase and 48 seconds for the portal venous phases. It is usual to employ dual-chamber programmable contrast injectors that can deliver a saline flush after the intravenous injection.

Contrast Injection Rate and Intravenous Access

With the use of power injectors for intravenous delivery of contrast media for all examination types including CT angiography, appropriate intravenous access is essential to maintain a desired injection rate and optimal iodine flux. For examinations mandating higher flow rates (i.e., of up to 5 mL/s for angiographic studies and 7 mL/s for perfusion studies) it is important to obtain an adequate-gauge intravenous access to sustain the intended iodine flux but also to prevent the unintended adverse event of contrast media extravasation. It is generally agreed that an intravenous cannula of 22 gauge is sufficient for most diagnostic examinations and low flow rate CT angiograms and that injection rates up to 3.5 mL/s are feasible, whereas the intravenous access of 20- and 18-gauge cannulas can facilitate higher injection rates up to 5 and 7 mL/s, respectively. In situations of disparity in the intravenous access and desired injection rate, the scan delay is adjusted, the scan delay is adjusted to time the data acquisition with the contrast circulation time of the organ of interest.

Technical Parameters

Scan Coverage

The scan length for a routine abdominopelvic CT extends from the dome of the diaphragm to the lower border of symphysis pubis. In multiphase CT examinations, the scan length of each phase may vary. In patients who have repeated CT examinations, such as for urolithiasis or pancreatitis, a targeted CT examination encompassing only relevant limited anatomic areas helps to significantly reduce radiation dose.[20]

Tube Potential

Most CT studies in adults are performed with a tube potential of 120 kVp. This parameter has a complex relationship with image noise, CT attenuation values (contrast), and radiation dose. A decrease in kVp increases noise and decreases radiation dose if other parameters are held constant but leads to higher attenuation values (except for water) and image contrast irrespective of other scanning parameters. Scanning at low kVp can help reduce the volume of intravenous contrast media administered for CT due to the high contrast-to-noise ratio. Low kVp CT examinations are also widely used as an approach for radiation dose reduction for indications ranging from diagnosis of urolithiasis to characterization of hypervascular liver tumors (Fig. 13-8).[21,22] To avoid inadvertently high image noise with low kVp CT studies, tube current must be correspondingly raised.[21,22] However, kVp reduction in obese or large patients must be avoided to ensure adequate signal-to-noise ratio for acceptable diagnostic interpretation.

Tube Current

Appropriate tube current (milliampere [mA]) selection for abdomen and pelvis can be achieved either by fixed tube current or automated tube current modulation (ATCM) techniques. ATCM customizes the tube current delivery to the patient's size and tissue density and permits a significant reduction in radiation dose. The techniques and nomenclature of ATCM software available from various manufacturers are different. ATCM relies on operator-defined parameters, such as noise index with General Electric CT scanners and reference tube current/time product (mAs) with Siemens CT scanners. ATCM techniques are discussed in detail in the section on radiation

TABLE 13-5 CT Scan Protocol Details of the Common Abdomen and Pelvic CT Examinations

Scanning* Protocol	Phases	Slice Thickness (mm)	kV/mAs/ Rotation Time	Contrast Medium	Volume	Flow Rate	Delay	Multiplanar Reconstructions	Oral Contrast Media
Renal colic	NCT	5	100-120 kVp ATCM TR: 0.5 s	None	-	-	-	2.5 to 3-mm coronal reformatted images	None
Routine abdomen	CECT: PV ± DP (2-5 min)	5	120-140 kVp ATCM TR: 0.5 s	370 mg I/mL	80-120 mL	3 mL/s	65-70 s (bolus tracking/ Smart Prep, 60 HU threshold liver)	2.5 to 3-mm coronal reformatted images	Positive oral contrast: over 45 min to 1 hr
Renal malignancy/ hematuria	NCT; CECT: NP + PY	15/2.5/5	120-140 kVp ATCM TR: 0.5 s	370 mg I/mL	80-120 mL	3 mL/s	NP: 90 s PY: 5 min	MIP, coronal reformatted images	None
Liver mass	NCT; CECT: ART + PV + DP	5/2./2.5/5	120-140 kVp ATCM TR: 0.5 s	370 mg I/mL	80-120 mL	4-5 mL/s	Arterial: 6-8 s Aorta (150 HU) PV: 65 s Liver (60 HU) DP: 5 min (10 min for cholangiocarcinoma)	Coronal reformatted images	None
Adrenal mass	NCT; CECT: PV + DP	2.5/2.5	120-140 kVp ATCM TR: 0.5 s	370 mg I/mL	80-120 mL	3 mL/s	PV: 65 s DP: 10 min	Coronal	None
Pancreatic mass	NCT; CECT: AR + PV	5/2.5/2.5	120-140 kVp ATCM TR: 0.5 s	370 mg I/mL	80-120 mL	3 mL/s	Early arterial: 12-15 s (PNET) Late arterial (40-45 s) (Other masses) PV: 70-75 s	Coronal, sagittal, and curved reformatted images CT pancreatography	Neutral oral contrast
CT enterography	CECT: PV	2.5	120-140 kVp ATCM TR: 0.5 s	370 mg I/mL		4 mL/s	PV: 65 s Liver (60 HU)	Coronal and sagittal reformatted images	Neutral oral contrast (VoLumen)

*All the CT examinations are performed with breath-hold at end of expiration.
NCT, noncontrast CT; CECT, contrast-enhanced CT; ART, arterial phase; PV, portovenous phase; DP, delayed phase; NP, nephrographic phase; PY, pyelographic phase; ATCM, automated tube current modulation; PNET, pancreatic neuroendocrine tumors.

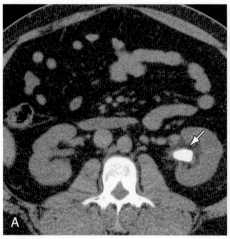
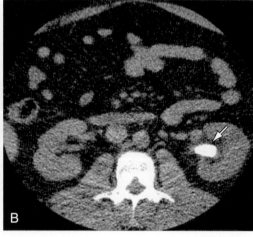

■ **FIGURE 13-8** Follow-up CT scans in a 55-year-old man with left midpole staghorn calculus. **A,** Axial unenhanced CT scan (120 kVp, 240 mAs) shows the left midpole renal calculus (*arrow*). **B,** Follow-up CT scan was performed with reduced technique (100 kVp, 100 mAs). Confident diagnosis of the renal calculus (*arrow*) can be made on the low-dose CT in spite of increased noise in the image.

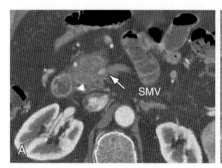
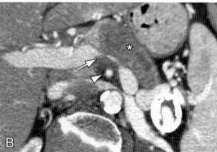
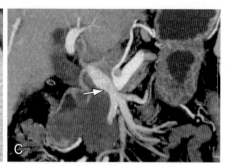

■ **FIGURE 13-9** Pancreatic adenocarcinoma. **A,** MDCT image of patient with hypoattenuating lesions in the head and neck of the pancreas, corresponding to adenocarcinoma, encasing the superior mesenteric vein (SMV). **B,** Reformatted image along the portal vein. Note encasement and narrowing of the lumen of the portal vein (*arrow*) secondary to invasion from pancreatic adenocarcinoma located in the body and neck (*asterisk*). Encasement of the superior mesenteric artery is also noted (*arrowhead*). **C,** Coronal MIP image in a patient with invasive adenocarcinoma of the head and neck of the pancreas with encasement of the portal confluence (*arrow*).

dose. Change in the tube current does not affect image contrast or CT attenuation values, and reduction in the tube current remains one of the most common approaches for radiation dose reduction.

Pitch

In order to prevent the increase in noise as pitch is increased, or the increase in radiation dose as pitch is decreased, modern MDCT has mechanisms for automatic adjustment of the tube current. The mAs is changed in proportion to the pitch. When the effective mAs (which is the ratio of mAs to pitch) is unchanged, both dose and noise remain constant. For a routine abdominal study, a pitch of approximately 1.0 unit is used.[23]

Reconstructed Slice Thickness

The reconstructed slice thickness for routine abdominal and pelvic applications is generally 2.5 to 5.0 mm.[13] Thinner reconstructed axial slices are not normally used for rendering diagnostic interpretation but are mainly obtained for coronal and sagittal reformations.[13] However, in certain abdominal CT angiographic studies, particularly those of the liver, kidneys, and pancreas, thinner slice thickness (0.625 to 2.5 mm) is used for axial viewing.[13] As the section thickness reduces, the images become noisier but have higher spatial resolution and less partial volume averaging. Moreover, the radiation dose also increases as the sections become thinner. To avoid the radiation excess resulting from thinner slices, a preferred option is to obtain thicker sections and then reconstruct thinner images from the volumetric data.

Volume Acquisition and Postprocessing

The postprocessing techniques routinely employed in the CT studies of the abdomen and pelvis include standard reformatting, curved reformatting, maximum intensity projection (MIP), and volume rendering techniques (Fig. 13-9). A detailed discussion of the various postprocessing techniques is provided elsewhere in this book.

USE OF CT IN SPECIFIC SITUATIONS

CT in the Pregnant Patient

The potential risks of radiation dose during pregnancy include spontaneous abortion, teratogenesis, and carcinogenesis. Spontaneous abortion may occur with irradiation of greater than 100 mGy in the first 2 weeks of embryogenesis. However, there is no further risk if the embryo survives (all or none phenomenon).[24]

The potential teratogenic effects of radiation, given between 2 and 20 weeks of gestation, include mental retardation, behavioral abnormalities, and cataracts.[25,26] The risk of mental retardation is more likely with radiation given between 8 and 15 weeks of gestation. These effects are believed to occur beyond a threshold dose. Although this threshold is not known with certainty, it is estimated to be between 50 and 150 mGy.[24] The estimated dose of maternal pelvic CT varies from about 25 mGy in the first trimester to about 45 mGy in the third trimester.[24,26] Thus, it is highly unlikely that a single pelvic CT evaluation will induce teratogenesis.

The risk of carcinogenesis does not have a threshold dose. The baseline risk of cancer is about 1 in 2000 pregnancies, and this risk is doubled if there is exposure to a radiation dose of 50 mGy, which is in the range of a single pelvic CT examinaton. Although this risk is small, every effort must be made to reduce radiation dose, such as decreasing the mAs, using z-axis modulation, and increasing scan pitch. Intravenous contrast media may be used if clinically indicated because the risk of neonatal hyperthyroidism after its use is thought to be negligible.[27] It is also unnecessary to withhold breast feeding in lactating women receiving intravenous contrast media.[28]

CT in Very Large Patients

When obese patients are scanned, the principal change in CT parameters is an increase in tube current. This is required to reduce noise to diagnostically acceptable levels. Other parameters that may be changed include lowering the pitch to about 0.75, increasing the gantry rotation time to 0.8 to 1.0 second, and changing detector configurations. For example, with a 16-slice CT scanner (Brilliance 16, Philips Medical Systems; Best, The Nether-

lands) a detector configuration of 8×3 mm may be chosen instead of the standard configuration of 16×1.5 mm. These effects will increase scan time and radiation dose.[29,30] However, for the same absorbed dose, the effective radiation dose will be lower in an obese patient, compared with a normal sized patient, owing to the photon-attenuating effects of subcutaneous adipose tissue.[29]

CONCLUSION

CT has made a huge impact in the imaging of the abdomen and pelvis since its introduction in 1972. The continuing advancements in the CT technology coupled with introduction of better contrast agents has empowered MDCT as the modality of choice for evaluation of the entire range of abdominal pathologic processes. It is important to understand the fundamentals of MDCT and the basics of various CT protocols to derive the maximum benefit from this exciting technology.

KEY POINTS

■ MDCT protocol optimization is essential to enable accurate diagnosis and staging.

■ Appropriate use of oral and intravenous iodinated contrast media should be considered to meet the clinical objectives of the ordered MDCT examination.

■ Contrast media protocol optimization and coordinating scan timing is considered the most important part of a good-quality MDCT examination.

■ Image reconstruction in off-axial plane (coronal/sagittal/oblique) is considered essential for rendering an accurate diagnosis in the abdomen and pelvis.

■ 3D images are considered integral for planning complex surgeries in the abdomen and monitoring treatment effects.

SUGGESTED READINGS

Cahir JG, Freeman AH, Courtney HM. Multislice CT of the abdomen. Br J Radiol 2004; 77:S64-S73.

Maher MM, Kalra MK, Sahani DV, et al. Techniques, clinical applications and limitations of 3D reconstruction in CT of the abdomen. Korean J Radiol 2004; 5:55-67.

Prokop M. General principles of MDCT. Eur J Radiol 2003; 45(Suppl 1):S4-S10.

Rogalla P, Kloeters C, Hein PA. CT technology overview: 64-slice and beyond. Radiol Clin North Am 2009; 47:1-11.

Saini S. Multi-detector row CT: principles and practice for abdominal applications. Radiology 2004; 233:323-327.

REFERENCES

1. Berther R, Patak MA, Eckhardt B, et al. Comparison of neutral oral contrast versus positive oral contrast medium in abdominal multidetector CT. Eur Radiol 2008; 18:1902-1909.

2. Macari M, Megibow AJ, Balthazar EJ. A pattern approach to the abnormal small bowel: observations at MDCT and CT enterography. AJR Am J Roentgenol 2007; 188:1344-1355.

3. Megibow AJ, Babb JS, Hecht EM, et al. Evaluation of bowel distention and bowel wall appearance by using neutral oral contrast agent for multi-detector row CT. Radiology 2006; 238:87-95.

4. Anderson SW, Soto JA, Lucey BC, et al. Abdominal 64-MDCT for suspected appendicitis: the use of oral and IV contrast material versus IV contrast material only. AJR Am J Roentgenol 2009; 193:1282-1288.

5. Johnson PT, Horton KM, Kawamoto S, et al. MDCT for suspected appendicitis: effect of reconstruction section thickness on diagnostic accuracy, rate of appendiceal visualization, and reader confidence using axial images. AJR Am J Roentgenol 2009; 192:893-901.

6. Lee SY, Coughlin B, Wolfe JM, et al. Prospective comparison of helical CT of the abdomen and pelvis without and with oral contrast in assessing acute abdominal pain in adult emergency department patients. Emerg Radiol 2006; 12:150-157.

7. Mun S, Ernst RD, Chen K, et al. Rapid CT diagnosis of acute appendicitis with IV contrast material. Emerg Radiol 2006; 12:99-102.

8. Allen TL, Cummins BF, Bonk RT, et al. Computed tomography without oral contrast solution for blunt diaphragmatic injuries in abdominal trauma. Am J Emerg Med 2005; 23:253-258.

9. Holmes JF, Offerman SR, Chang CH, et al. Performance of helical computed tomography without oral contrast for the detection of gastrointestinal injuries. Ann Emerg Med 2004; 43:120-128.

10. Stafford RE, McGonigal MD, Weigelt JA, Johnson TJ. Oral contrast solution and computed tomography for blunt abdominal trauma: a randomized study. Arch Surg 1999; 134:622-626.

11. Stuhlfaut JW, Soto JA, Lucey BC, et al. Blunt abdominal trauma: performance of CT without oral contrast material. Radiology 2004; 233:689-694.

12. Tsang BD, Panacek EA, Brant WE, Wisner DH. Effect of oral contrast administration for abdominal computed tomography in the evaluation of acute blunt trauma. Ann Emerg Med 1997; 30:7-13.

13. Harieaswar S, Rajesh A, Griffin Y, et al. Routine use of positive oral contrast material is not required for oncology patients undergoing follow-up multidetector CT. Radiology 2009; 250:246-253.

14. Delorme S, van Kaick G. Imaging of abdominal nodal spread in malignant disease. Eur Radiol 1996; 6:262-274.

15. Korobkin M. Computed tomography of the retroperitoneal vasculature and lymph nodes. Semin Roentgenol 1981; 16:251-267.

16. Baid SK, Lai EW, Wesley RA, et al. Brief communication: radiographic contrast infusion and catecholamine release in patients with pheochromocytoma. Ann Intern Med 2009; 150:27-32.

17. Bessell-Browne R, O'Malley ME. CT of pheochromocytoma and paraganglioma: risk of adverse events with I.V. administration of nonionic contrast material. AJR Am J Roentgenol 2007; 188:970-974.

18. Mukherjee JJ, Peppercorn PD, Reznek RH, et al. Pheochromocytoma: effect of nonionic contrast medium in CT on circulating catecholamine levels. Radiology 1997; 202:227-231.

19. Thoeni RF, Cello JP. CT imaging of colitis. Radiology 2006; 240:623-638.

20. Kalra MK, Maher MM, Toth TL, et al. Radiation from "extra" images acquired with abdominal and/or pelvic CT: effect of automatic tube current modulation. Radiology 2004; 232:409-414.

21. Marin D, Nelson RC, Samei E, et al. Hypervascular liver tumors: low tube voltage, high tube current multidetector CT during late hepatic arterial phase for detection—initial clinical experience. Radiology 2009; 251:771-779.

22. Schindera ST, Nelson RC, Yoshizumi T, et al. Effect of automatic tube current modulation on radiation dose and image quality for low tube voltage multidetector row CT angiography: phantom study. Acad Radiol 2009; 16:997-1002.

23. Primak AN, McCollough CH, Bruesewitz MR, et al. Relationship between noise, dose, and pitch in cardiac multi-detector row CT. RadioGraphics 2006; 26:1785-1794.

24. Chen MM, Coakley FV, Kaimal A, Laros RK Jr. Guidelines for computed tomography and magnetic resonance imaging use during pregnancy and lactation. Obstet Gynecol 2008; 112:333-340.

25. De Santis M, Di Gianantonio E, Straface G, et al. Ionizing radiations in pregnancy and teratogenesis: a review of literature. Reprod Toxicol 2005; 20:323-329.

26. Patel SJ, Reede DL, Katz DS, et al. Imaging the pregnant patient for nonobstetric conditions: algorithms and radiation dose considerations. RadioGraphics 2007; 27:1705-1722.

27. Bona G, Zaffaroni M, Defilippi C, et al. Effects of iopamidol on neonatal thyroid function. Eur J Radiol 1992; 14:22-25.

28. Ito S. Drug therapy for breast-feeding women. N Engl J Med 2000; 343:118-126.

29. Schindera ST, Nelson RC, Lee ER, et al. Abdominal multislice CT for obese patients: effect on image quality and radiation dose in a phantom study. Acad Radiol 2007; 14:486-494.

30. Israel GM, Herlihy S, Rubinowitz AN, et al. Does a combination of dose modulation with fast gantry rotation time limit CT image quality? AJR Am J Roentgenol 2008; 191:140-144.

Magnetic Resonance Imaging

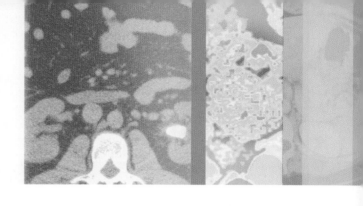

CHAPTER 14

Principles of MRI Physics

Garry Choy

TECHNICAL ASPECTS

The principles of magnetization and physics allow us to create images via MRI noninvasively. In this chapter an overview is provided on how images are created, illustrating the concepts of protons, radiofrequency (RF) excitation, T1 and T2 relaxation, image acquisition, spatial encoding, and Fourier transform analysis and k-space.

Magnetization and Protons

The nucleus of choice for imaging is hydrogen because the human body consists of an abundance of water as well as hydrogen. Every water molecule contains two hydrogen atoms, and lipids or proteins frequently contain numerous hydrogen atoms. Hydrogen atoms, also referred to as protons, precess at the Larmor frequency (Fig. 14-1). The Larmor frequency can be calculated from the gyromagnetic ratio and also the magnetic field strength of the magnet. All the spins comprise the net magnetization as aligned to B_0. The Larmor frequency is the frequency at which the RF excitation pulse must be in order to alter magnetization to generate a signal and, subsequently, images.

Radiofrequency Excitation

To use principles of magnetization to generate signals and anatomic information, an excitation RF pulse is generated. The frequency of this pulse will correspond to the center frequency of the system, whether it is a 1.5-Tesla (T) or 3.0-T system. The net RF pulse can change the net magnetization from 1 to 180 degrees; this angle is referred to as the flip angle.

T1 and T2 Relaxation

All proton spins reach equilibrium and in the process result in the release of measurable RF signal. In essence, after the RF excitation phase, the net magnetization realigns with the z-axis of the magnet.

There are two types of proton spin relaxations that can be described by the time constants T1 or T2. The T1 relaxation time constant refers to the recovery of longitudinal magnetization. The T2 relaxation time constant refers to the recovery of the transverse magnetization. By enabling the discrimination of anatomic structures via magnetic resonance, each tissue exhibits a different T1 or T2 relaxation time because all protons interact differently in their respective environments depending on whether the tissue is, for example, fat, muscle, or bone. T1 and T2 relaxation times are essentially determinants of tissue contrast (Figs. 14-2 and 14-3).

T1 relaxation, also known as spin-lattice relaxation, occurs in the z-axis of the magnet. A hydrogen proton may be bound tightly, in fat, for example, when compared with in water. More tightly bound protons release energy in a shorter period of time.

On the other hand, T2 relaxation, known as spin-spin relaxation, is an independent process in a perpendicular x-y plane. When the RF excitation pulse is applied, the protons are all spinning in phase. Eventually, protons will return to their out-of-phase initial pre-RF excitation state, as measured by the T2 relaxation time. The rate of dephasing is different for each tissue, resulting in further tissue contrast. T2 relaxation also occurs at a much faster rate than T1 relaxation, which can impact the design of sequences in abdominal MRI.

Image Acquisition

The acquisition of images occurs during T1 and T2 relaxation as protons return to equilibrium while energy is released simultaneously. To measure signals in all three orthogonal planes, the receive coil must be present orthogonally located to the main magnetic field B_0. The orthogonal positioning enables the induction of measurable electric currents in the coil. The receive coil in many systems is actually the same transmit coil for the initial RF frequency excitation pulse. Many types of coils can be used and are optimized for different body parts.

$$\omega_0 = \gamma \times B_0$$

■ **FIGURE 14-1**   Equation for Larmor frequency.

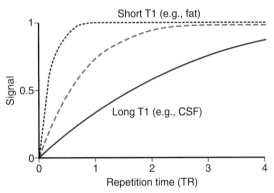

■ **FIGURE 14-2**   T1 and T2 relaxation times are essentially determinants of tissue contrast. For example, fat has a short T1 relaxation time and cerebrospinal fluid (CSF) has a long T1 relaxation time.

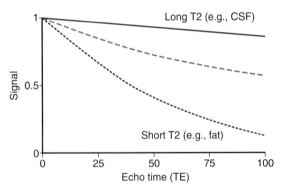

■ **FIGURE 14-3**   T1 and T2 relaxation times are essentially determinants of tissue contrast. For example, cerebrospinal fluid (CSF) has a long T2 relaxation time and fat has a short T2 relaxation time.

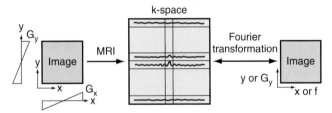

■ **FIGURE 14-4**   Illustration of mathematical transformation analysis known as k-space. *(From Hashemi RH, Bradley WG, Lisanti CJ [eds]. MRI: The Basics, 2nd ed. Philadelphia, Lippincott Williams & Wilkins, 2003, p 153.)*

Spatial Encoding

A significant advance that has made MRI possible is the ability to perform 3D localization. To accomplish this, the location of the signal can be determined using gradient coils that overlay a superimposed magnetic field. This subsequently enables the analysis of amplitude, phase, and frequency of the RF wave associated with proton spins in a specific voxel. The amplitude of an RF wave is dependent on the amount of proton spins.

Gradient coils are placed in all three orthogonal axes and allow for the 3D generation of signal. Slice encoding or selection can therefore be accomplished in the z-axis along the bore of the magnet and B_0 and can be referred to as the G_z gradient. On each slice, additional spatial localization can be accomplished by utilizing the G_y (phase-encoding gradient) and G_x (frequency-encoding gradient).

Fourier Transform Analysis and k-Space

The data acquired before processing and mathematical transformation analysis are known as k-space (Fig. 14-4). k-Space is best explained and represented by a 2D matrix, often referred to as the time domain. Depending on the frequency of signals, raw data are mapped into k-space. Low-frequency data predominantly include signal and contrast, and high-frequency data include data regarding resolution. In other words, the center of k-space contains values that are responsible for contrast and the periphery of k-space determines resolution. As a map of imaging data, when Fourier transform analysis is applied to k-space, an image of physical space is subsequently generated.

KEY POINTS

■ The nucleus of choice for imaging is hydrogen because the human body consists of an abundance of water as well as hydrogen.

■ All proton spins reach equilibrium and in the process result in the release of a measurable radiofrequency signal.

■ The data acquired before processing and mathematical transformation analysis are known as k-space.

■ As a map of imaging data, when Fourier transform analysis is applied to k-space, an image of physical space is subsequently generated.

SUGGESTED READINGS

Edelman ER, et al (eds). Clinical Magnetic Resonance Imaging. Philadelphia, Elsevier, 2006.

Elster AD. Questions and Answers to MRI. St. Louis, CV Mosby, 2000.

Haaga JR, Lanzieri CF, Gilkeson RC. CT and MR Imaging of the Whole Body. St. Louis, CV Mosby, 2003.

Martin DR, Brown MA, Semelka RC. Primer of MR Imaging of the Abdomen and Pelvis. New York, Wiley, 2005.

McRobbins DW, et al. MRI from Picture to Proton, 2nd ed. New York, Cambridge University Press, 2007.

Mitchell DG, Cohen MS. MRI Principles, 2nd ed. Philadelphia, WB Saunders, 1999.

Schild HH. MRI Made Easy (…Well Almost). Berlin, Schering AG, 1990.

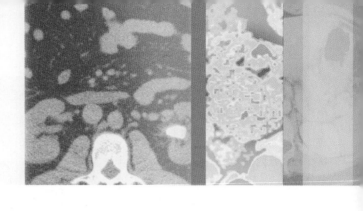

CHAPTER 15

MRI Instrumentation and Safety

Garry Choy

TECHNICAL ASPECTS

Instrumentation

MRI Magnets

There are a number of different types of configurations of clinical MR magnets. The choice of magnet depends on the type of imaging applications and other factors such as economic constraints, because some magnets are more expensive than others.

Permanent Magnets

A permanent magnet is typically used in "open MRI" units and consists of a material that generates a fixed magnetic field. The field strength is usually low, ranging between 0.064 to 0.3 T. The advantage of this type of magnet includes a lower cost, relatively low energy costs, decreased operating expenses, and patient comfort in open designs. However, this type of magnet has a low field strength, thus limiting imaging quality in certain applications.

Resistive Magnets

Resistive magnets are another type of magnet that relies on electric current–generated magnetic fields. Like permanent magnets, they are of low field strength (up to 0.3 T) and usually have an open design that increases patient comfort and decreases claustrophobia. In addition, significant amounts of heat are generated by this type of magnet. The disadvantages of resistive magnets include high power consumption costs, limited field strength, and extensive cooling requirements.

Superconducting Magnets

The most commonly used magnets are superconducting, as opposed to permanent, magnets. A superconducting magnet is also known as a bore-type magnet (Fig. 15-1), in contrast to the open type. The magnetic field is primarily generated by wiring that is cooled by liquid helium. Liquid helium cools the wiring to as low as 4 Kelvin ($-270°C$) when the wiring loses its resistance, resulting in a sustained magnetic field. Superconducting magnets are clinically superior, producing higher-quality images via more homogeneous fields and higher field strengths. Currently, most clinical scanners are 1.5 T, but 3.0-T scanners are being increasingly used. Some of the issues of superconducting magnets include high installation cost, high maintenance costs, and high cryogen costs.

Radiofrequency Coils

Radiofrequency (RF) coils are the "antennas" that perform the transmission and reception of RF waves used in generating MR images. There are a wide range of various RF coils for different body parts. Ideally, the coil optimizes image quality by producing a uniform magnetic field and allows for the best signal-to-noise ratio. The closer the coil is to the body, the better the image. As applied to the abdomen and pelvis, phased-array coils are mainly used (Fig. 15-2). Phased-array coils are essentially a combination of multiple surface coils, resulting in a large sensitive area needed for image creation. Specialized multichannel coils for the parallel imaging technique have been a recent development, resulting in decreased scanning time and better signal-to-noise quality.

Radiofrequency System ("Radiofrequency Chain")

The RF system comprises hardware that is responsible for sending and receiving the RF signal, slice selection, gradient application, signal acquisition, and signal analysis. Analog-digital converters and spectrometers are examples of components vital to this system.

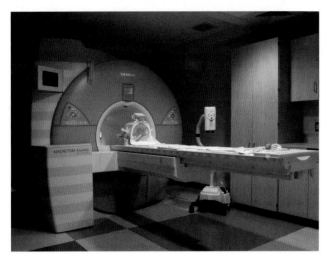

■ **FIGURE 15-1** Superconducting magnet.

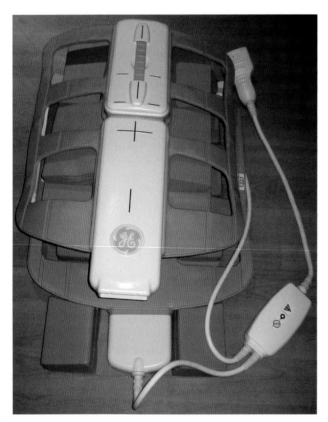

■ **FIGURE 15-2** Phased-array surface coils for body imaging.

Computer and Software

Computer hardware and software are required for the coordination and control of RF pulse transmission, acquisition, spectrometer, image reconstruction, and postprocessing. Speed and reliability are important issues in choosing computer systems. In addition, an ergonomic control room with a logical layout is important for safe and effective clinical imaging. Effective, proper training of MR technicians and comprehensive vendor-specific maintenance contracts are also essential for reliable, efficient, and high-quality operations management.

TABLE 15-1 Summary of Safety Issues in MRI
Cryogen safety
Eddy currents and acoustic noise
Ferromagnetic objects and materials
Specific absorption rate (SAR)
Sedation
Pregnancy and fetus risk
Gadolinium and nephrogenic systemic fibrosis

Safety

Unique safety challenges exist during MRI. With the proliferation of available MR scanners and increase in volume of imaging, a number of safety issues must be considered. Patients should be screened for risk factors or contraindications to MRI with a comprehensive clinical evaluation and history.[1] The primary safety issues are summarized in Table 15-1.

Cryogen Safety

Most often, superconducting magnets are used clinically, and the cryogen is helium. Under certain circumstances, if a magnet is quenched, that is, if liquid helium evaporates after heating, there is a large production of the gaseous form of helium. In a closed room, a large amount of helium can displace ambient levels of oxygen, resulting in asphyxiation or also cause thermal burns. Therefore, there must be special care in the design and adaptation of the MR examination room. Adequate ventilation systems and safety arrangements must be made.

Eddy Currents and Acoustic Noise

Constant switching of gradients results in the production of induced currents, also known as eddy currents. For example, in imaging echoplanar sequences, patients may cite symptoms from peripheral nerve stimulation.

Acoustic noise is also an important consideration. The source of noise from any magnet is the vibration of the MR components such as the gradient coils and conductors from generation of the magnetic gradient. The noise ranges between 60 to 100 dB, depending on the pulse sequence. Rapid gradient-echo sequences such as those used in abdominal and pelvic imaging are known to generate the highest amplitude sound. Therefore, sponge foam, wax ear plugs, or protective headphones are essential for patient safety. A spectrum of consequences including mild transient hearing loss to permanent hearing loss has been reported in the literature.[2]

Ferromagnetic Materials and Objects

Ferromagnetic materials carry two risks when in proximity to an MR scanner. The first arises from the generation of RF pulses and electromagnetic field resulting in severe heating of an object that could subsequently pose potential harm to the patient. The second is projectile risk, the displacement and movement of an object inside the MR scanner. Therefore, there are a variety of intraocular metallic materials, neurostimulators, bullet fragments, metal pins, nonremovable piercings, intrauterine birth control devices, skull plates, intracranial aneurysm clips, cochlear implants, pacemakers, and automatic implantable cardioverter-defibrillators (AICDs) that are contraindicated in MRI. Proper history must be obtained from family members, the referring physician, and the patient to assess for the presence of any ferromagnetic materials in the patient. At some centers, a hand-held metal detector has been documented to be effective as a final check before the patient is scanned. If there is uncertainty regarding MRI compatibility of any device or object, one should contact the manufacturer or use resources on the Internet as well as printed materials, such as those published by the American Society for Testing and Materials International, to assess MR compatibility before scanning. Larger objects containing ferromagnetic materials should never be moved in close proximity to an MR scanner, given the projectile risk; incidents involving chairs and oxygen tanks have been known to cause injuries and fatalities. A summary of devices and associated relative and absolute contraindications is presented in Table 15-2.

Specific Absorption Rate

The specific absorption rate (SAR) is the amount of energy per second absorbed per kilogram of body mass (measured in watts per kilogram) from the application of RF pulses. Essentially, the application of RF pulses can cause tissue heating. The U.S. Food and Drug Administration (FDA) has set limits on SAR where it is particularly of concern in imaging infants and pregnant women. SAR is a function of the electric field, pulse duty cycle, tissue density, patient body habitus/size, and net conductivity.

TABLE 15-2 Relative and Absolute Contraindications Associated with Various Medical Devices and Foreign Bodies

Level of Contraindication	Device or Foreign Body
Absolute	Implantable cardioverter-defibrillators and cardiac pacemakers
Absolute	Metallic heart valves (and bioprosthetic valves with metallic frames)
Absolute	Metallic cochlear implants
Absolute	Orbital implants/devices with metallic clips*
Absolute	Vagal nerve stimulators*
Absolute	Aneurysm clips*
Absolute	Any metallic foreign body or any foreign body with an unknown ferromagnetic composition
Relative	Orthopedic hardware (most hardware is now MRI safe but consultation of a comprehensive list and obtaining information such as time of implantation would be recommended)
Relative	Prior exposure to metallic debris to eyes or other body parts (pre-scan screening for history of exposure is required)
Relative	Permanent metallic body piercings

*Check with manufacturer because newer devices may be built to be MRI compatible.

SAR is proportional to the square of the field strength and significantly greater in scanners with high magnetic field. The FDA currently has limitations regarding SAR, and the reader is referred to its website or printed materials. In the design of any imaging sequence as well as for each imaging session, the SAR limit must not be exceeded. Parameters that can be adjusted include mainly, but are not limited to, the coil used, repetition time, number of sequences, flip angle, and echo train.

Sedation

Often patients may require sedation; those particularly affected include children, agitated adults, and patients who have claustrophobia.[3] Proper clinical history and monitoring of vital signs are critical. The risk of aspiration from sedation must be weighed before imaging. The availability of experienced clinical staff who can handle emergencies also should be arranged before imaging. If necessary, anesthesiology or critical care personnel should be readily available if a high-risk patient who requires sedation is scanned.

Pregnancy and Fetus Risk

In abdominal and pelvic MRI, at times the patient may be pregnant. To date, there has been no definite evidence that supports the claim that short-term exposure to electromagnetic fields poses any harm to the developing fetus. However, there are studies that have cited that prolonged exposure to electromagnetic radiation and an elevated SAR have resulted in chromosomal damage, alteration in fetal development, or abnormalities in mitosis. It is important to discuss with the patient the current known risks and obtain informed consent as per an institution's policy.

Gadolinium should be used with extreme caution in lactating women and pregnant women. Gadolinium has been shown to cross the placenta and therefore is used only when the benefit of MRI outweighs any potential risk. There is currently uncertain risk and lack of definitive data pertaining to the effects of gadolinium on a fetus during pregnancy as well as on the newborn during lactation. Caution is typically advised by many radiologists against administering gadolinium during pregnancy unless absolutely necessary.[4] Hence, many radiology departments undertake precautions with women who breast-feed by requiring that they stop breast-feeding at least 24 hours after gadolinium administration.[4]

Gadolinium and Nephrogenic Systemic Fibrosis

Gadolinium use should be performed with careful patient screening of renal dysfunction. Many abdominal MRI techniques rely on contrast enhancement with gadolinium; therefore, it is important to understand the risk of administering gadolinium in certain patient populations. Nephrogenic systemic fibrosis is a newly recognized condition that involves widespread cutaneous and systemic fibrosis. Initially termed nephrogenic fibrosing dermopathy, this condition is a debilitating disease that has been observed and cited by the FDA to be associated with gadolinium administration in patients with severely reduced renal function, specifically those who are undergoing dialysis.[5] The true cause of nephrogenic systemic fibrosis is still unclear and is actively being investigated. Its onset can be rapid, and it can result in severe debilitating contractures as quickly as within weeks. No therapy currently exists; therefore, active screening of patients for renal insufficiency is recommended. If possible, in patients at highest risk, active selection of appropriate imaging sequences is required; for example, for MR vascular studies, MRI techniques such as time-of-flight–based sequences can be used instead. As described by Kuo and colleagues,[6] if patients have stage 4 or 5 chronic renal disease or an estimated glomerular filtration rate of less than 30 mL/min/1.73 m², gadolinium contrast studies should be avoided when possible and the clinical decision to administer gadolinium should be discussed with the ordering physician.

CONTROVERSIES

At times there may be controversy as to what may constitute a relative versus absolute contraindication to MRI. For example, in the case of implantable hardware, although it is widely accepted that there are absolute contraindications to MRI, with the development of newer MRI-compatible implantable devices, certain patients can now be imaged. A detailed list of relative and absolute contraindications is described in Table 15-2. As newer devices are being developed, it is therefore important to prescreen patients to identify the exact year, make, and model of implantable hardware before imaging.

Imaging pregnant patients is also an ongoing area of debate. To date, no definite evidence supports the claim that short-term exposure to electromagnetic fields poses any harm to the developing fetus. However, there are studies that have cited prolonged exposure to electromagnetic radiation, and elevated SAR has resulted in chromosomal damage, alteration in fetal development, or abnormalities in mitosis. It is important to discuss with the patient the current known risks and obtain informed consent as per an institution's policy. Gadolinium should also be used with extreme caution in lactating and pregnant women.

Gadolinium use should be performed with careful patient screening of renal dysfunction because of the emerging gadolinium-associated illness nephrogenic systemic fibrosis discussed earlier.

KEY POINTS

- Patients must be screened for risk factors or contraindications to MRI via comprehensive clinical evaluation and history before imaging.
- Absolute contraindications to MRI include implantable defibrillators, pacemakers, metallic heart valves, metallic cochlear implants, metallic orbital implants, various vagal nerve stimulators, metallic aneurysm clips, or any metallic foreign body with unknown ferromagnetic composition.
- Relative contraindications to MRI include some orthopedic hardware (most are MRI compatible), prior exposure to metallic debris in body parts or eyes, and permanent metallic body piercings.

REFERENCES

1. Elster AD, Link KM, Carr JJ. Patient screening prior to MR imaging: a practical approach synthesized from protocols at 15 U.S. medical centers. AJR Am J Roentgenol 1994; 162:195-199.
2. Brummett RE, Talbot JM, Charuhas P. Potential hearing loss resulting from MR imaging. Radiology 1988; 169:539-540.
3. Quirk ME, et al. Anxiety in patients undergoing MR imaging. Radiology 1989; 170:463-466.
4. Webb JA, Thomsen HS, Morcos SK. The use of iodinated and gadolinium contrast media during pregnancy and lactation. Eur Radiol 2005; 15:1234-1240.
5. Cowper SE, Rabach M, Girardi M. Clinical and histological findings in nephrogenic systemic fibrosis. Eur J Radiol 2008; 66:191-199.
6. Kuo PH, et al. Gadolinium-based MR contrast agents and nephrogenic systemic fibrosis. Radiology 2007; 242:647-649.

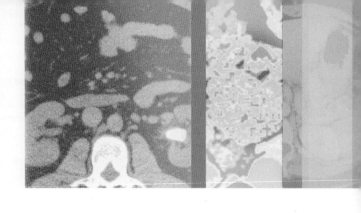

CHAPTER 16

MRI Pulse Sequences

Garry Choy

TECHNICAL ASPECTS

The cornerstone of MRI is its ability to distinguish pathologic tissue from normal tissue as well as to characterize soft tissues. Over the years, many sequences have been developed for imaging various organ systems and tissue types. Regardless of organ system, imaging sequences are tailored to optimizing quality and reproducibility for the best performance in identifying pathologic processes. Specific to the abdomen and pelvis, however, there has been the development of unique imaging sequences that have evolved to overcome a significant number of artifacts that in the past limited high contrast and quality MRI of these regions. Today's imaging sequences effectively aim to minimize the artifacts commonly seen in the abdomen as related to breathing, cardiac motion, arterial pulsations, vascular flow, chemical shift, and peristalsis. In addition, there have been advances and new uses of gadolinium enhancement for various applications and detection of disease.

Fundamentally, MRI of the abdomen and pelvis, as in other anatomic structures, relies on contrast between tissues obtained between differences in T1 and T2 relaxation times and proton densities (Table 16-1). Sequences obtained after gadolinium administration in the arterial, portal venous, and delayed phases also play an important role in characterizing lesions. In essence, techniques of abdominal MRI include the use of variations of spin-echo (SE) and gradient-recalled-echo (GRE) sequences (Table 16-2). In addition, most abdominal imaging sequences rely on breath-holding and patient cooperation, with the relative exception of single-shot techniques.

T1-Weighted Techniques

T1-weighted (T1W) sequences are useful sequences for abdominal imaging. Anatomic information can be derived simply from T1W images. Fat-containing structures are of high signal intensity on T1W sequences. Commonly used T1W fat-suppressed sequences can provide further infor-

mation on soft tissues present in the abdomen. Fluid content or fibrous tissue appears as low signal intensity, whereas fat, fluids high in protein concentration, or subacute blood products will appear as high signal intensity.

Gradient-Recalled-Echo Sequences

GRE sequences are very important in abdominal imaging. Of the T1W sequences, there are multiple pathologic processes that can be identified using GRE sequences. GRE sequences are faster than the basic T1W SE sequence. An SE sequence is produced by pairs of radiofrequency (RF) pulses, whereas a GRE sequence is produced by a single RF pulse with gradient reversal. Because only one RF pulse is applied, the echo is recorded very quickly and the echo time (TE) is shorter. To optimize the signal-to-noise ratio (SNR) and to maximize the number of slices acquired at any one time, GRE sequences utilize longer repetition times (TRs) at approximately 150 ms and short TEs at 4.2 to 4.5 ms. As a result of short TE and TR values, signal acquisition can be rapid and particularly useful in body imaging. Of the GRE sequences, "spoiled" GRE (SPGR) sequences are specifically used to disrupt transverse T2 coherences to ensure that prior to RF excitation pulses the steady-state magnetization has no transverse component. As a result, images do not have significant true T2 weighting but instead mainly incorporate T2* effects. Partial flip angles that are utilized in GRE techniques also take advantage of appreciable transverse magnetization that can be achieved via a partial flip angle.

Spoiled GRE sequences include, but are not limited to, FLASH (fast low-angle shot), SPGR, RF-FAST, and T1-FAST, as used by multiple manufacturers. MR angiography, echoplanar imaging, 3D imaging, and dynamic contrast-enhanced MRI also utilize GRE techniques. There are also faster techniques, namely, turbo-FLASH, MP-RAGE (magnetization-prepared rapid gradient-echo), and inversion recovery (IR)-prepared fast SPGR in which the TR is extremely short (i.e., when TR < T2*).

TABLE 16-1   Appearance of Various Tissues on MRI in Abdomen/Pelvis

Tissue	T1-Weighted Imaging	T2-Weighted Imaging
Fat	Hyperintense	Hypointense to isointense (hyperintense on fast spin-echo images)
Cystic collections predominantly water	Hypointense	Hyperintense
Cystic collections with high protein content	Hyperintense	Hyperintense
Bone marrow (yellow)	Hyperintense	Isointense to hypointense
Bone marrow (red)	Isointense	Hypointense
Cortical bone	Hypointense	Hypointense
Liver (normal)	Isointense to hyperintense	Hypointense
Liver (metastatic disease)	Isointense to hypointense	Hyperintense or isointense
Liver (hemangioma)	Hypointense	Hyperintense
Liver (fatty infiltration)	Hyperintense	Hypointense
Liver (iron deposition)	Hypointense to isointense	Hypointense
Pancreas	Hyperintense	Hypointense
Spleen	Hypointense	Hyperintense
Blood/hematoma (hyperacute, <6 hr)	Isointense	Isointense
Blood/hematoma (Acute, 6-24 hr)	Isointense to hypointense	Hypointense
Blood/hematoma (subacute, 1 day to 1 mo)	Hyperintense	Hyperintense or hypointense on susceptibility sequences
Blood/hematoma (chronic, >1 mo)	Isointense to hyperintense	Isointense to hyperintense
Muscle	Isointense to hypointense	Hypointense

TABLE 16-2   Commonly Used Parameters for Abdominal Imaging Pulse Sequences

	T1-Weighted Images	T2-Weighted Images
Spin-Echo Sequences		
Echo time (TE)	<25 ms	>50 ms
Repetition time (TR)	<500 ms	>1500 ms
Gradient-Echo Sequences		
TE	10-20 ms	20-40 ms
TR	20-200 ms	100-200 ms
Flip angle	45 to 90 degrees	10 to 25 degrees
Inversion-Recovery Sequences		
TE	15-30 ms	
TR	1000-2000 ms	
Inversion time (TI)	Variable: 300-500 ms; Short tau inversion recovery is in range of <200 ms	

Fat Suppression

Very helpful in identifying pathologic processes, fat suppression is used on nearly all studies of the abdomen. As precontrast images, fat-suppressed sequences enable the minimization of T1 signal from fat but enable the detection of subacute blood, melanin, and fluids high in protein concentration. There are several different techniques of reducing the fat signal, including those based on phase evolution, frequency-selective excitation and saturation, and T1-dependent suppression (commonly known as short tau inversion recovery [STIR]).

Phase evolution was used on earlier scanners but in modern MRI is not generally used. Frequency selective techniques are now generally preferred, including frequency selective excitation and saturation. Because water and fat resonance frequencies are distinct, fat suppression can be accomplished by selectively exciting the slower precessing of fat hydrogen protons followed by spoiler gradients to saturate the peak of fat before imaging, thereby reducing its signal during acquisition.

STIR is a technique that is applicable at all field strengths and is another method used for fat suppression. STIR techniques take advantage of the relatively short T1 relaxation times of fat within the body. In STIR, the longitudinal magnetization is inverted by a 180-degree pulse followed by a time delay; when the longitudinal magnetization of fat is at the null point, image formation is performed by inverting the negative values of longitudinal magnetization of all other tissues; therefore, combined T1 and T2 effects result in bright signal from tissues with long T1 relaxation times such as cerebrospinal fluid and tumors. Fat suppression techniques are certainly useful on contrast-enhanced studies, improving the contrast between intra-abdominal fat and diseases within tissues and vascular structures.

Out-of-Phase Imaging

Out-of-phase imaging is another type of GRE technique that helps elucidate disease processes where there is the presence of both fat and water in the same voxel. Voxels that contain both fat and water will demonstrate signal dropoff on out-of-phase sequences. Typically, a TE of 2.3 ms is used at 1.5 T. This technique relies on chemical shift, involving the different precessional frequencies of protons in fat and water. The shorter the TE, the higher the signal and faster the sequence, with the advantage of significantly less susceptibility effect. The TE is set such that the proton spins in fat and water are 180 degrees apart, thereby resulting in destructive interference. A signal drop is visualized when there is a mixture of fat/water, with a 50%/50% composition requiring complete signal dropoff. If the tissues are all water or all fat, then there is no significant signal dropoff and there is an equal ratio. The most commonly used applications of out-of-phase techniques are in the evaluation of the degree of fatty infiltration within the liver and of adrenal masses, when signal dropoff from out-of-phase images compared with in-phase images can help distinguish lipid-rich adenomas from adrenal malignancies.

Contrast-Enhanced Sequences

Contrast-enhanced GRE sequences are commonly used in abdominal imaging to evaluate the solid organs and malignancies. T1W fat suppression is typically used for contrast-enhanced sequences. Although this topic is discussed in more detail in Chapter 18, it is important to note that data acquisition must be fast enough for the entire dataset to be generated from a distinct phase of enhancement. Precontrast sequences should also be performed to adequately evaluate postgadolinium images. Obtaining images at various time points for dynamic contrast-enhanced MRI is also very useful clinically.

T2-Weighted Techniques

Much of MRI is based on T2-weighted (T2W) imaging techniques. T2W imaging is highly sensitive to pathologic processes within the abdomen. The characterization of T2 signal in tissues allows for the determination of water content, degree of fibrotic change, diffuse liver disease, and presence of iron or calcium deposition. T2W sequences, particularly the fast SE (FSE) techniques, delineate fluid-filled structures such as the biliary system, pancreatic ducts, stomach, bowel, and other cystic or fluid-filled collections.

Spin-Echo Sequences

There are both breath-hold and non–breath-hold T2W techniques. Standard T2W SE sequences last several minutes and thus are vulnerable to motion artifacts from breathing and bowel peristalsis. Even if respiratory gating is used, mild blurring of edges occurs and gating results in significant increase in scan time. By shortening the typical MR scan time, fast scanning techniques therefore have gained significant practical popularity and are used increasingly.

Fast Spin-Echo Sequences and Single-Shot Fast Spin-Echo Sequences

More practical and faster than traditional spin-echo techniques, the introduction of FSE sequences has played a significant role in abdominal and pelvic MRI. Typical scan times for FSE sequences range between 5 and 15 minutes. A pitfall of FSE sequences is motion degradation. Therefore, faster techniques have been developed.

Analogous to single-shot echoplanar techniques, the single-shot FSE (SSFSE) sequence is a method that enables the rapid acquisition of an image in one excitation pulse. SSFSE sequences are relatively motion insensitive and are very useful in abdominal and pelvic imaging (Fig. 16-1). Total scan times for SSFSE sequences can be reduced to as low as 2 to 4 minutes. These techniques are typically also classified as echo-train SE sequences, rapid SE, turbo

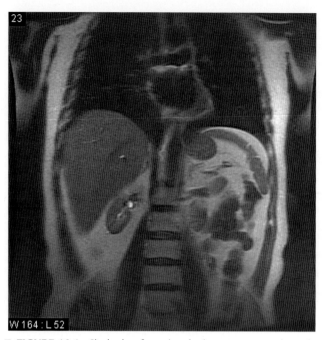

■ **FIGURE 16-1** Single-shot fast spin-echo image, a commonly used and effective imaging sequence for abdominal MRI.

SE, single-shot turbo SE, or rapid acquisition with refocused echoes (RARE) techniques. FSE imaging is based on the acquisition of multiple echoes within a given repetition time (TR), where the number of echoes in a given TR is known as the echo train length (ETL). Multiple 180-degree refocusing pulses, typically between 80 and 100, after a single 90-degree pulse generate the train of echoes. Unlike standard multiple-echo techniques, FSE techniques change the phase-encoding gradient between echoes such that k-space can be filled faster. Basically, multiple lines of k-space with multiple phase-encoding steps are then acquired within a given repetition time in a relatively short period of time. A disadvantage of FSE and echo-train–based SE techniques includes slightly decreased T2 contrast, but this is generally not substantial because the conspicuity of pathologic processes in the abdomen and pelvis is prominent. Of note, fat also demonstrates significantly higher signal on FSE compared with conventional SE techniques due to intermolecular interactions known as J-coupling. In conventional SE sequences, fat is indeterminant in signal intensity in contrast to high T2 signal found in pathologic processes. Therefore, for FSE techniques, fat suppression is an important aspect of abdominal MRI to better identify pathologic processes.

Fat-Suppressed T2-Weighted Sequences

In the abdomen and pelvis, fat suppression on T2W sequences should be applied to maximize contrast between intra-abdominal fatty tissue from high T2 signal in pathologic processes, cysts, or other fluid collections. In addition, fat-suppressed T2 images may be helpful for identifying lesions in the background of diffuse fatty infiltration of the liver. Fat-suppressed FSE and STIR sequences are useful methods to consider.

Fast Advanced Spin Echo

The fast advanced spin-echo technique, also on some scanners referred to as HASTE (half-Fourier single-shot turbo spin-echo), uses long ETLs, resulting in ultrashort scan times. HASTE relies on acquiring only half of k-space in one RF excitation pulse. This MR technique is used to perform a study known widely as MR cholangiopancreatography (MRCP). MRCP is based on modified echo-train sequences in which the TE is lengthened to produce heavily T2W images to clearly accentuate the biliary system, gallbladder, and pancreatic duct (Fig. 16-2). For MRCP, the TE is increased to 250 to 500 ms and performed in thin sections for higher resolution, but it can also be acquired in thick slabs to encompass the entire biliary system and pancreatic ducts.

General Strategies

The optimal strategy for abdominal and pelvic MRI relies on standardization of protocols and proper training of

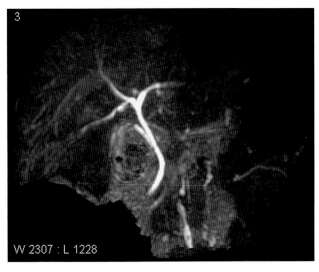

■ **FIGURE 16-2**   MR cholangiopancreatography. Heavily T2W images are useful for imaging the biliary tree.

personnel. Routine protocols for disease processes or organ systems should be established as standard departmental protocols. Immediate access and open communication with the radiologist for customization and fine tuning of sequences is also extremely important.

Because MRI scan time has decreased significantly over the past few years, abdominal imaging examinations typically average between 20 to 40 minutes.

Patients must also be properly coached before beginning the scan. Proper breath-hold instructions must be clearly stated to obtain the highest quality images. For sedated or uncooperative patients, sequences such as breath-hold independent single-shot FSE sequences are useful. In patients who are moving and/or agitated, single-shot techniques become highly useful and should be employed.

KEY POINTS

- Very helpful in identifying pathologic processes, fat suppression is used on nearly all studies of the abdomen. As precontrast images, fat-suppressed sequences minimize T1 signal from fat and enable the detection of subacute blood, melanin, and fluids with high protein concentration.
- More practical and faster than traditional spin-echo techniques, the introduction of fast spin-echo (FSE) sequences has played a significant role in abdominal and pelvic MRI.
- T2W sequences, particularly the FSE techniques, delineate fluid-filled structures such as the biliary system, pancreatic ducts, stomach, bowel, and other cystic or fluid-filled collections.
- In the abdomen and pelvis, fat suppression on T2W sequences should be applied to maximize contrast between intra-abdominal fatty tissue from high T2 signal in pathologic processes, cysts, or other fluid collections.
- The optimal strategy for abdominal and pelvic MRI relies on standardization and proper training of personnel. Proper breath-hold instructions must be clearly stated to obtain the highest quality images. For sedated or uncooperative patients, sequences such as breath-hold independent single-shot FSE sequences are useful.

SUGGESTED READINGS

Edelman ER, et al (eds). Clinical Magnetic Resonance Imaging. Philadelphia, Elsevier, 2006.

Elster AD. Questions and Answers to MRI. St. Louis, CV Mosby, 2000.

Haaga JR, Lanzieri CF, Gilkeson RC. CT and MR Imaging of the Whole Body. St. Louis, CV Mosby, 2003.

Martin DR, Brown MA, Semelka RC. Primer of MR Imaging of the Abdomen and Pelvis. New York, Wiley, 2005.

McRobbins DW, et al. MRI from Picture to Proton, 2nd ed. New York, Cambridge University Press, 2007.

Mitchell DG, Cohen MS. MRI Principles, 2nd ed. Philadelphia, WB Saunders, 1999.

Schild HH. MRI Made Easy (...Well Almost). Berlin, Schering AG, 1990.

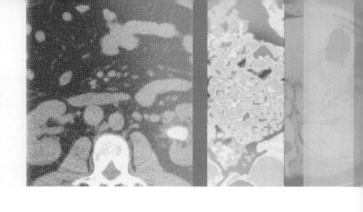

CHAPTER 17

MRI Artifacts

Garry Choy

TECHNICAL ASPECTS

Artifacts are found on nearly all MR images. It is important in the diagnostic evaluation of MR images to be aware of the many MR artifacts and their causes. Understanding the reason for MR artifacts enables better interpretation of images. Basic and commonly found artifacts such as motion artifact, chemical shift artifact, susceptibility and paramagnetic artifacts, phase-related artifacts, and frequency-related artifacts are discussed in this chapter (Table 17-1).

Types of Artifacts

Motion Artifacts

Phase direction determines the axis and appearance of motion artifacts. Motion on MRI is phase related because motion artifact is created when a proton spin moves between the radiofrequency (RF) excitation and signal acquisition. This results in essentially "mismapping" of spins. In abdominal MRI, motion artifacts commonly can be a result of breathing artifacts, cardiac motion, bowel peristalsis, or patient motion (Figs. 17-1 to 17-3). A certain amount of artifact may be unavoidable in many cases as long as the motion artifact does not completely obscure the detection of a pathologic process or drastically reduce image quality in the region of interest. Proper instruction of the patient by the MR technologist is one of the most important factors. In addition, technical solutions by various vendors have been developed, including flow compensation, respiratory triggering, and cardiac triggering techniques. In the abdomen, high-quality imaging is highly dependent on breath-hold techniques and fast imaging sequences to minimize motion artifact.

Chemical Shift Artifact

Chemical shift artifact is seen at fat/water interfaces, and although at times can result in image distortion, sometimes it can be helpful for diagnostic purposes. For example, chemical shift artifacts are used via in-phase and out-of-phase imaging to determine the presence of micro-scopic fat content within adrenal glands and lesions. Chemical shift artifact can also be commonly seen at the vertebral body end plates, around abdominal visceral organs, and in the orbits. This artifact appears as a dark contour along the fat/water interface on one border and a bright contour along the fat/water interface at the opposite border. The cause of chemical shift artifact arises from the different resonance frequencies of protons in water and fat, resulting in a frequency difference interpreted as a spatial position difference. Therefore, because this artifact is most related to frequency, fat-containing tissues are shifted in the frequency direction. Chemical shift artifacts are greater at higher field strengths and might be an issue to be considered when deciding between using a scanner at 3.0 T or 1.5 T.

Phase-Wrap Artifact/Aliasing Artifact

When the field of view (FOV) is smaller than the object being scanned, wrap-around artifact or "phase wrap" occurs in the phase-encoding direction (Fig. 17-4). In the FOV specified, the phase encoding is divided into steps within the phase direction of the FOV from 1 to 360 degrees. Once beyond 360 degrees, the phase-encoding process will start again outside the FOV. During the acquisition of signal, the system will therefore receive signal from both *inside* and *outside* the FOV, resulting in a wrap-around artifact. To avoid this artifact, the images could be acquired by scanning a larger FOV but then reconstructing the image in the desired FOV. This technique is effective but requires significantly more scan time. Similarly, aliasing artifact can occur in the frequency direction. This artifact can be reduced by applying frequency-specific filters or by sampling the signal twice as fast.

Frequency-Encoding Artifacts

Frequency artifacts occur in the frequency-encoding direction. This type of artifact occurs as noise or snow on the image in the frequency direction. The etiology of frequency artifacts is usually due to hardware issues such as defective electronics, faulty transmitters, nonshielded or MRI-compatible equipment adjacent to the MR scanner,

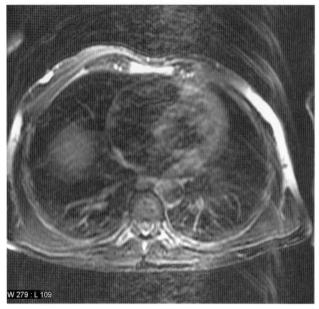

■ **FIGURE 17-1** Motion artifact due to respiratory motion in the anteroposterior plane.

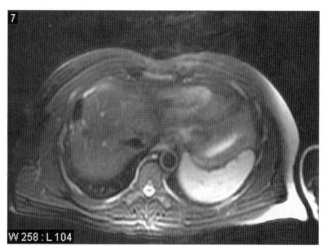

■ **FIGURE 17-2** Cardiac motion artifact.

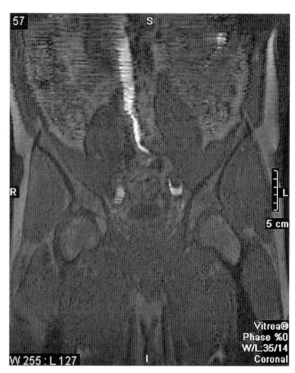

■ **FIGURE 17-3** Aortic pulsatile artifact.

TABLE 17-1 Common MRI Artifacts and Corresponding Image Quality Improvement Strategy

Motion Artifacts	Provide proper patient instruction for breathing instructions and minimization of body movement.
	Maintain cooperation between radiology technologist and patient.
	Choose fast scan sequences.
	Optimize respiratory gating.
Aliasing/Phase-Wrap Artifacts	Acquire images by scanning using a larger field of view but then reconstructing in the desired field of view.
Frequency Artifacts	Ensure proper hardware maintenance and minimization of failure of hardware.
	Ensure shielding of MRI-compatible equipment adjacent to the MR scanner.
	Reduce RF cage leak by closing door to MR scanner.
	Remove any metal near the patient.
Susceptibility Artifacts	Properly screen patients before scan for implantable hardware or prior surgery.
	Attempt to center the bore away from metal but balanced with required coverage region.
	Use fast spin-echo instead of gradient-recalled-echo sequences, which are more sensitive to susceptibility artifact.

an open door resulting in RF-cage leak, metal within or near the patient, or interference from outside a poorly caged room.

Susceptibility Artifact (T2* Effect) and Paramagnetic Effects

Susceptibility artifacts on MRI occur when there is a significant gradient or alteration of the magnetic field due to interfaces between substances of very different magnetic susceptibilities. For example, significant artifact is seen surrounding ferromagnetic objects within the soft tissues of the human body. In turn, shifts of frequency and dephasing occur, resulting in degradation of the image with dark or bright pixels displayed. Gradient-recalled-echo–based sequences and sequences with very long echo times are most vulnerable to susceptibility artifact.

Metal, in particular, alters the magnetic field, changing the resonance frequency beyond the range of MRI. These protons of the metal will not be excitable by RF pulses and therefore will not be able to be imaged. Not all metals cause severe artifacts; the degree of image distortion depends on the iron concentration (Fig. 17-5). Surgical clips or even metallic foreign bodies, no matter how small, can cause image distortion. In addition to distorting the

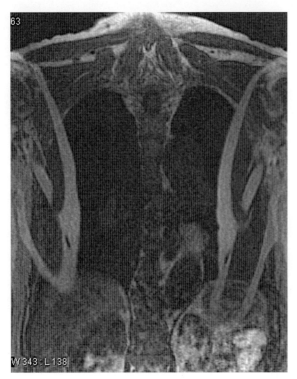

■ **FIGURE 17-4** Phase-wrap artifact.

images, metals with high iron content can also result in severe heating and internal organ damage. Therefore, all patients must be screened for metal implants or history of metallic foreign bodies. Metals such as titanium and aluminum are examples of MRI-safe metals. Many manufacturers of implantable devices are using titanium and aluminum.

Patient Compliance and Capacity for Cooperation

Adequate and proper patient cooperation is important in nearly all cases to determine image quality. Imaging of adults differs significantly from that of pediatric patients. In pediatric populations, age determines the ability of patients to follow breath-hold instructions. Also, children often become agitated or have shorter patience duration for long imaging sequences; therefore, single-shot sequences become quite useful. In any population, the ability and will to comply with breath-hold instructions are key issues to resolve. It is here that a competent and diligent MRI technologist plays a vital role in obtaining the highest quality diagnostic MR images. It may be difficult to obtain images in patients with agitation, stroke, or dementia. Hence, proper sedation and personnel may also be required and should be planned in advance of the scan.

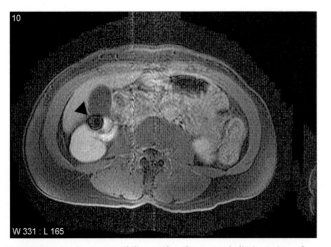

■ **FIGURE 17-5** Susceptibility artifact from metal clip in region of right kidney.

KEY POINTS

- Properly screen patients before the scan for implantable hardware or prior surgery; attempt to center the bore away from metal but balanced with required coverage region; use fast spin-echo instead of gradient-recalled-echo sequences, which are more sensitive to susceptibility artifact.
- Minimize motion artifacts with proper patient instruction for breath-holding and minimization of body movement; maintain the cooperation of the patient; choose fast scan sequences; optimize respiratory gating.
- Decrease aliasing and phase-wrap artifacts by acquiring data in a larger field of view; ensure proper hardware maintenance and minimization hardware failure; ensure shielding of MRI-compatible equipment adjacent to the MR scanner; reduce RF cage leak by closing door to MR scanner; remove any metal near the patient critical to decreasing frequency-based artifacts.

SUGGESTED READINGS

Edelman ER, et al (eds). Clinical Magnetic Resonance Imaging. Philadelphia, Elsevier, 2006.

Elster AD. Questions and Answers to MRI. St. Louis, CV Mosby, 2000.

Haaga JR, Lanzieri CF, Gilkeson RC. CT and MR Imaging of the Whole Body. St. Louis, CV Mosby, 2003.

Martin DR, Brown MA, Semelka RC. Primer of MR Imaging of the Abdomen and Pelvis. New York, Wiley, 2005.

McRobbins DW, et al. MRI from Picture to Proton, 2nd ed. New York, Cambridge University Press, 2007.

Mitchell DG, Cohen MS. MRI Principles, 2nd ed. Philadelphia, WB Saunders, 1999.

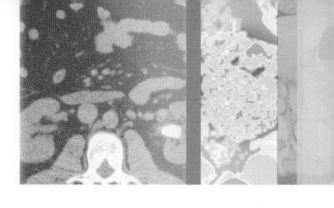

18

Contrast Media and Contrast-Enhanced MRI

Garry Choy

TECHNICAL ASPECTS

A significant number of abdominal and pelvic MR images are obtained after intravenous administration of a contrast agent. Contrast agents enhance the visualization of vascular structures as well as pathologic tissues, which appear more prominent against the background of normal tissue. Development of novel contrast agents continues to be an exciting area, with new targeted agents, blood pool agents, and agents based on nanoparticle technologies. The discussion here is focused on water-soluble gadolinium chelates used in abdominal and pelvic MRI.

Principle of Relaxivity

The current use of gadolinium is based on paramagnetism. Gadolinium has more orbitals than electron pairs, an odd number, resulting in a net electron spin, and is therefore classified as paramagnetic. Its magnetic moment in addition with unpaired electrons makes gadolinium a useful compound for MRI. Although any agent that alters the local magnetic field can alter both T1 and T2 relaxation, gadolinium predominantly shortens T1 relaxation.

Chemical Structure of Currently Approved Chelates of Gadolinium

Gadolinium-DTPA (gadopentetate) was first approved in 1988. Table 18-1 summarizes the currently approved agents for use in Europe and the United States. All of these agents contain a gadolinium ion centrally, an octadentate ligand, and a coordinated water molecule in their chemical structure. The octadentate ligand is responsible primarily for safety because it provides thermodynamic stability. Unchelated gadolinium is severely toxic to human tissues and cells. The coordinated water molecule allows for rapid chemical exchange with other water molecules

in the solution that gadolinium is in, resulting in shortening of relaxation time of the water environment.

Biodistribution

The human body can be divided into extracellular and intracellular compartments. All currently approved gadolinium chelates are extracellular space agents. The extracellular compartment can be simplified into the intravascular and interstitial spaces, which then are linked to the kidneys and liver, where there is hepatobiliary or renal excretion. Agents are initially distributed within the intravascular space and then diffuse into the interstitial space. As an extracellular agent, gadolinium chelates are very hydrophilic and thereby shorten the T1 relaxation time of the molecules around them. Although gadolinium chelates are nonspecific and their distribution is governed by perfusion, tissues that have a larger extracellular or interstitial space, increased capillary breakdown, or increased permeability will also receive a higher concentration of contrast agent, thereby appearing brighter on T1-weighted (T1W) sequences.

Phases of Vascular and Tissue Enhancement

As soon as gadolinium is injected intravenously, the agent is distributed into the pulmonary circulation, aorta, systemic arteries, capillaries, interstitial space, and kidneys for excretion into the urinary collecting system. The phases of enhancement in the vessels and tissues can be divided into arterial, blood pool, and extracellular phases.

The *arterial phase* is best imaged using fast pulse sequences that allow for capturing the initial arrival of contrast agent into arteries before venous filling. Temporal resolution maximization is critical for good arterial phase imaging. Arterial phase imaging is useful for

TABLE 18-1 MRI Contrast Agents Currently Approved for Use in the United States and Europe

Gd-DTPA (Magnevist)
Gd-DO3A-butrol (Gadovist)
Gd-DOTA (Dotarem)
Gd-DTPA-BMA (Omniscan)
Gd-DTPA-BMEA (OptiMARK)
Gd-HPDO3A (ProHance)

evaluating arteries and arterially enhancing lesions within the liver or pancreas. Faster techniques such as those utilizing parallel imaging techniques have enabled better quality arterial phase imaging. The best time for arterial phase imaging usually occurs at 20 to 40 seconds after injection.

The *blood pool phase* or *portal venous phase* follows 60 to 80 seconds after injection and is characterized by contrast agent distributed throughout the vessels. Tumors within the abdomen and pelvis are commonly more prominent during this phase. This is also the phase of highest liver parenchymal enhancement. In many cases, malignancies may be less intense in the portal venous phase. As a result, the portal venous phase is an important component for any evaluation of liver neoplasm.

The *extracellular phase* follows 120 to 150 seconds after intravenous injection. During this phase, contrast agent begins to diffuse into the interstitial component of the extracellular space. Pathologic processes such as malignancy demonstrate increased interstitial space or abnormal capillary structure with increased permeability, thereby appearing hyperintense with contrast enhancement during this phase. It is also during this phase that the contrast agent begins to undergo filtration in the kidneys and accumulates in the collecting system and bladder.

PROS AND CONS

Contrast agents improve the visualization of vascular structures as well as pathologic tissues, which appear more prominent against the background of normal tissue.

Sensitivity and specificity of lesion detection can be improved if these agents are used properly, depending on the clinical indication.

With the emerging risk of nephrogenic systemic fibrosis, gadolinium-based agents should be used only after careful patient screening for renal dysfunction. Many abdominal MRI techniques rely on contrast enhancement with gadolinium; therefore, it is important to understand the risk of administering gadolinium in certain patient populations. Nephrogenic systemic fibrosis is a newly recognized condition that involves widespread cutaneous and systemic fibrosis. Initially termed nephrogenic fibrosing dermopathy, this condition is a debilitating disease that has been observed and cited by the U.S. Food and Drug Administration to be associated with gadolinium administration in patients with severely reduced renal function, specifically those who are undergoing dialysis.[1] The true cause of nephrogenic systemic fibrosis is still unclear and is actively being investigated. As described by Kuo and colleagues, if patients have stage 4 or 5 chronic renal disease or an estimated glomerular filtration rate of less than 30 mL/min/1.73 m^2, gadolinium-based contrast studies should be avoided when possible and the clinical decision to administer gadolinium should be discussed with the ordering physician.[2]

KEY POINTS

- Contrast agents enable the visualization of vascular structures as well as pathologic tissues, which appear more prominent against the background of normal tissue.
- Although any agent that alters the local magnetic field can alter both T1 and T2 relaxation, gadolinium predominantly shortens T1 relaxation.
- Development of novel contrast agents continues to be an exciting area, with new targeted agents, blood pool agents, and agents based on nanoparticle technologies.
- With the emerging risk of nephrogenic systemic fibrosis, gadolinium-based agents should be used only after careful patient screening for renal dysfunction.

SUGGESTED READINGS

Edelman ER, et al (eds). Clinical Magnetic Resonance Imaging. Philadelphia, Elsevier, 2006.
Elster AD. Questions and Answers to MRI. St. Louis, CV Mosby, 2000.
Haaga JR, Lanzieri CF, Gilkeson RC. CT and MR Imaging of the Whole Body. St. Louis, CV Mosby, 2003.
Martin DR, Brown MA, Semelka RC. Primer of MR Imaging of the Abdomen and Pelvis. New York, Wiley, 2005.

McRobbins DW, et al. MRI from Picture to Proton, 2nd ed. New York, Cambridge University Press, 2007.
Mitchell DG, Cohen MS. MRI Principles, 2nd ed. Philadelphia, WB Saunders, 1999.
Schild HH. MRI Made Easy (…Well Almost). Berlin, Schering AG, 1990.

REFERENCES

1. Cowper SE, Rabach M, Girardi M. Clinical and histological findings in nephrogenic systemic fibrosis. Eur J Radiol 2008; 66:191-199.

2. Kuo PH, et al. Gadolinium-based MR contrast agents and nephrogenic systemic fibrosis. Radiology 2007; 242:647-649.

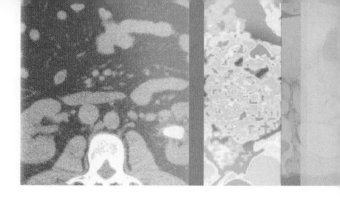

CHAPTER 19

MR Angiography

Garry Choy

TECHNICAL ASPECTS

The imaging of vessels and blood flow remains an active area in both research and clinical settings. A wide variety of techniques for MR angiography (MRA) have been studied and implemented in body imaging as well as brain imaging to diagnose vascular abnormalities. Current clinical techniques for MRA are based on the time-of-flight (TOF) technique, phase-contrast imaging, and contrast enhancement. Each technique has its strengths and limitations.

Time-of-Flight MRA

TOF sequences are often used in conjunction with contrast-enhanced MRA or as an alternative if there are contraindications to gadolinium administration. TOF techniques work by the saturation and suppression of background tissue signal in a region of interest while preserving high signal from protons in flowing blood (bright blood technique). Figure 19-1 is an example of TOF imaging.

TOF Principles

To saturate or suppress the signal from background tissue in a region of interest, TOF sequences utilize a series of rapid slice-selection radiofrequency (RF) excitation pulses such that the longitudinal magnetization is kept at a minimum. Saturated spins therefore appear dark on imaging in contrast to unsaturated spins, which appear bright. Inflow of blood that was outside the imaging slice and unaffected by RF excitation pulses therefore would be unsaturated and appear bright on imaging. The vascular signal actually appears brighter with increasing velocity and volume.

Imaging Parameters

Repetition time, flip angle, slice orientation, and voxel size are additional parameters that can be adjusted to further optimize resolution and signal-to-noise ratio. Presaturation bands upstream and outside the region of interest can also be used to negate the signal from inflow of venous blood. This same technique can also be used to reduce flow-related artifacts or artifacts from respiratory or cardiac motion.

2D versus 3D Sequences

TOF techniques can be performed as a 2D or 3D sequence. The 2D TOF technique involves sequential acquisition of thin sections perpendicular to blood inflow. This technique maximizes inflow effects. On the other hand, 3D TOF techniques have better spatial resolution than those of 2D TOF techniques. The 3D TOF techniques divide the region of interest into partitions that are contiguous with one another and require a longer acquisition time. They also work best only with moderate to high rates of flow. The 2D TOF techniques are more sensitive to slow blood flow, such as that in veins and peripheral arteries. Breath-hold techniques can be better accomplished using 2D TOF techniques. The 3D TOF techniques are less sensitive to loss of signal from turbulent flow than the 2D TOF techniques.

Phase-Contrast MRA

Phase-contrast angiography utilizes phase shift of moving spins relative to stationary spins. Images can be acquired as 2D or 3D images, where 2D is used for scout views or rapid projections and 3D is used for higher resolution. A velocity-encoding gradient is needed to quantitate phase shifts into velocities; the adjustment of the parameters for this gradient is important to tailor imaging of slow or fast flow and to therefore avoid aliasing if velocities are out of range.

Phase-Contrast Imaging Principles

One advantage of phase-contrast imaging is that all motion is used to depict flow and there is better suppression of background images. Phase-contrast images are usually obtained via acquisition of multiple datasets, where the differences between the datasets are due to phase changes

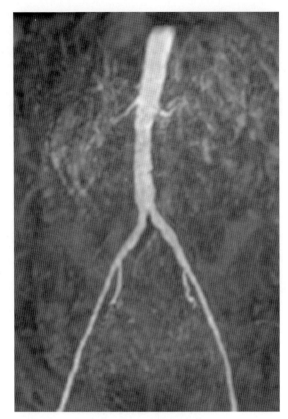

■ FIGURE 19-1 Example of time-of-flight imaging.

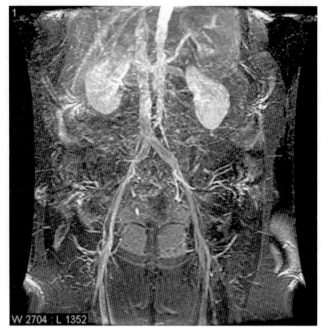

■ FIGURE 19-2 Example of gadolinium contrast-enhanced MRA.

by motion along a chosen axis. To obtain motion along one axis, two datasets must be obtained; and to obtain motion in three dimensions, four datasets must be acquired. The multiple datasets then allow for better depiction of motion, namely, that of spins within flowing blood. In interpreting images produced by phase-contrast techniques, the higher the signal intensity, the higher the velocity. The measurement of phase changes is best if the image is perpendicular to the axis of flow.

2D and 3D Phase-Contrast Imaging

2D phase-contrast imaging is often performed via thick slabs to obtain a fast assessment of flow and used in scout images. Spatial resolution is not optimal given the thick slab but yields important information regarding flow velocities and direction. Background tissue is usually isointense to hypointense. In addition, flow in one direction is hyperintense and flow in the opposite direction is hypointense, yielding directional information.

Imaging using the 3D phase-contrast method offers advantages in demonstrating flow with a higher signal-to-noise ratio and higher spatial resolution. The 3D acquisition of data also allows for reformatted and maximal intensity projection (MIP) images from along any plane and axis, a very useful option in angiography. Thus, 3D phase-contrast imaging can be useful in cerebral artery angiography, peripheral arterial angiography, and visceral/abdominal angiography.

Advantages and Disadvantages

When compared with TOF techniques, phase-contrast imaging has both advantages and disadvantages. Phase-contrast techniques can detect small vessels due to superior background suppression. In TOF imaging, soft tissue structures are often still visible and hematomas or blood products may still appear bright, thereby mimicking blood flow, but in phase-contrast imaging, stationary materials no matter their T1 relaxivity, including fat and blood products (methemoglobin), are dark on imaging. In addition, phase-contrast imaging is also superior for imaging of low-velocity blood flow, which can be seen in venous structures and in aneurysms. Disadvantages of phase-contrast imaging include longer acquisition times; sensitivity to inhomogeneity in the magnetic field, resulting in lower background suppression; and greater sensitivity to complex flow than TOF, resulting in more artifacts in high-grade stenosis or aneurysms.

Contrast-Enhanced MRA

Gadolinium shortens the T1 relaxation of surrounding protons, particularly blood, when injected intravenously, thereby making blood appear bright on T1-weighted images. Gadolinium essentially increases the signal from the intravascular space. In MRA, a bolus of contrast agent is injected and images are acquired serially over a region of interest. Figure 19-2 illustrates an example of gadolinium contrast-enhanced MRA.

Pulse Sequences

Contrast-enhanced MRA is typically performed using 3D Fourier transform gradient-echo techniques. Repetition time (TR) and echo time should be as short as possible when selecting a sequence for contrast-enhanced MRA. The use of the shortest echo time increases coherence of phase and allows for optimal image acquisition. Short TR ensures that the background tissue is as saturated as possible to emphasize the brightness of vessels. Short TR also enables faster imaging and less motion artifact. In addition, because there is a narrow time window to capture the arterial phase, imaging requires fast acquisition times. The flip angle is another parameter that must be adjusted such that the background tissue is saturated; it is usually kept at between 30 and 60 degrees.

Addressing T1 signal from fat is an important principle in MRA. Fat suppression must be performed because fat demonstrates a short T1 relaxation, as do gadolinium-based contrast agents. Postprocessing can also be performed in which unenhanced images can be subtracted from enhanced images to better illustrate vessel enhancement.

Contrast Injection and Bolus Timing

The contrast agent should be injected in a sufficient dose and rate, usually at 2 mL/s, and of variable volume and depends on recommended doses per kilogram of weight by the manufacturer. Generally, higher doses at faster injection rates result in better image quality.

Timing of image acquisition after bolus injection is critical and is typically performed manually depending on the technologist's experience, standard delay timings defined by departmental protocols, or bolus tracking techniques, such as SmartPrep (GE Medical Systems). Scanning too late may result in opacification of the venous vasculature, obscuring the arterial system. Given the emerging risk of nephrogenic systemic fibrosis, proper screening of the patient population must be performed. Techniques such as TOF imaging often can be a useful alternative to contrast-enhanced MRA.

Dynamic or Time-Resolved MRA

Time-resolved MRA involves the serial rapid acquisition of images such that different phases of enhancement can be seen. Images are continually obtained before, during, and after phases of contrast enhancement. The optimal images

---

TABLE 19-1 Advantages of Phase-Contrast Imaging over Time-of-Flight Imaging in Abdominal Imaging Applications

- Phase-contrast imaging has excellent background suppression in the abdomen for better visualization of vessels.
- Phase-contrast imaging allows for quantification: velocity encoding, volume measurements, and directional information.
- 3D and 2D phase-contrast imaging is available; 2D imaging can be used for major vascular structures to assess for patency; 3D acquisitions have an advantage over 2D acquisitions because any plane can be assessed, which is useful to evaluate small to medium-sized abdominal vessels.
- Time-of-flight imaging is not ideal, given the tortuosity of the vessels in the abdomen.

---

can then be retrospectively selected and used for diagnostic interpretation.

PROS AND CONS

Both TOF and phase-contrast techniques can be applied in abdominal MRI. Each technique has its own pros and cons (Table 19-1).

KEY POINTS

■ Current clinical techniques for MR angiography are based on the time-of-flight technique, phase-contrast imaging, and contrast enhancement.

■ Phase-contrast imaging has excellent background suppression in the abdomen for better visualization of vessels.

■ Phase-contrast imaging allows for quantification: velocity encoding, volume measurements, and directional information.

■ 3D and 2D phase-contrast imaging is available; 2D imaging can be used for major vascular structures to assess for patency; 3D acquisitions have an advantage over 2D acquisitions because any plane can be assessed, which is useful to evaluate small to medium-sized abdominal vessels.

■ Time-of-flight imaging is not ideal, given the tortuosity of the vessels in the abdomen.

SUGGESTED READINGS

Edelman ER, et al (eds). Clinical Magnetic Resonance Imaging. Philadelphia, Elsevier, 2006.

Elster AD. Questions and Answers to MRI. St. Louis, CV Mosby, 2000.

Haaga JR, Lanzieri CF, Gilkeson RC. CT and MR Imaging of the Whole Body. St. Louis, CV Mosby, 2003.

Martin DR, Brown MA, Semelka RC. Primer of MR Imaging of the Abdomen and Pelvis. New York, Wiley, 2005.

McRobbins DW, et al. MRI from Picture to Proton, 2nd ed. New York, Cambridge University Press, 2007.

Mitchell DG, Cohen MS. MRI Principles, 2nd ed. Philadelphia, WB Saunders, 1999.

Schild HH. MRI Made Easy (...Well Almost). Berlin, Schering AG, 1990.

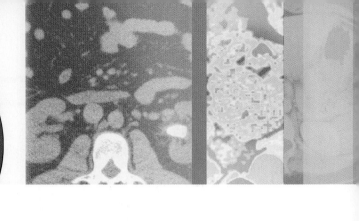

CHAPTER 20

Advanced MRI Applications

Garry Choy

TECHNICAL ASPECTS

MRI has evolved significantly since its infancy, with major advances in hardware, software, coil developments, sequence development, and contrast agents. Industry and academia continue to advance the field with continued exciting emerging technologies. The discussion in this chapter focuses on the recent emergence of parallel imaging, high field strength 3.0-T clinical scanners, dedicated contrast agents, perfusion and dynamic contrast-enhanced MRI, and diffusion-weighted imaging techniques.

Parallel Imaging

Parallel MRI techniques have been introduced by most vendors. Parallel MRI methods allow for faster imaging. In parallel imaging, multiple independent receiver (phase-array) coils placed in a configuration around the subject enable acquisition of fewer data to avoid aliasing in order to generate an image. In addition to reducing scan time, the advantages of parallel imaging include higher spatial resolution, less motion artifact on single-shot sequences, and reduced specific absorption rate. Parallel imaging techniques can be particularly utilized on higher field strength magnets to reduce the specific absorption rate.

Clinical High Field Strength Imaging with 3.0-T Imaging

In the past few years, there have been numerous installations of the latest high field strength 3.0-T clinical scanners at various institutions around the world. In addition to research purposes, there has been increasing use of 3.0-T scanners in clinical settings. High field strength imaging with 3.0 T offers significantly higher signal-to-noise ratio in abdominal tissues, particularly when compared with currently widely available 1.5-T scanning.[1,2] In 3.0-T imaging, there is approximately a twofold increase in signal-to-noise ratio.[2,3] Many studies have examined the use of 3.0-T

scanners in musculoskeletal and neurologic imaging applications.

Various technical issues are unique to 3.0 T imaging. For example, there is an increased specific absorption rate of approximately four times the radiofrequency deposition when compared with 1.5 T. Chemical and susceptibility artifacts are also increased significantly. Given that there is an increased field strength, the T1 relaxation time is also increased for most tissues. The T2* relaxation of tissues is shorter, and that of T2 is nearly identical. Studies are still ongoing in high field strength body imaging and show significant promise.

Novel Tissue-Specific Contrast Agents

Liver-Specific MRI Contrast Agents

In recent years, liver-specific MRI contrast agents have been developed specifically targeted to hepatocytes or reticuloendothelial cells, providing either positive or negative enhancement after intravenous administration. Hepatocyte-specific contrast agents include mangafodipir trisodium and two gadolinium chelates: gadoxetic acid and gadobenate dimeglumine. Reticuloendothelial cell–specific agents include superparamagnetic iron oxides (SPIOs): ferumoxides and ferucarbon. The currently available liver-specific MRI contrast agents and their availability globally are listed in Table 20-1.

Mangafodipir Trisodium

Manganese (mangafodipir trisodium [Mn-DPDP; Teslascan]) is similar to gadolinium and is strongly paramagnetic. Manganese is cleared from the body primarily by biliary or intestinal secretion. It appears to have an affinity for metabolically active tissues, including primarily the liver, and has been marketed with U.S. Food and Drug Administration (FDA) approval for liver lesion characterization. Mangafodipir trisodium contains Mn^{2+}, a transitional element that exhibits paramagnetic properties due to five unpaired electrons and shortens the T1 relaxation

123

TABLE 20-1 Liver-Specific MR Contrast Agents

Name	Cell Specificity	Current Status
Mangafodipir trisodium [Mn-DPDP] (Teslascan)	Hepatocyte	Approved in United States and European Union
Gadoxetic acid [Gd-EOB-DTPA] (Primovist)	Hepatocyte	Approved in Sweden; completed phase 3 trials in United States
Gadobenate dimeglumine [Gd-BOPTA] (MultiHance)	Hepatocyte	Approved in European Union
Ferumoxides (Feridex)	Reticuloendothelial cell	Approved in United States
Ferucarbotran (Resovist)	Reticuloendothelial cell	Approved in European Union

time. Because of its chemical similarity to vitamin B_6, it is specifically taken up by hepatocytes. However, evidence exists that metabolic products of this compound are also responsible for selective uptake into liver, pancreas, and cardiac muscle.[4] This compound is administered through slow intravenous infusion over 2 to 5 minutes, and the effect is seen within a few minutes (about 15 minutes) and lasts for 24 hours. The adverse events commonly reported include facial flushing and a sensation of heat. The prolonged imaging window makes this agent a good choice for imaging the liver. The signal intensity of normal liver parenchyma is increased, providing high lesion-to-liver contrast. This helps in detecting small liver lesions.[5] This agent may be taken up by well-differentiated hepatocellular carcinoma and thus may mask the tumor. Mangafodipir trisodium is best used for the detection of metastases. During the later phases, it is excreted into bile and provides excellent details of the biliary ducts and aids in the diagnosis of various biliary pathologic processes such as biliary obstruction and bile leaks.

Gadolinium Chelates

Two gadolinium chelates exhibit liver specificity owing to their selective uptake by hepatocytes through a carrier-mediated transport across the cell membrane. These include gadoxetic acid (Gd-EOB-DTPA; Primovist) and gadobenate dimeglumine benzyloxy-propionic tetraacetic acid (Gd-BOPTA; MultiHance). These agents are excreted into the bile unaltered and are ultimately excreted through urine and feces. After intravenous administration, these agents have an initial intravascular phase similar to that of other gadolinium chelates and during the later phase they accumulate in the liver parenchyma and increase the signal intensity of the liver. Thus, the lesion-to-liver contrast is increased and these agents aid in the detection of small liver lesions. The initial intravascular phase helps in characterization of liver lesions similar to that obtained with any other gadolinium chelate. Similar to mangafodipir trisodium, these agents provide excellent details of the biliary ducts during the delayed phase.

Ferumoxides

SPIO nanoparticles are the basis for agents known as ferumoxides (Feridex, Combidex).[6] Ferumoxides are composed of a central iron oxide particle—Fe_2O_3—which is a superparamagnetic compound surrounded by a dextran coating. These agents have a greater magnetic susceptibility than conventional gadolinium-based contrast agents. Their dominant effect is preferentially on T2 and T2* shortening rather than T1 shortening. Water near these particles therefore becomes dephased by local inhomogeneities, resulting in signal loss and thus acting as a negative contrast agent.

Of note, these agents should be infused slowly over a period of 30 minutes to avoid cardiovascular effects and lumbar pain. Specificity of particles depends on the size of the particle because the amount of contrast depends on the degree of uptake by the Kupffer cells. For instance, SPIOs are preferentially taken up by Kupffer cells in the liver, whereas ultra-small iron oxide particles (USPIOs) are taken up by macrophages in lymph nodes, liver, lung, and spleen. Similar to mangafodipir trisodium, these agents provide prolonged periods of time for imaging after intravenous infusion, facilitating higher-resolution thin-section imaging.

One agent, Feridex, approved by the FDA since 1996, acts as a negative contrast agent when imaging hepatic lesions and may enable detection of smaller lesions.[7,8] Ferumoxtran-10 (Combidex) is another type of investigational SPIO-based agent that aims to differentiate normal lymph nodes from lymph nodes with metastatic cancer involvement.[9] With potential applications in breast cancer and prostate cancer, clinical studies have thus far demonstrated that Combidex uptake occurs preferentially in normal lymph nodes; as a result, any lymph node with retained signal intensity would be of concern for metastatic disease.

Ferucarbotran

Similar to ferumoxides, ferucarbotran (Resovist) contains both a polycrystalline iron oxide core (Fe_2O_3 and Fe_2O_4) and a carbodextran coating. Unlike ferumoxides, this agent can be safely injected as a bolus with significantly fewer adverse cardiovascular events or back pain. Ferucarbotran improves focal liver lesion detection on T2- and T2*-weighted sequences.

Blood-Pool Contrast Agents

Macromolecular contrast agents, namely, blood pool agents, are also being developed for vascular and perfusion imaging. Another dedicated contrast agent, gadobenate dimeglumine (Gd-BOPTA), is used in the imaging of liver malignancies.[10,11] The structure of gadobenate dimeglumine is similar to that of the commonly used gadolinium diethylenetriamine pentaacetic acid (Gd-DTPA), with the addition of a benzene ring and short carbon chain, allowing the agent to be preferentially localized to hepatocytes. Gadobenate dimeglumine is typically seen to demonstrate uptake into hepatocytes and excretion into the biliary system at 30 to 120 minutes.

Because gadobenate meglumine circulates in the intravascular space for a longer period of time, there is a significant reduction in T1 relaxation time of blood containing the agent. Therefore, MR angiography has become a useful application for this contrast agent. Although these agents do not diffuse through normal capillary wall, they can diffuse through defective capillaries commonly found in tumor vasculature, possibly playing a role in measuring the permeability of tumor microvasculature. For example, Gadomer-17 is a polymeric compound with a high molecular weight that due to its hydration properties has already demonstrated utility in measuring myocardial perfusion and in tumor imaging. Interestingly, although not yet ready for clinical use, novel agents involving the chelation of ligands such as antibodies to gadolinium for targeted imaging are undergoing active preclinical development.

Lymph Node–Specific MRI Contrast Agents

Lymph node–specific contrast agents are also actively being developed. Although not yet approved, these agents demonstrate significant promise in the evaluation of lymph node involvement in the setting of malignancies. For example, much promise has already been demonstrated in differentiating benign from malignant lymph nodes in prostate cancer using USPIO agents. The smaller size of USPIOs compared with SPIOs as well as their hydrophilic coating results in longer circulation in the intravascular space and rapid accumulation in the reticuloendothelial system. Therefore, as these particles are phagocytosed by macrophages, they accumulate in the lymphatic system, resulting in signal drop on T2* images in normal lymph node tissue. However, malignant involvement is devoid of macrophages, resulting in a higher signal intensity. Typically, it takes 24 to 36 hours for the contrast agent to accumulate in lymph nodes and, thus, postcontrast imaging is usually obtained 24 hours after its administration. The currently available contrast agent in this group for research use is ferumoxtran/AMI-227. Another agent also under investigation is gadofluorine-M.

Diffusion-Weighted Imaging in the Abdomen

Until recently, diffusion-weighted imaging (DWI) has been implemented mainly in brain imaging and has made a significant impact on imaging in stroke patients. Introduction of DWI techniques in the body have recently demonstrated potential. For example, DWI techniques have been applied to differentiate benign from malignant lesions in the liver.[12,13] Malignant liver tumors, probably due to increased cellular density and to altered nuclear-to-cytoplasmic ratios, exhibit restricted water molecule diffusion and therefore reduced apparent diffusion coefficients (ADCs) when compared with benign lesions. Because of the variation of sequences available by vendors and the extremely high sensitivity of DWI measurements

to motion, this technique is extremely operator dependent.

Perfusion Imaging and Dynamic Contrast-Enhanced MRI

Whereas standard cross-sectional imaging techniques solely focus on morphology, another technique that moves beyond anatomy and into physiologic or functional assessment includes the use of dynamic contrast-enhanced MRI (DCE-MRI).[14,15] In the literature and various investigations, this technique has been applied to the evaluation of tumor neovasculature. Kinetic modeling of imaging data plays an important role for DCE-MRI, because quantitative parameters allow for the characterization of physiologic data such as blood volume, vascular permeability, and vessel density. DCE-MRI holds significant promise in monitoring the effect of antiangiogenic agents because morphologic changes in tumor size often lag behind physiologic changes, which can be better characterized by enhancement characteristics.

CONTROVERSIES

In addition to the emerging risk of nephrogenic systemic fibrosis related to gadolinium-based agents, newer contrast agents are not without potential risks. Iron oxide nanoparticles are taken up by macrophages in the reticuloendothelial system involving the liver, spleen, and bone marrow. The long-term effects of nanoparticle presence in the reticuloendothelial system are not completely clear at this time, but preclinical evaluations of SPIOs and USPIOs showed satisfactory and safe clinical profiles according to current pharmacologic and toxicologic tests. Reported symptoms have included, but are not limited to, rash, dyspnea, chest pain, and back pain, but no serious adverse effects have been reported thus far. Many of these promising nanoparticle-based agents are currently undergoing FDA evaluation.

KEY POINTS

- Parallel imaging allows for faster imaging, higher spatial resolution, less motion artifact, and lower specific absorption rate.
- Novel tissue-specific contrast agents serve as new tools to characterize tissues.
- Lymph node–specific contrast agents are also actively being developed. Although not yet approved, these agents demonstrate significant promise in the evaluation of lymph node involvement in malignancy.
- Perfusion and dynamic contrast-enhanced MRI enables physiologic and functional assessment of tissues, such as in monitoring the effects of antiangiogenic agents on tumor vasculature.

SUGGESTED READINGS

Edelman ER, et al (eds). Clinical Magnetic Resonance Imaging. Philadelphia, Elsevier, 2006.

Elster AD. Questions and Answers to MRI. St. Louis, CV Mosby, 2000.

Haaga JR, Lanzieri CF, Gilkeson RC. CT and MR Imaging of the Whole Body. St. Louis, CV Mosby, 2003.

Martin DR, Brown MA, Semelka RC. Primer of MR Imaging of the Abdomen and Pelvis. New York, Wiley, 2005.

REFERENCES

1. Fenchel M, Nael K, Seeger A, et al. Whole-body magnetic resonance angiography at 3.0 Tesla. Eur Radiol 2008; 18:1473-1483.
2. Schindera ST, et al. Abdominal magnetic resonance imaging at 3.0 T: what is the ultimate gain in signal-to-noise ratio? Acad Radiol 2006; 13:1236-1243.
3. Merkle EM, Dale BM. Abdominal MRI at 3.0 T: the basics revisited. AJR Am J Roentgenol 2006; 186:1524-1532.
4. Toft KG, Hustvedt SO, Grant D, et al. Metabolism of mangafodipir trisodium (MnDPDP), a new contrast medium for magnetic resonance imaging, in beagle dogs. Eur J Drug Metab Pharmacokinet 1997; 22:65-72.
5. Oudkerk M, Torres CG, Song B, et al. Characterization of liver lesions with mangafodipir trisodium-enhanced MR imaging: multicenter study comparing MR and dual-phase spiral CT. Radiology 2002; 223:517-524.
6. Saokar A, Braschi M, Harisinghani M. Lymphotrophic nanoparticle enhanced MR imaging (LNMRI) for lymph node imaging. Abdom Imaging 2006; 31:660-667.
7. Wen G, et al. Superparamagnetic iron oxide (Feridex)-enhanced MRI in diagnosis of focal hepatic lesions. Di Yi Jun Yi Da Xue Xue Bao 2002; 22:451-452.
8. Clement O, et al. Liver imaging with ferumoxides (Feridex): fundamentals, controversies, and practical aspects. Top Magn Reson Imaging 1998; 9:167-182.
9. Harisinghani MG, et al. Noninvasive detection of clinically occult lymph-node metastases in prostate cancer. N Engl J Med 2003; 348:2491-2499.
10. Kirchin MA, Pirovano GP, Spinazzi A. Gadobenate dimeglumine (Gd-BOPTA): an overview. Invest Radiol 1998; 33:798-809.
11. Pavone P, et al. Improvement of vascular signal intensity in contrast-enhanced MRA with Gd-BOPTA: comparison with Gd-DTPA. Acad Radiol 2002; 9(Suppl 1):S134.
12. Ichikawa T, et al. Diffusion-weighted MR imaging with a single-shot echoplanar sequence: detection and characterization of focal hepatic lesions. AJR Am J Roentgenol 1998; 170:397-402.
13. Yoshikawa T, et al. ADC measurement of abdominal organs and lesions using parallel imaging technique. AJR Am J Roentgenol 2006; 187:1521-1530.
14. Rosen MA, Schnall MB. Dynamic contrast-enhanced magnetic resonance imaging for assessing tumor vascularity and vascular effects of targeted therapies in renal cell carcinoma. Clin Cancer Res 2007; 13:770s-776s.
15. Taylor JS, et al. MR imaging of tumor microcirculation: promise for the new millennium. J Magn Reson Imaging 1999; 10:903-907.

SECTION

FIVE

Positron Emission Tomography and Co-Registered PET/CT

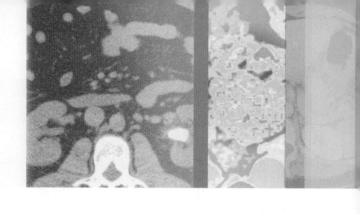

CHAPTER 21

PET/CT Technique and Instrumentation

Michael Blake and Michael Moore

TECHNICAL ASPECTS

PET/CT represents the successful technical combination of multidetector computed tomography (MDCT) and positron emission tomography (PET) into a single scanner. PET with the fluorine-18 (^{18}F)–labeled glucose analog fluorodeoxyglucose (FDG) provides metabolic imaging of tissues, both normal and diseased. FDG-PET provides valuable qualitative and quantitative metabolic information for both diagnosis and management. PET has been shown to be of value in diagnosing and staging malignant tumors as well as in follow-up oncologic imaging after surgical, radiation, or chemotherapeutic treatment.[1] However, the sensitivity of PET at detecting hypermetabolic foci is compromised in large part by the low background FDG uptake when attempting accurate anatomic localization.[2] The lack of readily identifiable and reliable anatomic structures on PET is particularly true for abdominal and pelvic imaging regions in which variable physiologic FDG uptake also poses issues.

Current CT provides rapidly acquired datasets of high spatial resolution. This gives multiplanar information regarding the morphologic features and attenuation values of both normal anatomy and pathologic lesions. The clinical use of CT is burgeoning, and it is the modality of choice for much cross-sectional imaging, particularly of oncologic entities. A major weakness of CT, however, is its dependence on changes in the size, shape, or attenuation values of a structure to detect pathologic processes.

Separate CT and PET scans of the same patient acquired on different scanners can certainly be aligned using a number of available software methods, but the algorithms are often labor intensive and, particularly in the abdomen, may fail to provide a satisfactory overlap. However, combined imaging with PET/CT allows for the precise structural information provided by CT to accurately locate the hypermetabolic foci identified with PET and thereby improve the overall diagnostic performance (Fig. 21-1). The information from combined PET/CT also facilitates identification of physiologic from pathologic uptake and diminishes the false-negative and false-positive interpretations of the individual components. Both modalities have individual strengths that are also highly complementary. Indeed, it has been shown that PET/CT is more accurate for many oncologic entities than either CT or PET alone.[3] Furthermore, PET has the potential to be used with different radiotracers other than FDG to provide other useful biologic information, whereas CT provides useful information about the behavior of orally and intravenously administered contrast agents.

Instrumentation Considerations

The first PET/CT prototype scanner was revealed in 1998.[4] Subsequently, the first clinical scanners appeared in 2001, and by early 2007 more than 800 combined PET/CTs had been installed in clinical institutions worldwide. Essentially all new PET machine sales are now as PET/CT scanners.[3] Although there are technical differences between the various commercial manufacturers, the basic PET/CT format has generally remained similar, namely, a single unit containing aligned separate diagnostic PET and CT scanners, usually with a single common patient bed.

The automatic and more accurate co-registration of the structural and metabolic data is just one of the inherent advantages of hybrid PET/CT machines. PET-only whole-body scans traditionally required up to 45 to 60 minutes to complete. The transmission scan that is required for attenuation correction to improve the qualitative and quantitative accuracy of PET is a major contributor to this long scan time.[5] However, CT-based attenuation correction is significantly quicker than traditional PET transmission methods and can provide almost noise-free information and allows for total PET/CT scanning durations of 20 to 30 minutes or less. This greatly reduced scanning time enhances patient comfort and convenience and also allows a greater patient throughput. The current emission PET scan time may now also be decreased by the use of

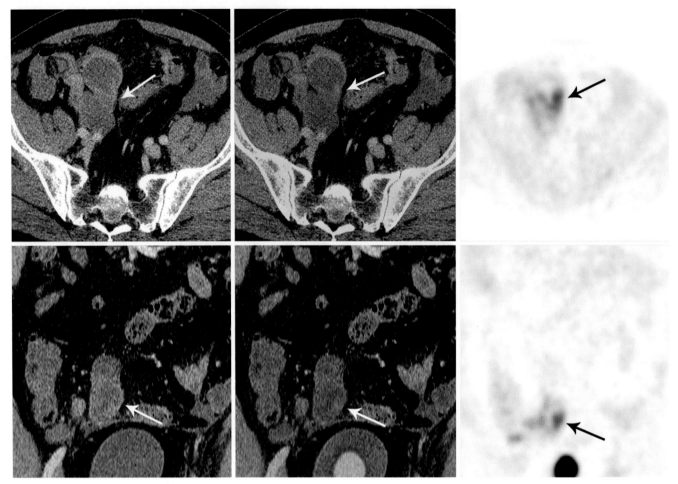

■ **FIGURE 21-1** Value of precise localization and complementary strengths. Appendiceal adenocarcinoma. Markedly dilated appendix with thick wall and communication with cecum shows increased FDG uptake (*arrows*) along its wall. Without the PET findings, the CT finding might have been overlooked with the dilated appendix mimicking a large bowel loop. Without the CT findings, the PET activity would not have been precisely localized and may have possibly been misinterpreted as physiologic bowel activity.

time-of-flight (TOF) technology, which shortens scan time and improves signal-to-noise ratio.[6]

Feasible TOF can now be applied owing to the newer fast scintillators with high stopping power such as lutetium oxyorthosilicate (LSO) and LYSO (which is LSO with the addition of a small percentage of yttrium).[7] TOF makes use of the ability of the new scanners to measure the arrival time difference between the two positron annihilation-generated photons reaching the detectors to within a certain resolution. Recent detector and scintillator developments allow sub-nanosecond coincidence timing resolution, which provides a rapid, TOF-based and back-projection-free, 3D reconstruction algorithm that, combined with real-time data acquisition and a quick detector encoding scheme, permits high-quality images to be obtained in a significantly reduced time, particularly in nonobese patients.[8] The stability of these new scanners in practice has yet to be confirmed; and although encouraging and interesting, the precise clinical contribution of TOF PET has yet to be determined. Certainly, high spatial resolution PET detectors appear to optimize the conspicuity of FDG uptake in small lesions.

From the late 1980s until recently, the bismuth germanate (BGO) block detector was the standard for PET. However, the introduction of new faster scintillators with greater light output and shorter decay time than BGO such as gadolinium oxyorthosilicate (GSO) and LSO (and LYSO) has recently improved the performance of PET scanners for clinical imaging. The faster scintillators decrease the coincidence timing window and thus the random coincidence rate. The improved light output of the new scintillators makes the energy resolution more accurate by reducing the statistical uncertainty of the measurement. This higher light output also improves the positioning accuracy of a block detector, with potential spatial resolution benefits.

The block design developed by Casey and Nutt has been the basic detector component in all multi-ring PET scanners for the past 2 decades. The first multi-ring PET scanners incorporated septa between the detector rings to shield the detectors from scattered photons out of the transverse plane, thus not allowing 3D reconstruction algorithms. The first multi-ring PET scanners with retractable septa that included the capability to acquire data in either the 2D or 3D mode appeared in the early 1990s. The advantages of 3D imaging for the brain are widely accepted, but 3D imaging for the rest of the body has posed more problems. Recently, however, statistically based reconstruction algorithms, more accurate scatter correction methods,[9] and faster scintillators have significantly improved the achievable whole-body 3D imaging quality; 2D imaging may still be more suitable for large patients, however. Increased axial coverage makes better use of the emitted radiation for a given volume of scintillator. For most PET/CT scanners, axial PET coverage is about 15 cm, ranging up to a recently extended 21.6 cm, with resulting imaging advantages.

Technique Considerations

PET/CT continues to be an evolving new modality and, as such, accepted optimal protocols are not yet established. There is still debate, for example, regarding the use of oral and intravenous contrast material and the optimal respiratory phase to scan as well as the most appropriate CT scanning parameters.[10-12] FDG-PET provides quantitative information in the form of the standardized uptake value (SUV). SUV estimation requires attenuation correction to avoid the variability in FDG uptake depending on the tumor depth beneath the skin. As mentioned earlier, CT images are used for attenuation correction of the PET emission data, eliminating the need for a separate lengthy PET transmission scan with much less statistical noise. However, there is also a potential risk of overestimating the true FDG activity with this technique. In normal structures, including bone and soft tissues, this is unlikely to be problematic.[10] However, very dense structures on CT such as metallic prostheses, surgical clips, and devices as well as high-density oral and intravenous contrast can result in overcorrection with subsequent artifact formation. As a consequence, the corresponding photopenic areas on PET may manifest artifactually as hypermetabolic foci. This can usually be recognized by reviewing the nonattenuation corrected PET images. These artifacts, however, may also obscure true foci of abnormal activity on the attenuation-corrected images, although they are most intense at areas of contrast influx, such as the subclavian vein, outside the abdomen. A saline flush after intravenous injection of a contrast agent may reduce attenuation correction PET artifacts. Recent reports have suggested that the changes in attenuation correction wrought by intravenous contrast agents are neither statistically or clinically significant.[11] This is reassuring because intravenous contrast agents are regularly used in CT to augment the contrast between normal and abnormal tissues and thus increase the ease of interpretation. They give useful information about the patency (Fig. 21-2), course, and relations of vessels (Fig. 21-3) and also dynamic data regarding tissue enhancement, perfusion, and de-enhancement.

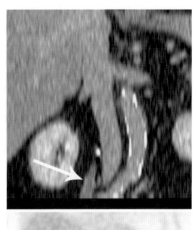
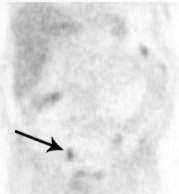

■ **FIGURE 21-2** Value of intravenous contrast: patency. Dilated nonenhancing gonadal vein (*arrow*) consistent with gonadal vein thrombosis, which may have been overlooked if an intravenous contrast agent had not been given because there is no corresponding FDG uptake. *Arrow* indicates ureteric-excreted FDG activity on PET alone.

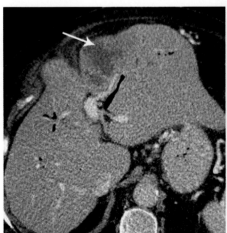
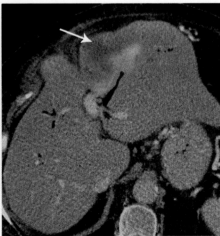
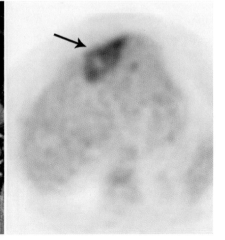

■ **FIGURE 21-3** Intravenous contrast value: vascular relationships. FDG-positive hepatic cholangiocarcinoma with the CT images precisely showing the tumor's relationship to the portal vein and its branches (*arrow*). The PET image cannot provide this high spatial resolution information regarding lesion location and the relationships necessary for surgical planning.

Modifications to the basic scaling algorithm[13] have been introduced to distinguish oral contrast enhancement from bone, and strategies have been developed that minimize problems due to both intravenous and oral contrast material. The modified algorithm can also somewhat reduce artifacts due to metallic objects in the patient. Because the attenuation values are energy dependent, the correction factors derived from a CT scan at mean photon energy of 70 keV must be scaled to the PET energy of 511 keV. Scaling algorithms typically use a bilinear function to transform the attenuation values above and below a given threshold with different factors. The scaled CT images are then interpolated from CT to PET spatial resolution, followed by re-projection of the interpolated images. Alternatively, fully optimized contrast-enhanced CT can be performed after initial low-mAs PET/CT without intravenous contrast agent administration for attenuation correction, although this may increase radiation exposure to the patient.

Oral contrast agents are also routinely used in CT to assist the CT diagnosis of both gastrointestinal tract–related and neighboring pathologic conditions. In the past, these were generally positive, dense substances including barium and Gastrografin compounds. This again leads to the potential production of erroneous hypermetabolic foci after CT-based attenuation correction. Furthermore, the distribution of such agents may change position owing to peristalsis between the CT used for attenuation correction and the PET components, a further potential confounding phenomenon. Accordingly, some authors support the use of water-attenuation oral contrast agents[14] or even not using any oral agent at all. However, clearly, oral contrast is helpful for CT interpretation and, as with intravenous contrast agents, there is growing consensus that dilute concentrations of even positive oral contrast agents do not significantly alter PET/CT attenuation correction.[15] Optimal PET/CT allows for the ability to delineate the bowel on the CT component and thus differentiate FDG uptake in the colon from adjacent tumor sites (Fig. 21-4).

Diagnostic CT carries with it a significant radiation dose to patients. When integrating a full-dose CT, with a tube current of 100 to 140 mA, the radiation dose for a scan from the head to the top of the thighs is 15 to 20 mSv. It has been shown that much lower tube currents, with a range of 10 to 40 mA, are adequate for CT-based attenuation correction.[16] Such low-dose scans confer a significantly lower radiation dose, 3 to 4 mSv, to patients, but it

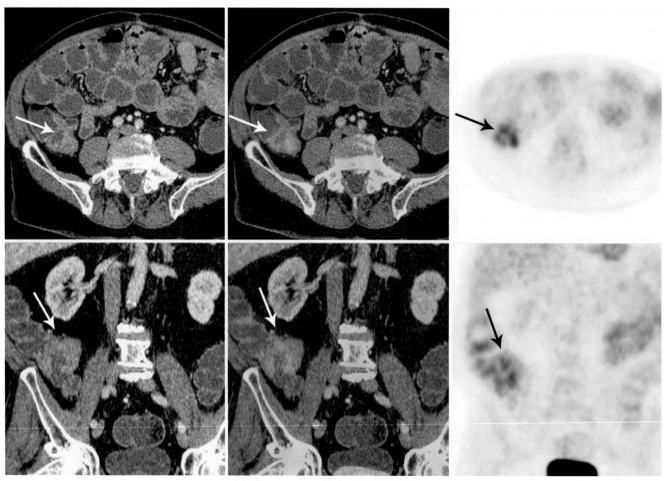

■ **FIGURE 21-4** Oral contrast value. Marked focal uptake in the right lower quadrant corresponding to circumferential mural soft tissue thickening in the colon due to a colorectal carcinoma (*arrow*). Orally administered contrast agent helps with the identification of the cause of the focal FDG uptake.

is doubtful if such scans are sufficient to allow accurate CT-based interpretation owing to the increased noise level and suboptimal image quality.

As discussed earlier, a major benefit of PET/CT over its individual components is the ability to more accurately localize a focus of hypermetabolic activity. When the individual PET and CT components are superimposed or co-registered on the workstation, there should be appropriate alignment of the two datasets. The advantage of combined imaging is that potential misregistration due to patient motion, bowel motility, and urinary tract distention is minimized by the single examination. However, differing respiratory phases may lead to significant misregistration. Standard diagnostic CT studies are usually performed during a maximal inspiration breath-hold, a technique ideal for chest imaging. Although some patients may not be able to breath-hold sufficiently long for a whole-body CT, resulting in motion artifact in the later scanned body parts, modern multislice CT scanners, including 64-slice machines, are capable of faster whole-body scan times and should allow scan durations within a single breath-hold in the majority of cases. PET studies have average bed acquisition times of 3 to 5 minutes, which are too long for a single breath-hold and are thus acquired with the patient quietly breathing. Employing these two differing techniques usually results in marked misregistration of the diaphragm and adjacent organs. The most prominent respiratory artifact causes a scalloped appearance of the superior hepatic and splenic borders, generating problems of lesion localization in the lung base or liver dome. Respiratory misregistration can also affect the inferior margins of the upper abdominal organs, resulting in lesion misregistration between the inferior margins of the liver, kidney, and spleen and adjacent bowel. Respiratory artifacts can be exacerbated with older scanners that utilize a slower CT component. Again with faster 16-slice or higher CT units, these artifacts are usually less marked.

The most appropriate CT breathing protocol remains to be agreed upon. During quiet free breathing, the diaphragm is most commonly in the position of end-tidal volume, and it has been shown that performing CT during a suspended end-tidal breath-hold allows for the most accurate image registration.[17] Technologists must instruct and practice with the patient so that breathing instructions are understood before the CT component is performed. However, others, including pulmonary imaging investigators at our institution, have demonstrated that good PET and CT alignment is also possible with mid-suspended breath-hold and quiet breathing, as well as end-expiration, without statistical difference.[18] However, an inspiratory scan is indeed optimal for chest parenchymal evaluation, and manual and mental adjustment of registration is certainly possible during interpretation if the primary scan is obtained during inspiration and, if necessary, additional selected chest images may also be obtained. In addition to respiratory artifacts, misregistration artifacts can also occur in the abdomen as a result of shifting positions of bowel over the course of the PET portion of the study. One must be aware of these potential misregistration artifacts when interpreting the examination. In the future, respiratory gating software may help to eliminate many of these artifacts.

Having acquired the desired PET and CT datasets, it is then mandatory that the scans be interpreted on a dedicated PET/CT workstation. An accurate interpretation of the study requires the ability to simultaneously review the CT data, including multiplanar reconstructions with various window settings, together with both the non-attenuation-corrected and attenuation-corrected PET data as well as with the superimposed co-registered images. All this, as well as the ability to compare with prior PET or PET/CT studies, generally requires a dedicated PET/CT workstation.

Protocols in Practice

Given the multiple variables to decide on for a protocol for an abdominopelvic PET/CT evaluation, ranging from low-radiation dose nonenhanced CT to a fully diagnostic CT study employing both oral and intravenous contrast, and given the issues and potential artifacts from these various factors, it is apparent why a definitive, standardized protocol has not yet been agreed upon in the literature or practice. In our institution, we combine the two aforementioned approaches.[19] We first acquire a low-radiation dose, nonenhanced CT image mainly to provide attenuation correction for the PET images. Then the PET is performed, followed by a fully diagnostic standard radiation dose, intravenous contrast–enhanced CT with a neutral density oral contrast.[20] We believe that this approach optimizes the diagnostic information from the study and reduces the potential artifact risk.

Patients are kept fasting for a minimum of 6 hours before the test. Because FDG is a glucose analog, its uptake and its distribution in tissues are affected by serum glucose and insulin levels such that low levels of both are desirable. An elevated blood glucose level has been shown to decrease FDG uptake within tumors. Water intake is, however, encouraged, together with regular bladder voiding, to aid renal tract excretion because FDG, unlike glucose, is excreted by the urinary tract. In addition to fasting, patients with diabetes should not receive regular insulin within the 4-hour period before the study. The serum glucose level should be less than 200 mg/dL, and if it is higher than this level then available options include gentle exercise and then a recheck, administration of subcutaneous insulin and rechecking the serum glucose value after approximately 3 hours, or rescheduling the examination.

After an appropriate glucose range is confirmed, FDG is administered intravenously at a dose of 140 μCi/kg. Patients are given up to 1350 mL of neutral density oral contrast to drink over 45 minutes.

While waiting the 60 minutes (some centers wait 90 minutes) between FDG administration and subsequent imaging, patients are encouraged to rest and activities including talking, chewing, and walking are discouraged. Then the PET/CT scan is obtained as described earlier with the following additional details. The patient is positioned in the scanner with arms up (except for scanning head and neck cancer patients). If a patient is unable to tolerate the arms-up position for imaging, the arms may then be positioned in front of the body, resting on the thighs or abdomen. Above-head hand grips, as commonly used in radiation therapy practice, can facilitate the arms-up position for PET/CT. These can also help keep the patient immobile and comfortable throughout the scan. The PET scan is performed as a series of acquisitions at discrete bed positions. For high-resolution imaging of lung disease, respiratory gating can be applied to the PET scan. The CT scan from the base of the brain to the upper thigh can be acquired in less than 20 seconds, and the PET scan with an extended field of view (FOV) system requires just five bed positions at 2 to 3 minutes per position, depending primarily on patient weight. The practical advantages of an FOV scanner include fewer bed positions needed, reduced scan times, and overall better image quality for larger patients owing to the 78% increase in sensitivity. These faster scanning protocols with extended FOV scanners lead to improved patient compliance with less reported claustrophobia and reduced movement, with the added advantage of increased patient throughput. The extended FOV is particularly beneficial when scanning the entire body, as is desirable when scanning patients with melanoma. This range can be covered in less than 25 minutes and only 11 bed positions with an extended FOV.[21] Injected dose can then be reduced with an up to 50% radiation exposure decrease to the patient.

Specific pelvic imaging–oriented technical details need to address the issues related to physiologic bowel and urinary FDG uptake and their dynamic patterns on both PET and CT. The patient should be well hydrated for the study and have voided completely immediately before starting image acquisition to reduce the FDG/high urinary content as much as possible. The administration of diuretics or placement of Foley catheters is not commonly performed at present. Particularly in patients with specific clinical pelvis-related questions, the pelvis should be imaged at the beginning of the study to achieve the shortest time interval between the CT and PET components at this level, to best achieve similar bladder size, volume, and shape on both imaging modalities (Fig. 21-5).

PROS AND CONS

As we have discussed, there are, in general, many major advantages and few disadvantages with PET/CT compared with the separate performance of both individual components. The convenience to the patient and the referring physician of a single setting examination is clear. The integration of nuclear medicine and radiology is welcome for improved patient care although it poses some logistic issues regarding interpretation and reports.

CONTROVERSIES

PET/CT continues to be an evolving new modality, and accepted optimal protocols are not yet established. As discussed earlier, there is ongoing debate regarding the use of oral and intravenous contrast material and the optimal respiratory phase to scan as well as the most

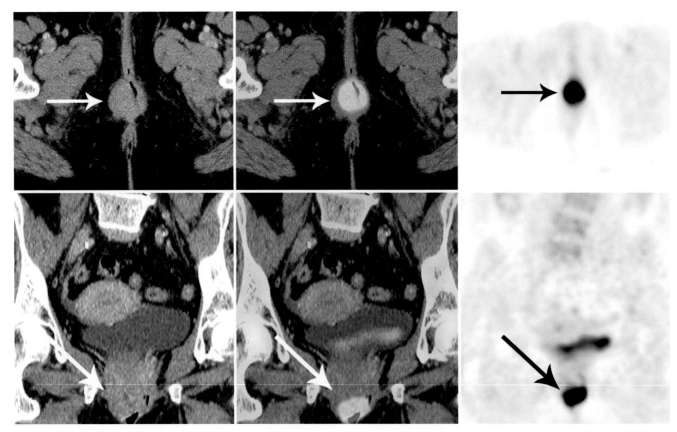

■ **FIGURE 21-5** Pelvic PET/CT considerations. Intense FDG uptake (*arrow*) in lower pelvis corresponding to soft tissue mass on CT and PET/CT images in this postmenopausal woman with a vaginal carcinoma. Ideally, the pelvis should be imaged at the beginning of the PET study to achieve the shortest time interval between the noncontrast CT and PET components at this level and to best achieve similar bladder size, volume, and shape on both imaging modalities. On occasion, bladder catheterization may be helpful to keep the bladder empty throughout the PET and both the noncontrast and contrast-enhanced CT acquisitions.

appropriate CT scanning quality. There are also logistic controversies regarding PET/CT, including billing, training required for interpretation, and the desirable number of reports. We believe that both components of PET/CT should be optimized while mutually not compromising the performance of the other.

SUMMARY

The first commercial PET/CT scanner was put into clinical use just several years ago, and the technology is still evolving. However, advances in both PET and CT can fortunately be relatively easily applied to the combined scanner design. For PET, the recent introduction of new scintillator materials, detector strategies, and electronics has led to overall enhanced PET performance. Concurrently, the spiraling number of detector rows, reduction in rotation time, and resulting benefits in speed and resolution have revolutionized CT performance. PET/CT allows for easier recognition of normal variants and better character-

ization of subtle findings on both components of the examination. The combination of state of the art PET and CT in PET/CT results in a powerful oncologic imaging modality.

KEY POINTS

■ Combined imaging with PET/CT scanners enables fusion of the CT-acquired morphologic information with the PET-provided functional imaging.
■ The recent introduction of new scintillator materials, detector strategies, and electronics has led to overall enhanced PET performance.
■ The reduction in rotation time with resulting benefits in speed and resolution has revolutionized CT performance.
■ Together, combined PET/CT imaging results in a powerful imaging modality for oncologic patients.

SUGGESTED READINGS

Alessio AM, Kinahan PE, Cheng PM, et al. PET/CT scanner instrumentation, challenges, and solutions. Radiol Clin North Am 2004; 42: 1017-1032.

Beyer T, Townsend DW, Brun T, et al. A combined PET/CT scanner for clinical oncology. J Nucl Med 2000; 41:1369-1379.

Blodgett TM, Meltzer CC, Townsend DW. PET/CT: form and function. Radiology 2007; 242:360-385.

Carney JP, Townsend DW. CT-based attenuation correction for PET/CT scanners. In von Schulthess G (ed). Molecular Anatomic Imaging: PET-CT and SPECT-CT Integrated Molecular Imaging. Philadelphia, Lippincott Williams & Wilkins, 2007, pp 55-62.

Kapoor V, McCook BM, Torok FS. An introduction to PET-CT imaging. RadioGraphics 2004; 24:523-543.

Rohren EM, Turkington TG, Coleman RE. Clinical applications of PET in oncology. Radiology 2004; 231:305-332.

Townsend DW. Physics and instrumentation for PET. In Wahl RL (ed). RSNA Syllabus: Categorical Course in Diagnostic Radiology: Clinical PET and PET/CT imaging. Oak Brook, IL, Radiological Society of North America, 2007.

Wong TZ, Paulson EK, Nelson RC, et al. Practical approach to diagnostic CT combined with PET. AJR Am J Roentgenol 2007; 188:622-629.

REFERENCES

1. Kapoor V, McCook BM, Torok FS. An introduction to PET-CT imaging. RadioGraphics 2004; 24:523-543.
2. Wahl RL. Why nearly all PET of abdominal and pelvic cancers will be performed as PET/CT. J Nucl Med 2004; 45(Suppl 1):82S-95S.
3. Blodgett TM, Meltzer CC, Townsend DW. PET/CT: form and function. Radiology 2007; 242:360-385.
4. Beyer T, Townsend DW, Brun T, et al. A combined PET/CT scanner for clinical oncology. J Nucl Med 2000; 41:1369-1379.
5. Rohren EM, Turkington TG, Coleman RE. Clinical applications of PET in oncology. Radiology 2004; 231:305-332.
6. Conti M, Bendriem B, Casey M, et al. First experimental results of time-of-flight reconstruction on an LSO PET scanner. Phys Med Biol 2005; 50:4507-4526.
7. Surti S, Kuhn A, Werner ME, et al. Performance of Philips Gemini TF PET/CT scanner with special consideration for its time-of-flight imaging capabilities. J Nucl Med 2007; 48:471-480.
8. Crespo P, Shakirin G, Fiedler F, et al. Direct time-of-flight for quantitative, real-time in-beam PET: a concept and feasibility study. Phys Med Biol 2007; 52:6795-6811.
9. Watson CC. New, faster image-based scatter correction for 3D PET. IEEE Trans Nucl Sci 2000; 47:1567-1594.
10. Nakamoto Y, Osman M, Cohade C, et al. PET/CT: comparison of quantitative tracer uptake between germanium and CT transmission attenuation-corrected images. J Nucl Med 2002; 43:1137-1143.
11. Antoch G, Freudenberg LS, Beyer T, et al. To enhance or not to enhance? 18F-FDG and CT contrast agents in dual-modality 18F-FDG PET/CT. J Nucl Med 2004; 45(Suppl 1):56S-65S.
12. Wong TZ, Paulson EK, Nelson RC, et al. Practical approach to diagnostic CT combined with PET. AJR Am J Roentgenol 2007; 188:622-629.
13. Carney JP, Townsend DW. CT-based attenuation correction for PET/CT scanners. In Von Schulthess G (ed). Molecular Anatomic Imaging: PET-CT and SPECT-CT Integrated Molecular Imaging. Philadelphia, Lippincott Williams & Wilkins, 2007, pp 55-62.
14. Antoch G, Kuehl H, Kanja J, et al. Dual-modality PET/CT scanning with negative oral contrast agent to avoid artifacts: introduction and evaluation. Radiology 2004; 230:879-885.
15. Cohade C, Osman M, Nakamoto Y, et al. Initial experience with oral contrast in PET/CT: phantom and clinical studies. J Nucl Med 2003; 44:412-416.
16. Kamel E, Hany TF, Burger C, et al. CT vs 68Ge attenuation correction in a combined PET/CT system: evaluation of the effect of lowering the CT tube current. Eur J Nucl Med Mol Imaging 2002; 29:346-350.
17. de Juan R, Seifert B, Berthold T, et al. Clinical evaluation of a breathing protocol for PET/CT. Eur Radiol 2004; 14:1118-1123. Epub 2003; Dec 16.
18. Gilman MD, Fischman AJ, Krishnasetty V, et al. Optimal CT breathing protocol for combined thoracic PET/CT. AJR Am J Roentgenol 2006; 187:1357-1360.
19. Blake MA, Singh A, Setty BN, et al. Pearls and pitfalls in interpretation of abdominal and pelvic PET-CT. RadioGraphics 2006; 26:1335-1353.
20. Moore M, Blake MA. PET/CT in abdominal and pelvic malignancies: principles and practices. In Kalra MK, Saini S, Rubin GR (eds). MDCT from Protocols to Practice. New York, Springer, 2008, pp 166-208.
21. Townsend DW. Physics and instrumentation for PET. In Wahl RL (ed). RSNA Syllabus: Categorical Course in Diagnostic Radiology: Clinical PET and PET/CT Imaging. Oak Brook, IL, Radiological Society of North America, 2007.

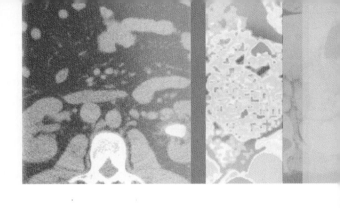

22

Pearls and Pitfalls in PET and PET/CT Interpretation

Michael Blake, Michael Moore, and Ajay Singh

TECHNICAL ASPECTS

Accurate anatomic localization of foci of fluorine-18–labeled fluorodeoxyglucose (FDG) uptake signifying increased metabolic activity on PET can be difficult or impossible. This is particularly so in the abdomen and pelvis where there is a lack of reliable identifiable landmarks and variable physiologic FDG uptake. CT, in contradistinction, provides valuable multiplanar information regarding the morphologic features and attenuation values of lesions, as well as demonstrating oral and intravenous contrast behavior. The advent of PET/CT has successfully combined the metabolic information obtained by FDG-PET with the morphologic imaging information of CT.[1-3] Although the fusion of the two separate datasets results in more accurate localization of abnormalities and improved overall performance, it has also brought its own potential pitfalls and difficulties in interpretation. This, again, is particularly the case in the abdomen and pelvis, where physiologic FDG uptake can be challenging and CT has tissue characterization limitations, especially in postoperative patients.

Artifacts and pitfalls related to interpretation of separate PET and CT images are well documented and are being increasingly recognized as clinical experience grows.[4-8] Hybrid PET/CT provides its own specific pitfalls and artifacts.[1,9,10] Physicians interpreting the combined examination should be aware of both the combined and individual modality artifacts. Indeed, it is mandatory that a working knowledge of these potential problems be acquired to optimize both image interpretation and patient care. In this chapter, we emphasize some of the challenges and solutions regarding abdominal/pelvic PET and PET/CT interpretation. We highlight both general and specific interpretative issues in abdominal/pelvic PET/CT.

PRINCIPLES

General Interpretation

False-positive FDG uptake with respect to malignancy can, in general, occur in PET/CT from infectious or inflammatory processes. Some benign tumors such as colonic adenomas and uterine cellular fibroids may also demonstrate marked FDG uptake. False-negative FDG-PET examinations can occur in malignancies that are either too small (Fig. 22-1) or non-FDG avid. These include some neuroendocrine tumors, renal cell carcinoma, and certain types of lymphoma. Generally, most lymphomas show increased FDG uptake. Indeed, previous studies have demonstrated that PET is usually more specific than CT for staging in patients after treatment of lymphoma. However, some subtypes of lymphoma often show poor FDG uptake, including marginal zone lymphoma (of which mucosa-associated lymphoid tissue [MALT] lymphoma is a subtype) and peripheral T-cell lymphoma. Therefore, CT is particularly important in the staging of these lymphoma subtypes at diagnosis and follow-up. Some mucinous and low-grade tumors are also known to sometimes show poor FDG uptake.[5] High adjacent background activity can also mask pathologic FDG uptake.

Misregistration between the PET and CT images in the pelvis is caused in particular by changes in content and variations in distention of the urinary bladder and, to a lesser extent, by changes in the amount of bowel gas and movement. These may potentially lead to incorrect superimposition of foci of increased FDG activity on erroneous anatomic structures. Misinterpretation may generally be avoided by the ability to correctly attribute FDG activity to the corresponding abdominal structure on the concurrent CT examination. A dedicated PET/CT workstation is essential for optimal interpretation of the overlaid images.

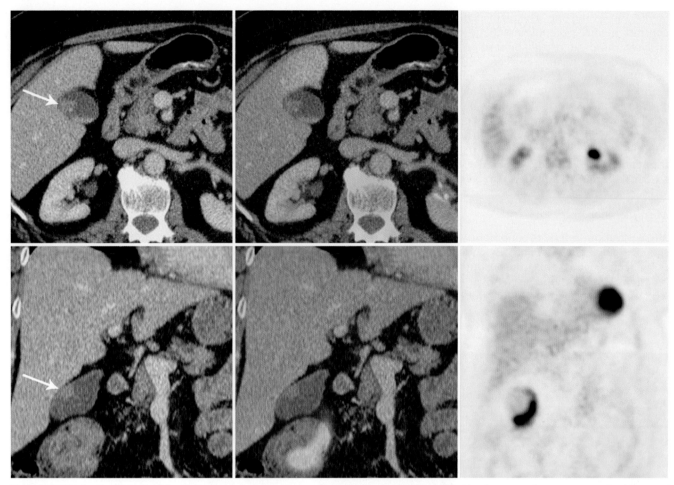

■ **FIGURE 22-1** Size limitations for FDG uptake. Patient with a small enhancing mass of the gallbladder due to a melanoma metastasis without corresponding FDG activity likely owing to the small size of the metastasis because large melanoma metastasis to the colon shows intense uptake (see also Fig. 23-1).

Choosing appropriate window settings for both CT and PET and reviewing both the attenuation-corrected and noncorrected PET data displays allows a complete, integrated interpretation.

Specific Interpretation

Artifacts

Attenuation Correction

Conventional PET examinations require a relatively lengthy transmission scan to perform attenuation correction of the emission data for reliable radiotracer uptake quantitation. In PET/CT scanners, the FDG emission data can be corrected for photon attenuation using the CT image to generate an attenuation map. This confers the following major advantages: First, there is less statistical noise from the CT, compared with germanium (^{68}Ge) transmission data in conventional PET scanners. Second, the CT scan time is much shorter than for radionuclide sources, thus reducing overall examination duration by 15 to 20 minutes. Finally, there is no longer a need for PET transmission hardware or the replacement of germanium source rods.[11]

There is, however, a risk of overestimating the FDG activity with CT-based attenuation correction. Nakamoto and colleaagues reported that the measured activity with CT-based attenuation correction was higher by an average of 11% in bone and 2.1% in soft tissue when compared with ^{68}Ge-based radionuclide attenuation correction.[11] Attenuation correction using CT data may lead to errors by overcorrection of photopenic areas corresponding to very high density structures on CT. This falsely renders such areas of intense uptake on the attenuation-corrected PET images. Certain studies have shown that the use of very high density positive oral and intravenous contrast media may lead to attenuation correction artifacts in the corrected PET image, particularly if the contrast media move between the acquisitions of the PET and the CT used for attenuation correction. Metallic prosthetic implants such as hip replacements, intrauterine contraceptive devices, or surgical clips can also produce beam hardening on CT, with resulting attenuation correction artifact on the PET image.

It is important to be aware of this overcorrection phenomenon on the attenuation correction PET images when interpreting PET/CT. In clinical practice, Dizendorf and colleagues reported only a 4% overestimation of standardized uptake values (SUVs) owing to positive oral contrast media, suggesting only a negligible effect.[12] If positive oral contrast media accumulate and raise the possibility of artifacts, these can usually be resolved by viewing the CT and the non–attenuation-corrected PET images, which are not affected by the high-density material. The use of neutral attenuation oral contrast media also essentially eliminates the issue.[13] Algorithms have being developed to allow for this overestimation of activity by CT attenuation correction and may minimize these effects. Yau and colleagues have reported that co-registration with contrast-enhanced CT images does not result in significant artifacts after CT attenuation correction.[14]

Misregistration

Misregistration refers to imprecise superimposition of the FDG activity over apparently equivalent normal structures seen on CT. This can be due to patient motion, breathing, bowel motility, or urinary bladder distention. It can cause erroneous PET/CT interpretation by super-imposing radiotracer activity on the wrong anatomic structure (Fig. 22-2).[15]

Quiet "free" breathing or normal expiratory phase for acquisition of CT images has been found to be more suitable than maximum inspiratory or maximum expiratory phases for co-registration. Breath-hold imaging, however, clearly confers significant advantages in CT image quality. Some patients may not be able to breath-hold long enough for a whole-body CT, resulting in motion artifact in the lower parts of the body, but modern multislice CT scanners, including 64-slice machines, are capable of faster whole-body scan times and enable study completion within a single breath-hold in the majority of cases. Reducing or minimizing the time delay between the PET and CT scans is beneficial, as is preventing patient motion between the scans. The interpreting physician must be alert to both recognizing misregistration and correcting it via software co-registration. Awareness of potential misregistration and its causes are important in accurate interpretation of PET/CT.

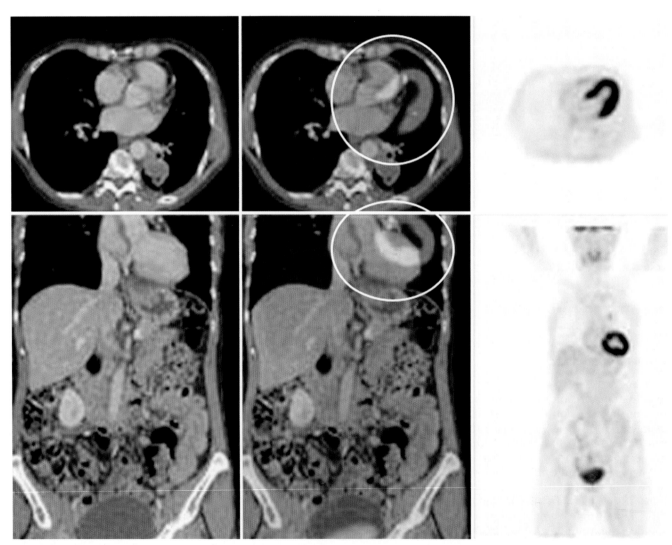

■ **FIGURE 22-2** PET/CT misregistration artifact. Fused PET/CT image shows misregistered physiologic cardiac radiotracer activity (*circle*) in relation to cardiac positioning by CT, secondary to respiration differences between the CT and PET acquisitions. Manual registration correction available with dedicated PET/CT workstations may be helpful in such cases.

PROS AND CONS

We have highlighted in the preceding section some of the general pearls and pitfalls of CT, PET, and PET/CT imaging of the abdomen and pelvis and will cover some of the specific issues peculiar to the various abdominal organs and anatomic areas in the sections to follow. The two modalities comprising PET/CT are generally highly complementary and in combination usually lead to higher accuracy and greater confidence. However, learning the pertinent clinical history of the individual patient and being aware of both general and specific PET/CT issues, variants, and artifacts are important to avoid pitfalls in interpretation.

CONTROVERSIES

Although some of the PET/CT contrast attenuation correction issues have been or are being resolved as we have discussed, the recommendation by some to use contrast-enhanced CT instead of noncontrast CT for attenuation correction has not yet been generally adopted in clinical practice. This would have the added benefit of reducing the overall radiation dose by eliminating the need for noncontrast CT for attenuation correction, although this is usually now of low radiation dose in any event. Furthermore, there are logistic issues of interpretation still to

be resolved regarding who should report these studies. In time, there will be more physicians with dual training in both PET and CT, but, currently, at our institution and some other academic centers, PET/CT reporting is done as a consensus between the nuclear medicine department and the chest and abdominal divisions of the radiology department. The most practical method of reporting, however, clearly depends on the staffing and areas of expertise in individual imaging centers. Nonetheless, we do not agree with the attempts of some to render the CT component of PET/CT "nondiagnostic" so as to merely provide attenuation correction only because this does not extract the full benefits of PET/CT. Other protocol issues still to be resolved are discussed elsewhere (see Chapter 21).

IMAGING OF SPECIFIC LESIONS OR REGIONS

Nonmalignant Hypermetabolic Lesions

As we have discussed earlier, hypermetabolic lesions do not always indicate malignancy. False-positive FDG uptake can occur in PET and PET/CT due to abscess, surgical changes, granulomatous disease, foreign body reaction, or inflammatory processes, such as with diverticulitis, gastritis, and arteriosclerosis (Fig. 22-3). A commonly

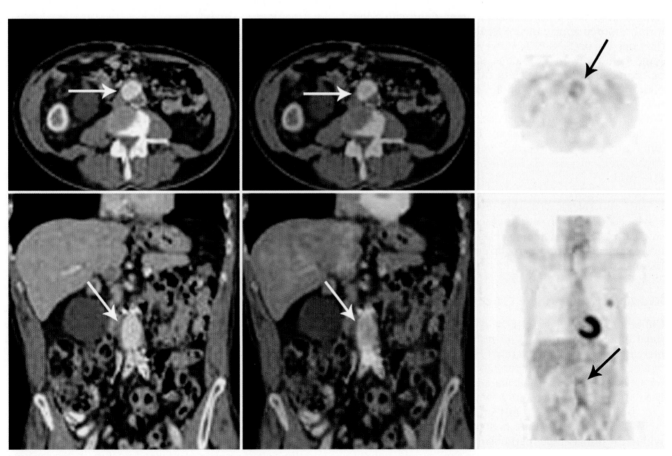

■ **FIGURE 22-3** Non-neoplastic hypermetabolic activity on PET/CT. PET image shows FDG uptake by aortic graft (*arrows*) secondary to re-endothelialization of the graft or a sterile inflammatory response, with corresponding CT and PET/CT overlaid images showing the extent of the graft (*arrows*) from the lower abdominal aorta to the common iliac arteries.

encountered inflammatory process in the pelvis is associated with an intrauterine device. Some benign tumors may also demonstrate intense FDG uptake. On the other hand, high adjacent background activity can obscure nonintense malignant FDG uptake.

The concurrent diagnostic CT from the PET/CT can readily reveal clinically pertinent non-neoplastic conditions such as aortic aneurysms, inflammatory/infectious processes, and bowel obstruction. In addition, the use of oral and intravenous contrast media can enhance CT performance to often allow detection of the responsible non-neoplastic hypermetabolic conditions and thus prevent false-positive interpretation.[13] CT will furthermore often provide complementary diagnostic information when there is high background FDG activity masking a malignancy. Allowing a long enough time interval between radiation or surgical treatment and PET or PET/CT is important in preventing false-positive interpretation owing to persistent post-treatment FDG activity. It is best to wait at least 6 weeks after surgery or radiation treatment and preferably longer before performing PET or PET/CT if recurrence of tumor is suspected in the surgical or irradiated bed. Interpreting physicians should be cognizant of any pertinent clinical symptoms and signs such as fever, pain and leukocytosis, which may point to an underlying inflammatory/infectious pathologic process.

Liver and Spleen

Hepatic FDG activity is usually mildly intense with a uniformly mottled appearance. Splenic activity is usually less than hepatic on FDG-PET. However, splenules can cause some confusion on PET alone. Liver dome lesions can be erroneously projected into the lung base due to respiratory artifact.[15] In addition, up to 36% to 50% of hepatomas are reported to lack significant FDG avidity. Well-differentiated hepatocellular carcinomas in particular lack significant FDG avidity in contrast to less well differentiated ones. Necrotic and mucinous metastatic adenocarcinomas are also known to generally be poorly FDG avid.

The co-registered CT images can help clarify both hepatic and splenic FDG-avid lesions. Dynamic contrast-enhanced CT can provide the necessary information for surgical planning, including relationships to vessels and liver segments. It also helps correctly identify intrasplenic lesions and splenules.

Kidney and Urinary Tract

Unlike its analog glucose, FDG is not reabsorbed by the renal tubules, and thus all of the urinary tract can show increased activity from excreted FDG. This can cause difficulties in identifying a pathologic process of the urinary tract because it may be obscured by the excreted FDG. Dilated or redundant ureters as well as bladder diverticula can also lead to pitfalls in PET or PET/CT interpretation.

It is therefore generally beneficial to minimize stasis within the urinary tract, particularly when there is a pelvic lesion. Good hydration and regular voiding are helpful. Some also advocate the intravenous use of diuretics or bladder catheterization. Caution must be taken when interpreting PET images in the context of renal cell carcinoma because studies have demonstrated only about 60% sensitivity. When no intravenous contrast agent is given, the FDG excretion gives some helpful renal physiologic information and can usually distinguish parapelvic cysts from hydronephrosis. CT is a well-recognized leading modality for assessing genitourinary pathologic processes in general and, for example, can readily distinguish the PET interpretation pitfalls of lymphadenopathy in the peri-aortic and periureteral regions from horseshoe kidney and ureteral activity, respectively (Fig. 22-4).

Pancreas

Small and early-stage pancreatic cancers can be falsely negative on FDG-PET, a major limitation of FDG-PET alone in detection of pancreatic cancer. Furthermore, false-positive FDG-PET results for pancreatic cancer can occur in active pancreatitis and autoimmune pancreatitis. Such uptake of the tracer by inflamed parenchyma or irradiated tissues may be indistinguishable from pancreatic malignancy. Increased FDG uptake has also been reported due to portal vein thrombosis, retroperitoneal fibrosis, hemorrhagic pseudocysts, and peripancreatic lymph nodes.[16] PET/CT improves the independent performances of its component PET and CT modalities in diagnosing pancreatic cancer by allowing both greater recognition of false-positive PET findings and greater confidence in making the correct diagnosis on CT (Fig. 22-5).

Adrenal Gland

Characterization of adrenal lesions by FDG-PET is dependent on increased glucose metabolism in malignancy. Several studies have reported on the excellent ability of FDG-PET to distinguish between benign and malignant adrenal lesions. Lesions with activity lower or much greater than liver activity could be confidently diagnosed as benign or malignant, respectively. Lesions with slightly increased activity relative to liver are often classed as indeterminant. Authors have reported up to 90% to 100% sensitivity and specificity for FDG-PET in distinguishing benign from malignant lesions.[17-19]

However, false-positive scans do occur in FDG-PET adrenal imaging, particularly in relation to pheochromocytoma, adrenal hyperplasia, as well as approximately 5% of adenomas (probably due to functioning tumors) and, rarely, myelolipomas.[17-20] Brown fat occurring in a suprarenal distribution is another potential pitfall of PET/CT in adrenal imaging owing to increased brown fat FDG uptake.[21] The characteristic brown fat pattern is more commonly seen in the neck and supraclavicular regions but can also extend to the paraspinal and periadrenal regions (Fig. 22-6). Brown fat is a vestigial organ of thermogenesis, which utilizes increased glucose and is sympathetically innervated. The distinctive FDG-PET pattern is more common in thin patients and during the winter months.[21] Brown fat uptake is usually diagnosable by its characteristic distribution, co-registration to areas of fat, and the lack of a corresponding adrenal mass. Knowledge of this entity together with accurate CT correlation usually results in the correct diagnosis.[21]

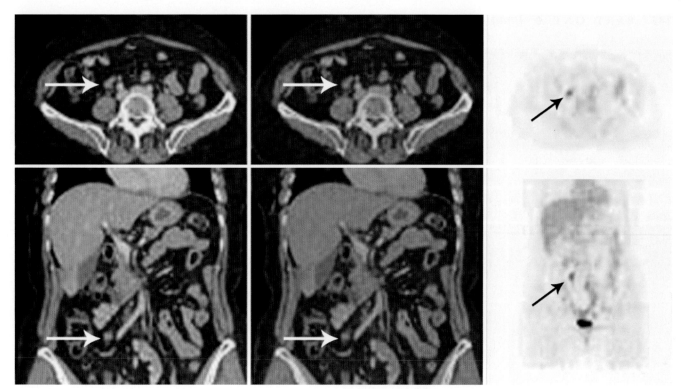

■ **FIGURE 22-4** Retroperitoneal lymphadenopathy mimicking ureteral activity on FDG-PET. PET image shows focal increased FDG activity (*arrows*) in the right retroperitoneum. Without PET/CT superimposition, the hypermetabolic activity may be mistaken for physiologic activity in the right ureter but the CT shows enlarged right retroperitoneal lymph nodes (*arrows*) adjacent to the right mid ureter in this patient with lymphoma.

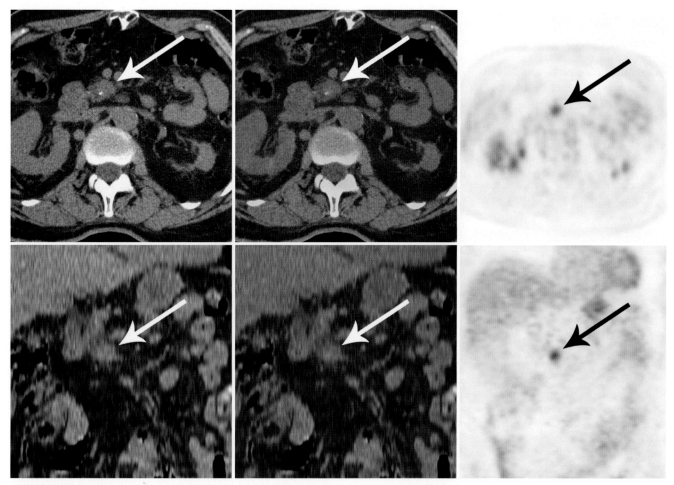

■ **FIGURE 22-5** Pancreatic carcinoma. PET and PET/CT image shows hypermetabolic focus in the pancreatic head (*arrows*), corresponding to a pancreatic adenocarcinoma. Nonenhanced CT shows a small mass (*arrows*) in the pancreatic head, not optimally seen on unenhanced CT alone. Some small pancreatic cancers are not FDG avid, and an inflammatory process involving the pancreas or peripancreatic regions can falsely mimic pancreatic tumor on PET.

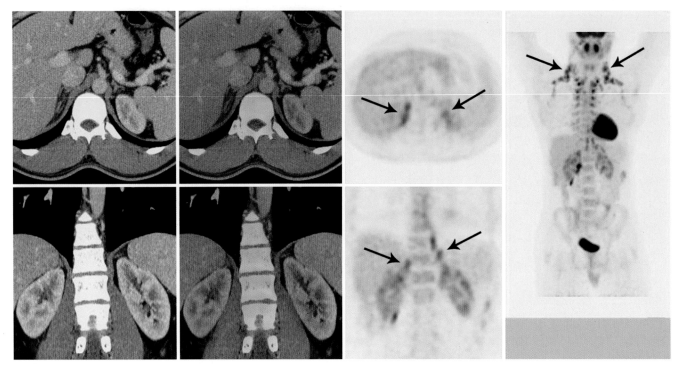

■ **FIGURE 22-6**   Brown fat. Increased FDG uptake in the periadrenal region on axial and coronal PET images but no abnormal masses in these regions with normal-appearing adrenal glands. MIP image shows characteristic pattern of uptake of brown fat in the neck (*arrows*) extending in this case to the retroperitoneum.

Adrenal PET/CT provides both the attenuation characteristics and the metabolic activity of adrenal lesions in one examination and should be diagnostic for the majority of adrenal lesions encountered. CT can also be helpful in circumstances when non-neoplastic lesions cause increased FDG uptake, by identifying the cause of the increased FDG uptake. Indeed the majority of adrenal lesions can be characterized by CT criteria alone if a noncontrast CT of adequate image quality is acquired. Approximately 70% of adrenal adenomas contain enough intracytoplasmic fat to produce a CT attenuation of 10 Hounsfield units or less.[22] Adrenal lesions can be even further characterized by wash-out characteristics on delayed postcontrast CT if acquired.[23-25] Both components of PET/CT thus provide helpful information for adrenal lesion characterization. The integrated PET/CT information may be invaluable in the rare event of collision tumors when an adenoma and metastasis arise in the same adrenal gland.

Hypometabolic Lesions

Although PET has good sensitivity for the detection of a number of neoplasms such as lung, esophageal, colorectal, breast, thyroid, and head and neck cancers, as well as lymphoma, melanoma, and sarcoma, there are a number of malignancies that are not hypermetabolic and thus not FDG avid. These cancers include certain renal cell cancers, some lymphoma subtypes, neuroendocrine tumors, bronchoalveolar carcinomas, mucinous adenocarcinomas in general, prostate carcinomas, and carcinoid tumors.[5-7] The information provided by the diagnostic CT component of PET/CT is clearly extremely valuable when the

malignancy does not show significant FDG uptake. Contrast-enhanced diagnostic-quality CT allows for tumor detection and characterization. Alternate agents are possible for more specific PET, and these are being further investigated but, too, will likely greatly benefit from being part of a PET/CT examination because reliable PET landmarks with these new agents are even more lacking. The use of FDG-PET for follow-up is generally not advisable when the pre-chemotherapy PET fails to show FDG uptake, although it can sometimes reveal transformation to higher-grade tumors, for example, in some patients with lymphoma. PET is also clearly less helpful when one of the known hypometabolic histologic types is being staged.

Gastrointestinal Tract

Gastrointestinal tract FDG uptake particularly from the colon is highly variable, and this can create difficulty in diagnosing a malignancy in the vicinity of bowel loops.[26] The normal esophagus, however, generally does not demonstrate marked increased uptake. Homogeneous increased uptake in the stomach wall and gastroesophageal junction is relatively common. Small bowel uptake is somewhat variable but usually of low grade. However, uptake within the colon may be quite avid, especially in the cecum/ascending colon and in the anal sphincter region. Postsurgical changes can also show increased FDG uptake over the first 6 to 8 weeks after the operation. Superficial FDG activity can be due to herniated bowel loops at sites of a weakened abdominal wall after surgery. Increased FDG uptake in a colostomy with a diffuse low-level pattern is related, in general, to postoperative inflammatory changes.

Risk of misinterpretation may be minimized by the ability to correctly attribute FDG activity to the equivalent abdominal structure. Focal large bowel activity greater than hepatic activity should suggest the possible presence of a pathologic process. A diligent regional review of the corresponding CT images is warranted to search for focal masses or adjunct signs of inflammation, bearing in mind that bowel peristalsis and patient breathing and motion may lead to misregistration artifact. Ideally, this should be a fully diagnostic CT with oral and intravenous contrast media. Even in the absence of corresponding CT findings, focal intense colonic activity on PET still warrants further investigation because true colonic lesions may not be visible on CT given the colon's unprepped, nondistended state. Animal studies claim that the majority of physiologic intestinal activity is from intestinal mucosa or bowel contents. Bowel uptake usually has a recognizable linear appearance. Physiologic FDG uptake in pelvic organs is the primary cause for false-positive interpretations in patients being evaluated for rectal cancer recurrence because the organs are displaced posteriorly after abdominoperineal resection. The number of false-positive results is reduced with PET/CT image co-registration.[27] Indeed, PET/CT has been reported to be an accurate technique in the detection of pelvic recurrence after surgical removal of rectal cancer after at least a 6-month interval after surgery and is reported in those circumstances to allow differentiation of a benign lesion from a neoplastic abnormality with a sensitivity of 100% and a specificity of 96%.[26]

Reproductive Tract

FDG-PET is capable of visualizing lymph nodal and distant metastases in the staging of reproductive tract malignancies sometimes before these changes can be visualized or recognized as malignant on CT. To date, FDG-PET has been used for the evaluation of patients with prostate, ovarian, cervical, and testicular cancer. CT is also helpful, however, for all of these indications and again provides useful complementary information to PET in combined PET/CT.[1,9,10]

Uterus

The endometrial uptake of FDG changes cyclically in premenopausal women, increasing during the ovulatory and menstrual phases; however, any postmenopausal endometrial uptake is abnormal. The patient's pertinent menstrual history is thus extremely helpful for informed interpretation, with expected increased activity during the ovulatory and menstrual phases. Increased endometrial uptake beside a cervical tumor therefore does not necessarily represent endometrial tumor invasion.[28] Uterine fibroids, especially the cellular subtype, can sometimes show increased FDG activity. Saksena and associates found 18% of fibroids to be hypermetabolic in their series.[29]

FDG-PET has been reported to be accurate and sensitive (>95%) in detecting recurrence of endometrial cancer and evaluating therapeutic response in the limited studies available to date. FDG also accumulates reliably in cervical cancer. Concurrent CT allows localization of the focus of abnormal FDG to the corresponding gynecologic structure in PET/CT.

Ovary

Increased ovarian uptake may be functional in premenopausal women because corpus luteum cysts can transiently increase the ovarian uptake of FDG (Fig. 22-7). However, increased ovarian uptake in postmenopausal patients is again associated with malignancy.

Postsurgical changes in the pelvis can make CT interpretation challenging. Again, menstrual history is extremely helpful for interpretation with expected increased activity from corpus luteal cysts, which also have a characteristic appearance on contrast-enhanced CT as small, rim-enhancing cystic lesions (see Fig. 22-7). FDG-PET is helpful in differentiation between residual or recurrent disease and for diagnosis when CT is inconclusive owing to anatomic distortion. PET performance is limited, however, in assessing for microscopic metastases and peritoneal disease. FDG-PET has higher specificity as compared with CA-125 level and conventional CT/MRI for detecting recurrent ovarian cancers. Combining the PET and CT information in PET/CT further enhances accuracy.[1,9,10] The CT component of PET/CT is particularly useful for recognition of transposed ovaries in women of reproductive age. These may appear on integrated PET/CT studies as lower abdominal or high lateral pelvic masses showing increased FDG uptake owing to the presence of preserved ovarian function in an ectopic location, which should not be misinterpreted as a site of malignancy. Surgical information regarding a history of ovarian transposition is helpful, especially when there is a history of a previous malignancy treated by pelvic irradiation.

Prostate

Primary prostate cancers are generally hypometabolic and therefore show only faint FDG uptake, but their metastases are more FDG avid. Currently ^{11}C-acetate seems more useful than FDG in the detection of local recurrences and regional lymph node metastases, but its role is still under investigation. A positive correlation has been shown between serum prostate-specific antigen (PSA) level and both ^{11}C-acetate uptake and FDG uptake.[30] Fluorocholine PET/CT is also a promising imaging modality for detecting local recurrence and lymph node metastases in patients with recurrent prostate cancer. The search for nodal disease and distant metastases by CT can again be enhanced with the addition of PET in PET/CT.

SUMMARY

FDG-PET poses interpretative challenges especially because high-intensity focal physiologic uptake can mimic cancer, and malignant sites themselves may also be missed when FDG activity in normal structures overlies or neighbors malignant lesions. Accurate PET and PET/CT interpretation requires knowledge of the pitfalls associated with the two imaging components individually and, furthermore, as a result of their fusion.

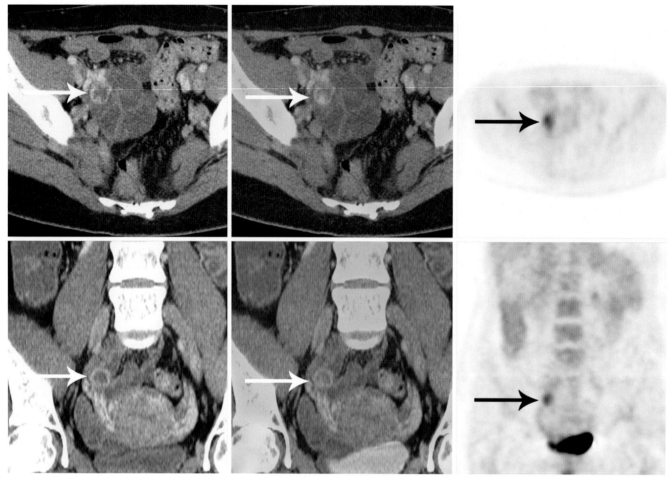

■ **FIGURE 22-7** Physiologic ovarian uptake of FDG in the corpus luteum in the postovulation phase of the menstrual cycle. PET, CT, and PET/CT images show focal increased FDG activity corresponding to a rim-enhancing cyst consistent with a corpus luteum (*arrows*) seen in the right ovary. CT can readily recognize corpus luteal cysts especially if the date of the patients' last menstrual period is known.

KEY POINTS

■ FDG-PET and CT are highly complementary modalities whose combined individual strengths fortunately tend to overcome their respective separate weaknesses.

■ PET/CT publications to date have been highly encouraging but optimal hybrid scanning protocols are not yet established; larger prospective studies will provide more answers.

■ In practice, knowing the pertinent clinical history, adhering to sound imaging principles, and being aware of advances in this powerful developing modality are necessary requirements for optimal interpretation of abdominal PET/CT.

SUGGESTED READINGS

Agress H, Wahl RL. PET and PET/CT artifacts: variants and approaches to image interpretation. In Wahl RL (ed). RSNA Syllabus: Categorical Course in Diagnostic Radiology: Clinical PET and PET/CT imaging. Oak Brook, IL, Radiological Society of North America, 2007.

Blake MA, Singh A, Setty BN, et al. Pearls and pitfalls in interpretation of abdominal and pelvic PET-CT. RadioGraphics 2006; 26:1335-1353.

Blodgett TM, Meltzer CC, Townsend DW. PET/CT: form and function. Radiology 2007; 242:360-385.

Cook GJ, Wegner EA, Fogelman I. Pitfalls and artifacts in ^{18}FDG PET and PET/CT oncologic imaging. Semin Nucl Med 2004; 34:122-133.

Israel O. FDG PET/CT of the pelvis: normal anatomy, pitfalls and pelvic malignancies. In Wahl RL (ed). RSNA Syllabus: Categorical Course in Diagnostic Radiology: Clinical PET and PET/CT imaging. Oak Brook, IL, Radiological Society of North America, 2007.

Moore M, Blake MA. PET/CT in abdominal and pelvic malignancies: principles and practices. In Kalra MK, Saini S, Rubin GR (eds). MDCT from Protocols to Practice. New York, Springer, 2008, pp 166-208.

Mosley CK, Schuster DM. Practical PET/CT of the abdomen. In Wahl RL (ed). RSNA Syllabus: Categorical Course in Diagnostic Radiology:

Clinical PET and PET/CT Imaging. Oak Brook, IL, Radiological Society of North America, 2007.

Prabhakar HB, Sahani DV, Fischman AJ, et al. Bowel hot spots at PET-CT. RadioGraphics 2007; 27:145-159.

Sureshbabu W, Mawlawi O. PET/CT imaging artifacts. J Nucl Med Technol 2005; 33:156-161; quiz 163-164.

Wong TZ, Paulson EK, Nelson RC, et al. Practical approach to diagnostic CT combined with PET. AJR Am J Roentgenol 2007; 188:622-629.

REFERENCES

1. Kapoor V, McCook BM, Torok FS. An introduction to PET-CT imaging. RadioGraphics 2004; 24:523-543.
2. Blodgett TM, Meltzer CC, Townsend DW. PET/CT: form and function. Radiology 2007; 242:360-385.
3. Antoch G, Kuehl H, Kanja J, et al. Dual-modality PET/CT scanning with negative oral contrast to avoid artifacts: introduction and evaluation. Radiology 2004; 230:879-885.
4. Rohren EM, Turkington TG, Coleman RE. Clinical applications of PET in oncology. Radiology 2004; 231:305-332.
5. Agress H, Wahl RL. PET and PET/CT artifacts, variants and approaches to image interpretation. In Wahl RL (ed). RSNA Syllabus: Categorical Course in Diagnostic Radiology: Clinical PET and PET/CT imaging. Oak Brook, IL, Radiological Society of North America, 2007.
6. Gordon BA, Flanagan FL, Dehdashti F. Whole-body positron emission tomography: normal variations, pitfalls, and technical considerations. AJR Am J Roentgenol 1997; 169:1675-1680.
7. Shreve PD, Anzai Y, Wahl RL. Pitfalls in oncologic diagnosis with FDG PET imaging: physiologic and benign variants. RadioGraphics 1999; 19:61-77; quiz 150-151.
8. Shirkoda A. Variants and Pitfalls in Body Imaging. Philadelphia, Lippincott Williams & Wilkins, 2000.
9. Blake MA, Singh A, Setty BN, et al. Pearls and pitfalls in interpretation of abdominal and pelvic PET-CT. RadioGraphics 2006; 26:1335-1353.
10. Subhas N, Patel PV, Pannu HK, et al. Imaging of pelvic malignancies with in-line FDG PET-CT: case examples and common pitfalls of FDG PET. RadioGraphics 2005; 25:1031-1043.
11. Nakamoto Y, Osman M, Cohade C, et al. PET/CT: comparison of quantitative tracer uptake between germanium and CT transmission attenuation-corrected images. J Nucl Med 2002; 43:1137-1143.
12. Dizendorf E, Hany TF, Buck A, et al. Cause and magnitude of the error induced by oral CT contrast agent in CT-based attenuation correction of PET emission studies. J Nucl Med 2003; 44:732-738.
13. Antoch G, Kuehl H, Kanja J, et al. Dual-modality PET/CT scanning with negative oral contrast agent to avoid artifacts: introduction and evaluation. Radiology 2004; 230:879-885.
14. Yau YY, Chan WS, Tam YM, et al. Application of intravenous contrast in PET/CT: does it really introduce significant attenuation correction error? J Nucl Med 2005; 46:283-291.
15. Osman MM, Cohade C, Nakamoto Y, et al. Clinically significant inaccurate localization of lesions with PET/CT: frequency in 300 patients. J Nucl Med 2003; 44:240-243.
16. Vesselle HJ, Miraldi FD. FDG-PET of the retroperitoneum: normal anatomy, variants, pathologic conditions, and strategies to avoid diagnostic pitfalls. RadioGraphics 1998; 18:805-823; discussion 823-824.
17. Yun M, Kim W, Alnafisi N, et al. ^{18}F-FDG PET in characterizing adrenal lesions detected on CT or MRI. J Nucl Med 2001; 42:1795-1799.
18. Boland GW, Goldberg MA, Lee MJ, et al. Indeterminate adrenal mass in patients with cancer: evaluation at PET with 2-(F-18)-fluoro-2-deoxy-D-glucose. Radiology 1995; 194:131-134.
19. Shulkin BL, Thompson NW, Shapiro B, et al. Pheochromocytomas: imaging with 2-(fluorine-18) fluoro-2-deoxy-D-glucose PET. Radiology 1999; 212:35-41.
20. Erasmus JJ, Patz EF Jr, McAdams HP, et al. Evaluation of adrenal masses in patients with bronchogenic carcinoma using ^{18}F-fluorodeoxyglucose positron emission tomography. AJR Am J Roentgenol 1997; 168:1357-1360.
21. Yeung HW, Grewal RK, Gonen M, et al. Patterns of (18) F-FDG uptake in adipose tissue and muscle: a potential source of false-positives for PET. J Nucl Med 2003; 44:1789-1796.
22. Boland GW, Lee MJ, Gazelle GS, et al. Characterization of adrenal masses using unenhanced CT: an analysis of the CT literature. AJR Am J Roentgenol 1998; 171:201-204.
23. Szolar DH, Kammerhuber FH. Adrenal adenomas and nonadenomas: assessment of washout at delayed contrast-enhanced CT. Radiology 1998; 207:369-375.
24. Korobkin M, Brodeur FJ, Francis IR, et al. Delayed enhanced CT for differentiation of benign from malignant adrenal masses. Radiology 1996; 200:737-742.
25. Blake MA, Kalra MK, Sweeney AT, et al. Distinguishing benign from malignant adrenal masses: multi-detector row CT protocol with 10-minute delay. Radiology 2006; 238:578-585.
26. Even-Sapir E, Parag Y, Lerman H, et al. Detection of recurrence in patients with rectal cancer: PET/CT after abdominoperineal or anterior resection. Radiology 2004; 232:815-822.
27. Prabhakar HB, Sahani DV, Fischman AJ, et al. Bowel hot spots at PET-CT. RadioGraphics 2007; 27:145-159.
28. Lerman H, Metser U, Grisaru D, et al. Normal and abnormal ^{18}F-FDG endometrial and ovarian uptake in pre- and postmenopausal patients: assessment by PET/CT. J Nucl Med 2004; 45:266-271.
29. Saksena MA, Blake MA, Brachtel E, et al. Uterine fibroid ^{18}F-fluorodeoxyglucose (FDG) uptake on combined PET/CT. Reston, VA, American Roentgen Ray Society Scientific Abstracts (Abstract 082).
30. Fricke E, Machtens S, Hofmann M, et al. Positron emission tomography with ^{11}C-acetate and ^{18}F-FDG in prostate cancer patients. Eur J Nucl Med Mol Imaging 2003; 30:607-611.

CHAPTER 23

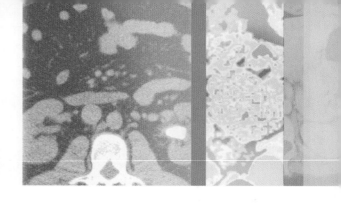

PET and PET/CT Clinical Applications

Michael Blake and Michael Moore

The focus of this chapter is on PET and PET/CT applications specific to the tumors arising in the gastrointestinal tract and female gynecologic organs, excluding systemic malignancies such as lymphoma and melanoma, which can manifest in the abdomen (Fig. 23-1), as well as other approved extra-abdominal malignancies that can metastasize to the abdomen, such as lung and breast cancers.

IMAGING OF SPECIFIC AREAS

Gastrointestinal Tract

Esophageal Carcinoma

Because it is mainly an intrathoracic organ, the esophagus will not be discussed except to note that the incidence of adenocarcinoma of the distal esophagus and gastroesophageal junction has increased dramatically in recent years, currently accounting for the majority of new cases of esophageal cancer.[1] The Centers for Medicare and Medicaid (CMS) guidelines in the United States approve FDG-PET, and thus PET/CT, for the diagnosis, staging, and restaging of patients with esophageal cancer, including both squamous cell carcinoma and adenocarcinoma subtypes (Fig. 23-2).

Colorectal Carcinoma

Colorectal cancer is the malignant abdominal tumor that has been extensively investigated with FDG-PET and PET/CT. The CMS guidelines in the United States have approved Medicare coverage for FDG-PET, and thus PET/CT, for the diagnosis, staging, and restaging of patients with colorectal cancer.

Diagnosis

FDG-PET is sensitive for detecting primary colorectal carcinoma (95% to 100%), but it has unacceptably lower specificity than conventional modalities at initial staging. In practice, FDG-PET is therefore rarely specifically used for the diagnosis of colorectal cancer, although it may incidentally detect such a tumor as PET, and especially PET/CT, becomes more extensively used. At the primary site, however, the positive predictive value of PET is lower than the negative predictive value, owing to the false-positive FDG-PET findings of both physiologic bowel activity and inflammatory processes.[2]

Staging

In staging patients with colorectal cancer, FDG-PET and PET/CT are mainly used to assess regional lymph node involvement and distal metastases. However, FDG-PET has been shown to have a very low sensitivity of between 22% and 29% for regional lymph node metastases, with CT also demonstrating low values (29%). However, FDG-PET specificity was superior (96% vs. 85%).[3] False-negative findings in regional metastatic lymph nodes on FDG-PET are considered to be due to low sensitivity for microscopic involvement of small lymph nodes or occasionally due to the increased FDG uptake by the primary tumor, which masks the immediately neighboring structures. CT has known limitations in characterizing lymph nodes by essentially size criteria alone.

Most patients with colorectal cancer at initial staging have disease limited to the colon or to regional pericolic or mesenteric lymph nodes. For patients with early colorectal cancer, surgery is usually performed with the intention to achieve cure. However, distant metastatic disease may necessitate the surgery for complications, which include hemorrhage, obstruction, and perforation. Given this role of surgery in both regional and advanced disease, surgical and pathologic criteria define the colorectal cancer staging classification.[4]

The standard TNM classification is currently advocated by the American Joint Committee on Cancer. Because of inherent technologic limitations, imaging modalities of

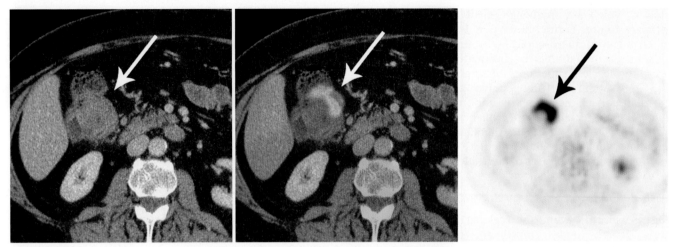

■ **FIGURE 23-1** Melanoma metastasis. PET image shows intense focal uptake in the right upper quadrant (*arrow*), which co-registers to a large colonic soft tissue mass (*arrows*) on CT and PET/CT images, representing a melanoma metastasis to the bowel wall.

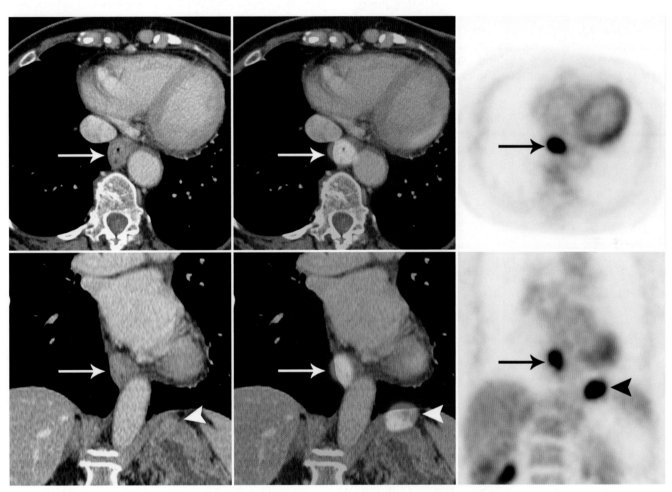

■ **FIGURE 23-2** Esophageal cancer. Focal FDG uptake in lower esophagus corresponding to esophageal thickening (*arrows*), representing an esophageal adenocarcinoma with a left diaphragmatic FDG-avid metastatic lymph node (*arrowheads*).

today are generally unable to match the diagnostic staging information provided by surgical and pathologic findings. PET cannot provide an accurate T stage determination necessary for TNM nomenclature, in which exact depth of invasion is the primary parameter. PET is usually only accurate in cases of gross serosal penetration and invasion of neighboring structures. CT gives more exact structural information but, unfortunately, usually also cannot adequately resolve the bowel wall layers. N staging necessitates evaluation of mesenteric nodes as well as pericolic nodes, which are frequently small and lie beside the primary tumor. Furthermore, pericolic nodes again are often involved microscopically by tumor, which usually can be diagnosed only by histopathologic evaluation.[5] Despite the clear superiority of surgery and histopathology at TNM staging, preoperative imaging detection of nodal or organ metastases is important in guiding the general management toward palliation or curative tumor resection. Despite its staging limitations, PET/CT offers combined metabolic and structural information that is particularly useful in cases of more advanced local disease.

Metastatic Disease

Disease spread beyond the regional pericolic or mesenteric lymph nodes represents metastatic disease. Lymphatic spread usually involves internal iliac or retroperitoneal nodes whereas hematogenous spread of colorectal cancer usually involves the lungs or liver (Fig. 23-3). Metastases to other sites in the absence of pulmonary or hepatic involvement are relatively unusual. A major advantage of PET as well as PET/CT is the accurate detection of distant metastases.[3]

Liver metastases, if recognized early enough, may be treated by neoadjuvant chemotherapy and resection, which may lengthen survival for patients with colorectal cancer, and both PET and CT are accurate for diagnosis of metastases to the liver. Multidetector row CT after intravenous administration of a contrast agent is a standard primary imaging modality for the assessment of focal liver lesions, with uncertain liver lesions generally evaluated with enhanced MRI. In a meta-analysis performed by Kinkel and colleagues, PET was considered to be superior to older CT technology for the detection of liver metastases[6] but appears limited in its ability to demonstrate subcentimeter lesions.[7] In a study by Kantorová and colleagues,[8] FDG-PET had a sensitivity, specificity, and accuracy of 78%, 96%, and 91%, respectively, for the identification of hepatic metastases compared with 67%, 100%, and 91%, respectively, for CT. Sahani and associates showed that gadolinium-enhanced MRI outperformed PET in assessing liver metastases from colorectal and pancreatic cancer, again particularly for small lesions.[9] In addition, PET alone does not provide adequate anatomic information for satisfactory surgical planning regarding the precise localization of metastases according to hepatic segments or with respect to the positioning of lesions in relationship to or involvement of vessels or gallbladder. There are, in general, very few studies comparing PET or PET/CT with modern CT or MRI technique, but a relatively recent study by Chua and coworkers[10] compared PET/CT with CT with intravenous contrast for the evaluation of patients with hepatic metastases. In patients with colorectal carcinoma, PET/CT had 94% sensitivity and 75% specificity compared with inferior values of 91% and 25%, respectively, for CT. Furthermore, PET/CT may be particularly helpful in patients with fatty liver and hypodense or hypoenhancing liver lesions that are not clearly characterized by CT alone and in patients with an increasing carcinoembryonic antigen (CEA) value in whom CT fails to detect metastases. In such circumstances, PET/CT can directly affect patient care by guiding biopsies or directing surgical resection or ablation of liver metastases.

The most important role of PET in patients with hepatic metastases is in the diagnosis of extrahepatic metastatic foci that would preclude a curative tumor resection. CT

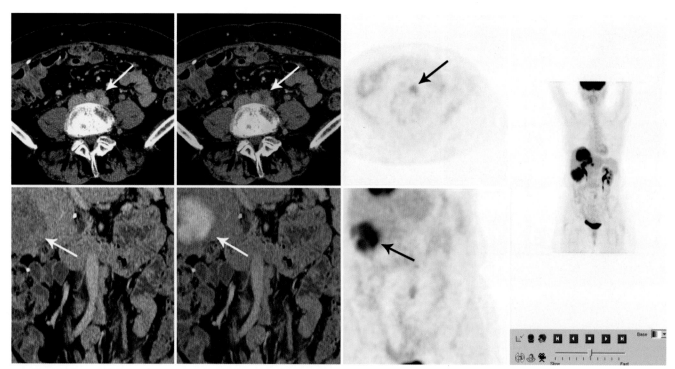

■ **FIGURE 23-3**   Metastatic colorectal cancer. FDG-positive liver masses (*arrows*) with left para-aortic lymph node also showing increased uptake (*arrows*) due to hepatic metastases and para-aortic metastatic adenopathy.

is an accepted imaging modality for depiction of extrahepatic disease before an attempt at a curative procedure. However, owing to its reliance on primarily morphologic changes to depict disease, interpretation of CT alone may falsely report a lesion as malignant that is, in fact, unrelated to malignancy or indeed not realize the significance of a finding because CT pathologic size criteria are not met. Moreover, the abnormality may indeed be visible on the CT but overlooked on interpretation, perhaps sometimes owing to the high volume of CT data that now routinely needs to be reviewed. Several investigators have examined the incremental value of PET as a supplement to CT and found that PET offers significant management information beyond that from CT alone. Investigators have found that when PET is added to CT in preoperative planning for patients with hepatic metastases, additional extrahepatic metastatic foci are identified in 11% to 23% of patients and can result in prolonged patient survival after institution of appropriate patient management. This is often due to a treatment change to a systemic approach with chemotherapy rather than localized therapy.

In patients with elevated CEA levels, FDG-PET can identify metastases previously unrecognized on conventional diagnostic modalities. Indeed, imaging with FDG in patients with colorectal cancer has been proven to be a cost-effective technique that often leads to a change in patient management. Valk and coworkers[11] found that an average of $3,003 was saved per patient when PET was added to the preoperative diagnostic workup; FDG scanning was able to differentiate patients with unresectable disease rather than resectable disease, thus avoiding futile operations. This reduction in unnecessary procedures was supported by a study by Park and colleagues.[12] Management was altered in 27 patients based on PET/CT results; 9 had intermodality changes, 10 received more extensive surgery, and 8 avoided futile procedures. PET/CT improved the management plan in 24% of patients with primary colorectal cancer.

Restaging

As during the initial staging of colorectal cancer, FDG-PET has been reported to be more accurate overall than CT for the presence of metastatic disease. An early study by Hung and colleagues[13] compared FDG-PET, CT, and serum CEA for the evaluation of recurrent colorectal disease. They reported sensitivity and specificity of FDG-PET to be 100% and 83%, respectively, compared with 33% and 86%, respectively, for CEA. Abdominal CT had a lower sensitivity and specificity of 78% and 61% for detecting local recurrence and detected one lymphatic and one hepatic metastasis. They concluded that FDG-PET was more accurate than CT and CEA for the detection of recurrent colorectal cancer. In a recurrent colorectal carcinoma meta-analysis study by Wiering and colleagues,[14] pooled sensitivity and specificity were 88% and 96%, respectively, for FDG-PET in the detection of hepatic metastases compared with lower values of 83% and 84%, respectively, for CT. For extrahepatic disease, pooled sensitivity and specificity for PET were 92% and 95%, respectively, in comparison to 61% and 91% for CT. Clinical management changed in 32% based on the PET findings.

The imaging distinction of postoperative inflammation, scarring, radiation fibrosis, and other sequelae of prior therapy from recurrence is challenging in patients with prior colorectal carcinoma. This is most problematic with rectal tumors, in which presacral scarring and pelvic desmoplastic changes are common findings. With conventional imaging, serial examinations are frequently required before slowly developing malignant changes can be appreciated. When PET is performed more than 6 months after surgery, a time when postsurgical change is not hypermetabolic unless there is a leak causing persistent inflammation, increased FDG uptake in the presacral space generally indicates tumor recurrence.[4] PET/CT at this time has been shown to be highly accurate for differentiation of benign from malignant presacral changes, with reported sensitivity, specificity, and positive and negative predictive values of 100%, 96%, 88%, and 100%, respectively (Fig. 23-4).[4] PET has a further advantage in that a single study is sufficient for the diagnosis, rather than the serial studies usually required with more conventional imaging. The first published study of PET/CT of colorectal cancer reported that the staging and restaging accuracy improved from 78% with PET alone to 89% with PET/CT. The frequency of equivocal and probable lesion characterization was halved,[15] and the superiority of PET/CT over CT or PET alone has become more established with numerous studies demonstrating improved results.[16,17] Furthermore, PET/CT as a single study is more accurate for recurrent colorectal cancer than co-registration of two separately acquired PET and CT studies.[17] There is a growing consensus that PET/CT is the preferred imaging modality in these patients, because it restages the disease in one setting and can appropriately guide patient care.

Future PET/CT Applications for the Patient with Colorectal Disease

PET/CT will continue to play an important role in determining the resectability status of patients with recurrent rectal carcinoma before surgery and in the planning of aggressive procedures (Fig. 23-5) but is limited in defining local invasion of rectal tumors to adjacent tissues. Assessment of neoadjuvant therapy and guidance for radiation therapy are other applications that may be particularly suited to PET/CT. CT colonography (virtual colonoscopy) is a recently approved approach for the evaluation of patients at risk for colon cancer. It is possible combined PET/CT colonography will add specificity by selectively identifying hypermetabolic polyps, likely carrying a higher risk for malignant degeneration. Studies using the PET/CT colonography approach have reported encouraging results, showing this modality to be at least equivalent to PET plus CT for staging of colorectal cancer as well as detecting premalignant lesions.

Other Gastrointestinal Malignancies

PET and PET/CT have been used to assess patients with a number of other malignancies associated with the gastrointestinal tract and other abdominal organs. Although many of these are not currently covered by the CMS in

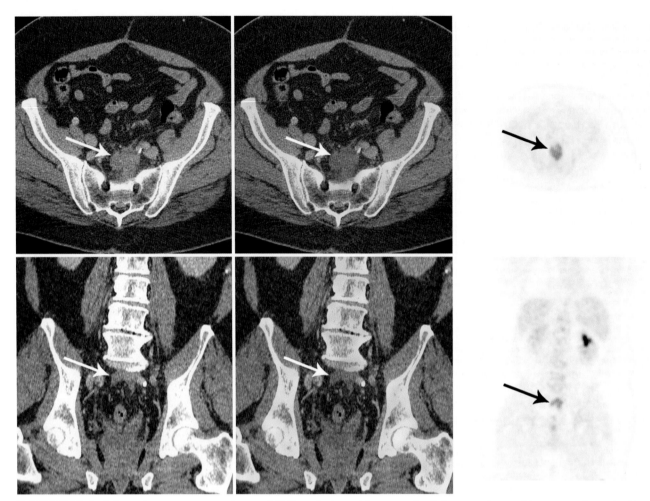

■ **FIGURE 23-4** Colorectal cancer recurrence. Increased FDG uptake (*arrows*) in presacral soft tissue consistent with recurrent disease in this patient with colorectal cancer.

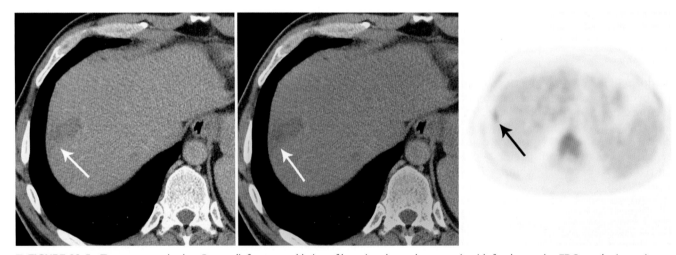

■ **FIGURE 23-5** Treatment monitoring. Post-radiofrequency ablation of hepatic colorectal metastasis with focal posterior FDG uptake (*arrows*) corresponding to an irregularly enhancing focus, consistent with recurrent disease at the edge of the low-density zone of ablation.

the United States, the National Oncologic PET Registry (NOPR) has allowed their use for such diseases if patients are suitably enrolled and with time many of these malignancies may gain full coverage.[18] Some of these will therefore be briefly discussed here.

Gastric Cancer

Early-stage gastric carcinoma has a relatively good prognosis, but unfortunately patients usually present late with advanced disease and, as a result, it is the second leading cause of cancer death worldwide. Where screening for

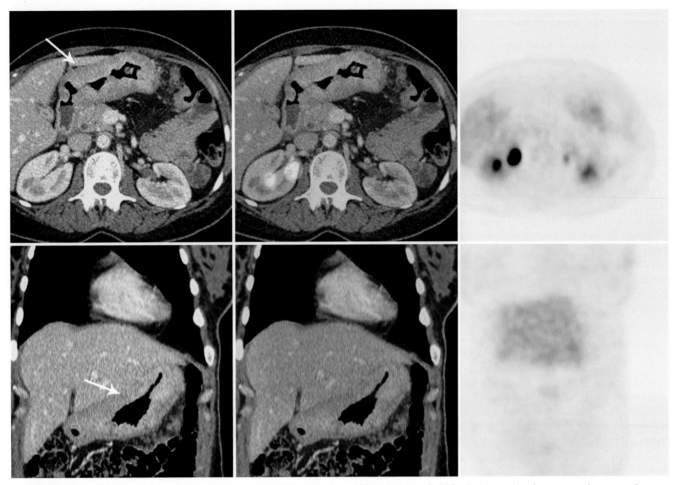

■ **FIGURE 23-6** Mucinous tumor with poor FDG uptake. CT images show diffuse gastric wall thickening (*arrows*) owing to a mucinous gastric adenocarcinoma that does not show significant FDG uptake.

gastric cancer occurs, the prognosis is better because the malignancy is detected at an earlier stage.

The role of FDG-PET and PET/CT in gastric cancer remains controversial. Despite a positive initial study by Yeung and colleagues,[19] most subsequent studies have demonstrated poorer rates of primary lesion detection, including a study by Shoda and coworkers,[20] which reported just 10% sensitivity and 99% specificity for early gastric cancer. This has led some authors to conclude that FDG-PET is not a suitable first-line diagnostic procedure in the detection of gastric cancer and is not helpful in tumor staging. There are a number of reasons for the relatively poor performance of FDG-PET in gastric cancer. First, normal physiologic FDG uptake in the stomach and gastroesophageal junction is variable and can have a focal appearance, especially if the stomach is empty and collapsed or after partial gastrectomy for malignancy. Benign inflammatory conditions show increased uptake, which can result in false-positive results. It has been proposed that the sensitivity of PET/CT may be improved upon with the ingestion of water or neutral density contrast to distend the stomach at the time of scanning. Stahl and associates[21] reported variable FDG uptake to be dependent on differing histopathologic findings, which may help explain the variable results for FDG-PET

in gastric carcinoma. They reported overall 60% sensitivity for the detection of locally advanced gastric cancers. Within this group, the detection rate was higher for intestinal type at 83% versus just 41% for the diffuse type. The mean standard uptake value was also significantly lower for mucus- versus non–mucus-containing tumors (Fig. 23-6).

Although unlikely to be highly accurate in local staging of gastric cancer, it is generally expected that PET/CT may play a useful role in the detection of distant metastases, such as those of the liver, lungs, adrenal glands, ovaries, and skeleton. FDG-PET may also be helpful in the assessment of chemotherapy, allowing for the identification of early response to treatment. More recently, there has been some interest in PET using different radiotracers. Herrmann and associates[22] reported on a comparison of 3-deoxy-3-^{18}F-fluorothymidine (FLT) with FDG for the detection of gastric cancer and reported 100% sensitivity for FLT and 69% for FDG. Further studies are needed to determine the efficacy of FDG and other novel PET radiotracers in the detection of local nodal metastases and peritoneal dissemination. Nevertheless, the combined use of CT and PET can be helpful in the preoperative staging of patients with stomach cancer and in their therapeutic monitoring.

Tumors of the Small Intestine

Adenocarcinoma, a rare tumor of the small intestine, mostly occurs in the duodenum. The more common small intestinal tumors include neuroendocrine tumors and sarcomas occurring mainly in the jejunum and ileum. Metastases may also occur especially from breast or melanoma and may be detected with PET/CT. FDG-PET has been used successfully in the detection of duodenal tumors, with one study reporting a 100% sensitivity. PET of neuroendocrine tumors has been successful with the use of FDG and with novel radiotracers such as 6-fluoro-L-dopa (FDOPA) and ^{68}Ga-DOTA-D Phe(1)-Tyr(3)-Octreotide (DOTATOC). FDG-PET has also been useful in the evaluation of both bone and soft tissue sarcomas. Bastiaannet and colleagues reported pooled sensitivity, specificity, and accuracy of 91%, 85%, and 88%, respectively, for PET detection of sarcoma in a meta-analysis.[23] They demonstrated its ability to discriminate between low- and high-grade sarcomas, and it is also expected that PET/CT would be of even greater benefit.

Gastrointestinal Stromal Tumors

Gastrointestinal stromal tumors (GISTs) are uncommon, accounting for less than 6% of all sarcomas and 3% of all gastrointestinal neoplasms. Most (70% to 80%) GISTs are benign. There is, however, a spectrum from benign to malignant that can be generally predicted according to tumor size and mitotic frequency. GISTs originate most commonly in the stomach and small bowel but can arise from anywhere along the gastrointestinal tract. They usually arise in the bowel wall, generally from or between the muscularis mucosa and propria. They may also originate in the mesentery or omentum. Metastatic disease can occur locally by direct invasion of adjacent structures or less typically by involvement of regional lymph nodes. Distant metastatic disease can involve the peritoneum as well as liver, lung, and bones.

There is variable FDG uptake by GISTs. FDG-PET was performed on eight patients, and the primary lesion was identified in just 50% of cases in a study by Hersh and coworkers.[24] The false-negative results were in smaller lesions, with a mean diameter of 6 cm and a homogeneous appearance on CT. The PET-positive cases were larger and heterogeneous on CT, and all had metastatic disease. The superior ability of contrast-enhanced CT over FDG-PET in the detection of GIST was confirmed by Goerres and associates,[25] who reported variable FDG uptake and a greater sensitivity for contrast-enhanced CT for lesion detection as compared with PET. The varied reported accuracy of PET at GIST staging may be due to the varied nature of the neoplasm itself. Although the majority of GISTs are benign, there is essentially a histologic continuum between benign and malignant lesions. There is higher FDG uptake in more malignant lesions, and it is possible that this may be used preoperatively to assess malignant potential. Goerres and coworkers concluded that single-stage PET/CT was superior to either PET and/or CT.[25] Comprehensive surgical removal offers the best chance of cure, and the tyrosine kinase inhibitor imatinib has shown good response rates. Heinicke and colleagues[26] reported that

FDG-PET can assess the response to imatinib at just 1 week after starting therapy. In another study, PET/CT was found to be superior to separate PET and CT at tumor response to imatinib treatment characterization, demonstrating 95% accuracy at 1 month and 100% accuracy at 3- and 6-month follow-up.[27] Not only can PET and PET/CT provide information on treatment response, but it has also been shown that the degree of FDG uptake at both initial staging and follow-up provides important prognostic information.[25]

Hepatic metastases from GIST can be isointense to liver on the portal venous phase of contrast-enhanced CT and may be better visualized on a non–contrast-enhanced CT for the initial PET/CT staging of GIST. Furthermore, treatment with imatinib may result in liquefaction of hepatic metastases. Patients who subsequently develop disease recurrence may manifest a new soft tissue nodule within a liquefied metastasis. This nodule-within-a-mass appearance is best appreciated with contrast enhancement, and therefore intravenous contrast should always be included in the follow-up PET/CT protocol for patients with GIST.

Gynecologic Malignancy

CMS guidelines in the United States approve the use of FDG-PET, and thus PET/CT, for use in staging patients with cervical cancer with conventional imaging negative for extrapelvic metastatic disease. CMS guidelines also approve the use of PET, and thus PET-CT, for patients with ovarian cancer in certain circumstances. PET and PET/CT have also been used to assess patients with endometrial and prostate cancer.

In premenopausal women, the endometrium shows biphasic FDG uptake peaks during the ovulatory and menstrual phases. The patient's menstrual history is thus useful for accurate interpretation, because increased endometrial uptake adjacent to a cervical malignancy does not necessarily represent tumor invasion. In addition, FDG uptake has been demonstrated in uterine fibroids (up to 18% in one series) but only in premenopausal women. Increased ovarian FDG uptake may transiently be seen in premenopausal patients owing to uptake in a corpus luteal cyst. However, ovarian uptake in postmenopausal women is not physiologic and is indicative of malignancy.

Cervical Cancer

Cervical cancer, although decreasing, is still estimated to be the third most common gynecologic malignancy in the United States. PET/CT is valuable in the primary staging of untreated advanced cervical cancer, for evaluation of unexplained tumor marker elevation post treatment, and for restaging of potentially curable recurrent cervical cancer, although it is of limited value in assessing early-stage cervical cancer. PET is approved in the evaluation of asymptomatic cervical patients with high tumor markers and negative conventional imaging.

A meta-analysis of 15 studies of FDG-PET in cervical cancer reported a pooled sensitivity and specificity of 84% and 95%, respectively, for aortic node metastases and 79% sensitivity and 99% specificity for pelvic node metastases.[28]

In the evaluation of cervical cancer recurrence, PET has been shown to be 90.3% sensitive and 76.1% specific for the detection of disease recurrence in patients with otherwise no evidence of cervical cancer after treatment. The meta-analysis of data from 15 studies on FDG-PET in cervical cancer reported a pooled sensitivity and specificity of 96% and 81%, respectively, for recurrent cervical cancer with clinical suspicion.[28] The results for combined PET/CT in the evaluation of disease recurrence are even better, with one study reporting sensitivity, specificity, and accuracy rates of 90.3%, 81.0%, and 86.5%, respectively.[29]

The use of PET/CT alters patient management, by up to 23% of cases in one study.[29] Assessment of para-aortic lymph node metastases is prognostically important and is related to progression-free survival in advanced cervical cancer. PET has high sensitivity and specificity and is more sensitive than MRI or CT for the detection of para-aortic lymphadenopathy from advanced cervical cancer.[28] A positive PET study post treatment for cervical cancer is associated with a significantly worse outcome, with subsequent development of metastatic disease and death.

Ovarian Cancer

Ovarian cancer is responsible for more than half of gynecologic malignancy–related deaths, and the overall 5-year survival for advanced disease is only 17%.

Reports of PET and PET/CT in ovarian cancer show mixed results. One study demonstrated CT to have a 53% accuracy rate for staging of newly diagnosed ovarian cancer in comparison with surgical staging. When the CT studies were evaluated conjointly with FDG-PET, the accuracy rate for combined imaging was 87%.[30] The overall FDG-PET sensitivity rates for detection of recurrent ovarian cancer range between 45% and 100%, with specificity rates of 40% to 99% (Fig. 23-7).[30] Currently, PET is considered to be beneficial for patients with leveled off or increasing abnormal serum CA-125 values and for patients with CT- or MRI-defined localized recurrence for whom biopsy is not possible. Second-look laparotomy or laparos-

copy is sometimes performed on patients after treatment who do not have clinical evidence of disease to assess disease response. FDG-PET with second-look laparotomy can decrease unnecessary laparotomies from 70% to 5% and also reduce health care costs. Further studies are needed to clarify the precise role of PET and PET/CT in patients with ovarian cancer.

Endometrial Cancer

Endometrial carcinoma is the fourth most common cancer in women and most common female pelvic malignancy. It is treated and staged by surgery, but, because adjuvant radiation therapy is given in most cases, assessment of nodal involvement is important. There is some evidence supporting the use of PET and PET/CT in patients with endometrial carcinoma.

One prospective study assessing preoperative evaluation of patients with endometrial carcinoma reported 96.7% sensitivity for PET (Fig. 23-8). However, PET detected none of the five cases of lymph node metastases less than 1 cm in diameter and, excluding retroperitoneal lymph nodes, PET proved to be 83.3% sensitive for the detection of extrauterine lesions.[31]

Belhocine and colleagues[32] assessed the usefulness of FDG-PET in the post-therapy surveillance of endometrial cancer and found 96% sensitivity, 78% specificity, and 90% accuracy for the detection of residual or recurrent disease. These results have been supported by other studies, again highlighting the superior nature of PET over conventional imaging with CT or MRI in the detection of recurrent disease. Most of these studies have highlighted that the performance of PET is improved upon when combined with a morphologic imaging modality. Sironi and associates[33] specifically evaluated the role of PET/CT in patients with uterine cancer, either cervical or endometrial, for the detection of tumor recurrence. They reported patient-based sensitivity, specificity, and accuracy for the detection of tumor recurrence of 93%, 100%, and 96%, respectively. The positive and negative predictive values were 100% and 92%.

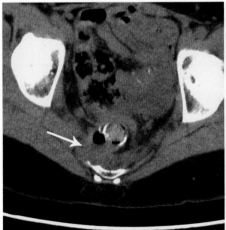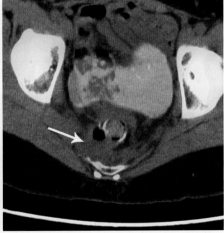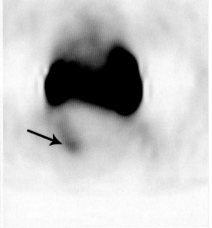

■ **FIGURE 23-7** Ovarian cancer recurrence. Focal FDG uptake in the posterior pelvis (*arrow*) corresponding to asymmetric soft tissue thickening on CT and PET/CT images consistent with recurrent disease in this patient status post surgery for ovarian cancer.

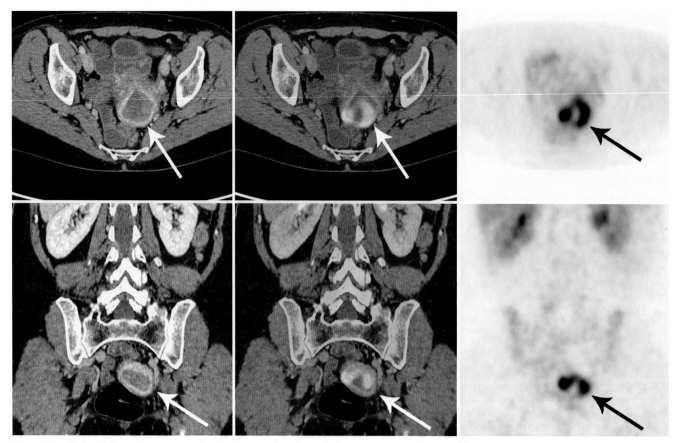

■ **FIGURE 23-8** Endometrial cancer staging. Large central uterine soft tissue mass on CT (*arrows*) with increased FDG uptake on the PET images (*arrows*) representing endometrial cancer.

These results emphasize the benefits of PET and PET/CT in endometrial carcinoma, but further larger studies will be necessary to clarify its role. Early results have shown that the addition of PET to CT may have important prognostic capabilities and may also affect patient management in up to a third of cases. PET/CT guides pelvic radiation portals and helps direct intensity-modulated radiotherapy to this area, as well as elsewhere in the body, by defining nodal sites of tumor involvement. This enables tailored radiation doses with increased sparing of normal tissues.

KEY POINTS

- PET/CT has been demonstrated to be the imaging modality of choice for many abdominopelvic malignancies.
- PET/CT plays a particularly important role in the management of patients with colorectal cancer and cervical cancer.
- The current and future results of the National Oncologic PET Registry may provide evidence to further expand approved PET and PET/CT indications and applications.
- Combined PET/CT is superior to later co-registered images for diagnostic accuracy.
- New radiotracers may help to improve the performance of PET/CT in those tumors that currently are better imaged with CT or MRI.

SUGGESTED READINGS

Blodgett TM, Meltzer CC, Townsend DW. PET/CT: form and function. Radiology 2007; 242:360-385.

Chao A, Chang TC, Ng KK, et al. ^{18}F-FDG PET in the management of endometrial cancer. Eur J Nucl Med Mol Imaging 2006; 33:36-44.

Hersh MR, Choi J, Garrett C, Clark R. Imaging gastrointestinal stromal tumors. Cancer Control 2005; 12:111-115.

Kapoor V, McCook BM, Torok FS. An introduction to PET-CT imaging. RadioGraphics 2004; 24:523-543.

Moore M, Blake MA. PET/CT in abdominal and pelvic malignancies: principles and practices. In Kalra MK, Saini S, Rubin GR (eds). MDCT from Protocols to Practice. New York, Springer, 2008, pp 166-208.

Pandit-Taskar N. Oncologic imaging in gynecologic malignancies. J Nucl Med 2005; 46:1842-1850.

Rohren EM, Turkington TG, Coleman RE. Clinical applications of PET in oncology. Radiology 2004; 231:305-332.

Subhas N, Patel PV, Pannu HK, et al. Imaging of pelvic malignancies with in-line FDG PET-CT: case examples and common pitfalls of FDG PET. RadioGraphics 2005; 25:1031-1043.

Wahl RL. Why nearly all PET of abdominal and pelvic cancers will be performed as PET/CT. J Nucl Med 2004; 45(Suppl 1):82S-95S.

Yen TC, Lai CH. Positron emission tomography in gynecologic cancer. Semin Nucl Med 2006; 36:93-104.

REFERENCES

1. Cerfolio RJ, Bryant AS, Ohja B, et al. The accuracy of endoscopic ultrasonography with fine-needle aspiration, integrated positron emission tomography with computed tomography, and computed tomography in restaging patients with esophageal cancer after neo-adjuvant chemoradiotherapy. J Thorac Cardiovasc Surg 2005; 129:1232-1241.
2. Gutman F, Alberini JL, Wartski M, et al. Incidental colonic focal lesions detected by FDG PET/CT. AJR Am J Roentgenol 2005; 185:495-500.
3. Kamel IR, Cohade C, Neyman E, et al. Incremental value of CT in PET/CT of patients with colorectal carcinoma. Abdominal Imaging 2004; 29:663-668.
4. Even-Sapir E, Parag Y, Lerman H, et al. Detection of recurrence in patients with rectal cancer: PET/CT after abdominoperineal or anterior resection. Radiology 2004; 232:815-822.
5. Rohren EM, Turkington TG, Coleman RE. Clinical applications of PET in oncology. Radiology 2004; 231:305-332.
6. Kinkel K, Lu Y, Both M, et al. Detection of hepatic metastases from cancers of the gastrointestinal tract by using noninvasive imaging methods (US, CT, MR imaging, PET): A meta-analysis. Radiology 2002; 224:748-756.
7. Rohren EM, Paulson EK, Hagge R, et al. The role of F-18-FDG PET in preoperative assessment of the liver in patients being considered for curative resection of hepatic metastases from colorectal cancer. Clin Nucl Med 2002; 27:550-555.
8. Kantorová I, Lipská L, Bělohlávek O, et al. Routine (18)F-FDG PET preoperative staging of colorectal cancer: comparison with conventional staging and its impact on treatment decision making. J Nucl Med 2003; 44:1784-1788.
9. Sahani DV, Kalva SP, Fischman AJ, et al. Detection of liver metastases from adenocarcinoma of colon and pancreas: comparison of mangafodipir trisodium enhanced liver MRI and whole body FDG-PET. AJR Am J Roentgenol 2005; 185:239-246.
10. Chua SC, Groves AM, Kayani I, et al. The impact of (18)F-FDG PET/CT in patients with liver metastases. Eur J Nucl Med Mol Imaging 2007; 34:1906-1914.
11. Valk PE, Abella-Columna E, Haseman MK, et al. Whole-body PET imaging with (^{18}F)fluorodeoxyglucose in management of recurrent colorectal cancer. Arch Surg 1999; 134:503-511.
12. Park IJ, Kim HC, Yu CS, et al. Efficacy of PET/CT in the accurate evaluation of primary colorectal carcinoma. Eur J Surg Oncol 2006; 32:941-947.
13. Hung GU, Shiau YC, Tsai SC, et al. Value of ^{18}F-fluoro-2-deoxyglucose positron emission tomography in the evaluation of recurrent colorectal cancer. Anticancer Res 2001; 21:1375-1378.
14. Wiering B, Krabbe PF, Jager GJ, et al. The impact of fluor-18-deoxyglucose-positron emission tomography in the management of colorectal liver metastases. Cancer 2005; 104:2658-2670.
15. Cohade C, Osman M, Leal J, Wahl RL. Direct comparison of (18) F-FDG PET and PET/CT in patients with colorectal carcinoma. J Nucl Med 2003; 44:1797-1803.
16. Chen LB, Tong JL, Song HZ, et al. (18)F-FDG PET/CT in detection of recurrence and metastasis of colorectal cancer. World J Gastroenterol 2007; 13:5025-5029.
17. Kim JH, Czernin J, Allen-Auerbach MS, et al. Comparison between 18F-FDG PET, in-line PET/CT, and software fusion for restaging of recurrent colorectal cancer. J Nucl Med 2005; 46:587-595.
18. Hillner BE, Liu D, Coleman RE, et al. The National Oncologic PET Registry (NOPR): design and analysis plan. J Nucl Med 2007; 48:1901-1908.
19. Yeung HW, Macapinlac H, Karpeh M, et al. Accuracy of FDG-PET in gastric cancer. Preliminary experience. Clin Positron Imaging 1998; 1:213-221.
20. Shoda H, Kakugawa Y, Saito D, et al. Evaluation of (18)F-2-deoxy-2-fluoro-glucose positron emission tomography for gastric cancer screening in asymptomatic individuals undergoing endoscopy. Br J Cancer 2007; 97:1493-1498.
21. Stahl A, Ott K, Weber WA, et al. FDG PET imaging of locally advanced gastric carcinomas: correlation with endoscopic and histopathological findings. Eur J Nucl Med Mol Imaging 2003; 30:288-295.
22. Herrmann K, Ott K, Buck AK, et al. Imaging gastric cancer with PET and the radiotracers 18F-FLT and 18F-FDG: a comparative analysis. J Nucl Med 2007; Nov 15 (Epub ahead of print).
23. Bastiaannet E, Groen H, Jager PL, et al. The value of FDG-PET in the detection, grading and response to therapy of soft tissue and bone sarcomas; a systematic review and meta-analysis. Cancer Treat Rev 2004; 30:83-101.
24. Hersh MR, Choi J, Garrett C, Clark R. Imaging gastrointestinal stromal tumors. Cancer Control 2005; 12:111-115.
25. Goerres GW, Stupp R, Barghouth G, et al. The value of PET, CT and in-line PET/CT in patients with gastrointestinal stromal tumours: long-term outcome of treatment with imatinib mesylate. Eur J Nucl Med Mol Imaging 2005; 32:153-162.
26. Heinicke T, Wardelmann E, Sauerbruch T, et al. Very early detection of response to imatinib mesylate therapy of gastrointestinal stromal tumours using ^{18}fluoro-deoxyglucose-positron emission tomography. Anticancer Res 2005; 25:4591-4594.
27. Antoch G, Kanja J, Bauer S, et al. Comparison of PET, CT, and dual-modality PET/CT imaging for monitoring of imatinib (STI571) therapy in patients with gastrointestinal stromal tumors. J Nucl Med 2004; 45:357-365.
28. Havrilesky LJ, Kulasingam SL, Matchar DB, Myers ER. FDG-PET for management of cervical and ovarian cancer. Gynecol Oncol 2005; 97:183-191.
29. Chung HH, Jo H, Kang WJ, et al. Clinical impact of integrated PET/CT on the management of suspected cervical cancer recurrence. Gynecol Oncol 2007; 104:529-534.
30. Yoshida Y, Kurokawa T, Kawahara K, et al. Incremental benefits of FDG positron emission tomography over CT alone for the preoperative staging of ovarian cancer. AJR Am J Roentgenol 2004; 182:227-233.
31. Suzuki R, Miyagi E, Takahashi N, et al. Validity of positron emission tomography using fluoro-2-deoxyglucose for the preoperative evaluation of endometrial cancer. Int J Gynecol Cancer 2007; 17:890-896.
32. Belhocine T, De Barsy C, Hustinx R, Willems-Foidart J. Usefulness of (18)F-FDG PET in the post-therapy surveillance of endometrial carcinoma. Eur J Nucl Med Mol Imaging 2002; 29:1132-1139.
33. Sironi S, Picchio M, Landoni C, et al. Post-therapy surveillance of patients with uterine cancers: value of integrated FDG PET/CT in the detection of recurrence. Eur J Nucl Med Mol Imaging 2007; 34:472-479.

Postprocessing

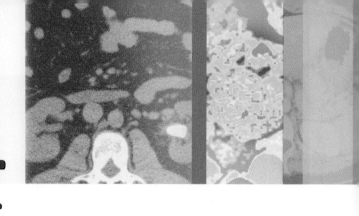

CHAPTER 24

Principles of 3D Postprocessing

Anand Singh, Gordon J. Harris, Wenli Cai, Dushyant V. Sahani, and Hiroyuki Yoshida

TECHNICAL ASPECTS

Two-dimensional (2D) and three-dimensional (3D) image processing has become an integral part of the current radiology work flow. With respect to abdominal imaging, image postprocessing not only provides a much-desired finesse to the multidetector CT (MDCT), ultrasonography, and MRI protocols but also has been frequently discussed and applied to extract important clinical information in oncology practice. Some examples of 3D benefits in oncology include generation of tumor volumes for treatment planning and assessing responses and for screening precancerous colonic polyps. Whereas the role of advanced 3D applications has been increasingly realized, the improvements in MDCT and MRI technology have made 3D more popular because it is now possible to apply 3D algorithms on thin-section datasets of higher resolution.

Before a 3D image is presented to the ordering clinician or the radiologist, it undergoes processing at various levels, which includes data acquisition at the scanner, the transfer of the required images to picture archiving and communication systems [PACS], transfer to the 3D laboratory, and application of the desired postprocessing algorithm in the 3D laboratory. Before we discuss the details of advanced postprocessing algorithms such as segmentation and image fusion, it is important to understand the technical basis of data handling before applying postprocessing algorithms on them.

Data Handling

MDCT

The 16- and 64-channel detector collimation scanners have tremendously boosted the capabilities of present-day 3D workstations, because it is now possible to employ various postprocessing algorithms on thin axial sections of high isotropic voxel resolution. More so, these scanners provide fast scan speed and thus have reduced the number of motion artifacts. This has immensely propelled the confidence of radiologists, who now have the option of viewing high-quality 3D-rendered images (Fig. 24-1).[1] With improvement in the quality of source data, even the simple reformatted images generated at various angles at the workstations are of good quality and resolution.[2,3] From the abdominal imaging perspective, recent advances in MDCT have been heavily used because coronal and sagittal reformatted images postprocessed with quality-enhancing filters are the mainstay in the diagnosis of pathologic processes of the bowel and are mostly generated for interpretation along with the source axial images (Fig. 24-2).

However, as the advantages of 3D postprocessing with thin sections of MDCT data become more evident, issues such as appropriate alterations of CT protocols and reduction in radiation dose are becoming increasingly important. This is especially applicable for those scans in which protocols employ the use of biphasic or triphasic acquisitions. The two pitfalls for thin-section acquisitions are longer time of scan and, more importantly, increased radiation dose to the subject. In our institution, we usually employ thin acquisitions only to those phases of pancreatic and liver MDCT protocols that will enable postprocessing of desired information (e.g., thin arterial phase acquisitions for mapping arterial anatomy of liver and kidney donors and image postprocessing for aortic aneurysms).

Recent improvements in contrast injection technology have provided reasonable assurance of perfection and setting up of contrast timing with the use of bolus tracking technologies. Recent research has also focused on improvements in the quality of images by using higher concentration contrast media, whereas the advent of dual-source MDCT has opened avenues for future improvements in protocol.

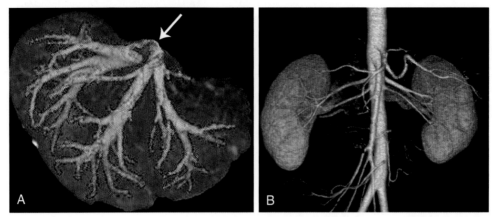

■ **FIGURE 24-1**   **A,** Volume-rendered CT liver image of a 35-year-old female donor showing hepatic venous confluence (*white arrow*). **B,** Volume-rendered CT image of a 46-year-old male donor showing renal arterial anatomy.

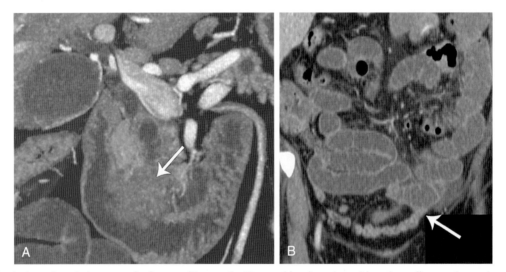

■ **FIGURE 24-2**   **A,** A good-resolution coronal reformatted image of a 49-year-old male patient with periampullary carcinoma (*arrow*) obtained on a 16-slice MDCT scanner. **B,** Coronal reformatted image obtained on an 8-slice CT scanner showing a stricture from Crohn's disease (*arrow*) in a 39-year-old man.

CT of Liver and Biliary Tree

The most useful and commonly employed postprocessing applications to liver MDCT protocols are for mapping of liver vascular anatomy before liver donor hepatic resection, placement of intra-arterial pumps, and tumor resection (Fig. 24-3). Other advanced postprocessing algorithms are useful for estimation of tumor volume and total and partial liver volume.

The knowledge of the hepatic arterial variants and the hepatic venous and portal venous anatomy is essential for the surgeon preoperatively, and image postprocessing done on such arterial and venous phase datasets helps to increase the surgeon's confidence. It is essential that the arterial and portal venous phase datasets be acquired at 1.25- and 2.5-mm sections, respectively, to ensure optimal quality of the postprocessed images (Table 24-1). The arterial phase acquisitions should be of thin collimation because hepatic arterial variants are of narrow caliber and sections of more than 2.0 mm may lead to image distortion by causing stair-stepping artifacts.

Usually 5-mm portal venous phase acquisitions are sufficient for follow-up scans or patients who undergo CT for monitoring treatment response, as 3D imaging is not of much use in such cases. However, thinner portal venous phase acquisitions are imperative to facilitate good quality 3D mapping of hepatic tumors as they are better characterized on the portal venous phase data. Thinner acquisitions can facilitate generation of tumor volumes without stair-stepping artifacts and calculation of total and partial liver volumes, especially useful before planning liver transplantation.

CT of Pancreas

One of the early postprocessing applications in our institute was generation of peripancreatic arterial and main portal vein maps for assessing vascular invasion by aggressive tumors such as pancreatic adenocarcinoma and curvilinear reformatted images for characterization of intraductal papillary mucinous neoplasms.

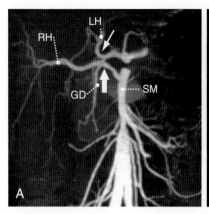
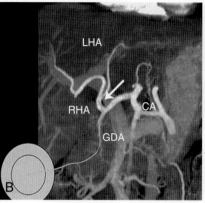
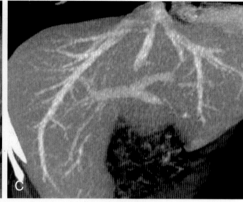

■ **FIGURE 24-3** **A,** A volume MR-MIP image displaying arterial anatomy of a 31-year-old male liver donor. Accessory right hepatic artery (RH) (*thick arrow*) is seen originating from the superior mesenteric artery (SM) while the left hepatic (LH) and gastroduodenal (GD) arteries originate from the celiac artery (*thin arrow*). **B,** A volume CT MIP image showing hepatic arterial anatomy from a 57-year-old female patient. The tip of the intra-arterial chemotherapy pump line is seen in the right hepatic artery (RHA, *thin arrow*). CA, celiac artery; GDA, gastroduodenal artery; LHA, left hepatic artery. **C,** A CT coronal volume MIP image from a 29-year-old male donor showing hepatic venous anatomy.

TABLE 24-1 Liver CT Angiography Protocol and Recommended Postprocessing Techniques

Parameters	16-Channel MDCT	64-Channel MDCT	Postprocessing Protocol
Range	Dome to L4		1. Batch MIP reformatted images: axial + coronal reformatted images – arterial and venous phase acquisitions: 3 mm (covering entire liver)
Detector collimation (mm)	1.25	0.625	
Table speed (mm/s)	13.75	55	
Slice: arterial (mm)	1	0.625	2. Manually generated oblique volume MIPs and VRs: 10-mm thick MIPs displaying hepatic arterial variants at various angles and 10- to 15-mm volume-rendered images of hepatic vascular anatomy with a subtracted background (enhanced display of arterial branch to segment IV of liver)
Slice: venous (mm)	2.5	1.25	
Injection rate (mL/s)	3-4	4-5	
Delay: arterial (s)	Bolus track/automated trigger: 25 seconds		
Delay: venous (s)	60 seconds		
120-150 mL of 300 mg/mL nonionic contrast medium at 4 mL/s or 80-100 mL of 370 mg/mL at 5 mL/s			

MIP, Maximum intensity projection; VR, volume rendering.

TABLE 24-2 Pancreas CT Angiography Protocol and Recommended Postprocessing Techniques

Parameters	16-Channel MDCT	64-Channel MDCT	Postprocessing Protocol
Range	Dome to L4		1. Batch MIP reformatted images:
Detector collimation (mm)	1.25	0.625	Axial + coronal reformatted images – arterial and venous phase acquisitions: 3 mm (covering entire pancreas)
Table speed (mm/s)	13.75	55	Oblique coronal reformatted images: slab oriented parallel to body of pancreas
Slice: arterial (mm)	1.25	0.625	Oblique reformatted images: slab oriented perpendicular to course of portal vein (useful for adenocarcinoma involving pancreatic head to assess circumference of portal vein involvement.)
Slice: venous (mm)	2.5	2.5	
Injection rate (mL/s)	3-4	4-5	
Delay: arterial (s)	Bolus track/automated trigger: 35 seconds		2. Manually generated oblique volume MIPs and VRs:
Delay: venous (s)	60 seconds		10-mm thick MIPs displaying peripancreatic arterial and venous relationship to pancreatic tumor at various angles. Volume-rendered images (15 mm) of hepatic and pancreatic vascular anatomy with a subtracted background displaying celiac trunk and superior mesenteric artery (enhanced zoomed display of relationship of portal vein to pancreatic tumor [oblique coronal images] + curvilinear MinIP reformatted images of pancreatic duct for pancreatic cystic neoplasms).
120-150 mL of 300 mg/mL nonionic contrast medium at 4 mL/s or 80-100 mL of 370 mg/mL at 5 mL/s			

MIP, Maximum intensity projection; VR, volume rendering; MinIP, minimum intensity projection.

A dedicated pancreatic CT angiography protocol is used for staging of pancreatic malignancies (Table 24-2). Because of the complex peripancreatic vascular anatomy, thin acquisitions for both the arterial phase and portal venous phase are justified because involvement of narrow arteries like the common hepatic artery and celiac trunk with or without the portal vein involvement can make a tumor unresectable. However, we are supportive of previous established study conclusions that pancreatic tumor is best evaluated by reviewing the pancreatic phase and

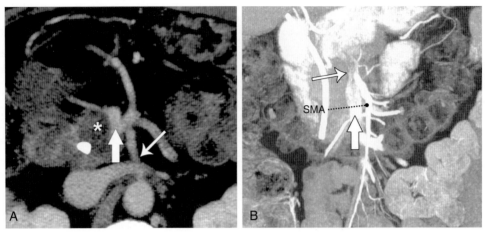

■ **FIGURE 24-4** **A,** Axial CT image of a 53-year-old male patient with pancreatic adenocarcinoma showing contrast medium in the portal vein (*arrow*) that is involved by the pancreatic head mass (*asterisk*) and the superior mesenteric artery (*arrow*). **B,** A coronal volume MIP image from a 62-year-old man showing contrast opacification of both superior mesenteric vein (*thick arrow*) and superior mesenteric artery (SMA). Narrowing of SMV caliber by the pancreatic mass is seen (*thin arrow*).

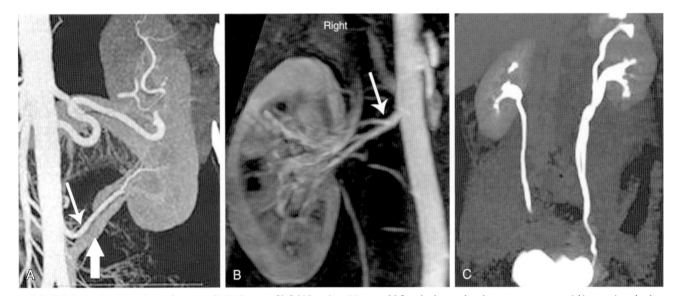

■ **FIGURE 24-5** **A,** CT angiography coronal MIP image of left kidney in a 32-year-old female donor showing accessory artery (*thin arrow*) and vein (*thick arrow*) at the lower pole. Accessory venous origin is from the left common iliac vein. **B,** MR angiography image of right kidney in a 45-year-old male donor showing early arterial branching of right main renal artery (*thin arrow*). **C,** CT urography coronal MIP image in a 29-year-old man showing incomplete duplication of the left collecting system. (*A and C reprinted with permission from Singh AK, Sahani DS, Kagay CR, et al. Semiautomated MIP images created directly on 16-section multidetector CT console for evaluation of living renal donors. Radiology 2007; 244:583-590.*)

the portal venous phase scans because it ensures optimal pancreatic parenchymal enhancement.[4,5] Some authorities prefer to increase the scan delay time (35 to 40 seconds) after contrast agent injection in such a manner that the initial acquisition is midway between the arterial phase (25 seconds' delay) and pancreatic phase (50 seconds) (Fig. 24-4). Such applications and trial alterations in protocols are only in their evolution since the advent of bolus triggering technique, which ensures optimal contrast opacification of the desired vessels in a particular phase. In addition, scan acquisition for four phases—noncontrast, arterial, pancreatic, and portal venous—can raise concerns with respect to radiation dose. We encourage such trials when increasing scan delay time after contrast injection can lead to reduction in radiation dose without compromising the scan information.

CT of Urinary Tract

The benefits of postprocessing have been explored in imaging of renal donors because knowledge of renal vascular variants is an important preoperative requisite for the surgeon to decide on the donor kidneys and because 3D maps of renal arteries and veins prove extremely useful (Fig. 24-5). Maximum intensity projections (MIPs) and volume-rendered images provide an elegant display of the renal arterial and venous variants and also the abnormalities of the donor kidney collecting system. Postprocessing applications have also proven useful for displaying the extent of renal vein thrombosis and quantification of renal tumor volumes, but it is imperative that protocols be planned to suit the postprocessed image quality. Because of extensive realization of postprocessing benefits for

TABLE 24-3 CT Angiography of Renal Donor and Recommended Postprocessing Techniques

Parameters	16-Channel MDCT	64-Channel MDCT	Postprocessing Protocol
Range	Dome to L4		1. Batch MIP reformatted images:
Detector collimation (mm)	1.25	0.625	Coronal + oblique coronal reformatted images for
Table speed (mm/s)	13.75	55	vascular phase (slab oriented parallel to renal
Slice: arterial + venous (mm) – single phase acquisition	1.25	0.625	vessels on axial images for both sides): 3 mm
Slice: delayed (mm)	2.5	2.5	Oblique coronal: for delayed phase with slab oriented parallel to lumbar spine
Injection rate (mL/s)	3-4	4-5	2. Manually generated oblique volume MIPs and
Delay: arterial (s)	Bolus tracking/automated trigger: 25 seconds		VRs:
120-150 mL of 300 mg/mL nonionic contrast medium at 4 mL/s or 80-100 mL of 370 mg/mL at 5 mL/s			10-mm thick MIPs displaying renal arterial and venous anatomy at various angles and volume-rendered images (enhanced zoomed display of early arterial renal artery branching and annotations displaying length of renal vein on both sides)

MIP, Maximum intensity projection; VR, volume rendering.

imaging renal donors, CT protocol is standardized at most centers that obtain 1.25-mm sections for vascular-phase acquisitions and 2.5-mm sections for CT urography (Table 24-3).

CT in Lower Abdominal Pain

In most patients with presentation of acute right lower abdominal pain, a specific diagnosis of acute appendicitis can be made with CT, leading to prompt surgical intervention. However, in most cases, there is an existing differential diagnosis (e.g., pancreatitis, cholecystitis, diverticulitis, typhlitis, intussusception) (Fig. 24-6).[6] Because the diagnosis is unknown, we usually restrict the protocol to a single postcontrast phase acquisition in which 1.25-mm or 0.625-mm scan acquisitions on the 16- and 64-channel detector MDCT are reconstructed to 2.5-mm thin sections at 2.5-mm intervals. In an emergency setting the value of coronal and sagittal reformatted images for diagnosis of pathologic processes of the bowel is indispensable; however, we prefer to keep our acquisitions thin to maintain the optimal quality of reformatted images and facilitate further postprocessing if needed.

CT Enterography

Optimal evaluation of the bowel segment can only be achieved if the small bowel is well distended, intravenous contrast has been administered, and thin 1- to 2-mm sections have been obtained. The most important factor to be considered for a CT enterography is the type of oral contrast media that is used. Many centers have still retained the use of positive oral contrast materials for evaluation of pathologic processes of the bowel. However, when the small bowel is distended with positive contrast media, the wall is thin and may be imperceptible but should not measure more than 1 to 2 mm.[7] The potential limitation of using positive oral contrast agents in evaluation of the small bowel is obscuration of mucosal enhancement by the intravenous contrast agent, which is a reliable finding to differentiate normal from an abnormal bowel wall. This fact justifies the use of neutral oral contrast such as

a commercially available, low-density barium solution in most institutions.[8,9]

For imaging the small bowel we encourage the use of 16- and 64-channel detector scanners, which ensures thin acquisitions and generates good-quality coronal and sagittal reformatted images.

Ultrasonography

It is only in the past few years that 3D ultrasonography has gained more importance due to the progress in computer technologies and visualization applications. With such advances, it is now possible to obtain a volumetric picture in a single image with automated compiling of numerous image acquisitions.[10] Such techniques have established increasing popularity in obstetric imaging, where they are useful to detect congenital anomalies and for guidance of surgical procedures.

An essential prerequisite to ensure optimal quality of 3D images is data acquisition such that the acquisition geometry is known to avoid distortions, and this is made possible by rapid image acquisitions that are free from motion artifacts. Another requirement is that the mechanism that manipulates the transducer or localizes its position in space must not interfere with the regular performance of the ultrasonographic examination.

The four types of ultrasound data acquisition systems that facilitate 3D data generation are mechanical, tracked freehand, untracked freehand, and 2D transducer arrays.

In mechanical scanning systems, the linear or annular transducer array is positioned on a mechanical assembly that enables precision in transducer movement by a computer-controlled motor. The 3D image generation by mechanical transducers is dependent on three basic types of transducer motions: linear, tilting, and rotational.[11] The linear scanning requires that the transducer be moved by a stepping motor in a linear fashion along the surface of the patient's skin so that the 2D images are obtained parallel to each other. This facilitates determination of spatial sampling interval along with a majority of the parameters needed for reconstruction that can lead to shortening of reconstruction time. With tilt and rotational scanning, the

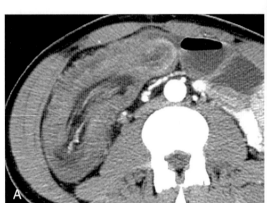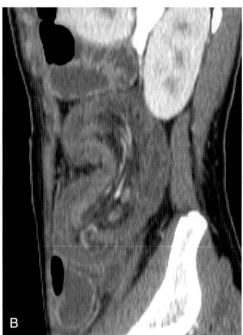

■ **FIGURE 24-6** **A,** Axial CT image from a 39-year-old woman showing incarceration of the bowel in intussusception. **B,** Sagittal CT reformatted image from the same patient showing the same pathologic process.

image acquisition is usually in a fan-like geometry or around the center axis, respectively. With tracked free-hand systems, the operator holds the assembly composed of the transducer and a position-sensor device and manipulates it over the anatomic area under evaluation. They are of three types: acoustic tracking, optical tracking, and magnetic field tracking; and discussion of their technical details is beyond the scope of this chapter.[12-14] Magnetic field tracking is relatively new and utilizes a tracked free-hand technique in which magnetic localizers are used to measure transducer positions and angles in space. With such techniques, minimizing electromagnetic interference and placing the transducer close to the receiver can achieve high 3D reconstruction accuracy.

Image fusion is a process of aligning and superimposing images obtained using two different imaging modalities. It is a rapidly evolving field of interest in abdominal imaging with its own specific operational conditions. At present, such techniques have found a useful role for imaging-guided interventions on liver lesions. The basic concept is to combine the real-time imaging of ultrasonography with the resolution provided by MDCT and produce the image volume. Such fusion equipment is expensive, yet given the cost-effectiveness, can be valuable to perform thermal tumor ablations that require positioning of multiple applicators and puncture of multiple lesions, thus reducing the puncture risk and procedure time.

MRI

Unlike CT, MRI has distinct advantages because it provides images in all three orthogonal planes, is radiation free, and has inherent 3D generation capabilities. Although MDCT is more commonly used in preoperative imaging of renal

donors due to its isotropic voxel resolution, some centers still prefer MRI, which provides a remarkable display of renal vascular anatomy (Table 24-4). However, better post-processing benefits of MRI have been realized in imaging of pancreaticobiliary and hepatic pathologic processes and imaging of liver donors because narrow hepatic arterial variants can easily be seen and pancreatic cystic neoplasms can be better displayed (Fig. 24-7). One of the most popular pulse sequences, especially in abdominal imaging today, is volumetric interpolated breath-hold examination (VIBE), which is basically a fast low-angle shot (FLASH) sequence with 3D Fourier transformation imaging and fat saturation prepulses.[15] This sequence provides near-isotropic data with a breath-hold of nearly 20 seconds. The combination of gadolinium bolus injection followed by running VIBE sequences has proven extremely beneficial in characterization of focal liver lesions such as benign and malignant tumors and hemangiomas by revealing characteristic enhancement patterns. It may also be possible to map the vasculature inside the lesion because maximum intensity projection (MIP) algorithms can then be applied to the VIBE sequence data and images can be generated.

In evaluation of the bowel, volumetric T1-weighted FLASH sequences with fat saturation in combination with oral paramagnetic contrast agent administration provide high-resolution images from which virtual endoscopic views can be generated by application of volume-rendering algorithms.[16] It is imperative to maintain a high signal-to-noise ratio for thin-slice acquisition because this can lead to better delineation of bowel lumen and bowel wall from the surrounding tissues. With the presence of water in the intestinal lumen and with intravenous gadolinium administration, different bowel wall enhancement patterns can be well appreciated, which

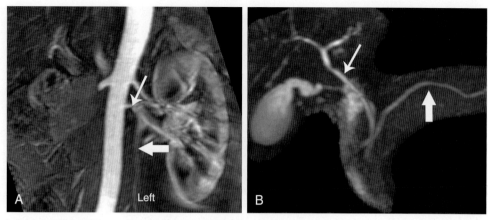

■ **FIGURE 24-7** **A,** Coronal MRA volume-rendered image of the left kidney from a 41-year-old man showing accessory left renal artery (*thin arrow*) and left lumbar vein (*thick arrow*). **B,** An MRCP MIP image showing the biliary (*thin arrow*) and pancreatic (*thick arrow*) ductal anatomy.

TABLE 24-4 MR Protocol for Imaging of Renal Donors

MR Sequences	TR (ms)	TE (ms)	Fat Suppression ±	Breath-hold ±
Axial T2W fast spin-echo	2500	90	+	+
Axial T1W gradient-echo (in-phase & out-phase)	170	4.7/2.3	−	+
Coronal T2W fast spin-echo (HASTE)	1500	105	−	−
*Postcontrast-3D (VIBE)	5.0	2.3	−	+
Axial-fat saturated (bolus timing + 20-30 mL IV gadolinium)				

*Immediate acquisition after injection followed by acquisitions at 30, 70, and 120 seconds.

distinguishes inflammatory or malignant wall pathologic processes from a normal bowel wall, and thus this method can be used for detection of colonic polyps.[17]

Presently, 3D Fourier transformation volume studies have been conducted with gradient-echo sequences and they offer pure T2-weighted volumetric images without susceptibility artifacts. These sequences offer superb T2 contrast and are extremely useful in MR cholangiopancreatography (MRCP).[18] Because this sequence employs a relatively long echo time value, only the fluid-filled pancreatic and biliary ducts appear highlighted while the surrounding soft tissue expresses moderate to short T2 relaxation times. Special prepulses have been proposed to make this sequence more efficient in terms of time acquisition.

Segmentation of Abdominal Viscera

Image segmentation provides quantitative information about relevant anatomy, such as estimation of the volume and size of a particular organ. Presently, segmentation techniques are becoming increasingly popular in abdominal imaging, where the preoperative knowledge of total and partial liver and kidney volumes before transplantation is essential. Splenic volume estimation in infiltrative disorders such as Gaucher's disease, ongoing research on pancreatic segmentation, and abdominal fluid quantification are some important areas in which segmentation is likely to establish its importance from a clinical standpoint. Various segmentation techniques include manual

segmentation, thresholding, edge-based segmentation, region-based segmentation, and automated segmentation.

Manual segmentation is basically plotting the points with mouse clicks or performing tracing along the borders of the organ or area that needs to be segmented (Fig. 24-8). Plotting of points is basically done on either consecutive or every alternate or third axial section, and then the software can compile all the points together on the stack of images and generate a volume of the organ. This method is more popular on the research front and is more reliable in terms of accuracy because it is operator controlled.

Segmentation based on thresholding is basically selection of a certain value (range of Hounsfield units), which the computer recognizes as the area to be highlighted and calculated. When using such methods, it is important to define the exact range of Hounsfield units in which the desired structure will fall. Such techniques are usually applied to segment abdominal fat and quantify it, because it is more useful for structures that have generalized distribution, as manual tasks for such segmentation are usually tedious.

Edge-based segmentation is dependent on discontinuities in the image data at the border of the organ that is to be segmented. The main method of identifying an organ by this method is the difference in pixel values at the border of the organs. In this way, each organ is outlined along its border by means of a gradient operator such as a Sobel or Roberts filter. However, this method of segmentation has proved to be more difficult in the past and is not very popular in current practice.

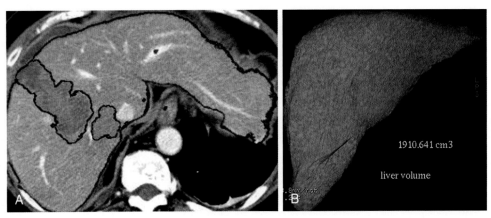

■ **FIGURE 24-8** **A,** Manual tracings of the liver (*red*) and tumor borders (*blue*) performed in a 52-year-old man with hepatocellular carcinoma. **B,** An image showing generated liver volume of a 30-year-old female donor after having performed segmentation on every alternate axial CT slice obtained on a 16-MDCT scanner.

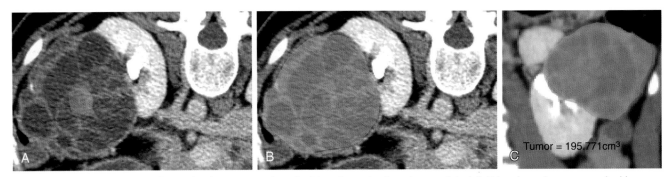

■ **FIGURE 24-9** **A,** A prone CT image showing segmentation of solid-cystic renal cell carcinoma of the left kidney by region: grow method by means of a computer mouse click. **B,** Region tracing includes the whole tumor on the axial slice. **C,** A coronal reformatted image showing the same finding along with volume estimation of the tumor.

One of the most popular methods that is gaining increasing importance is segmentation of an organ by growth of a plotted seed point. In this method, a seed point is plotted in the desired organ parenchyma and then the growth of the point is initiated by a computer mouse click. The point spread is based on identifying similar pixels in the vicinity (Hounsfield units on CT) and then establishing a growth pattern (Fig. 24-9). This method is much quicker and allows operator maneuverability through much sophisticated and automated erasers to facilitate edits and increase accuracy. In addition, the seed point growth method offers more comfort to the operator, who just has to press the mouse button and monitor the growth of points to prevent leaks rather than plotting points along the desired organ boundaries on multiple axial images.

Various other methods for segmentation are evolving, namely, the level set method and segmentation by active contouring and deformable models. However, traditional methods such as manual segmentation and region growing by seed points are more popular because they allow more operator control, with the latter method being much more comfortable and automated.

Filtering of 3D Images

There are various preprocessing steps in medical image processing at workstations. The idea is to get rid of the image noise that gives a generalized fuzziness to the 3D image from its presence in the originally acquired axial datasets. Various filters have been developed using gradient maps and vector field physics formulas for elimination of such image noise and creating a better delineation between two object boundaries. Smoothening of the image often has a blurring effect on the image boundaries, and it is imperative that the recent filters should possess the ability to reduce image noise proportionally while ensuring sharp transition margins between tissues.

An anisotropic filter is one of the proposed solutions to achieve smoothening of images without affecting object boundaries.[19] This basically works on different regions of the image as a diffusive process that can be applied to the whole image except the boundaries between two objects where the filter displays suppressed activity due to selection of appropriate diffusion strengths. Thus, the filter is able to perform intraparenchymal smoothening without smoothening the edges and displaying organ details with relative clarity. Such filtering techniques have assumed important roles and are under further development because their role is extremely vital in cardiac and abdominal image postprocessing in which images have variable degrees of motion artifacts.

Various other filters such as the gradient vector flow (GVF) snake model (deformable model) and fuzzy C/mean cluster segmentation are more sophisticated techniques to achieve optimal quality, and description of their technical principles is beyond the scope of this chapter.[20]

Visualization of 3D Image

Some of the algorithms for visualization of a 3D image are surface rendering, volume rendering, and projection algorithms such as maximum intensity projection (MIP) and minimum intensity projection (MinIP). Postprocessing techniques for evaluation of various abdominal pathologic processes are given in Table 24-5.

Surface rendering is generation of apparent surfaces from the dataset, which are suitably visualized. Either a triangular algorithm or a marching cube algorithm can generate the desired surface. In a triangular algorithm, contours defined on two adjacent slices are divided in the same number of equiangular sectors, which are then joined by points connected by obtaining a series of triangles that will define the surface.

Volume rendering is a process that visualizes sample functions of 3D data volume by computing 2D projections of a semi-transparent volume from a desired point of view, that is, it preserves any information contained in the data volume. Typically, for each voxel in the data volume a color and transparency is assigned. Then rays are traced into volume and are attenuated and colored depending on their route through the volume.

More simple and quicker ways of postprocessing are the application of projection algorithms like MIP and MinIP. In MIPs, the maximum value of the gray scale in the image is chosen and brighter structures are highlighted, whereas for MinIPs the lower gray scale values form the image. Therefore, for most of the CT angiography protocols in the abdomen, MIP projection algorithms are used for postprocessing to achieve optimal vessel prominence, which is opacified after contrast agent injection. MinIPs are usually helpful for better delineation of thin fluid-filled structures such as the pancreatic duct and therefore are invaluable in characterization of tiny cystic pancreatic neoplasms.

Virtual Endoscopy

Virtual endoscopy is simply a computer-generated endoscopic view of a lumen. Basically, the intention behind virtual endoscopy would be to achieve the same perspective and views of the lumen that an actual endoscope can provide to the clinician.

However, because of the demand for better image quality and resolution, which are essential prerequisites for production of virtual endoscopy images, appropriate alteration to MDCT protocol is essential.

Colon

One of the most important and frequently used applications in abdominal imaging is virtual colonoscopy, which is now an emerging screening tool for detection of precancerous colonic polyps. Ideal CT data for colonography should be of thinner-section acquisition and be devoid of breathing artifacts. The procedure should ensure optimal colonic cleansing and patient comfort. Bowel preparation should be tailored with proper cathartic cleansing and tagging of stool or fluid. Distention is achieved by rectal air or carbon monoxide insufflations, and CT localizer (scout) images are acquired before thin-section acquisitions to confirm optimal bowel distention. The new-generation scanners such as 16- and 64-slice MDCT have helped immensely to improve patient comfort and reduce the breathing artifacts.[21,22] Scan protocol should be tailored in such a way that polyps less than 5 mm in diameter are also included. Most places prefer thinner 1.25- to 2.00-mm acquisitions to obtain better image quality with about the same reconstruction intervals. Obtaining double acquisitions is a good idea because the positions of bowel loops vary and two images from different acquisitions of

TABLE 24-5 Recommended Postprocessing for Common Abdominal Pathologic Processes

Process	Reformatted MIPs: Coronal + Axial	Volume MIP + VR-Manually Created	Advanced Applications
Liver			
Donor	+	+ (hepatic vasculature)	Segmentation and volumetry (total and partial liver)
Tumor	+	+ (hepatic vasculature)	Segmentation + tumor volume
Pancreas			
Tumors	+	+ (peripancreatic vasculature)	–
IPMN	+	+ (peripancreatic vasculature)	Curvilinear reformatted image of pancreatic duct (MinIP)
Kidneys			
Donors and recipients	+	+ (renal vasculature)	Segmentation + kidney volume
Stone	+ (average algorithm; no MIPs)	–	–
Bowel			
Suspected obstruction	+ (average algorithm; no MIPs)	–	–
Virtual colonoscopy	+ (average algorithm; no MIPs)	–	Segmentation, virtual navigation, computer-aided detection for polyp detection and electronic cleansing

MIP, Maximum intensity projection; VR, volume rendering; MinIP, minimum intensity projection; IPMN, intraductal papillary mucinous neoplasm.

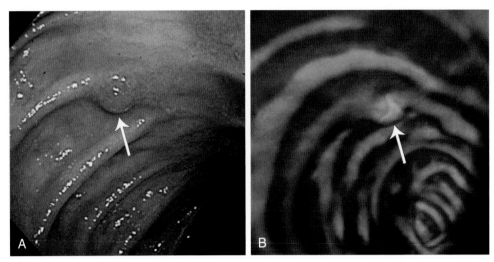

■ **FIGURE 24-10** **A,** A screening optical colonoscopy image showing a polyp in the descending colon (*arrow*) of a 56-year-old man. **B,** A virtual CT colonoscopy image confirming the same finding (*arrow*).

the same area help to differentiate polyps from fecal material (Fig. 24-10).

Vessels

Dedicated angiography protocols with appropriate scan delays from contrast injection are vital to enable desired image postprocessing of abdominal aortic aneurysms. Virtual angioscopy has allowed better assessment of intimal flaps in cases of intimal tears in aortic dissection and also maps the origin of the renal arteries and celiac trunk. Additionally, it can be valuable in assessment of intra-stent stenosis. We recommend thin-scan acquisitions (1 mm) to improve the quality of virtual angioscopy pictures, especially when evaluation of intimal flap origin and relationship of true and false lumen need to be established.[23] MR angiography can also be performed for the purpose of evaluating dissecting aneurysms but with the better contrast resolution and time savings offered by MDCT.

Computer-Aided Detection

Effective automated detection of colonic polyps has provided computer-aided detection with a much-needed boost and has highlighted its importance as a potential solution for future work flow.[24] With extensive research data available, computer-aided detection in CT colonography has been established as an effective screening tool for detection of precancerous colonic polyps.[25] The main idea is to train a computer such that it locates a desired point, which can then be presented to the radiologist for assessing whether the area is normal or abnormal. The problem, which still remains unsolved, is the higher number of false-positive detections by computer-aided detection, which a radiologist has to eventually assign as normal or abnormal.

Recent research at prominent conferences has focused on the vital role that computer-aided detection may have to offer for automated detection of tiny lymph nodes in lymphomas or detection of bleeding or tiny liver metastases. However, whether it is feasible to direct the research on computer-aided detection toward such perspectives or retain the present methods of diagnosis is debatable.

PROS AND CONS

With respect to abdominal imaging, image postprocessing is becoming increasingly popular among radiologists and referring clinicians. Certain important considerations such as volume calculations of tumor mass, segmentation of abdominal viscera such as liver and kidney for presurgical planning, MIP algorithms for vascular mapping, and computer-aided detection for colonic polyps have helped boost the role of 3D imaging immensely. Moreover, with the advent of newer-generation CT and MRI scanners, thin axial sections have increased further the postprocessing benefits.

It is important to draw a vital balance between acquisitions of MDCT datasets and optimal control of radiation dose delivery to the patients. Certain technical alterations such as acquiring thin sections for enabling postprocessing of a desired phase and relatively thicker sections for other phases while ensuring optimal information in the rest of the datasets are some recommendations to enhance the role of postprocessing in MDCT.

With similar concepts applying for MRI, higher detector-row MDCT scanners and higher Tesla-strength MRI scanners help to reduce scanning time, thereby reducing the motion artifacts. However, protocols for CT and MRI enterography and colonoscopy need improvement in terms of bowel preparation, thinness of acquisitions, and speed of scan.

With respect to presurgical planning of hepatic and pancreatic tumor resections, appropriate thinness of datasets for multiple scan phases is essential for generation of 3D vascular maps and also for reliable calculations of liver tumor volumes. With respect to MRI in abdominal imaging, 3D Fourier transformation gradient-recalled-echo sequences for MRCP and VIBE sequences for characterization of liver lesions are among the most discussed. Although various ultrasound data acquisition systems are available, ultrasound data capture is more automated with recent ultrasound scanners that permit 3D postprocessed views on the monitor.

Various methods for organ segmentation have been developed, namely, the edge-based segmentation, region segmentation by point spread, and deformable modeling. However, for segmentation purposes and organ volume estimations, the method of manually segmenting every alternate or third axial slab allows the most operator maneuverability and improves accuracy. The experiences with newer workstations have projected a promising role of region segmentation by point spread because it is relatively quick and still provides the much desired operator control.

Application of various filters to reduce image noise and fuzziness in image postprocessing is gaining widespread popularity because it helps the display of the interface between two objects in a more clear and distinct fashion. Volumetry, organ segmentation, and computer-aided detection are recent advances in 3D imaging that have established their crucial roles in imaging of liver, kidney, and colon. However, the older methods of displaying vascular maps by use of projection algorithms such as MIP and volume rendering still remain the most commonly performed and asked-for techniques from the clinical standpoint in abdominal imaging.

With respect to ongoing developments in computer-aided detection, virtual colonoscopy has received recognition as a screening tool for colon cancer, but other projected roles of computer-aided detection such as automated mapping and quantification of abdominal lymph node burden in lymphoma, location of bleeding, and detection of abdominal collections are still in evolutionary stages.

KEY POINTS

- Recent advances in ultrasonography, MDCT, and MRI scanners have propelled the benefits in imaging, because thin sections of artifact-free datasets allow better postprocessing of datasets.
- MDCT, which is the most frequently ordered modality of choice for staging pathologic processes, provides thin axial datasets of isotropic voxel resolution, which has helped immensely in exploring various postprocessing options.
- Although postprocessing has justified its usefulness for CT angiography protocols in the abdomen, tailoring of remaining abdominal CT protocols that ensure good postprocessed image quality while ensuring optimal control over the patient's radiation dose needs consideration.
- Manual control over advanced postprocessing techniques such as segmentation and volume estimations of liver, spleen, and kidney offers more reliability and accuracy, pending further developments in computer automation.
- MIP, which employs the use of maximum value of gray scale in the image, and volume rendering, which generates 3D data volume using 2D projections, are simple projection algorithms that still are the mainstays of CT angiography and MR angiography protocols in the abdomen.

SUGGESTED READINGS

Harris GJ. Three-dimensional imaging in radiology. In Dreyer K, Hirschorn D, Thrall JT, Mehta A (eds). PACS: A Guide to the Digital Revolution, 2nd ed. New York, Springer, 2006, pp 447-465.

Li G, Citrin D, Camphausen K, et al. Advances in 4D medical imaging and 4D radiation therapy. Technol Cancer Res Treat 2008; 7:67-82.

Maher MM, Kalra MK, Sahani DV, et al. Techniques, clinical applications and limitations of 3D reconstruction in CT of the abdomen. Korean J Radiol 2004; 5:55-67.

Vosshenrich R, Fischer U. Contrast-enhanced MR angiography of abdominal vessels: is there still a role for angiography? Eur Radiol 2002; 12:218-230.

Yoshida H, Näppi J. CAD in CT colonography without and with oral contrast agents: progress and challenges. Comput Med Imaging Graph 2007; 31:267-284.

REFERENCES

1. Rastogi N, Sahani DV, Blake MA, et al. Evaluation of living renal donors: accuracy of three-dimensional 16-section CT. Radiology 2006; 240:136-144.
2. Singh AK, Sahani DV, Kagay CR, et al. Semiautomated MIP images created directly on 16-section multidetector CT console for evaluation of living renal donors. Radiology 2007; 244:583-590.
3. Singh AK, Sahani DV. Imaging of the renal donor and transplant recipient. Radiol Clin North Am 2008; 46:79-93.
4. Goshima S, Kanematsu M, Kondo H, et al. Pancreas: optimal scan delay for contrast-enhanced multi-detector row CT. Radiology 2006; 241:167-174.
5. Vargas R, Nino-Murcia M, Trueblood W, Jeffrey RB Jr. MDCT in pancreatic adenocarcinoma: prediction of vascular invasion and resectability using a multiphasic technique with curved planar reformations. AJR Am J Roentgenol 2004; 182:419-425.
6. O'Malley ME, Halpern E, Mueller PR, Gazelle GS. Helical CT protocols for the abdomen and pelvis: a survey. AJR Am J Roentgenol 2000; 175:109-113.
7. Macari M, Balthazar EJ. CT of bowel wall thickening: significance and pitfalls of interpretation. AJR Am J Roentgenol 2001; 176:1105-1116.
8. Hara AK, Leighton JA, Sharma VK, et al. Imaging of small bowel disease: comparison of capsule endoscopy, standard endoscopy, barium examination, and CT. RadioGraphics 2005; 25:697-711; discussion 711-718.
9. Megibow AJ, Babb JS, Hecht EM, et al. Evaluation of bowel distention and bowel wall appearance by using neutral oral contrast agent for multi-detector row CT. Radiology 2006; 238:87-95.
10. Brandl H, Gritzky A, Haizinger M. 3D ultrasound: a dedicated system. Eur Radiol 1999; 9(Suppl 3):S331-S333.

11. Fenster A, Downey DB, Cardinal HN. Three-dimensional ultrasound imaging. Phys Med Biol 2001; 46:R67-R99.

12. Ofili EO, Nanda NC. Three-dimensional and four-dimensional echocardiography. Ultrasound Med Biol 1994; 20:669-675.

13. King DL, King DL Jr, Shao MY. Three-dimensional spatial registration and interactive display of position and orientation of real-time ultrasound images. J Ultrasound Med 1990; 9:525-532.

14. West BJ, Maurer CR Jr. Designing optically tracked instruments for image-guided surgery. IEEE Trans Med Imaging 2004; 23:533-545.

15. Rofsky NM, Lee VS, Laub G, et al. Abdominal MR imaging with a volumetric interpolated breath-hold examination. Radiology 1999; 212:876-884.

16. Papanikolaou N, Prassopoulos P, Grammatikakis J, et al. Optimization of a contrast medium suitable for conventional enteroclysis, MR enteroclysis, and virtual MR enteroscopy. Abdom Imaging 2002; 27:517-522.

17. Lauenstein TC, Herborn CU, Vogt FM, et al. Dark lumen MR-colonography: initial experience. Rofo 2001; 173:785-789.

18. Chrysikopoulos H, Papanikolaou N, Pappas J, et al. MR cholangiopancreatography at 0.5 T with a 3D inversion recovery turbo-spin-echo sequence. Eur Radiol 1997; 7:1318-1322.

19. Perona P, Malik J. Scale space and edge detection using anisotropic diffusion: on pattern analysis and machine intelligence. IEEE Trans 1990; 12:629-639.

20. Udupa JK, Samarasekera S. Fuzzy connectedness and object definition: theory, algorithm and application in image segmentation. Graphical Models and Image Processing 1996; 58:246-261.

21. Laghi A, Catalano C, Panebianco V, et al. [Optimization of the technique of virtual colonoscopy using a multislice spiral computerized tomography]. Radiol Med (Torino) 2000; 100:459-464.

22. Hara AK, Johnson CD, MacCarty RL, et al. CT colonography: single-versus multi-detector row imaging. Radiology 2001; 219:461-465.

23. Sbragia P, Neri E, Panconi M, et al. [CT virtual angioscopy in the study of thoracic aortic dissection]. Radiol Med (Torino) 2001; 102:245-249.

24. Doi K. Diagnostic imaging over the last 50 years: research and development in medical imaging science and technology. Phys Med Biol 2006; 51:R5-R27.

25. Yoshida H, Näppi J. CAD in CT colonography without and with oral contrast agents: progress and challenges. Comput Med Imaging Graph 2007; 31:267-284.

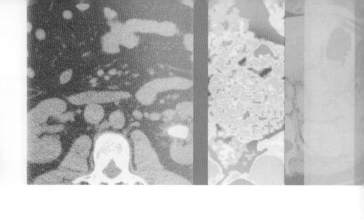

25

Advanced Applications in Postprocessing

Anand Singh, Gordon J. Harris, Dushyant V. Sahani, Wenli Cai, and Hiroyuki Yoshida

TECHNICAL ASPECTS

The advances in the newer-generation multidetector computed tomography (MDCT) and MRI scanners have increased the usefulness of advanced 3D applications and have brought certain important applications to the epicenter of research. Use of certain advanced postprocessing techniques were restricted in the previous decade because of unavailability of thinner sections of an axial dataset with appropriate resolution. With the availability of newer scanners, the feasibility and accuracy of certain advanced postprocessing applications such as virtual endoscopy, organ segmentation, and volumetry have acquired reasonable momentum. The basic principles governing the performance of such applications were discussed in Chapter 24. Here we describe the techniques of such applications more comprehensively, focusing on the present and projected future roles of such applications in a clinical setting.

Virtual Endoscopy

Virtual endoscopy is an advanced postprocessing application technique that is more geared to provide an endoscopy-like feel to clinicians by generation of a fly-through image through a lumen. The idea is to provide a picture that simulates a view that is obtained by an invasive endoscopy procedure (Fig. 25-1). The research on feasibility of such virtual navigation techniques and its clinical applications was questionable until the advent of higher-generation MDCT and MRI scanners that facilitated the availability of thin-section axial data, which are essential for generation of fly-through images. Although still in its evolutionary stages in the diagnosis of certain abdominal pathologic processes of bile and pancreatic ducts and vascular details, virtual endoscopy has established a role in the detection of precancerous colonic polyps.[1,2]

Scan Parameters

Thin-section axial images of isotropic voxel resolution (0.625 to 2 mm) that are artifact free with optimal distention of the desired lumen to be visualized, provide ideal preprocessed data that can ensure the generation of high-quality virtual fly-through images. CT protocol considerations in regard to certain applications of virtual endoscopy such as virtual colonoscopy call for alterations of scan protocols such that they are more suited to feasible and efficient generation of navigation images (Fig. 25-2). Apart from the proven usefulness of virtual colonoscopy as a screening tool for detection of colonic polyps, the clinical application of virtual endoscopy in abdominal imaging is still being explored; its use has been found to be encouraging for detection of some pancreatic and stomach pathologic processes. A more feasible proposition is that virtual endoscopy be reserved as an add-on postprocessing tool apart from routine CT and MRI datasets until its importance is proven effective by multiple studies. Therefore, effective research may encourage alterations of CT and MRI protocols to enhance the quality of the virtual endoscopy images and its performance.

Colon

For performing virtual colonoscopy, scan parameters should be optimized in such a way that they pose no hindrance for detection of polyps that are greater than 5 mm in diameter with appropriate tailoring of the kV and mAs settings (Fig. 25-3). Initially with single-slice CT, collimation of 3 to 5 mm was used. However, with 8- to 64-channel multidetector row CT (MDCT) scanners, fast artifact-free scan of 0.5 to 1.0 mm is possible, which has tremendously enhanced the per-polyp and per-patient sensitivity of detection of polyps.[3] Because distention of segments is influenced by position, it is essential to obtain

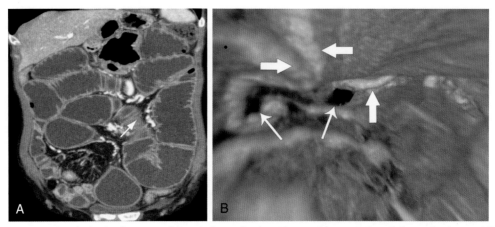

■ **FIGURE 25-1** **A,** Mesenteric volvulus leading to small bowel obstruction in a 39-year-old man. Point of obstruction is seen (*thin arrow*). **B,** Endoscopy image through the small intestine shows narrowing of lumen (*thin arrows*) and convergence of folds (*thick arrows*). (*Reprinted with permission from Singh AK, Hiroyuki Y, Sahani DV. Advanced postprocessing and the emerging role of computer-aided detection. Radiol Clin North Am 2009; 47(1):59-77.*)

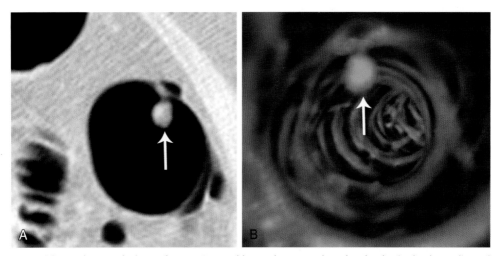

■ **FIGURE 25-2** **A,** An axial CT colonography image from a 49-year-old man shows a pedunculated polyp in the descending colon (*arrow*). **B,** A virtual CT colonoscopy image confirms the same finding (*arrow*). (*Reprinted with permission from Singh AK, Hiroyuki Y, Sahani DV. Advanced postprocessing and the emerging role of computer-aided detection. Radiol Clin North Am 2009; 47(1):59-77.*)

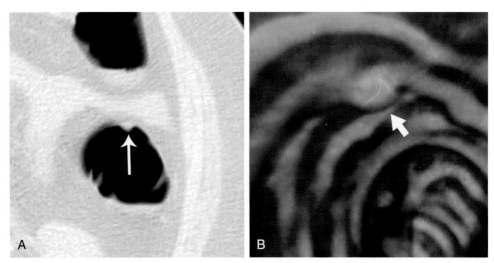

■ **FIGURE 25-3** **A,** An axial CT colonography image from a 50-year-old woman shows a flat polyp in the descending colon (*arrow*). **B,** A virtual CT colonoscopy image confirms the same finding (*arrow*).

TABLE 25-1 CT Colonography Protocol

Indications: Incomplete conventional colonoscopy; patient clinically unfit to undergo conventional colonoscopy; screening asymptomatic individuals for colorectal polyps/neoplasms
Rectal CO_2: Inflate colon with 4.0 L CO_2—mechanical inflation.

Plain Supine Scout Films and Series

Scan Parameters	16-MDCT	64-MDCT
Slice thickness	2.5 mm	2.5 mm
Pitch	1.375	1.375
Speed	13.75 mm/s	55 mm/s
Interval	1.25 mm	0.625 mm
Kilovoltage	120	120
Auto mA	50 (minimum) to 100 (maximum)	50 (minimum) to 100 (maximum)
Noise index	35	35

Plain Prone Scout Films and Series

Scan Parameters	16-MDCT	64-MDCT
Slice thickness	2.5 mm	2.5 mm
Pitch	1.375	1.375
Speed	13.75 mm/s	55 mm/s
Interval	1.25 mm	0.625 mm
Kilovoltage	120	120
Auto mA	150 (minimum) to 400 (maximum)	150 (minimum) to 400 (maximum)
Noise index	15	15

scans with the patient in both supine and prone positions. The CT colonography protocol is given in Table 25-1.

No definite MR protocols have been defined for exploring the colon. As it applies for CT, optimal colonic distention is essential before performing MR examinations for which liquid enema techniques are most suited, as opposed to air and carbon dioxide insufflations.[4] Different liquid enema techniques that are used to visualize the colon on MRI are bright lumen, black lumen, and fecal tagging. Whereas a 3D spoiled T1-weighted gradient-recalled-echo (GRE) sequence is used to visualize the bright lumen based on water gadolinium enema completely filling the colonic lumen, the 2D half-Fourier single-shot turbo spin-echo sequence can be used for delineation of the colonic wall. Fecal tagging techniques refer to ingestion of a diet before a CT/MRI examination that contains barium to give stools the same Hounsfield unit or signal intensity, which can decrease false-positive detection of colonic polyps.[5]

Vascular Imaging

The role of virtual angioscopy has so far been restricted to vessels that have a larger luminal diameter, such as the aorta, and thus has been useful for visualization of the intimal flap and rent of aortic dissections and for the relationship of the vessel with a false lumen. The prerequisites for a good-quality angioscopy image include presence of bright and homogeneous contrast medium in the vessel lumen and clear delineation of vessel boundaries. Thin-section acquisitions of 0.5 to 1.0 mm allow optimal postprocessing of data, provided scan acquisitions have been efficiently performed after a 20- to 30-second scan delay in MDCT and after dynamic gadolinium injection in MRI. However, the current role of virtual angioscopy has

been restricted to abdominal aortic aneurysms as an alternative method of 3D dataset evaluation, and so far MRI has been considered superior to MDCT for navigation of the aortic lumen.[6]

Biliary and Urinary Tracts

It can be rightfully said that as with the navigation of the aortic lumen, MRI is also more popular among clinicians for virtual endoscopy of the biliary and urinary tracts. No specific alterations to protocols have been suggested apart from the routine MR urography and cholangiopancreatography sequences. However, thin dataset acquisitions, optimal signal-to-noise ratio, and heavy T2-weighted acquisitions in axial, coronal, and sagittal planes covering the region of interest are certain prerequisites that should be strictly adhered to. The idea is to improve the contrast between the intraluminal bile/urine and structures surrounding it by fat saturation while maintaining an optimal signal-to-noise ratio.[7]

Segmentation of the Desired Volume

The technical details and physics involved in segmentation and fly-through techniques are beyond the scope of this chapter. In simple terms, for any navigation to be made possible, segmentation of the structure of interest is the first essential step. The newer-generation MDCT and MRI scanners offer numerous advantages in terms of scan speed and image quality along with thin sections of isotropic voxel resolution. The present workstations are more compatible with the Digital Imaging and Communications in Medicine (DICOM) format of datasets, and most can perform automated segmentation of the structures if the appropriate range of thin axial datasets is chosen. The segmented volume can be visualized by either surface renderings or more sophisticated volume-rendering techniques (Fig. 25-4). With surface rendering, differentiation between two structures with different intensity of density can be done, and before starting this display the operator should be aware of the different threshold values that are used. Volume rendering is more advanced in terms of quality of image display, entails use of transfer property functions so that structures having different voxel values are attenuated and progressively increased or decreased by linear scale of values, and is considered more user interactive.

Creating a Fly-Through Path

Creation of a fly-through path is a critical issue with virtual endoscopy. Basically, it is essential that a center line through the tubular lumen be delineated for the purposes of performing a fly-through. This central navigation path is simple to create for luminal structures that are anatomically straight in orientation like the aorta. However, creation of this straight navigation path is a challenge for convoluted structures such as colon and small bowel loops. Various techniques have been suggested for automated generation of such navigation paths.[8] However, the basic requisite still remains acquisition of thin-section and artifact-free axial datasets. The other important

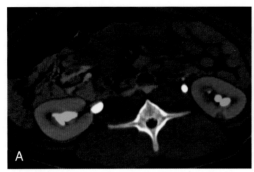
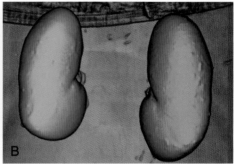

■ **FIGURE 25-4** **A,** An axial CT image shows segmentation of porcine kidneys. **B,** A volume-rendered coronal image shows the kidneys generated from axial segmentation. (*Reprinted with permission from Cai W, Holalkere N, Narris G, et al. Dynamic-threshold level set method for volumetry of porcine kidney in CT images: In vivo and ex vivo assessment of the accuracy of volume measurement. Acad Radiol 2007; 14(7):890-896.*)

consideration behind design of such a technique is establishing a direct interaction with the objects displayed in the endoscopic views. Especially with respect to screening for precancerous colonic polyps, the present fly-through techniques are very promising for detection of true polyps, but concern remains about the number of false-positive results, that is, misrepresentation of various objects such as colonic folds and fecal material as polyps. To overcome this shortcoming, most software now provides the corresponding axial and coronal reformatted images for a fly-through image where the target object is encountered.

Virtual Endoscopy of Upper Gastrointestinal Tract

The scope and application of virtual endoscopy of the esophagus is restricted because mostly the esophagus is found to be collapsed, which poses severe restrictions in generating navigation views because an air-filled lumen is a prerequisite. In addition, invasive endoscopy offers the only means of obtaining tissue diagnosis in cases of esophageal carcinoma; thus the virtual navigation methods have not received much encouragement in research.

However, because the stomach is usually well distended with air and a large structure, virtual gastroscopy has been recognized as a complementary tool for diagnosis of various stomach disorders. Some authorities have encouraged the use of virtual gastroscopy for measuring gastric tumors as opposed to conventional endoscopy in which lesions can also be categorized and classified based on the Bormann classification.[9] However, because it is easier to perform conventional gastroscopy than colonoscopy, virtual gastroscopy is still considered an add-on postprocessing technique to other reformatted imaging. With existing controversies about its feasibility, virtual gastroscopy has shown better promise for evaluation of gastric ulcers and differentiating benign and malignant gastric ulcers. Like conventional endoscopy of the small bowel, applications of virtual endoscopy have received negligible focus until now, considering the length and complexities in bowel position. Conventional radiography and barium follow-through studies are still relied on for diagnostic purposes.

Virtual Endoscopy of the Colon

Virtual colonoscopy is an imaging technique that uses thin-section CT of the colon to generate a 3D "endoluminal view" of the entire colon comparable to that seen with optical colonoscopy. In this visualization mode, radiologists can perform virtual "fly through" in the colon, from the rectum to the cecum and back. The need for a full bowel preparation with rigorous cathartic colon cleansing is believed to be one of the major sources of restricted patient compliance in colon cancer screening.[10] Computer-aided detection for CT colonography is attractive, but perceptual errors may be caused by the presence of normal structures that simulate polyps. Another problem of CT colonography is the need for bowel cleansing, and various studies are now focusing on techniques to remove fecal material that lessen patient discomfort, such as minimal preparation, reduced preparation, laxative-free preparation, or noncathartic preparation. Some studies conclude that a combination of dietary fecal tagging by orally administered contrast agents such as barium, iodine, or Gastrografin and reduced or noncathartic bowel cleansing could be a viable alternative to full cathartic colon cleansing.[11,12] Presently, the major focus of computer-aided detection is on CT images acquired by cathartically cleansed CT colonography without and with fecal tagging (see later).

Bowel Preparation

The role of spasmolytic agents for achieving adequate colonic distention is controversial because they are contraindicated in patients with prostatic hyperplasia, glaucoma, and cardiac disorders. A more feasible option of mechanical bowel distention has proven to be more acceptable so far. Insufflation of room air in the colon leads to optimal colonic distention or even more at times, which may cause pain until the air is expelled by peristalsis (see Table 25-1). CO_2 is a better-tolerated option because it is passively absorbed by the colonic mucosa and can be eliminated by respiration. Advantages of new approaches such as automatic CO_2 insufflation have been highlighted recently in which much better distention of the left colon is achieved, especially on supine scans.[13]

Interpretation

In spite of ongoing developments with 3D imaging and virtual navigation, 2D viewing of colonic dimensions on axial and coronal datasets is still popular. Most authorities, however, recommend simultaneous evaluation of 3D navigation datasets along with the 2D data to maximize the accuracy in reporting. Newer workstations are now equipped with user-interactive platforms in which corresponding 2D datasets are available while navigation through the colonic lumen is done.

The CT colonography reports should include size, location, and appearance of the polyps, if present. They should be further classified according to their shape, namely, sessile (broad-base), flat, or pedunculated (has a stalk). The location of each polyp should be assigned to any of the six colonic segments: rectum, sigmoid, descending colon, transverse colon, ascending colon, and cecum. It is generally believed that polyps less than 5 mm in diameter have a very low malignant potential and should not be reported because this may increase the number of false-positive findings in an examination.[14] Polyps that range between 6 and 9 mm in diameter have an intermediate grade of malignant potential and should be mentioned, in which case multiplicity of lesions and family history should necessitate referral to optical colonoscopy. Patients with lesions greater than 3 cm in diameter should be referred to a surgeon.

Virtual Cholangioscopy

Optical cholangioscopy is an advanced application in endoscopy that is under investigation for its usefulness in diagnosis and management of biliary duct calculi, stenosis, and malignancies.[15] However, there are certain limitations such as cost, operator dependence, and relative likelihood of complications (e.g., hemorrhage in ducts, laceration, nausea, fever, and vagal reactions). Virtual cholangioscopy provides a very close simulation to optical cholangioscopy, in which virtual navigation images are generated by software using axial MR or MDCT datasets, taking into account volume rendering and surface rendering algorithms for generation of an endoluminal view.

Such virtual endoscopy was first used on the aorta and its branches when navigational views were generated for the bright-contrast, opacified vessel lumen. MRI datasets have been more popular with attempts at virtual

endoscopy studies in the past because the lumen of interest usually appears very bright and well complements the software requirements for generation of views. In addition, MR cholangiopancreatography datasets are more preferred for cholangioscopy than MDCT because they provide a higher contrast difference between the bright-appearing bile ducts and the dark surrounding structures. Previous studies have established various appearances of the common bile duct by virtual cholangioscopy, namely, endoluminal polyp-like appearances and stenosis (narrowing of duct) and occlusion.[16] The polyp-like appearance of common bile duct stones is by far the most commonly encountered (85%) pathologic process on virtual cholangioscopy. The endoluminal views, when used in conjunction with axial datasets, have been shown to improve detection sensitivity of common bile duct stones.

Virtual Pancreatoscopy

The applicability and usefulness of CT and MR virtual pancreatoscopy are recently emerging because various studies have proved the effectiveness of virtual navigation through the pancreatic duct. It is a useful tool for characterization of an intraductal papillary mucinous neoplasm (IPMN). Advances in MDCT have well complemented the requirements for virtual pancreatoscopy because thinner collimation slices (1 to 3 mm) of better resolution are now available for segmentation of pancreatic duct and generation of endoluminal pancreatic duct views through software (Fig. 25-5). CT and MRI datasets have both been popular in the characterization of IPMNs in which virtual pancreatoscopy images have proven either more useful or have been shown to yield the same results as optical endoscopies.[17] Another extended application of virtual pancreatoscopy has been the visualization of ductal details in cases of chronic pancreatitis in which various strictures and narrowing of the duct can be encountered while performing navigation. However, future applicability of virtual pancreatoscopy remains in question, because findings of chronic pancreatitis are usually evident on routine CT/MRI datasets.

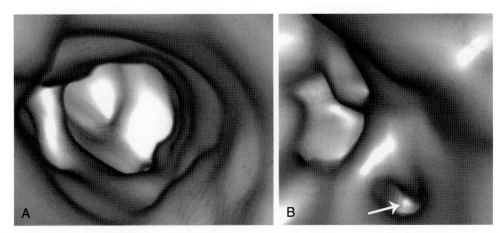

■ **FIGURE 25-5** **A,** A virtual endoscopy image of a normal main pancreatic duct shows the pancreatic duct lumen. **B,** A pancreatic duct navigation image shows opening of a side-branch duct (*arrow*). (*Reprinted with permission from Singh AK, Hiroyuki Y, Sahani DV. Advanced postprocessing and the emerging role of computer-aided detection. Radiol Clin North Am 2009; 47(1):59-77.*)

Volumetry

The recent scanners have opened new avenues for advancement of segmentation techniques, which is essentially the first step for volume estimation of any organ or pathology. Volumetry is becoming increasingly popular in abdominal imaging because diagnosis of various pathologic processes, treatment planning, and follow-up information can be revealed for volume estimations of abdominal visceral organs such as the liver, spleen, and kidneys. Newer MDCT and MRI protocols are now tailored to increase the accuracy of organ segmentations followed by automated volume estimation of the segmented region by employment of advanced software tools. (The technique of organ segmentation is discussed in Chapter 24.) The manual method of organ segmentation ensures better accuracy but remains unsuitable for a busy work flow. More modern means such as segmentation by the region-growing method or slice interpolation techniques are now commonly used in a busy practice.

Liver and Spleen

Provision of total and partial lobar liver volumes is an essential prerequisite for planning partial liver resection in a liver donor. It is extremely crucial to leave a major portion of liver volume in the donor while simultaneously ensuring optimal needed volume for the recipient who has hepatic compromise secondary to cirrhosis.[18] It is therefore essential to divide the total liver followed by further subsegmentation into its right and left lobes, thus obtaining total and partial liver volumes on scans (Fig. 25-6).

The MDCT angiography and MR angiography liver donor scanning protocols are better for 3D depiction of the vascular anatomy of liver donors, the knowledge of which is another essential prerequisite in planning the transplant. These angiography protocols consist of thin-slice axial datasets (1 to 3 mm) for the arterial and venous phase that not only complement the need for 3D maps but also ensure better accuracy in segmentation and subsequently their volume estimations. The recipient with end-stage liver disease will need liver graft volume that is 1% of the recipient's body mass (calculated by the graft-

to-recipient's body weight ratio). The advances in MDCT and MRI have facilitated postprocessing applications such as 3D volumetry in a transplant setting. In addition, there is some element of liver regeneration in donors and recipients after surgery in which volumetric estimation can play a further role. In select centers, liver volumetry on CT/MRI is also done for assessment of liver regeneration in recipients after transplant surgery.

Spleen volumetry has not been very popular in the 3D laboratory as a sole indicator for monitoring the progression of disease and for treatment planning.[19] Although there is always some proportion of increase of splenic volume in donors after partial liver lobe resection, estimation of splenic volume has not been felt to be important in diagnosis because splenomegaly can be judged by browsing through routine axial CT/MRI datasets.

Kidney

Estimation of kidney volume is becoming popular with transplant surgeons. Various segmentation techniques have been tried recently for segmentation of kidneys, of which segmentation by the region-growing method has proven particularly beneficial for segmentation of the entire kidney, owing to less variability in attenuation values in the renal parenchyma.[20] The areas where kidney volumetry can prove useful are renal transplants, prognostic assessment of adult polycystic kidneys, and monitoring response of renal tumors to radiofrequency ablation and chemotherapy.[21] As far as establishment of volumetry as a standard of care is concerned, previous studies have effectively justified the role of renal volume estimations for polycystic kidneys and, to a lesser extent, in transplants where estimation of kidney volume of donors helps in preoperative planning.

Tumor Volumes

A fair amount of research efforts has now been diverted to ways in which accuracy of tumor volume estimations can be achieved. One such extensively investigated area is volume estimation of primary liver tumors and meta-

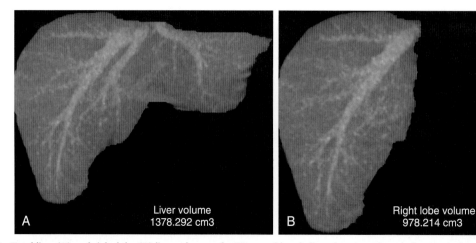

■ **FIGURE 25-6**   Total liver (**A**) and right lobe (**B**) liver volumes of a 37-year-old male liver donor generated after manual segmentation performed on axial MDCT datasets. (*Reprinted with permission from Singh AK, Hiroyuki Y, Sahani DV. Advanced postprocessing and the emerging role of computer-aided detection. Radiol Clin North Am 2009; 47(1):59-77.*)

TABLE 25-2 Overview of Advanced Postprocessing Applications and Their Present Role in Clinical Practice

Application	Clinical Significance	Established ±	Under Investigation ±	Computer-Aided Detection Assisted ±
Virtual Endoscopy				
Stomach and duodenum	Tumor detection, ulcers	–	+	–
Aorta	Aortic aneurysm	–	+	–
Colon	Colonic polyps, colonic tumors.	++	+ (Electronic bowel cleansing)	++
Pancreatic duct and common bile duct	Intraductal papillary mucinous neoplasm, common bile duct calculi and stenosis	–	++	–
Upper ureters	Calculi	–	+	–
Volumetry				
Liver (partial lobe + total)	Pretransplantation surgical planning	+	–	+
Kidney	Pretransplantation surgical planning	–	++	+
Liver tumors	Monitoring treatment response, radiation therapy planning	+	–	++
Renal tumors	Monitoring treatment response post radiofrequency ablation and chemotherapy	+	++	–
Spleen (MRI)	Glycogen and lipid storage disorders	–	+	–

static lesions, which is used to monitor response to chemotherapy and irradiation and predict long-term survival of such patients.[22] The requirements for liver tumor segmentations are fulfilled by modern MDCT and MRI protocols, which provide thin axial slices of optimal resolution that are devoid of artifacts. Ideally, the total liver volume is calculated after determination of total tumor burden by software upgrades that sum up the multiple tumor volumes that are generated. Further software sophistication provides total tumor burden in right and left lobes, which helps in radiation therapy planning and resection. Estimation of renal tumor volume after radiofrequency ablation is another area in which the role of volumetry is being investigated. The software sophistication required for automation of software has highlighted the future role of computer-aided applications and detection of pathologic processes, which is a fast-evolving science with a promising potential. Computer-aided segmentation techniques for liver and tumor recognition methods by computer-aided detection have been in discussion in recent conferences.

Computer-Aided Techniques

Computer-aided detection is gradually gaining practical value in diagnostic radiology and has become one of the major research focuses in the past few years.[23] It has been universally agreed that computer applications should be generally used as an adjunctive tool by radiologists rather than as an independent diagnostic aid. The synergism between the radiologist's performance and computerized detection for improving diagnosis has highlighted the importance of computer-aided detection in various clinical settings and thus the realization of the benefits of computer-aided detection on a much wider scale. The clinical significance and current standing of advanced postprocessing applications are given in Table 25-2.

One of the most important concerns of existing computer-aided detection programs is their merger with the current work flow. Any technologic upgrade or advancement in computer-aided detection should be easily compatible with the picture archiving and communication systems (PACS). In spite of significant advances in computer-aided detection tools for detection of colonic polyps and pulmonary nodules, its easy merger with PACS is still an unresolved issue that needs to be addressed. However, recent promise has emerged with the development of software packages that have the ability to convert a screen-captured image of a computer-aided detection result to a DICOM file so that it is available in PACS immediately. DICOM-SC (Secondary Capture) and DICOM-IHE (Integrating the Health Enterprise) are recent software tools that ensure smooth incorporation of computer-aided detection results with PACS.[24]

The recent advances in MDCT and MRI have markedly propelled the developments in computer-aided detection. The advent of 16-, 64-, and higher-channel detector-row scanners have immensely boosted the ongoing developments in postprocessing, because artifact-free CT data of better resolution are now available. This allows better detection of lesions and performance of computer-aided detection on the whole owing to clear delineation of lesion margins, their conspicuity, and better characterization of tiny lesions. With this emerging picture, one should not underestimate the extent of exploration of MDCT and MRI capabilities in the future and the pace of growth of computer-assisted applications.

Colon

One of the most thoroughly investigated computer-aided detection applications is that for detection of colonic polyps. CT colonography is now a recognized screening tool for detection of precancerous colonic polyps, and computer-aided detection has established its role with CT colonography for detection of colonic polyps because it provides methods for automated colonic segmentations and electronic cleansing of the bowel to eliminate residual

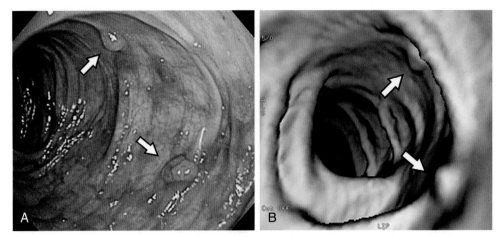

■ **FIGURE 25-7** **A,** A screening optical colonoscopy image shows polyps in the splenic flexure (*arrows*) of a 53-year-old man. **B,** Automated detection of polyps by computer-aided detection (*arrows*) shown on a virtual CT colonoscopy image. (*Reprinted with permission from Singh AK, Hiroyuki Y, Sahani DV. Advanced postprocessing and the emerging role of computer-aided detection. Radiol Clin North Am 2009; 47(1):59-77.*)

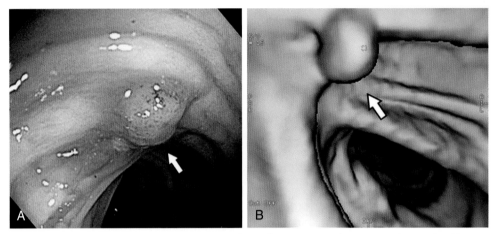

■ **FIGURE 25-8** **A,** A screening optical colonoscopy image shows a polyp in the transverse colon (*arrow*) of a 49-year-old man. **B,** Automated detection of a polyp by computer-aided detection (*arrow*) shown on a virtual CT colonoscopy image.

fecal matter and decrease false-positive detection of colonic polyps. The recent workstations are fully equipped with incorporated software and algorithms, which provide computer-aided detection, thus aiding the detection of colonic polyps after selection of the CT colonography dataset. Although CT colonography is a promising alternative screening tool for colon cancer, variable sensitivity for polyp detection across studies, the expertise and time required of the readers for interpreting the CT colonography images, in particular, for detection of small polyps, and the need for a full bowel preparation with rigorous colon cleansing are some problems that need to be addressed.[25]

Computer-aided detection for CT colonography is attractive because it has the potential to overcome the just-mentioned problems (Figs. 25-7 and 25-8). The false-positive interpretations may be caused by the presence of normal structures that mimic polyps or problems with the display method.

Use of computer-aided detection can overcome this lack of consistency by radiologists, and thus it is useful for reducing variability among readers in identifying polyps in CT colonography. Also, cathartic bowel cleansing is

required for removal of residual fecal materials in the colon because such materials mimic or obscure polyps. Such fecal materials can be "tagged" by orally administered contrast agents such as barium, iodine, or Gastrografin before CT colonography. The orally administered contrast agent thus opacifies residual solid stool and fluid in the colon while keeping polyps and folds unopacified and untagged. This technique of fecal tagging is a promising method for differentiating between residual feces and polyps and improves accuracy of polyp detection. This technique can be used, and has been shown to be effective, for cathartically cleansed colons as well.[26] Most CT colonographic examinations are still performed without fecal tagging. However, an increasing number of fecal tagging CT colonographic examinations are performed with varying degrees of bowel preparation; thus, fecal-tagging CT colonography with a cathartically cleansed colon appears to form the second major group of CT colonographic examinations. Other preparations such as reduced and noncathartic CT colonography are still in experimental stages. Thus, currently, the major targets of computer-aided detection are CT images acquired by

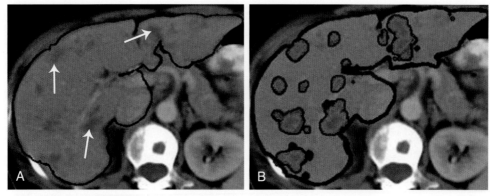

■ **FIGURE 25-9** Automated detection of liver metastases by computer-assisted detection in a 37-year-old woman with breast cancer. **A,** Mapping of the liver boundaries is seen, which is the first step in segmentation to generate right and left lobe tumor volumes. Metastatic lesions are unmarked (*arrows*). **B,** Automated mapping of liver metastases after application of a computer-assisted design algorithm. (*Reprinted with permission from Cai W, Harris G, Yoshida H. Computer-aided volumetrics of liver tumor in hepatic CT images. Computed Assisted Radiology and Surgery 2006; June: 375-377.*)

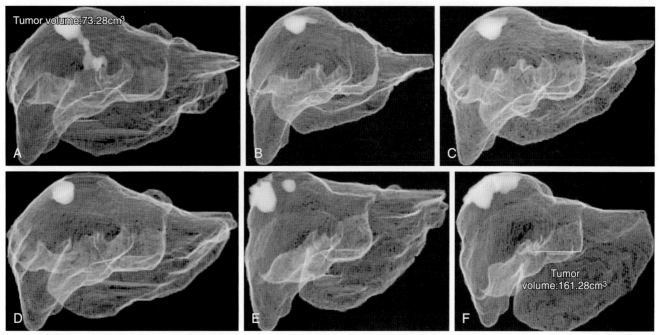

■ **FIGURE 25-10** Volumetry in monitoring response to therapy. Serial volumetry images from a 63-year-old man with hepatocellular carcinoma treated with chemotherapy for 10 months. Tumor volumes obtained at 0 (**A**), 2.3 (**B**), 5.7 (**C**), 13.8 (**D**), 18.6 (**E**), and 19.6 (**F**) months after start of treatment. Pretreatment (**A**) and post-treatment (**F**) tumor volumes are given. (*Reprinted with permission from Cai W, Yoshida H, Harris G. Dynamic-thresholding level set: a novel computer-aided volumetry method for liver tumors in hepatic CT images. SPIE Medical Imaging, San Diego. 2007; 6514.*)

cathartically cleansed CT colonography without and with fecal tagging. Electronic bowel cleansing of the tagged stools by computer-aided detection is a benchmark advancement for detection of polyps in the colon.

Liver

Various computer-aided detection algorithms have replaced manual methods of total liver and partial liver lobe segmentations, which have made the postprocessing a task that complements the work flow needs. Some studies have targeted the accuracy of computer-aided detection applications for automated detection and quantification of liver tumors and have gone to the extent of implementing it into their routine work flow (Figs. 25-9 and 25-10).[27] The newer workstations are now available with tools that allow minor edits such as shrinkage or

expansion of the segmented tumor or organ by computer-aided detection, which makes the process of manual editing of computer-aided detection points a much simpler task. The computer-aided detection software performance is basically dependent on the range of pixel or voxel identification, which is assigned values with range of either liver parenchyma or tumor substance, depending on the software application to be used. Further upgrades in computer-aided detection software have been made to incorporate the results of total liver volume and tumor burden volumes, which are then projected in percentages in respective liver lobes. However, the incidence of false-positive findings does exist, and manual corrections to erase or include some regions are still an unresolved problem, which is relatively decreased by automations of maneuvering tools available at modern workstations.

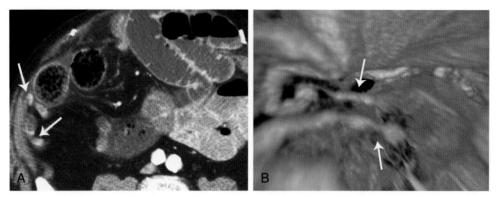

■ **FIGURE 25-11** **A,** False-positive detection (*arrows*) by computer-aided detection near the abdominal wall of transition site in a 42-year-old man with small bowel obstruction due to Crohn's stricture. **B,** Navigation view in the same patient showing a true-positive luminal narrowing with convergence of folds (*top arrow*) along with false-positive detection of luminal narrowing (*bottom arrow*).

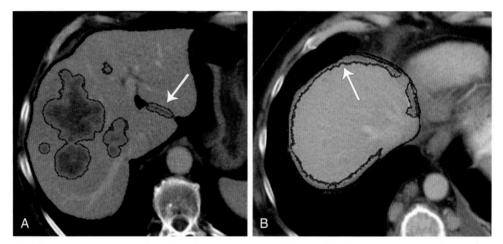

■ **FIGURE 25-12** **A,** A fat plane between two lobes of liver (*arrow*) as a cause of false-positive liver tumor detection by computer-aided detection in a 54-year-old man with multicentric hepatocellular carcinoma. **B,** Low CT attenuation values at the liver edges (*arrow*) as a cause of false-positive tumor detection in the same case.

Small Bowel

Some recent investigators have explored further benefits of computer-aided detection in detection of transition points for small bowel obstruction, and such work has been presented at international meetings (Fig. 25-11).[28] These computer-aided detection upgrades have been designed on the same principles of colon computer-aided detection in which the small bowel is segmented and software is trained to detect points where relative narrowing of small bowel is present. The known challenges are the number of high false-positive detections, which fortunately can be easily ruled out by readers, and segmentation of entire small bowel, which is a challenging task considering its length.

Kidney

Some studies have highlighted techniques in which automated segmentation and volume estimations of kidneys are possible with fairly good accuracy except in cases of false-positive/false-negative detection of parenchyma, which also remains a problem for computer-aided segmentation of the liver (Fig. 25-12). Computer-aided detec-

tion applications, which work on level-set methods, have been discussed recently for exploring options of quick and automated kidney segmentation.[29] Computer-aided detection for renal tumor segmentation works on the same principles as designed for liver tumor segmentation, but its role in clinical practice is yet to be investigated, unlike quantification of adult polycystic kidney volume, which has been proven to be a useful prognostic indicator of the disease (Fig. 25-13).

SUMMARY

The newest MDCT and MRI scanners have immensely advanced the techniques in postprocessing and 3D image quality owing to the availability of datasets of near isotropic voxel resolution that are devoid of artifacts. This has led to exploration of advanced postprocessing applications such as virtual endoscopy, volumetry, and computer-aided advances in postprocessing.

A significant benefit of virtual colonoscopy has been established and is now a standard of care for screening of precancerous colonic polyps. Scan protocols are now tailored such that good-quality virtual fly-through views are

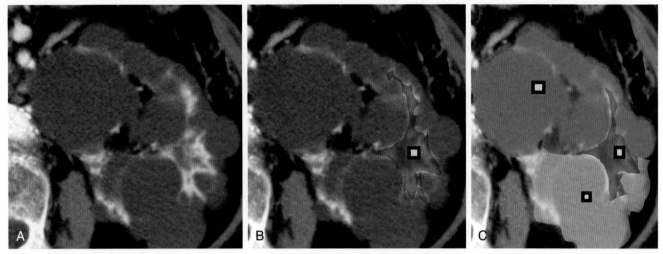

■ **FIGURE 25-13** Challenges in segmentation of a polycystic left kidney by point-spread method in a 33-year-old man. **A,** Contrast enhancement of renal parenchymal components amid the cystic components. **B,** Segmentation of bright structures by point-spread method. **C,** Segmentation of other left renal cystic components. (*Reprinted with permission from Singh AK, Hiroyuki Y, Sahani DV. Advanced postprocessing and the emerging role of computer-aided detection. Radiol Clin North Am 2009; 47(1):59-77.*)

available after automated colonic segmentation by computer software. The scan datasets of 0.625- to 2.0-mm thickness are adequate for such purposes. Optimal colonic distention is of paramount importance before any CT colonographic examination, which also ensures a good performance of the computer-aided detection software with decrease in number of false-positive polyp detections. The feasibility and importance of other applications of virtual navigation technique such as visualization of the intimal flap in cases of aortic aneurysm, tumors and ulcers in the stomach and duodenum, characterization of IPMNs through the pancreatic duct, and detection of calculi and stenosis in the common bile duct are being investigated.

Volumetry of organs has seen advances in recent segmentation software and is gaining considerable importance and recognition. Estimation of total liver and partial liver lobe volumes is essential for preoperative planning of liver transplants. The importance of kidney volume estimation as a prognostic indicator of adult polycystic kidney disease has been established. Estimation of tumor burden in the liver is crucial for determination of radiation dose in cases of radiation therapy to the liver.

The role of computer-aided detection has been established in CT colonography where automated detection of colonic polyps by workstation-incorporated software has been recently recognized as a standard screening procedure for colonic cancer. Electronic bowel cleansing is another potential advancement of computer-aided detection application and is being actively investigated. Computer-aided techniques for automated liver and partial liver lobe segmentations and volume estimations ensure good accuracy and efficient performance. Other com-

puter-aided detection applications such as determination of transition points in small bowel obstructions and automated kidney segmentation and volume estimation have received much focus at recent meetings and conferences.

KEY POINTS

- The advancements in MDCT and MRI scanners have complemented the dataset requirements of advanced postprocessing applications such as virtual endoscopy, volumetry, and computer-aided detection.
- The application of virtual navigation has been more prominently recognized in screening CT colonography for precancerous colonic polyps.
- Feasibility of other applications of virtual endoscopy such as detection of gastric and duodenal tumors and ulcers, virtual cholangiopancreatoscopy, and virtual angioscopy for aortic aneurysms is being investigated.
- Volumetry is an extended arm of organ and tumor segmentation in which the importance of liver volumes and liver tumor volumes has been established in preoperative planning of liver transplantation and monitoring response to chemotherapy and radiation therapy for liver tumors.
- Computer-aided detection is well suited to provide results of automated polyp detection in CT colonography, and recent research studies are focused on improving polyp detection sensitivity and enhancing the performance of electronic bowel cleansing.
- Computer-aided sophistication of existing workstation tools for segmentation of abdominal visceral organs and tumors has proven effective in terms of accuracy of volume estimation and saving time.

SUGGESTED READINGS

Bartolozzi C, Neri E, Caramella D. CT in vascular pathologies. Eur Radiol 1998; 8:679-684.

Fujimoto J, Yamanaka J. Liver resection and transplantation using a novel 3D hepatectomy simulation system. Adv Med Sci 2006; 51:7-14.

Perumpillichira JJ, Yoshida H, Sahani DV. Computer-aided detection for virtual colonoscopy. Cancer Imaging 2005; 5:11-16.

Sugawara Y, Makuuchi M. Living donor liver transplantation: present status and recent advances. Br Med Bull 2006; 75-76:15-28.

Taylor SA, Suzuki N, Beddoe G, Halligan S. Flat neoplasia of the colon: CT colonography with CAD. Abdom Imaging 2009; 34:173-181.

Yoshida H, Dachman AH. Computer-aided diagnosis for CT colonography. Semin Ultrasound CT MR 2004; 25:419-431.

Yoshida H, Näppi J. CAD in CT colonography without and with oral contrast agents: progress and challenges. Comput Med Imaging Graph 2007; 31:267-284.

REFERENCES

1. White TJ, Avery GR, Kennan N, et al. Virtual colonoscopy versus conventional colonoscopy in patients at high risk of colorectal cancer—a prospective trial of 150 patients. Colorectal Dis 2009; 11:138-145.

2. Kalapala R, Sunitha L, Nageshwar RD, et al. Virtual MR pancreatoscopy in the evaluation of the pancreatic duct in chronic pancreatitis. J Pancreas (Online) 2008; 9:220-225.

3. Arnesen RB, von Benzon E, Adamsen S, et al. Diagnostic performance of computed tomography colonography and colonoscopy: a prospective and validated analysis of 231 paired examinations. Acta Radiol 2007; 48:831-837.

4. So NM, Lam WW, Mann D, et al. Feasibility study of using air as a contrast medium in MR colonography. Clin Radiol 2003; 58:555-559.

5. Lauenstein TC, Goehde SC, Ruehm SG, et al. MR colonography with barium-based fecal tagging: initial clinical experience. Radiology 2002; 223:248-254.

6. Carrascosa P, Capuñay C, Vembar M, et al. Multislice CT virtual angioscopy of the abdomen. Abdom Imaging 2005; 30:249-258.

7. Prassopoulos P, Papanikolaou N, Maris T, et al. Development of contrast-enhanced virtual MR cholangioscopy: a feasibility study. Eur Radiol 2002; 12:1438-1441.

8. Jolesz FA, Lorensen WE, Shinmoto H, et al. Interactive virtual endoscopy. AJR Am J Roentgenol 1997; 169:1229-1235.

9. Kim HJ, Kim AY, Oh ST, et al. Gastric cancer staging at multidetector row CT gastrography: comparison of transverse and volumetric CT scanning. Radiology 2005; 236:879-885.

10. Dykes C, Cash BD. Key safety issues of bowel preparations for colonoscopy and importance of adequate hydration. Gastroenterol Nurs 2008; 31:30-35; quiz 36-37.

11. Taylor SA, Slater A, Burling DN, et al. CT colonography: optimisation, diagnostic performance and patient acceptability of reduced-laxative regimens using barium-based faecal tagging. Eur Radiol 2008; 18:32-42.

12. Gryspeerdt S, Lefere P, Herman M, et al. CT colonography with fecal tagging after incomplete colonoscopy. Eur Radiol 2005; 15:1192-1202.

13. Burling D, Halligan S, Taylor S, et al. Polyp measurement using CT colonography: agreement with colonoscopy and effect of viewing conditions on interobserver and intraobserver agreement. AJR Am J Roentgenol 2006; 186:1597-1604.

14. Zalis ME, Barish MA, Choi JR, et al. CT colonography reporting and data system: a consensus proposal. Radiology 2005; 236:3-9.

15. Picus D. Percutaneous biliary endoscopy. J Vasc Interv Radiol 1995; 6:303-310.

16. Neri E, Caramella D, Boraschi P, et al. Magnetic resonance virtual endoscopy of the common bile duct stones. Surg Endosc 1999; 13:632-633.

17. Sata N, Kurihara K, Koizumi M, et al. CT virtual pancreatoscopy: a new method for diagnosing intraductal papillary mucinous neoplasm (IPMN) of the pancreas. Abdom Imaging 2006; 31:326-331.

18. Tu R, Xia LP, Yu AL, Wu L. Assessment of hepatic functional reserve by cirrhosis grading and liver volume measurement using CT. World J Gastroenterol 2007; 13:3956-3961.

19. Mazonakis M, Damilakis J, Maris T, et al. Estimation of spleen volume using MR imaging and a random marking technique. Eur Radiol 2000; 10:1899-1903.

20. Cai W, Holalkere NS, Harris G, et al. Dynamic-threshold level set method for volumetry of porcine kidney in CT images: in vivo and ex vivo assessment of the accuracy of volume measurement. Acad Radiol 2007; 14:890-896.

21. van der Veldt AA, Meijerink MR, van den Eertwegh AJ, et al. Sunitinib for treatment of advanced renal cell cancer: primary tumor response. Clin Cancer Res 2008; 14:2431-2436.

22. Pech M, Mohnike K, Wieners G, et al. Radiotherapy of liver metastases: comparison of target volumes and dose-volume histograms employing CT- or MRI-based treatment planning. Strahlenther Onkol 2008; 184:256-261.

23. Fujita H, Uchiyama Y, Nakagawa T, et al. Computer-aided diagnosis: the emerging of three CAD systems induced by Japanese health care needs. Comput Methods Programs Biomed 2008; 92:238-248.

24. Zhou Z, Liu BJ, Le AH. CAD-PACS integration tool kit based on DICOM secondary captures, structured report and IHE workflow profiles. Comput Med Imaging Graph 2007; 31:346-352.

25. Petrick N, Haider M, Summers RM, et al. CT colonography with computer-aided detection as a second reader: observer performance study. Radiology 2008; 246:148-156.

26. Näppi J, Yoshida H. Adaptive correction of the pseudo-enhancement of CT attenuation for fecal-tagging CT colonography. Med Image Anal 2008; 12:413-426.

27. Graham KC, Ford NL, MacKenzie LT, et al. Noninvasive quantification of tumor volume in preclinical liver metastasis models using contrast-enhanced x-ray computed tomography. Invest Radiol 2008; 43:92-99.

28. Sainani NI, Näppi J, Sahani DV, Yoshida H. Computer-aided detection of small bowel strictures in CT enterography (CTE) in an emergency setting: a pilot study. In Proceedings of the 93rd assembly and annual meeting of the Radiological Society of North America (RSNA), Chicago, November 25-30, 2007. Chicago, RSNA Press, 2007, p 256.

29. Singh AK, Sahani DV. Imaging of the renal donor and transplant recipient. Radiol Clin North Am 2008; 46:79-93, vi.

PART TWO

Nontraumatic Acute Abdomen

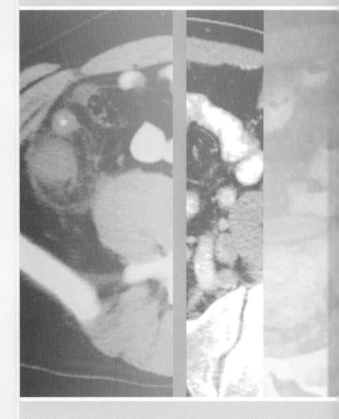

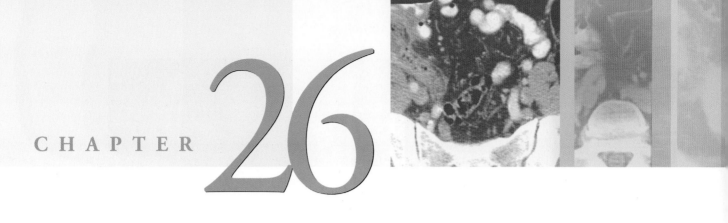

CHAPTER 26

Ureteral and Kidney Stones

Jorge A. Soto

ETIOLOGY

Renal calculi are typically caused by crystallization of supersaturated stone-forming materials in the urine. Calcium, in the form of calcium oxalate, calcium phosphate, and calcium urate, is the most common stone-forming material. Uric acid is the second most common component. Numerous other less common components include xanthine, cystine, struvite, as well as precipitation of medications such as the protease inhibitor indinavir sulfate in persons infected with human immunodeficiency virus (HIV). Alternatively, renal pathology may initiate crystal formations within the renal tubules that are extruded into the renal collecting system to undergo further growth. Urinary stasis secondary to chronic obstruction or reflux, urinary pH abnormalities, and chronic infections may also contribute to stone formation. Ureteral calculi are most commonly renal calculi that have passed distally into the ureters.

PREVALENCE AND EPIDEMIOLOGY

Nephrolithiasis and ureterolithiasis represent a significant cause of urinary obstruction and abdominal pain. Infections, such as pyelonephritis, pyonephrosis, or renal abscess, may complicate stone disease and may be difficult to differentiate clinically. Imaging evaluation is usually necessary to confirm the diagnosis of stone disease and to detect possible complications.

The lifetime risk of forming renal stones differs in various parts of the world: it is 1% to 5% in Asia, 5% to 9% in Europe, and 13% in North America. The composition of stones and their location in the urinary tract, bladder, or kidneys may also significantly differ in different countries. Renal stone disease is slightly more common in males than in females and in whites than in blacks. Stones in the upper urinary tract are related to lifestyle and are more frequent among affluent people, those living in developed countries, and in those with diets high in animal protein. A high frequency of stone formation occurs among hypertensive patients and among those with a high body mass index.

CLINICAL PRESENTATION

Nephrolithiasis and ureterolithiasis present as often severe colicky pain in the region of the flanks that may radiate into the groin, especially with distal progression of the stones into the ureters. Nausea and vomiting, costovertebral angle tenderness, and hematuria are commonly present with obstruction of a ureter with urinary calculi.

PATHOPHYSIOLOGY

The vast majority of patients with symptomatic renal or ureteral stones seek medical attention because of flank pain caused by acute ureteral obstruction. The most common location of the stone is in one of the three areas of narrowing in the course of the ureter: the ureteropelvic junction, the pelvic brim as the ureter crosses into the pelvis, and the ureterovesical junction.

IMAGING

Radiography

On abdominal radiographs, nephrolithiasis may be identified as focal calcific densities projecting over the renal shadows.[1] The expected course of the ureters should be analyzed for evidence of ureteral calculi. Also, bladder calculi may be identified on plain radiographs. In patients with a known history of renal calculi who have undergone lithotripsy, plain radiographs may be used to evaluate for residual renal or ureteral calculi. When multiple ureteral calculi are identified after lithotripsy, this is termed *steinstrasse*, the translation of this German term being "stone street."

Although CT has replaced the intravenous pyelogram (IVP) in the vast majority of patients, some institutions still

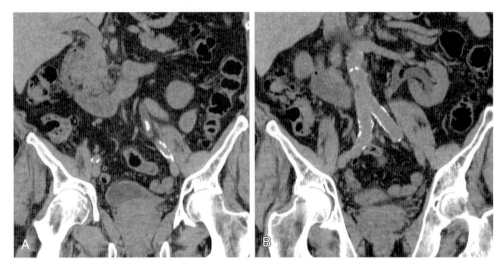

■ **FIGURE 26-1** **A,** Coronal reformatted image of axial CT data demonstrates a dense stone within the middle area of the left ureter. **B,** A slightly more posterior reformatted view than in **A** shows the dilated collecting system and proximal ureter.

perform IVP for this indication. In acute ureteral obstruction, the IVP demonstrates delayed transit of contrast medium through the affected kidney, with delayed images showing the dilated collecting system and the site of the obstructing stone.[1] The main disadvantage of IVP, in addition to the requirement of iodinated contrast material, is the potential delay in diagnosis from having to wait for the delayed radiographs.

CT

Typically, renal stone CT protocols are acquired without the use of oral or intravenous contrast media, which may obscure the underlying stones. CT has a high diagnostic accuracy in the detection of renal and ureteral calculi and may be used to differentiate among stones of various chemical composition.[1-7] Recently, ultra-low-dose CT with a radiation dose equivalent to a kidney-ureter-bladder (KUB) radiograph has been shown to be sufficiently diagnostically accurate in evaluating renal and ureteral calculi.[8,9] The most common forms of renal stones are all readily identified by routine CT techniques (Figs. 26-1 and 26-2). However, urinary stones formed by crystallized protease inhibitors used for HIV therapy are more difficult to identify on CT (Fig. 26-3).

Secondary CT signs of acute ureteral obstruction include enlargement of the kidney (Fig. 26-4), which often demonstrates diffusely decreased attenuation secondary to edema, perinephric stranding, as well as dilatation of the ureter and collecting system (see Figs. 26-1 and 26-2). Stones are most commonly evident in the three areas of ureteral narrowing: the ureteropelvic junction, the pelvic brim, and the ureterovesical junction. Ureteral stones may demonstrate a "soft tissue rim" sign surrounding the calculus (Fig. 26-5), distinguishing a ureteral calculus from adjacent pelvic vein phleboliths. Large intrarenal stones occupying most of the renal pelvis and some of the calyces, known as staghorn calculi, can also be seen on CT (Fig. 26-6). CT may also show renal parenchymal calcifications in cases of nephrocalcinosis (Fig. 26-7).

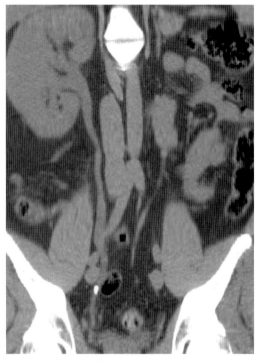

■ **FIGURE 26-2** Distal right ureteral stone with hydroureter demonstrated on a coronal reformatted CT image.

MRI

Occasionally, ureteral or kidney stones may be detected on MRI examinations. On T2-weighted (typically breath-hold half-Fourier acquisition single-shot turbo spin-echo [HASTE]) images, stones typically appear as low-signal intensity foci partially or completely surrounded by the high signal fluid in the dilated collecting system and/or ureter.[10-14] However, differentiation between an obstructed ureter secondary to a stone and the physiologic dilatation of the ureter and collecting system commonly seen in

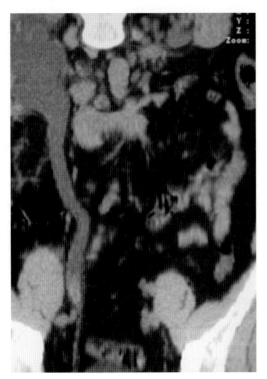

■ **FIGURE 26-3** Coronal reformatted CT image shows hydronephrosis and hydroureter on the right side with a distal ureteral stone. The stone is only slightly hyperattenuating relative to the urine-filled ureter. The patient was undergoing therapy with indinavir for HIV infection.

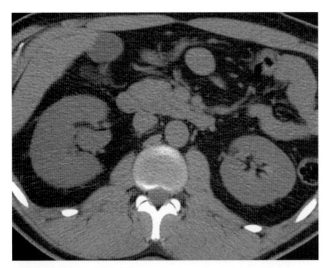

■ **FIGURE 26-4** Axial CT image demonstrates an enlarged right kidney with hydronephrosis, secondary to a distal ureteral stone (not shown).

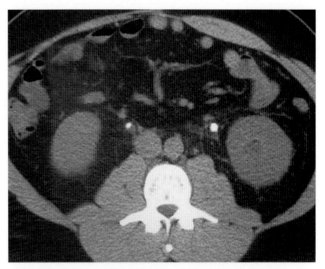

■ **FIGURE 26-5** Axial CT image shows bilateral ureteral stones. There is a small crescent of soft tissue partially surrounding the right ureteral stone known as the "soft tissue rim" sign.

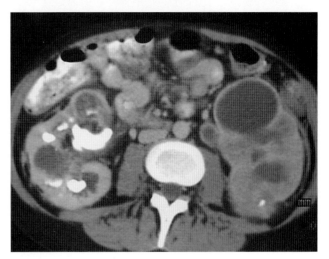

■ **FIGURE 26-6** Staghorn calculus. The CT image demonstrates a large calculus occupying most of the collecting system of the right kidney.

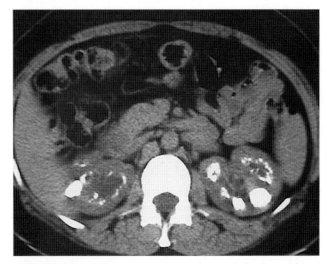

■ **FIGURE 26-7** Noncontrast CT image shows calcifications within the pyramids of both kidneys. Nephrocalcinosis was secondary to medullary sponge kidney in this patient. Parenchymal calcifications can be associated with ureteral stones.

pregnancy during the second and third trimesters may be difficult.

Ultrasonography

Ultrasonography is often employed in patients presenting with acute renal failure. Renal calculi are echogenic foci that typically demonstrate posterior acoustic shadowing.[1,15-17] Also, signs of hydronephrosis and hydroureter

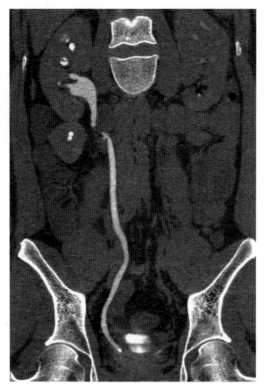

■ **FIGURE 26-8**   Delayed phase of the contrast-enhanced CT scan (coronal reformatted image) demonstrates the dilated right ureter and a distal obstructing stone.

may be identified on ultrasound images in patients with acute obstruction. Proximal and distal ureteral stones may be clearly identified on ultrasonography, but bowel gas usually obscures a large part of the ureter; therefore, the sensitivity of ultrasonography for ureteral calculi is significantly less than that of CT. Peristaltic activity of the patent ureter creates ureteral "jets" in the urinary bladder, and these can be readily identified with color Doppler imaging. The presence of bilateral ureteral jets excludes high-grade ureteral obstruction.

Imaging Algorithm

Overall, CT is the preferred method when a diagnosis of ureteral stones is suspected. When a calcification cannot be classified confidently as a ureteral stone, excretory images after intravenous contrast are useful to delineate the stone and the obstructed ureter (Fig. 26-8). Ultrasonography is useful as a screening modality because the

presence of bilateral jets of urine arising from the ureteral orifices rules out significant obstruction. MRI has little role in the evaluation of ureteral stones. IVP has little role at institutions where rapid access to CT is available (Table 26-1).

Classic Signs

■ *Radiography:* calcified stone
■ *CT:* "soft tissue rim" sign
■ *Ultrasonography:* intraureteral echogenic focus with hydro-ureter and hydronephrosis

---

DIFFERENTIAL DIAGNOSIS

Acute ureteral obstruction secondary to an impacted stone should be differentiated from pyelonephritis, acute diverticulitis, and other gastrointestinal causes of acute abdominal pain as well as from acute gynecologic conditions, including ectopic pregnancy and rupture or torsion of ovarian cysts. Depending on the specific clinical presentation, ureteral stones can mimic a ruptured abdominal aortic aneurysm, aortic dissection, renal or splenic infarction, acute cholecystitis, or acute pancreatitis.

If all the signs of acute ureteral obstruction are present, including direct visualization of the stone, the diagnosis can be made with certainty in the vast majority of cases. However, if the stone has already passed at the time of CT imaging, findings may be confused with acute pyelonephritis or other causes of acute obstruction. On plain radiographs and CT scans, calcifications in the pelvis are very common. Phleboliths typically have a radiolucent center. Calcified atheromas can usually be localized to the wall of an arterial branch. The "soft tissue rim" sign is most useful for making a confident diagnosis of a ureteral stone on CT.

TREATMENT

Medical Treatment

Obstruction in the absence of infection can be managed with analgesics and hydration. The stone will likely pass if its diameter is smaller than 5 to 6 mm (larger stones are more likely to require surgical measures).

TABLE 26-1   Accuracy, Limitations, and Pitfalls of Modalities Used in Imaging of Ureteral and Renal Stones

Modality	Accuracy	Limitations	Pitfalls
Radiography	Sensitivity 70%	Does not assess degree of obstruction	Calcifications can be confused with phleboliths or gallstones.
CT	Sensitivity 92%-98%	Function not evaluated	Stones and phleboliths may be difficult to differentiate.
MRI	Insufficient data	Time consuming	Interpretation can be difficult.
Ultrasonography	Relatively insensitive	Operator dependent	Bowel gas often precludes evaluation of the pelvic region.

Surgical Treatment

The primary indications for surgical treatment include persistent pain, uncontrolled infection, and persistent obstruction. Extracorporeal shock wave lithotripsy is the least invasive of the surgical methods of stone removal. Approximately 85% of urinary tract calculi that require treatment are currently managed with lithotripsy. Ureteroscopic manipulation of a stone is the next most commonly applied modality. Often, a ureteral stent must be placed after this procedure to prevent obstruction from ureteral spasm and edema. Other options include percutaneous nephrostolithotomy and open extraction.

What the Referring Physician Needs to Know

■ Where is the stone located?
■ How large is the stone?
■ Is there associated obstruction?
■ Is there associated infection?

KEY POINTS

■ CT is the preferred imaging method for diagnosis of acute ureteral obstruction.
■ CT is highly sensitive for urinary calculi.

SUGGESTED READINGS

Chen MY, Scharling ES, Zagoria RJ, et al. CT diagnosis of acute flank pain from urolithiasis. Semin Ultrasound CT MR 2000; 21:2-19.

Dalrymple NC, Casford B, Raiken DP, et al. Pearls and pitfalls in the diagnosis of ureterolithiasis with unenhanced helical CT. RadioGraphics 2000; 20:439-447.

Goldman SM, Sandler CM. Genitourinary imaging: The past 40 years. Radiology 2000; 215:313-324.

Heidenreich A, Desgrandschamps F, Terrier F. Modern approach of diagnosis and management of acute flank pain: review of all imaging modalities. Eur Urol 2002; 41:351-362.

Novelline RA, Rhea JT, Rao PM, Stuk JL. Helical CT in emergency radiology. Radiology 1999; 213:321-339.

Sandhu C, Anson KM, Patel U. Urinary tract stones: I. Role of radiological imaging in diagnosis and treatment planning. Clin Radiol 2003; 58:415-421.

Smith RC, Levine J, Rosenfeld AT. Helical CT of urinary tract stones: epidemiology, origin, pathophysiology, diagnosis, and management. Radiol Clin North Am 1999; 37:911-952.

Tamm EP, Silverman PM, Shuman WP. Evaluation of the patient with flank pain and possible ureteral calculus. Radiology 2003; 228:319-329.

Vieweg J, Teh C, Freed K, et al. Unenhanced helical computerized tomography for the evaluation of patients with acute flank pain. J Urol 1998; 160:679-684.

REFERENCES

1. Yilmaz S, Sindel T, Arslan G, et al. Renal colic: comparison of spiral CT, US and IVU in the detection of ureteral calculi. Eur Radiol 1998; 8:212-217.

2. Smith RC, Rosenfield AT, Choe KA, et al. Acute flank pain: comparison of non-contrast-enhanced CT and intravenous urography. Radiology 1995; 194:789-794.

3. Smith RC, Verga M, McCarthy S, Rosenfield AT. Diagnosis of acute flank pain: value of unenhanced helical CT. AJR Am J Roentgenol 1996;166:97-101.

4. Preminger GM, Vieweg J, Leder RA, Nelson RC. Urolithiasis: detection and management with unenhanced spiral CT—a urologic perspective. Radiology 1998; 207:308-309.

5. Smith RC, Verga M, Dalrymple N, et al. Acute ureteral obstruction: value of secondary signs of helical unenhanced CT. AJR Am J Roentgenol 1996; 167:1109-1113.

6. Boridy IC, Kawashima A, Goldman SM, Sandler CM. Acute ureterolithiasis: nonenhanced helical CT findings of perinephric edema for prediction of degree of ureteral obstruction. Radiology 1999; 213:663-667.

7. Boridy IC, Nikolaidis P, Kawashima PA, et al. Ureterolithiasis: Value of the tail sign in differentiating phleboliths from ureteral calculi at nonenhanced helical CT. Radiology 1999; 211:619-621.

8. Paulson EK, Weaver C, Ho LM, et al. Conventional and reduced radiation dose of 16-MDCT for detection of nephrolithiasis and ureterolithiasis. AJR Am J Roentgenol 2008; 190:151-157.

9. Tack D, Sourtzis S, Delpierre I, et al. Low-dose unenhanced multidetector CT of patients with suspected renal colic. AJR Am J Roentgenol 2003; 180:305-311.

10. Regan F, Kuszyk B, Bohlman ME, Jackman S. Acute ureteric calculus obstruction: unenhanced spiral CT versus HASTE MR urography and abdominal radiograph. Br J Radiol 2005; 78:506-511.

11. Reuther G, Kiefer B, Wandl E. Visualization of urinary tract dilatation: value of single-shot MR urography. Eur Radiol 1997; 7: 1276-1281.

12. Regan F, Bohlman ME, Khazan R, et al. MR urography using HASTE imaging in the assessment of ureteric obstruction. AJR Am J Roentgenol 1996; 167:1115-1120.

13. O'Malley ME, Soto JA, Yucel EK, Hussain S. MR urography: evaluation of a three-dimensional fast spin-echo technique in patients with hydronephrosis. AJR Am J Roentgenol 1997; 168:387-392.

14. Sudah M, Vanninen R, Partanen K, et al. Patients with acute flank pain: comparison of MR urography with unenhanced helical CT. Radiology 2002; 223:98-105.

15. Patlas M, Farkas A, Fisher D, et al. Ultrasound vs CT for the detection of ureteric stones in patients with renal colic. Br J Radiol 2001; 74:901-904.

16. Sheafor DH, Hertzberg BS, Freed KS, et al. Nonenhanced helical CT and US in the emergency evaluation of patients with renal colic: prospective comparison. Radiology 2000; 217:792-797.

17. Fowler KAB, Locken JA, Duchesne JH, Williamson MR. US for detecting renal calculi with nonenhanced CT as a reference standard. Radiology 2002; 222:109-113.

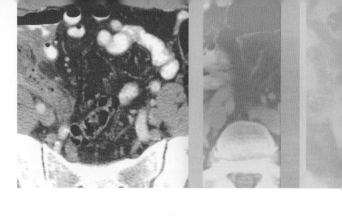

CHAPTER 27

Acute Appendicitis

Stephan W. Anderson and Jorge A. Soto

ETIOLOGY

Acute appendicitis results from obstruction of the appendiceal lumen from any cause (most commonly a fecalith), leading to overdistention and superinfection and, if not treated promptly, to perforation and peritonitis.

EPIDEMIOLOGY

Acute appendicitis is a very common clinical concern in patients presenting to the emergency department with abdominal pain, with a lifetime risk of 5% to 7%. The mortality rate is less than 1% but may be as high as 20% in certain populations, such as the elderly. In the clinical evaluation and diagnostic investigation of patients with acute right lower quadrant pain, other conditions should be considered in the differential diagnosis. These include right-sided diverticulitis, acute cholecystitis, epiploic appendagitis, renal or ureteral stones, omental infarction, bowel obstruction, and, in females, acute gynecologic conditions.

CLINICAL PRESENTATION

Patients typically present with gradual onset of anorexia, nausea/vomiting, and nonspecific abdominal pain that worsens progressively and eventually localizes in the right lower quadrant with clinical evidence of peritoneal irritation, leukocytosis, and fever. If all these symptoms and signs are present, imaging may not be necessary. However, in patients with less typical presentations or those requiring further characterization of the suspected diagnosis, imaging is often employed.

PATHOPHYSIOLOGY

The appendiceal orifice is located at the tip of the cecum. However, given the mobility of the cecum itself and the variable length (5 to 12 cm or more) and course of the appendix, the pain can be localized almost anywhere in the abdomen or pelvis.

PATHOLOGY

Initially, the appendiceal lumen occludes secondary to a number of causes, including fecaliths and lymphoid hyperplasia. Once occluded, intraluminal fluid continues to accumulate, distending the appendix and eventually increasing the intraluminal and intramural pressures to the point of vascular and lymphatic obstruction. Ineffective venous and lymphatic drainage allows bacterial invasion of the appendiceal wall and lumen. If this bacterial infection is not treated, perforation of the appendix and peritonitis may ensue.

IMAGING

Radiography

Currently, abdominal radiographs have very limited clinical utility in patients with suspected appendicitis. A calcified fecalith (appendicolith) may be identified in the right lower quadrant (Fig. 27-1), or there may be a focally dilated loop of small bowel ("sentinel loop" sign).

CT

CT is the preferred method for diagnosing appendicitis,[1-5] either after a nonconclusive ultrasound examination or directly as the first imaging test. On CT, the appendix appears enlarged, often with surrounding inflammatory changes, fascial thickening, and small amounts of free intraperitoneal fluid (Figs. 27-2 and 27-3). Appendicoliths are also readily identified on CT (Fig. 27-4). There may be edema at the origin of the appendix, as evidenced by thickening of the adjacent cecum, the "arrowhead" sign. There is a wide variation in the diameter of the appendix in normal patients, with sizes ranging up to 1 cm. However, mean values range between 5 and 7 mm depending on whether the appendix is distended with air. Therefore, when the appendix measures slightly greater than the standard cutoff value of 6 mm, secondary signs of inflammation should be sought to determine whether appendicitis is present. Filling of the appendix by orally or rectally introduced positive contrast material is a useful imaging finding in excluding obstruction of the appendix and, therefore, acute appendicitis. However, isolated involvement of the distal segment of the appendix ("tip" appendicitis) is seen occasionally. In patients in whom the appendix is not visualized, this finding, in the absence of right lower quadrant inflammation, carries a high negative predictive value of appendicitis.

The most important complication of acute appendicitis that should be recognized with CT is focal appendiceal rupture. Signs of rupture include periappendiceal abscess (Fig. 27-5), extraluminal gas (localized or free), free peritoneal fluid, and focal poor enhancement of the appendiceal wall.[6-9] Other, less common complications include diffuse peritonitis (with free gas in the peritoneal cavity) and portal vein thrombosis.

MRI

Pregnant females with abdominal pain often present a diagnostic challenge. Typically, an ultrasound examination is completed to rule out other causes of abdominal pain in this patient population, such as ectopic pregnancy or ovarian torsion. However, as the gravid uterus enlarges, the appendix is displaced from its expected location in the right lower quadrant and it becomes very difficult to visualize. In those patients with an inconclusive ultrasound examination, both CT and MRI are often employed. The findings of acute appendicitis on CT in pregnant

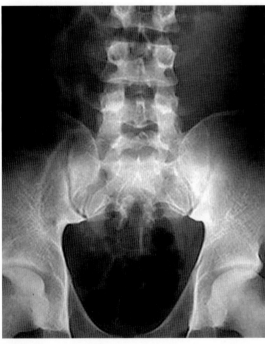

■ **FIGURE 27-1** Abdominal radiograph in a patient with acute appendicitis demonstrates a calcification in the right side of the pelvis representing an appendicolith.

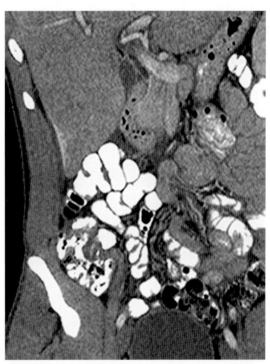

■ **FIGURE 27-3** Coronal reformatted image from axial CT data (CT scan performed with oral and intravenous contrast) clearly demonstrates the inflamed appendix in its longitudinal axis.

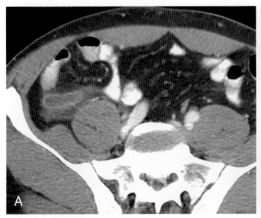

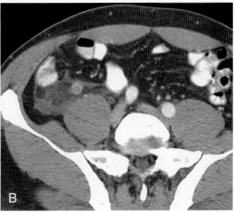

■ **FIGURE 27-2** **A,** Axial CT image performed after oral and intravenous administration of contrast agents demonstrates the typical appearance of acute appendicitis: a blind-ending tubular structure with enhancing walls and periappendiceal inflammation. The inflamed appendix is seen in its longitudinal axis. **B,** CT image at a slightly different level demonstrates a cross section of the inflamed appendix.

patients are similar to those in the nonpregnant population. Given concerns regarding radiation dose to the fetus, MRI is frequently used to evaluate for suspected appendicitis in pregnant patients.[10-12] MRI offers high diagnostic accuracy and is an excellent modality for excluding appendicitis. The appendix may be considered normal when it is less than or equal to 6 mm in diameter or is filled with air or oral contrast material. As on CT, MRI findings of appendicitis include enlargement of the appendix and associated secondary findings such as periappendiceal inflammation (Fig. 27-6). As the gravid uterus enlarges, the cecum, and therefore the appendix, may be in atypical locations, displaced superiorly. Therefore, it is helpful to identify the landmarks of the terminal ileum and cecum in attempting to localize the appendix on MRI.

Ultrasonography

In the younger population, and especially in females, ultrasonography may be used as an initial imaging evaluation to avoid ionizing radiation.[13-18] The typical ultrasound findings of appendicitis include the visualization of a noncompressible, blind-ending tubular structure that is distended with fluid and measures more than 6 mm in diameter during graded compression (Fig. 27-7). Appendicoliths may also be visualized as echogenic, shadowing foci within the lumen of the appendix (Fig. 27-8). Color

Doppler imaging may demonstrate increased vascularity of the inflamed appendiceal wall. Technical limitations of ultrasonography include difficulties imaging obese patients, and the wide variety of locations of the appendix, especially those located more posteriorly within the peritoneal cavity, poses increased difficulty for evaluation.

Imaging Algorithm

Overall, CT is the preferred method when the diagnosis of acute appendicitis is entertained. Ultrasonography is used mainly in pediatric patients, young women, and patients with small amounts of intraperitoneal fat. MRI is generally reserved for pregnant patients with acute right lower quadrant pain (Table 27-1).

Classic Signs

- *Radiography:* calcified appendicolith and sentinel loop
- *Ultrasonography:* noncompressible blind-ending tubular structure measuring more than 6 mm in diameter
- *CT:* distended appendix with adjacent inflammatory changes and thickening of adjacent cecum ("arrowhead" sign)
- *MRI:* distended appendix with high T2 signal

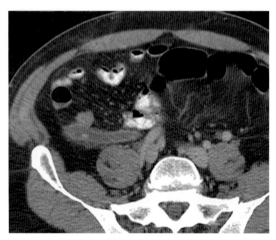

■ **FIGURE 27-4**   Dilated, inflamed appendix with an intraluminal high-attenuation focus, representing the appendicolith.

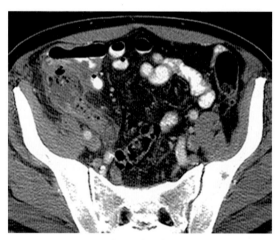

■ **FIGURE 27-5**   CT scan after oral and intravenous administration of contrast agents shows acute appendicitis with perforation. The lateral wall of the dilated, inflamed appendix is interrupted, and there is extraluminal gas and fluid, representing the periappendiceal abscess.

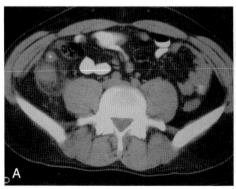

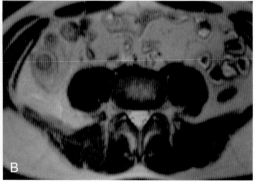

■ **FIGURE 27-6**   **A,** Axial image of a CT scan performed with oral contrast but without intravenous contrast depicts the dilated appendix with periappendiceal fat inflammation and fascial thickening. These findings are typical of acute appendicitis. **B,** Axial T2-weighted MR image obtained at the same level as in **A** again shows the dilated appendix and inflammation of the periappendiceal fat.

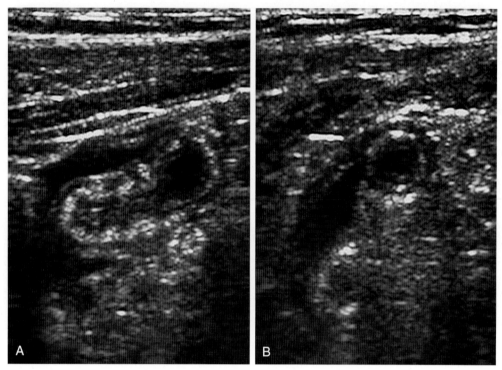

■ **FIGURE 27-7** Acute appendicitis. **A,** A longitudinal ultrasound image of the blind-ending appendix is distended with fluid and was not compressible on the real-time examination. There is a small amount of periappendiceal fluid as well. **B,** On cross section, the inflamed appendix has the typical "target" appearance, with fluid within the lumen and also adjacent to the appendix.

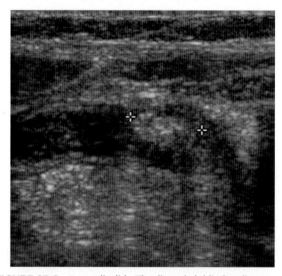

■ **FIGURE 27-8** Appendicolith. The distended, blind-ending appendix contains an intraluminal echogenic focus at the tip, with some associated acoustic shadowing. This is the appendicolith.

TABLE 27-1 Accuracy, Limitations, and Pitfalls of Modalities Used in Imaging the Appendix

Modality	Accuracy	Limitations	Pitfalls
Radiography	<10%	Appendix not seen	Rarely used in practice
CT	92-98%	Ionizing radiation	Early appendicitis
MRI	95%	Time consuming	Difficult study to interpret
Ultrasonography	80-85%	Operator dependent	Appendix may be difficult to find

DIFFERENTIAL DIAGNOSIS

Acute appendicitis should be differentiated from pyelonephritis, acute cholecystitis, diverticulitis of the cecum and ascending colon, and, in females, from ectopic pregnancy and ruptured or torsed ovarian cysts. Epiploic appendagitis can also produce similar clinical findings.

On ultrasonography the appendix should be differentiated from loops of small bowel. On CT the main difficulty arises when trying to separate a normal appendix from a minimally inflamed one. However, alternative diagnoses are often made with CT and should be readily identified. Epiploic appendagitis is recognized as an ovoid lesion containing fat that abuts the colon and has surrounding inflammatory stranding, often with a central high-attenuation focus representing a thrombosed vein. In acute diverticulitis, the epicenter of the inflammatory process is an inflamed or perforated diverticulum in the ascending colon or cecum. These may be difficult to differentiate from acute appendicitis, and follow-up imaging may be necessary if the patient does not undergo surgical intervention. Other conditions, such as ureteral stones, acute biliary processes, and gynecologic diseases are discussed elsewhere in this text.

TREATMENT

The vast majority of patients with acute appendicitis are treated with surgery, increasingly performed via a laparoscopic approach.

What the Referring Physician Needs to Know

- Is the appendix present and is it inflamed?
- Is there evidence of appendiceal rupture?
- Is there an alternative diagnosis?

KEY POINTS

- CT is the preferred imaging method for diagnosis of acute appendicitis.
- Ultrasonography is preferred in young, thin, and female patients of reproductive age. However, the appendix may be difficult to identify.
- MRI is a good diagnostic alternative for pregnant patients.

SUGGESTED READINGS

Birnbaum BA, Wilson SR. Appendicitis at the millennium. Radiology 2000; 215:337-348.

Hayes R. Abdominal pain: general imaging strategies. Eur Radiol 2004; 14(Suppl 4):L123-L137.

Kosaka N, Sagoh T, Uematsu H, et al. Difficulties in the diagnosis of appendicitis: review of CT and US images. Emerg Radiol 2007; 14:289-295.

Macari M, Balthazar EJ. The acute right lower quadrant: CT evaluation. Radiol Clin North Am 2003; 41:1117-1136.

Pedrosa I, Zeikus EA, Levine D, Rofsky NM. MR imaging of acute right lower quadrant pain in pregnant and nonpregnant patients. RadioGraphics 2007; 27:721-743; discussion 743-753.

Puylaert JB. Ultrasonography of the acute abdomen: gastrointestinal conditions. Radiol Clin North Am 2003; 41:1227-1242, vii.

Yu J, Fulcher AS, Turner MA, Halvorsen RA. Helical CT evaluation of acute right lower quadrant pain. I. Common mimics of appendicitis. AJR Am J Roentgenol 2005; 184:1136-1142.

Yu J, Fulcher AS, Turner MA, Halvorsen RA. Helical CT evaluation of acute right lower quadrant pain. II. Uncommon mimics of appendicitis. AJR Am J Roentgenol 2005; 184:1143-1149.

REFERENCES

1. Lane MJ, Liu DM, Huynh MD, et al. Suspected acute appendicitis: nonenhanced helical CT in 300 consecutive patients. Radiology 1999; 213:341-346.

2. Rhea JT, Halpern EF, Ptak T, et al. The status of appendiceal CT in an urban medical center 5 years after its introduction: experience with 753 patients. AJR Am J Roentgenol 2005; 184:1802-1808.

3. Keyzer C, Zalcman M, De Maertelaer V, et al. Comparison of US and unenhanced multi-detector row CT in patients suspected of having acute appendicitis. Radiology 2005; 236:527-534.

4. Rao PM, Novelline RA, McCabe CJ, et al. Helical CT technique for the diagnosis of appendicitis: prospective evaluation of a focused appendix CT examination. Radiology 1997; 202:139-144.

5. Rao PM, Rhea JT, Novelline RA, et al. Effect of computed tomography of the appendix on treatment of patients and use of hospital resources. N Engl J Med 1998; 338:141-146.

6. Oliak D, Sinow R, French S, et al. Computed tomography scanning for the diagnosis of perforated appendicitis. Am Surg 1999; 65:959-964.

7. Foley TA, Earnest F, Nathan MA, et al. Differentiation of nonperforated from perforated appendicitis: accuracy of CT diagnosis and relationship of CT findings to length of hospital stay. Radiology 2005; 235:89-96.

8. Horrow MM, White DS, Horrow JC. Differentiation of perforated from nonperforated appendicitis at CT. Radiology 2003; 227:46-51.

9. Yeung KW, Chang MS, Hsiao CP. Evaluation of perforated and non-perforated appendicitis with CT. Clin Imaging 2004; 28:422-427.

10. Birchard KR, Brown MA, Hyslop WB, et al. MRI of acute abdominal and pelvic pain in pregnant patients. AJR Am J Roentgenol 2005; 184:452-458.

11. Pedrosa I, Levine D, Eyvazzadeh AD, et al. MR imaging evaluation of acute appendicitis in pregnancy. Radiology 2006; 238:891-899.

12. Oto A, Srinivasan PN, Ernst RD, et al. Revisiting MRI for appendix location during pregnancy. AJR Am J Roentgenol 2006; 186:883-887.

13. Birnbaum BA, Jeffrey RB. CT and sonographic evaluation of acute right lower abdominal pain. AJR Am J Roentgenol 1998; 170:361-371.

14. Jeffrey RB Jr, Laing FC, Townsend RR. Acute appendicitis: sonographic criteria based on 250 cases. Radiology 1988; 167:327-329.

15. Balthazar EJ, Birnbaum BA, Yee J, et al. Acute appendicitis: CT and US correlation in 100 patients. Radiology 1994; 190:31-35.

16. Wise SW, Labuski MR, Kasales CJ, et al. Comparative assessment of CT and sonographic techniques for appendiceal imaging. AJR Am J Roentgenol 2001; 176:933-941.

17. Puylaert JB. Acute appendicitis: US evaluation using graded compression. Radiology 1986; 158:355-360.

18. Lim HK, Lee WJ, Kim TH, et al. Appendicitis: usefulness of color Doppler US. Radiology 1996; 201:221-225.

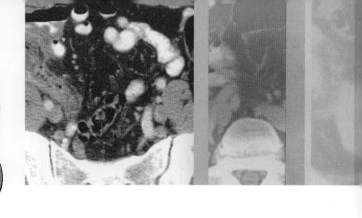

CHAPTER 28

Hollow Viscus Perforation

Jorge A. Soto and Stephan W. Anderson

ETIOLOGY

The presence of extraluminal air in an acutely ill patient with abdominal pain is an ominous sign that usually indicates perforation of a hollow viscus. Common causes include gastroduodenal peptic ulcer disease, perforation of a gastrointestinal neoplasm, acute appendicitis with perforation, and acute colonic or (less often) small bowel diverticulitis, including Meckel's diverticulitis.[1] Other considerations include iatrogenic perforations caused by catheters or endoscopes, perforations caused by foreign bodies, or spontaneous rupture of the distal esophagus (Boerhaave's syndrome), as well as ischemia leading to necrosis and resultant loss of bowel wall integrity.

PREVALENCE AND EPIDEMIOLOGY

The epidemiology of hollow viscus perforation depends on the underlying cause. Although the prevalence of the various causes varies greatly, the morbidity and mortality of hollow viscus perforation are significant in all cases, given the possibility of progression to peritonitis and its resultant complications.

The most common cause of hollow viscus perforation is gastroduodenal peptic ulcer disease. Peptic ulcer disease is exceedingly common, with a lifetime prevalence of approximately 10% in the United States and with variable prevalence internationally, depending mainly on its association with the use of nonsteroidal anti-inflammatory drugs (NSAIDs) or *Helicobacter pylori* infection. The incidence of perforation has been reported to be 2% to 5% in patients with peptic ulcer disease.[2] Perforated peptic ulcer disease carries significant morbidity and mortality, especially because many patients are elderly and have associated comorbidities. Overall postoperative mortality has been reported to be 19% but exceeds 40% in patients older than 79 years of age.[3]

A second common cause of nontraumatic hollow viscus perforation is perforated colonic diverticulitis. The prevalence of diverticulosis is significantly associated with age

and is reported to affect 65% of patients older than 65 years of age; 10% to 25% of patients with diverticular disease are reported to develop diverticulitis.[4] Of these, approximately 10% to 15% of patients develop free perforation. Interestingly, the incidence of perforated diverticulitis has been reported to be increasing in certain populations secondary to aging and dietary influences.[5] The mortality of perforated sigmoid diverticulitis has been reported to be approximately 8%.[6]

CLINICAL PRESENTATION

Because the signs and symptoms of hollow viscus perforation are typically related to the underlying cause, there are a variety of clinical presentations. Initially, symptoms will typically be localized to the area of disease; for example, patients with peptic ulcers may complain of intermittent or constant epigastric pain, sometimes radiating to the back. Although myriad initial clinical presentations exist, once free perforation into the peritoneal cavity is achieved, many patients will have generalized peritonitis with peritoneal guarding, shock, and prostration.

PATHOPHYSIOLOGY

Anatomic considerations are dependent on the underlying cause of the hollow viscus perforation. In considering the imaging findings associated with the various causes, one must consider the anatomic locations of the various portions of the gastrointestinal tract. Patients with esophageal perforation typically present with pneumomediastinum, which may dissect into the neck, pleural space, pericardial space, as well as the retroperitoneum and intraperitoneal cavity. The short, intra-abdominal portion of the esophagus is within the retroperitoneum. The second and third portions of the duodenum, ascending and descending colon (in most patients), as well as the rectum are considered retroperitoneal structures (Fig. 28-1). The remainder of the gastrointestinal tract is considered intraperitoneal. Typically, free air will be found within the abdominal

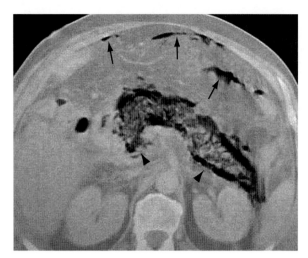

■ **FIGURE 28-1** Axial CT image reveals foci of free intraperitoneal air (*arrows*) as well as significant retroperitoneal air, predominantly within the anterior pararenal space around the pancreas (*arrowheads*). At surgery, the patient was found to have perforated ulcers within both the first and third portion of the duodenum, accounting for the intraperitoneal and retroperitoneal air, respectively.

cavity containing the portion of the gastrointestinal tract that is perforated. However, air may track within from the peritoneal cavity into the retroperitoneum and vice versa as well as caudad into the thorax, including the mediastinum and pleural spaces.

Anatomic considerations in patients with esophageal rupture secondary to Boerhaave's syndrome relate to failure of the cricopharyngeus muscle to relax in coordination with vomiting. The esophageal tears are typically within the posterolateral aspect of the distal esophagus, several centimeters proximal to the gastroesophageal junction. This area has been shown to be an anatomically relatively weak point.[7]

In patients with peptic ulcer disease, the duodenum is more commonly affected than the stomach. Within the duodenum, the ulcers are most commonly found within the first portion of the duodenum.[8] Based on preoperative imaging, the sites of gastroduodenal ulcer perforation are typically within the duodenum or are juxtapyloric in location.[9]

In patients with small bowel diverticulosis, the diverticula may be categorized as congenital or acquired.[10] In acquired, or true, diverticula, the more common type, all three layers of the bowel wall are involved. Like pulsion diverticula elsewhere, acquired diverticula contain protrusions of portions of the bowel wall through an area of focal mural weakness. Meckel's diverticula are true diverticula in that they contain all three layers of the intestinal wall and arise along the antimesenteric border of the small bowel. They are commonly found 40 to 100 cm proximal to the ileocecal valve, and the length of the diverticulum ranges from 1 to 10 cm in 90% of patients.[11] Colonic diverticula represent pulsion diverticula and present as outpouchings of mucosa, muscularis mucosa, or submucosa through focal weaknesses of the colonic wall.

PATHOLOGY

The pathology of hollow viscus perforation depends on the underlying cause. As noted earlier, patients with Boerhaave's syndrome have a failure of the proper timing of cricopharyngeal relaxation with vomiting. This causes a significant increase in the intraluminal pressures of the esophagus, leading to full-thickness rupture.

In patients with peptic ulcer disease, failure of gastroduodenal mucosal mechanisms secondary to *H. pylori* infection, NSAID use, and hypersecretory states, among others, results in a defect in the muscularis mucosa.[12] If the ulceration continues beyond the muscularis mucosa, free perforation of the stomach or duodenum may occur.

In diverticulitis of the small bowel or colon, once the mucosa-lined outpouching through the bowel wall is obstructed, distention results secondary to ongoing secretion of mucus and bacterial overgrowth. Vascular compromise of these mucosal outpouchings may occur, leading to perforation. Similar to the pathophysiology of perforated diverticulitis, appendicitis results from obstruction of the appendiceal lumen with subsequent distention from mucosal secretions. Capillary perfusion pressures are outstripped, and venous and lymphatic drainage is obstructed. The influx of bacteria into the appendiceal wall as well as the decreasing arterial flow and tissue necrosis result in an appendiceal perforation.

In patients with colonic perforation secondary to colorectal carcinoma, the perforation may occur proximal to the tumor, related to obstruction and distention, or occur directly at the site of the tumor. In cases of perforation related to obstruction, the pathophysiology is similar to that of the aforementioned examples of increasing luminal distention and decreasing venous return followed by decreasing arterial inflow, resulting in tissue necrosis and loss of mural integrity. In cases of perforation directly at the site of the tumor, transmural tumor invasion and necrosis are underlying mechanisms resulting in loss of mural integrity.

IMAGING

Radiography

Plain radiography is useful in the initial evaluation of suspected hollow viscus perforation to detect the secondary signs of extraluminal air. However, the precise location and underlying cause of perforation are unlikely to be detected with radiography.

Plain radiographs are often initially employed to detect pneumoperitoneum (Fig. 28-2). Often, this includes the acquisition of both a supine radiograph of the abdomen and an upright view of the chest to evaluate for free intraperitoneal air. Other options include left lateral decubitus views of the abdomen or lateral chest radiographs. Upright radiographs or left lateral decubitus views should be acquired with the central ray of the x-ray beam at the highest level of the peritoneal cavity to increase the sensitivity of detection of intraperitoneal air.[13] Numerous signs of pneumoperitoneum on abdominal radiographs have been described, including Rigler's sign, in which

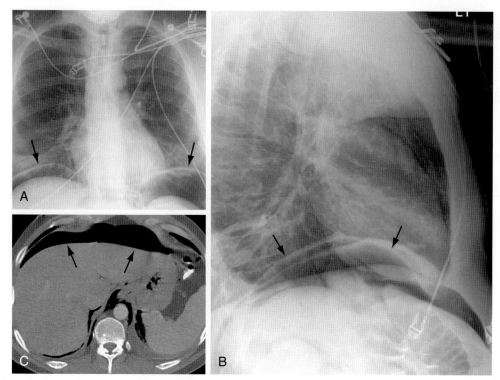

■ **FIGURE 28-2** **A,** Anteroposterior chest radiograph reveals significant free intraperitoneal air as evidenced by the lucency beneath the diaphragms bilaterally (*arrows*). **B,** Lateral chest radiograph reveals significant free intraperitoneal air, as evidenced by the lucency beneath the diaphragms (*arrows*). **C,** Axial CT image confirms the presence of significant free intraperitoneal air (*arrows*). Air is also seen tracking into the mediastinum about the aortic hiatus. The patient was diagnosed with perforated diverticulitis at operative exploration.

air is seen on both sides of the bowel wall; the falciform ligament sign, in which air outlines the falciform ligament; the football sign, in which air outline the confines of the peritoneal cavity; the inverted-"V" sign, in which air outlines the medial umbilical folds; and the right upper quadrant air sign, in which a focal, typically triangular, collection of gas is seen in the right upper quadrant.[14] Visualization of air outlining the median subphrenic space, the so-called cupola sign, has also been described in a minority of patients with pneumoperitoneum on supine radiographs.

Because esophageal rupture as well as dissection of air from intra-abdominal perforations may lead to pneumomediastinum, chest radiography may be employed for initial evaluation. Various radiographic findings have been described, including the visualization of air superolateral to the heart on the left on an upright chest radiograph, lucent streaks of air outlining the aorta or great vessels, the continuous diaphragm sign with air outlining the superior portions of the diaphragm, and many others.[15]

Finally, because hollow viscus perforation may be associated with retroperitoneal air, abdominal radiographs may be useful in the initial diagnosis. Retroperitoneal air may be identified as linear or bubbly lucencies overlying the expected location of the retroperitoneum. Alternatively, air may be seen along fascial planes of known retroperitoneal structures such as the psoas muscles, kidneys and adrenal regions, or muscles of the diaphragm.[16]

CT

CT is the most sensitive modality in detecting small volumes of extraluminal air. In cases of hollow viscus perforation, CT has been shown to be highly accurate in the localization of the site of perforation, especially when thin collimation images and multiplanar reformatted images are viewed.[17,18] The findings of focal bowel wall thickening, localized air bubbles, and direct visualization of a rent within the wall of the bowel have been shown to be accurate predictors of the site of perforation.[17]

Findings of esophageal rupture on CT include pneumomediastinum, periesophageal fluid, and esophageal thickening as well as the possibility of direct visualization of the esophageal rent.[19] Additional findings associated with esophageal rupture on CT include esophageal hematoma, extravasation of oral contrast media, as well as an aberrant course of a nasogastric tube. Also, in cases of foreign body ingestion, direct CT visualization of the foreign body may be possible.[19]

CT findings in patients with perforation related to peptic ulcer disease include extraluminal gas as well as extravasation of oral contrast media (Figs. 28-3 and 28-4).[20] In addition, focal thickening of the gastrointestinal tract about the site of perforation as well as inflammatory stranding of the adjacent abdominal structures may be seen.

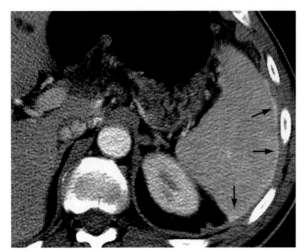

■ **FIGURE 28-3** Axial CT image reveals extravasated oral contrast medium within the peritoneal cavity surrounding the spleen (*arrows*). The patient was found to have a perforated gastric ulcer at operative exploration.

The CT findings related to perforation of small bowel diverticulitis are typically somewhat nonspecific.[21] Pneumoperitoneum as well as an inflammatory phlegmon or associated fluid are typically identified. Underlying small bowel diverticulosis may or may not be identified. In most cases of perforation due to Meckel's diverticulitis, direct visualization of the inflamed diverticulum is described, in addition to the pneumoperitoneum.[22] On CT, Meckel's diverticulum appears as a blind-ending pouch that is typically several centimeters in length with surrounding inflammatory changes.

In patients with perforated colonic diverticulitis, the findings of pneumoperitoneum or retroperitoneal gas as well as extravasation of oral contrast medium are typically identified (Fig. 28-5).[23] In addition, the affected segment of colon is typically inflamed and thickened, with diverticula visualized in the area. In the minority of patients with perforated colonic diverticulitis, the defect within the wall of the colon may be directly visualized on CT (Fig. 28-6).

In cases of hollow viscus perforation due to gastrointestinal obstruction, the pathophysiology involves a component of ischemia. Therefore, in addition to extraluminal gas and dilated loops of bowel, secondary signs of ischemia may be seen. These include pneumatosis intestinalis, air within the portal and mesenteric veins, as well as decreased enhancement of the affected bowel. Ischemia unrelated to bowel obstruction may also result in perforation. In these cases, the cause of ischemia, such as mesenteric venous or arterial thrombosis, may be directly visualized on CT.

Finally, in patients with cancer as the underlying cause of the hollow viscus perforation, direct visualization of the mass lesion is typically achieved.[24] In these cases, the resultant perforation may be due to transmural extension of tumor with necrosis or obstruction with upstream dilatation and ischemia; these causes may be differentiated on CT based on the presence of bowel distention and secondary findings of ischemia as described earlier.

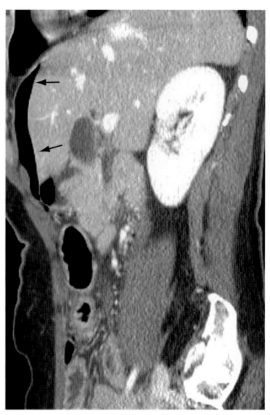

■ **FIGURE 28-4** Sagittal reformatted image from axial CT data reveals significant intraperitoneal air along the nondependent aspect of the peritoneal cavity anterior to the liver (*arrows*). The patient was diagnosed with a perforated duodenal ulcer at operative repair.

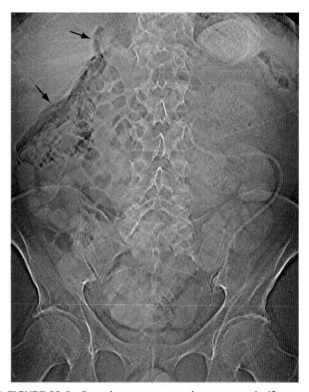

■ **FIGURE 28-5** Frontal scout topogram demonstrates significant free intraperitoneal air about the inferior edge of the liver (*arrows*). The patient had perforated right-sided diverticulitis.

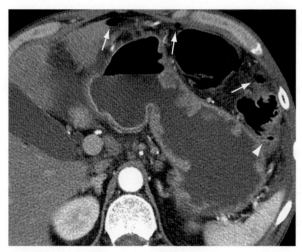

■ **FIGURE 28-6** Axial CT image demonstrates multiple foci of free intraperitoneal air (*arrows*) with evidence of moderate thickening of the distal transverse colon (*arrowhead*). The patient was successfully treated conservatively for perforated diverticulitis.

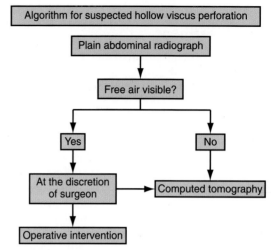

■ **FIGURE 28-7** Algorithm for suspected hollow viscus perforation.

Imaging Algorithm

The initial imaging evaluation in patients with suspected hollow viscus perforation includes plain radiography. If esophageal rupture is suspected, anteroposterior and lateral chest radiographs are commonly acquired. If an intra-abdominal perforation is suspected, supine and upright abdominal radiographs are typically acquired, possibly along with an upright anteroposterior radiograph of the chest for the evaluation of pneumoperitoneum. If there is evidence of hollow viscus perforation based on the initial plain radiographic findings such as pneumoperitoneum, depending on the clinical status of the patient the surgical team may decide to proceed directly to operative exploration.

Alternatively, patients with radiographic evidence of hollow viscus perforation may undergo CT evaluation for localization and further characterization of the underlying cause. However, because patients with hollow viscus perforation may present with nonspecific signs and symptoms, CT may be the initial diagnostic evaluation (Fig. 28-7 and Table 28-1).

DIFFERENTIAL DIAGNOSIS

The clinical signs and symptoms of hollow viscus perforation, especially once peritonitis ensues, are nonspecific. Therefore, differential diagnostic considerations include other causes of peritonitis, such as spontaneous bacterial peritonitis, systemic infections involving the peritoneum, such as tuberculosis, as well as sterile irritants of the peritoneal cavity, such as blood, bile, and pancreatic secretions.

In addition to perforation of a hollow viscus, other causes of extraluminal air include iatrogenic causes such as recent surgery as well as intercourse. Also, dissection of air from the thorax in cases of pneumothorax or pneumomediastinum from various causes are differential considerations in cases of extraluminal, intra-abdominal gas.

TABLE 28-1 Accuracy, Limitations, and Pitfalls of the Modalities Used in Imaging of Hollow Viscus Perforation

Modality	Accuracy	Limitations	Pitfalls
Radiography	<40%	Etiology, site of perforation not evaluated	Insensitive for small volumes of extraluminal gas
CT	>95%	Ionizing radiation	Alternative, benign causes of extraluminal gas (e.g., recent surgery)

Classic Signs

- Rigler's sign: air is seen on both sides of the bowel wall (pneumoperitoneum).
- Falciform ligament sign: air outlines the falciform ligament (pneumoperitoneum).
- Football sign: air outlines the confines of the peritoneal cavity (pneumoperitoneum).
- Inverted-"V" sign: air outlines the medial umbilical folds (pneumoperitoneum).
- Right upper quadrant air sign: a focal, typically triangular, collection of gas is seen in the right upper quadrant (pneumoperitoneum).
- Cupola sign: air outlines the median subphrenic space (pneumoperitoneum).
- Continuous diaphragm sign: air tracks along the superior layers of the diaphragm; the diaphragm appears continuous across the midline (pneumomediastinum).

In cases of pneumoperitoneum related to prior surgery, one should expect appropriate resolution during the postoperative period. The majority of cases are noted to resolve within 2 days based on radiography, but many patients may have minute areas of free air for several days and even up to several weeks on postoperative CT scans.

TREATMENT

Medical Treatment

The appropriate therapy in patients with hollow viscus perforation is highly dependent on the underlying cause and typically involves emergent surgical management. However, in a subgroup of patients with perforated diverticulitis, when there is no evidence of gross free intraperitoneal air and fluid, conservative medical management, including intravenous antibiotics, may be indicated. Also, in selected patients with perforated appendicitis, medical management including intravenous antibiotics may be employed before definitive operative management. In patients with hollow viscus perforation managed conservatively, radiology may be a critical facet of non-operative management via the use of image-guided percutaneous placement of drainage catheters to manage intra-abdominal fluid collections.

Surgical Treatment

The vast majority of patients with hollow viscus perforation undergo emergent surgical intervention. The preferred treatment in patients with esophageal perforation has traditionally been surgical intervention, although less invasive interventions are evolving.[25] In patients with perforated peptic ulcer disease, surgical intervention is typically employed, with laparoscopic techniques increasing in prevalence.[26] Patients with severe diverticulitis and gross perforation are typically managed surgically, often employing two-stage procedures.[27] In hollow viscus perforation related to ischemia, surgical intervention is employed, typically with resection of the segments of necrotic bowel. Finally, in patients with perforation secondary to underlying cancer, surgical intervention with resection of the underlying mass lesion is done.[28]

What the Referring Physician Needs to Know

- Is extraluminal gas visualized? How much?
- Where is the site of perforation?
- What is the underlying cause of the perforation?

KEY POINTS

- There are many causes of hollow viscus perforation.
- Although plain radiography may be employed initially, CT is the modality of choice for diagnosis and characterization of hollow viscus perforation.
- Generally, hollow viscus perforation represents a surgical emergency; clinical teams should be immediately notified.

SUGGESTED READINGS

Cho KC, Baker SR. Extraluminal air: diagnosis and significance. Radiol Clin North Am 1994; 32:829-844.

Espinoza R, Rodríguez A. Traumatic and nontraumatic perforation of hollow viscera. Surg Clin North Am 1997; 77:1291-1304.

Furukawa A, Sakoda M, Yamasaki M, et al. Gastrointestinal tract perforation: CT diagnosis of presence, site, and cause. Abdom Imaging 2005; 30:524-534.

Marincek B. Nontraumatic abdominal emergencies: acute abdominal pain: diagnostic strategies. Eur Radiol 2002; 12:2136-2150.

Shaffer HA Jr. Perforation and obstruction of the gastrointestinal tract: assessment by conventional radiology. Radiol Clin North Am 1992; 30:405-426.

REFERENCES

1. Espinoza R, Rodríguez A. Traumatic and nontraumatic perforation of hollow viscera. Surg Clin North Am 1997; 77:1291-1304.
2. Cocks JR. Perforated peptic ulcer: the changing scene. Dig Dis 1992; 10:10-16.
3. Uccheddu A, Floris G, Altana ML, et al. Surgery for perforated peptic ulcer in the elderly: evaluation of factors influencing prognosis. Hepatogastroenterology 2003; 50:1956-1958.
4. Comparato G, Pilotto A, Franzè A, et al. Diverticular disease in the elderly. Dig Dis 2007; 25:151-159.
5. Mäkelä J, Kiviniemi H, Laitinen S. Prevalence of perforated sigmoid diverticulitis is increasing. Dis Colon Rectum 2002; 45:955-961.
6. Mäkelä JT, Kiviniemi H, Laitinen S. Prognostic factors of perforated sigmoid diverticulitis in the elderly. Dig Surg 2005; 22:100-106.
7. Korn O, Oñate JC, López R. Anatomy of the Boerhaave syndrome. Surgery 2007; 141:222-228.
8. Al-Bahrani ZR, Kassir ZA, Al-Doree W. The location and multiplicity of chronic duodenal ulcer (a study of 1320 patients in Iraq). Gastroenterol Jpn 1980; 15:539-542.
9. Grassi R, Romano S, Pinto A, Romano L. Gastro-duodenal perforations: conventional plain film, US and CT findings in 166 consecutive patients. Eur J Radiol 2004; 50:30-36.
10. Pearl MS, Hill MC, Zeman RK. CT findings in duodenal diverticulitis. AJR Am J Roentgenol 2006; 187:W392-W395.
11. Ludtke FE, Mende V, Kohler H, Lepsien G. Incidence and frequency of complications and management of Meckel's diverticulum. Surg Gynecol Obstet 1989; 169:537-542.
12. Mertz HR, Walsh JH. Peptic ulcer pathophysiology. Med Clin North Am 1991; 75:799-814.
13. Miller RE, Becker GJ, Slabaugh RD. Detection of pneumoperitoneum: optimum body position and respiratory phase. AJR Am J Roentgenol 1980; 135:487-490.
14. Levine MS, Scheiner JD, Rubesin SE, et al. Diagnosis of pneumoperitoneum on supine abdominal radiographs. AJR Am J Roentgenol 1991; 156:731-735.
15. Bejvan SM, Godwin JD. Pneumomediastinum: old signs and new signs. AJR Am J Roentgenol 1996; 166:1041-1048.

16. Hill MC, Bieber WP, Koch RL, Coulson W. Extraperitoneal perforations of the gastrointestinal tract. AJR Am J Roentgenol 1967; 101:315-321.
17. Hainaux B, Agneessens E, Bertinotti R, et al. Accuracy of MDCT in predicting site of gastrointestinal tract perforation. AJR Am J Roentgenol 2006; 187:1179-1183.
18. Ghekiere O, Lesnik A, Millet I, et al. Direct visualization of perforation sites in patients with a non-traumatic free pneumoperitoneum: added diagnostic value of thin transverse slices and coronal and sagittal reformations for multi-detector CT. Eur Radiol 2007; 17:2302-2309.
19. De Lutio di Castelguidone E, Pinto A, Merola S, et al. Role of spiral and multislice computed tomography in the evaluation of traumatic and spontaneous oesophageal perforation: our experience. Radiol Med (Torino) 2005; 109:252-259.
20. Jacobs JM, Hill MC, Steinberg WM. Peptic ulcer disease: CT evaluation. Radiology 1991; 178:745-748.
21. Greenstein S, Jones B, Fishman EK, et al. Small-bowel diverticulitis: CT findings. AJR Am J Roentgenol 1986; 147:271-274.
22. Bennett GL, Birnbaum BA, Balthazar EJ. CT of Meckel's diverticulitis in 11 patients. AJR Am J Roentgenol 2004; 182:625-629.
23. Lohrmann C, Ghanem N, Pache G, et al. CT in acute perforated sigmoid diverticulitis. Eur J Radiol 2005; 56:78-83.
24. Hulnick DH, Megibow AJ, Balthazar EJ, et al. Perforated colorectal neoplasms: correlation of clinical, contrast enema, and CT examinations. Radiology 1987; 164:611-615.
25. Wu JT, Mattox KL, Wall MJ Jr. Esophageal perforations: new perspectives and treatment paradigms. J Trauma 2007; 63:1173-1184.
26. Kirshtein B, Bayme M, Mayer T, et al. Laparoscopic treatment of gastroduodenal perforations: comparison with conventional surgery. Surg Endosc 2005; 19:1487-1490.
27. Floch MH, White JA. Management of diverticular disease is changing. World J Gastroenterol 2006; 28:12:3225-3228.
28. Cuffy M, Abir F, Audisio RA, Longo WE. Colorectal cancer presenting as surgical emergencies. Surg Oncol 2004; 13:149-157.

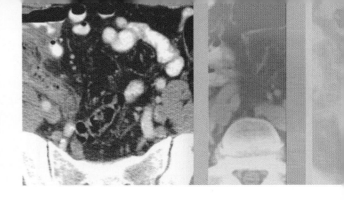

CHAPTER 29

Acute Gastrointestinal Bleeding

Jorge A. Soto and Stephan W. Anderson

ETIOLOGY

The causes of upper gastrointestinal bleeding include esophageal or gastric varices, Mallory-Weiss tears, gastritis, and gastric or duodenal ulcers. Common causes of lower gastrointestinal tract bleeding include colonic diverticulosis, ischemic and infectious colitis, colonic neoplasm, benign anorectal disease, arteriovenous malformations, ischemia, and Meckel's diverticulum.

PREVALENCE AND EPIDEMIOLOGY

Acute gastrointestinal bleeding is a major clinical problem and is often classified into upper and lower gastrointestinal categories based on the site of hemorrhage (proximal or distal to the ligament of Treitz). Any loss of blood occurring throughout the gastrointestinal tract requires immediate medical attention. Acute lower gastrointestinal hemorrhage is a common cause of hospital admission, with significant associated morbidity and mortality. Rapid stabilization of and therapy for patients with acute gastrointestinal bleeding is critical, because the mortality rate is reported to be up to 20% in cases of upper gastrointestinal hemorrhage, depending on the cause.[1] Mortality in patients with acute lower gastrointestinal bleeding is also reported to approach 20%.[2]

CLINICAL PRESENTATION

Patients with upper gastrointestinal hemorrhage present clinically with hematemesis, hematochezia, or melena. Patients with acute lower gastrointestinal hemorrhage report melena or hematochezia. When hematochezia occurs from an upper tract source, the acute blood loss can be estimated at greater than 1000 mL. The signs and symptoms are somewhat dependent on the underlying cause. Abdominal pain and diarrhea may be associated with infectious and inflammatory colitis. When severe, gastrointestinal hemorrhage may result in hemodynamic

instability and shock. Importantly, the amount of blood passed in vomitus or stool does not serve as a reliable indicator of the severity of the event, because large amounts of blood can be sequestered in the intestines.

In addition to the total amount of blood lost, the rate of bleeding and the overall health of the patient are other factors determining the clinical presentation and the need for emergent intervention. Healthy patients have a tremendous capacity to compensate for acute blood losses. In young individuals with no cardiovascular disease, up to 2 units of blood can be lost with minimal or no hemodynamic changes. Blood flow can be diverted from the skin, splanchnic circulation, and kidneys to maintain perfusion of essential organs such as the brain and heart. Hypotension and tachycardia indicate a larger volume of blood loss, whereas confusion and oliguria develop when bleeding loss reaches 3 to 4 units. Finally, although there is usually a rush to intervene, up to 75% or 80% of the patients will experience spontaneous cessation of bleeding before any therapy is initiated.

PATHOPHYSIOLOGY

The pathophysiology of gastrointestinal hemorrhage depends on the underlying cause. In considering the common causes of upper gastrointestinal hemorrhage, peptic ulcer disease results in a defect in the gastroduodenal mucosa with eventual exposure and damage to the underlying arteries, including arteritis, aneurysmal dilatation, and eventual rupture and hemorrhage.[3] The larger the underlying, ruptured vessel, the more significant the hemorrhage becomes. Mallory-Weiss tears result spontaneously from the marked increase in intraluminal pressures associated with retching and are associated with the presence of a hiatal hernia.[4] Linear tears within the mucosa of the distal esophagus, cardioesophageal junction, or cardia result in injury to the underlying vasculature with subsequent hemorrhage. In patients with varices, increasing hepatic venous pressure gradients result in enlarged varices and the increased risk of rupture and hemorrhage. Additionally, the concurrent presence of a bacterial infection is known to increase the risk of variceal hemorrhage, possibly by decreasing hemostatic function and the presence of systemic endotoxins.[5]

Diverticular hemorrhage results from rupture of the vasa recta at the dome of the diverticulum.[6] These vessels have been shown to have eccentric intimal thickening with asymmetric rupture, suggesting that trauma to these vessels results in intimal proliferation and scarring, leading to subsequent rupture and hemorrhage. Angiodysplasia is typically located within the lower gastrointestinal tract, specifically the right colon. Although the pathophysiology is incompletely understood, angiodysplastic lesions are thought to be acquired through the degenerative process of aging.[7]

IMAGING

Radiography

Abdominal radiographs have very limited clinical utility in patients with acute gastrointestinal bleeding. Clinical criteria including a history of lung disease and abnormal pulmonary findings on physical examination may be useful in selecting a subset of patients with acute gastrointestinal bleeding to receive chest radiographs on admission.[8] Abdominal radiographs have been shown not to affect clinical outcomes or management decisions in patients admitted to an intensive care unit with gastrointestinal hemorrhage.[9]

CT

Recently, CT has been shown to have a high diagnostic accuracy in both the detection and the localization of massive gastrointestinal bleeding (Fig. 29-1).[10-13] Optimal results necessitate the distention of the bowel with a contrast agent with neutral attenuation, such as water or low-density barium suspensions (Fig. 29-2). Both unenhanced and arterial-phase intravenous contrast-enhanced acquisitions should be acquired. CT diagnosis relies on the visualization of an area of active arterial contrast extravasation. In the majority of cases, CT may diagnose the underlying cause of acute hemorrhage, such as in the case of small bowel or colonic neoplasms.[10,12,13] The efficiency and ease of acquisition as well as reported diagnostic accuracies of multidetector CT in the evaluation of acute gastrointestinal bleeding make this a promising first-line imaging modality.

Nuclear Medicine

Both technetium-99m (^{99m}Tc)–labeled red blood cells and ^{99m}Tc sulfur colloid are applied in the evaluation of acute gastrointestinal hemorrhage.[14] However, ^{99m}Tc-labeled red blood cells offer the possibility for delayed imaging in cases of intermittent bleeding. The use of nuclear scintigraphy has been demonstrated to be sensitive in the detection and accurate in the localization of the source of acute gastrointestinal hemorrhage. The diagnosis of gastrointestinal bleeding on nuclear scintigraphy depends on the visualization of an area of tracer localization that persists and should be seen to move through the lumen of the bowel secondary to peristalsis. Both antegrade and retrograde transit is observed, but localization is dependent on the initial area of visualization (Fig. 29-3). The localization of the site of bleeding has been shown to be highly accurate with nuclear scintigraphy and clinically useful in guiding subsequent transcatheter therapies or surgical resection.[15]

Imaging Algorithm

There is no consensus regarding the initial imaging evaluation of patients presenting with acute gastrointestinal bleeding. Endoscopy, ^{99m}Tc-labeled red blood cell scintigraphy, CT, and conventional mesenteric angiography are

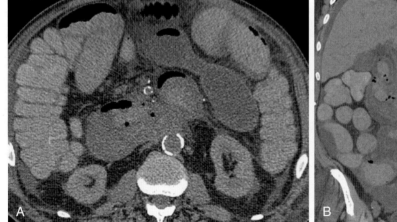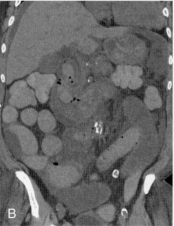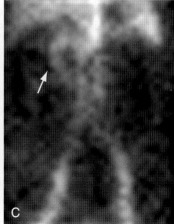

■ **FIGURE 29-1** **A,** Axial unenhanced CT image reveals diffuse hyperattenuation throughout the bowel lumen. The lack of intravenous use of a contrast agent precludes the localization of the hemorrhage; however, CT demonstrates its significant volume. **B,** Coronal reformatted axial CT image reveals the extent of intraluminal hemorrhage as evidenced by hyperattenuation throughout the bowel. **C,** ^{99m}Tc-labeled red blood cell scan localizes the area of active hemorrhage to the duodenum (*arrow*). The patient's acute hemorrhage, which was related to underlying peptic ulcer disease, was successfully treated with coil embolization.

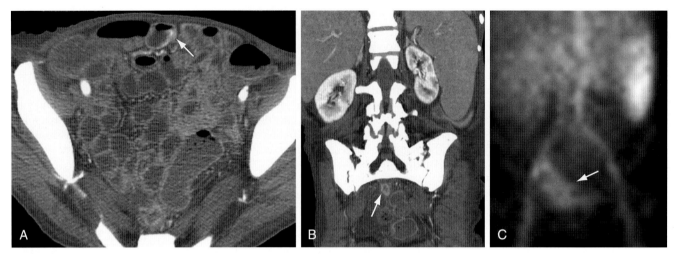

■ **FIGURE 29-2** **A,** Axial CT image reveals a punctuate area of hyperattenuation in the distal ileum consistent with active extravasation (*arrow*). This image demonstrates the importance of adequate oral preparation with a neutral attenuation contrast agent to optimize the contrast between active hemorrhage and the bowel lumen. **B,** Coronal reformatted axial CT image demonstrates the area of active hemorrhage within the distal ileum (*arrow*). **C,** ⁹⁹ᵐTc-labeled red blood cell scan reveals ongoing hemorrhage in the distal ileum (*arrow*). The patient underwent digital subtraction angiography twice without evidence of ongoing hemorrhage before receiving definitive partial small bowel resection.

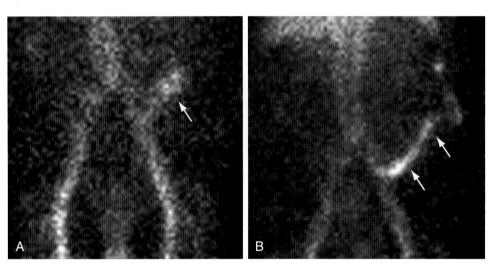

■ **FIGURE 29-3** **A,** ⁹⁹ᵐTc-labeled red blood cell scan reveals an initial area of active hemorrhage in the proximal sigmoid colon (*arrow*). **B,** Note ongoing hemorrhage with retrograde transit within the descending colon (*arrows*). Localization is dependent on initial visualization and in this case is secondary to sigmoid diverticulosis.

TABLE 29-1   Accuracy, Limitations, and Pitfalls of the Modalities Used in Imaging of Acute Gastrointestinal Bleeding

Modality	Accuracy	Limitations	Pitfalls
CT	>95% for localization	Ionizing radiation exposure, intermittent bleeding	Hypervascular gastrointestinal neoplasms
Nuclear medicine	>90% for localization	Poor localization of bleeding site	Vascular organs interfere with interpretation.
Angiography	>95% for localization	Rate of bleeding, intermittent bleeding	

all successfully applied, depending on the given scenario (Table 29-1).[10-17] Upper endoscopy is very valuable in patients with upper gastrointestinal bleeding to determine the exact source and cause and as a means of therapy in many instances. For patients with hematochezia and/or unclear sources of bleeding, nuclear scintigraphy is a valuable technique, although CT enterography is gaining acceptance in this situation as well. In cases of severe,

massive upper or lower gastrointestinal hemorrhage, catheter angiography of the mesenteric circulation is often necessary as a means for catheter-directed therapy, such as injection of vasopressin and, more currently, for superselective embolization techniques that have been shown to be an effective method of treatment (Fig. 29-4). In general, it is believed that a critical rate of hemorrhage of approximately 0.5 mL/min is necessary for a bleeding

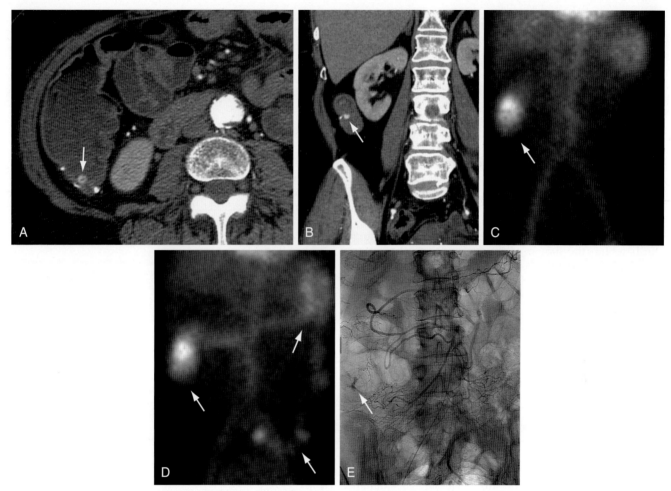

■ **FIGURE 29-4** **A,** Axial CT image shows a punctuate area of hyperattenuation in the ascending colon, consistent with active hemorrhage (*arrow*). **B,** Coronal reformatted axial CT image demonstrates the area of active hemorrhage within the ascending colon (*arrow*). **C,** ^{99m}Tc-labeled red blood cell scan reveals active hemorrhage with initial localization to the ascending colon, as on CT (*arrow*). **D,** Note the ongoing active hemorrhage with antegrade transit into the transverse, descending, and sigmoid colon (*arrows*). **E,** Digital subtraction angiogram shows an area of active extravasation within the ascending colon (*arrow*) that was subsequently successfully treated with coil embolization.

focus to be detected with angiography, whereas 0.05 mL/min can be detected with state of the art scintigraphic techniques.[18]

An algorithm for the evaluation of acute gastrointestinal bleeding is presented in Figure 29-5.

Classic Signs

■ On CT, the area of gastrointestinal hemorrhage is identified as a contrast blush seen on the contrast-enhanced images within the lumen of the gastrointestinal tract.
■ On nuclear scintigraphy, bleeding is seen as a focus of activity that either increases in intensity or changes in location over time secondary to peristalsis.
■ On catheter angiography, active hemorrhage is seen as a focus of active extravasation of contrast-enhanced blood that persists and may grow over time and is not washed out on delayed images.

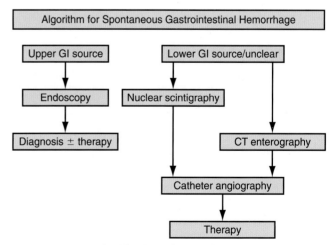

■ **FIGURE 29-5** Algorithm for evaluation of spontaneous gastrointestinal hemorrhage.

DIFFERENTIAL DIAGNOSIS

Differential considerations from clinical data depend on the severity of the gastrointestinal bleeding and its underlying etiology. In the presence of hematemesis, melena, or hematochezia, gastrointestinal hemorrhage, by definition, is the diagnosis. However, if these signs are not evident and the patient is presenting with syncope or signs of hypotension, myriad differential considerations may be entertained. This would include sources of hemorrhage elsewhere, including intra-abdominal, retroperitoneal, or intramuscular locations. However, patients with acute gastrointestinal bleeding typically present with hematemesis, melena, or hematochezia, allowing for the diagnosis to be made.

Using CT, the differential considerations of a contrast blush within the lumen of the gastrointestinal tract are limited. Potential considerations include small, hypervascular tumors, such as neuroendocrine tumors. A second contrast-enhanced phase of imaging would potentially be useful in differentiating active arterial extravasation from a hypervascular mass lesion. On nuclear scintigraphy, abnormal accumulations of the radiotracer potentially representing foci of hemorrhage must be differentiated from other sources of activity such as ectopic or accessory spleens, uterine leiomyomas, or a vascular mass lesion, among other potential sources.[19]

TREATMENT

Medical Treatment

Patients with acute gastrointestinal hemorrhage should be admitted to the hospital for observation and evaluation. Initial resuscitation includes correction of volume loss with crystalloids and blood products. Continuous monitoring with electrocardiographic lead placement, pulse oximeters, and automatic blood pressure cuffs is advised.

Invasive, nonsurgical techniques include transcatheter-directed therapies and endoscopy. Currently, transcatheter-directed embolotherapy is commonly applied in cases of acute gastrointestinal hemorrhage.[17,20] Various forms of therapy are also available with endoscopy, including sclerotherapy, laser coagulation, and banding.[16,21,22]

Surgical Treatment

Although conservative, endoscopic and transcatheter means of therapy are preferred, emergent surgery is necessary for patients who do not respond or in whom bleeding recurs rapidly after several attempts of control with less-invasive methods. Morbidity and mortality rates are high in these patients.

What the Referring Physician Needs to Know

- Is there a source of active bleeding?
- What is the location of the active bleeding?
- What is the cause of bleeding?
- Is the patient a candidate for transcatheter therapy?

KEY POINTS

- Sources of acute bleeding should be separated into those affecting the upper and lower gastrointestinal tract, using the ligament of Treitz as the boundary.
- After initial resuscitation and stabilization, diagnostic methods commonly used include upper and lower endoscopy, nuclear scintigraphy, catheter angiography, and, more recently, CT.
- Many patients can be successfully treated with transcatheter interventional techniques.

SUGGESTED READINGS

Anthony S, Milburn S, Uberoi R. Multi-detector CT: review of its use in acute GI haemorrhage. Clin Radiol 2007;62:938-949.

Funaki B. Microcatheter embolization of lower gastrointestinal hemorrhage: an old idea whose time has come. Cardiovasc Intervent Radiol 2004;27:591-599.

Howarth DM. The role of nuclear medicine in the detection of acute gastrointestinal bleeding. Semin Nucl Med 2006;36:133-146.

Laing CJ, Tobias T, Rosenblum DI, et al. Acute gastrointestinal bleeding: emerging role of multidetector CT angiography and review of current imaging techniques. RadioGraphics 2007;27:1055-1070.

REFERENCES

1. Abraldes JG, Bosch J. The treatment of acute variceal bleeding. J Clin Gastroenterol 2007; 41(10 Suppl 3):S312-S317.
2. Anthony T, Penta P, Todd RD, et al. Rebleeding and survival after acute lower gastrointestinal bleeding. Am J Surg 2004; 188:485-490.
3. Swain CP, Storey DW, Bown SG, et al. Nature of the bleeding vessel in recurrently bleeding gastric ulcers. Gastroenterology 1986; 90:595-608.
4. Knauer CM. Mallory-Weiss syndrome: characterization of 75 Mallory-Weiss lacerations in 528 patients with upper gastrointestinal hemorrhage. Gastroenterology 1976; 71:5-8.
5. Husová L, Lata J, Husa P, et al. Bacterial infection and acute bleeding from upper gastrointestinal tract in patients with liver cirrhosis. Hepatogastroenterology 2005; 52:1488-1490.
6. Meyers MA, Alonso DR, Gray GF, Baer JW. Pathogenesis of bleeding colonic diverticulosis. Gastroenterology 1976; 71:577-583.
7. Foutch PG. Colonic angiodysplasia. Gastroenterologist 1997; 5:148-156.
8. Tobin K, Klein J, Barbieri C, Heffner JE. Utility of routine admission chest radiographs in patients with acute gastrointestinal hemorrhage admitted to an intensive care unit. Am J Med 1996; 101:349-356.

9. Andrews AH, Lake JM, Shorr AF. Ineffectiveness of routine abdominal radiography in patients with gastrointestinal hemorrhage admitted to an intensive care unit. J Clin Gastroenterol 2005; 39:228-231.

10. Yoon W, Jeong YY, Shin SS, et al. Acute massive gastrointestinal bleeding: detection and localization with arterial phase multi-detector row helical CT. Radiology 2006; 239:160-167.

11. Laing CJ, Tobias T, Rosenblum DI, et al. Acute gastrointestinal bleeding: emerging role of multidetector CT angiography and review of current imaging techniques. RadioGraphics 2007; 27:1055-1070.

12. Scheffel H, Pfammatter T, Wildi S, et al. Acute gastrointestinal bleeding: detection of source and etiology with multi-detector-row CT. Eur Radiol 2007; 17:1555-1565.

13. Jaeckle T, Stuber G, Hoffmann MH, et al. Detection and localization of acute upper and lower gastrointestinal (GI) bleeding with arterial phase multi-detector row helical CT. Eur Radiol 2008; 18:1406-1413.

14. Howarth DM. The role of nuclear medicine in the detection of acute gastrointestinal bleeding. Semin Nucl Med 2006; 36:133-146.

15. Suzman MS, Talmor M, Jennis R, et al. Accurate localization and surgical management of active lower gastrointestinal hemorrhage with technetium-labeled erythrocyte scintigraphy. Ann Surg 1996; 224:29-36.

16. Green BT, Rockey DC. Lower gastrointestinal bleeding—management. Gastroenterol Clin North Am 2005; 34:665-678.

17. Kuo WT, Lee DE, Saad WE, et al. Superselective microcoil embolization for the treatment of lower gastrointestinal hemorrhage. J Vasc Interv Radiol 2003; 14:1503-1509.

18. Alavi A, Ring EJ. Localization of gastrointestinal bleeding: superiority of ^{99m}Tc sulfur colloid compared with angiography. AJR Am J Roentgenol 1981; 137:741-748.

19. Angelides S, Gibson MG, Kurtovic J, Riordan S. Abdominal wall hematomata and colonic tumor detected on labeled red blood cell scintigraphy: case report. Ann Nucl Med 2003; 17:399-402.

20. Lee CW, Liu KL, Wang HP, et al. Transcatheter arterial embolization of acute upper gastrointestinal tract bleeding with *N*-butyl-2-cyanoacrylate. J Vasc Interv Radiol 2007; 18:209-216.

21. Ramirez FC, Colon VJ, Landan D, et al. The effects of the number of rubber bands placed at each endoscopic session upon variceal outcomes: a prospective, randomized study. Am J Gastroenterol 2007; 102:1372-1376.

22. Olmos JA, Marcolongo M, Pogorelsky V, et al. Argon plasma coagulation for prevention of recurrent bleeding from GI angiodysplasias. Gastrointest Endosc 2004; 60:881-886.

Stomach

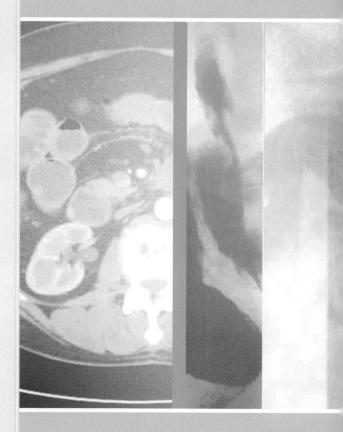

Stomach Imaging Techniques

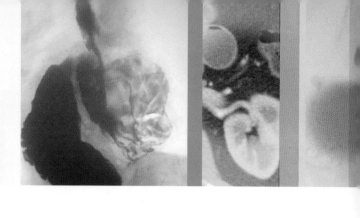

CHAPTER 30

Conventional Imaging of the Stomach and Duodenum

Sukanya Ghosh, Sujit Vaidya, and Niall Power

TECHNICAL ASPECTS

The development of fiberoptic endoscopy has provided an accurate tool to assess the upper gastrointestinal tract. Endoscopic experience has shown that the majority of small lesions and even a disturbing number of large lesions can be missed on conventional barium studies.

Conventional barium studies can be used as first-line noninvasive diagnostic studies in patients with dyspepsia, weight loss, anemia, an upper abdominal mass, unexplained gastrointestinal hemorrhage, and partial obstruction.

The most common radiologic investigation of the stomach and duodenum is the barium meal. The barium meal examination typically comprises four components: double contrast, compression, mucosal relief, and barium filling.[1]

The Double-Contrast Examination

The barium meal is a double-contrast study that demonstrates good anatomic and mucosal detail, provided that there is adequate distention, mucosal coating with a contrast agent, and use of the proper projection.

Technique

The patient is given Carbex granules (sodium bicarbonate/dimethicone), a gas-producing agent, to swallow and then drinks the E-Z HD 250% w/v 60 mL barium. Spot views of the esophagus are taken at the beginning (anteroposterior and right anterior oblique positions) while barium is being swallowed (if clinically indicated), and then the patient is asked to lie down on the left side (thus preventing the barium reaching the distal duodenum too quickly and obscuring views of the greater curvature and antrum of the stomach). A gastroparetic agent such as Glucagon or Buscopan may be employed to delay filling

of the small bowel during the study. The patient then is asked to lie slightly on the right so that the barium is against the gastroesophageal junction to check for reflux while screening. If reflux is not elicited, then the patient may be asked to cough, swallow water, or tip the head down while being observed fluoroscopically and spot films are taken. Then the following maneuvers are performed quickly so that the barium does not enter the duodenum and gas is maintained within the stomach. The patient is turned to the right side and then quickly prone, to the left, and supine again, finishing in a right anterior oblique position (completing a circle). This is repeated until a good coating of the stomach is achieved by the barium, which is evident when the areae gastricae in the antrum are seen.[2]

Stomach Views

- Antrum and greater curvature—right anterior oblique (Fig. 30-1)
- Body and antrum—supine (Fig. 30-2)
- Lesser curvature en face—left anterior oblique (Fig. 30-3)
- Left lateral with head tilted up at 45 degrees

Throughout this procedure it is vital to ensure the barium does not flood into the duodenum, and thus the patient is asked to roll onto the left side as soon as the fundus view has been taken.

Duodenum Views

- Duodenal loop—the patient lies prone on the compression pad to prevent barium flooding into the duodenum (additional views of the anterior wall of the duodenal loop can be taken in the right anterior oblique position).
- Duodenal cap—the following spot views can help: prone, right anterior oblique, supine, and left anterior

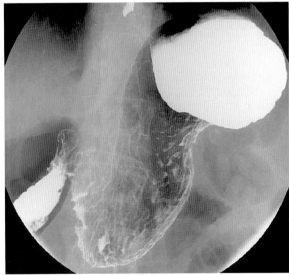

■ **FIGURE 30-1**   Right anterior oblique view.

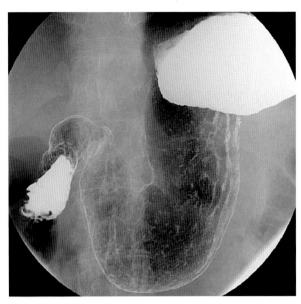

■ **FIGURE 30-2**   Supine view.

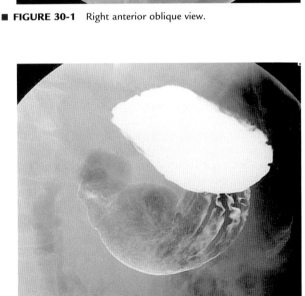

■ **FIGURE 30-3**   Left anterior oblique view.

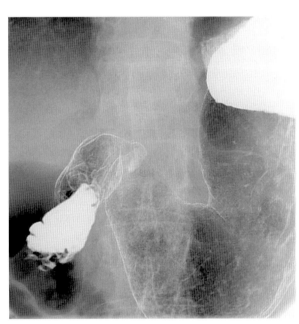

■ **FIGURE 30-4**   Duodenal view.

oblique (occasionally tilting the head up and allowing the air bubble to rise into the coated duodenal cap) (Fig. 30-4). The appearance of the duodenum varies according to the patient's body habitus, and the gallbladder often indents the duodenal cap.

Erect views of the fundus can be taken at the end of the study.

Single-Contrast Examination

A single-contrast examination can emphasize mucosal relief, compression, and barium filling. This includes spot views of the barium-filled stomach with the patient recumbent: prone, left posterior oblique, right lateral, and right anterior oblique. *Mucosal relief* radiographs are per-

formed by giving the patient 60 to 90 mL of barium to drink, and then prone and supine spot views are taken to correctly demonstrate the gastric fold pattern. The anterior gastric wall is better seen on the single-contrast study than the double-contrast examination. *Compression views* require compression of the stomach, which is moderately distended with a small amount of barium to spread on the rugal folds. Overdistention makes it impossible to penetrate the barium radiographically, and the amount of barium used can be controlled by patient rotation or tilting the table. The views seen vary according to patient body habitus, and compression can only be performed below the rib cage; hence, often only the distal stomach can be identified. The compression view often demonstrates ulcers and masses, although small flat lesions can be missed and wall rigidity may occur from scarring or infiltration.

PROS AND CONS

The double-contrast technique provides excellent detail of the stomach mucosa, allowing identification of ulceration and decreasing the use of invasive endoscopy. The shallow barium pool fills small ulcerations and allows small protrusions to appear as filling defects.[3] Detail is usually maximal at the distal stomach, and anterior wall lesions are difficult to identify, necessitating compression and mucosal relief imaging. Shallow ulcers, otherwise known as gastric erosions, do not penetrate the muscularis mucosa; thus the best modality to identify these is the double-contrast barium meal.

The double-contrast examination of the stomach was perfected in Japan to diagnose early gastric cancer,[4] thus permitting curative management not only by surgical[5,6] but also by endoscopic mucosal resection or minimally invasive laparoscopic gastrectomy.[7,8] In Japan, the mass screening by barium meal examination has significant survival benefits at an acceptable financial cost.[9]

Because of the interest in surface detail, the radiographic exposures in a double-contrast study are considerably lighter and can be exposed at a lower kilovoltage than a single-contrast study. The exposures are shorter, and there is less scatter.[10]

CONTROVERSIES

The technical quality of a double-contrast study is highly dependent on the skill and commitment of the radiologist and on the quality of the materials. With the emergence of endoscopy and multidetector CT, the "art" of producing a high-quality double-contrast study is slowly diminishing.

NORMAL ANATOMY

The stomach is the widest part of the gastrointestinal tract and can vary in size and shape depending on body habitus. It lies in the left upper abdomen just below the dome of the diaphragm. When fully distended it forms a "J"-shaped configuration and is divided into cardia, fundus, body, pyloric antrum, and pylorus (Fig. 30-5). Proximally the stomach is attached to the distal gastroesophageal junction (which is technically below the hemidiaphragm), and distally the gastric outlet is continuous with the duodenum via the pylorus. This muscular cavity is fixed at the two ends as described, and the remainder is quite mobile, allowing a maximum capacity of approximately 1500 mL.

The stomach has two surfaces: anterosuperior and posteroinferior, bounded by two borders, the lesser and greater curvatures, respectively. This hollow organ is completely covered by peritoneum, which passes as a double layer from the lesser curve (as the lesser omentum) and from the greater curve (as the greater omentum).[11] The stomach is composed of four layers: the outer serosa layer, muscularis externa, submucosa, and mucosa. The outer serosal layer consists of layers of connective tissue continuous with the peritoneum. The muscularis externa con-

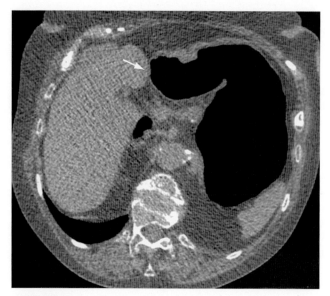

■ **FIGURE 30-5** CT with air contrast within the stomach demonstrating the axial configuration (*arrow*).

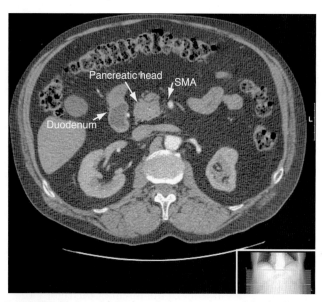

■ **FIGURE 30-6** Axial CT through the second part of the duodenum. SMA, superior mesenteric artery.

sists of three layers: the inner oblique layer (thicker at the antrum to perform forceful contractions); a middle circular layer that is thickest at the pylorus, forming a pyloric sphincter; and an outer longitudinal layer. The stomach is lined by columnar cells (for acid protection), unlike the esophagus, which is lined with squamous cells.

The duodenum has a "C"-shaped configuration and is divided into four parts. The first (superior) portion extends from the pylorus to the neck of the gallbladder and consists primarily of the duodenal bulb. The second part (Fig. 30-6) lies to the right of the second/third lumbar vertebrae, running inferiorly lateral to the head of the pancreas and medial to the hilum of the right kidney. Posteromedially at the junction of the upper two thirds and the lower third of the duodenum lies the opening of the duodenal papilla or ampulla of Vater (opening of the bile and pancreatic ducts).

The third part runs from right to left below the lower margin of the head of the pancreas, whereas the fourth portion is 4 cm and runs craniad and lies medial to the left psoas muscle, fixed by the ligament of Treitz (a peritoneal fold that ascends to the right crus of the diaphragm). This is an important landmark when distinguishing malrotation of the small intestine in children. The first part of the duodenum is the only part that is intraperitoneal, whereas the rest are retroperitoneal structures, again an important point for localizing a pathologic process.

The mucous membrane of the first part of the duodenum is smooth, whereas the remainder of the small bowel and duodenum is broken up into plicae circulares or valvulae conniventes, which are circular folds that encircle two thirds of the inner mucosal wall.

Anatomic Relationships of the Stomach and Duodenum

The anterior surface of the stomach lies in contact with the left dome of the diaphragm, the anterior abdominal wall, and the caudate lobe of the liver. The remainder of the stomach is situated posteriorly and collectively known as the "stomach bed." This relates to the diaphragm, the left adrenal gland, the upper pole of the left kidney, the splenic artery, the pancreas, the transverse mesocolon, and sometimes the transverse colon.

The first part of the duodenum is the only intraperitoneal part of the duodenum and is important in localizing a pathologic process. Anteriorly, there is the caudate lobe of the liver and the gallbladder. The lesser sac when seen posteriorly is related to the gallbladder. The gastroduodenal artery (from the hepatic artery) runs inferiorly behind the first part of the duodenum, whereas the bile duct often runs posteriorly, opening at the ampulla of Vater. The portal vein, formed by the splenic and the superior mesenteric veins, runs above the duodenum. The inferior vena cava lies posteriorly, whereas the pancreatic head lies inferiorly.

The second part of the duodenum (see Fig. 30-6) is 8 cm long. It lies in front of the hilum of the right kidney and to the right of the second and third lumbar vertebral bodies. The ampulla of Vater opens posteromedially, draining the biliary and pancreatic ducts. There may also be an additional accessory duct from the pancreas that opens proximally. Anteriorly lies the fundus of the gallbladder, the right lobe of the liver, and small bowel intestinal loops. Posteriorly, the hilum of the right kidney and the ureter are seen. Laterally, the ascending colon, hepatic flexure, and the right lobe of the liver are noted. The head of the pancreas is seen medially; and if there is an inflammatory process (e.g., pancreatitis) or neoplastic lesion (e.g., a large head of pancreas tumor), the second part of the duodenum and the ampulla of Vater are often involved. Consequently, the common bile duct and the pancreatic duct are dilated and seen as secondary signs on CT.

The third part of the duodenum (Fig. 30-7) is also approximately 8 cm long, running from the patient's right to left and curving forward over the psoas muscle, inferior vena cava, and aorta but following the lower margin of

the body of the pancreas. Running obliquely along the third part of the duodenum are the superior mesenteric vein and artery. Posteriorly from right to left are the ureter and right psoas muscle, inferior vena cava, and the aorta.

The fourth part of the duodenum ascends craniad by 4 cm, lying medially to the left psoas muscle, the left gonadal and renal vessels, and the inferior mesenteric vein. Anteriorly it is covered by jejunal loops and the beginning of the mesentery of the small bowel loops.

Blood Supply

Arterial Supply to the Stomach

Multiple branches from the celiac trunk supply the stomach and extensively interconnect with each other. The celiac trunk (Fig. 30-8) divides into left gastric, hepatic, and splenic arteries. The hepatic artery gives rise

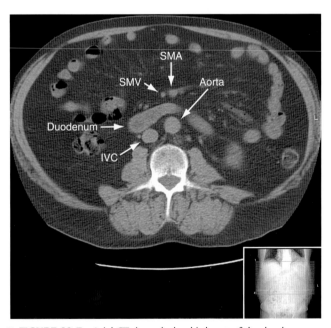

■ **FIGURE 30-7** Axial CT through the third part of the duodenum. SMV, superior mesenteric vein; SMA, superior mesenteric artery; IVC, inferior vena cava.

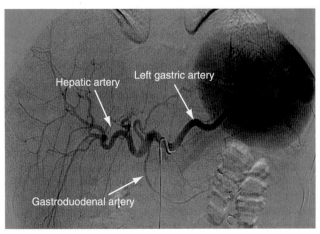

■ **FIGURE 30-8** Celiac axis.

to the right gastric and the gastroduodenal arteries. The gastroduodenal artery, in turn, branches to form the right gastroepiploic artery. The lesser curve is supplied superiorly by the left gastric artery and inferiorly by the right gastric artery (branch of hepatic artery). The right gastric artery arises above the first part of the duodenum and runs to the left within the lesser omentum anastomosing with the left gastric artery. The right gastroepiploic artery (branch of gastroduodenal artery from the hepatic artery) supplies the inferior part of the greater curvature, whereas the left gastroepiploic artery (branch of the splenic artery) supplies the superior portion. The fundus is supplied by the short gastric arteries. Several gastric branches pass to the greater curvature from the splenic artery via the gastrosplenic ligament.

Venous Drainage of the Stomach

The veins of the stomach follow the gastric arteries, draining into the portal venous system. The portal vein receives the right and left gastric veins, whereas the short gastric and the left gastroepiploic veins drain into the splenic vein. Meanwhile, the right gastroepiploic vein drains into the superior mesenteric vein. This is an important point because it demonstrates why gastric varices (seen with portal hypertension) are formed if there is resistance to the portal venous flow.

Lymphatic Drainage of the Stomach

The lymphatic drainage follows the arteries supplying the stomach. All the gastric lymphatic vessels eventually drain into the celiac lymph nodes surrounding the origin of the celiac artery.

Arterial Supply of the Duodenum

The duodenum is essentially supplied by two arteries: the gastroduodenal artery and the pancreaticoduodenal artery. The hepatic artery descends behind the first part of the duodenum and divides into right gastroepiploic and the superior pancreaticoduodenal branches. The superior pancreaticoduodenal artery supplies the proximal first and second part of the duodenum up to the major duodenal ampulla, and the remainder of the duodenum is supplied by the inferior pancreaticoduodenal artery, a branch of the superior mesenteric artery.

Venous Drainage of the Duodenum

Venous drainage follows the arteries draining into the portal system, either directly or indirectly through the splenic or superior mesenteric vein.

Lymphatic Drainage of the Duodenum

Lymphatic drainage follows the arterial supply. The proximal duodenum is drained via the pancreaticoduodenal nodes to the gastroduodenal nodes and thus to the celiac nodes. The remainder of the duodenum drains into the pancreaticoduodenal nodes to the superior mesenteric nodes just at the origin of the superior mesenteric artery.

PATTERNS AND APPEARANCES ON BARIUM STUDIES
Gastric Ulcers

The detection of gastric ulcers and the decision regarding whether these represent benign or malignant processes are a major part of the barium meal study.

Helicobacter is a gram-negative bacteria that is recognized as an important cause of 70% of peptic ulcer disease and 95% of duodenal ulcers in the United States.[12] Patients infected with *H. pylori* have a six times risk of developing gastric carcinoma and a 90% association with mucosal-associated lymphoid tissue (MALT). Other causes of infectious gastritis include tuberculosis, histoplasmosis, and syphilis.

Ulcers are best identified on double-contrast studies. Often they are common on the posterior wall of the stomach and least common on the fundus.[12] Ulcers secondary to nonsteroidal anti-inflammatory drugs and alcohol are often seen on the greater curvature of the antrum, possibly owing to the direct toxic effects.[13]

The en face radiologic signs of gastric ulcers are best seen on double-contrast studies. Primarily, the signs include pooling of barium within the ulcer crater (on the dependent wall). A thin radiolucent line is often seen separating the barium in the lumen from that in the crater and is referred to as Hampton's line. If the ulcer is on the nondependent wall, the barium coats the "rim," causing a ring-like effect. The patient can be turned prone or supine to fill the middle part of the crater. Often a small mound of edema is seen surrounding the crater causing a circular filling defect. The folds radiating from this should be smooth and symmetric with normal areae gastricae, suggesting benignity. Classically, benign ulcers are seen on the lesser curvature (Fig. 30-9). Giant ulcers (>3 cm) are virtually almost always benign. A healed ulcer is identified when folds converge to the site of the ulcer, whereas incomplete healing, irregularity of the folds, residual mass, or loss of mucosal pattern suggests malignancy.

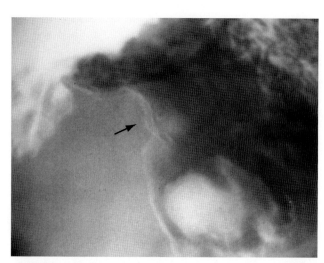

■ **FIGURE 30-9** Note the irregular edge of a benign gastric ulcer on the lesser curvature (*arrow*).

Carman's meniscus sign is diagnostic of a specific type of ulcerated neoplasm. When examined in profile with compression, the ulcer has a semicircular (meniscoid) configuration. The combination of this characteristic type of barium-filled ulcer and a radiolucent shadow of the elevated ridge of neoplastic tissue surrounding it is called the Carman-Kirklin complex. The inner margin of the barium trapped in the ulcer is usually irregular. It is always convex toward the lumen, in contrast to the "crescent sign" of a benign gastric ulcer in which the inner margin is concave toward the lumen.[14]

An abrupt transition between the normal mucosa and the abnormal tissue surrounding a gastric ulcer is characteristic of a neoplastic lesion, in contrast to the diffuse, almost imperceptible transition between the mound of edema surrounding a benign ulcer and normal gastric mucosa. Nodularity, clubbing, and amputation of normal radiating folds also suggest a malignant lesion.

Superficial Gastric Erosions

These are defects in the epithelium of the stomach that do not penetrate beyond the muscularis mucosa. They are hard to demonstrate on radiographic examinations. The classic radiographic appearance is a tiny fleck of barium surrounded by a radiolucent halo.

Duodenal Ulcers

Duodenal ulcers also can be identified by double-contrast studies, and sometimes complications are seen, for example, formation of a fistula with the biliary tree (Fig. 30-10).

Narrowing of the Stomach (Linitis Plastica Pattern)

A linitis plastica pattern refers to any condition in which marked thickening of the gastric wall causes the stomach to resemble a rigid tube. The most common cause is scirrhous carcinoma of the stomach (Fig. 30-11). The tumor invades the gastric wall, resulting in a desmoplastic reaction that leads to diffuse thickening and fixation of the stomach wall. At fluoroscopy, peristalsis does not pass through the tumor site.

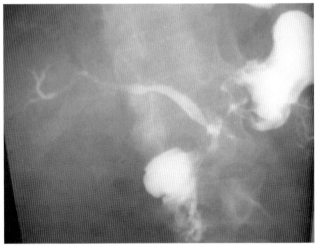

■ **FIGURE 30-10**   Note that the biliary tree is opacified, suggesting fistulation with a duodenal ulcer.

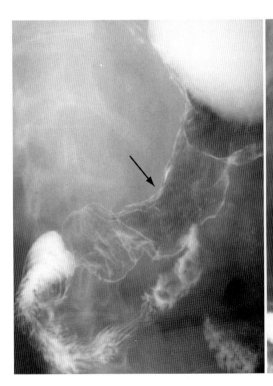
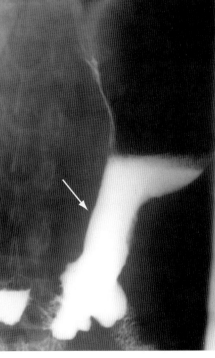

■ **FIGURE 30-11**   Linitis plastica pattern. Note the marked narrowing of the body and antrum of the stomach due to lymphatic infiltration (*arrows*).

Other lesions that can mimic this appearance are lymphoma, Kaposi's sarcoma, and metastases. Sometimes benign causes such as ulcer disease, Crohn's disease, sarcoidosis, and tuberculosis can also cause these appearances.

Filling Defects in the Stomach

Areae gastricae are normal anatomic features of the gastric mucosa. On a double-contrast study they are seen as a fine reticular pattern surrounded by barium-filled grooves. This appearance simulates multiple filling defects.

Hyperplastic polyps are the most common causes of discrete filling defects in the stomach, accounting for up to 90% of all gastric polyps. Most hyperplastic polyps appear as sharply defined, round or oval filling defects measuring less than 1 cm. They have smooth contours and no evidence of contrast material within them. They tend to be multiple and are clustered in the fundus or body of the stomach.

An adenomatous polyp is a true neoplasm and shows a definite tendency to malignant transformation. It is therefore vital to identify it. Characteristic features include size greater than 1 cm, lobulated or pedunculated shape, and a variation in size over time.

Other lesions that can present as filling defects include lymphoma, carcinoid tumor, and metastases.

Thickening of Gastric Folds

Longitudinal folds traverse the stomach in the direction of its long axis. Folds in the fundus are thicker and more tortuous than distally. Folds in the antrum measuring more than 5 mm are considered abnormal. These folds may appear prominent in a nondistended stomach.

Extrinsic Lesions

Lesions outside the gastric walls could indent on the stomach and cause extrinsic impressions or apparent filling defects. Cysts arising from the kidney, spleen, and pancreas can produce these appearances.

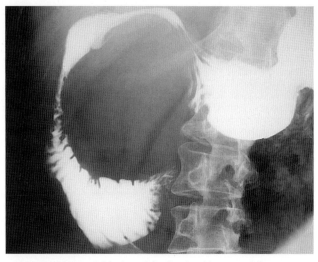

■ **FIGURE 30-12** Widening of the duodenal loop secondary to a large pancreatic head tumor.

Widening of the Duodenal "C" Loop

Although this finding is often taken to represent a pancreatic malignancy, benign conditions such as pseudocyst may also cause such an appearance. It is advisable to resort to cross-sectional imaging to resolve this diagnostic issue (Fig. 30-12).

KEY POINTS

■ Endoscopy is the gold standard in evaluating the upper gastrointestinal tract, and the role of the barium examination is diminishing.

■ A double-contrast study can help detect ulcers and characterize them.

■ A malignant ulcer does not protrude beyond the gastric outline, demonstrates the "meniscus sign," and shows focal nodularity and distortion of adjacent areae gastricae with amputated folds.

■ On barium studies, other important findings such as linitis plastica, filling defects, and thickening of the folds could point to disease.

SUGGESTED READINGS

Eisenberg RL. Clinical Imaging: An Atlas of Differential Diagnosis, 4th ed. Philadelphia, Lippincott Williams and Wilkins, 2002.

Grainger RG, Allison D, Adam D, et al (eds). Grainger and Allison's Diagnostic Radiology: A Textbook of Medical Imaging, 4th ed. New York, Churchill Livingstone, 2001.

REFERENCES

1. Stevenson GW, Somers S, Virjee J. Routine double-contrast barium meal: appearance of normal duodenal papillae. Diagn Imaging 1980; 49:6-14.
2. Chapman S, Nakielny R. A Guide to Radiological Procedures, 4th ed. London, Saunders, 2001, pp 57-59.
3. Megibow AJ. Duodenum. In Megibow AJ (ed). Computed Tomography of the Gastrointestinal Tract. St. Louis, Mosby, 1986, pp 175-216.
4. Tominaga S. Cancer mortality and morbidity statistics: Japan and the world—1994. Gann Monog Cancer Res 1994; 41:175-177.
5. Arai J, Yamada H, Maruyama M. Initial radiographic findings of early gastric cancer detected in health check programs and human "dry dock" (multiphasic screening) collective health checks and treated by endoscopic mucosal resection. Gastric Cancer 2002; 5:35-42.

6. Kondo H, Gotoda T, Ono H, et al. Percutaneous traction-assisted EMR by using an insulation-tipped electrosurgical knife for early stage gastric cancer. Gastrointest Endosc 2004; 59:284-288.

7. Kitano S, Shiraishi N, Kakisako K, et al. Laparoscopy-assisted Billroth-I gastrectomy (LADG) for cancer: our 10 years' experience. Surg Laparosc Endosc Percutan Tech 2002; 12:204-207.

8. Kitano S, Shiraishi N. Current status of laparoscopic gastrectomy for cancer in Japan. Surg Endosc 2004; 18:182-185.

9. Kunisaki C, Ishino J, Nakajima S, et al. Outcomes of mass screening for gastric carcinoma. Ann Surg Oncol 2006; 13:221-228.

10. Laufer I. Double Contrast Gastrointestinal Radiology with Endoscopic Correlation. Philadelphia, Saunders 1979, pp 1-8.

11. Robbins SE, Virjee J. The gastrointestinal tract. In Butler P, Mitchell AWM, Ellis H. Applied Radiological Anatomy. Cambridge University Press, 1999, pp 211-214.

12. Nolan DJ. The duodenum. In Grainger RG, Allison D, Adam D, et al (eds). Grainger and Allison's Diagnostic Radiology: A Textbook of Medical Imaging. 4th ed. New York, Churchill Livingstone, 2001, pp 1063-1073.

13. Kottler RE, Tuft RJ. Benign greater curve gastric ulcer: the sump-ulcer. Br J Radiol 1981; 54:651-654.

14. Eisenberg RL. Clinical Imaging: An Atlas of Differential Diagnosis, 4th ed. Philadelphia, Lippincott Williams and Wilkins, 2003, p. 326.

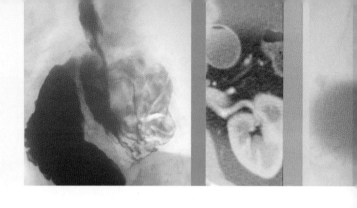

CHAPTER

31

CT of the Stomach and Duodenum

Sukanya Ghosh, Niall Power, and Sujit Vaidya

TECHNICAL ASPECTS

Endoscopy is usually the first test performed to assess symptoms or signs referable to the stomach or duodenum because it allows direct visualization of the mucosa and biopsy if indicated. If this is not well tolerated, an upper gastrointestinal study with barium contrast is a second-line investigation. CT is usually reserved to further investigate abnormal findings after either of these tests or for evaluation of vague symptoms such as anemia, abdominal pain, or weight loss. To optimize assessment of the stomach and duodenum with CT, it is essential that both organs be optimally distended. This is usually accomplished by having the patient drink 800 to 1000 mL of water in the 15 to 20 minutes before the procedure. Water is preferred to positive oral contrast material because it does not obscure subtle gastric or duodenal wall enhancement. Optimal distention can also be facilitated by the intravenous administration of a smooth muscle relaxant, typically 1 mg of hyoscine butylbromide (Buscopan), immediately before the procedure, although this product is not licensed for use in the United States. Assessment of wall thickness of a collapsed stomach or duodenum may be unreliable, but if the organs are well distended any wall thickness of more than 5 mm should be regarded with suspicion and attention paid to the nature of wall thickening, be it focal, diffuse, or circumferential, the degree of enhancement, any evidence of abnormality in the surrounding fat, and any local lymphadenopathy. Scans are typically obtained in the portovenous phase after intravenous administration of a contrast agent (at 60 to 70 seconds). At our institution raw data are reconstructed at 1.5- and 5-mm intervals with 1.5-mm coronal reformatted images routinely generated. Further generation of multiplanar reconstructed or 3D volume-rendered images is at the discretion of the radiologist. *Virtual gastroscopy* is a term used to describe 3D multidetector CT images of the gastric mucosa, simulating the type of views obtained at endoscopy, following the administration of gas-forming granules orally and intravenous contrast media. It is gaining in popularity in parts of the world such as Japan where gastric cancer is common as a means of detecting early cancerous lesions. Provided gastric and duodenal distention is optimized, multidetector CT can be a very useful tool in the evaluation of a range of benign and malignant conditions.

CT OF THE STOMACH

Inflammatory Disease

Helicobacter pylori is a gram-negative bacteria that is recognized as an important cause of 70% of peptic ulcer disease and 95% of duodenal ulcers in the United States.[1] Patients infected with *H. pylori* have a six times risk of developing gastric carcinoma and a 90% association with mucosa-associated lymphoid tissue (MALT). Other causes of infectious gastritis include tuberculosis, histoplasmosis, and syphilis. Organisms that can affect the stomach in immunocompromised patients include cytomegalovirus, *Cryptosporidium,* and *Toxoplasma.* CT findings are nonspecific and may include complications of deep ulcerations, including fistulization.

Gastric Ulcer

A gastric ulcer is a very common cause of upper gastrointestinal tract symptoms and is amenable to reliable radiologic detection. An upper gastrointestinal study with barium contrast is a reliable, noninvasive investigation used to identify ulcers and early mucosal lesions in the stomach.[2]

CT findings of gastritis include the following[3]:

- Thickened gastric folds
- Focal wall thickening, particularly at the antrum
- A three-layered wall appearance that may enhance during the arterial phase due to hyperemia. Maintenance of normal wall layering may distinguish benign and malignant conditions.

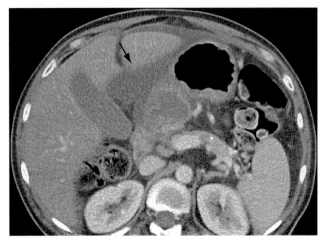

■ **FIGURE 31-1** On this CT image note the secondary sign of periantral fluid (*arrow*) most likely secondary to the perforated peptic ulcer.

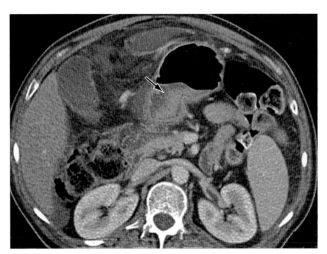

■ **FIGURE 31-2** Axial CT slice through the gastric antrum with high density within it (*arrow*) demonstrating active extravasation of blood from a peptic ulcer.

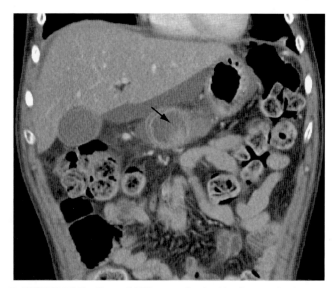

■ **FIGURE 31-3** Coronal CT image of active bleeding peptic ulcer (*arrow*).

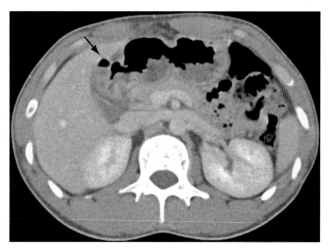

■ **FIGURE 31-4** The small locule of air (*arrow*) is a secondary CT sign of perforated peptic ulcer.

● Life-threatening emphysematous gastritis, which, although rare, is characterized by air within the stomach wall secondary to invasion by gas-producing organisms (*Escherichia coli*) through the gastric wall

A gastric ulcer may be suggested on CT by the presence of a focal area of wall thickening with an associated defect in the mucosa. Edema of the submucosa may also be seen. Although the sensitivity of CT for detecting gastritis and ulceration is less than that of the upper gastrointestinal study with barium contrast, it is excellent at identifying complications such as bleeding or perforation due to gastric antral or duodenal ulcers. CT signs of perforation include tiny locules of fluid (Figs. 31-1 to 31-3) and/or air (Fig. 31-4) around the organ concerned. Giant gastric ulcers are almost always greater than 3 cm and benign but have a higher rate of complications.

Generalized Gastric Wall Thickening

Thickening of the stomach including the gastroesophageal junction is often difficult to interpret. It is an important but not a specific sign. On CT, the gastric wall can appear "thickened" because the mucosal folds are collapsed. It gives the appearance of "pseudo thickening," which can often be mistaken for tumor infiltration.

Pseudotumor at the gastroesophageal junction in patients with hiatal hernia or apparent thickening due to underdistention of the stomach needs to be excluded. It is essential to ensure aggressive distention of the stomach and gastroesophageal junction with water or air as a contrast agent.

Focal or diffuse thickening of the gastric wall (with adequate distention of the stomach) that exceeds 5 mm suggests the following differential diagnosis: carcinoma, lymphoma, gastric inflammation (peptic ulcer/Crohn's disease), perigastric inflammation (e.g., pancreatitis), and radiation.[4-6]

Gastric wall thickening is commonly focal and in the antrum. Often, the mucosal wall may enhance avidly during the arterial phase of scanning due to hyperemia, causing a "three-layered wall appearance" suggesting possible malignant change. It may help to identify secondary

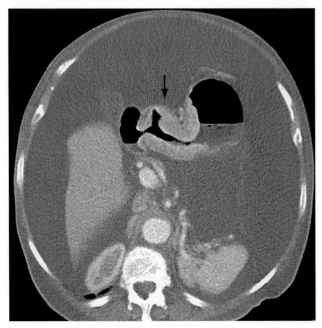

■ **FIGURE 31-5** On this CT image note the diffuse fibrotic thickening of the gastric antrum causing luminal narrowing (*arrow*).

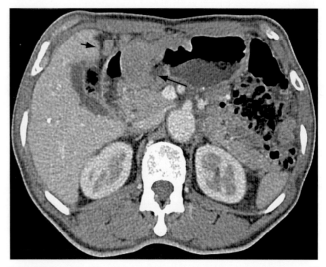

■ **FIGURE 31-6** The gross antral thickening greater than 1 cm on this CT image suggests malignancy (*long arrow*). There also is a small periantral node (*short arrow*).

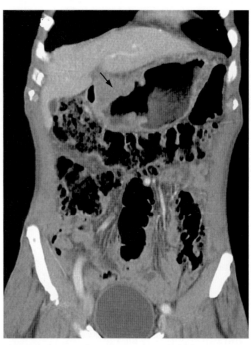

■ **FIGURE 31-7** Coronal CT image of antral thickening suggesting malignancy (*arrow*).

signs such as stranding at the gastroesophageal junction or around the stomach, celiac axis lymphadenopathy, and metastasis to other organs such as the liver.

Neoplasms

CT can be used to determine whether a lesion is likely to be malignant or benign and whether further follow-up/ investigation is necessary.

Primary Malignant Neoplasms

The highest prevalence of gastric cancer is seen in Japan and thus a lot of work has been performed there for early gastric cancer screening. Ninety-five percent of gastric carcinoma is adenocarcinoma.[7] The remainder includes lymphoma, sarcoma (malignant gastrointestinal stromal tumors [GISTs]), carcinoid, and metastasis. Most early gastric carcinomas manifest on CT as focal, nodular, or irregular segmental thickening of the gastric wall or as a polypoid intraluminal mass. Diffuse thickening with narrowing of the lumen suggests appearances of "scirrhous carcinoma" (linitis plastica) (Fig. 31-5). It has been proven that in a well-distended stomach, a wall thickness of more than 1 cm that is focal, eccentric, and enhancing after intravenous administration of a contrast agent has a sensitivity of 100% and a specificity of 98% in detecting a malignant or potentially malignant lesion, warranting further investigation by upper gastrointestinal study with barium contrast or endoscopy.[8] Perigastric fat involvement is nearly always present when the wall thickness is more than 2 cm. Blurring of the serosal surfaces, fat stranding, and peritoneal deposits are often seen. Perigastric lymph nodes with the short-axis diameter greater than 6 mm, particularly near the tumor and the celiac axis or gastrohepatic ligament, are suggestive of malignant infiltration (Figs. 31-6 and 31-7). Nodal involvement is likely if the nodes are heterogeneous or enhance markedly after administration of a contrast agent.

Advanced tumors frequently present as large, irregular masses that may ulcerate (Fig. 31-8). There may be transgastric spread, occasionally with direct invasion of adjacent structures (namely, liver, spleen, pancreas, transverse colon); hematogenous spread to liver, lung, adrenal glands, kidneys, bones and brain; or diffuse intraperitoneal spread.

The following CT features are therefore important if resection is considered:

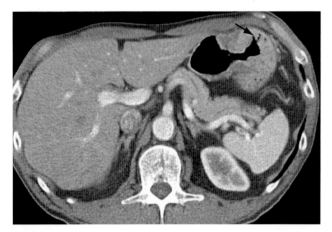

■ FIGURE 31-8 Note the gastric wall thickening with thin linear pocket of air suggesting possible ulceration (*arrow*) on this CT image.

TABLE 31-1	TNM Classification for Staging of Gastric Cancer

T1	Tumor limited to mucosa/submucosa
T2	Tumor involves serosa
T3	Tumor penetrates through serosa
T4a	Invasion of adjacent contiguous tissues
T4b	Invasion of adjacent contiguous organs, diaphragm, abdominal wall
N1	Perigastric nodes within 3 cm along lesser/greater curvature
N2	Regional nodes >3 cm along celiac axis
N3	Para-aortic, hepatoduodenal, retropancreatic, mesenteric nodal involvement
M0	No other organ involvement
M1	Distant metastasis

- Site and size of tumor
- Involvement of serosa
- Lymph node spread
- Metastasis

Staging of Gastric Cancer

Most centers perform staging using CT, although endoscopic ultrasonography is also used, primarily for evaluating depth of gastric wall invasion. The TNM (tumor, node, metastasis) staging classification of gastric cancer is shown in Table 31-1.

Local recurrence of gastric carcinoma appears as focal gastric wall thickening at the anastomotic site or remnant stomach. Recurrence presenting as nodal disease often involves nodes along the hepatic artery or in the para-aortic region.

Gastric Lymphoma

The most frequent site of lymphoma in the gastrointestinal tract is the stomach (Fig. 31-9),[9] and 90% to 95% are non-Hodgkin's lymphoma. Gastric lymphoma can present as diffuse wall infiltration that involves at least 50% of the length of the stomach, as segmental focal or nodular thickened folds, or as a polypoid mass associated with an ulcer.

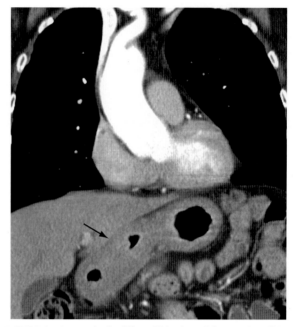

■ FIGURE 31-9 Markedly diffuse thickening of the gastric wall is seen on this CT image of a patient with lymphoma (*arrow*).

Additionally, widespread lymphadenopathy may be present. The CT features that favor a diagnosis of lymphoma rather than carcinoma include marked gastric wall thickening, often more than 4- to 5-cm, bulkier nodes that may extend below the renal hilum, and involvement of more than one region of the gastrointestinal tract.[10] Whereas carcinoma typically causes luminal narrowing, in lymphoma the lumen is preserved and may be dilated.

The differentiating features of lymphoma from adenocarcinoma are summarized in Table 31-2.

Other Tumors

Submucosal Lesions

Gastrointestinal Stromal Tumors

Gastrointestinal stromal tumors are the most common nonepithelial tumors of the gastrointestinal tract, with an estimated incidence of 4500 to 6000 per year in the United States.[11] Sixty to 70 percent arise in the stomach (Fig. 31-10) from the interstitial cells of Cajal and lack the features of smooth muscle or Schwann cells and thus are entirely different from leiomyomas, leiomyosarcoma, and leiomyoblastomas. They characteristically express tyrosine kinase, which is the rationale behind the use of imatinib, a new molecularly targeted tyrosine kinase receptor blocker that can result in a dramatic response and markedly improved long-term survival in patients with GISTs. However, for localized primary GISTs, surgical therapy is the mainstay of therapy. Thus, it is vital to detect and differentiate these tumors from other types and be able to monitor the treatment and tumor progression, for which CT is the imaging modality of choice.

GISTs smaller than 2 cm are usually benign with a very low rate of recurrence. Clinical features of GISTs depend

TABLE 31-2 Comparison of the Features of Adenocarcinoma and Lymphoma

Feature	Adenocarcinoma	Lymphoma
Wall thickness	Focal thickness, usually <2 cm	Usually >3-4 cm, homogeneously thick
Fat planes	Usually blurred	Preserved
Lymph node involvement	Peritumor; does not extend below renal vein, less bulky	Common, large, bulky, extensive and may extend below the renal hilum
Extent	May involve duodenum	Does not commonly involve duodenum
Metastasis	Direct invasion or hematogenous spread to liver, lung, spleen, and adrenals Intraperitoneal deposits	Discrete lymphomatous deposits can be seen in other organs, e.g., kidneys, spleen, and small bowel.

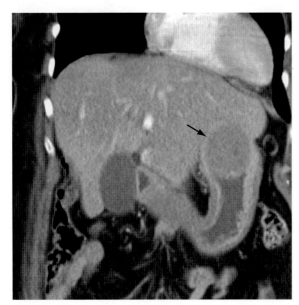

■ **FIGURE 31-10** CT image demonstrates localized GIST (*arrow*) in the fundus of the stomach.

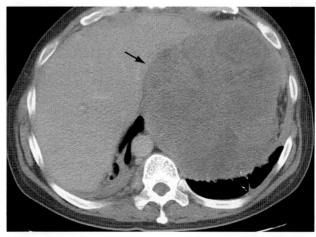

■ **FIGURE 31-11** This CT image shows a primary GIST of mixed attenuation (*arrow*) suggesting necrosis and hemorrhage.

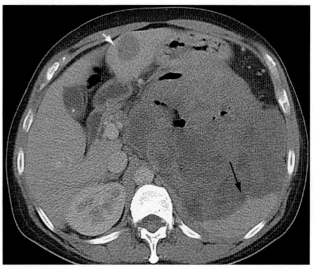

■ **FIGURE 31-12** An advanced GIST with invasion to adjacent organs such as the spleen (*long arrow*) and liver metastasis (*short arrow*) is shown on this CT scan.

on the size and aggressiveness of the tumor at the time of presentation. Small GISTs are typically intramural, polypoid, and localized lesions that are usually homogeneous, and may be an incidental finding on CT or endoscopy. Primary GISTs may be hypervascular with peripheral enhancement on contrast-enhanced CT images. Larger tumors are often heterogeneous because of necrosis, hemorrhage, or cystic degeneration (Fig. 31-11)[12,13] and may displace organs and vessels. Direct invasion of adjacent structures is rare and seen in advanced cases. The likelihood of malignancy increases in tumors that arise outside the stomach, if they are more than 5 cm with or without the presence of an ulcer, or if there is mesenteric fat infiltration, direct organ invasion, or metastasis (Fig. 31-12).[14] Often the tumor can ulcerate into the lumen of the gastrointestinal tract, and hence the most common presentation of symptomatic GIST is gastrointestinal bleeding.[13] Fifty percent of GISTs metastasize,[15] commonly by hematogenous spread, usually to the liver, or by peritoneal seeding. Lymph node metastasis is rare and more commonly seen with adenocarcinoma. Monitoring GISTs after treatment with imatinib is important and evaluated with decrease in tumor size, according to the RECIST (Response Evaluation Criteria In Solid Tumours) criteria. This may

take several months. After treatment a GIST may change from a hyperattenuating to a homogeneously hypoattenuating appearance with reduction in size of tumor bulk and a decrease in tumor vascularity. The reduction in attenuation may be secondary to myxoid degeneration and occasionally hemorrhage or necrosis and may be seen as early

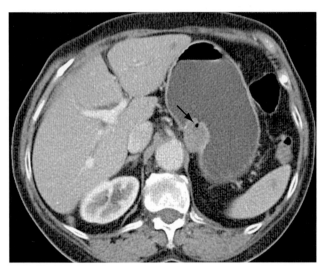

■ **FIGURE 31-13** CT image demonstrates a leiomyoma with a pocket of air (*arrow*), possibly representing superinfection or perforation.

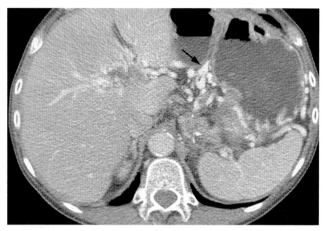

■ **FIGURE 31-14** This CT image shows a cluster of collateral vessels around the lesser curvature (*arrow*) and splenomegaly secondary to splenic vein thrombosis.

as 5 days after treatment or even earlier. Hence, use of the term *cystic degeneration* should be avoided in treated tumors.

Fluorodeoxyglucose (FDG)-labeled PET/CT is an alternative means of following up a GIST after treatment and is indicated when CT findings are inconclusive.

Leiomyosarcoma

Leiomyosarcoma is an uncommon tumor, accounting for 1% of gastric lesions. However, it is the second most common type of polypoid lesion in the stomach after hyperplastic polyps. It is a smooth muscle tumor arising from the muscularis propria, and growth is often exophytic and exogastric or dumbbell shaped. The tumor is usually larger than 5 cm at presentation. These lesions can be submucosal and thus often not seen by endoscopy. Therefore, CT is important to detect and characterize the mass and to evaluate spread. Leiomyosarcoma is often heterogeneous with areas of low attenuation suggestive of necrosis and with primarily exophytic growth.[16] Complications include ulceration (suggested by the presence of air within the lesion) and perforation. Another cause of air within the lesion may be superinfection of the necrotic tumor (Fig. 31-13). Leiomyosarcoma can invade adjacent organs directly (e.g., the left lobe of the liver, spleen, lesser sac, pancreas, and kidney) or metastasize hematogenously to the liver or lung.

Metastasis

The most common primary tumors metastasizing to the stomach are breast cancer, malignant melanoma, and lung cancer. Hematogenous spread to the stomach may manifest as submucosal masses that may appear nonspecific. Breast cancer metastasis can present as a linitis plastica–like appearance, indistinguishable from primary gastric cancer.

Miscellaneous Disorders

Gastric Varices

Gastric varices are often seen secondary to portal hypertension or splenic vein thrombosis. CT findings include clusters of round and/or tubular structures in or adjacent to the stomach. The risk of gastrointestinal hemorrhage is increased in the presence of varices (Fig. 31-14).[17] Other signs of liver disease are frequently seen, including a nodular heterogeneous appearance of the liver suggestive of cirrhosis, splenomegaly, and splenic varices. Splenic vein thrombosis often presents as gastric varices without esophageal varices.

Gastric Distention

Gastric distention can be seen secondary to diabetic neuropathy or secondary to gastric outlet obstruction, causes of which include pyloric gastritis with scarring, gastric or duodenal tumors, or extrinsic compression (Fig. 31-15).

CT OF THE DUODENUM

It is important to identify and recognize the pancreaticoduodenal groove because multiple disease processes may affect this region. For example, inflammatory processes, such as pancreatitis, can affect the surrounding peripancreatic fat and the second, third, and fourth parts of the duodenum, resulting in an associated duodenitis.

Tumors of the pancreatic head can grow and invade the surrounding structures, namely, the second and/or third parts of the duodenum.

Duodenal tumors, too, can be aggressive, such as leiomyosarcoma (although this tumor comprises only 10% of duodenal tumors). These tumors tend to infiltrate adjacent structures such as the pancreas. Hence when reviewing a CT, it is essential to inspect the pancreaticoduodenal groove to assess involvement and spread of disease processes.[18]

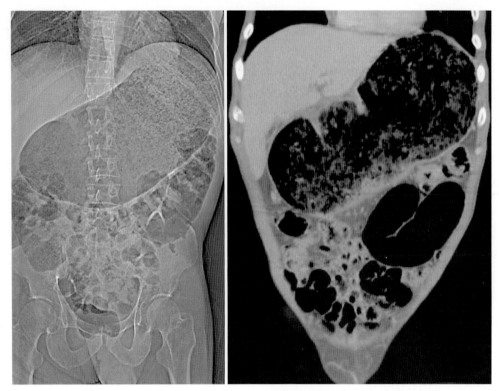

■ **FIGURE 31-15** Gastric distention in scanogram (*left*) and coronal CT scan (*right*).

Inflammatory Conditions

As in the stomach, *H. pylori* is the most common cause of peptic duodenal ulcer. There are weak associations of duodenal ulcers with smoking and alcohol intake. Most patients with peptic ulcers can be investigated endoscopically; however, the upper gastrointestinal study with barium contrast is excellent at demonstrating duodenal ulcers. CT helps to distinguish complications, such as perforation (Fig. 31-16).

Giant duodenal ulcers are defined as a benign ulcer crater of more than 2 cm in diameter and have a tendency to bleed.[1]

Pancreatitis is the most common cause of inflammatory change in the duodenum (Figs. 31-17 and 31-18). In pancreatitis, there is typically periduodenal retroperitoneal fat stranding. Peripancreatic fluid collections may be seen. The release of the pancreatic enzymes causes reactive edema of the duodenum, the extent of which may be severe enough to cause gastric outlet obstruction. Disruption of the intramural vasculature by the digestive pancreatic enzyme elastase can result in intramural hematoma.

Severe cholecystitis can result in inflammation of the duodenum, and if this is of long standing it can result in a gallstone eroding through the gallbladder wall into the duodenum, eventually causing gallstone ileus. Bouveret's syndrome is gastric outlet obstruction due to a gallstone.

Duodenal Diverticulum

The incidental finding of a duodenal diverticulum is frequent on CT. These lesions are typically seen in the second

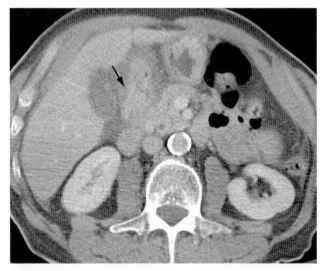

■ **FIGURE 31-16** CT image of perforated duodenal ulcer with free fluid around the duodenal wall (*arrow*).

part of the duodenum, with 85% arising from the medial surface (Figs. 31-19 and 31-20).[19] They are lined with intestinal epithelium, the majority causing no symptoms. However, occasionally a diverticulum can be lined by aberrant pancreatic, gastric, or other functioning mucosa and can be the site of ulceration or perforation. Retention of food or foreign body occasionally can cause symptoms. Aberrant insertion of the common bile duct into a duodenal diverticulum may cause cholangitis or pancreatitis.[20]

CT features of duodenal diverticulum include saccular outpouching, which may resemble a mass-like structure

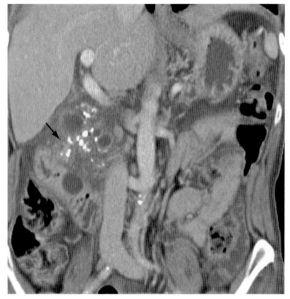

■ **FIGURE 31-17** Gross calcification of pancreatitis involving the first, second, and third part of the duodenum (*arrow*) can be seen on this CT image.

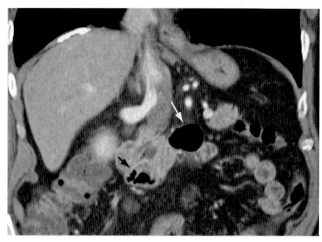

■ **FIGURE 31-20** The most common region for a diverticulum is the medial aspect of the second part of the duodenum (*arrows*).

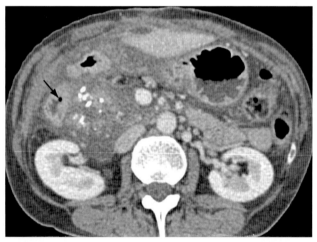

■ **FIGURE 31-18** Axial CT image of pancreatitis and duodenitis. Note the duodenal wall thickening (*arrow*), fat stranding, and extensive inflammatory change.

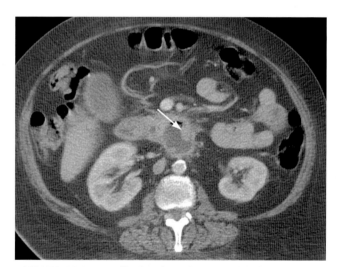

■ **FIGURE 31-21** Small enhancing soft tissue within the duodenal lumen (*arrow*) is evident on this CT image. Histologic evaluation confirmed adenocarcinoma.

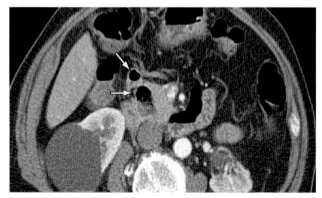

■ **FIGURE 31-19** Axial CT image through the second part of the duodenum demonstrating two air-filled, saccular diverticula (*arrows*).

between the duodenum and the pancreas containing air; air-fluid level; contrast material; or debris. However, the features of duodenal diverticulitis are similar to those seen in the colon, with wall thickening and retroperitoneal fat stranding. Perforation is a rare complication.[21]

Neoplasm

Malignant Tumors

Malignant tumors of the duodenum are uncommon, the most common being primary adenocarcinoma (Fig. 31-21) or tumor of the papilla of Vater (Fig. 31-22). Presentation of these tumors can vary and include obstruction or the appearance of peptic ulcer disease. CT often demonstrates a mass within the duodenum, causing obstruction proximally (Fig. 31-23); or if it is at the ampulla of Vater there may be evidence of dilatation of the bile ducts or pancreatic duct.

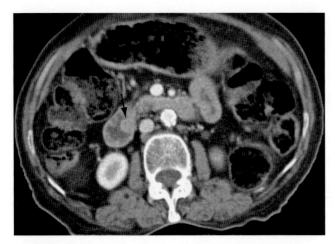

■ **FIGURE 31-22** Small, enhancing papillary carcinoma (*arrow*).

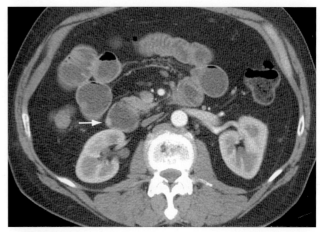

■ **FIGURE 31-24** Small, round, enhancing carcinoid tumor within the duodenal wall (*arrow*).

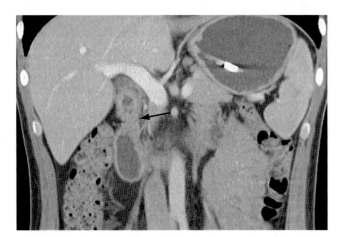

■ **FIGURE 31-23** Circumferential duodenal tumor (*arrow*) causing gastric outlet obstruction.

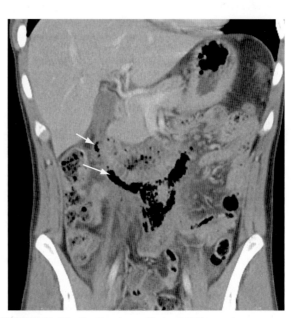

■ **FIGURE 31-25** Duodenal tear. Coronal CT image demonstrates free retroperitoneal air (*arrows*) adjacent to the duodenum and extending into the root of the small bowel mesentery. The duodenum is noted to be thick walled. A tear in the third part of the duodenum was confirmed at laparotomy.

Secondary Involvement

The most common tumors that can involve the duodenum include gastric carcinoma and lymphoma; in both cases, duodenal involvement is typically secondary to direct spread across the pylorus. Carcinoma of the head of the pancreas often involves the duodenum. Owing to its close proximity to the duodenum, the tumor may cause widening of the "C" shape of the duodenal loop. It may present as bleeding, perforation, or duodenal obstruction.

Metastatic deposits to the duodenum may arise from primary tumors of the colon, kidney, uterus, or breast or from malignant melanoma.

Other Tumors

Gastrointestinal carcinoid tumors are neuroendocrine in origin located within the mucosa or submucosa. Carcinoid tumors are most common in the ileum. Duodenal carcinoids are rare and often asymptomatic; however, they may be associated with Zollinger-Ellison syndrome, multiple endocrine neoplasia type 1, and neurofibromatosis type 1.

These tumors can present as small focal masses that enhance during the arterial and portovenous phases of intravenous contrast-enhanced CT and wash out during the equilibrium phase (Fig. 31-24).[13]

Trauma

CT plays a vital role in the diagnosis of duodenal injury. Duodenal trauma may be caused by direct penetrating trauma or indirect injury causing contusion or transection. It is vital to diagnose duodenal perforation because this is a surgical emergency. Duodenal injury should be suspected in patients when (1) pockets of air are adjacent to the duodenum within the retroperitoneum (Fig. 31-25),

(2) there is extravasation of oral contrast material in the retroperitoneum, (3) retroperitoneal fluid is seen, (4) edema of the duodenal wall is noted, (5) peripancreatic fat stranding is noted, and (6) there is pancreatic transection.[22]

Iatrogenic perforation is a rare complication of endoscopy due to direct endoscopic trauma or extended sphincterotomy and is identified by pockets of retroperitoneal air or fluid around the duodenum.

KEY POINTS

- The best modality to identify peptic/duodenal ulcers is the upper gastrointestinal study with barium contrast, whereas CT demonstrates complications such as perforation.
- Gastric cancer and lymphoma can be difficult to distinguish.
- Staging of gastric carcinoma by CT is very useful for planning treatment.
- GISTs are often large and exophytic but can respond dramatically to therapy.
- Duodenal trauma is a surgical emergency and is identified by secondary signs of small pockets of air or fluid adjacent to the duodenum.

SUGGESTED READINGS

Gore RM, Levine SL. Textbook of Gastrointestinal Radiology, 2nd ed. Philadelphia, WB Saunders, 2000, pp 546-657.

Grainger RG, Allison DJ, Adam A, Dixon AK: Grainger and Allison's Diagnostic Radiology: A Textbook of Medical Imaging, 4th ed. Edinburgh, Churchill Livingstone, 2004, vol 2, pp 1063-1073.

Scatarige JC. CT of the stomach and duodenum. Radiol Clin North Am 1989; 27:687-706.

REFERENCES

1. Grainger RG, Allison DJ, Adam A, Dixon AK. Grainger and Allison's Diagnostic Radiology: A Textbook of Medical Imaging, 4th ed. Edinburgh, Churchill Livingstone, 2004, vol 2, pp 1063-1073.
2. Shirakabe H, et al. Atlas of the X-ray Diagnosis of Early Gastric Cancer. Tokyo, Igaku Shoin, 1966.
3. Webb R, Brant W, Major N. Fundamentals of Body CT, 3rd ed. Philadelphia, WB Saunders, 2006, pp 324-328.
4. Desai RK, Tagliabue JR, Wegryn SA, et al. CT evaluation of wall thickening in the alimentary tract. RadioGraphics 1991; 11:771-783.
5. Gossios KJ, Tsianos EV, Demou LL, et al. Use of water or air as oral contrast media for computed tomographic study of the gastric wall: comparison of the two techniques. Gastrointest Radiol 1991; 16:293-297.
6. Scatarige JC. CT of the stomach and duodenum. Radiol Clin North Am 1989; 27:687-706.
7. Howson CP, Hiyama T, Wynder EL. The decline in gastric cancer: epidemiology of an unplanned triumph. Epidemiol Rev 1986; 8:1-27.
8. Insko EK, Levine MS, Birnbaum BA, Jacobs JE. Benign and malignant lesions of the stomach: evaluation of CT criteria for differentiation. Radiology 2003; 228:166-171.
9. Enhlich AN. Gastrointestinal manifestations of malignant lymphoma. Gastroenterology 1968; 54:1115-1121.
10. Megibow AJ. Gastrointestinal lymphoma: the role of CT in diagnosis of gastric lymphoma. AJR Am J Roentgenol 1982; 138:859-865.
11. Demetri GD, Benjamin RS, Blanke CD, Blay JY. NCCN Task Force report: management of patients with gastrointestinal stromal tumor (GIST)—update of the NCCN clinical practice guidelines. J Natl Compr Canc Netw 2007; 5(Suppl 2):S1-29; quiz S30. Erratum in J Natl Compr Canc Netw 2007; 5.
12. Burkill GJC, Badran M, Al-Muderis O, et al. Malignant gastrointestinal stromal tumour: distribution, imaging features and pattern of metastatic spread. Radiology 2003; 226:527-532.
13. Levy AD, Taylor LD, Abbott RM, Sobin LH. Duodenal carcinoids: imaging features with clinical-pathologic comparison. Radiology 2005; 237:967-972.
14. Kim HC, Lee JM, Kim KW, et al. Gastrointestinal stromal tumors of the stomach: CT findings and prediction of malignancy. AJR Am J Roentgenol 2004; 183:893-898.
15. Nilsson B, Bümming P, Meis-Kindblom JM, et al. Gastrointestinal stromal tumors: the incidence, prevalence, clinical course, and prognostication in the pre-imatinib mesylate era—a population-based study in western Sweden. Cancer 2005; 103:821-829.
16. Pannu HK, Hruban RH, Fishman EK. CT of gastric leiomyosarcoma: patterns of involvement. AJR Am J Roentgenol 1999; 173:369-373.
17. Chang D, Levine MS, Ginsberg GG, et al. Portal hypertensive gastropathy: radiographic findings in eight patients. AJR Am J Roentgenol 2000; 175:1609-1612.
18. Gore RM, Levine SL. Textbook of Gastrointestinal Radiology, 2nd ed. Philadelphia, WB Saunders, 2000, pp 546-657.
19. Levene G. The clinical significance of duodenal diverticula. Am J Dig Dis 1962; Oct: 7:877-885.
20. Rose PG. Clinical and radiological features of aberrant insertion of the common bile duct. Clin Radiol 1975; 26:121-127.
21. Pearl MS, Hill MC, Zeman R. CT findings in duodenal diverticulitis. AJR Am J Roentgenol 2006; 187:W392-W395.
22. Jayaraman MV, Mayo-Smith WW, Movson JS, et al. CT of the duodenum: an overlooked segment gets its due. RadioGraphics 2001; 21:S147-S160.

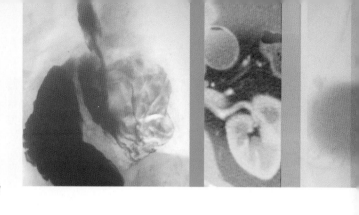

CHAPTER 32

Anatomic Variants of the Stomach and Duodenum

Sukanya Ghosh, Niall Power, and Sujit Vaidya

The normal anatomy of the stomach and duodenum is discussed in Chapter 30, so the focus in this chapter is on anatomic variants. It is important that radiologists recognize some of the congenital abnormalities of the stomach and duodenum and appreciate postoperative changes when interpreting images.

CONGENITAL ABNORMALITIES

Microgastria

Microgastria is a rare anomaly.[1,2] The stomach is small and vertically orientated and has a tubular or slightly fusiform configuration. Microgastria is usually associated with several multisystem malformations that are incompatible with life.

Isolated Dextrogastria

Isolated dextrogastria is a rare anomaly of the stomach in which during embryologic development the stomach grows and descends normally but rotates to the right rather than the left. This anomaly is usually detected in asymptomatic individuals during routine barium studies.[3]

Gastric Duplication

Seven percent of gastrointestinal tract duplications involve the stomach. Most duplications are discovered in infants and present as abdominal pain and vomiting, although often they may be asymptomatic. The anatomic variants of gastric duplication include noncommunicating (most common) and spherical/ovoid closed cysts.[4]

The most common site of these anomalies is the greater curvature. Because of abnormal development of the endoderm and notochord separation, the mucosal lining is often seen lying outside the normal stomach wall. Barium studies demonstrate a perigastric mass displacing the stomach and the bowel, whereas CT and ultrasonography show a well-defined fluid-filled cystic mass lying close to the greater curvature of the stomach. The signs of duplication are the presence of an echogenic inner rim and hypoechoic outer muscle layers.[5,6]

Duodenal Duplication

Duplication often occurs along the first and second part of the duodenum and is usually noncommunicating. Clinically it presents as obstruction, but because of its location there may be biliary obstruction and pancreatitis. Barium studies usually demonstrate the duodenum to be compressed by a mass in the concavity of the duodenal C-loop. Ultrasonography, CT, or MRI shows the cystic nature of the lesion, which should be differentiated from a choledochal cyst or pancreatic pseudocyst.[7]

Duodenal Diverticulum

Duodenal diverticula are incidental findings often seen on both CT and barium studies. There is often a defect of the muscular wall causing the sac of mucosal and submucosal layer to herniate. The duodenal diverticula fill or empty secondary to gravity, resulting from the pressure of the duodenal peristalsis. On barium studies, duodenal diverticula are recognized by smooth outpouchings from the medial border of the descending duodenum. Often they are multiple, and patients are asymptomatic. Rarely do they cause serious complications such as duodenal diverticulitis or upper gastrointestinal bleeding. They may enlarge and cause gastric outlet obstruction as a result of compression of the pylorus.[8]

ACQUIRED POSITIONAL ABNORMALITIES

Gastric Hernia

Acquired positional abnormalities of the stomach generally arise by two different mechanisms. Extreme laxity of

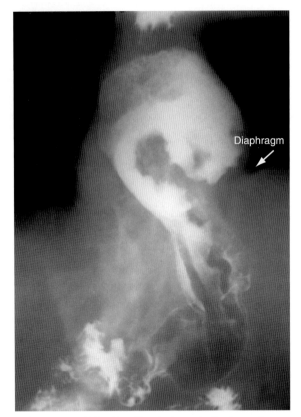

■ **FIGURE 32-1** Sliding hiatal hernia. Note the fundus and esophageal junction are herniating through the diaphragmatic hiatus.

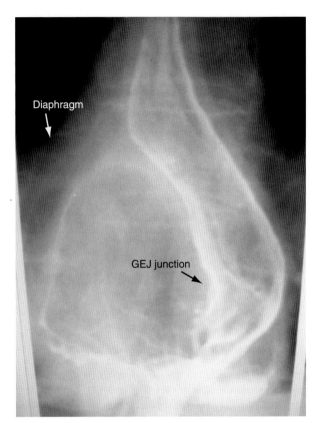

■ **FIGURE 32-2** Rolling hiatal hernia is when the gastroesophageal junction remains below the hemidiaphragm.

the peritoneal attachments can lead to greater mobility of the organ. This is commonly associated with an accessible potential space for gastric herniation through either the diaphragm or the anterior abdominal wall. Additionally, space-occupying lesions of the upper abdomen can compress and displace the stomach.

Herniations

Gastric herniation can occur through the anterior abdominal wall and extremely rare. Hiatal hernia (Fig. 32-1) is a gastric herniation through the esophageal hiatus. It is common in the elderly population. The herniation is usually partial. It involves the gastric fundus, which migrates through the diaphragmatic hiatus into the lower mediastinum. Sometimes a large portion of the stomach or even the entire organ migrates.

There are two types of gastric hiatal hernias. A sliding hiatal hernia (see Fig. 32-1) is present when both the esophagogastric junction and the stomach herniate into the stomach. These sliding hiatal hernias are common and often slide in and out of the thorax. A rolling or paraesophageal hernia (Fig. 32-2) is one in which the gastroesophageal junction remains below the diaphragmatic hiatus. This hernia is rare.

Volvulus

The normal stomach is suspended and tightly secured by the gastric ligaments, namely, the *gastrohepatic* ligament along the lesser curvature, the *gastrocolic* and *gastro-*

splenic ligaments along the greater curvature, and the *gastrophrenic* ligament along the posterior aspect of the fundus. Along with these supporting ligaments the esophagus holds the stomach in place superiorly, while the fixed duodenum tends to hold the pylorus/antrum inferiorly. The abnormal position, laxity, or absence of these ligaments, whether congenital or pathologic, causes herniation and volvulus of the stomach.

The intrathoracic volvulus is a major complication of a large hiatal hernia. In an unobstructed hiatal hernia the fundus lies above the diaphragm. In torsion, the fundus, which was previously within the hernial sac,[9] descends to a normal position within the abdomen, and the antrum undergoes organoaxial torsion into the vacated hernial sac.

Gastric volvulus can be a surgical emergency because it can result in gastric outlet obstruction or, more importantly, vascular compromise. The stomach twists itself between the points of normal anatomic fixation. It can occur at any age but occurs commonly in the elderly and is often associated with a large sliding or paraesophageal hiatal hernia.[10,11]

There are at least two types of gastric volvulus, depending on the plane of torsion: organoaxial and mesoaxial (Fig. 32-3).[12]

Predisposing factors that can cause gastric volvulus include phrenic nerve palsy, eventration of the diaphragm, traumatic diaphragmatic hernia, and gastric distention. Interestingly, gastric volvulus also is associated with "wandering spleen" due to the congenital absence of intraperitoneal visceral ligaments. Defective and lax gas-

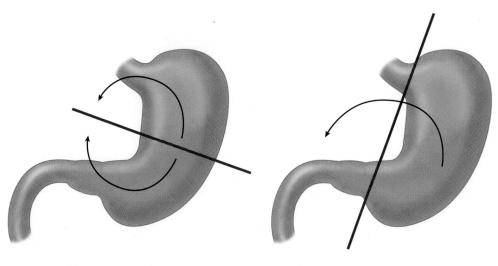

■ **FIGURE 32-3**   Organoaxial and mesoaxial volvulus.

Mesenteroaxial volvulus

Organoaxial volvulus

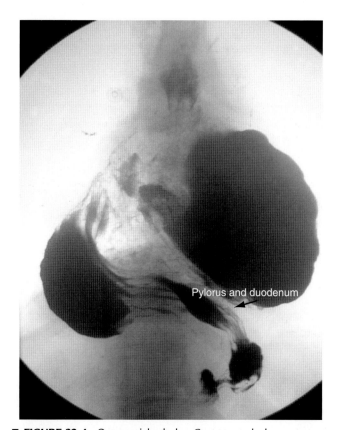

Pylorus and duodenum

■ **FIGURE 32-4**   Organoaxial volvulus. Contrast study demonstrates that the first and second part of the duodenum has flipped to the left along the axis between the cardia and the pylorus.

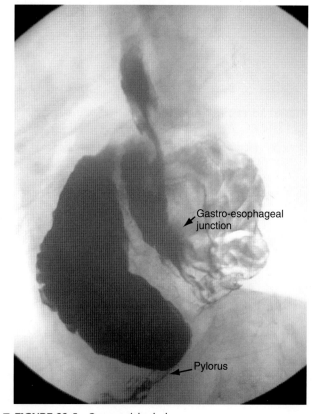

Gastro-esophageal junction

Pylorus

■ **FIGURE 32-5**   Organoaxial volvulus.

trosplenic ligaments allow the spleen to move freely in the abdomen and twist on its own pedicle. Consequently, the stomach, too, can twist and present as a volvulus.[13]

Organoaxial Volvulus

Fifty-nine percent of cases of volvulus are of this type (Figs. 32-4 to 32-6).[14] The axis for this volvulus is marked as a line drawn between the cardia and the pylorus. In the

organoaxial volvulus the stomach rotates along this long axis. If the stomach was horizontal initially, the volvulus flips the greater curvature superior to the lesser curvature. If the stomach, however, was vertically aligned originally, then the volvulus causes a right-left twist (see Fig. 32-6).

Mesoaxial Volvulus

Mesoaxial volvulus, although less common, has more significant consequences. In this type of volvulus, the axis is

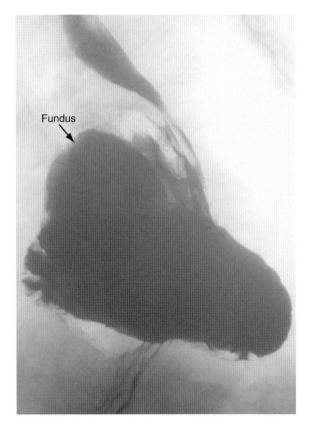

■ **FIGURE 32-6** Organoaxial volvulus in which the stomach is vertically aligned, causing a right-left twist (note the fundus has rotated to the right).

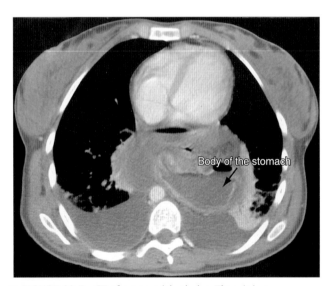

■ **FIGURE 32-7** CT of a mesoaxial volvulus. The axis is a perpendicular line between the midpoint of the lesser and greater curvatures. Hence the body of the stomach is seen craniad.

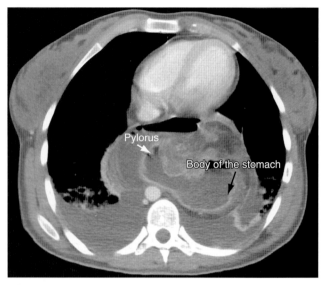

■ **FIGURE 32-8** CT of a mesoaxial volvulus.

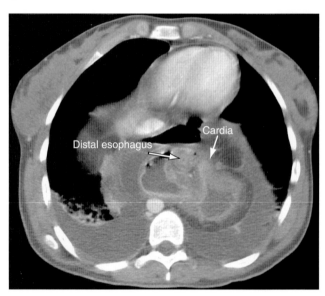

■ **FIGURE 32-9** CT of a mesoaxial volvulus. Axial CT image shows that the position of the cardia is below the fundus.

a line joining the middle part of the lesser and greater curvatures perpendicular to the stomach (Fig. 32-7). The axis corresponds to the mesenteric attachments of the greater and lesser omentum,[15] causing an appearance of an "upside-down stomach." The fundus and proximal stomach are distal to the antrum and pylorus (Figs. 32-8 and 32-9). This increases the risk of traumatic diaphragmatic injuries.

On plain radiographs, a gastric volvulus is seen as a double air-fluid level of the stomach in the mediastinum and upper abdomen on an upright film. Barium studies demonstrate the abnormalities well, with evidence of complications such as gastric outlet obstruction.

Malrotation

Embryologically, the bowel rotates along the superior mesenteric artery as the axis until it resumes its correct position. The process involves rotation of the two ends of the alimentary canal, namely, the proximal duodenojejunal loop and the cecocolic loop. This is quite a complex process and involves at least three stages, resulting in the

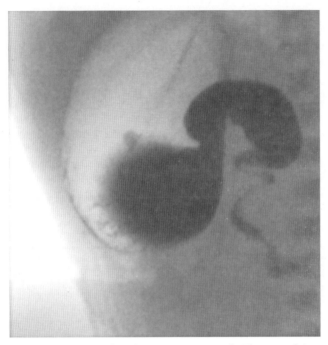

■ **FIGURE 32-10** Malrotation on a contrast study. The stomach is on the right side, and the duodenojejunal junction is not at the level of the ligament of Treitz (left lateral aspect of the vertebral bodies).

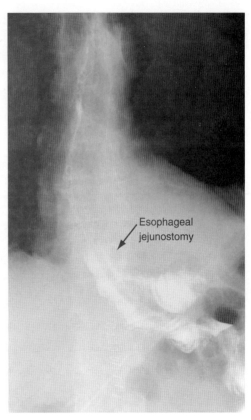

Esophageal jejunostomy

■ **FIGURE 32-12** Gastrectomy with esophagojejunal anastomosis.

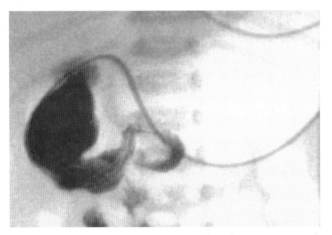

■ **FIGURE 32-11** Malrotation of the small bowel on a contrast study.

correct position of the duodenojejunal junction lying lateral and to the left of the ligament of Treitz.

Intestinal malrotation is defined by abnormal positioning of the duodenojejunal junction, which may then lead to midgut volvulus, a potentially life-threatening complication (Figs. 32-10 and 32-11). Any malrotation can cause compromise to the superior mesenteric artery, resulting in an ischemic small bowel. There are various degrees and types of malrotation that are often associated with a congenital abnormality. Malrotation is unusually diagnosed in 75% of symptomatic neonates (presenting with bilious vomiting), and up to 90% of cases occur in the first year of life.[16]

The Postoperative Stomach

Gastric surgery is often performed for malignancies, for weight reduction, or to bypass obstruction. It is important to recognize the surgical appearance of these operations and also to identify any complications.

Partial or total gastrectomies are performed for malignancies. Total gastrectomies include removal of the stomach and anastomosis of the distal esophagus to the duodenum/jejunum, depending on the extent of surgery (Fig. 32-12). Partial gastrectomy is the partial removal of the stomach with anastomosis of the duodenum to the gastric remnant.

Another procedure is the laparoscopic Roux-en-Y gastric bypass surgery, which is a bariatric surgery used to treat obesity. It is being performed more and more owing to its shortened hospital stay, faster recovery, and decreased wound complications. The procedure involves construction of a 15- to 30-mL gastric pouch, a Roux limb, and enteroenteric anastomosis; placement of the Roux limb; and creation of the gastrojejunostomy.[17]

Initially the stomach is stapled, and a pouch is created. Then the Roux loop and the enteroenteric anastomosis is constructed. The jejunum is divided 25 to 50 cm distal to the ligament of Treitz, creating two limbs: a biliopancreatic limb and the Roux limb. The biliopancreatic limb is joined 75 cm distal to the Roux limb via side-to-side anastomosis, thus bypassing most of the jejunum (Fig. 32-13).[18,19] Then the pouch is anastomosed to 75 to 150 cm of the Roux limb that is brought to the pouch through the transverse mesocolon.[20]

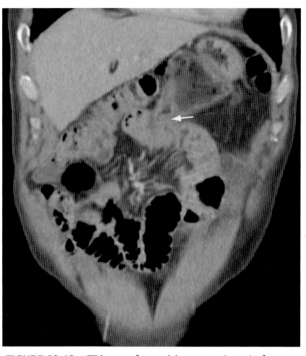

■ **FIGURE 32-13**   CT image of gastrojejunostomy (*arrow*) after a Whipple procedure.

Another operation often seen is the Whipple procedure, which is performed on patients with carcinoma of the head of pancreas, pancreatic ducts, or vessels near the pancreas. It involves removal of the distal half of the stomach (antrectomy), gallbladder (cholecystectomy), distal portion of the common bile duct (choledochectomy), head of the pancreas, duodenum, proximal jejunum, and regional lymph nodes. Then reconstruction consists of attaching the pancreas to the jejunum (pancreaticojejunostomy), attaching the common bile duct to the jejunum (choledochojejunostomy), and attaching the stomach to the jejunum (gastrojejunostomy) to allow food to pass through.

KEY POINT

■ It is important for radiologists to recognize anatomic variants of both the stomach and the duodenum when interpreting images.

SUGGESTED READINGS

Blachar A, Federle MP, Pealer KM, et al. Gastrointestinal complications of laparoscopic roux-en-y gastric bypass surgery: clinical and imaging findings. Radiology 2002; 223:625-632.

Eisenberg RL. Miscellaneous abnormalities. In Gore RN, Levine MS, Laufer I (eds). Textbook of Gastrointestinal Radiology. Philadelphia, WB Saunders, 1994, vol 1, p 717.

Gore RM, Levine SL. Textbook of Gastrointestinal Radiology, 2nd ed. Philadelphia, WB Saunders, 2000, pp 546-657.

REFERENCES

1. Shackleford GD, McAlister WH, Brodeur AE, et al. Congenital microgastria. AJR Am J Roentgenol 1975; 123:72-76.
2. Kessler H, Smulewicz JJ. Microgastria associated with agenesis of the spleen. Radiology 1973; 107:393-396.
3. Teplick JG, Wallner RJ, Levine AH, et al. Isolated dextrogastria: report of two cases. AJR Am J Roentgenol 1979; 132:124-126.
4. Berrocal T, Torres I, Gutierrez J, et al. Congenital anomalies of the upper gastrointestinal tract. RadioGraphics 1999; 19:855-872.
5. Barr LL, Hayden CK, Stansberry SD, et al. Enteric duplication cysts in children: are their ultrasonographic wall characteristics diagnostic? Paediatr Radiol 1990; 20:326-330.
6. Segal SR, Sherman NH, Rosenberg HK, et al. Ultrasonographic features of gastrointestinal duplications. J Ultrasound Med 1994; 13: 863-870.
7. Teele RL, Henshke CI, Tapper D. The radiographic and ultrasonographic evaluation of enteric duplication cysts. Pediatr Radiol 1980; 10:9-12.
8. Gore RM, Levine SL. Textbook of Gastrointestinal Radiology, 2nd ed. Philadelphia, WB Saunders, 2000, pp 546-657.
9. Blatt ES, Schneider HJ, Wiot JF, Felson B. Roentgen findings in obstructed diaphragmatic hernia. Radiology 1962; 79:648-657.
10. Eisenberg RL. Miscellaneous abnormalities. In Gore RN, Levine MS, Laufer I (eds). Textbook of Gastrointestinal Radiology. Philadelphia, WB Saunders, 1994, vol 1, p 717.
11. Wastell C, Ellis H. Volvulus of the stomach: a review with a report of 8 cases. Br J Surg 1971; 58:557-562.

12. Caroline DF, Evers K. The stomach. In Grainger RG, Allison D, Ellis D. et al. Grainger and Allison's Diagnostic Radiology: A Textbook of Medical Imaging, 4th ed. New York, Churchill Livingstone, 2001, pp 1049-1050.
13. Uc A, Kao SC, Sanders KD, Lawrence J. Gastric volvulus and wandering spleen. Am J Gastroenterol 1998; 93:1146-1148.
14. Wastell C, Ellis H. Volvulus of the stomach: a review with a report of 8 cases. Br J Surg 1971; 58:557-562.
15. Gerson DE, Lewicki AM. Intrathoracic stomach: when does it obstruct? Radiology 1976; 119:257-264.
16. Strouse PJ. Disorders of intestinal rotation and fixation ("malrotation"). Pediatr Radiol 2004; 34:837-851.
17. Christopher D, Scheirey CD, Scholz FJ, et al. Radiology of the laparoscopic Roux-en-Y gastric bypass procedure: conceptualization and precise interpretation of results. RadioGraphics 2006; 26: 1355-1371.
18. Nguyen NT, Goldman C, Rosenquist CJ, et al. Laparoscopic versus open gastric bypass: a randomized study of outcomes, quality of life, and costs. Ann Surg 2001; 234:279-289; discussion 289-291.
19. Lujan JA, Frutos MD, Hernandez Q, et al. Laparoscopic versus open gastric bypass in the treatment of morbid obesity: a randomized prospective study. Ann Surg 2004; 239:433-437.
20. Blachar A, Federle MP, Pealer KM, et al. Gastrointestinal complications of laparoscopic Roux-en-Y gastric bypass surgery: clinical and imaging findings. Radiology 2002; 223:625-632.

Stomach Lesions

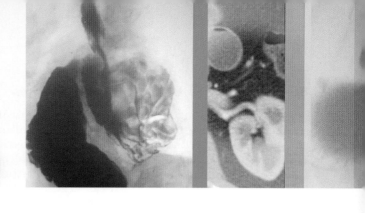

CHAPTER 33

Benign Mucosal Diseases of the Stomach

Hima B. Prabhakar

ETIOLOGY

A wide range of benign disease processes can affect the mucosa of the stomach, including inflammatory, infectious, hereditary, and autoimmune processes. What all of these processes have in common is that they affect one of the primary defenses of the stomach wall—the mucosal layer.

In considering the radiologic appearance of these many entities, it is helpful to divide them into their primary mucosal manifestations—ulcers, polyps/masses, and diffuse mucosal processes. Some of the more common processes include:

Ulcers: infections (*Helicobacter pylori,* cytomegalovirus), erosive gastritis (nonsteroidal anti-inflammatory drugs [NSAIDs], alcohol, stress, radiation, direct trauma), Crohn's disease, autoimmune (Behçet's) disease, sarcoidosis[1]

Polyps/masses: hyperplastic and adenomatous polyps (also seen in Cronkhite-Canada syndrome and familial polyposis of the colon), hamartomas (Peutz-Jeghers syndrome, Cowden disease), heterotopic pancreatic tissue, lymphoid hyperplasia[2]

Diffuse mucosal processes: acute gastritis, atrophic gastritis, eosinophilic and lymphocytic gastritis, Zollinger-Ellison syndrome, Ménétrier's disease, and those that cause a linitis plastica appearance (corrosives, radiation, Crohn's disease, tuberculosis, sarcoidosis, syphilis)[2]

In this chapter, the discussion is tailored to each of these categories, with a description of the most common entities.

PREVALENCE AND EPIDEMIOLOGY

Benign Diseases Causing Mucosal Ulcerations

The most common benign cause of mucosal ulcerations is peptic ulcer disease. Although decreasing in overall incidence with the routine use of histamine-2 (H_2) blockers, the overall death rate from peptic ulcer disease has remained stable. The vast majority of cases of gastric ulcers (70% to 90%) and duodenal ulcers (up to 90%) are due to *H. pylori* infection, which was discovered to be a causative agent in the 1980s.[3] Many subsequent studies have shown that treating patients with antibiotics for *H. pylori* decreases the rate of ulcer recurrence to less than 20%. Fifteen to 20 percent of patients colonized with *H. pylori* do not develop peptic ulcer disease, demonstrating that other factors play a role.[2]

Other causes of gastric ulcers include NSAIDs and aspirin.[4] Chronic NSAID users have a prevalence of peptic ulcer disease of 25%. Additionally, because these drugs affect platelets, these patients tend to have a higher incidence of complications, including hemorrhage and perforation. It is recommended that any patient at high risk for developing NSAID-associated peptic ulcer disease should receive acid-suppressive medication, misoprostol, or an alternative treatment such as with a cyclooxygenase-2 (COX-2) inhibitor.[1]

Less common causes of benign gastric mucosal ulcers include stress ulcers in burn patients (Curling ulcers) and head trauma patients (Cushing ulcer), crack cocaine and alcohol abuse,[1] Crohn's disease,[5,6] sarcoidosis,[7] cytomegalovirus infection, and Behçet's disease.

Benign Diseases Causing Polyps/Masses

Polypoid lesions of the stomach include hyperplastic (regenerative), adenomatous, hamartomatous, and inflammatory polyps as well as heterotopic pancreatic tissue. The most common benign polyps are hyperplastic polyps, which can commonly occur in the setting of gastritis. Unlike adenomatous polyps, which can degenerate in a similar fashion as colonic adenomas, hyperplastic polyps have almost no malignant potential.[2]

Hamartomatous polyposis syndromes are rare and include Peutz-Jeghers syndrome, multiple hamartoma/Cowden disease,[8] juvenile polyposis, Cronkhite-Canada syndrome, and Bannayan-Riley-Ruvalcaba syndrome. Whereas hamartomatous polyps are themselves without malignant potential, they are frequently associated with adenomatous polyps. More importantly, these syndromes can also be associated with extraintestinal malignancies, and it is essential to make the diagnosis so that the patient can be screened for these tumors.[9]

Benign Diseases Causing Diffuse Mucosal Abnormalities

The most common diseases that affect the gastric mucosa diffusely are acute gastritis and chronic/atrophic gastritis. Acute gastritis, most commonly secondary to *H. pylori* infection, can progress to a chronic state if left untreated. Other causes of acute gastritis include NSAID-induced gastritis, caustic ingestion,[1] and granulomatous disease (sarcoidosis,[7] tuberculosis), as well as less common causes such as cytomegalovirus infection, herpesvirus infection, and syphilis.[10]

Chronic gastritis can progress to atrophic gastritis, which is characterized by loss of the normal mucosal glands and is categorized by the portion of the stomach involved. Type A chronic/atrophic gastritis, which affects predominantly the fundus/body, has been termed *autoimmune gastritis* and is the least common of the two types. This form is associated with pernicious anemia, which is caused by destruction of the parietal cells and loss of intrinsic factor, which leads to vitamin B_{12} deficiency and megaloblastic anemia. More common is type B chronic/atrophic gastritis, which affects predominantly the antrum and is associated with chronic *H. pylori* infection.[1]

Other causes of gastritis are less common. Eosinophilic gastritis is characterized by blood eosinophilia as well as eosinophilic infiltrates within the gastric wall. The antrum is predominantly involved, and mucosal fold thickening can become severe enough to cause gastric outlet obstruction.[11] Bowel involvement can also occur and is termed *eosinophilic gastroenteritis*.[1]

Diffuse gastric fold thickening can occur as a result of inflammation or infiltration. In Ménétrier's disease there is hypertrophy of the mucus-producing cells of the stomach mucosa, causing marked fold thickening. This rare disorder is of unknown etiology and can mimic malignancy as well as severe gastritis or an infiltrative process.[2] In addition to the usual clinical presentation of pain, weight loss, and occasional bleeding, the disorder is characterized by hypoalbuminemia secondary to loss of proteins.[1]

CLINICAL PRESENTATION

Epigastric pain and weight loss are common presenting symptoms in patients with stomach mucosal ulcerations from a variety of causes. Pain that worsens with eating is a classic description for gastric ulcers. Additionally, weight loss can be seen secondary to food avoidance. The chronicity can vary depending on the underlying etiology—acute in cases of gastritis caused by *H. pylori* and alcohol/caustic ingestion to chronic in patients with Crohn's disease, Behçet's disease, and eosinophilic gastroenteritis. Patients may also present with gastrointestinal bleeding or anemia, which is the most common complication seen in peptic ulcer disease. Finally, any acute change in severity of symptoms may reflect ulcer perforation, which is the second most common ulcer-related complication. The least common complication, gastric outlet obstruction, is discussed in Chapter 36.[2]

Benign gastric polyps are usually incidentally detected during barium upper gastrointestinal study or endoscopy. Rarely, if they are pedunculated and outgrow their blood supply, they can ulcerate and bleed. If the polyps are present as part of a syndrome, for example in Cowden syndrome, Peutz-Jeghers syndrome, or familial polyposis, patients may present principally with signs and symptoms of these disorders.[2]

There is a wide variety of causes of benign diffuse mucosal abnormalities, and the clinical presentation varies just as widely. Chronic processes causing a linitis plastica physiology such as Crohn's disease can be accompanied by weight loss and early satiety. Also, because Ménétrier's disease is a protein-losing gastropathy, patients will have hypoproteinemia and diarrhea.[1]

NORMAL ANATOMY

There are four layers of the gastric wall: mucosa, submucosa, muscularis propria, and serosa. The mucosa is the innermost layer and is lined with columnar glandular epithelium. Depending on the location within the stomach there are different types of epithelial cells that line the gastric glands as well as endocrine cells. Additionally, there are mucus-secreting cells that extend into the glands and produce bicarbonate to protect the stomach from acid injury. Overall, the layers that make up the gastric mucosa are the epithelium, lamina propria, and muscularis mucosa. The mucosa and submucosa comprise the gastric rugae, which stretch out as the stomach distends.[2]

PATHOLOGY

In general, entities that affect the stomach mucosa can be broken down into a few broad categories: infectious, inflammatory, infiltrative, autoimmune, and hereditary. Those processes causing ulcers can fall into any of these categories, but polypoid lesions tend to represent either inflammatory or hereditary causes.[2]

Infectious causes, including most commonly *H. pylori*, all begin by circumventing the stomach mucosa's natural defenses. Because of its highly acidic environment, the stomach is able to withstand infection from a wide range of ingested bacteria. However, in the case of *H. pylori,* the bacteria have adapted mechanisms to neutralize the acidic environment by creating sodium bicarbonate and ammonia from the enzyme urease. Once it has colonized the stomach, *H. pylori* causes an increase in gastric acid production through a variety of mechanisms, including inhibition of the production of somatostatin by the antral D cells. Because somatostatin is a potent inhibitor of antral G cell gastrin production, this leads to an overall increase in acid secretion. This acid hypersecretion is thought to be the primary mechanism for *H. pylori*-induced gastritis and ulcer formation.[2]

Other infectious agents, including herpesvirus and cytomegalovirus, involve direct viral infection of the mucosal cells. Clinically, these affect immunocompromised patients such as those with the acquired immunodeficiency syndrome. Cytomegalovirus infection is characterized by intranuclear inclusions seen on biopsy.[1] Syphilitic involvement of the stomach is rare but has been seen with increasing frequency in immunocompromised patients. In early disease, gastritis is characterized pathologically by perivascular and mucosal mononuclear infiltration. In later stages of the disease, gummatous involvement of the stomach can occur, as well as scarring and stricture.[10]

Inflammatory causes of gastritis include NSAID-induced gastritis, as well as caustic ingestion. The most common of these disorders is NSAID-induced gastritis. NSAIDs cause a decrease in stomach mucus and bicarbonate production by inhibiting prostaglandins. This leads to a breakdown in the defensive barrier of the stomach lining to gastric acid, which in turn leads to gastritis and ulcer disease.[1]

Infiltrative causes tend to cause a diffuse abnormality of the stomach mucosa. These include eosinophilic and lymphocytic gastritis, Ménétrier's disease, sarcoidosis, and tuberculosis. The pathologic hallmark is infiltration of mucosa or submucosa with abnormally increased cells (in the case of eosinophilic and lymphocytic gastritis, as well as Ménétrier's disease) or reactive tissue (in the case of granulomas of sarcoidosis and tuberculosis).[11]

Benign polypoid and mucosal mass lesions of the stomach are most commonly hyperplastic and are frequently seen in the setting of gastritis. These have a low potential for malignancy.[12] Adenomatous polyps, which can be seen in the setting of polyposis syndromes mentioned previously, have a higher potential for malignancy and can be either tubular or villous.[13] Finally, hamartomatous polyps, also seen in the setting of polyposis syndromes, are the least common of the subtypes.[14]

IMAGING

Ulcers

Gastric ulcer disease typically presents as symptoms of epigastric/abdominal pain, which is worse with eating. These clinical symptoms are nonspecific and can be seen in a wide variety of abdominal pathologic processes, not just referable to the stomach.[15] MRI, ultrasonography, and PET/CT are not generally useful in the diagnosis.

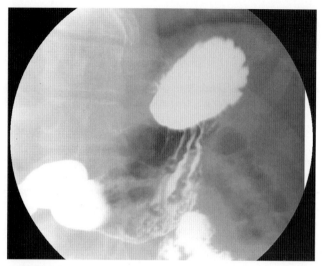

■ **FIGURE 33-1** Double-contrast barium upper gastrointestinal examination of the stomach reveals thickened gastric folds with multiple ulcers lined along the gastric folds. Endoscopic sampling revealed gastritis, negative for *H. pylori.* This case was thought to be most likely secondary to use of NSAIDs.

Radiography

Evaluation of mucosal disease is best seen with double-contrast barium evaluation. Gastric ulcers appear as abnormal accumulations of contrast media that persist on different views. Within the stomach, these collections are most often round, as opposed to in the esophagus where they can also appear as linear defects. In benign ulcers, the ulcer crater projects outside the gastric lumen. Additionally, mucosal folds are typically thin and extend to the margin of the ulcer (this is not seen with malignant ulcers or ulcerated masses).[16] The pattern of mucosal ulcerations can also be useful. In the case of erosive gastritis caused by NSAID use, small ulcers are aligned along thickened folds (Fig. 33-1).[4] Peptic ulcers tend to be solitary or few, but aphthous ulcers of Behçet's disease and Crohn's disease are often multiple.[6]

CT

Recent studies have shown that multidetector CT with virtual gastroscopy is a useful way to distinguish benign from malignant gastric ulcers. Using criteria such as ulcer shape and margin (regular vs. irregular), gastric fold changes, and enhancement of the ulcer base, Lee and colleagues have shown 80% to 90% sensitivity and 77% to 78% specificity for the differentiation of benign from malignant ulcers.[17]

More commonly, CT is used to generally evaluate patients with abdominal pain. In these cases, gastric wall thickening/edema can be seen at the site of ulcers. Importantly, some of the complications of gastric ulcers can be readily detected by CT, including perforation (Fig. 33-2) and gastric outlet obstruction. Bleeding ulcers are less likely to be detected as a cause of gastrointestinal bleeding with CT.[2]

Nuclear Medicine

In general, nuclear medicine studies are not useful in the detection of gastric ulcer disease. However, in two specific scenarios, in patients presenting with known Zollinger-Ellison syndrome or gastrointestinal bleeding of unknown etiology, nuclear medicine tests may be useful in the diagnosis.[18]

In Zollinger-Ellison syndrome, it is important to detect the underlying location of the gastrinoma, which is typically less than 1 cm and difficult to detect at surgery. Approximately 80% lie in the region of the proximal duodenum and pancreas and are easily seen by CT and MRI when larger. The current imaging modality of choice for detecting gastrinomas is the octreotide scan (indium-labeled somatostatin receptors), which binds somatostatin.[2]

In the evaluation of gastrointestinal bleeding, bleeding within the stomach should typically be diagnosed clinically with the placement of a nasogastric tube. However, if not diagnosed this way, the patient may go on to receive a nuclear medicine bleeding scan, with either red blood cells or sulfur colloid labeled with technetium-99m. In these cases, gastric hemorrhage may be detected, but the imaging pitfall of free pertechnetate, which causes gastric activity, should be excluded.[19]

Polyps/Masses

Gastric polyps and benign masses are generally clinically occult unless they cause bleeding or gastric outlet obstruction. These are typically incidentally detected with endoscopy or barium radiography. MRI, ultrasonography, nuclear medicine studies, and PET/CT are not generally useful in diagnosis.

Radiography

The radiographic evaluation of benign mucosal polyps/masses again rests on the double-contrast barium upper gastrointestinal evaluation. Gastric polyps appear as filling defects on barium studies and can be pedunculated/tubular (Fig. 33-3) or villous. When numerous, the possibility of a polyposis syndrome is raised. Additionally, mucosal masses such as heterotopic pancreatic rests can have a characteristic appearance, typically with a centrally umbilicated mass located in the pylorus.[20-22]

CT

CT is not generally useful when imaging mucosal lesions unless there is a large mass or a complication such as gastric outlet obstruction.[23]

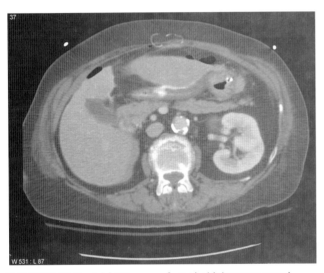

■ **FIGURE 33-2** Axial CT scan performed with intravenous and oral contrast media demonstrates a defect in the gastric wall, with oral contrast medium entering the peritoneal cavity. At surgery this was found to be a perforated gastric ulcer.

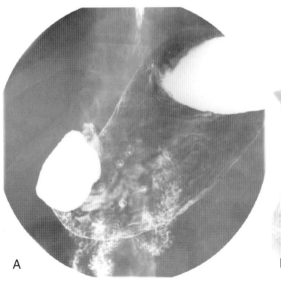

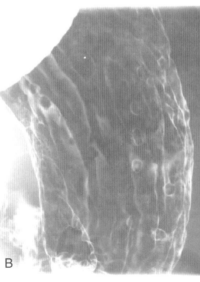

■ **FIGURE 33-3** **A,** Double-contrast barium upper gastrointestinal examination of the stomach reveals multiple polypoid lesions. **B,** Endoscopic biopsy revealed hyperplastic polyps, the most common type.

A   B

TABLE 33-1 Accuracy, Limitations, and Pitfalls of the Modalities Used in Imaging of Benign Mucosal Diseases of the Stomach

Modality	Accuracy	Limitations	Pitfalls
Radiography	With an experienced radiologist, double-contrast barium upper gastrointestinal studies can identify different patterns of mucosal involvement.	Wide differential considerations for the variety of patterns	Small ulcers or diffuse disease may be difficult to detect.
CT	MDCT with virtual gastroscopy may be useful in differentiating benign and malignant ulcers.	Not sensitive or specific for gastric mucosal disease; better for evaluation of late complications	
Nuclear medicine	Gold standard for detection of gastrinomas seen in Zollinger-Ellison syndrome		

Diffuse Mucosal Disease

Again, abdominal pain is the most common presenting symptom in these cases and is nonspecific. If a patient has scarring/fibrosis, early satiety may be a symptom that would prompt evaluation of the stomach. Additionally, patients with Ménétrier's disease present with hypoalbuminemia, which may prompt a search for an underlying cause.[18]

Radiography

Double-contrast barium radiography may be ordered in the patient with early satiety to evaluate for underlying neoplasm or mass. Barium studies may instead show nondistensibility of the stomach, or segmental scarring, such as in Crohn's disease. The differential considerations for this appearance are wide, and close evaluation of the patient's history may be useful to narrow the diagnostic possibilities.[5]

CT

CT is generally not useful without a distended stomach. Wall thickening of the stomach can be simulated by underdistention.

Nuclear Medicine

In cases with gastric scarring/fibrosis there can be delayed gastric emptying. Nuclear medicine gastric emptying studies, performed with technetium-99m–labeled sulfur colloid, may be useful in the evaluation and management of these select cases.[19]

PET/CT

PET/CT is not useful in the diagnosis of diffuse gastric mucosal disease. In patients who have PET/CT for other reasons, incidental detection of inflammatory processes such as gastritis may be seen with increased fluorodeoxyglucose uptake.[24]

Imaging Algorithm

In patients presenting with abdominal pain, the first-line imaging study is typically CT. If CT does not yield a diagnosis, such as complications related to underlying ulcer disease, the patient should proceed to double-contrast barium upper gastrointestinal study or endoscopy for further evaluation. The choice of these two procedures most often depends on the patient's clinical status and pretest likelihood of disease (Table 33-1).

Classic Signs

- Hampton's line (benign ulcer): thin straight line at the base of the ulcer seen in profile indicating thin rim of undermined mucosa[16]
- Ram's horn sign (Crohn's disease): deformity, nondistensibility, narrowing, and poor peristalsis of the stomach antrum, leading to configuration similar to a ram's horn[5]
- Linear/serpiginous gastric ulcers (aspirin/NSAID-induced erosive gastritis)[4]
- Heterotopic pancreatic rests: a centrally umbilicated mass located in the pylorus[20-22]

DIFFERENTIAL DIAGNOSIS

Abdominal and epigastric pain are the classic symptoms of gastritis and ulcer disease. These are nonspecific symptoms and may only prompt evaluation of the stomach with the appropriate clinical history (e.g., NSAID use, history of Crohn's disease or sarcoidosis).[15,18]

As discussed previously, the differential diagnosis rests on categorizing mucosal diseases into their primary manifestations: ulcers, polyps/masses, and diffuse processes. The differential diagnostic considerations were listed previously under Etiology.

TREATMENT

Medical Treatment

The advent of effective drug therapy for gastritis and ulcer disease has led to a marked improvement in patient outcomes as well as a decrease in the frequency of acute complications (e.g., bleeding, obstruction). The primary treatments include antibiotic therapy for infection with *H. pylori,* as well as antacids, H$_2$ receptor antagonists, and proton pump inhibitors. Additionally, mucosal protective agents such as misoprostol, bismuth agents, and sucralfate have been useful.[1]

With regard to other causes of ulcer disease as well as diffuse mucosal processes such as Crohn's disease, sarcoidosis, and tuberculosis, medical management focuses on treatment of the underlying cause. For polypoid lesions of the stomach, treatment involves endoscopic polypectomy for pathologic evaluation and to exclude malignancy.[14]

Surgical Treatment

Surgical management is generally focused on patients who have failed medical management or have complications related to underlying ulcer disease. These include intractable bleeding, perforation, obstruction, or nonhealing ulcers. Depending on the clinical situation, ulcer location, and type of complication, procedures such as vagotomy, vagotomy with antrectomy, or distal gastrectomy can be performed. In patients with Zollinger-Ellison syndrome, surgical management involves localization and removal of the gastrinoma. Finally, in Ménétrier's disease, gastric resection may be indicated for cases of intractable bleeding, severe hypoproteinemia, or, rarely, concomitant malignancy.[2]

What the Referring Physician Needs to Know

- Benign mucosal diseases of the stomach typically present as nonspecific symptoms, including epigastric/abdominal pain.
- The most common causes include peptic ulcer disease as well as infection with *H. pylori* and NSAID-induced gastritis.
- Endoscopy and double-contrast barium upper gastrointestinal studies are the most likely to detect an underlying abnormality.
- When a patient has a known diagnosis (e.g., gastric ulcer disease or Zollinger-Ellison syndrome), other imaging modalities may be useful.

KEY POINTS

- The most useful imaging technique for the diagnosis of gastric mucosal disease is the double-contrast barium upper gastrointestinal study.
- CT can be useful in further evaluating known ulcers as well as in imaging the acute complications such as perforation and gastric outlet obstruction.

SUGGESTED READINGS

Cello JP. *Helicobacter pylori* and peptic ulcer disease. AJR Am J Roentgenol 1995; 164:283-286.

Chen CY, Wu DC, Kuo YT, et al. MDCT for differentiation of category T1 and T2 malignant lesions from benign gastric ulcers. AJR Am J Roentgenol 2008; 190:1505-1511.

Harned RK, Buck JL, Sobin LH. The hamartomatous polyposis syndromes: clinical and radiologic features. AJR Am J Roentgenol 1995; 164: 565-571.

Levine MS, Ekberg O, Rubesin SE, Gatenby RA. Gastrointestinal sarcoidosis: radiographic findings. AJR Am J Roentgenol 1989; 153: 293-295.

Levine MS, Laufer I. The upper gastrointestinal series at a crossroads. AJR Am J Roentgenol 1993; 161:1131-1137.

Levine MS, Verstandig A, Laufer I. Serpiginous gastric erosions caused by aspirin and other nonsteroidal antiinflammatory drugs. AJR Am J Roentgenol 1986; 146:31-34.

Rourke JA, Tomchik FS. Diffuse gastric abnormality—benign or malignant? Am J Roentgenol Radium Ther Nucl Med 1966; 96: 400-407.

Thompson G, Somers S, Stevenson GW. Benign gastric ulcer: a reliable radiologic diagnosis? AJR Am J Roentgenol 1983; 141:331-333.

REFERENCES

1. Valle JD. Peptic ulcer disease and related disorders. In Fauci AS, Braunwald E, Kasper DL, et al (eds). Harrison's Principles of Internal Medicine, 17th edition. New York, McGraw-Hill, 2008.

2. Dempsey DT. Stomach. In Brunicardi FC, Andersen DK, Billiar TR, et al (eds). Schwartz's Principles of Surgery, 8th ed. New York, McGraw-Hill, 2008.

3. Cello JP. *Helicobacter pylori* and peptic ulcer disease. AJR Am J Roentgenol 1995; 164:283-286.

4. Levine MS, Verstandig A, Laufer I. Serpiginous gastric erosions caused by aspirin and other nonsteroidal antiinflammatory drugs. AJR Am J Roentgenol 1986; 146:31-34.

5. Farman J, Faegenburg D, Dallemand S, Chen CK. Crohn's disease of the stomach: the "ram's horn" sign. Am J Roentgenol Radium Ther Nucl Med 1975; 123:242-251.

6. Nelson SW. Some interesting and unusual manifestations of Crohn's disease ("regional enteritis") of the stomach, duodenum and small intestine. Am J Roentgenol Radium Ther Nucl Med 1969; 107: 86-101.

7. Levine MS, Ekberg O, Rubesin SE, Gatenby RA. Gastrointestinal sarcoidosis: radiographic findings. AJR Am J Roentgenol 1989; 153:293-295.

8. Gold BM, Bagla S, Zarrabi MH. Radiologic manifestations of Cowden disease. AJR Am J Roentgenol 1980; 135:385-387.

9. Harned RK, Buck JL, Sobin LH. The hamartomatous polyposis syndromes: clinical and radiologic features. AJR Am J Roentgenol 1995; 164:565-571.

10. Jones BV, Lichtenstein JE. Gastric syphilis: radiologic findings. AJR Am J Roentgenol 1993; 160:59-61.

11. Burhenne HJ, Carbone JV. Eosinophilic (allergic) gastroenteritis. Am J Roentgenol Radium Ther Nucl Med 1966; 96:332-338.

12. Joffe N, Antonioli DA. Atypical appearances of benign hyperplastic gastric polyps. AJR Am J Roentgenol 1978; 131:147-152.

13. Miller JH, Gisvold JJ, Weiland LH, McIlrath DC. Upper gastrointestinal tract: villous tumors. AJR Am J Roentgenol 1980; 134:933-936.

14. Wong-Kee-Song L, Topazian M. Gastrointestinal endoscopy. In Fauci AS, Braunwald E, Kasper DL, et al (eds). Harrison's Principles of

Internal Medicine, 17th ed. New York, McGraw-Hill, 2008, pp 1836-1846.

15. Spiller RC. ABC of the upper gastrointestinal tract: anorexia, nausea, vomiting, and pain. BMJ 2001; 323:1354-1357.

16. Thompson G, Somers S, Stevenson GW. Benign gastric ulcer: a reliable radiologic diagnosis? AJR Am J Roentgenol 1983; 141: 331-333.

17. Chen CY, Wu DC, Kuo YT, et al. MDCT for differentiation of category T1 and T2 malignant lesions from benign gastric ulcers. AJR Am J Roentgenol 2008; 190:1505-1511.

18. Hasler WL, Owyang C. Approach to the patient with gastrointestinal disease. In Fauci AS, Braunwald E, Kasper DL, et al (eds). Harrison's Principles of Internal Medicine, 17th ed. New York, McGraw-Hill, 2008, pp 1847-1854.

19. Thrall JH, Zeissman HA. Nuclear Medicine, The Requisites. St. Louis, CV Mosby, 2001.

20. Stone DD, Riddervold HO, Keats TE. An unusual case of aberrant pancreas in the stomach: a roentgenographic and gastrophotographic demonstration. Am J Roentgenol Radium Ther Nucl Med 1971; 113:125-128.

21. Rohrmann CA Jr, Delaney JH Jr, Protell RL. Heterotopic pancreas diagnosed by cannulation and duct study. AJR Am J Roentgenol 1977; 128:1044-1045.

22. Besemann EF, Auerbach SH, Wolfe WW. The importance of roentgenologic diagnosis of aberrant pancreatic tissue in the gastrointestinal tract. Am J Roentgenol Radium Ther Nucl Med 1969; 107:71-76.

23. Cherukuri R, Levine MS, Furth EE, et al. Giant hyperplastic polyps in the stomach: radiographic findings in seven patients. AJR Am J Roentgenol 2000; 175:1445-1448.

24. Prabhakar HB, Sahani DV, Fischman AJ, et al. Bowel hot spots at PET-CT. RadioGraphics 2007; 27:145-159.

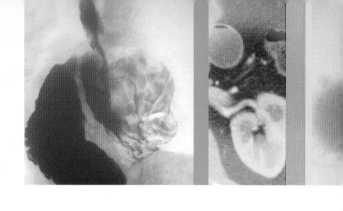

CHAPTER 34

Malignant Mucosal Diseases of the Stomach

Hima B. Prabhakar and Anand M. Prabhakar

ETIOLOGY

Malignant mucosal processes can have similar manifestations as benign disease, and it is helpful to categorize them according to their most common presentations. Overall, there is considerable overlap in the presentation of malignant gastric diseases because the major diseases—gastric adenocarcinoma, lymphoma, and metastatic disease—can all present as any of the radiologic manifestations described here. Classifying these processes by their different mucosal manifestations—ulcer, polyp/mass, and diffuse mucosal processes—yields the following causes:

Ulcers: Malignant gastric ulcer secondary to gastric adenocarcinoma, lymphoma, carcinoid, metastatic disease from melanoma, lung, adenocarcinoma, Kaposi's sarcoma
Polyps/masses: Gastric carcinoma, carcinoid
Diffuse mucosal processes: linitis plastica (gastric carcinoma, lymphoma, metastatic disease especially from breast cancer), Ménétrier's disease with associated adenocarcinoma

PREVALENCE AND EPIDEMIOLOGY

Both primary and metastatic malignancy can affect the stomach. Primary malignancies include adenocarcinoma (95%), lymphoma (4%), and gastrointestinal stromal tumors (GIST) (1%). Of metastatic malignancies, direct invasion from adjacent tumors of the pancreas or colon is more common than hematogenous metastases such as those from carcinoma of the breast and melanoma. Of these, malignancies that can affect the gastric mucosa include adenocarcinoma, lymphoma, and hematogenous metastases.[1]

Overall, the incidence of gastric malignancy has decreased over the past century. In the early 1900s, gastric cancer was the leading cause of death in men in the United States, whereas today it is not in the top 10. However, while the incidence has decreased in the West, gastric cancer is still relatively common in Asia and Eastern Europe, representing the second most common cancer. The highest prevalence occurs in Costa Rica, Japan, and the republics of the former Soviet Union, whereas the lowest prevalence is in the United States and parts of Africa and Southeast Asia.[2] Overall, prognosis is poor, with 5-year survival at 22%, a statistic that has not changed significantly in the past 30 years.[1,2]

Causes of gastric adenocarcinoma are unclear, but epidemiologic studies have pointed to diet (low in fruits/vegetables, high in nitrates/salt) as a factor. Additionally, *Helicobacter pylori* infection has been implicated in the increased risk of both adenocarcinoma and lymphoma. Genetic mutations, including those seen with Li-Fraumeni syndrome and hereditary nonpolyposis colorectal cancer, increase the risk for gastric malignancy.[1-3]

Unlike adenocarcinoma, the incidence of gastric lymphoma has been increasing. Similar to adenocarcinoma, infection with *H. pylori* is a risk factor and there can be significant regression of lymphomatous involvement with antibiotic treatment. Staging for gastric lymphoma, which is almost always the B-cell non-Hodgkin's type, is the same as for non-Hodgkin's lymphoma.[2]

CLINICAL PRESENTATION

Epigastric pain and weight loss are common presenting symptoms in patients with stomach mucosal disease from a variety of causes, both benign and malignant. In general, symptomatic patients present with advanced disease. Patients may also present with occult gastrointestinal bleeding or anemia, but overt bleeding is seen in only 20% of patients.[1,2,4,5]

NORMAL ANATOMY

There are four layers of the gastric wall: mucosa, submucosa, muscularis propria, and serosa. The mucosa is the innermost layer and is lined with columnar glandular epithelium. Depending on the location within the stomach, there are different types of epithelial cells that line the gastric glands as well as endocrine cells. Additionally, there are mucus-secreting cells that extend into the glands and produce bicarbonate to protect the stomach from acid injury. Overall, the layers that make up the gastric mucosa are the epithelium, lamina propria, and muscularis mucosa. The mucosa and submucosa comprise the gastric rugae, which stretch out as the stomach distends.[1]

PATHOLOGY

Gastric adenocarcinoma, which comprises 95% of gastric malignancies, is generally divided into two broad categories: type I (intestinal) and type II (diffuse). Type I adenocarcinoma is generally well differentiated, contains distinct glandular elements, is typically found in older male patients, and carries a better prognosis. Type II adenocarcinoma is poorly differentiated, is infiltrative, is found in younger/female patients, and carries a worse prognosis.[2]

Gastric lymphoma, although less common, is the most common extranodal site for lymphomatous involvement. Almost all cases of gastric lymphoma are B-cell non-Hodgkin's type. These can include both well-differentiated superficial mucosa-associated lymphoid tissue (MALT) type lymphoma as well as high-grade large cell lymphoma.[3]

IMAGING

Malignant Mucosal Disease

There is considerable overlap in the clinical presentation of benign and malignant mucosal processes of the stomach. As stated previously, these symptoms most commonly include epigastric pain, weight loss, food avoidance, and anemia. Depending on risk factors, which are themselves poorly understood, the clinician can decide whether initial testing will involve double-contrast barium radiography or endoscopic evaluation. Generally, because it is easier and less invasive to perform double-contrast barium radiography, this is often the initial test ordered.[3,4]

Radiography

Double-contrast barium radiography is often recommended as the first method of evaluation for patients presenting with a wide variety of epigastric/abdominal complaints. When mucosal abnormalities are present, they generally fall into one of three main categories: ulcers, polyps/masses, or diffuse mucosal disease. These three categories include numerous benign and malignant causes in the differential diagnosis, and most often the patient must undergo endoscopic evaluation and biopsy for definitive diagnosis. There are, however, classically described findings in benign and malignant ulcers that may suggest a cause.

The goal of double-contrast barium radiography in the evaluation of mucosal ulcerations is to distinguish benign from malignant ulcers. As stated in Chapter 33, benign ulcers have been classically described as round, with thin mucosal folds radiating to the crater surface as well as projecting outside the gastric lumen. In contrast, malignant ulcers have nodular, irregular radiating folds that do not extend to the ulcer crater (ulcerated mass) and lie within the stomach wall. Using these criteria, those ulcers that clearly fall within the benign category do not need endoscopic confirmation according to the radiology literature.[6,7] However, it is still recommended in the internal medicine literature that all ulcers undergo endoscopic evaluation to confirm benignity.[3,4]

In patients with mucosal polyps or masses seen on double-contrast barium radiography, the majority are benign hyperplastic/inflammatory polyps (see Chapter 33). However, because a percentage of these polyps are adenomatous and cannot be distinguished from hyperplastic polyps, endoscopic removal is recommended to exclude premalignant lesions. Villous polyps have a higher rate of malignancy (55%) and are removed endoscopically or surgically when found.[8]

Thickened gastric folds and other diffuse mucosal presentations can have a variety of causes. In general, thickened, irregular, tortuous folds invoke an infiltrative etiology, such as adenocarcinoma (Fig. 34-1), lymphoma, or metastatic disease. However, there is overlap with other conditions such as Ménétrier's disease, which can be benign or associated with other malignancies (Fig. 34-2). Nondistensibility of the stomach is not helpful because it can be seen with scirrhous carcinoma and metastatic disease as well as benign causes such as Crohn's disease and syphilis. When any of these findings are seen at double-contrast barium radiography, they should trigger further evaluation for the underlying cause.[9-11]

CT

Although most useful in the staging and follow-up for gastric malignancy, multidetector CT with virtual gastroscopy has been used to differentiate benign from malignant ulcers. Using ulcer shape, wall thickness, and enhancement as criteria, in conjunction with multiplanar reconstruction images, Chen and colleagues were able to demonstrate 80% sensitivity and 100% specificity in differentiating benign from malignant ulcers.[12]

More commonly, CT is used in the staging of known gastric malignancy or in the evaluation of complications. When a patient presents acutely with abdominal pain, CT is often the first test ordered. In these cases, patients who demonstrate perforation, obstruction (Figs. 34-3 and 34-4), or hemorrhage are surgically treated and the underlying cause (malignant or benign) can be determined. In patients with diffuse disease, such as extensive gastric wall thickening, the presence of extragastric disease will point to a malignant cause over a benign one (Fig. 34-5).[13-15] Additionally, when the primary gastric cancer is not evident, multidetector CT can be useful in excluding advanced disease and allow for a less invasive treatment to be considered.[16]

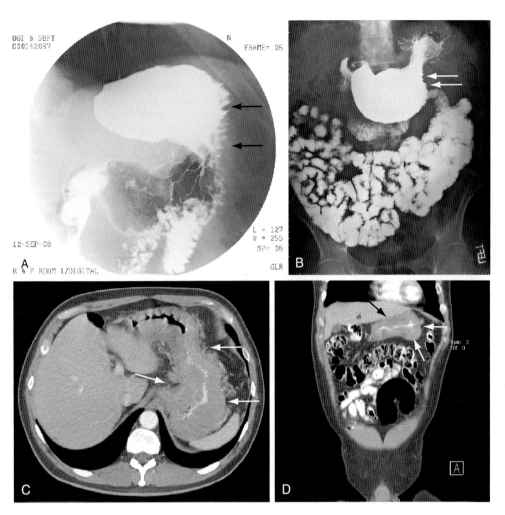

■ **FIGURE 34-1** Linitis plastica appearance of the stomach secondary to gastric adenocarcinoma. **A** and **B,** Double-contrast barium radiography demonstrates limited distensibility and thickened gastric folds (*arrows*). **C** and **D,** Axial and coronal CT images enhanced with intravenous and oral contrast agents show marked gastric wall thickening (*arrows*) with limited gastric distensibility.

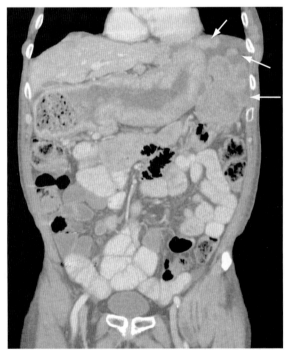

■ **FIGURE 34-2** Ménétrier's disease associated with nongastric adenocarcinoma. Coronal CT image enhanced with intravenous and oral contrast agents shows marked gastric wall thickening and associated enhancing soft tissues masses (*arrows*) in the left upper quadrant. Biopsy revealed gastric changes consistent with Ménétrier's disease, and the adjacent mass was consistent with adenocarcinoma.

MRI

MRI can be useful in evaluating indeterminate hepatic lesions in patients with known malignancy.

Ultrasonography

Ultrasonography can play a role in the evaluation of gastric metastases to the liver as well as in ultrasound-guided biopsy of suspected parenchymal or lymph node metastases.

Ultrasound evaluation of the patient with gastric lymphoma may be useful in defining different patterns of disease. For example, ultrasonographic patterns that have been described include circumferential, segmental, bulky, and extranodal. Unfortunately, these patterns have limited utility in staging.[17]

Nuclear Medicine

Whereas gallium-67 has been used in the past for staging lymphoma and abdominal/pelvic tumors, its sensitivity is low and it has been mostly replaced by fluorodeoxyglucose (FDG)-labeled PET.[18]

PET/CT

FDG-PET has been shown to be sensitive in the detection of gastric malignancy as well as in the staging of both

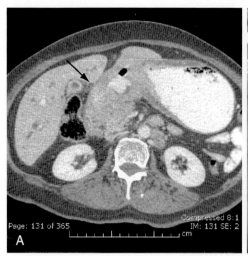 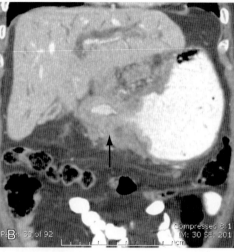

■ **FIGURE 34-3** Gastric adenocarcinoma causing gastric outlet obstruction. **A** and **B,** Axial and coronal CT images enhanced with intravenous and oral contrast agents show marked gastric wall thickening of the distal stomach (*arrows*), with distention of the proximal stomach, consistent with gastric outlet obstruction. Currently, malignancy is the most common cause of gastric outlet obstruction.

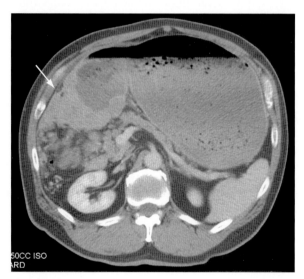

■ **FIGURE 34-4** Gastric lymphoma causing gastric outlet obstruction. Axial CT image enhanced with intravenous and oral contrast agents shows distal gastric wall thickening (*arrow*) with gastric outlet obstruction. This case is not easily distinguishable from that in Figure 34-3 and demonstrates the importance of biopsy.

adenocarcinoma and lymphoma. It is not useful in the initial detection of disease unless the patient is undergoing staging for another malignancy, and gastric metastatic involvement is not suspected.[19] Additionally, after treatment, FDG-PET is useful in evaluating for recurrence, lymph node metastases, and distant metastatic disease. Specificity is increased when FDG-PET/CT is used.[20-23]

Imaging Algorithm

Patients presenting with nonspecific complaint of epigastric pain/weight loss should undergo double-contrast barium radiography or CT for further evaluation, depending on the clinical suspicion for underlying disease (Table 34-1). If an abnormality is detected, the patient should undergo endoscopic evaluation to exclude malignancy, unless the radiographic signs of benignity are all characteristically present.

DIFFERENTIAL DIAGNOSIS

Abdominal pain and weight loss are typical presenting symptoms of gastric malignancy, but these can also be

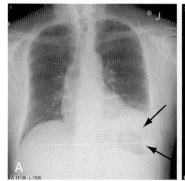 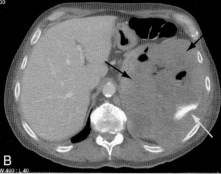 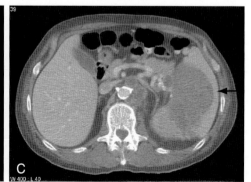

■ **FIGURE 34-5** Gastric lymphoma invading the spleen. **A,** Posteroanterior view of the chest shows nodular gastric wall thickening (*arrows*). **B** and **C,** Axial CT images enhanced with intravenous and oral contrast show marked gastric wall thickening, with invasion of the spleen (*arrows*). Note the small amount of oral contrast agent within the stomach lumen, which is grossly distorted (*yellow arrow*).

TABLE 34-1 Accuracy, Limitations, and Pitfalls of the Modalities Used in Imaging of Malignant Mucosal Diseases of the Stomach

Modality	Accuracy	Limitations	Pitfalls
Radiography	With an experienced radiologist, double-contrast barium upper gastrointestinal studies can identify different patterns of mucosal involvement.	Benign and atypical/malignant causes can be difficult to differentiate.	Small ulcers or diffuse disease may be difficult to detect.
CT	MDCT with virtual gastroscopy may be useful in differentiating benign and malignant ulcers. CT is important in staging gastric malignancy and follow-up for treatment.	CT is not sensitive or specific for gastric mucosal disease and is better for evaluation of late complications.	Benign and malignant causes can have similar appearance, especially if there is significant edema or late complications.
PET/CT	Excellent modality for the staging and follow-up of gastric malignancies such as adenocarcinoma and lymphoma, as well as metastatic disease.		

Classic Signs

- Carman's meniscus sign (malignant ulcer): semicircular (meniscoid) configuration of a gastric ulcer seen in profile with compression[6]
- Bull's-eye ulcer (metastatic melanoma, lymphoma): mass with central ulceration in a bull's-eye configuration that may be solitary or multiple[11]

---

seen in benign disorders (gastritis, benign ulcer disease, gastroparesis/gastric outlet obstruction). Clinical diagnosis rests on patient symptom correlation with risk factors, such as chronic gastritis/*H. pylori* infection, family history, smoking, and a diet rich in nitrates.[1]

As with benign mucosal diseases, differential diagnoses can be categorized by the primary radiologic manifestations: ulcers, polyps/masses, and diffuse mucosal processes. The differential diagnosis was listed previously under Etiology.

TREATMENT

Medical Treatment

Adjuvant chemotherapy with 5-fluorouracil and leucovorin, in conjunction with irradiation and gastrectomy, has been shown to increase survival in patients with stage II and III gastric adenocarcinoma. Chemotherapeutic agents that have some effectiveness against gastric adenocarcinoma include 5-fluorouracil, methotrexate, doxorubicin, and cisplatin.[2] Additionally, in Japan, there has been some success with endoscopic resection of small (<2 cm) malignancies confined to the mucosa and without evidence of metastatic disease. Palliative chemotherapy and/or irradiation has not been shown to improve survival but may alleviate pain and bleeding.[1]

In patients with gastric lymphoma there has been some recent success with primary chemotherapy and irradiation. Bleeding and perforation complications are higher with this approach than when it is done in conjunction with surgery.[1]

Surgical Treatment

Surgery (gastric resection) can be curative in patients with localized gastric adenocarcinoma who are good surgical candidates, although this accounts for less than a third of patients.[3] Even in patients with progressive disease, those experiencing complications such as ulcer perforation or gastric outlet obstruction or requiring palliative treatment will benefit from surgical management. The goal of surgical management is to remove all of the tumor and perform lymphadenectomy to assess for metastases. Frozen section evaluation of tumor margins is important because many gastric tumors are infiltrative.[1]

In patients with gastric lymphoma, gastrectomy is useful in the treatment of bulky disease. Interestingly, however, treatment for *H. pylori* disease can lead to regression of 75% of cases of gastric MALT lymphoma. In these cases, patients should be treated with antibiotics before consideration of surgery, chemotherapy, and irradiation.[3] More recently, however, primary chemotherapy with radiation has shown good results, but there is increased risk of perforation and bleeding. Typically, surgery with adjuvant chemotherapy has been the main treatment.[1]

What the Referring Physician Needs to Know

- Presenting clinical symptoms of gastric malignancies are nonspecific and can mimic benign disease.
- Although radiologic diagnosis may be possible in select cases, the role of imaging is more important in the staging and follow-up of malignancy, as well as in the evaluation of potential complications.

KEY POINTS

- The double-contrast barium upper gastrointestinal series may be the initial test in patients presenting with epigastric pain.
- Once a gastric mucosal process is diagnosed, the patient should undergo endoscopic evaluation/biopsy because malignant mucosal disease can mimic benign ulcers/masses. Additionally, benign causes of linitis plastica are not distinguishable from malignant causes.

SUGGESTED READINGS

Chen CY, Wu DC, Kuo YT, et al. MDCT for differentiation of category T1 and T2 malignant lesions from benign gastric ulcers. AJR Am J Roentgenol 2008; 190:1505-1511.

Kanne JP, Mankoff DA, Baird GS, et al. Gastric linitis plastica from metastatic breast carcinoma: FDG and FES PET appearances. AJR Am J Roentgenol 2007; 188:W503-W505.

Levine MS, Laufer I. The upper gastrointestinal series at a crossroads. AJR Am J Roentgenol 1993; 161:1131-1137.

Prabhakar HB, Sahani DV, Fischman AJ, et al. Bowel hot spots at PET-CT. RadioGraphics 2007; 27:145-159.

Rourke JA, Tomchik FS. Diffuse gastric abnormality—benign or malignant? Am J Roentgenol Radium Ther Nucl Med 1966; 96:400-407.

Yoshioka T, Yamaguchi K, Kubota K, et al. Evaluation of ^{18}F-FDG PET in patients with advanced, metastatic, or recurrent gastric cancer. J Nucl Med 2003; 44:690-699.

REFERENCES

1. Dempsey DT. Stomach. In Brunicardi FC, et al (eds). Schwartz's Principles of Surgery, 8th ed. New York, McGraw-Hill, 2005, pp 181-188.

2. Phan AT, Yao JC, Allam SR, et al. Carcinoma of the esophagus and gastric carcinoma. In Kantarjian HM, Wolff RA, Koller CA (eds). MD Anderson Manual of Medical Oncology. New York, McGraw-Hill, 2006.

3. Mayer RJ. Gastrointestinal tract cancer. In Fauci AS, Braunwald E, Kasper DL, et al (eds). Harrison's Principles of Internal Medicine, 17th ed. New York, McGraw-Hill, 2008, pp 570-579.

4. Hasler WL, Owyang C. Approach to the patient with gastrointestinal disease. In Fauci AS, et al (eds). Harrison's Principles of Internal Medicine, 17th ed. New York, McGraw-Hill, 2008, pp 1831-1835.

5. Spiller RC. ABC of the upper gastrointestinal tract: anorexia, nausea, vomiting, and pain. BMJ 2001; 323:1354-1357.

6. Low VH, Levine MS, Rubesin SE, et al. Diagnosis of gastric carcinoma: sensitivity of double-contrast barium studies. AJR Am J Roentgenol 1994; 162:329-334.

7. Thompson G, Somers S, Stevenson GW. Benign gastric ulcer: a reliable radiologic diagnosis? AJR Am J Roentgenol 1983; 141:331-333.

8. Miller JH, Gisvold JJ, Weiland LH, McIlrath DC. Upper gastrointestinal tract: villous tumors. AJR Am J Roentgenol 1980; 134:933-936.

9. Balthazar EJ, Davidian MM. Hyperrugosity in gastric carcinoma: radiographic, endoscopic, and pathologic features. AJR Am J Roentgenol 1981; 136:531-535.

10. Bragg DG, Seaman WB, Lattes R. Roentgenologic and pathologic aspects of superficial spreading carcinoma of the stomach. Am J Roentgenol Radium Ther Nucl Med 1967; 101:437-446.

11. Rourke JA, Tomchik FS. Diffuse gastric abnormality—benign or malignant? Am J Roentgenol Radium Ther Nucl Med 1966; 96:400-407.

12. Chen CY, Wu DC, Kuo YT, et al. MDCT for differentiation of category T1 and T2 malignant lesions from benign gastric ulcers. AJR Am J Roentgenol 2008; 190:1505-1511.

13. Balthazar EJ, Siegel SE, Megibow AJ, et al. CT in patients with scirrhous carcinoma of the GI tract: imaging findings and value for tumor detection and staging. AJR Am J Roentgenol 1995; 165:839-845.

14. Buy JN, Moss AA. Computed tomography of gastric lymphoma. AJR Am J Roentgenol 1982; 138:859-865.

15. Park MS, Kim KW, Yu JS, et al. Radiographic findings of primary B-cell lymphoma of the stomach: low-grade versus high-grade malignancy in relation to the mucosa-associated lymphoid tissue concept. AJR Am J Roentgenol 2002; 179:1297-1304.

16. Yu JS, Choi SH, Choi WH, et al. Value of nonvisualized primary lesions of gastric cancer on preoperative MDCT. AJR Am J Roentgenol 2007; 189:W315-W319.

17. Goerg C, Schwerk WB, Goerg K. Gastrointestinal lymphoma: sonographic findings in 54 patients. AJR Am J Roentgenol 1990; 155:795-798.

18. Thrall JH, Zeissman HA. Nuclear Medicine, The Requisites. St. Louis, Mosby, 2001.

19. Kanne JP, Mankoff DA, Baird GS, et al. Gastric linitis plastica from metastatic breast carcinoma: FDG and FES PET appearances. AJR Am J Roentgenol 2007; 188:W503-W505.

20. Lim JS, Yun MJ, Kim MJ, et al. CT and PET in stomach cancer: preoperative staging and monitoring of response to therapy. RadioGraphics 2006; 26:143-156.

21. McAteer D, Wallis F, Couper G, et al. Evaluation of ^{18}F-FDG positron emission tomography in gastric and oesophageal carcinoma. Br J Radiol 1999; 72:525-529.

22. Prabhakar HB, Sahani DV, Fischman AJ, et al. Bowel hot spots at PET-CT. RadioGraphics 2007; 27:145-159.

23. Yoshioka T, Yamaguchi K, Kubota K, et al. Evaluation of ^{18}F-FDG PET in patients with advanced, metastatic, or recurrent gastric cancer. J Nucl Med 2003; 44:690-699.

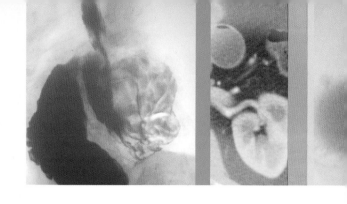

35

Gastric Stromal Tumors

Anand M. Prabhakar and Hima B. Prabhakar

INTRODUCTION

Stromal tumors of the stomach are rare tumors that arise from the mesenchymal tissue of the stomach. The mesenchyma represents the connective tissue and blood vessels that support an organ. The parenchyma, on the other hand, represents the functional tissue of the organ. Within the stomach, the parenchyma includes the epithelial glandular tissue within the mucosa and the mesenchyma consists of the supporting tissues, or stroma. The components of the stroma include smooth muscle cells, nerve cells, lipocytes, vascular structures, and epithelioid cells. Gastric stromal tumors arise from each of these cell types.

PREVALENCE AND EPIDEMIOLOGY

The prevalence of gastric stromal tumors varies by type. The most common is the gastrointestinal stromal tumor (GIST), with 10 to 20 cases per million persons, representing 5000 to 6000 cases in the United States annually. GISTs make up 2% to 3% of all gastric tumors.[1] Lipomas represent 2% to 3% of benign gastric tumors, neurogenic tumors account for 4%, and vascular tumors comprise 2%. The remainder of the gastric stromal tumors are exceedingly rare.

There is an increased risk of GIST with neurofibromatosis, Carney's syndrome, and germline mutations of *KIT*. No other specific associations have been described.[1]

CLINICAL PRESENTATION

Gastrointestinal bleeding (33%) and abdominal pain (19%) are the most common presenting symptoms associated with GIST.[2] Anemia, hematochezia, hematemesis, abdominal bloating, abdominal pain, palpable mass, and abdominal distention are additional features.

PATHOLOGY

Historically, GISTs were referred to as leiomyoma, leiomyosarcoma, epithelioid leiomyosarcoma, and leiomyoblastomas, based on the thought that the tumors arise from smooth muscle cells.[1] However, it is now felt that GISTs arise from the interstitial cell of Cajal, which is a primitive gut stem cell in the muscularis propria that expresses KIT, a tyrosine kinase receptor. Distinguishing GIST from other stromal tumors is by the expression of KIT and 95% of GISTs express KIT. Mutations in KIT are felt to be responsible for cell proliferation and resistance to apoptosis. Immunohistochemistry stains are positive for KIT (CD117) and are diagnostic of GIST.[1] The expression of KIT in GIST is the premise behind medical therapy.

GISTs can be benign or malignant. The determination of a benign or malignant GIST is based on the number of mitoses observed per high-power field. Malignant GISTs can recur and metastasize to the liver and peritoneal surface, with distant metastasis being rare. Metastatic GIST do not present with lymphadenopathy.[1] Therefore, if lymphadenopathy is present, other malignant tumors, such as adenocarcinoma and lymphoma, should be considered.

Other gastric stromal tumors are diagnosed histologically. Schwannomas stain positive for S-100 protein.[3] True leiomyomas and leiomyosarcomas arise from smooth muscle cells and are rare in the stomach.[1]

IMAGING

Seventy percent of GISTs are found in the stomach (Fig. 35-1), and 75% of these are found in the body. GISTs can also be found anywhere from the esophagus to the anus and also can arise from the mesentery, retroperitoneum, and omentum. The second most common site of presentation is within the small bowel representing 20% to 30% of cases.[1] Other stromal tumors mimic the appearance of GIST and should be considered in the differential diagnosis.

Radiography

GISTs may present on plain radiographs as abdominal mass effect and only rarely calcification can be appreciated. Stromal tumors are submucosal masses on barium studies of the stomach and are smoothly marginated and form obtuse angles with the stomach wall.[1]

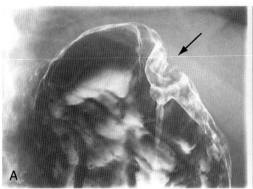
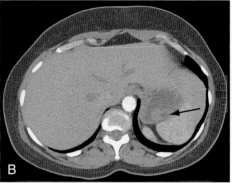

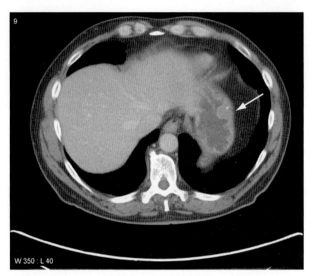

■ **FIGURE 35-2** Contrast-enhanced CT shows an intraluminal stomach mass with a punctate focus of calcification (*arrow*), later determined to be a GIST.

CT

On CT, GISTs are usually peripherally contrast enhancing and will often have extragastric and intragastric components. Given their size, it is often difficult to determine which portion of the bowel the GIST arises from, but subtle bowel wall thickening can be a clue. Cavitation and calcification can be present, but are not common (Fig. 35-2).[1]

No definite imaging criteria have been established to distinguish benign from malignant GIST. Initially, it was found that besides evidence of metastatic disease, only size greater than 5 cm was predictive of malignancy.[4] Recently, however, it has been suggested that heterogeneous enhancement and a cystic-necrotic component can be found with a GIST with malignant potential.[5] Metastatic disease from GISTs are often confined to the liver and mesentery, with predominantly hypervascular metastasis.[5]

Gastric adenocarcinoma and lymphoma do not often have extragastric components and that can be used as a clue for diagnosis. Other benign stromal tumors are much rarer, and imaging characteristics are nonspecific, but are also on the differential diagnosis. However, gastric schwannomas, for example, may be suspected if there is homogenous enhancement of a well-circumscribed mass.[3]

A smooth, well-circumscribed mass measuring −70 to −120 Hounsfield units is diagnostic of gastric lipoma.[6]

MRI

The MRI appearance of GISTs mimics that of CT. The lesions will usually have increased T1 signal in the solid areas and increased T2 signal in the cystic areas. The mass can be heterogeneous due to the presence of hemorrhage. GISTs usually enhance with intravenous administration of gadolinium and also demonstrate hypervascular metastases.[7]

Uniformly high T1 signal in a submucosal mass is consistent with a lipoma.[8] Only a single case of MRI of gastric schwannoma has been reported, which described uniform enhancement of a lobulated, low T1 signal, high T2 signal well-circumscribed mass.[9]

PET/CT

GISTs and metastases generally demonstrate high fluorodeoxyglucose (FDG) activity.[10] PET has been utilized for both staging and follow-up for treatment of GIST (Fig. 35-3).[10] PET is especially helpful in monitoring the response to imatinib (Gleevac). In patients treated with imatinib, marked decrease in FDG activity has been observed shortly after treatment is initiated, further described in the medical treatment section.

TREATMENT

Medical Treatment

Historically, the medical treatment for metastatic or unresectable GIST involved cytotoxic chemotherapy. However, results generally have been poor. Currently, the mainstay of medical therapy is with imatinib. Imatinib is a tyrosine kinase inhibitor that selectively inhibits KIT, as well as certain other tyrosine kinases. It has been used classically in the treatment of chronic myeloid leukemia. Because many GISTs overexpress KIT, targeted medical therapy with imatinib is now being utilized. This drug has been shown to cause significant tumor regression with only mild to moderate side effects.[11] Imatinib is indicated in patients with KIT and GISTs that are metastatic or surgically unresectable.[12] Currently, imatinib is being investigated for utility in post-resection adjuvant therapy, based

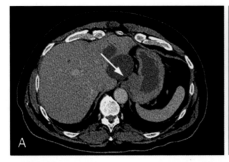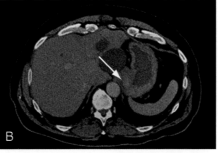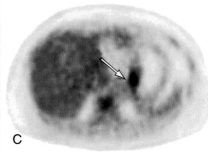

■ **FIGURE 35-3** Gastric mass. A 67-year-old man presented with an incidentally detected gastric mass on upper endoscopic evaluation for a guaiac-positive stool. Axial CT (**A**), axial fused PET/CT (**B**), and axial PET (**C**) images show increased FDG uptake corresponding to a proximal soft tissue gastric mass seen on CT (*arrows*). Biopsy of the mass revealed a GIST.

on the grading of the tumor.[11] Recently, it has been found that patients can show resistance to imatinib. In these patients, another tyrosine kinase inhibitor, sunitinib (Sutent) has been approved for treatment.[13]

After treatment with imatinib, primary tumor and metastatic lesions can become cystic.[14,15] On follow-up CT examinations, enhancing nodules or peripheral thickening, even without an increase in size, can represent progression and may suggest lack of response to imatinib.[16] PET/CT shows a marked reduction in activity of primary and malignant GISTs even after one dose of imatinib, months before CT changes are detected. Response has even been shown on PET/CT even after 24 hours of a single dose.[17-19] A lack of decrease in activity suggests that the tumors are resistant to imatinib.[10]

Surgical Treatment

Despite the medical therapy advances, the main treatment of GIST continues to be surgery, especially in localized, resectable cases.[20] Complete surgical resection can be accomplished in 40% to 60% of patients. The location of the tumor often determines the surgical approach. Tumors near the gastric cardia or pylorus are treated with open surgical resection, whereas tumors from other areas of the stomach are often treated with laparoscopic resection. CT gastrography may help in defining the location of the

tumor.[21] Neoadjuvant therapy with imatinib can be considered in patients where reducing the size of the tumor would improve surgical morbidity.[22] Adjuvant therapy with imatinib is utilized in patients with high-grade tumors. Patients should be observed at regular intervals to detect recurrence. Current research is aimed at stratifying patients into surgical and medical treatment based on tumor status and new targeted agents.

What the Referring Physician Needs to Know

■ Radiologic staging of GIST may impact the surgical and medical management, especially with regard to metastatic disease.

KEY POINTS

■ GISTs are exophytic masses that may occur anywhere from the esophagus to the anus and predominantly arise from the stomach.
■ Surgery is the usual treatment modality with adjuvant therapy with imatinib if indicated. Follow-up imaging with PET/CT and CT is helpful for determining the response to therapy.

SUGGESTED READINGS

Levy AD, Remotti HE, Thompson WM, et al. Gastrointestinal stromal tumors: radiologic features with pathologic correlation. RadioGraphics 2003; 23:283-304.

REFERENCES

1. Levy AD, Remotti HE, Thompson WM, et al. Gastrointestinal stromal tumors: radiologic features with pathologic correlation. RadioGraphics 2003; 23:283-304.
2. Scarpa M, Bertin M, Ruffolo C, et al. A systematic review on the clinical diagnosis of gastrointestinal stromal tumors. J Surg Oncol 2008; 98:384-392.
3. Levy AD, Quiles AM, Miettinen M, Sobin LH. Gastrointestinal schwannomas: CT features with clinicopathologic correlation. AJR Am J Roentgenol 2005; 184:797-802.
4. Kim HC, Lee JM, Kim KW, et al. Gastrointestinal stromal tumors of the stomach: CT findings and prediction of malignancy. AJR Am J Roentgenol 2004; 183:893-898.
5. Ulusan S, Koc Z, Kayaselcuk F. Gastrointestinal stromal tumours: CT findings. Br J Radiol 2008; 81:618-623.
6. Thompson WM, Kende AI, Levy AD. Imaging characteristics of gastric lipomas in 16 adult and pediatric patients. AJR Am J Roentgenol 2003; 181:981-985.
7. Sandrasegaran K, Rajesh A, Rushing DA, et al. Gastrointestinal stromal tumors: CT and MRI findings. Eur Radiol 2005; 15:1407-1414.
8. Regge D, Lo Bello G, Martincich L, et al. A case of bleeding gastric lipoma: US, CT and MR findings. Eur Radiol 1999; 9:256-258.
9. Yang M, Martin DR, Karabulut N. Gastric schwannoma: MRI findings. Br J Radiol 2002; 75:624-626.

10. Van den Abbeele AD, Annick D. The lessons of GIST-PET and PET/CT: a new paradigm for imaging. Oncologist 2008; 13:8-13.
11. Patel SR, Peters PWT. Gastrointestinal stromal tumors: current management. J Surg Oncol. Accessed online (early view) Jan 8, 2010.
12. Demetri GD, Von Mehren M, Blanke CD, et al. Efficacy and safety of imatinib mesylate in advanced gastrointestinal stromal tumors. N Engl J Med 2002; 347:472-480.
13. Demetri GD, Van Oosterom AT, Garrett CR. Efficacy and safety of sunitinib in patients with advanced gastrointestinal stromal tumour after failure of imatinib: a randomised controlled trial. Lancet 2006; 368:1329-1338.
14. Chen MY, Bechtold RE, Savage PD. Cystic changes in hepatic metastases from gastrointestinal stromal tumors (GISTs) treated with Gleevec (imatinib mesylate). AJR Am J Roentgenol 2002; 179:1059-1062.
15. Gong JS, Zuo M, Yang P, et al. Value of CT in the diagnosis and follow-up of gastrointestinal stromal tumors. Clin Imaging 2008; 32:172-177.
16. Mabille M, Vanel D, Albiter M, et al. Follow-up of hepatic and peritoneal metastases of gastrointestinal tumors (GIST) under imatinib therapy requires different criteria of radiological evaluation (size is not everything!!!) Eur J Radiol 2008; Nov 27 [Epub].
17. Holdsworth CH, Badawi RD, Manola JB, et al. CT and PET: early prognostic indicators of response to imatinib mesylate in patients with gastrointestinal stromal tumor. AJR Am J Roentgenol 2007; 189:W324-W330.
18. Shinto A, Nair N, Dutt A, Baghel NS. Early response assessment in gastrointestinal stromal tumors with FDG PET scan 24 hours after a single dose of imatinib. Clin Nucl Med 2008; 33:486-487.
19. Van den Abbeele AD, Badawi RD, Tetrault RJ, et al. FDG-PET as a surrogate marker for response to Gleevec (imatinib mesylate) in patients with advanced gastrointestinal stromal tumors (GIST). J Nucl Med 2003; 44(suppl):24P.
20. Hueman MT, Schulick RD. Management of gastrointestinal stromal tumors. Surg Clin North Am 2008; 88:599-614.
21. Lee MW, Kim SH, Kim YJ, et al. Gastrointestinal stromal tumor of the stomach: preliminary results of preoperative evaluation with CT gastrography. Abdom Imaging 2008; 33:255-261.
22. Eisenberg BL, Judson I. Surgery and imatinib in the management of GIST: emerging approaches to adjuvant and neoadjuvant therapy. Ann Surg Oncol 2004; 11:465-475.

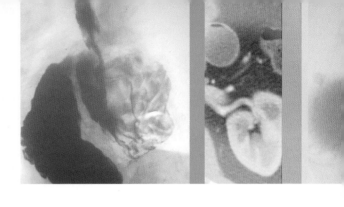

36

Gastric Outlet Obstruction

Hima B. Prabhakar and Priya D. Prabhakar

ETIOLOGY

Gastric outlet obstruction is an uncommon clinical consequence that has a wide range of causes. Benign and malignant as well as gastric and extragastric causes have been described throughout the literature. It was once relatively common to see patients present with gastric outlet obstruction secondary to inflammation and/or scarring from peptic ulcer disease (up to 12%).[1] Although it is difficult to define with certainty the incidence of gastric outlet obstruction, it is thought to have likely declined as treatments have improved for gastritis/peptic ulcer disease. Since the introduction of histamine-2 (H_2) blockers, malignant causes now represent the most common etiology of gastric outlet obstruction overall.[2]

Peptic ulcer disease remains the most common benign cause of gastric outlet obstruction.[3] Other benign causes include gastric/gastroduodenal bezoars,[4,5] Crohn's disease, hyperplastic[6] or eosinophilic gastroenteritis,[7] heterotopic pancreatic tissue within the antrum or duodenal bulb,[8] gastric volvulus, obstructing gallstone (also known as Bouveret's syndrome),[9-11] and pancreatitis/pancreatic pseudocysts.[12] Unusual benign causes that have been described in the literature include Brunner's gland hyperplasia (Fig. 36-1),[13] gastroduodenal tuberculosis,[14,15] and neurofibromatosis.[16] Gastric outlet obstruction is rare in the pediatric population and includes such benign causes as antral/pyloric atresia, antral/pyloric webs,[17] gastric/gastroduodenal lactobezoars,[18] and pyloric duplication cysts.[1]

Malignant causes now represent the most common cause of gastric outlet obstruction in the adult population.[2] Neoplasms that can cause gastric outlet obstruction include gastric adenocarcinoma, lymphoma, pancreatic adenocarcinoma,[19] and gallbladder carcinoma.[20] In these cases, gastric outlet obstruction may represent a presenting manifestation of the disease or may be caused by inflammation/scarring from treatments such as radiation therapy.[20]

The role of imaging/interventional radiology in the diagnosis and treatment of gastric outlet obstruction depends on the underlying etiology. Most commonly, when a patient presents with symptoms of gastric outlet obstruction, including intractable vomiting, "food fear," and cachexia,[21] some of the first diagnostic studies are abdominal radiography and CT. It is relatively straightforward to make a diagnosis of gastric outlet obstruction using these modalities, but the more difficult task remains in determining which one of the previously listed causes may be the culprit in any individual patient. Some of the causes have classic imaging findings on CT (e.g., gastric bezoar[4]), and some will likely be easy to diagnose (e.g., advanced pancreatic neoplasm). However, it is also likely that the underlying causes may not be readily ascertained by the initial imaging study (e.g., as in the case of gastric lymphoma). For this reason, it is important to keep in mind not only the different causes of gastric outlet obstruction but also the epidemiology of these entities to better tailor a differential diagnosis.

PREVALENCE AND EPIDEMIOLOGY

The overall prevalence of gastric outlet obstruction is difficult to determine secondary to the wide variety of underlying causes. It may be easier to consider how often each of the possible causes, both benign and malignant, present as gastric outlet obstruction.

In the adult population, malignant causes are the most common, followed by benign peptic ulcer disease. Studies have indicated that the incidence of people presenting with advanced peptic ulcer disease has decreased with the advances in treatment, including H_2 blockers. Presumably, as this once-common entity and presentation has become rarer, the overall incidence of gastric outlet obstruction has also likely decreased. This, however, has not been studied in the literature.[22]

Currently, the most common causes of gastric outlet obstruction in the adult are malignant.[2] Up to 35% of patients with gastric cancer present with gastric outlet obstruction, but the incidence of this is thought to be decreasing in the developed world. Fifteen to 25 percent of patients with pancreatic cancer present with gastric outlet obstruction, and typically these patients will also have signs and symptoms of biliary obstruction.[23]

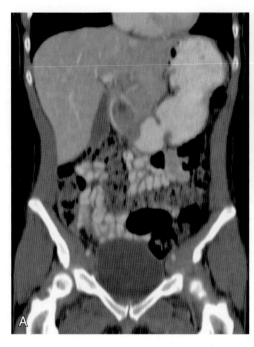

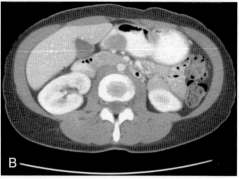

■ **FIGURE 36-1** **A,** Coronal CT reconstructed image after intravenous and oral contrast agent administration demonstrates a markedly distended stomach. **B,** Axial CT image shows a mass in the distal stomach/antrum. Biopsy of this lesion demonstrated Brunner's gland hyperplasia to be the cause of the gastric outlet obstruction.

In the pediatric population, malignant causes are unlikely. Benign causes that may be seen in younger patients include congenital causes (pyloric stenosis, antral webs, and duplication cysts),[17] inflammatory processes (pancreatitis/pancreatic pseudocyst), and acquired obstruction (foreign body, bezoar).[18]

CLINICAL PRESENTATION

The clinical hallmark of gastric outlet obstruction is nausea and intractable vomiting. Typically, the vomiting is nonbilious and may contain undigested food particles.[1] Depending on the underlying cause, the patient may present with pain, particularly in peptic ulcer disease,[22] pancreatitis,[12] or Bouveret's syndrome.[10] In patients with malignancy as a cause for gastric outlet obstruction, early satiety and weight loss are frequent symptoms.[19] These can also be seen in patients with chronic causes such as gastric bezoars.

With severe gastric outlet obstruction, the abdomen may be distended with a tympanic left upper quadrant. Depending on the underlying cause, physical examination may yield additional clues. Patients with underlying progressive malignancies may be cachectic or jaundiced in the case of pancreatic/biliary malignancies. In patients with peptic ulcer disease, pancreatitis, or obstruction caused by gallstones, there will be associated pain to palpation. In the infant with pyloric stenosis, the classically described physical examination finding is an "olive" in the upper abdomen. Finally, in patients with trichobezoars, hair loss from constant pulling may be found.[24]

Abnormal laboratory values may be associated with gastric outlet obstruction if the patient has had long-standing vomiting causing dehydration or malnutrition. Vomiting causes loss of hydrochloric acid and can lead to metabolic alkalosis. Additionally, if the patient has progressed to dehydration, abnormalities of blood urea nitrogen and creatinine may be present. Finally, any laboratory abnormalities associated with the underlying cause of the

gastric outlet obstruction may also be seen. These include a positive test for *Helicobacter pylori* in cases of peptic ulcer disease, elevated amylase and lipase levels in pancreatitis, an elevated bilirubin level in cases of obstructive jaundice secondary to pancreatic neoplasm, and anemia in patients with bleeding peptic ulcer disease, underlying malignancy, or chronic disease such as Crohn's disease or tuberculosis.[1,12,22]

ANATOMY

The stomach is the most capacious segment of the gastrointestinal tract. From proximal to distal, it is divided into the following segments: cardia, fundus, body, antrum, and pylorus. The distal portion of the stomach, including the antrum and pylorus, is typically the location of a gastric obstructive pathologic process that can lead to gastric outlet obstruction. Additionally, any pathologic process within the duodenum or the proximal small bowel can cause secondary gastric outlet obstruction.[1]

The duodenum is divided into four segments. The first portion includes the duodenal bulb, which is the site for duodenal ulcers, heterotopic pancreatic tissue, and Brunner's gland hypertrophy. The second portion is composed of the descending segment of the duodenum. This segment is closely opposed to the head of the pancreas, and any mass (benign or malignant) that affects the pancreatic head can impinge on the medial aspect. The third (transverse) and fourth (ascending) portions of the duodenum can also cause obstructive pathophysiology leading to gastric outlet obstruction, but this is less common given the causes already discussed.[1]

PATHOLOGY

A discussion of the specific pathologic findings of each of the causes of gastric outlet obstruction is beyond the scope of this chapter.

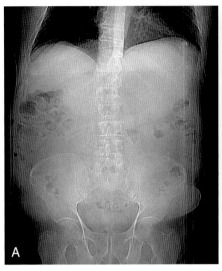

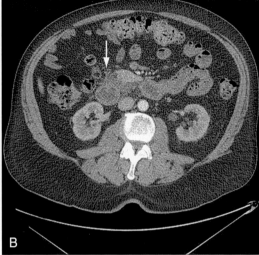

■ **FIGURE 36-2** **A,** Preliminary scout image from a CT scan demonstrates marked distention of the stomach, which displaces the transverse colon inferiorly. **B,** CT scan performed after intravenous contrast agent administration shows a hypodense mass at the head of the pancreas, which causes gastroduodenal obstruction (*arrow*).

IMAGING

The general manifestations of gastric outlet obstruction are nausea and intractable vomiting. In more severe or chronic cases, cachexia and food aversion may be seen. Differential considerations for this broad spectrum of symptoms can be narrowed with evaluation of patient age, physical examination, laboratory data, diagnostic imaging, and endoscopic evaluation if necessary.[25]

Radiography

Abdominal radiography may show a dilated stomach, which can displace bowel inferiorly (see Fig. 36-1). Barium upper gastrointestinal studies may show the site of obstruction. Narrowing of the distal portion of the stomach can help differentiate gastric outlet obstruction from functional gastroparesis/delayed gastric emptying. In the acute setting, barium upper gastrointestinal studies are rarely performed. In more chronic cases, if a double-contrast barium study is performed, an ulcer or intrinsic mass that is large enough to cause gastric outlet obstruction should be readily seen.

CT

CT is the most useful imaging modality for both the diagnosis of gastric outlet obstruction and the differentiation of its many underlying causes. On CT, gastric outlet obstruction is seen as a large dilated stomach.[4,11] If an oral contrast agent has been administered, little of it will have progressed past the site of obstruction.

More useful is CT's role in differentiating the underlying causes of gastric outlet obstruction. Malignant processes such as pancreatic cancer can be diagnosed using CT, particularly if it progressed enough to cause gastric outlet obstruction (Fig. 36-2). Benign causes such as pancreatitis/pancreatic pseudocyst (Fig. 36-3), bezoar,[4] and Bouveret's syndrome[11] can also be differentiated.

MRI

MRI is of limited utility in the diagnosis of gastric outlet obstruction. Although some of the previously described

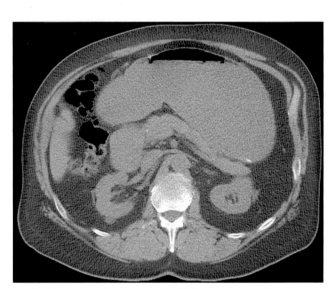

■ **FIGURE 36-3** Axial noncontrast CT demonstrates a dilated stomach consistent with gastric outlet obstruction. Stranding is seen in the region of the pancreatic head, with a small focus of calcification, consistent with pancreatitis.

entities can be seen with MRI, including pancreatic neoplasm, pancreatitis/pancreatic pseudocyst, and gastric cancer, MRI is rarely used for the initial diagnosis in cases that have progressed to gastric outlet obstruction.

Ultrasonography

In the pediatric population, ultrasonography is often one of the first imaging modalities to be used, because of the absence of ionizing radiation. Ultrasound evaluation is useful in the diagnosis of pyloric stenosis, in which the criteria for the thickness and length of the pylorus are well described. Additionally, the ultrasonographic findings of obstructing bezoars have been described and include an intraluminal mass with a hyperechoic surface and marked posterior acoustic shadowing.[4] Ultrasonography can show pancreatic pseudocysts, but if the size of the cyst is large enough to cause gastric outlet obstruction it may be difficult to clearly determine the origin of the cystic lesion.

Nuclear Medicine

Although not generally used in the diagnosis of acute gastric outlet obstruction, patients with more chronic cases may obtain a nuclear medicine gastric emptying study to evaluate for gastroparesis.[26]

PET/CT

PET/CT is useful in the staging of gastric cancer and lymphoma but not typically used for the initial diagnosis of gastric outlet obstruction. In patients with a chronic gastric outlet obstruction secondary to a known malignancy, PET/CT may demonstrate these findings.

Imaging Algorithm

If abdominal radiographs demonstrate the presence of gastric dilatation, CT should be obtained to further evaluate for an underlying cause (Table 36-1).

Classic Signs

- Bouveret's syndrome: calcified gallstone in the distal stomach/duodenum with air in the gallbladder from cholecystoduodenal fistula (seen on CT).[11]
- Obstructing gastric bezoar: well-defined intraluminal mass with air within the interstices (seen on CT)[4]
- Pyloric stenosis in the infant: shoulder sign (collection of barium in the dilated antrum on upper gastrointestinal study). On ultrasonography, pyloric muscle thickness greater than 4 mm and a length greater than 16 mm may be seen.
- Crohn's disease of the stomach: ram's horn sign, a tubular narrowing, and deformity of the antrum, with poor distensibility[27]

DIFFERENTIAL DIAGNOSIS

Based on the clinical presentation of nausea, vomiting, anorexia, and pain, the differential considerations are broad. Most importantly, the clinician needs to take into account the patient's age to come to a more focused differential list. In fact, given the relatively low incidence of gastric outlet obstruction, it is likely not to be one of the differential considerations. The likelihood of an underlying pathologic process rises with age, with fewer than half of patients younger than the age of 40 having an organic cause for their symptoms.[25]

The most common differential considerations based on clinical presentation include functional dyspepsia, gallstones, gastric and duodenal ulcer (not necessarily causing gastric outlet obstruction), irritable bowel syndrome, gastroesophageal reflux, and gastric cancer. These can be further narrowed based on patient characteristics. Gallstones are more common in women, whereas the incidence of ulcer disease and gastric cancer is higher in men. If the patient presents with painless jaundice, nausea, vomiting and anorexia, pancreatic cancer becomes higher in the differential diagnosis and gastric outlet obstruction may be the presenting symptom.[25]

In summary, there is nothing specific in the typical clinical presentation that will point exclusively to gastric outlet obstruction. However, when considered in conjunction with demographic clues, physical examination, and possibly laboratory values, an underlying etiology for gastric outlet may be suggested.

Based on imaging studies, gastric outlet obstruction is a relatively straightforward diagnosis to make. More importantly, using imaging techniques can help the gastroenterologist or surgeon narrow the differential diagnosis and allow for the appropriate treatment methods, either medical or surgical management.

TREATMENT
Medical Treatment

In the acute setting, patients presenting with gastric outlet obstruction should be treated symptomatically. A nasogas-

---

TABLE 36-1 Accuracy, Limitations, and Pitfalls of the Modalities Used in Imaging of Gastric Outlet Obstruction

Modality	Accuracy	Limitations	Pitfalls
Radiography	Depends on the severity of the obstruction	Generally cannot differentiate underlying causes	
CT	High, excellent for differentiating most underlying causes	Difficult to differentiate benign and malignant gastroduodenal inflammation and thickening	Difficult to differentiate benign versus malignant gastric ulcers/inflammation
MRI	Not generally used for diagnosis; may be useful for staging underlying gastric or pancreatic neoplasm	Difficult to differentiate inflammation from malignancy in the acute setting	Gadolinium enhancement can be seen in both benign and malignant causes
Ultrasonography	Modality of choice for imaging pyloric stenosis in the infant; can see large masses/cysts causing obstruction	Limited utility in the diagnosis of other causes; will generally need CT to define extent of underlying disease/obstruction	Excessive gas from bowel obstruction will limit utility of this modality.
PET/CT	Not used in primary diagnosis; useful in the secondary staging of gastric cancer and lymphoma	Not used in primary diagnosis	

tric tube should be inserted to decompress the stomach, and the patient should receive intravenous fluids and supplemental nutrition if dehydration and malnutrition are issues.[21]

Once the acute symptoms have lessened, medical treatment consists of treating the underlying cause. In patients with malignant causes of gastric outlet obstruction, a palliative stent can be placed by endoscopy or under fluoroscopic guidance.[28] In patients with peptic ulcer disease, medical treatment can be used if it is thought that the obstruction was caused by inflammation rather than scarring.[22] Endoscopic balloon dilatation can be used in patients with benign pyloric stenosis from a variety of causes.[3]

Surgical Treatment

Traditionally, the palliative treatment of malignant gastric outlet obstruction was gastrojejunostomy; however, stenting is now more commonly used because there is less associated morbidity. Surgical treatment may be used in patients with peptic ulcers (vagotomy and antrectomy or distal gastrectomy), pyloric stenosis (pyloroplasty), and pancreatitis/pancreatitic pseudocyst (débridement

as necessary). Additionally, if the patient fails stenting in cases of malignant causes, gastrojejunostomy can be considered.[1]

What the Referring Physician Needs to Know

■ Gastric outlet obstruction is caused by a wide variety of causes, both benign and malignant.

■ In patients with gastric outlet obstruction, a search for an underlying cause should begin once the acute presentation has been stabilized.

KEY POINTS

■ Gastric outlet obstruction is a clinical manifestation of a wide range of benign and malignant causes.

■ The most common cause in adults is malignancy (gastric and pancreatic).

■ The most common benign cause in adults is peptic ulcer disease.

■ Once gastric outlet obstruction is diagnosed, CT can be helpful to determine an underlying cause.

SUGGESTED READINGS

Lopera JE, Brazzini A, Gonzales A, Castaneda-Zuniga WR. Gastroduodenal stent placement: current status. RadioGraphics 2004; 24:1561-1573.
Ripolles T, Garcia-Aguayo J, Martinez MJ, Gil P. Gastrointestinal bezoars: sonographic and CT characteristics. AJR Am J Roentgenol 2001; 177:65-69.

Shone DN, Nikoomanesh P, Smith-Meek MM, Bender JS. Malignancy is the most common cause of gastric outlet obstruction in the era of H_2 blockers. Am J Gastroenterol 1995; 90:1769-1770.
Tuney D, Cimsit C. Bouveret's syndrome: CT findings. Eur Radiol 2000; 10:1711-1712.

REFERENCES

1. Dempsey DT. Stomach. In Brunicardi FC, et al (eds). Schwartz's Principles of Surgery, 8th ed. New York, McGraw-Hill, 2005, pp 933-995.
2. Shone DN, Nikoomanesh P, Smith-Meek MM, Bender JS. Malignancy is the most common cause of gastric outlet obstruction in the era of H_2 blockers. Am J Gastroenterol 1995; 90:1769-1770.
3. Yusuf TE, Brugge WR. Endoscopic therapy of benign pyloric stenosis and gastric outlet obstruction. Curr Opin Gastroenterol 2006; 22:570-573.
4. Ripolles T, Garcia-Aguayo J, Martinez MJ, Gil P. Gastrointestinal bezoars: sonographic and CT characteristics. AJR Am J Roentgenol 2001; 177:65-69.
5. Sodhi KS, Khandelwal N, Khandelwal S, Suri S. Gastric bezoar: an uncommon yet important cause of abdominal pain. J Emerg Med 2005; 28:467-468.
6. Dean PG, Davis PM, Nascimento AG, Farley DR. Hyperplastic gastric polyp causing progressive gastric outlet obstruction. Mayo Clin Proc 1998; 73:964-967.
7. Burhenne HJ, Carbone JV. Eosinophilic (allergic) gastroenteritis. Am J Roentgenol Radium Ther Nucl Med 1966; 96:332-338.
8. Haj M, Shiller M, Loberant N, et al. Obstructing gastric heterotopic pancreas: case report and literature review. Clin Imaging 2002; 26:267-269.
9. Cappell MS, Davis M. Characterization of Bouveret's syndrome: a comprehensive review of 128 cases. Am J Gastroenterol 2006; 101:2139-2146.
10. Kaushik N, Moser AJ, Slivka A, et al. Gastric outlet obstruction caused by gallstones: case report and review of the literature. Dig Dis Sci 2005; 50:470-473.

11. Tuney D, Cimsit C. Bouveret's syndrome: CT findings. Eur Radiol 2000; 10:1711-1712.
12. Greenberger N, Toskes P. Acute and chronic pancreatitis. In Fauci A, Braunwald E, Kasper D, et al (eds). Harrison's Principles of Internal Medicine, 17th ed. New York, McGraw-Hill, 2008.
13. Krishnamurthy P, Junaid O, Moezzi J, et al. Gastric outlet obstruction caused by Brunner's gland hyperplasia: case report and review of literature. Gastrointest Endosc 2006; 64:464-467.
14. Rao YG, Pande GK, Sahni P, Chattopadhyay TK. Gastroduodenal tuberculosis management guidelines, based on a large experience and a review of the literature. Can J Surg 2004; 47:364-368.
15. Amarapurkar DN, Patel ND, Amarapurkar AD. Primary gastric tuberculosis—report of 5 cases. BMC Gastroenterol 2003; 3:6.
16. Bakker JR, Haber MM, Garcia FU. Gastrointestinal neurofibromatosis: an unusual cause of gastric outlet obstruction. Am Surg 2005; 71:100-105.
17. Brandon FM, Weidner WA. Antral mucosal membrane: a congenital obstructing lesion of the stomach. Am J Roentgenol Radium Ther Nucl Med 1972; 114:386-389.
18. DuBose TM, Southgate WM, Hill JG. Lactobezoars: a patient series and literature review. Clin Pediatr 2001; 40:603-606.
19. Molinari M, Helton WS, Espat NJ. Palliative strategies for locally advanced unresectable and metastatic pancreatic cancer. Surg Clin North Am 2001; 81:651-666.
20. Mogavero GT, Jones B, Cameron JL, Coleman J. Gastric and duodenal obstruction in patients with cholangiocarcinoma in the porta hepatis: increased prevalence after radiation therapy. AJR Am J Roentgenol 1992; 159:1001-1003.

21. Hasler WL, Owyang C. Approach to the patient with gastrointestinal disease. In Fauci A, Braunwald E, Kasper D, et al (eds). Harrison's Principles of Internal Medicine, 17th ed. New York, McGraw-Hill, 2008.
22. Valle JD. Peptic ulcer disease and related disorders. In Fauci AS, et al (eds). Harrison's Principles of Internal Medicine, 17th ed. Access Medicine.
23. Chua YJ, Cunningham D. Pancreatic cancer. In Fauci AS, et al (eds). Harrison's Principles of Internal Medicine, 17th ed. Access Medicine.
24. Carr JR, Sholevar EH, Baron DA. Trichotillomania and trichobezoar: a clinical practice insight with report of illustrative case. J Am Osteopath Assoc 2006; 106:647-652.
25. Spiller RC. ABC of the upper gastrointestinal tract: Anorexia, nausea, vomiting, and pain. BMJ 2001; 323:1354-1357.
26. Thrall JH, Zeissman HA. Nuclear Medicine, The Requisites. St. Louis, CV Mosby, 2001.
27. Farman J, Faegenburg D, Dallemand S, Chen CK. Crohn's disease of the stomach: the "ram's horn" sign. Am J Roentgenol Radium Ther Nucl Med 1975; 123:242-251.
28. Lopera JE, Brazzini A, Gonzales A, Castaneda-Zuniga WR. Gastroduodenal stent placement: current status. RadioGraphics 2004; 24:1561-1573.

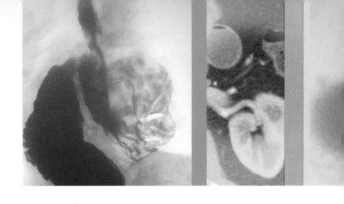

CHAPTER 37

Abnormal Positions of the Stomach

Priya D. Prabhakar and Hima B. Prabhakar

ETIOLOGY

Although there are a number of causes for altered position of the stomach, many are related to abnormalities of the diaphragm. A defect in the diaphragm, which may be congenital, acquired, or traumatic, allows movement of the stomach from its usual location into the thoracic cavity. The most common change in position of the stomach is the hiatal hernia.

DEFINITIONS, PREVALENCE, AND EPIDEMIOLOGY

A *hiatal hernia* is defined as displacement of the stomach through the esophageal hiatus of the diaphragm into the mediastinum (Fig. 37-1). There are two general varieties of hiatal hernias: sliding hiatal hernia and paraesophageal hernias. The most common type is the sliding hiatal hernia, which occurs when the gastroesophageal junction and cardia move upward through a widened esophageal hiatus of the diaphragm. The prevalence of sliding hiatal hernias is estimated to be between 10% and 80% owing to the difficulty of objectively diagnosing this entity, which is most commonly associated with gastroesophageal reflux disease. Age, obesity, and general muscular weakening contribute to the development of this entity.[1]

Paraesophageal hernias constitute between 5% and 15% of hiatal hernias and are defined as upward movement of the gastric fundus through a diaphragmatic defect with a normal position of the gastroesophageal junction (Fig. 37-2). The paraesophageal hernia may progress to an intrathoracic stomach with enlargement of the hernia, allowing for rotation of the stomach that can lead to gastric volvulus. These hernias may also occur as a post-surgical complication of antireflux procedures, esophago-myotomy, and gastrectomy.[1]

Gastric volvulus is defined as abnormal rotation of the stomach either along its longitudinal (organoaxial) axis or along a perpendicular axis crossing the lesser and greater curvature of the stomach (mesenteroaxial) axis (Figs. 37-3 and 37-4). Organoaxial volvulus or "upside-down stomach" accounts for approximately two thirds of all gastric volvulus. Gastric volvulus is uncommon and may be primary or secondary in etiology. Subdiaphragmatic or primary volvulus accounts for 30% of gastric volvulus cases and is due to congenital or acquired laxity of the suspensory ligaments that maintain the position of the stomach, allowing for rotation of the stomach without a diaphragmatic defect. The remainder of the volvulus cases are mostly supradiaphragmatic and are secondary to paraesophageal hernias, acquired diaphragmatic defects, diaphragmatic paralysis, abdominal bands, or adhesions. Most cases affect patients in their 50s and are associated with paraesophageal hernias. Twenty percent of cases occur in infants related to congenital diaphragmatic defects.[2]

Congenital diaphragmatic hernias (CDHs) occur in 1 in 2500 live births and result from either delayed fusion of the diaphragm or inhibited or delayed gut migration that results in lack of closure of the diaphragm. There is a high mortality of this condition, with up to 35% in live births due to pulmonary complications as well as associated anomalies. CDHs can occur through diaphragmatic defects that are posterolateral (Bochdalek hernias) or anterome-dial (Morgagni hernias), through the esophageal hiatus, or in the septum transversum. Bochdalek hernias are the most common, constituting 95% of all CDH cases. The stomach can occasionally herniate through one of these openings.[3]

Traumatic diaphragmatic hernia (Figs. 37-5 and 37-6) occurs most commonly after blunt injury but can occur from direct penetrating injury. Injuries to the diaphragm occur in 0.8% to 8% of patients after blunt trauma, and 90% of diaphragmatic rupture occurs in young men after a motor vehicle collision. Bowel, including stomach, and abdominal organs can then move upward through the diaphragmatic tear.[4]

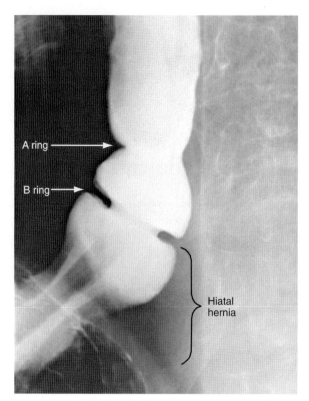

■ **FIGURE 37-1** A barium double-contrast study performed on a young patient with symptoms of epigastric burning and reflux demonstrates a small sliding hiatal hernia (type I). *Arrows* point to the muscular A ring and the B ring.

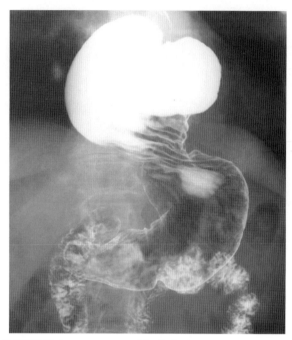

■ **FIGURE 37-3** A mesenteroaxial volvulus is seen partially above the level of the diaphragm on this barium upper gastrointestinal series.

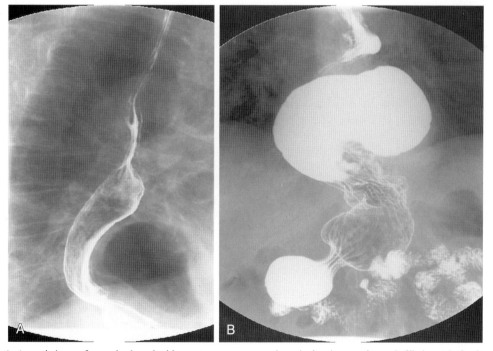

■ **FIGURE 37-2** A, An early image from a barium double-contrast upper gastrointestinal series reveals an air-filled gastric fundus above the level of the diaphragm consistent with a paraesophageal hernia. B, A delayed supine image demonstrates filling of the gastric fundus in this type II hiatal hernia.

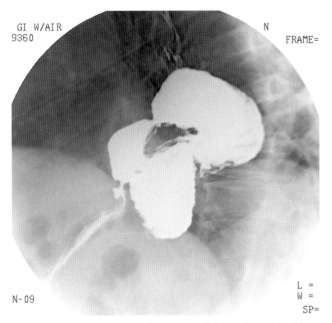

GI W/AIR
9360   N
                                    FRAME=

N-09
                                    L =
                                    W =
                                    SP=

■ **FIGURE 37-4** A patient with a history of chest pain and vomiting presented with an organoaxial gastric volvulus as seen on a barium gastrointestinal study.

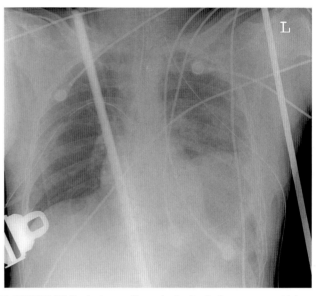

■ **FIGURE 37-5** A chest radiograph obtained after a motor vehicle accident shows opacity overlying the left lower lobe above the location of the diaphragm with a lucency that extends over the left lower chest and upper abdomen. A nasogastric tube is seen overlying the left lower lobe, consistent with traumatic left diaphragmatic rupture with herniation of the stomach into the left hemithorax.

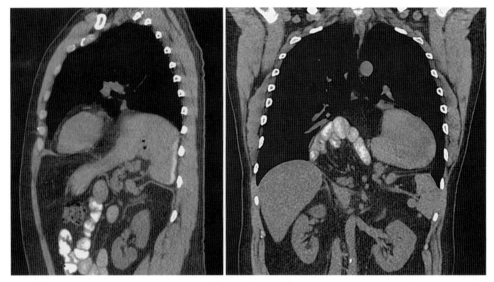

■ **FIGURE 37-6** A male patient presented with a chronic, large diaphragmatic defect and hernia containing stomach, jejunum, pancreas, and a mesenteric vessel. This was thought to be related to remote trauma and is well demonstrated on sagittal (*left*) and coronal (*right*) CT reformatted images.

CLINICAL PRESENTATION

Patients with sliding hiatal hernias may present with acid reflux, epigastric burning pain, or pain similar to angina pectoris, dysphagia, or dyspnea. Those with paraesophageal hernias may experience chest pain or pressure after eating, nausea, and retching. The classic symptoms of acute gastric volvulus are known as Borchardt's triad: severe epigastric pain and distention, vomiting followed by nonproductive retching, and inability or difficulty passing a nasogastric tube. Symptoms are also localized to the upper abdomen in primary volvulus and to the chest

in secondary volvulus. Without early detection, poor outcome is a major concern because mortality rates of acute gastric volvulus range between 30% and 50% due to strangulation, necrosis, perforation, and hypovolemic shock.[5]

CDHs are often detected in utero through ultrasound fetal surveys or shortly after birth. Neonates with a Bochdalek type hernia present with a scaphoid abdomen and respiratory symptoms that vary depending on the degree of pulmonary hypoplasia caused by the presence of abdominal contents in the chest during development.

Morgagni hernias are uncommon and are usually asymptomatic. They are often detected incidentally but can be associated with mild respiratory or gastrointestinal symptoms.[3]

Traumatic diaphragmatic hernias are frequently not recognized at the time of injury (see Fig. 37-6), with an early diagnosis made in less than 50% of cases. All patients have a history of abdominal trauma and can present with respiratory distress and chest pain with diaphragmatic rupture. Many cases do not present for months to years after an injury with symptoms consistent with acute bowel strangulation.[6]

PATHOPHYSIOLOGY

The diaphragm is a musculotendinous structure made up of three parts. A sternal portion attaches to the xiphoid and lower sternum, the costal portion attaches to the inner aspect of the 6th to 12th ribs, and the lumbar part attaches to the arcuate ligaments and the periosteal surface of the upper lumbar vertebral bodies. The three parts converge into a central tendon. There are three naturally occurring openings in the diaphragm: the aortic hiatus, the esophageal hiatus, and the foramen vena cava. The thoracic surface is covered with pleura, and the abdominal surface is covered by peritoneum except for over the bare area of the liver. There is usually a pressure difference between the abdominal and thoracic cavities, with higher pressure in the abdomen.[3] The stomach position is maintained in the abdominal cavity by the gastrocolic, gastrohepatic, gastrophrenic, and gastrosplenic ligaments.[7]

The distal portion of the esophagus that appears normal and slightly dilated is termed the *vestibule*. At the superior aspect of the vestibule is a broad muscular ring, the A ring. The more inferiorly located gastroesophageal junction occurs at the B ring (see Fig. 37-1). B rings are seen radiographically in only about 15% of patients.

PATHOLOGY

A sliding hiatal hernia results from upward movement of the gastroesophageal junction through an enlarged esophageal hiatus into the posterior mediastinum and is defined as a separation greater than or equal to 2 cm between the B ring and the diaphragm. Paraesophageal hernias are due to a defect in the phrenoesophageal membrane that anchors the esophagus to the diaphragm such that the gastroesophageal junction remains fixed but the gastric fundus is able to move upward through the defect.[1]

The diaphragm normally closes the space between the pleural and peritoneal cavities at 8 weeks' gestation. CDHs result from late or incomplete development of the diaphragm or premature return of bowel to the abdomen before the diaphragm develops. Bochdalek and Morgagni hernias arise from failure of development of either the posterolateral or the anteromedial aspect of the diaphragm, respectively.[3]

Failure in one or more of the ligaments that fix the position of the stomach results in primary gastric volvulus, whereas disorders of adjacent structures or function of the stomach can lead to secondary volvulus.[2]

Traumatic diaphragmatic defects and hernias most commonly occur on the left, probably owing to protection of the right side of the diaphragm by the liver. Blunt trauma causes increased pressure in the abdominal cavity that tears the diaphragm and forces abdominal contents into the thorax.[4]

CDHs lead to pulmonary hypoplasia, which can result in varying degrees of decreased respiratory function in the neonate and has a high associated mortality. Hiatal hernias, gastric volvulus, and traumatic diaphragmatic hernias with herniated abdominal contents are associated with pulmonary symptoms depending on the size of the hernia and can cause dyspnea and possible aspiration.[3]

IMAGING

The main imaging modalities for diagnosis and detection of hernias, gastric volvulus, and traumatic diaphragmatic injuries include plain radiographs, barium/fluoroscopic studies, CT, MRI, and ultrasonography.

Radiography

Large hernias and supradiaphragmatic volvulus may sometimes be seen on plain radiographs of the chest, especially when there is an air-fluid level. One may see an intestinal air pattern or opacity in the thorax with any of the hernias discussed in this chapter. A lateral view of the chest can help localize the hernia. This is also true with CDHs in the neonate when radiographs show a hemithoracic opacity with deviation of the mediastinum and a paucity of bowel gas.[3]

Small hiatal hernias are often only detected with barium/fluoroscopic studies that enable visualization of the position of the gastroesophageal junction and stomach relative to the diaphragm. However, diagnosis of sliding hiatal hernias is difficult owing to mobility of the gastroesophageal junction that occurs at different phases in the peristaltic wave and the use of abdominal compression.[1] Barium studies may reveal barium-filled stomach or bowel within the hemithorax or can define altered orientation of the stomach in the case of gastric volvulus.[2] Fluoroscopic studies can also be used to evaluate diaphragmatic motion in cases of traumatic injury. Those patients with diaphragmatic rupture usually show abnormalities on chest radiographs, including opacity or lucency at the lung base, elevation of the left hemidiaphragm, absent diaphragmatic contour, and nasogastric tube above the level of the diaphragm.[6]

Ultrasonography

Prenatal fetal ultrasound survey can demonstrate abdominal organs in the chest in the case of CDH, with the unaerated bowel appearing as a mass in the thorax, absence of a fluid-filled stomach below the diaphragm, and a small abdominal circumference. Up to 80% of pregnancies with CDH also demonstrate polyhydramnios.

Adult-onset hernia is difficult to evaluate with ultrasound owing to air-filled bowel, air-filled lungs, and the ribs. Moderate to large hernias and those containing abdominal organs can be detected relative to the position

TABLE 37-1 Accuracy, Limitations, and Pitfalls of Modalities Used in Imaging of Abnormalities of the Stomach

Modality	Accuracy	Limitations	Pitfalls
Upper gastrointestinal study with barium	High	Patient must be able to ingest oral contrast agent.	Small hernias are difficult to evaluate objectively.
Radiography	Low to moderate	Depends on presence of air-fluid levels of intestinal gas pattern in the chest	
CT	High	Best accompanied by coronal, sagittal, and 3D reformatted images	
MRI	Low	Best for diaphragm anatomy and injuries	Motion; long time of imaging
Ultrasonography	Low	Mostly useful only for prenatal diagnosis of congenital diaphragmatic hernia	Adult evaluation limited by air-filled bowel, lungs, and ribs

of the diaphragm with ultrasonography. Diaphragmatic paralysis and eventration can also be detected after acute trauma.[3]

CT

CT is extremely useful for evaluating all types of hernias, gastric volvulus, and injuries to the diaphragm, especially with sagittal, coronal, and 3D reformatted images. The position of the gastroesophageal junction and stomach can be well visualized with oral contrast images. Diaphragmatic injuries and defects are often clearly defined, as is the relative position of stomach, bowel, and abdominal organs relative to the diaphragm. CT findings include discontinuity of the diaphragm, visualization of the site of herniation, and constriction of the herniating viscus at the site of diaphragmatic tear. The anatomy, abnormalities, and complications of the entities discussed in this chapter, including obstruction and ischemia, are best evaluated with CT.[4]

MRI

MRI is not practical for imaging of gastric hernias and volvulus but can be useful in evaluating the diaphragm. The normal openings in the diaphragm and areas of injury can be seen with sagittal and coronal images and are most suitable for chronic and complex post-traumatic injuries.[4]

Imaging Algorithm

In the case of suspected sliding hiatal hernia, an upper gastrointestinal study with barium contrast is the procedure of choice because certain techniques such as the Valsalva maneuver can be used to better visualize displacement of the gastroesophageal junction and gastroesophageal reflux. Paraesophageal hernias and gastric volvulus are best evaluated with barium studies or CT. CDHs are usually detected during prenatal ultrasonography or in the neonate may be first detected with radiographs. Traumatic diaphragmatic injuries and associated hernias may be incidentally detected on early radiographs of the chest with an intestinal gas pattern or opacity in the chest; however, if they are suggested, they are best evaluated with CT (Table 37-1).

Classic Signs

- Sliding hiatal hernia: B ring greater than or equal to 2 cm above the diaphragm
- Intrathoracic stomach: can be seen with paraesophageal or traumatic hernias
- Gastric volvulus: organoaxial volvulus along the longitudinal axis of the stomach is also known as upside-down stomach; mesenteroaxial volvulus occurs along the axis perpendicular to a line crossing the greater and lesser curvatures of the stomach.
- Acute gastric volvulus: classically presents as Borchardt's triad—severe epigastric pain and distention, vomiting followed by nonproductive retching, and inability or difficulty passing a nasogastric tube

---

DIFFERENTIAL DIAGNOSIS

Diseases presenting as epigastric or chest pain, nausea, and vomiting can be attributed to a number of other processes, including but not limited to coronary or cardiac disease, pulmonary infection/inflammatory disease, chest or abdominal malignancy, gastric or esophageal ulcer disease, and pancreatitis.

Mediastinal, esophageal, or chest processes can mimic intrathoracic stomach or volvulus with plain radiographs demonstrating an air-fluid level, such as achalasia, esophageal malignancy with obstruction, esophageal perforation, pulmonary cavitary disease, and medially located hydropneumothorax. The differential diagnosis for traumatic diaphragmatic hernias includes hydropneumothorax or pneumothorax. Opacity in the hemithorax of a neonate may alternatively be due to congenital cystic adenomatoid malformation or pulmonary sequestration.[8]

TREATMENT

Medical Treatment

Medical therapy for hiatal hernias is usually considered only for sliding hiatal hernias in patients with mild to moderate gastroesophageal reflux disease. Treatment consists of medication to reduce gastric acid and alteration of lifestyle and diet. Patients should try to avoid acidic meals and foods that relax the lower esophageal sphincter and should not eat too close to bedtime.[9]

Surgical Treatment

A sliding hiatal hernia associated with severe gastroesophageal reflux and erosive esophagitis may indicate surgical fundoplication, which can be done laparoscopically and is successful in 85% of patients in significantly reducing symptoms and healing esophagitis. Type II to IV hiatal hernias, or paraesophageal hernias, should be repaired, owing to the risk of development of gastric volvulus. Anterior gastropexy is performed for paraesophageal hernias, and the enlarged hiatus is closed.[3] Traumatic hernias and diaphragmatic defects are also surgically corrected with sutures or synthetic grafts used to repair diaphragmatic defects. Gastric volvulus is surgically repaired in asymptomatic patients as well as symptomatic patients because of the risk of ischemia and mortality. Reduction of the stomach and repair of the hiatal hernia with or without gastropexy is performed for gastric volvulus and can be done laparoscopically.[5]

What the Referring Physician Needs to Know

- Upper gastrointestinal studies with barium contrast and CT are the most useful diagnostic tools for gastric hernias and volvulus.
- It is important to recognize acute clinical and radiologic findings in paraesophageal hernias and gastric volvulus and that there is a risk for strangulation and mortality.

KEY POINTS

- Hiatal hernias become more common with age and obesity owing to laxity of supportive ligaments and widening of the diaphragmatic hiatus. Imaging plays a key role in detection and determination of the type of hernia.
- Gastric volvulus is a potentially life-threatening entity in which imaging can help make the diagnosis.
- Traumatic diaphragmatic hernias often go undiagnosed and should be excluded in cases of blunt or penetrating abdominal trauma.

SUGGESTED READINGS

Eren S, Ciriş F. Diaphragmatic hernia: diagnostic approaches with review of the literature. Eur J Radiol 2005; 54:448-459.

Godshall D, Mossallam U, Rosenbaum R. Gastric volvulus: case report and review of the literature. J Emerg Med 1999; 17:837-840.

Gourgiotis S, Vougas V, Germanos S, Baratsis S. Acute gastric volvulus: diagnosis and management over 10 years. Dig Surg 2006; 23:169-172.

Iochum S, Ludig T, Walter F, et al. Imaging of diaphragmatic injury: a diagnostic challenge? RadioGraphics 2002; 22:S103-S116; discussion S116-S118.

Kahrilas PJ, Kim HC, Pandolfino JE. Approaches to the diagnosis and grading of hiatal hernia. Best Pract Res Clin Gastroenterol 2008; 22:601-616.

REFERENCES

1. Kahrilas PJ, Kim HC, Pandolfino JE. Approaches to the diagnosis and grading of hiatal hernia. Best Pract Res Clin Gastroenterol 2008; 22:601-616.
2. Godshall D, Mossallam U, Rosenbaum R. Gastric volvulus: case report and review of the literature. J Emerg Med 1999; 17:837-840.
3. Eren S, Ciriş F. Diaphragmatic hernia: diagnostic approaches with review of the literature. Eur J Radiol 2005; 54:448-459.
4. Iochum S, Ludig T, Walter F, et al. Imaging of diaphragmatic injury: a diagnostic challenge? RadioGraphics 2002; 22:S103-S116; discussion S116-S118.
5. Gourgiotis S, Vougas V, Germanos S, Baratsis S. Acute gastric volvulus: diagnosis and management over 10 years. Dig Surg 2006; 23:169-172.
6. Worthy SA, Kang EY, Hartman TE, et al. Diaphragmatic rupture: CT findings in 11 patients. Radiology 1995; 194:885-888.
7. Cribbs RK, Gow KW, Wulkan ML. Gastric volvulus in infants and children. Pediatrics 2008; 122:752.
8. Davis S. Aids to Radiologic Differential Diagnosis, 5th ed. Philadelphia, Elsevier Saunders, 2009.
9. McQuaid KR. Gastrointestinal disorders. In McPhee SJ, Papadakis MA, Tierney LM Jr (eds): Current Medical Diagnosis & Treatment 2009. Available at http://www.accessmedicine.com/content.aspx?aID=6395.

Gastric Function Imaging

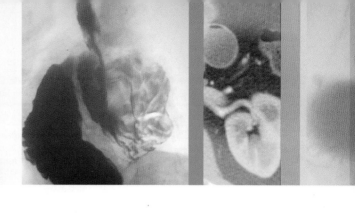

CHAPTER 38

Gastric Function Imaging Techniques

Rivka R. Colen and Johannes B. Roedl

TECHNICAL ASPECTS

Radionuclide gastric emptying studies (scintigraphy) remain the most widely used methods for evaluation of gastric function.

Radiopharmaceuticals

Gastric emptying scintigraphy is most commonly performed with technetium-99m (^{99m}Tc) sulfur colloid dispersed in a solid bolus and/or liquid bolus to evaluate one or both bolus phases. The properties of ^{99m}Tc sulfur colloid include 140 keV and a half-life of 6 hours.

To qualify as a tracer for gastric function, a radioactive marker must meet certain principal criteria. The principal criteria for a good liquid-phase marker includes the ability to equilibrate rapidly and be nonabsorbable. ^{99m}Tc sulfur colloid in water meets these criteria. The solid-phase radioactive marker for evaluation of solid gastric emptying requires the ability to bind tightly to the solid food particle. The reason is that liquids empty faster than solids, thereby producing an erroneously shortened solid emptying time. Two well-accepted in-vitro methods for radioactive labeling include cooking injected or surface-labeled liver cubes or paté or frying eggs with ^{99m}Tc sulfur colloid, resulting in tight binding to the egg albumin. The latter is the most widely used and is administered as an egg sandwich.[1]

In dual (solid/liquid) phase studies, indium-111–labeled diethylenetriaminepentaacetic acid (^{111}In-DTPA) is the liquid marker and ^{99m}Tc sulfur colloid is the solid marker.

Pharmacologic Adjuncts

Although not a common practice, multiple prokinetic drugs have been used in cases of delayed gastric emptying because these drugs improve emptying by increasing the amplitude of antral contractions.[2] The two most common include (1) metoclopramide, which has both central and peripheral antidopaminergic properties and causes release of acetylcholine from the myenteric plexus, and (2) erythromycin, which is a motilin agonist.

Technique

Gastric emptying scintigraphy requires the patient to be fasting for 8 to 12 hours.[3,4] Medications that affect gastric motility should be stopped, if possible. These include, but are not limited to, calcium channel blockers, anticholinergics, antidepressants, narcotics, gastric acid suppressants, and aluminum-containing antacids. Alcohol consumption and use of tobacco products should be stopped for a minimum of 24 hours.

On the morning of the study, the radiolabeled meal is prepared (Table 38-1). ^{99m}Tc sulfur colloid (1 mCi) is added to solidifying scrambling eggs and mixed until completely solidified. Salt and pepper is added and then placed between two pieces of toasted bread to make a sandwich. Once prepared, the ^{99m}Tc sulfur colloid radiolabeled egg should be consumed within 5 to 10 minutes. Promptly after ingestion, a continuous data acquisition with a frame rate of 30 to 60 seconds per image is performed for a duration of 90 minutes (64×64 pixels) with the patient positioned in the supine position. Additional imaging at 3 and 4 hours can be performed to identify patients with delayed emptying but a normal 90-minute gastric emptying time.[5]

A region of interest (ROI) is drawn over the stomach, and the percent of gastric emptying is determined. The radioactive counts increase as the food travels from the

TABLE 38-1	Adult Dosimetry for Gastric Function	
Phase	**Adult Dosimetry for Gastric Scintigraphy**
Liquid	0.5-1 mCi ^{99m}Tc sulfur colloid
Solid	0.5-1 mCi ^{99m}Tc sulfur colloid ovalbumin
	0.5-1 mCi ^{99m}Tc sulfur colloid chicken liver

TABLE 38-2 Accuracy, Limitations, and Pitfalls of Gastric Function Imaging Modalities

Modality	Accuracy	Limitations	Pitfalls
Scintigraphy	Most accurate to assess gastric function	Radiation exposure Time consuming Poor interlaboratory standardization	Cannot always determine the etiology of delayed gastric emptying
MRI (echoplanar)	Correlates well with scintigraphy in both solid and liquid phase	Investigational Time consuming Patient-limiting factors: breath-holding, claustrophobia, pacemakers	
Ultrasonography		Patient-limiting factors: large body habitus and bowel gas	
Breath test		Patient-limiting factors: results can be altered by liver, pancreatic, pulmonary, and small intestinal disease	
Gastric intubation		Invasive Requires serial aspirations Patient discomfort	
Marker dilution		Invasive Patient discomfort Tubing can alter emptying	
SPECT	Investigational	Measures only gastric accommodation	

fundus, a posterior structure, to the antrum, an anterior structure. The attenuation effect is therefore one of the technical factors that can cause underestimation of gastric emptying and, therefore, a false-positive result. This is most commonly corrected with the accepted gold standard for correcting attenuation, the geometric mean measure.[6] Frequent image acquisition increases accuracy in determining rate of gastric emptying. An alternative method to decrease false-positive results is to acquire images in the left anterior oblique (LAO) position.

Measurements of gastric emptying can be derived by the determination of the time it takes to reach half of the peak counts. Because of the various radiolabeling meal options and variations within each laboratory, standardized protocols and references applicable and valid for each laboratory must be obtained to achieve reproducible results.

PROS AND CONS

Radionuclide gastric emptying studies have become the gold standard for evaluation of gastric function, reflected by the test's accuracy, sensitivity, both qualitative and quantitative abilities, and ease of performance (Table 38-2).

The major disadvantage is radiation exposure. It is also time consuming and has poor interlaboratory standardization. Each laboratory has its standardization values that

take into account both whether a liquid or solid substance is used as well as the type of food particle binding agent. It is because of this that competing nonradionuclide techniques have surged and investigative efforts have intensified.[7]

CONTROVERSIES

In addition to the alternative methods just described, there are many more, albeit predominantly investigational, methods that are being evaluated. However, radionuclide gastric scintigraphy remains the mainstay for evaluation of gastric emptying.

KEY POINTS

■ ^{99m}Tc sulfur colloid properties include 140 keV and a half-life of 6 hours.

■ ^{99m}Tc sulfur colloid–radiolabeled egg sandwich is the most widely used radiolabeled meal for gastric emptying studies. Geometric mean measurement or acquisition in the LAO projection must be obtained to decrease false-positive results.

■ Standardization protocols and value references must be obtained in each laboratory so that results are reproducible.

REFERENCES

1. Knight LC, Malmud LS. Tc-99m ovalbumin labeled eggs: comparison with other solid food markers in vitro. J Nucl Med 1981; 22:28.
2. Saremi F, Jadvar H, Siegel ME. Pharmacological interventions in nuclear radiology: indications, imaging protocols, and clinical results. RadioGraphics 2002; 22:477-490.
3. Donohue KJ, Maurer AH, Ziessman HA, et al. Society of Nuclear Medicine Procedure Guideline for Gastric Emptying and Motility. Reston, VA, Society of Nuclear Medicine, 2004, version 2.0.
4. Zeissman HA, Fahey FH, Atkins FB, Tall J. Standardization and quantification of radionuclide solid gastric-emptying studies. J Nucl Med 2004; 45:760-764.
5. Zeissman HA, Bonta DV, Goetz S, Ravich WJ. Experience of a simplified, standardized 4-hour gastric-emptying protocol. J Nucl Med 2007; 48:568-572.
6. Ford PV, Kennedy RL, Vogel JM. Comparison of left anterior oblique, anterior and geometric mean methods for determining gastric emptying times. J Nucl Med 1992; 33:127-130.
7. Brattern J, Jones MP. New direction in the assessment of gastric function: clinical applications of physiologic measurements. Dig Dis 2006; 24:252-259.

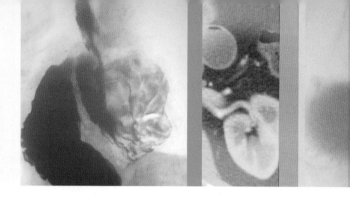

CHAPTER 39

Clinical Applications of Gastric Function Imaging

Rivka R. Colen and Johannes B. Roedl

EMBRYOLOGY

The stomach develops from the distal part of the foregut and initially is a simple tubular structure. At approximately the fourth week, a slight dilatation occurs indicating the site of the future stomach. As the stomach enlarges to take on the adult shape, it slowly rotates 90 degrees in a clockwise direction around its longitudinal axis (Fig. 39-1).

GASTRIC ANATOMY AND FUNCTION

There are three anatomic divisions of the stomach: the fundus, the body, and the antrum (Fig. 39-2). Functionally, the stomach is divided into two regions: the orad region, which includes the fundus and the proximal body, and the caudad region, which includes the distal portion of the body and antrum. The orad region functions to receive the food bolus by a process called receptive relaxation, which is controlled by a vagovagal reflex. The caudad region produces waves of contractions rippling from the proximal caudad region distally. Because these contractions close the pylorus, the gastric contents are propelled back and forth in the stomach for mixing and result in a further reduction in particle size, a process called retropulsion. During fasting, there are periodic gastric contractions called migrating myoelectric complexes that are mediated by motilin. These function to clear the stomach of residual food from the previous meal.

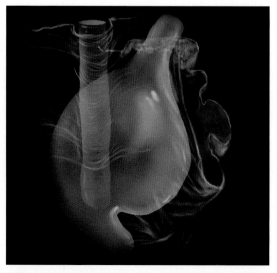

■ **FIGURE 39-1** Stomach embryology. A focal bulge is seen in the foregut region, the site that will eventually mature to be the normal stomach. *(Image courtesy of Alexander A. Ree, MD.)*

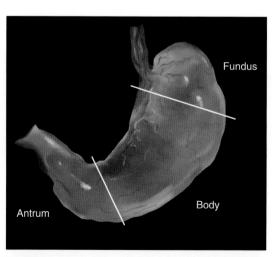

■ **FIGURE 39-2** Normal stomach anatomy. The stomach develops into a bottle-shaped structure that is anatomically divided into three regions: fundus, body, and antrum. *(Image courtesy of Alexander A. Ree, MD.)*

NORMAL GASTRIC ANALYSIS CURVES AND IMAGE

Liquids empty immediately in an exponential fashion, with no initial delay (lag phase). The dual-phase meal demonstrates exponential emptying as well, however at a slower rate relative to a liquid-only phase. In contrast, solid empty-ing demonstrates an initial lag phase, followed by a constant linear rate of gastric emptying (Fig. 39-3).[1-3]

PATHOPHYSIOLOGY

Causes of delayed gastric emptying can be divided into mechanical and functional causes. Mechanical causes of

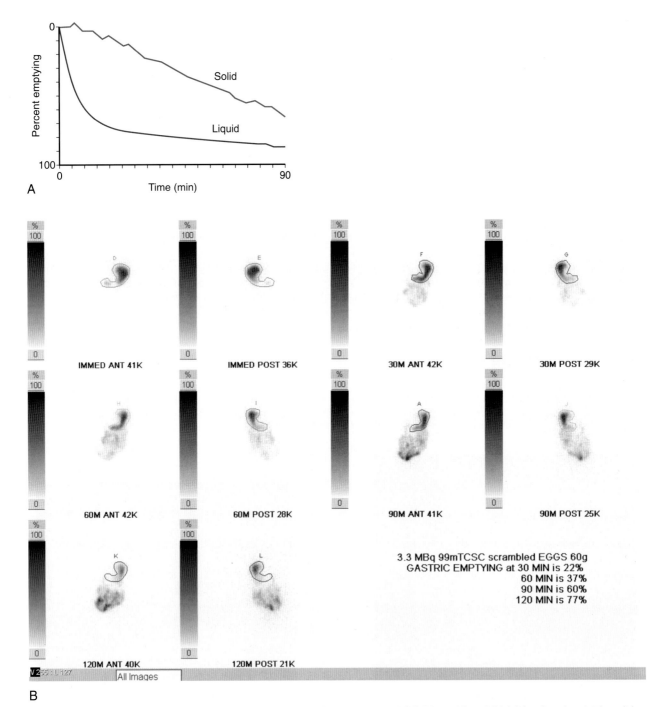

■ **FIGURE 39-3** **A,** Normal gastric function. Liquids empty immediately in an exponential fashion, with no initial delay (lag phase). The solid emptying demonstrates an initial lag phase, followed by a constant linear rate of gastric emptying. **B,** Normal gastric function. There is more than 50% gastric emptying at 60 minutes. (Values are standardized in each laboratory.) *(A courtesy of Alexander A. Ree, MD, and B courtesy of Ruth Lim, MD.)*

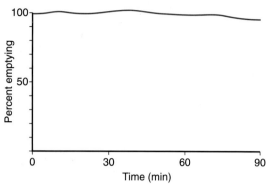

■ **FIGURE 39-4** Mechanical obstruction. A 68-year-old female patient presented with a complete pyloric obstruction due to an antral/pyloric gastric carcinoma. Preoperative radionuclide gastric emptying study demonstrates no gastric emptying. *(Courtesy of Alexander A. Ree, MD.)*

TABLE 39-1 Causes of Functional Delayed Gastric Emptying

Acute Dysfunction	Chronic Dysfunction
Gastroenteritis	Diabetes mellitus (most common)
Hyperalimentation	Post vagotomy
Acute uncontrolled hyperglycemia	Gastric ulcer (also a cause of mechanical delayed gastric
Trauma	emptying)
Postoperative ileus	Tumor, secondary to myenteric plexus invasion (also a cause
Metabolic disorders: hypokalemia, hypercalcemia, acidosis, myxedema,	of mechanical delayed gastric emptying)
hepatic coma	Hypothyroidism
Physiologic factors: Gastric distention, mental or physical stress,	Autoimmune diseases: systemic lupus erythematosus,
labyrinth stimulation	progressive systemic sclerosis, dermatomyositis
Drugs: antidepressants, anticholinergics, β-agonists, opiates, nicotine,	Myotonic dystrophy
opiates, progesterone, levodopa, alcohol, oral contraceptives	Familial dysautonomia
Physiologic hormones: progesterone, estrogen, gastrin, secretin,	Fabry's disease
somatostatin, glucagons, cholecystokinin	Pernicious anemia
	Anorexia nervosa
	Bulbar poliomyelitis
	Idiopathic

delayed gastric emptying include obstruction by tumor or pyloric ulcer. Functional causes of gastroparesis include acute dysfunction such as from acute gastroenteritis and metabolic derangements or, more commonly, chronic dysfunction, such as from diabetes mellitus.[3-5]

Factors Affecting Gastric Emptying

There are multiple physiologic and technical factors that affect gastric emptying (Table 39-1). The meal content is a primary factor. Large food volumes, weight, particle size, and caloric density slow the rate of gastric emptying. Solid food empties the slowest, followed by semisolid food, which empties slower than nutrient liquids. Clear liquids empty faster than nutrient liquids. Therefore, solid-phase analysis is more sensitive than liquid emptying to determine early abnormal gastric emptying.[3]

Mechanical Delayed Gastric Emptying

Mechanical obstruction can cause delayed gastric emptying (Fig. 39-4).

Functional Delayed Gastric Emptying

The most common clinical cause of chronic delayed gastric emptying is diabetes mellitus, which most commonly affects patients with type 1 insulin-dependent diabetes (Fig. 39-5).[4,5] It is thought to be due to vagal neuropathy, but no abnormality has been identified.

Uncontrolled hyperglycemia alone can also delay gastric emptying. Additionally, in diabetic patients, this can make glucose control difficult.

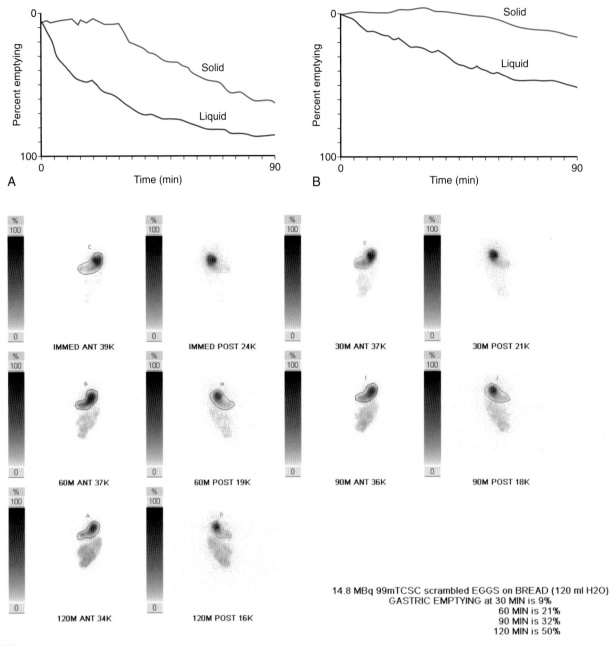

■ **FIGURE 39-5** Chronic functional gastroparesis. **A,** A 45-year-old patient presented with a history of insulin-dependent diabetes for 20 years. Radionuclide gastric emptying study demonstrates delayed solid emptying but normal liquid emptying consistent with early gastroparesis. (Of note, the solid meal is more sensitive for detection of less severe or early gastroparesis.) **B,** Same patient 10 years later. Radionuclide gastric emptying study demonstrates delayed solid and liquid emptying consistent with more severe gastroparesis. **C,** Same patient 5 years later. Radionuclide gastric emptying study with ^{99m}Tc-sulfur colloid mixed in a scrambled egg sandwich demonstrates delayed solid emptying consistent with gastroparesis. (**A** and **B** courtesy of Alexander A. Ree, MD; **C** courtesy of Ruth Lim, MD.)

KEY POINTS

- Liquids empty immediately in an exponential fashion.
- Solid emptying demonstrates an initial lag phase, followed by a constant linear rate of gastric emptying.

- The most common cause of delayed gastric emptying is functional from diabetic gastroparesis.

REFERENCES

1. Abell TL, Camiller M, Donohoe K, et al. Consensus recommendations for gastric emptying scintigraphy: a joint report of the American Neurogastric and Motility Society and the Society of Nuclear Medicine. Am J Gastroenterol 2008; 103:753-763.
2. Lartigue S, Bizais Y, Des Varannes SB, et al. Inter- and intrasubject variability of solid and liquid gastric emptying parameters: a scintigraphic study in healthy patients and diabetic patients. Dig Dis Sci 1994; 39:109-115.
3. Matolo NM, Stadalnik RC. Assessment of gastric motility using meal labeled with technetium-99m sulfur colloid. Am J Surg 1983; 146: 823-826.
4. Rothstein RD, Alavi A. The evaluation of the patient with gastroparesis secondary to insulin-dependent diabetes mellitus. J Nucl Med 1992; 33:1707-1709.
5. Urbain JL, Vekemans MC, Bouillon R, et al. Characterization of gastric antral motility disturbances in diabetes using a scintigraphic technique. J Nucl Med 1993; 34:576-581.

PART FOUR

Small Bowel and Colon

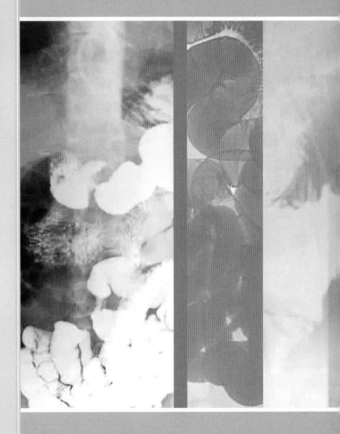

Small Bowel

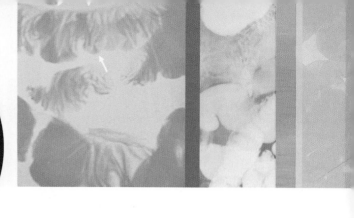

CHAPTER 40

Conventional Imaging of the Small Bowel

Senta Berggruen

TECHNICAL ASPECTS

Small bowel barium examinations are frequently used when imaging patients. Patients who may benefit from this imaging include those with abdominal pain, a history of inflammatory bowel disease, and malignancy. CT, including CT enterography, also increasingly is used for evaluating small bowel abnormalities.[1] However, barium examinations still play a vital role in assessing the small bowel, including providing functional information. Pathologic processes manifest as areas of luminal narrowing, a thickened bowel wall, and abnormal peristaltic activity. Early disease detection requires attention to radiologic technique and familiarity with the normal appearance of the small bowel and its variations.[2]

Because of bowel length and motility, imaging can take a long time. Intestinal loops overlap and change in size, shape, and position with peristalsis. Normal small bowel transit ranges from 30 to 120 minutes. Transit time can be lengthened dramatically in patients with obstruction or adynamic ileus. Fluoroscopy is a key component of any small bowel examination. The radiologist evaluates the barium column to assess overall small bowel location, course, and size as well as the luminal contour and searches for abnormalities that extend beyond the small intestine (e.g., diverticula, sacculations, ulcers) or lesions that protrude into the lumen (e.g., polyps and abnormal folds). The small bowel folds are best evaluated with a fully distended lumen. Fold width depends on the amount of luminal distention: the greater the distention, the thinner the folds appear. En face mucosal detail is seen during compression of the barium column or with use of the double-contrast technique. Visualization of the mucosa is necessary for detecting mucosal granularity/nodularity or small (e.g., aphthoid) ulcers. The radiologist also assesses bowel motility, distensibility, and pliability during the examination.[3,4]

Small Bowel Follow-Through

The small bowel follow-through (SBFT) is a single contrast examination of the esophagus, stomach, and small bowel that uses low density (30% to 50% w/v) barium (Fig. 40-1). The patient is advised to fast from 10 PM the day before the test. A single-contrast upper gastrointestinal series is often performed using 1 to 2 cups of low-density barium. The purpose is to show gross upper gastrointestinal involvement by diseases that affect the small bowel, such as Crohn's disease. A double-contrast upper gastrointestinal examination using high-density barium often prevents adequate visualization of pelvic small bowel loops. After the examination, the patient drinks an extra 1 to 2 cups of low-density barium. This is equivalent to ingesting 500 to 1000 mL of barium. A technologist obtains serial overhead radiographs for the radiologist to evaluate. The radiologist then performs fluoroscopy when an abnormality is suspected and/or when barium reaches the terminal ileum. An SBFT relies on fluoroscopic detection and spot image documentation of bowel abnormalities. Small bowel loops in each abdominal quadrant are palpated when they are optimally distended by barium. The radiologist should therefore evaluate the patient at least several times: 15 to 30 minutes after the upper gastrointestinal examination is performed and then at 15- to 45-minute intervals, depending on how fast the barium column is progressing through the small bowel. The patient is turned into various positions with manual palpation (including supine, lateral, and prone compression views) to splay out individual small bowel loops (Fig. 40-2).[3,4] The examination time can be shortened by using 20 mg of metoclopramide (Reglan) given orally 20 to 30 minutes before the study or 10 mg given intravenously at the start of the examination.[5,6] This accelerates gastric emptying and small bowel transit but also increases baseline muscle tone, producing incomplete

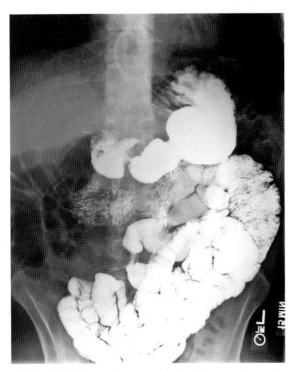

■ **FIGURE 40-1** Fifteen-minute overhead radiograph of normal small bowel follow-through examination.

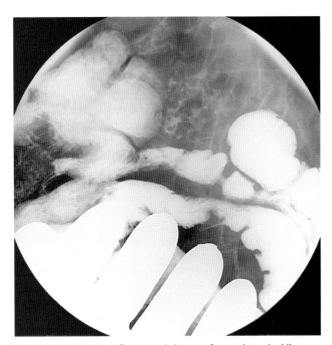

■ **FIGURE 40-2** Spot fluoroscopic image of normal terminal ileum with manual compression.

small bowel distention.[7] This technique produces a faster but less optimal examination.

Two to three doses of an effervescent agent (600 to 900 mL of CO_2) can be given when barium reaches the pelvic ileal loops or the terminal ileum. This shortens the examination and produces an air-contrast examination of one third to one half of the small bowel loops.[8] However, this can produce uncomfortable intestinal cramping.

A barium mixture of 24% w/v barium suspended in methylcellulose produces more luminal distention than a routine SBFT barium suspension.[9] However, the barium is not as dense, so it can be more difficult to detect filling defects in the barium.

Peroral Pneumocolon

A peroral pneumocolon examination may be done in conjunction with an SBFT. This is a double-contrast examination primarily used in patients with suspected Crohn's disease in the terminal ileum. The patient undergoes a barium enema preparation to clear the area of feces. After a routine SBFT, 1 mg of glucagon is given intravenously. Air is insufflated into the rectum via a Foley catheter to slowly distend the colon as the patient is turned to reflux air into the terminal ileum. Double-contrast spot images of the terminal ileum are then taken.[10,11]

Enteroclysis

The small bowel can be evaluated via intubation techniques, which involve placing a tube beyond the pylorus and overdistending the small bowel with various contrast agents. Patient discomfort during intubation precludes universal acceptance of this procedure. A bowel preparation is given to clear feces from the terminal ileum before the examination because fecal matter obscures mucosal detail and mimics polyps.[12] The preparation may include osmotic cathartics such as magnesium citrate and colonic stimulants such as bisacodyl. A clear liquid diet the day before combined with four 5-mg tablets of bisacodyl the evening before the examination is suggested. Nothing is ingested after 10 PM. On the examination day, the patient should temporarily stop medications such as narcotics that decrease small bowel peristalsis.[12] Metoclopramide is administered orally (20 mg) or intravenously (10 mg) before the examination and begins to take effect 1 to 3 minutes after the intravenous dose or 30 to 60 minutes after oral ingestion.[13] This drug helps the enteroclysis catheter pass by relaxing the pyloric sphincter and duodenal bulb and by increasing gastric antral contractions and duodenal peristalsis.[14,15] It is contraindicated in patients with pheochromocytoma because it may stimulate catecholamine release, precipitating a hypertensive crisis. It is also contraindicated in patients with epilepsy because it increases the frequency and severity of seizures. The intubation process is more comfortable with conscious sedation such as a combination of fentanyl or diazepam for analgesia and midazolam for an amnesic effect.[16] Multiple enteroclysis catheters are available. The catheters have a diameter of 8 to 13 Fr, an end hole or side holes, and a balloon attached to their tip.[17] The patient can drink a small amount of barium (15 to 30 mL) before intubation to coat the antrum, pylorus, and duodenal bulb, which provides a guide for the radiologist in passing the catheter.[12-14,18] The catheter is passed into the oropharynx via an oral or nasal route. The nasal route causes less gagging. However, nasal intubation may cause nasal bleeding and produce nasal discomfort as the catheter is manipulated during the examination. Nasal intubation is made easier using topical lidocaine jelly. The purpose of the catheter

TABLE 40-1 Key Points of Enteroclysis

Modality	Barium (w/v)	Amount (mL)	Pros	Cons
Single contrast	20-40%	600-1200	Easier to perform	Limited mucosal detail
Air	50-80%	300-600	Excellent mucosal detail	Patient discomfort
			Long-segment bowel disease evaluated	Overexposed bowel loops
Methylcellulose	50%	300-600	Excellent mucosal detail	Patient emesis/diarrhea
	80%	200-300	Short-segment bowel disease evaluated	

guidewire is to torque or guide the catheter tip along the longitudinal axis of the bowel. Sometimes, the guidewire is retracted, allowing the soft catheter tip to pass through the pylorus or to curve around tight bends, such as the duodenal bulb apex. Catheter passage into the duodenum can be guided with manual compression or by turning the patient on the fluoroscopic table. The catheter tip can be left in the second portion of the duodenum for single- or air-contrast enteroclysis. When methylcellulose is used, the catheter tip and inflated balloon should be placed in the first jejunal loop to limit the reflux of methylcellulose into the stomach.[19] If the patient complains of discomfort during balloon inflation, the balloon should be immediately deflated until the discomfort resolves. Duodenal perforation is a rare complication of intubation.[20]

Contrast material can be infused through the enteroclysis catheter with syringes or an electric pump. This enables the radiologist to accurately control the infusion rate. If the rate is too fast, jejunal overdistention can cause bowel hypotonia. If the infusion rate is too slow, however, the lumen may be suboptimally distended, prolonging the examination time. Flow rates are generally between 50 and 150 mL/min.[3] There are multiple ways to perform the enteroclysis, either single or double contrast, with varying density and amounts of barium (Table 40-1).

Single-Contrast Enteroclysis

Single-contrast enteroclysis can be performed with low-density (20% to 40% w/v) barium. Between 600 and 1200 mL of barium is injected at an initial rate of about 75 mL/min.[15] Water may then be instilled into the catheter to push barium into the distal ileum and obtain a moderate double-contrast effect. Multiple spot images are obtained, varying the patient position to define anatomy and identify a pathologic process. Single-contrast studies are easier to perform than other types of enteroclysis. Evaluation of mucosal detail en face depends on compression and analysis of fold morphology.[3]

Double-Contrast Enteroclysis

In patients with known or suspected malabsorption, however, double-contrast enteroclysis techniques are recommended, such as with air or methylcellulose.

Air-Contrast Enteroclysis

Air-contrast enteroclysis is performed with 300 to 600 mL of barium (50% to 80% w/v) instilled by gravity, syringe,

or pump.[12,21] The barium infusion rate is changed to preserve peristalsis and for uniform distention of the proximal and middle small bowel. Room air or carbon dioxide is administered when barium reaches the pelvic small bowel or terminal ileum. Small bowel hypotonia may be induced by 1 mg of glucagon given intravenously after barium has reached the right colon.[18]

Air-contrast enteroclysis produces excellent mucosal detail of bowel loops coated by barium and distended by gas. Air-contrast techniques are more likely to be of value for patients with intestinal disease involving long segments of small bowel (e.g., malabsorptive states or Crohn's disease).[3] However, it is more difficult to manipulate the barium pool, so that some loops are visualized only with dense barium, despite using various patient positions and compression. Overlap of barium-filled loops with air-filled loops also results in radiographic overexposure of some bowel loops. Distention of pelvic loops with air is also sometimes incomplete.[3] Another disadvantage of air-contrast enteroclysis is that injection of large amounts of air into the small bowel can cause considerable patient discomfort. Sedation of these patients is suggested.

Methylcellulose-Contrast Enteroclysis

The use of methylcellulose-contrast enteroclysis is more effective than air-contrast study for patients with adhesions or other lesions involving shorter segments of small bowel. During methylcellulose-contrast enteroclysis, a small amount of barium is propelled through the small bowel by a large volume of radiolucent liquid (methylcellulose). Medium density (50% to 80% w/v) barium coats the intestinal mucosa, and methylcellulose distends the lumen.[13] The radiologist fluoroscopically follows the barium column, looking for obstructing lesions or lesions in the barium pool. The small bowel folds and en face mucosal detail are then evaluated when the lumen is distended by methylcellulose. Full luminal distention by methylcellulose straightens the valvulae conniventes, better delineates en face mucosal detail, and overdistends the lumen, increasing the conspicuity of low-grade obstructing lesions.

Varying amounts and densities have been employed for methylcellulose-contrast enteroclysis, including 200 to 300 mL of 80% w/v barium with an infusion rate of 60 to 80 mL/min via a syringe until about one half of the expected intestinal loops are visualized.[14] Another technique uses 300 to 600 mL of 50% w/v barium infused until the pelvic loops of ileum are filled.[22] The amount of barium infused depends on the small bowel length and diameter.

With methylcellulose-contrast techniques, the mucosal surface of the small bowel is readily demonstrated en face. The methylcellulose allows visualization through overlapping small bowel loops to a greater degree than that allowed with a single- or air-contrast enteroclysis.[3] Once methylcellulose has reached the colon, uncontrollable diarrhea may ensue.[12-14] Methylcellulose-contrast enteroclysis usually produces excellent double-contrast images in the jejunum. With enough methylcellulose, a double-contrast examination of the terminal ileum may also be achieved. However, barium diffusion into the methylcellulose may result in a poor double-contrast effect in the ileum, resulting in a single-contrast examination of the distal ileum. To prevent this, compression of ileal loops should be limited.[13]

Small Bowel Studies Using Water-Soluble Contrast Agents

Water-soluble contrast agents are hyperosmolar agents, which draw fluid into the intestinal lumen and are further diluted by excess fluid in the lumen of obstructed patients. Thus, the radiographic density of water-soluble contrast agents is generally suboptimal for diagnostic purposes in obstructed patients. These contrast agents are not indicated for examining the small bowel, except in patients with suspected leaks. Leaks arising in the duodenum or proximal jejunum can be demonstrated by water-soluble contrast studies. Leaks arising in the mid or distal small bowel, however, are often missed because of contrast agent dilution. CT should be employed to assess suspected leaks in the mid small bowel. When distal small bowel leak is considered, particularly at an ileocolonic anastomosis, it may be preferable to perform a water-soluble contrast enema with reflux of contrast agent into the distal ileum.[3]

Retrograde Examinations of the Small Intestine

The barium enema is a good examination for imaging the terminal ileum and distal ileum.[23] If plain abdominal radiographs or CT cannot differentiate a distal small bowel obstruction from an adynamic ileus, a single-contrast barium enema may be helpful in these patients.[24] The study can rule out an obstructing lesion in the colon as a cause of dilated small bowel. Barium reflux into a dilated terminal ileum indicates the presence of an adynamic ileus, whereas reflux of barium into a narrowed terminal ileum (with dilated gas-filled ileal loops more proximally) indicates the presence of a small bowel obstruction.

Ileostomy Enema

The small bowel proximal to an ileostomy can be evaluated by a retrograde examination through the ileostomy stoma. If there is a clinical suspicion of leak or obstruction, no preparation is used. If there is clinical suspicion of recurrent inflammatory or malignant disease, an oral preparation with magnesium citrate or Phospho-Soda is used for clearing debris. A clear diet is suggested the day before the procedure. A Foley catheter is inserted into the ileostomy. If disease is suggested at the ileostomy site (e.g., Crohn's disease or a stricture or leak), the catheter balloon should not be inflated. If after contrast agent injection no disease is seen in the distal ileum at or near the peritoneal reflection, then the catheter balloon may be inflated with 3 to 5 mL of air or saline and the balloon retracted to the peritoneal reflection. If balloon inflation is contraindicated and barium leaks out from the ileostomy stoma, the catheter is withdrawn, the balloon distended outside the ostomy, and the distended balloon pushed against the outside of the ileostomy opening to seal it. If a leak from the distal small bowel is suspected, water-soluble contrast agents should be used. If a distal small bowel obstruction is suspected, a single-contrast ileostomy enema can be performed with 30% to 50% w/v barium. Thin barium is injected via a syringe until the site of obstruction is reached and characterized. If Crohn's disease or a tumor is suspected, a double-contrast ileostomy enema can be performed, first injecting 50% to 80% w/v barium into the proximal ileum, followed by air to visualize mucosal detail. Fluoroscopy and spot images in multiple obliquities are critical. The ileostomy and small bowel adjacent to the anterior abdominal wall are best seen with the patient in the lateral position. The ileostomy is best filled after the catheter is removed, the ileostomy bag is replaced, and the patient is turned to a steep oblique or lateral position.[3]

PROS AND CONS

Small Bowel Follow-Through

The SBFT has two important limitations. The pylorus delays barium emptying so that the small bowel may be incompletely distended, making it difficult to evaluate luminal contour or to detect filling defects in the barium column. Because of small bowel transit times of 30 to 120 minutes or more, the radiologist cannot remain with the patient for the entire examination. As a result, the small bowel is evaluated only intermittently and lesions may be missed, depending on the degree of small bowel filling and distention of individual loops at fluoroscopy.[3,4]

The major advantage of SBFT over enteroclysis is that it avoids intubation. Long segments of abnormal bowel are easy to see as long as frequent fluoroscopy is performed. As a result, diseases involving long segments of small bowel, such as Crohn's disease, ischemia, or radiation change, are easily detected on SBFT.

Single-Contrast Enteroclysis

Barium reflux into the stomach rarely induces vomiting, as sometimes occurs with use of methylcellulose. Evaluation of mucosal detail en face depends on compression and analysis of fold morphology. Although the single-contrast technique is inferior to double-contrast techniques for visualizing mucosal details, the diagnosis of many small bowel abnormalities (e.g., adhesions, tumors, hernias) is possible.[3] Because of the emphasis on fluoroscopic and spot image diagnosis, enteroclysis is associated with a higher radiation dose to the patient than the SBFT.[25]

Air-Contrast Enteroclysis

Air-contrast enteroclysis produces excellent mucosal detail of bowel loops coated by barium and distended by gas. However, it is more difficult to manipulate the barium pool, so that some loops are visualized only with dense barium, despite using various patient positions and compression. Overlap of barium-filled loops with air-filled loops also results in radiographic overexposure of some bowel loops. Distention of pelvic loops with air is also sometimes incomplete. Another disadvantage of air-contrast enteroclysis is that injection of large amounts of air into the small bowel can cause considerable patient discomfort. Sedation of these patients is suggested. Air-contrast techniques are more likely to be of value for patients with intestinal disease involving long segments of small bowel (e.g., malabsorptive states or Crohn's disease).[3]

Methylcellulose-Contrast Enteroclysis

The mucosal surface of the small bowel is readily demonstrated en face. The methylcellulose allows better visualization through overlapping small bowel loops than that allowed with single- or air-contrast enteroclysis.[3] However, methylcellulose-contrast enteroclysis also has some disadvantages. Bubbles will form if methylcellulose is shaken. Unless an electric pump is used, methylcellulose is difficult to instill and messy because it is a thick sticky substance. Methylcellulose reflux into the stomach may induce projectile vomiting. Also, once methylcellulose has reached the colon, uncontrollable diarrhea may occur.[12-14]

Methylcellulose-contrast enteroclysis usually produces excellent double contrast in the jejunum. With enough methylcellulose, a double-contrast examination of the terminal ileum may also be achieved. However, barium diffusion into the methylcellulose may result in poor double-contrast effect in the ileum, resulting in a single-contrast examination of the distal ileum. To prevent this, compression of ileal loops should be limited.[13] Overdistention of pelvic ileal loops during enteroclysis may cause overlap of bowel loops, which make it difficult to demonstrate the terminal ileum in isolation.

Enteroclysis has important advantages over SBFT, including improved luminal distention. Short lesions such as tumors or skip lesions of Crohn's disease are better demonstrated by enteroclysis because the lumen is overdistended, making subtle areas of focal narrowing more conspicuous.[3] The small bowel folds are also better evaluated by enteroclysis because the folds are straightened (Fig. 40-3). Major mucosal abnormalities such as cobblestoning can be demonstrated on single-contrast SBFT with compression, but demonstration of subtle mucosal abnormalities requires a double-contrast technique.[26]

NORMAL ANATOMY

The small bowel is extremely tortuous, beginning at the pylorus and extending about 11 feet to the ileocecal valve. Intestinal length varies, depending on neuromuscular tone, vascular flow, and surgical history. The mesenteric small bowel is divided into the jejunum (proximal 40%) and ileum (distal 60%). The jejunum typically resides in

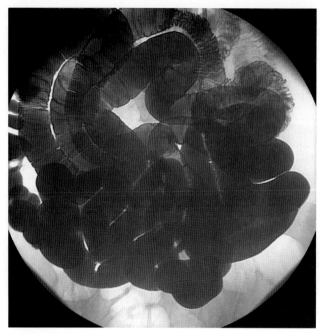

■ **FIGURE 40-3** Normal findings of small bowel enteroclysis.

the left upper quadrant; the ileum occupies the pelvis and right lower quadrant. The location of the jejunum and ileum varies, given the mobility of the bowel on the mesenteric root.[3]

Folds that encircle the lumen, known as the folds of Kerckring or valvulae conniventes, characterize the intestine. These folds are composed of mucosa and submucosa, increasing the surface area of the small intestine by 300%. The small bowel folds lie perpendicular to the longitudinal axis of the intestine and are thicker, taller, and more numerous in the jejunum than in the ileum. About 9 L of fluid, two thirds of these secretions, pours into the small bowel daily. These secretions contain proteins, fat, electrolytes, gastric juices, bile salts, mucus, and shed epithelial cells every day. The small bowel absorbs almost 8 of the 9 liters, with the remainder entering the colon. In the fasting state, this outpouring diminishes considerably. A mucous layer covers the entire surface of the small bowel mucosa. In this environment, barium may occasionally flocculate.[4] Normal variations of bowel can affect the radiologic appearance, showing the valvulae conniventes either as circular bands surrounding a wider lumen or as a feathery pattern in a decompressed small bowel.

SPECIFIC INDICATIONS

The clinician's differential diagnosis and patient's particular history will guide the diagnostic approach and choice of fluoroscopic examination.

Abdominal Pain

Unexplained abdominal pain can be evaluated by SBFT or enteroclysis. The SBFT is superior to enteroclysis for evaluating small bowel transit time and the motility disorders. In contrast, enteroclysis is superior for assessing the structural components of motor disorders (i.e., diverticula and sacculations or increased number of small bowel folds in scleroderma). Enteroclysis is also better for showing short lesions such as isolated adhesions or tumors that may account for abdominal pain.[3]

Chronic Diarrhea

SBFT is an adequate examination for the diagnosis of Crohn's disease or other inflammatory diseases involving long bowel segments.[14] The examination can demonstrate cobblestoning, mesenteric border ulcers, fissures, fistulas, and long narrowed segments. However, it can miss any short skip lesions in Crohn's disease as well as the aphthoid ulcers of early Crohn's disease. An enteroclysis is a better examination for disease extent and possible skip lesions. If a patient has a normal-appearing terminal ileum during an SBFT but there is a strong clinical suspicion of Crohn's disease, a peroral pneumocolon examination may be done for air-contrast views of the terminal ileum.[10]

Small Bowel Obstruction

CT has a major advantage over barium studies in that it does not rely on barium reaching the site of obstruction but rather uses intraluminal fluid to outline the transition zone.[24]

CT also is a shorter procedure than an antegrade barium study in patients with high-grade obstruction. An SBFT and enteroclysis are discouraged in patients with high-grade small bowel obstruction shown by plain abdominal radiographs or CT. Retrograde examination of the small bowel by barium enema is preferred in the setting of high-grade distal small bowel obstruction or if there is a question of whether the patient has an adynamic ileus, proximal colonic lesion, or distal small bowel obstruction. An antegrade study can be performed after decompressions by a nasogastric tube.

Unexplained Gastrointestinal Bleeding

An SBFT is quite limited for detecting causes of small intestinal bleeding.[22] Small tumors may be missed.[27] Methylcellulose-contrast enteroclysis is adequate for the demonstration of most small bowel tumors. However, it usually will not detect varices, arteriovenous malformations, or nonsteroidal anti-inflammatory drug–induced erosions. Air-contrast enteroclysis may allow diagnosis of subtle ulcerative lesions in the proximal small bowel in patients taking nonsteroidal anti-inflammatory drugs. An SBFT is indicated only when assessing for large structural causes of gastrointestinal bleeding. Methylcellulose- or air-contrast enteroclysis is satisfactory when searching for subtle lesions or small tumors. CT enterography is inferior to enteroclysis because it does not assess en face mucosal detail and has lower resolution than enteroclysis.[3]

Malabsorption

An SBFT detects large structural lesions that cause bacterial overgrowth (i.e., jejunoileal diverticulosis or Crohn's disease with obstruction). However, enteroclysis is superior for showing malabsorptive disorders involving the mucosa and submucosa of the bowel (e.g., celiac disease, Whipple's disease, and amyloidosis).[3]

KEY POINTS

- The unifying feature of all forms of barium examinations is palpation of each small bowel loop when the bowel loop is optimally distended to evaluate for mucosal abnormalities. Inadequate distention may mask a pathologic process.
- A single-contrast examination evaluates the luminal contour and filling defects in the barium column. A double-contrast examination evaluates the luminal contour, filling defects in the barium column or pool, and the mucosal detail en face.
- The major advantage of SBFT over enteroclysis is that it avoids intubation. Long segments of abnormal bowel are easy to see as long as frequent fluoroscopy is performed. As a result, diseases involving long segments of small bowel, such as Crohn's disease, ischemia, or radiation changes, are easily detected on SBFT.
- Enteroclysis has important advantages over SBFT, including improved luminal distention. Short lesions such as tumors or skip lesions of Crohn's disease are better demonstrated by enteroclysis because the lumen is overdistended, making subtle areas of focal narrowing more conspicuous. The small bowel folds are also better evaluated by enteroclysis because the folds are straightened.
- CT has a major advantage over barium studies in that it does not rely on barium reaching the site of obstruction but can use intraluminal fluid to outline the transition zone.

SUGGESTED READINGS

Hara AK, Leighton JA, Sharma VK, et al. Imaging of small bowel disease: comparison of capsule endoscopy, standard endoscopy, barium examination, and CT. RadioGraphics 2005; 25:697-718.

Herlinger H. Guide to imaging of the small bowel. Gastroenterol Clin North Am 1995; 24:309-329.

Maglinte DD. Small bowel imaging—a rapidly changing field and a challenge to radiology. Eur Radiol 2006; 16:967-971.

Maglinte DD, Balthazar EJ, Kelvin FM, et al. The role of radiology in the diagnosis of small-bowel obstruction. AJR Am J Roentgenol 1997;168: 1171-1180.

Maglinte DD, Howard TJ, Lillemoe KD, et al. Small-bowel obstruction: state-of-the-art imaging and its role in clinical management. Clin Gastroenterol Hepatol 2008; 6:130-139.

Maglinte DD, Kelvin FM, O'Connor K, et al. Current status of small bowel radiography. Abdom Imaging 1996; 21:247-257.

Maglinte DD, Sandrasegaran K, Lappas JC, et al. CT enteroclysis. Radiology 2007; 245:661-671.

Nolan DJ. Barium examination of the small intestine. Br J Hosp Med 1994; 52:136-141.

Nolan DJ, Trail ZC. The current role of the barium examination of the small intestine. Clin Radiol 1997; 52:809-820.

Saibeni S, Rondonotti E, Iozzelli A, et al. Imaging of the small bowel in Crohn's disease: a review of old and new techniques. World J Gastroenterol 2007; 13:3279-3287.

REFERENCES

1. Maglinte DD, Sandrasegaran K, Lappas JC, et al. CT enteroclysis. Radiology 2007; 245:661-671.
2. Lappas JC, Maglinte DD. Imaging of the small bowel. Curr Opin Radiol 1991; 3:414-421.
3. Rubesin SE. Barium examinations of the small intestine. In Gore RM (ed). Textbook of Gastrointestinal Radiology. Philadelphia, WB Saunders, 2008, pp 735-754.
4. Laufer I, Hreseel HY. Principles of double contrast diagnosis. In Levine MS (ed). Double Contrast Gastrointestinal Radiology. Philadelphia, WB Saunders, 2000, pp 8-46.
5. Howarth FH, Cockel R, Roper BW, et al. The effect of metoclopramide upon gastric motility and its value in barium progression meals. Clin Radiol 1969; 20:294-300.
6. Kreel L. The use of metoclopramide in the barium meal and follow-through examination. Br J Radiol 1970; 43:31-35.
7. Grumbach K, Herlinger H, Laufer I, et al. Metoclopramide-ceruletide–assisted small bowel examination. ROFO 1988; 149:47-51.
8. Fraser GM, Preston PG. The small bowel follow-through enhanced with an oral effervescent agent. Clin Radiol 1983; 34:673-679.
9. Fitch D. The small bowel follow-through: an improved method of radiographic small bowel visualization. Can J Med Radiat Tech 1995; 26:167-171.
10. Kressel HY, Evers KA, Glick SN, et al. The peroral pneumocolon examination: technique and indications. Radiology 1982; 144:414-416.
11. Fitzgerald EJ, Thompson GT, Somers SS, et al. Pneumocolon as an aid to small bowel studies. Clin Radiol 1985; 36:633-637.
12. Maglinte DDT, Lappas JC, Heitkamp DE, et al. Technical refinements in enteroclysis. Radiol Clin North Am 2003; 41:213-229.
13. Herlinger H. A modified technique for the double contrast small bowel enema. Gastrointest Radiol 1978; 3:201-207.
14. Herlinger H, Maglinte DDT, Tsuneyosi Y. Enteroclysis: technique and variations. In Herlinger H (ed). Clinical Imaging of the Small Intestine. New York, Springer-Verlag, 1999, pp 95-124.
15. Nolan DJ, Cadman PJ. The small bowel enema made easy. Clin Radiol 1987; 38:295-301.
16. Maglinte DDT, Lappas JC, Chernish SM, et al. Improved tolerance of enteroclysis by use of sedation. AJR Am J Roentgenol 1988; 151:951-952.
17. Taverner DS, Odurny A. Enteroclysis—the influence of tube design. Clin Radiol 1994; 49:176-178.
18. Rubesin SE, Levine MS: Principles of Performing a Small Bowel Examination. Westbury, NY, E-Z-EM, 2005.
19. Herlinger H. Small bowel. In Levine MS (ed). Double Contrast Gastrointestinal Radiology. Philadelphia, WB Saunders, 2000, pp 8-46.
20. Diner WC. Duodenal perforation during intubation for small bowel enema study. Radiology 1988; 168:39-41.
21. Shirakabe H, Kobayashi S. Air double-contrast barium study of the small bowel. In Herlinger H (ed). Clinical Radiology of the Small Intestine. Philadelphia, WB Saunders, 1989, pp 139-145.
22. Maglinte DDT, Lappas JC, Kevin FM, et al. Small bowel radiography: How, when and why? Radiology 1987; 163:297-305.
23. Miller RE. Complete reflux examination of the small bowel. Radiology 1986; 84:457-462.
24. Nicolaou S, Kai B, Ho S, et al. Imaging of acute small bowel obstruction. AJR Am J Roentgenol 2005; 185:1036-1044.
25. Jaffe TA, Gaca AM, Delaney S, et al. Radiation doses from small bowel follow-through and abdominopelvic MDCT in Crohn's disease. AJR Am J Roentgenol 2007; 189:1015-1022.
26. Taverne PP, Van der Jagt EJ. Small bowel radiography: a prospective comparative study of three techniques in 200 patients. ROFO 1985; 143:293-297.
27. Maglinte DDT, Burney BT, Miller RE. Lesions missed on small bowel follow through: analysis and recommendations. Radiology 1982; 144:737-739.

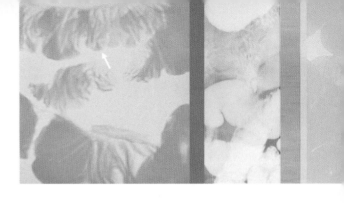

CHAPTER 41

CT of the Small Bowel

Maryam Rezvani and Vahid Yaghmai

Traditionally, evaluation of the small bowel has been an enigma—not accessible by the endoscope and only grossly evaluated by fluoroscopy. Despite the introduction of more invasive techniques such as enteroclysis, disease of the small bowel remained a diagnostic challenge. In recent years, enteroclysis has been further refined to include computed tomographic evaluation. A developing endoscopic technique is wireless capsule endoscopy.[1] With the advent of multidetector computed tomography (MDCT), CT enterography with neutral enteric contrast agents is emerging as the first-line imaging evaluation of the small bowel.[2]

TECHNICAL ASPECTS

"Routine" CT of the Abdomen and Pelvis

"Routine" CT of the abdomen and pelvis utilizes intravenous and positive oral contrast material. This allows for a general evaluation of the solid organs as well as the hollow viscera. With regard to the small bowel, the utility of this protocol is in the evaluation of small bowel obstruction and filling defects within the small bowel lumen.[3] In the setting of small bowel obstruction, CT is most useful in identifying the transition point and a possible cause, such as obstructive mass, bowel herniation, or closed-loop obstruction. In patients who cannot tolerate oral contrast material, small bowel obstruction may be detected without positive enteric contrast material because proximal bowel loops in these patients are usually fluid filled and distended. Although not essential, enhancement after oral administration of a contrast agent can be helpful if the substance is tolerated by the patient. It helps to differentiate small bowel loops from other fluid in the peritoneal cavity. Positive oral contrast material allows differentiation between complete and partial obstruction and can be helpful in distinguishing proximal from distal small bowel loops. Positive oral contrast material in more distal small

bowel loops will be less concentrated due to the dilutional effect of fluid accumulated proximal to the obstruction.[4] However, because transit time increases in such cases, it may be helpful to increase the routine 1- to 2-hour delay after the oral ingestion of a contrast agent.

Multiplanar reformatted images are extremely helpful in the evaluation of pathologic processes of the small bowel on CT. Coronal reformatted images are the most useful because they closely depict the anatomic lie of the bowel loops. They can help to identify normal structures and pathologic processes and have been shown to increase diagnostic confidence.[5] Small bowel obstruction, for example, can be detected on coronal reformatted images as well as the transverse reformatted images, and there are fewer images to evaluate.[6]

CT Enterography

CT enterography is emerging as the first-line modality for imaging of the small bowel.[2] MDCT technology with neutral oral contrast agents and intravenous contrast material has made complete noninvasive evaluation of the small bowel possible. Indications include evaluation of inflammatory bowel disease, small bowel tumors, mesenteric ischemia, as well as active and obscure gastrointestinal bleeding.[2,7-9] CT enterography can localize and evaluate the extent of inflammatory bowel disease as well as assess disease activity and response to therapy (Fig. 41-1). The American College of Radiology appropriateness criteria rate CT enterography as the most appropriate radiologic procedure in the evaluation of Crohn's disease both at initial presentation and with acute exacerbations.[2] Cross-sectional imaging is ideal for the evaluation of extraintestinal complications and manifestations of inflammatory bowel disease. Enhancing mucosal and submucosal masses are not obscured by a neutral oral contrast agent, allowing identification of small bowel tumors. Active gastrointestinal bleeding is evident as contrast extravasation into the bowel lumen and is best evaluated on multiphasic studies.[10]

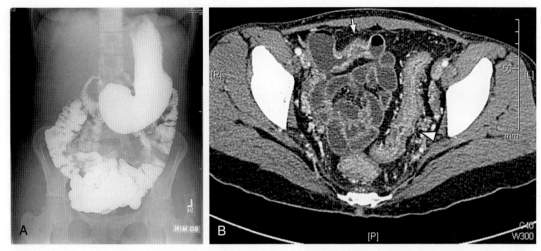

■ **FIGURE 41-1** Small bowel follow-through (SBFT) and CT enterography in a patient with Crohn's disease. **A,** SBFT cannot evaluate the colon or overlapping small bowel loops in the pelvis. **B,** CT enterography in the same patient performed after SBFT shows segmental mural thickening and hyperenhancement of an ileal loop (*arrow*) and acute colonic inflammation (*arrowhead*).

CT enterography is now being used to identify causes of obscure gastrointestinal bleeding such as vascular malformations.[10] It is noninvasive, rapid, readily available, and not operator dependent.

At its inception, CT enterography was performed with positive oral contrast material.[11] However, this was found to obscure the bowel wall, masses, mucosal detail, and adjacent vasculature. Consequently, neutral oral contrast agents with a density of 0 to 30 HU were adopted. Neutral oral contrast agents allow improved visualization of bowel wall enhancement, mural features, enhancing mucosal and submucosal masses, vascular malformations, and contrast extravasation into the bowel lumen. We use a commercially available neutral agent containing 0.1% w/v barium sulfate and sorbitol. Other neutral enteric contrast materials include methylcellulose, polyethylene glycol solution, or water. The commercially available very low density barium and sorbitol solution achieves better small bowel distention compared with water and methylcellulose.[12]

The diagnostic quality of CT enterography depends on optimal distention of small bowel loops. Slow administration of large volumes (1300 to 2000 mL) is necessary for achieving optimal distention. Patients are kept NPO for 6 hours before imaging. Enteric contrast material is ingested slowly over 60 minutes, with the last 225 mL given immediately before imaging. Glucagon has been used by some investigators to improve small bowel distention; however, its efficacy in CT enterography has not been validated as of yet. No medications are given in our practice.

Rapid intravenous administration of contrast material (4 mL/s) is necessary for adequate visualization of the bowel wall. Optimal mucosal enhancement is 45 seconds after rapid injection of intravenous contrast material and is referred to as the enteric phase.[13] Despite greater bowel wall enhancement, this early phase imaging has not been shown to yield additional diagnostic information over the portal venous phase.[14] A single phase of imaging or a multiphasic study may be performed depending on the indication. At our institution a single phase of imaging is performed at 45 seconds after the start of intravenous

contrast agent administration. Single-phase imaging is sufficient in the evaluation of inflammatory bowel disease and small bowel tumors. Examination for gastrointestinal bleeding and mesenteric ischemia requires a triphasic study with precontrast acquisition, in the arterial phase (30-second delay) and delayed phase (70-second delay). Precontrast images help to differentiate incidental hyperdense material in the bowel lumen from abnormal enhancement. A multiphasic study is necessary in the evaluation for vascular malformations and demonstration of the associated early draining vein, as well as evaluation of mesenteric arteries and veins in the setting of ischemia.

It is important to reconstruct images in the coronal and sagittal planes as well as prepare coronal maximum intensity projections. Coronal images allow a global view of the small bowel, help to identify the terminal ileum, and quantify the length of involved bowel segments. Closely apposed loops of small bowel and interloop abscesses are usually best evaluated on axial images. Sagittal images are particularly helpful in the evaluation of the rectum. Multiple planes are often useful for the identification and localization of fistulas. Maximum intensity projections are helpful for visualization of perienteric mesenteric stranding, engorged vasa recta, and the evaluation of vascular structures. Sagittal reformatted images are particularly useful for the detection of celiac or superior mesenteric artery stenosis. A combination of multiple planes may be necessary to detect all the manifestations of inflammatory bowel disease and identify a tumor or source of gastrointestinal bleeding on CT enterography.

CT Enteroclysis

CT enteroclysis is the gold standard in CT of the small bowel. There is a wide range of indications, including low-grade small bowel obstruction, inflammatory bowel disease, obscure gastrointestinal bleeding, and small bowel tumors (Fig. 41-2).[15,16] After nasojejunal intubation, a large volume of neutral enteric contrast medium is rapidly infused directly into the proximal jejunum by an

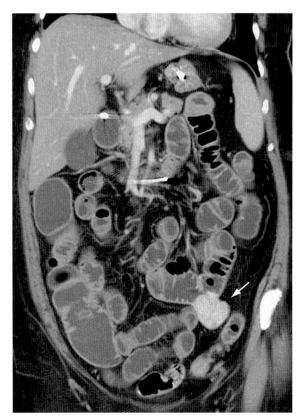

■ **FIGURE 41-2** CT enteroclysis with intravenous and neutral enteric contrast in a patient with a negative capsule endoscopy. There is an enhancing submucosal mass in a left lower quadrant small bowel loop (*arrow*). Pathologic diagnosis was gastrointestinal stromal tumor. (*Courtesy of Kumar Sandrasegaran, MD.*)

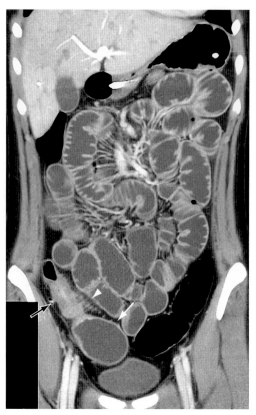

■ **FIGURE 41-3** CT enteroclysis with intravenous and neutral enteric contrast material in a patient with Crohn's disease. There is segmental mural thickening and hyperenhancement in the ileum (*black arrow*) with engorgement of the vasa recta (*white arrowhead*). Proximal ileal dilation (*white arrow*) indicates luminal stricture. Also note intrahepatic biliary dilation due to primary sclerosing cholangitis, which is an extraintestinal complication of Crohn's disease. (*Courtesy of Kumar Sandrasegaran, MD.*)

infusion pump, followed by thin-section CT with intravenous contrast material.[16] Compared with routine CT and CT enterography, the strength of this technique is the enteral volume challenge by nasojejunal intubation, which allows controlled rapid infusion of large volumes of enteric contrast material, thereby optimizing the degree and extent of small bowel distention. It is also advantageous compared with capsule endoscopy because it allows evaluation of the entire abdomen and is not affected by small bowel obstruction, which is an absolute contraindication in capsule endoscopy (Fig. 41-3). Because of the invasive nature of this examination, patients may require sedation. In addition to patient discomfort, there is a risk of bowel perforation with intubation, as well as the inherent risks of sedation. CT enteroclysis remains highly operator dependent and not widely available (Table 41-1).

PROS AND CONS

The strengths and weaknesses of each CT protocol must be considered in the context of the clinical scenario when deciding on the best study for a particular patient (Table 41-2).

CONTROVERSIES

Wireless capsule endoscopy is a revolutionary endoscopic technique for small bowel evaluation but has its limita-

tions. It is contraindicated in patients with strictures due to the risk of capsule retention and is a time-consuming examination. Imaging studies can complement wireless capsule endoscopy by identifying strictures and extraenteric disease. The enteral volume challenge in CT enteroclysis is ideal in the evaluation for strictures and low-grade small bowel obstruction; however, this is an invasive and costly study. Small bowel follow-through (SBFT) has been found to be insensitive before wireless capsule endoscopy in the evaluation of strictures. CT enterography has been shown to be more sensitive for the identification of strictures and inflammatory bowel disease compared with SBFT and is a noninvasive and more cost-efficient alternative to CT enteroclysis.[14,17] It is complementary to wireless capsule endoscopy both in the pre-capsule workup for strictures and in evaluation of patients with known or advanced inflammatory bowel disease (Fig. 41-4).[17,18]

Evaluation of obscure gastrointestinal bleeding was previously dominated by SBFT and enteroclysis. Wireless capsule endoscopy has brought endoscopy to the forefront of small bowel evaluation, allowing visualization of early Crohn's disease, vascular malformations, and small bowel tumors. Recent studies comparing wireless capsule endoscopy with multiphase CT enterography suggest a role for enterography in the evaluation of

TABLE 41-1 Characteristics of CT Protocols Used in Small Bowel Imaging

Protocol	Patient Preparation	Enteric Contrast	Medications	Intravenous Contrast	Scan Delay	Slice Thickness/ Reconstruction Interval	Reformed Images
Abdomen/ pelvis CT	Clamp nasogastric tube	Positive oral contrast 900 mL over 2 hr – 150 mL every 20 min	None	Optional 125 mL at 3 mL/s	70 s	5 mm/5 mm	Coronal – 2 × 2 mm
CT enterography	NPO 6 hr	Neutral oral contrast – 0.1% w/v barium 1350 mL over 1 hr – 450 mL in 20 min – 450 mL in next 20 min – 225 mL in next 20 min – 225 mL on CT table	None	Required 125 mL at 4 mL/s	Single-phase study – 45 s Multiphase study – precontrast – 30 s – 70 s	2 mm/2 mm	Coronal and sagittal – 2 × 2 mm Coronal MIP – 4 × 2 mm
CT enteroclysis	24 hr before the study – laxative and clear liquids Day of exam – NPO	Neutral or positive contrast via nasojejunal tube 3 L at an initial rate of 100 mL/min – 1.5 L–initially – 1.5 L on CT table – adjust rate as needed	IV glucagon	None with positive enteric contrast 125 mL at 4 mL/s with neutral enteric contrast	45 s	2 mm/1 mm	Multiplanar reformatted

TABLE 41-2 Comparison of CT Protocols Used in Small Bowel Imaging

Protocol	Indications	Pros	Cons
Abdomen/pelvis CT	Small bowel obstruction Patients with renal failure Patients with contrast allergy	Noninvasive Can be performed with or without intravenous contrast material Can differentiate complete from partial small bowel obstruction	Mural features and enhancing masses obscured by positive enteral contrast
CT enterography	*Single phase:* Inflammatory bowel disease Pre-wireless capsule endoscopy Small bowel mass *Multiphase:* Active gastrointestinal bleeding Obscure gastrointestinal bleeding Mesenteric ischemia (atherosclerotic disease, thrombosis, dissection, trauma, tumor)	Noninvasive Rapid and readily available Not operator dependent Can evaluate mural features and identify enhancing masses, vascular malformations, or bleeding	Requires intravenous contrast Requires patient compliance to drink a relatively large volume of oral contrast in the allotted time
CT enteroclysis	Low-grade small bowel obstruction Inflammatory bowel disease Small bowel mass Obscure gastrointestinal bleeding	Enteral volume challenge Can evaluate mural features or enhancing masses	Invasive Operator dependent Not widely available Requires sedation and nasojejunal intubation Logistical limitations (fluoroscopy and CT suites need to be in close proximity)

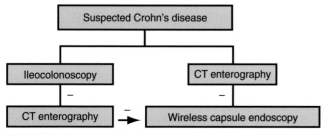

■ **FIGURE 41-4** Algorithm for the workup of patients with suspected Crohn's disease.

obscure gastrointestinal bleeding.[10] Preliminary studies show CT enterography is able to demonstrate small bowel abnormalities not identified by wireless capsule endoscopy and cecal abnormalities not seen on colonoscopy.[10] In the workup of obscure gastrointestinal bleeding, CT enterography is a promising complementary technique to wireless capsule endoscopy.

NORMAL ANATOMIC IMAGING FINDINGS

The mesenteric small bowel is approximately 6 meters in length and extends from the second portion of the

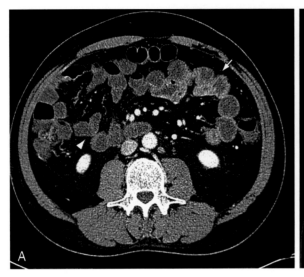
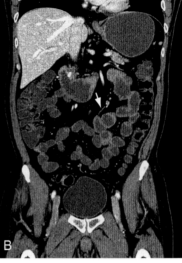

■ **FIGURE 41-5** Axial (**A**) and coronal (**B**) images of normal CT enterography. Enhancement of normal jejunal loops (*arrow*) is greater than that of normal ileal loops (*arrowhead*).

duodenum to the ileocecal valve. Normal small bowel wall thickness is less than 3 mm, and normal caliber is less than 3 cm. Optimal bowel wall enhancement is 45 seconds after bolus injection of intravenous contrast material.[13] Normal small bowel loops vary in their enhancement depending on the segment and degree of distention. Jejunal loops enhance more than ileal loops (Fig. 41-5). Collapsed small bowel loops enhance more than distended loops. It is important to compare loops of small bowel in the same region and with similar degrees of distention when assessing mural enhancement. Secondary signs of active disease are useful for distinguishing normal mucosal enhancement from abnormal mucosa.

KEY POINTS

- MDCT has made cross-sectional imaging of the small bowel possible.
- "Routine" CT of the abdomen and pelvis utilizes positive enteric contrast material with or without intravenous contrast material and is most useful for evaluation of small bowel obstruction.
- CT enterography is a noninvasive technique utilizing intravenous contrast and neutral enteric contrast material to visualize intrinsic small bowel abnormalities, as well as associated extraenteric pathologic processes.
- Indications for CT enterography include inflammatory bowel disease, acute gastrointestinal bleeding, obscure gastrointestinal bleeding, mesenteric ischemia, small bowel tumors, and pre-capsule endoscopy workup.
- Neutral enteric contrast material allows visualization of abnormal mucosal and mural enhancement, mucosal and submucosal small bowel masses, small bowel vascular mal-

formations, and extravasation of intravenous contrast material into the bowel lumen.
- Multiplanar reformatted images are an integral part of all imaging protocols, improving visualization of both normal structures and pathologic processes, as well as increasing diagnostic accuracy.
- With the advent of MDCT, imaging of the small bowel is complementary to endoscopic techniques, allowing identification of transmural or perienteric abnormalities and extraenteric complications.
- CT enteroclysis utilizes intravenous contrast material and nasojejunal intubation to volume-challenge the small bowel with neutral enteric contrast material.
- Indications for CT enteroclysis include low-grade small bowel obstruction, inflammatory bowel disease, obscure gastrointestinal bleeding, and small bowel tumors.

SUGGESTED READINGS

Horton KM, Fishman EK. Multidetector CT angiography in the diagnosis of mesenteric ischemia. Radiol Clin North Am 2007; 45:275.

Maglinte DD, et al. CT enteroclysis. Radiology 2007; 245:661-671.

Maglinte DD, Sandrasegaran K, Lappas JC. CT enteroclysis: techniques and applications. Radiol Clin North Am 2007; 45:389-401.

Paulsen SR, Huprich JE, Hara AK. CT enterography: noninvasive evaluation of Crohn's disease and obscure gastrointestinal bleed. Radiol Clin North Am 2007; 45:303-315.

Qalbani A, Paushter D, Dachman AH. Multidetector row CT of small bowel obstruction. Radiol Clin North Am 2007; 45:499-512.

Tochetto S, Yaghmai V. CT enterography: concept, technique and interpretation. Radiol Clin North Am 2009; 47:117-132.

REFERENCES

1. Maglinte DD. Capsule imaging and the role of radiology in the investigation of diseases of the small bowel. Radiology 2005; 236:763.
2. Huprich JE, Bree RL, Foley WD, et al. Expert Panel on Gastrointestinal Imaging. Crohn's disease. [online publication]. Reston, VA, American College of Radiology (ACR), 2005.
3. Nicolaou S, Kai B, Ho S, et al. Imaging of acute small-bowel obstruction. AJR Am J Roentgenol 2005; 185:1036.
4. Qalbani A, Paushter D, Dachman AH. Multidetector row CT of small bowel obstruction. Radiol Clin North Am 2007; 45:499.
5. Jaffe TA, Martin LC, Thomas J, et al. Small-bowel obstruction: coronal reformations from isotropic voxels at 16-section multidetector row CT. Radiology 2005; 238:135.
6. Yaghmai V, Nikolaidis P, Hammond NA, et al. Multidetector-row computed tomography diagnosis of small bowel obstruction: can coronal reformations replace axial images? Emerg Radiol 2006; 13:69.
7. Paulsen SR, Huprich JE, Fletcher JG, et al. CT enterography as a diagnostic tool in evaluating small bowel disorders: review of clinical experience with over 700 cases. RadioGraphics 2006; 26:641.
8. Paulsen SR, Huprich JE, Hara AK. CT enterography: noninvasive evaluation of Crohn's disease and obscure gastrointestinal bleed. Radiol Clin North Am 2007; 45:303.
9. Yoon W, Jeong YY, Shin SS, et al. Acute massive gastrointestinal bleeding: detection and localization with arterial phase multidetector row helical CT. Radiology 2006; 239:160.
10. Huprich JE, Fletcher JG, Alexander JA, et al. Obscure gastrointestinal bleeding: evaluation with 64-section multiphase CT enterography—initial experience. Radiology 2008; 246:562.
11. Raptopoulos V, Schwartz RK, McNicholas MM, et al. Multiplanar helical CT enterography in patients with Crohn's disease. AJR Am J Roentgenol 1997; 169:1545.
12. Megibow AJ, Babb JS, Hecht EM, et al. Evaluation of bowel distention and bowel wall appearance by using neutral oral contrast agent for multi-detector row CT. Radiology 2006; 238:87.
13. Schindera S, Nelson RC, DeLong DM, et al. Multi-detector row CT of the small bowel: peak enhancement temporal window—initial experience. Radiology 2007; 243:438.
14. Wold PB, Fletcher JG, Johnson CD, et al. Assessment of small bowel Crohn disease: noninvasive peroral CT enterography compared with other imaging methods and endoscopy—feasibility study. Radiology 2003; 229:275.
15. Maglinte DD, Sandrasegaran K, Lappas JC. CT enteroclysis: techniques and applications. Radiol Clin North Am 2007; 45:389.
16. Maglinte DD, Sandrasegaran K, Lappas JC, et al. CT enteroclysis. Radiology 2007; 245:661.
17. Hara AK, Leighton JA, Heigh RI, et al. Crohn disease of the small bowel: preliminary comparison among CT enterography, capsule endoscopy, small-bowel follow-through, and ileoscopy. Radiology 2006; 238:128.
18. Hara AK, Leighton JA, Sharma VK, et al. Small bowel: preliminary comparison of capsule endoscopy with barium study and CT. Radiology 2004; 230:260.

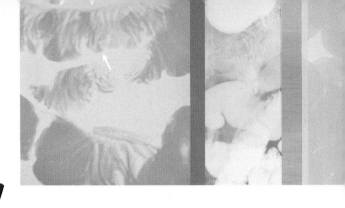

CHAPTER 42

Ultrasound Imaging of the Small Bowel

Thomas Grant

Ultrasonography is frequently used as the first imaging examination in patients with abdominal pain, primarily for the evaluation of solid abdominal viscera.[1] Bowel-related symptoms often necessitate numerous radiologic investigations, but ultrasonography is not often chosen as the initial imaging technique. Although radiologists performing abdominal imaging are familiar with the CT and barium study appearances of bowel abnormalities, they often underestimate the potential diagnostic strength of ultrasound imaging in the evaluation of bowel disease. Studies have also confirmed that ultrasonography has the ability to assess a wide variety of pathologic conditions related to the stomach, small bowel, colon, mesentery, and peritoneum. If performed by experts, ultrasonography has the potential to give excellent results.[2,3]

CT is usually the imaging procedure of choice in the assessment of suspected bowel, mesenteric, and peritoneal abnormalities. With the increasing awareness of potential adverse effects of ionizing radiation, alternate imaging techniques such as ultrasonography and MRI are more frequently being considered, especially in young patients and in women of child-bearing age.[4-6]

Ultrasonography can reveal important small bowel abnormalities that can have a profound impact on patient management. It is paramount for the sonographer and radiologist to be familiar with the normal location and appearance of the small bowel, so that alterations can be recognized. Many pathologic processes that affect the small bowel are amenable to ultrasound imaging. Infection, inflammatory diseases, neoplastic processes, and small bowel obstruction are all potential indications for ultrasonography.[7] These pathologic processes manifest as luminal narrowing, thickened bowel wall, and abnormal peristaltic activity. Familiarity with the ultrasound appearance and distribution of abnormalities may allow for a specific diagnosis.

TECHNICAL ASPECTS

The most important component of the ultrasound examination is constant interaction with the patient. It is imperative that the radiologist communicate with the patient because both the information provided by the patient and the ultrasound findings may lead to a specific diagnosis. The patient should be asked to place a finger on the area that is most tender. However, one should consider all possible differential diagnoses because the abnormality can also be found at locations other than the symptomatic region.

The ultrasound examination is an extension of the physical examination. Graded compression, first described by Puylaert,[8] is a technique using ultrasound-guided palpation. It is performed by applying uniform sustained gentle pressure with the transducer. When used appropriately, graded compression will displace normal gas-containing bowel away from narrowed, thickened, or fluid-filled small bowel. A fixed and noncompressible small bowel is the key to finding and characterizing a pathologic process. If, despite compression, gas continues to hinder the examination, the transducer can be placed at the mid or posterior axillary line so that ventrally located gas can be avoided. Decubitus or occasionally upright positioning may also be helpful.

It is beneficial to examine the small bowel with it in the resting state. Food and water can adversely affect the examination, so fasting by the patient before the evaluation is preferred. The choice of transducer for small bowel assessment largely depends on the patient's body habitus and the distance between the probe and the object of study. A 2.0- to 5.0-MHz curvilinear probe is used for a large patient. A 7.0- to 12.0-MHz linear transducer, which facilitates high-resolution ultrasonography, is used for an average-sized or thin patient and for assessment of superficial abnormalities. A multifrequency transducer allows for optimal visualization of a pathologic process using the highest frequency possible for better resolution. The field of view should be optimized so that all of the abdominal contents are included. The focal zone should be adjusted during the examination when looking for a bowel pathologic process or for finding normal landmarks.[9]

It is not unusual in women of child-bearing age to have nonspecific signs and symptoms, including pelvic pain, fever, or a pelvic mass, that make it difficult to differentiate gynecologic and gastrointestinal tract disease. Transvaginal ultrasonography is an excellent imaging method to assess the small bowel and to look for masses or ascites.[10] The perienteric fatty tissue is assessed for infiltration and the presence of fluid. The adjacent mesentery is checked for the presence of enlarged lymph nodes.

Color Doppler imaging can be used to differentiate edema or intramural hemorrhage from acute inflammation or infection.[11] Thus, mural thickening in conjunction with hyperemia of the small bowel seen on color or power Doppler imaging strongly suggests vasodilatation related to an infectious or inflammatory process. Similarly, a neoplastic mass can be differentiated from edema, ischemia, or an abscess by its hyperemic state.[12] However, the specificity of color Doppler imaging is unknown. The results of color Doppler imaging can also be misleading if the evaluation was performed incorrectly or if adequate clinical information is unavailable.

IMAGING

Normal Appearance

The multilayered ultrasonographic appearance of the wall of the stomach, small bowel, and colon is due to alternating hypoechoic and echogenic layers. These correspond to the histologic appearance of the bowel. There are five concentric rings (Fig. 42-1): the mucosa (most inner layer), submucosa, and serosal layers are echogenic; and the muscularis mucosa and the muscularis propria are hypoechoic. Although the lumen of the small bowel can vary in diameter, in normal patients the small bowel wall is 3 mm or less in thickness.

Small bowel peristalsis is a normal event. Peristalsis is also an important factor in diagnosing a small bowel pathologic process. One should always document the frequency of peristalsis and the amount of fluid or solid material within the small bowel lumen. In patients with bowel obstruction or gastroenteritis there is increased peristaltic activity and also a large amount of luminal fluid that makes the examination much easier to interpret. Normally, there is forward peristaltic movement. To-and-fro or reversed directional activity is always abnormal. Alternately, in patients with paralytic ileus there may be no peristaltic activity.

Ultrasonographic evaluation of the duodenum, jejunum, and ileum requires excellent knowledge of the anatomy. The duodenum, owing to its fixed location, is readily identified adjacent to the pancreas and surrounding vasculature. The terminal ileum can usually be identified by its location adjacent to the ascending colon and by detecting the ileocecal valve. The remainder of the small bowel is not seen in its entirety. The transition between the

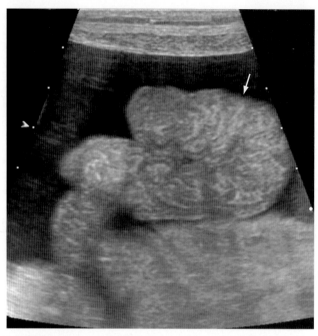

■ **FIGURE 42-1** Longitudinal ultrasound image of the small bowel, which is surrounded by ascites, shows the normal multilayered appearance (*arrow*).

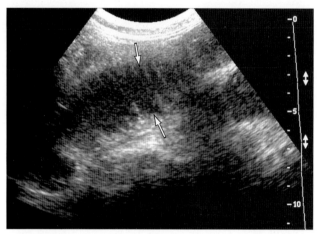

■ **FIGURE 42-2** Longitudinal ultrasound image of a 28-year-old pregnant patient with a small bowel obstruction from adhesions. The valvulae conniventes (*arrows*) are well demonstrated projecting into the fluid-filled small bowel.

jejunum and ileum is impossible to image because the small bowel is the most mobile portion of the gastrointestinal tract.

The small bowel is readily identified by its mucosal signature, the valvulae conniventes. Therefore, when this unique feature is imaged with ultrasound it should not be confused with other gastrointestinal structures. Although not present normally, the valvulae conniventes are readily identified when the small bowel is engorged or the wall is thickened (Fig. 42-2).

The Abnormal Small Bowel

Small bowel pathologic processes will manifest as wall thickening, a mass, luminal narrowing, abnormal peristalsis, or soft tissue abnormalities in the adjacent mesentery or peritoneum.[13] As a general rule, preservation of the bowel layers on ultrasonography suggests an infectious or inflammatory process (Fig. 42-3). Conversely, absence of such layering is more supportive of a neoplastic cause (Fig. 42-4). When examining the small bowel with ultrasound, it is imperative to note the thickness and length of the involved segment because that aids in differentiating the pathologic entities (Table 42-1). Attention to the shape and size of the local lymph nodes is essential. When an inflammatory process is present, the regional lymph nodes are usually not markedly enlarged, maintain their central echogenic hilum, and have an elliptical shape. Echogenic mesenteric fat adjacent to the abnormal bowel loops is an important finding and is secondary to mesenteric edema or neoplastic infiltration.[14-18]

There are several ultrasonographic signs that are specific and do not require additional imaging.[19-21] These are the "whirlpool" sign associated with midgut volvulus and the pseudokidney appearance of intussusception (Fig. 42-5). They are primarily found in children and are treated with surgery, nonsurgical intervention, or a follow-up ultrasound evaluation.

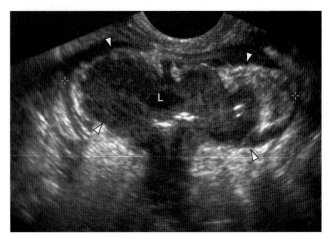

■ FIGURE 42-4 Transvaginal ultrasound image from a 45-year-old woman with non-Hodgkin's lymphoma. A huge mass with transmural destruction of the ileum (*arrowheads*) surrounds aneurysmal dilatation of the small bowel lumen (L).

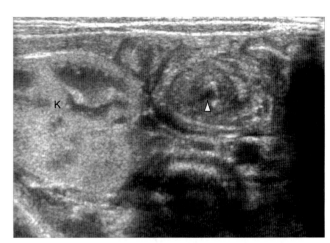

■ FIGURE 42-5 Transverse ultrasound image in the mid abdomen of a 6-month-old infant shows the whirlpool-like appearance of the superior mesenteric vein and mesentery twisted around the superior mesenteric artery (*arrowhead*). (*Courtesy of Tami Ben-Ami, MD, Childrens Memorial Hospital, Chicago, IL.*)

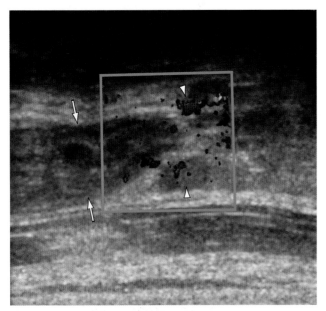

■ FIGURE 42-3 Transverse ultrasound image of the right lower quadrant of a 22-year-old woman with mesenteric adenitis. There is a thickened loop of ileum with a loss of normal stratification (*arrows*). Adjacent to the thickened bowel are slightly enlarged mesenteric lymph nodes showing hyperemia on color Doppler imaging (*arrowheads*). Although these findings are nonspecific, the patient recovered 2 days later.

TABLE 42-1 Diagnosis of Small Bowel Disease Based on Ultrasound Appearance of Small Bowel Thickening and Length of Involvement

	Type of Thickening		Length of Involvement	
Mild	*Marked*	*Symmetric*	*<10 cm*	*>10 cm*
Infectious enteritis	Adenocarcinoma	Infectious enteritis	Adenocarcinoma	Lymphoma
Crohn's disease	Gastrointestinal stromal	Crohn's disease	Gastrointestinal stromal	Infectious enteritis
Radiation injury	tumor	Radiation injury	tumor	Crohn's disease
Ischemia	Metastasis	Ischemia		Radiation injury
Edema—low protein	Lymphoma			Ischemia
	Systemic lupus			Diffuse infectious enteritis
				Edema-low protein
				Systemic lupus

CONTROVERSIES

The obvious advantages of ultrasonography in the assessment of the small bowel are lack of ionizing radiation and the need for intravenously administered contrast material and its cost-effectiveness. However, in clinical practice ultrasonography is usually not the favored modality, owing to inherent limitations, which include operator dependency, obscuration of pathologic bowel by gas, and abdominal pain that may limit the ability to perform graded compression. The sensitivity of ultrasonography to detect perforation, fistulas, abscesses, or the activity of the disease compared with the latest generation of CT and MR scanners is unknown.

KEY POINTS

■ The morphologic characteristic of the small bowel, the valvulae conniventes, must be identified to allow for correct localization of a pathologic process.

■ In mechanical small bowel obstruction there is a dilated, fluid-filled hyperactive small bowel with to-and-fro or reversed peristalsis. This is readily determined when the bowel contains a substantial fluid quantity. In a patient with a paralytic ileus there is no peristaltic activity.

■ The abnormal small bowel should be followed as far distally as possible. If there is no bowel wall thickening or luminal narrowing, the etiology is usually an adhesion. Thickened small bowel, luminal narrowing, or a mass at the site of obstruction suggests an inflammatory process, neoplasm, hernia, or intussusception.

REFERENCES

1. Wilson SR. Evaluation of the small intestine by ultrasonography. In Gourtsoyiannis NC (ed). Radiological Imaging of the Small Intestine. Heidelberg, Springer-Verlag, 2002, pp 73-86.
2. O'Malley ME, Wilson SR. US of gastrointestinal tract abnormalities with CT correlation. RadioGraphics 2003; 23:59-72.
3. Ledermann P, Borner N, Strunk H, Bongartz G. Bowel wall thickening on transabdominal sonography. AJR Am J Roentgenol 2000; 174:107-117.
4. Barloon TJ, Brown BP, Abu-Yousef MM, et al. Sonography of acute appendicitis in pregnancy. Abdom Imaging 1995; 20:149-151.
5. Pedrosa I, Levine D, Eyvazzadeh A, et al. MR imaging evaluation of acute appendicitis in pregnancy. Radiology 2006; 238:891-899.
6. Birchard KR, Brown MA, Hyslop WB, et al. MRI of acute abdominal and pelvic pain in pregnant patients. AJR Am J Roentgenol 2005; 184:452-458.
7. Puylaert J, van der Zant FM, Rijke AM. Sonography and the acute abdomen: practical. AJR Am J Roentgenol 1997; 168:179-186.
8. Puylaert JB. Acute appendicitis: US evaluation using graded compression. Radiology 1986; 158:355-360.
9. Chaubal N, Manjiri D, Shah M, Chaubal J. Sonography of the gastrointestinal tract. J Ultrasound Med 2006; 25:87-97.
10. Damani N, Wilson SR. Nongynecologic applications of transvaginal US. RadioGraphics 1999; 19:S179-S200.
11. Frisoli JK, Desser TS, Jeffrey RB. Thickened submucosal layer: A sonographic sign of acute gastrointestinal abnormality representing submucosal edema or hemorrhage. AJR Am J Roentgenol 2000; 175:1595-1599.
12. Hata J, Kamada T, Haruma K, Kusunoki H. Evaluation of bowel ischemia with contrast-enhanced US: initial experience. Radiology 2005; 236:712-715.
13. Hanbidge AE, Lynch D, Wilson SR. US of the peritoneum. RadioGraphics 2003; 23:663-685.
14. Rosch T, Classen M. Gastroenterologic Endosonography. New York, Thieme Medical Publishers, 1992, p 36.
15. Kimmey MB, Martin RW, Hagitt RC, et al. Histologic correlates of gastrointestinal ultrasound images. Gastroenterology 1989; 96:433-441.
16. Niclaou S, Kai B, Ho S, et al. Imaging of acute small-bowel obstruction. AJR Am J Roentgenol 2005; 185:1038-1044.
17. Retterbacher T, Hollerweger A, Macheiner P, et al. Abdominal wall hernias. AJR Am J Roentgenol 2001; 177:1061-1066.
18. Sarratiz J, Wilson SR. Manifestations of Crohn disease at US. RadioGraphics 1996; 16:499-520.
19. Sung T, Callahan M, Taylor GA. Clinical and imaging mimickers of acute appendicitis in the pediatric poplulation. AJR Am J Roentgenol 2006; 186:67-74.
20. Pracross JP, Sann L, Genin G, et al. Ultrasound diagnosis of midgut volvulus: the "whirlpool" sign. Pediatr Radiol 1992; 22:18-20.
21. del-Pozo G, Albillos JC, Tejedor D. Intussusception: US findings with pathologic correlation—the crescent-in-doughnut sign. Radiology 1996; 199:688-692.

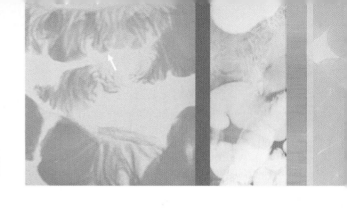

CHAPTER 43

MRI of the Small Bowel

Nancy A. Hammond and Paul Nikolaidis

TECHNICAL ASPECTS

Because of limited endoscopic techniques, radiologic studies play an important role in evaluating the small bowel. Traditionally, conventional small bowel follow-through (SBFT) examinations have been the technique utilized most frequently by radiologists and clinicians. Because of its invasive and time-consuming nature, conventional fluoroscopic enteroclysis has not been the first-line modality in evaluating small bowel pathology but has been reserved for cases in which SBFT examinations did not provide adequate assessment. However, SBFT and conventional enteroclysis allow only for indirect assessment of the small bowel wall and surrounding structures. As such, cross-sectional imaging including CT and MRI is playing an increasing role in evaluating pathologic processes of the bowel.

Whereas CT is widely used for evaluating the small bowel and the presence of extraluminal disease, MRI has played a limited role, owing to long examination times and motion artifacts caused by bowel peristalsis. However, with the advent of MR sequences that allow for rapid acquisition of high-resolution images, these limitations have been minimized and the role of MRI in evaluating the small bowel has increased.

Intraluminal Contrast Agents

Various oral contrast agents have been investigated in the use of MRI of the small bowel but no consensus on the ideal one has been reached. In fact, some authors have demonstrated that both the normal and abnormal small bowel can be adequately assessed utilizing heavily T2-weighted sequences and intrinsic intestinal fluid, thus eliminating the need for oral contrast administration.[1]

When exogenous oral contrast agents are indicated, important factors in agent selection include the ability to achieve homogeneous opacification of the bowel and adequate bowel distention, high contrast resolution between the lumen and bowel wall, no significant adverse effects, low artifact potential, and low cost. Agents with low absorption by the bowel are preferred to aid in achieving adequate bowel distention.

Intraluminal oral contrast agents are described as either negative, positive, or biphasic agents. Negative agents result in decreased signal in the bowel lumen, regardless of the sequence utilized. They include agents such as high weight per volume barium sulfate and supramagnetic iron oxide and other oral magnetic particles. Gas could also be potentially used as a negative contrast agent.[2] Bowel wall thickening and enhancement are nicely demonstrated with these agents. Side effects including nausea, vomiting, and rectal leakage may be seen in 5% to 15% of patients, however.[2] Other limitations of these agents include high cost, associated artifacts (most notable on low field strength MR systems), and paradoxical high signal intensity if not distributed evenly throughout the bowel.[2]

Positive agents result in increased signal in the bowel lumen. They include agents such as gadolinium chelates, manganese ions, ferrous ions, ferrous ammonium citrates, iron phytase, and natural food substances including milk or blueberry juice.[2] Bowel wall thickening is nicely demonstrated with these agents, but bowel wall enhancement may be obscured by the high signal intensity of the contrast agent within the bowel lumen.

Biphasic agents are hyperintense on T2-weighted sequences and hypointense on T1-weighted sequences. Water is the most basic form of a biphasic agent and can be employed as an oral contrast agent. However, because of its absorption by small bowel, water often results in unpredictable distention and is typically only effective for evaluating the stomach and proximal to mid small bowel.[3] Therefore, isosmolar biphasic agents are preferred owing to their decreased bowel absorption and improved bowel distention. Isosmolar biphasic agents to consider include dilute barium sulfate (98% water, 2% barium sulfate), psyllium fiber mixed with water, and mannitol with locust bean gum and polyethylene glycol (PEG).

A typical oral preparation includes patient fasting for 4 to 5 hours before the examination. Then 1.0 to 1.5 L of oral contrast is administered over 1 hour before the examination. If MR enteroclysis is being performed, the contrast agent is administered via a nasojejunal tube, allowing for more controlled bowel distention.

Pulse Sequences

Previously, MRI of the gastrointestinal tract was limited by motion artifact due to bowel peristalsis and respiratory motion. However, with the advent of fast and ultrafast sequences, the utility of MRI in assessing for pathologic processes in the small bowel has rapidly improved.

Currently, T2-weighted sequences commonly utilized in MR evaluation of the small bowel include half-Fourier acquired single-shot turbo spin echo (HASTE) and true fast imaging with steady precession (true FISP). HASTE and true FISP are vendor-specific acronyms. Depending on the vendor, HASTE-type sequences are also known as single-shot fast spin echo (SSFSE) and single-shot turbo spin echo (SSTE), whereas true FISP–like sequences are also referred to as steady-state free precession (SSFP), balanced field-echo (b-TFE), and fast imaging employing steady-state acquisition (FIESTA).

Both HASTE and true FISP are single-slice sequences with acquisition times of approximately 1 second per slice. The rapid acquisition time eliminates artifact due to respiratory motion and bowel peristalsis. HASTE and true FISP provide excellent image quality but have poor soft tissue resolution, limiting characterization of small bowel lesions.

Additional advantages of HASTE include insensitivity to susceptibility and black boundary artifact and high contrast between the lumen and the bowel wall. Disadvantages include relatively limited detail regarding the mesentery and bowel wall and high sensitivity to high-order motion artifacts, resulting in potential intraluminal flow voids (Fig. 43-1A). Additional advantages of true FISP include its insensitivity to motion artifact, resulting in homogeneous endoluminal opacification, the ability to evaluate the mesentery, and high contrast between the bowel lumen and bowel wall.[4] Disadvantages include sensitivity to susceptibility and black boundary artifact (see Fig. 43-1B). Black boundary artifact is defined as the thin

black line along the external surface of the bowel wall, which may mask subtle bowel wall thickening or pathology. This artifact can be eliminated by combining true FISP with fat suppression, which allows for better detection of subtle wall thickening.[5]

Fast low-angle shot (FLASH) and fast multiplanar spoiled gradient-recalled-echo (SPGR) sequences are the most commonly utilized T1-weighted sequences in evaluating the small bowel.[6] These are acquired as a stack of slices within one TR interval, requiring acquisition times of 15 to 20 seconds. The longer acquisition time makes these sequences more susceptible to motion and respiratory artifact. However, they provide superior soft tissue contrast compared with HASTE and true FISP, resulting in more accurate assessment of morphologic changes in the bowel wall and improved characterization of small bowel lesions. The use of fat suppression expands the dynamic range of intra-abdominal signal intensities and increases the conspicuity of gadolinium enhancement due to the elimination of the high signal of fat.[5]

Fat-suppressed, T2-weighted, fast spin-echo images have been advocated as an optional sequence to distinguish wall thickening due to mural edema from an acute inflammatory process versus wall thickening from chronic fibrosis.[7]

Because each of the MR sequences discussed earlier has its own strengths and weaknesses and provides unique information to the study, a protocol combining these characteristics provides the best way to effectively evaluate the small bowel with MRI. The multiplanar capability of MRI should also be utilized with these sequences obtained in multiple projections. The coronal plane demonstrates small bowel anatomy while the axial and sagittal planes aid in detecting and evaluating any underlying pathologic process.

Coil Selection

The use of a phased-array body coil provides for increased signal-to-noise ratio, resulting in excellent image quality but possibly at the expense of homogeneity. A body coil

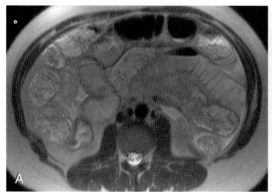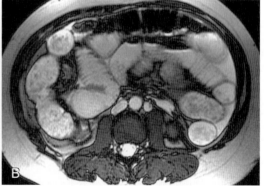

■ **FIGURE 43-1** **A,** Axial T2-weighted HASTE image in a patient with small bowel obstruction. Oral contrast was not administered. There is distention of the bowel by intrinsic enteric contents. Bowel is normal thickness and signal. However, note the apparent intraluminal filling defects confirmed to be artifactual on true FISP images. **B,** Axial true FISP image in the same patient again demonstrates fluid-filled, dilated loops of small bowel with more homogeneous intraluminal opacification lacking the apparent flow voids seen on the HASTE image. Additionally, black boundary artifact is also present and characterized by the black line along the external surface of the bowel wall. This artifact is frequently seen on true FISP sequences.

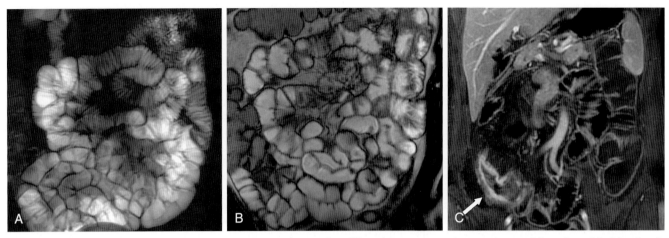

■ **FIGURE 43-2** **A,** Coronal thick SSFSE image in a patient with normal small bowel demonstrates the great degree of distention of the jejunal and ileal loops achieved with MR enteroclysis utilizing a hyperosmotic polyethylene glycol water solution. **B,** Coronal FIESTA sequence on the same patient shows the normal appearance of the intraluminal folds, the bowel wall, and the mesentery. Visualization of increased anatomic detail is aided by the significant degree of distention afforded by MR enteroclysis. **C,** Coronal post-gadolinium T1-weighted image in a patient with Crohn's disease who underwent MR enterography shows the abnormal terminal ileum with mural thickening and hyperenhancement of the mucosal and serosal surfaces and corresponding low signal intensity in muscularis and submucosa layers (*arrow*). Such a stratified pattern of enhancement to the bowel wall is indicative of active disease. This appearance results from hyperenhancement of the mucosa, with decreased enhancement of the submucosa and muscularis layers due to edema. *(All MR enteroclysis images courtesy of Dr. Gabriele Masselli, Umberto I Hospital, La Sapienza University, Rome, Italy.)*

may also be used, providing excellent image quality, homogeneity, and extended anatomic coverage.

MR Enteroclysis

MR enteroclysis combines the advantages of conventional enteroclysis with those of cross-sectional imaging and reliably achieves optimal small bowel distention (Fig. 43-2). However, it requires nasojejunal intubation, resulting in patient discomfort. The intubation is typically performed under fluoroscopic guidance, resulting in a longer procedure. The patient can then be transported to the MRI suite and the small bowel may be filled after the patient is placed on the scanner.[2] Patients are imaged in the prone position to achieve abdominal autocompression.[8] Then 1500 to 2000 mL of hyperosmotic water solution (PEG) is administered via the nasojejunal tube with an MR-compatible pump. If this pump is not available, either manual-injection or hand-held infusion pumps may be utilized.[2] Typically, the contrast agent is administered in two phases. Initially, a flow rate of 80 to 120 mL/min is utilized until the agent reaches the terminal ileum. The flow rate can then be increased to 300 mL/min to create reflex atony.[9] Small bowel filling may be monitored by use of MR fluoroscopy or intermittent imaging with a thick slab HASTE sequence.[2] Alternatively, the small bowel may be filled outside the scanner; however, less optimal distention may be attained without constant infusion.

PROS AND CONS

MRI is a rapidly emerging technique that may be successfully utilized to evaluate pathologic processes of the small bowel. With MRI now capable of the rapid acquisition of high-resolution images, limitations including long examination times and motion artifacts from bowel peristalsis and respiration have been minimized and its role in evalu-

ating the small bowel is increasing. MRI has several inherent advantages over CT, including lack of radiation exposure, eliminating the need for iodinated contrast material, outstanding soft tissue contrast, and its multiplanar capabilities. The lack of radiation exposure is particularly important in pregnant or pediatric patients or in patients undergoing serial follow-up examinations.

Practical disadvantages of MRI include higher examination costs and longer examination times compared with CT and known contraindications to MRI such as pacemakers. Gadolinium administration may be contraindicated in patients with renal insufficiency owing to nephrogenic systemic fibrosis.

Technically, MRI has decreased spatial resolution compared with CT, which may make superficial lesions difficult to detect. Additionally, the decreased temporal resolution of MRI may result in artifacts from bowel peristalsis, although this has been largely overcome by the use of fast T2-weighted sequences.

Diagnostically, pitfalls arise with incomplete distention of the bowel. Complete distention is most reliably achieved with MR enteroclysis. However, adequate results are generally obtained with MR enterography alone, obviating the need for nasojejunal intubation, and MR enteroclysis may be reserved for selected cases.[2] Subtle lesions can be masked by lack of distention, or, conversely, inadequately distended segments of small bowel can be mistakenly confused for areas of abnormal wall thickening (Fig. 43-3).

NORMAL ANATOMY

Anatomically, the small bowel is composed of the duodenum, jejunum, and ileum. The duodenum is divided into four parts including the duodenal bulb, the descending portion, the horizontal segment, and the ascending segment. The mesenteric small bowel begins at the jejunum, which is located in the left upper and left mid abdomen. The last portion, the ileum, predominantly occupies the right abdomen. Besides its location, the ileum can be distinguished from the jejunum by its fewer mucosal folds and narrower lumen.

IMAGING

Normal Appearance

On HASTE and true FISP sequences the small bowel appears as a tubular fluid-filled structure with the wall depicted as a thin line of intermediate signal.[7] Small bowel wall thickness should not exceed 3 mm, and the diameter of the small bowel should not exceed 3 cm (Fig. 43-4). On nonenhanced T1-weighted sequences (FLASH) with fat suppression, the small bowel has a feathery appearance.[10]

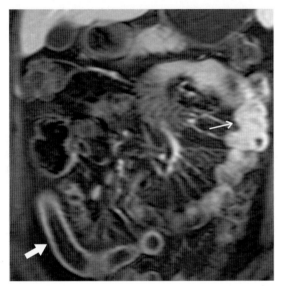

■ **FIGURE 43-3** Coronal, post-gadolinium, T1-weighted, gradient-recalled-echo, fat-saturation image demonstrates an abnormal segment of distal ileum in the right lower quadrant with mural thickening and hyperenhancement (*thick arrow*). Prominent perienteric vascularity is seen surrounding this segment. Adequate bowel distention allows for confident evaluation of the distal small bowel. This is in distinction to the jejunal loops in the left upper abdomen, which show apparent wall thickening due to lack of distention (*thin arrow*).

Biphasic intraluminal agents are hypointense. After the administration of gadolinium, the bowel wall should enhance moderately and uniformly. The degree of enhancement should be similar to, or less than that of, liver parenchyma. When evaluating the small bowel on MRI, it is important to note that areas of nondistention can falsely appear to have a thickened wall or be hyperenhancing. Conversely, areas of bowel wall thickening or abnormal enhancement can be obscured by lack of distention.

Small Bowel Obstruction

Although the diagnosis of small bowel obstruction can often be made clinically and with plain film radiographs, cross-sectional imaging is often utilized to determine the site and cause of obstruction. Traditionally, CT has been the modality of choice in evaluating suspected small bowel obstruction and identifying the cause of obstruction along with any extraluminal complications. With the advent of fast T2-weighted sequences, MRI has been shown to be capable of evaluating small bowel obstruction.[11] Additionally, MRI may also be utilized in instances in which limiting ionizing radiation is of importance or the administration of an iodinated contrast agent is contraindicated.

The multiplanar capability of MRI is crucial in evaluating the site and cause of obstruction (Fig. 43-5). The coronal plane provides a truer anatomic view of the abdomen and can be helpful to the surgeons.[12] Like CT, MRI depicts extraluminal complications or causes of obstruction. Post-gadolinium sequences are particularly important when there is concern for a malignant cause of small bowel obstruction. MRI has been shown to have an accuracy of 92% in distinguishing benign from malignant causes of bowel obstruction.[13]

MR enteroclysis has been shown to be useful in cases of low-grade partial small bowel obstruction by providing functional information via MR fluoroscopy.[12]

Crohn's Disease

Crohn's disease is a chronic inflammatory condition involving any portion of the gastrointestinal tract but is most commonly seen in the terminal ileum. Inflammatory

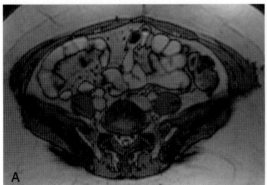
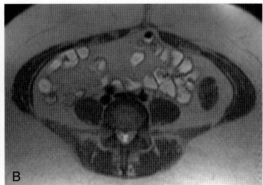

■ **FIGURE 43-4** Axial true FISP (**A**) and axial T2-weighted HASTE (**B**) images demonstrate normal small bowel with normal wall thickness (<3 mm) and signal. In this patient 1000 mL of dilute barium sulfate was administered over 1 hour just before the examination to achieve adequate bowel distention.

changes with transmural involvement of the bowel wall result in a spectrum of characteristic lesions, including aphthous ulcerations, cobblestoning, strictures, and fistula formation. In distinction to the contiguous areas of bowel involvement seen in ulcerative colitis, Crohn's disease results in the characteristic "skip lesions."

Traditionally, Crohn's disease has been evaluated with conventional SBFT, conventional enteroclysis, and endoscopy. However, MRI and CT are currently being used more frequently to assess the mural changes of Crohn's disease and to detect extraintestinal complications. Because radiation doses are quite high with MDCT, Jaffe

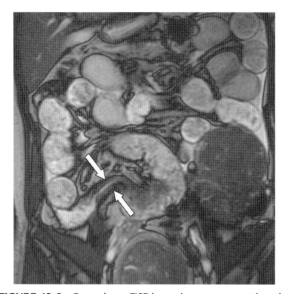

■ **FIGURE 43-5** Coronal true FISP image in a pregnant patient shows multiple dilated fluid-filled loops of small bowel consistent with a small bowel obstruction. A transition point is seen in the right lower quadrant (*arrows*). The coronal plane demonstrates a true anatomic depiction of the small bowel obstruction comparable to what the surgeon will encounter intraoperatively. The soft tissue mass in the left lower quadrant represented a subserosal uterine fibroid. The lack of ionizing radiation with MRI was particularly important in this pregnant patient.

and coworkers suggested that for the subset of patients who undergo numerous follow-up examinations, efforts should be made to minimize the number of CT examinations or MR enterography should be considered.[14] A study by Low and associates demonstrated MRI to be more sensitive in detecting earlier or milder forms of inflammatory bowel disease than CT.[15] Masselli and colleagues found MR enteroclysis to be the preferred initial study in patients with suspected Crohn's disease, whereas MR enterography plays a role in patients who refuse or fail nasojejunal intubation or as a follow-up study in patients with known Crohn's disease.[8]

MRI plays an important role in evaluating the presence and extent of active disease in patients with Crohn's disease. It assesses for the presence of wall thickening, mural changes, the degree and pattern of enhancement, and adjacent mesenteric inflammation. The degree and pattern of wall enhancement has been shown to correlate highly with the activity of disease. Actively inflamed bowel enhances to a greater extent than liver parenchyma.[16] A stratified pattern of enhancement to the bowel wall referred to as the "target sign" is also indicative of active disease. This appearance results from hyperenhancement of the mucosa, with decreased enhancement of the submucosa and muscularis layers due to edema. The target pattern can also be seen on T2-weighted sequences as a concentric pattern of layering in a thickened bowel wall. Central luminal high signal intensity is seen surrounded by a thin layer of low signal followed by a thicker layer of intermediate signal and a thin layer of low signal intensity (Fig. 43-6).[5] On T2-weighted sequences, high signal intensity and edema in the surrounding fat indicate active disease. T2-hypointense wall thickening combined with lack of enhancement on post-gadolinium sequences is seen with chronic or inactive disease.[2]

Extraluminal manifestations that can also be demonstrated by MRI include prominent perienteric vasculature, mesenteric lymphadenopathy, and extraintestinal complications. Fat-suppressed short tau inversion recovery (STIR) images and thin-section post-gadolinium images are

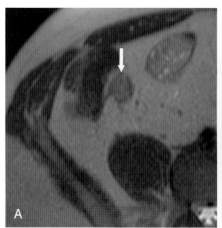
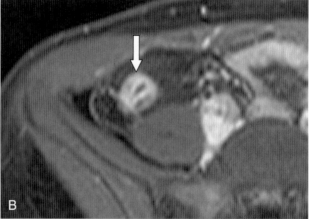

■ **FIGURE 43-6** **A,** Axial T2-weighted HASTE image shows concentric wall thickening with the characteristic appearance known as the target sign (*arrow*). This implies acute inflammation in this patient with active Crohn's disease. **B,** Axial, post-gadolinium, T1-weighted, gradient-recalled-echo, fat-saturation image in a different patient with active Crohn's disease again shows the characteristic target sign (*arrow*). Note the hyperenhancement of the mucosa and the decreased enhancement of the submucosa and muscularis layers due to edema.

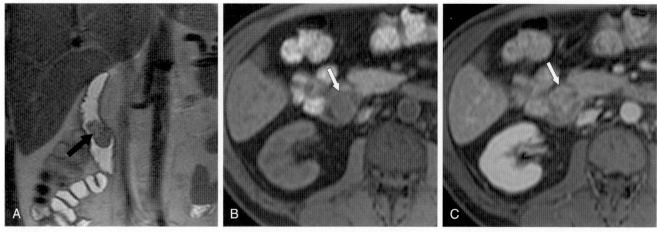

■ **FIGURE 43-7** A, Coronal T2-weighted HASTE image shows an intermediate signal mass arising from the descending portion of the duodenum. The mass (*arrow*) is well defined without associated wall thickening, suggesting a benign process. This lesion was proven to represent a duodenal adenoma. Pre- (**B**) and post- (**C**) gadolinium, fat-saturated, T1-weighted, gradient-recalled-echo images further characterize the lesion by demonstrating enhancement (*arrows*).

useful in evaluating for perirectal and perianal fistulas and abscesses.[7]

Small Bowel Neoplasms

Small bowel neoplasms are uncommon, accounting for less than 5% of all gastrointestinal tumors.[17,18] The most common benign tumors of the small bowel include adenomas, benign gastrointestinal stromal tumors, and lipomas. These occur most commonly in the distal small bowel. The most common malignant tumor of the small bowel is adenocarcinoma, which typically involves the duodenum. Gastrointestinal stromal tumor, lymphoma, carcinoid, and metastases are other malignant neoplasms found in the small bowel.

The role of MRI in evaluating small bowel tumors has not been fully evaluated. However, MRI can aid in characterizing a lesion's morphology, its internal constituents, and the extent of the lesion (Fig. 43-7).[6] Unlike inflammatory, infectious, or ischemic causes of wall thickening, small bowel tumors typically demonstrate asymmetric or focal wall thickening with homogeneous signal on T2-weighted images.[5] An abrupt transition from normal to abnormal bowel and lobulated or irregular contours are features more indicative of neoplastic lesions.[5] Wall thickening greater than 1 cm is unlikely to be seen in non-neoplastic lesions.[5]

> ### KEY POINTS
>
> ■ Adequate bowel distention is a crucial component of MRI of the small bowel and necessary in evaluating for mucosal abnormalities. Inadequate distention can mask subtle areas of bowel wall thickening or may falsely mimic wall thickening.
>
> ■ A variety of intraluminal oral contrast agents have been investigated. No consensus has been reached as to the ideal agent, but it should provide homogeneous opacification and adequate bowel distention. Agents with limited absorption allow for more consistent bowel distention.
>
> ■ MR enteroclysis results in reliable bowel distention but is invasive and time consuming.
>
> ■ Fast and ultrafast breath-hold sequences including HASTE and true FISP are commonly utilized T2-weighted sequences in evaluating the small bowel. These sequences limit respiratory and motion artifact and provide excellent-quality images. However, poor soft tissue resolution may limit characterization of lesions.
>
> ■ Pre- and post-gadolinium T1-weighted FLASH with fat suppression provides superior soft tissue contrast, allowing for assessment of bowel wall enhancement and lesion characterization based on enhancement pattern. The mesentery can also be accurately assessed.

SUGGESTED READINGS

Fidler J. MR imaging of small bowel. Radiol Clin North Am 2007; 45:317-331.

Kim KS, Ha HK. MRI for small bowel diseases. Magn Reson Imaging Clin North Am 2004; 12:637-650.

Malagò R, Manfredi R, Benini L. Assessment of Crohn's disease activity in the small bowel with MR-enteroclysis: clinico-radiological correlations. Abdom Imaging 2008; 33:669-675.

Prassopoulos P, Papanikolaou N, Grammatikakis J, et al. MR enteroclysis imaging of Crohn disease. RadioGraphics 2001; 21:S161-S172.

Umschaden HW, Gasser J. MR enteroclysis. Magn Reson Imaging Clin North Am 2004; 12:669-687.

REFERENCES

1. Lee J, Marcos H, Semelka R. MR imaging of the small bowel using the HASTE sequence. AJR Am J Roentgenol 1998; 170:1457-1463.
2. Fidler J. MR imaging of small bowel. Radiol Clin North Am 2007; 45:317-331.
3. Low R, Francis I. MR imaging of the gastrointestinal tract with IV gadolinium and diluted barium oral contrast media compared with unenhanced MR imaging and CT. AJR Am J Roentgend 1997; 169: 1051-1059.
4. Gourtsoyiannis N, Papnikolaou N, Grammatikakis J, et al. MR enteroclysis protocol optimization: comparison between 3D FLASH with fat saturation after intravenous gadolinium injection and true FISP sequences. Eur Radiol 2001; 11:908-913.
5. Umschaden HW, Gasser J. MR enteroclysis. Magn Reson Imaging Clin North Am 2004; 12:669-687.
6. Kim KS, Ha HK. MRI for small bowel diseases. Magn Reson Imaging Clin North Am 2004; 12:637-650.
7. Low R. Magnetic resonance imaging of the hollow viscera. In Gore R, Levine M (eds). Textbook of Gastrointestinal Radiology. Philadelphia, Saunders Elsevier, 2008, pp 91-106.
8. Masselli G, Casciani E, Polettini E, Gualdi G. Comparison of MR enteroclysis with MR enterography and conventional enteroclysis in patients with Crohn's disease. Eur Radiol 2008; 18:438-447.
9. Gourtsoyiannis N, Papanikolaou N. Magnetic resonance enteroclysis of the small bowel. In Gore R, Levine M (eds). Textbook of Gastrointestinal Radiology. Philadelphia, Saunders Elsevier, 2008, pp 765-774.
10. Semelka R, Pedro M, Armao D, et al. Gastrointestinal tract. In Semelka R (ed). Abdominal-Pelvic MRI. New York, Wiley-Liss, 2002, pp 527-649.
11. Regan F, Beall DP, Bohlman ME, et al. Fast MR imaging and the detection of small bowel obstruction. AJR Am J Roentgenol 1998; 170:1465-1469.
12. Umschaden HW, Szolar D, Gasser J, et al. Small bowel disease: comparison of MR enteroclysis images with conventional enteroclysis and surgical findings. Radiology 2000; 215:717-725.
13. Low RN, Chen SC, Barone R. Distinguishing benign from malignant bowel obstruction in patients with malignancy: findings at MR imaging. Radiology 2003; 228:157-165.
14. Jaffe TA, Gaca AM, Delaney S, et al. Radiation doses from small-bowel follow-through and abdominopelvic MDCT in Crohn's disease. AJR Am J Roentgenol 2007; 189:1015-1022.
15. Low RN, Francis IR, Politoske D, Bennett M. Crohn's disease evaluation: comparison of contrast-enhanced MR imaging and single phase helical CT scanning. J Magn Reson Imaging 1999; 11:127-135.
16. Low RN, Sebrechts CP, Politoske DA, et al. Crohn disease with endoscopic correlation: single-shot fast spin-echo and gadolinium-enhanced fat-suppressed spoiled gradient-echo MR imaging. Radiology 2002; 222:652-660.
17. Buckley JA, Fishman EK. CT evaluation of small bowel neoplasm: spectrum of disease. RadioGraphics 1998; 18:379-392.
18. Ashley SW, Wells SA. Tumors of the small intestine. Semin Oncol 1988; 15:116-128.

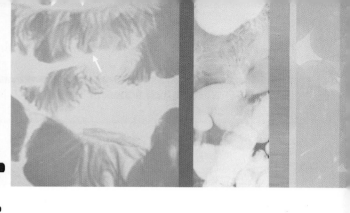

CHAPTER 44

Nuclear Medicine Techniques for the Small Bowel

Akash Joshi, Vahid Yaghmai, and Arti Gupta

The anatomic configuration and peristalsis of the small bowel make imaging of this organ a challenge. Radionuclide studies play a vital role in providing functional and metabolic information.

Certain scintigraphic studies play a pivotal role in the diagnosis of pathologic processes of the bowel. Technetium-99m (^{99m}Tc)-labeled red blood cell (RBC) scintigraphy offers a sensitive and noninvasive evaluation for gastrointestinal hemorrhage and is more sensitive than angiography for detecting hemorrhage of the lower gastrointestinal tract. A ^{99m}Tc-pertechnetate scintiscan is precise and accurate for the diagnosis of Meckel's diverticulum. Octreotide (indium-111 [^{111}In]-labeled pentetreotide) scanning can detect primary small bowel carcinoid and nodal metastasis that may not be visible on cross-sectional imaging. Newer techniques, such as positron emission tomography (PET), have widened the scope of nuclear medicine in the field of oncology.

Overall the scintigraphic evaluation of the small bowel can be divided into imaging studies and nonimaging studies (Box 44-1).

IMAGING STUDIES

Imaging of Inflammation and Infection

Assessment of disease extent in inflammatory bowel disease is very important for treatment planning, particularly when surgery is being considered. The true extent of the inflammation of the small bowel is difficult to assess in Crohn's disease and is often underestimated by conventional techniques.

Labeled leukocyte imaging is a noninvasive technique for the detection of occult inflammation and infection. Because leukocytes can be separated and labeled without significant loss of function, they can be used to image small bowel inflammation and disease complications, such as abscess and possibly fistula.[1]

Principle

White blood cells accumulate at the site of inflammation and mount a physiologic response. The labeled leukocytes marginate and then migrate to the inflamed lesion.

Several studies have examined the role of labeled leukocyte scintigraphy in the assessment of disease extent in patients with established inflammatory bowel disease.[2]

Scintigraphy is particularly useful in children[3] and very sick patients. Another advantage includes evaluation of the entire small and large bowel at the same time. The technique has the potential for verifying the presence of intra- and extra-abdominal abscesses and, possibly, fistulas.[1]

Technical Aspects

Of the many radioisotopes used to label leukocytes, ^{99m}Tc-hexamethyl propylene amine oxime (^{99m}Tc-HMPAO) and ^{111}In-tropolonate are the most widely used. Stable labeling of granulocytes can be achieved with either ^{111}In or ^{99m}Tc-HMPAO, with comparable labeling efficiency and sensitivity to detect infection.

Leukocytes are obtained from heparinized peripheral venous blood (40 to 60 mL) and then separated from erythrocytes and platelets by sedimentation. The patient's white blood cell count should be at least 2000/mL to have enough cells to label. Cell labeling is achieved by incubation with a lipophilic complex of radioisotope (oxime or tropolonate for ^{111}In and HMPAO for ^{99m}Tc) in plasma (or saline). ^{111}In labels and remains firmly bound to all cells in mixed leukocyte suspensions, whereas ^{99m}Tc is less tightly bound.[4] After washing, the labeled leukocytes are resuspended in the patient's own plasma and are injected intravenously. The injected labeled leukocytes marginate and then migrate into the inflamed lesion before being shed into the bowel lumen. Serial imaging is important to distinguish luminal from bowel wall activity. Some of the ^{99m}Tc-HMPAO is also released from the leukocytes and forms secondary hydrophilic complexes, which are excreted in bile.

With ^{111}In, images are most often obtained at 3 to 4 hours. Forward migration of luminal radioactivity[5] makes late (24 hours) scintiscans of little value, except when the technique is used to detect abscess, for which late imaging is required. With ^{99m}Tc-HMPAO, scanning at 30 to 60 minutes and at 2 hours is preferable. On delayed images, significant renal, biliary, and nonspecific bowel excretion of noncellular-bound ^{99m}Tc-labeled hydrophilic complexes is frequently seen. Although this may make scintiscan interpretation difficult, it can be circumvented by early (1 hour) and serial imaging.[6]

One of the main disadvantages of labeled leukocyte bowel imaging is the difficulty in accurately identifying the involved bowel segments, particularly in patients who have previously undergone bowel resection. This has been attributed to many factors, including absence of landmarks on bowel images and luminal migration of the shed white blood cells owing to the continuous peristalsis of the small bowel during imaging.[2] Thus, imaging within 1 hour, which minimizes small bowel movement and provides better image quality with ^{99m}Tc-HMPAO allows improved definition of affected bowel segments.

The effective radiation dose to the patient is higher with ^{111}In than with [99m]Tc. The effective dose equivalent is 6.7 mSv for ^{111}In scintiscans (injected dose of 18.5 MBq) and 4 mSv for ^{99m}Tc-HMPAO scintiscans (injected dose of 370 MBq).[7] The uterine and splenic absorbed dose is also higher with [111]In (2 mGy and 56 mGy, respectively) than ^{99m}Tc-HMPAO (0.8 mGy and 31.3 mGy, respectively).[8] The higher administered dose of ^{99m}Tc yields a much better signal-to-noise ratio. ^{99m}Tc-HMPAO is now preferred for leukocyte labeling owing to ready availability, superior image quality, ease of use, and radiation dosimetry.

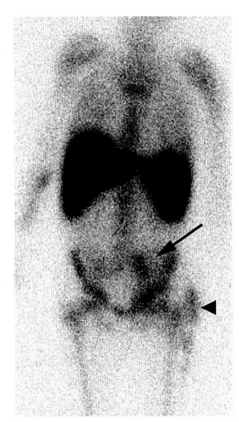

■ **FIGURE 44-1**   ^{111}In-labeled leukocyte scintiscan. Abnormal activity in left psoas abscess (*arrow*) and left gluteal inflammation (*arrowhead*) in a patient with methicillin-resistant *Staphylococcus aureus* (MRSA) septicemia.

Image Interpretation

[111]In WBC normal examination demonstrates activity in the spleen, liver, and bone marrow. Uptake in the spleen is most intense due to physiologic cell pooling. With ^{99m}Tc-HMPAO there is urinary excretion, and low-grade lung activity may be seen. Activity outside the normal expected distribution suggests infection (Fig. 44-1). Activity equal to that of the liver is considered clinically important. Uptake greater than that of the liver is typical for abscess. Activity less than marrow suggests a low-level inflammatory response.

Leukocyte scintigraphy has a high sensitivity for the detection of suspected inflammatory bowel disease and to assess disease activity in patients with known bowel inflammatory disease. A study comparing intraoperative small bowel enteroscopy and laparotomy findings in Crohn's disease concluded that the sensitivity of leukocyte scintigraphy for macroscopically evident small bowel inflammation was 85%, with specificity of 81% and accuracy of 84%.[9] Leukocyte scintigraphy can reliably differentiate between Crohn's disease and ulcerative colitis with an accuracy of 98% by the different patterns of involvement.[10]

Pros and Cons

Because of its low specificity, this technique may not be able to distinguish between infective enteritis and inflammatory or ischemic bowel conditions. Also, activity within the abdomen may be due to causes other than inflammation and has the potential for misinterpretation (Box 44-2).

Other Radiopharmaceuticals

^{99m}Tc-Fanolesomab (NeutroSpec)

This is a murine IgM antigranulocyte monoclonal antibody that binds to the surface CD15 antigens expressed on human neutrophils, monocytes, and eosinophils. It eliminates the need for in-vitro cell labeling.

NeutroSpec was approved in the United States for use in evaluation of acute appendicitis in June 2004. Its marketing was suspended in July 2007 because of serious safety concerns.

^{99m}Tc-Sulesomab (LeukoScan)

This is a Fab fragment of a murine IgG1 antigranulocyte antibody. The Fab fragments have less immunoreactivity as compared with whole antibodies. LeukoScan is commercially available in Europe.

^{18}F-Fluorodeoxyglucose (FDG)-PET

FDG-PET is commonly used clinically to detect tumors. It also can be used to detect inflammation or infection due to glucose uptake in the locally activated granulocytes. There is always a baseline low-level physiologic activity in the bowel. If the uptake in bowel is greater than that of bone, it is indicative of clinically important inflammation.

Gallium-67 Citrate

Gallium-67 (^{67}Ga) citrate has a limited role in abdominal infection and inflammation because of its physiologic uptake by bowel.

Imaging of Meckel's Diverticulum

Meckel's diverticulum occurs in about 2% of the population. It results from failure of closure of the omphalomesenteric duct. Almost 96% of Meckel's diverticula remain asymptomatic. Rarely, complications such as bleeding, intussusception, ulceration, obstruction, or torsion can occur. Heterotopic gastric mucosa is present in 10% to 30% of patients with Meckel's diverticula, in approximately 60% of symptomatic patients, and in 98% of those who bleed.

Principle

The principle of ^{99m}Tc-pertechnetate scintigraphy is that the pertechnetate anion is selectively taken up by the surface mucus-secreting cells that line the gastric mucosa whether it is located in the stomach or is ectopic.[11,12]

Technical Aspects

200 MBq of ^{99m}Tc-pertechnetate is given intravenously for the detection of the heterotopic gastric mucosa. Pentagastrin, cimetidine, and glucagon are pharmacologic agents that improve the sensitivity of the scintiscans. Pentagastrin enhances the uptake of pertechnetate in the gastric mucosa. It is associated with significant side effects and is no longer commercially available in the United States. Glucagon inhibits the peristaltic dilution and wash out of intestinal radioactivity. Cimetidine, a histamine-2 receptor antagonist, increases the activity in the gastric mucosa by inhibiting the release of pertechnetate into the lumen of Meckel's diverticulum.

Image Interpretation

The ^{99m}Tc-pertechnetate is taken up by the gastric mucosa. Meckel's diverticulum appears as a focal area of increased activity commonly in the right lower quadrant. The activity can be seen 5 to 10 minutes after tracer injection, increasing over time at a rate similar to gastric mucosa (Fig. 44-2).

Pertechnetate scintigraphy has a sensitivity of 80% to 90%, a specificity of 95%, and an accuracy of 90% in children.[13] In adults, the study is less reliable, with a sensitivity of 62.5%, a specificity of 9%, and an accuracy of 46%.[14]

Pros and Cons

It is important to be aware of the possible pitfalls involving scintigraphy in the evaluation of Meckel's diverticulum (Box 44-3). Most of the false-negative scintiscans are due to lack of gastric mucosa in the diverticulum.

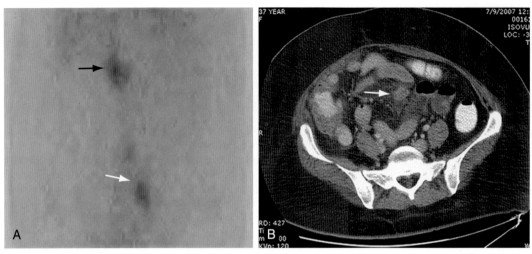

■ **FIGURE 44-2** ^{99m}Tc-pertechnetate scintiscan. **A,** Select anterior image shows abnormal activity left of the midline in the lower abdomen, appearing in the same temporal fashion as the stomach. **B,** CT scan in the same patient in the mid abdomen demonstrates an inflamed Meckel diverticulum (*arrow*).

BOX 44-3　Pitfalls of Meckel's Diverticulum Imaging

FALSE-NEGATIVE FINDINGS

■ Absent or minimal gastric mucosa
■ Very small diverticulum (<1 cm)
■ Necrosis of the mucosa
■ Rapid peristalsis and wash out

FALSE-POSITIVE FINDINGS

■ Renal or ureteric activity
■ Ectopic kidney
■ Vascular activity in hemangioma or angiodysplasia
■ Other ectopic gastric mucosa as in duplication cyst, Barrett's esophagus, pancreas, or duodenum
■ Hyperemia and inflammation in Crohn's disease, ulcerative colitis, appendicitis, abscess, and colitis
■ Neoplasm such as carcinoid, leiomyosarcoma, lymphoma, and carcinoma of sigmoid

Imaging for Gastrointestinal Bleeding

Gastrointestinal bleeding is usually classified as upper or lower, depending on its location in the gastrointestinal tract. Effective therapy will depend on accurate detection of the site of hemorrhage.

^{99m}Tc RBC scintigraphy plays an important role in the evaluation of lower gastrointestinal bleeding owing to the limited sensitivity of endoscopy and intermittent bleeding. Radionuclide studies have typically been used as a screening examination to identify patients who require targeted angiography or surgery.

Lower gastrointestinal tract bleeding is more frequent in the colon as opposed to the small bowel. The most common causes of colonic bleeding include mucosal vascular malformations such as angiodysplasia, diverticulum, adenomatous neoplasms, and polyps. Colonoscopy per-

formed within 24 hours of hospital admission will confirm a colonic bleeding site in 68% to 77% of cases. However, many patients may not be good candidates for colonoscopy.

Angiography will locate gastrointestinal bleeding sites in up to 65% of cases when hemorrhage occurs at a rate greater than 1 mL/min. The majority of gastrointestinal bleeding, however, is intermittent, and bleeding may not be occurring during contrast injection (20 to 30 seconds). Repeated angiographic studies are not practical. However with ^{99m}Tc-labeled RBCs, imaging can be performed over prolonged periods of time, which can be extremely useful in the setting of intermittent gastrointestinal bleeding. Also, a ^{99m}Tc RBC study can detect a bleeding rate of 0.04 mL/min.[15]

Principle

The principle of radionuclide gastrointestinal bleeding studies is that the blood pool agent normally remains confined in the vascular system. During active bleeding the radionuclide extravasates into the bowel lumen.

Technical Aspects

Intravascular blood pool agents such as ^{99m}Tc-labeled RBCs are the agents of choice, especially in cases of intermittent and slow bleeding. The agent remains in the vascular pool for over 24 hours. Any free technetium is excreted by the kidneys and is also taken up by the salivary glands and gastric mucosa and then secreted into the gastrointestinal tract. This can potentially result in misinterpretation, but effective labeling of the RBCs minimizes the percentage of free technetium. There are several methods of radiolabeling red blood cells.

The in-vivo method is the easiest with labeling efficiency of 75% to 80%. This technique involves intravenous injection of stannous pyrophosphate, then waiting for 20 minutes to allow its diffusion in the RBC, followed by intravenous administration of ^{99m}Tc sodium pertechnetate.

The modified in-vivo method has a labeling efficiency of 85% to 90%. This technique involves intravenous injection of stannous pyrophosphate, then waiting for 20 minutes to allow its diffusion in the RBC, followed by withdrawal of 5 mL of the blood into a shielded syringe with ^{99m}Tc-pertechnetate. The syringe is incubated for about 10 minutes to allow the ^{99m}Tc-pertechnetate to diffuse into the red cells and bind to the β chain of the hemoglobin. The RBCs are then washed with saline and resuspended and injected back into the patient.

The in-vitro method has the highest labeling efficiency of 97% to 98%. In this technique 1 to 3 mL of heparinized blood is mixed with 50 to 100 µg of stannous chloride and sodium citrate. After about 5 minutes, 0.6 mg of sodium hypochlorite is added to oxidize the extracellular tin, followed by citric acid, sodium citrate, and dextrose. Then ^{99m}Tc-pertechnetate is added to the vial and incubated for about 20 minutes. About 700 to 1000 MBq of ^{99m}Tc-labeled red blood cells is injected. An anterior flow is obtained at a rate of 2 to 5 seconds per frame for 1 to 2 minutes. This is followed by 60-second acquisitions per image for 60 to 90 minutes (cine scintigraphy). If cine scintigraphy is not possible, 750,000 to 1 million count static images can be acquired every 2 to 5 minutes for 60 to 90 minutes.

If bleeding is not detected, delayed images may be obtained at appropriate intervals between 2 to 6 hours and 18 to 24 hours. The more frequently images are taken, the higher the probability of detecting an intermittent hemorrhage.

[99m]Tc sulfur colloid can also be used for the detection of gastrointestinal bleeding but is less sensitive as compared with the ^{99m}Tc RBC scintiscan.[16] [99m]Tc sulfur colloid is rapidly cleared from the serum by the reticuloendothelial cells of the liver, spleen, and bone marrow (vascular half-life of 2.5 to 3.5 minutes). By 15 minutes it is completely cleared from the vascular system. If the bleeding is not actively occurring during this time, it will not be detected. However, the advantage is that it is easy to prepare, readily available, and inexpensive. It is beneficial in making a quick diagnosis in actively bleeding and clinically unstable patients.

Image Interpretation

A normal scintiscan shows activity confined to the blood pool, with activity in the heart, aorta, inferior vena cava, liver, and spleen. Activity is also seen in the genitalia, and there is some urinary excretion of free pertechnetate.

Gastrointestinal hemorrhage appears as a focal activity, not in the expected location of blood pool or urinary excretion. The activity should progressively increase over time and conform to an intestinal anatomy and show peristalsis, either antegrade or retrograde (Fig. 44-3).

Because of bowel peristalsis the hemorrhage may move antegrade or retrograde; therefore, it is important to review the 1-minute dynamic acquisition frames to accurately determine the site of bleeding (Fig. 44-4).

[99m]Tc RBC scintigraphy is 93% sensitive and 95% specific for detecting a bleeding site with active arterial or venous bleeding rates as low as 0.04 mL/min[15] anywhere within the gastrointestinal tract.

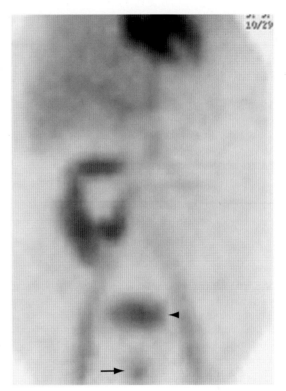

■ **FIGURE 44-3** Accumulation of ^{99m}Tc-labeled red blood cells in the expected location of the terminal ileum and colon in a patient with Crohn's disease. Physiologic activity is seen in the urinary bladder (*arrowhead*) and genitalia (*arrow*).

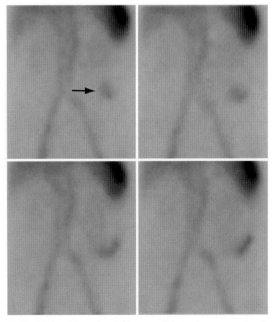

■ **FIGURE 44-4** Selected serial images from a cine sequence of a ^{99m}Tc-labeled RBC study demonstrating a focus of active small bowel bleeding as progressive tracer accumulation in the left lower quadrant (*arrow*).

The role of ^{99m}Tc RBC scintigraphy is limited in the evaluation of upper gastrointestinal bleeding owing to the widespread use of upper endoscopy as a first-line modality. Endoscopy of the upper gastrointestinal tract is reported to have an overall diagnostic accuracy of more than 90% in identifying duodenal and gastric ulcers, gastric erosions, varices, and Mallory-Weiss tears. However, ⁹⁹ᵐTc RBC scintigraphy can be useful when endoscopy is not readily available or in patients in whom endoscopy is difficult or impossible.

Pros and Cons

A ⁹⁹ᵐTc RBC study can be misinterpreted (Box 44-4).

Imaging of Tumors

Primary small bowel neoplasm is rare, representing less than 25% of all gastrointestinal neoplasms. Adenocarcinoma (usually in the proximal small bowel), carcinoid tumor (usually in the distal small bowel), lymphoma, and gastrointestinal stromal tumor (GIST) are the most common tumors of the small bowel. Cross-sectional imaging with CT and MRI forms the first line of evaluation.

Carcinoid tumors are of neuroendocrine origin and are the most common small bowel malignancy. Unlike adenocarcinoma, these more commonly affect the distal small bowel. The primary tumors are often very small and are slow growing. In approximately 30% of cases, multiple sites are demonstrated. A characteristic desmoplastic response can occur, with soft tissue infiltration and retraction of the adjacent mesentery. Calcifications are frequently present. Bulky lymphadenopathy can occur, with central low attenuation signifying necrosis. Pulmonary, hepatic, and osteoblastic skeletal metastases are common.

Principle

Somatostatin is a neuropeptide that is secreted and released by endocrine and nerve cells, especially by the hypothalamus. Somatostatin inhibits the release of growth hormone, insulin, glucagon, gastrin, serotonin, and calcitonin. Because carcinoid tumor is of neuroendocrine origin, high density of somatostatin receptors are present. Therefore, a radiolabeled somatostatin analog, that is, ¹¹¹In-labeled pentetreotide (Octreotide) can be used for imaging these tumors.

Technical Aspects

Before the examination the patient should be well hydrated, because the ¹¹¹In-labeled pentetreotide is primarily cleared by the kidneys. Bowel may be prepared with laxative and enema to decrease interfering bowel activity. If the patient is on Octreotide therapy, it may be discontinued for 3 to 7 days before the test. Then 6 mCi (222 MBq) of ¹¹¹In-labeled pentetreotide is injected intravenously and images are obtained at 4, 24, and 48 hours. Single photon emission CT of the abdomen and other areas may be obtained as clinically indicated.

Image Interpretation

In a normal scintiscan the activity is identified in the blood pool, thyroid gland, liver, gallbladder, spleen, kidneys, and bladder. As it is excreted by the kidneys significant activity is seen in the kidneys on the delayed images. Also on the delayed images activity can be normally seen in the bowel. Tumor is seen as a focal area of increased uptake, which persists on the delayed scintiscans. Eighty to 90% of tumors are visible by 4 hours. The conspicuity increases on the delayed images owing to background clearance (Fig. 44-5).

Octreotide scintigraphy serves as an efficient screening tool in patients with suspected carcinoid. It is useful in imaging of multifocal lesions and distant metastasis. For carcinoids the sensitivity of the Octreotide scintiscan is 85% to 95%.[17] Other neuroendocrine tumors, such as gastrinoma, pheochromocytoma, and neuroblastoma, which also have somatostatin receptors, can also be imaged with radiolabeled somatostatin analogs.

Pros and Cons

A false-positive scintiscan can occur in chronic inflammatory processes such as Crohn's disease, ulcerative colitis, and rheumatoid arthritis. Carcinoid tumors are small and can be easily missed on conventional imaging.

Imaging of Small Bowel Motility

Motility disorders can affect the stomach and small bowel. Chronic intestinal dysmotility is a syndrome of functional bowel obstruction in the absence of an obstructing anatomic lesion and bowel dilatation. A similar motor disorder, with dilatation of small bowel or colon, is referred to as chronic intestinal pseudo-obstruction. Constipation slows small bowel motility, increasing the bowel transit time.

Gastric emptying, quantitatively evaluated by a ⁹⁹ᵐTc sulfur colloid–tagged meal, has a proven clinical value. Normal range for gastric clearance is well documented, as opposed to small bowel transit.

Intestinal transit is usually assessed radiographically using barium studies. Scintigraphic small bowel transit studies are infrequently used to serially follow up patients with long-standing motility disorders and to assess the efficacy of a prokinetic agent in the long-term treatment of chronic intestinal dysmotility.

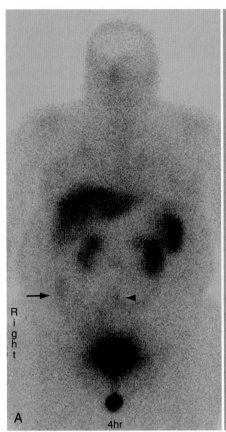
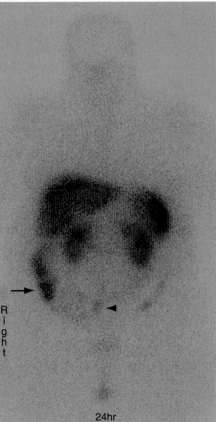
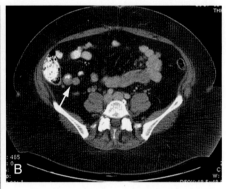

■ **FIGURE 44-5** **A,** Four-hour and 24-hour anterior ^{111}In-pentetreotide images of the abdomen show normal activity in the liver, kidneys, and spleen. Some bowel activity is seen on the 24-hour image. However, an abnormal focus of activity is seen in the right lower quadrant (*arrow*) and in the mesentery in the midline (*arrowhead*). These become more intense on the 24-hour delayed images. **B,** CT scan in the same patient in the mid abdomen demonstrating thickening of the terminal ileum (*arrow*) and an adjacent lymph node.

Principle

Slower intestinal transit results in prolonged retention of the intestinal contents. The transit time, therefore, is a measure of the small bowel motility.

Technical Aspects

The intestinal transit can be assessed with a liquid marker taken orally with or without a solid meal. [99m]Tc sulfur colloid, ^{99m}Tc-DTPA, or ^{111}In-DTPA can be used. None of these is absorbed in the gastrointestinal tract. Imaging is carried until the radioactivity reaches the colon. Activity not in the gastric and colonic region of interest is considered to be in the small bowel.[18]

Pros and Cons

Absolute normal values for the small bowel transit time are difficult to define because there is significant variation in the normal range. Difficulty in identifying cecum may result in inaccurate quantification.

NONIMAGING TECHNIQUES

Schilling Test

The Schilling test is used to evaluate absorption of vitamin B$_{12}$ in the small bowel, which requires the presence of intrinsic factor from the stomach.

Principle

Vitamin B$_{12}$ is absorbed in the ileum in the presence of intrinsic factor from the stomach. After absorption, vitamin B$_{12}$ is stored in the liver and various tissues. Once the body stores are saturated with normal unlabeled vitamin B$_{12}$, the excess absorbed cobalt-57 ([57]Co)-labeled vitamin B$_{12}$ is excreted in urine. Further discussion about the details of the Schilling test is beyond the scope of this textbook.

Breath Test for Small Bowel Bacterial Overgrowth

Patients with small bowel bacterial overgrowth typically develop signs and symptoms including nausea, bloating, vomiting, and diarrhea. Risk factors for the development of bacterial overgrowth include the use of medications including proton pump inhibitors; anatomic disturbances in the bowel, including fistulas, diverticula, and blind loops created after surgery; and resection of the ileocecal valve.

The diagnosis of bacterial overgrowth is made by a number of techniques, with the gold standard diagnosis being an aspirate from the jejunum that shows in excess of 10^5 bacteria per milliliter. Unlike the colon, which is rich with bacteria, the normal small bowel usually has less than 10^4 organisms per milliliter.

Principle

Breath tests have been developed to test for bacterial overgrowth, based on bacterial deconjugation of bile salts. The glycocholic acid breath test involves oral administration of the radiolabeled bile acid carbon-14 (^{14}C)-glycocholic acid. The bile acid is deconjugated by the bacteria, releasing ^{14}C-labeled CO_2. The CO_2 diffuses across the lining of the small bowel into the blood. It then is excreted from the lungs into the breath. Patients with small bowel bacterial overgrowth usually have increased level of ^{14}C-labeled CO_2. It compares well to jejunal aspirates in making the diagnosis of bacterial overgrowth. Further discussion about the details of breath tests is beyond the scope of this textbook.

Protein-Losing Enteropathy

Protein-losing enteropathy refers to any condition of the gastrointestinal tract that results in a net loss of plasma protein from the body.

^{99m}Tc-labeled albumin scintigraphy is a qualitative method to diagnose protein-losing enteropathy. Twenty-four-hour serial abdominal scanning after intravenous administration of ^{99m}Tc-labeled human serum albumin (^{99m}Tc-HSA) is reliable for intermittent protein loss. In a normal scan the majority of the activity is in the blood pool, with some normal excretion in the kidneys and bladder of the free pertechnetate. Patients with protein-losing enteropathy demonstrate significant activity in the abdominal cavity within 1 hour. Disadvantages of ^{99m}Tc-HSA include adverse effects such as nausea, vomiting, erythema, flushing, hypotension, dyspnea, tachycardia, dizziness, and abdominal pain. Active bleeding in the gas-trointestinal tract may result in a false-positive ^{99m}Tc-HSA scintigram because radiotracer is lost into the bowel lumen along with blood.

Chromum-51 (^{51}Cr)-labeled serum albumin can be administered intravenously, and stool can be collected as a measure of protein exudation into the gastrointestinal tract. Though sensitive and quantitative, it is cumbersome, time consuming, and also no longer commercially available.

Bile Salt Malabsorption

Bile acids normally undergo enterohepatic circulation. When this circulation is interrupted, bile acids enter the colon in increased concentrations, resulting in diarrhea with or without steatorrhea, and it may be complicated by gallstone disease and hyperoxaluria. Bile acid malabsorption is often due to a disease (most common is Crohn's disease) or partial resction of the terminal ileum.

23-^{75}Selena-25-homotaurocholic acid (^{75}SeHCAT) is a synthetic gamma-labeled analog of bile salt taurocholic acid. Metabolized similarly to natural bile acids, it provides a way of tracing the metabolism of bile acids and their enterohepatic circulation in vivo.

After oral administration, the majority of the ^{75}SeHCAT is absorbed by the distal ileum and enters the enterohepatic circulation. Baseline and day 7 whole-body activity is measured. Normal whole-body retention is greater than 15% from baseline in 7 days. Less than 10% retention in 7 days is suggestive of bile acid malabsorption.

KEY POINTS

Imaging Studies

- Inflammation and infection evaluation: detects intra- and extra-abdominal clinically occult inflammation and infection
- Meckel's diverticulum scintigraphy: Sensitivity of 80% to 90%, a specificity of 95%, and an accuracy of 90% in children (less in adults).
- Gastrointestinal bleeding studies: ^{99m}Tc-RBC study can detect a bleeding rate of 0.04 mL/min. The majority of gastrointestinal bleeding is intermittent.
- Neoplasm evaluation: Octreotide scintigraphy has an 85% to 95% sensitivity for carcinoids.
- Small bowel motility studies: There is significant variation in the normal range of small bowel motility.

Nonimaging Studies

- Schilling test: Two-stage test that evaluates absorption of vitamin B_{12} in the small bowel
- Breath test for bacterial overgrowth: Bacterial overgrowth in the small bowel, in excess of 10^5 bacteria per mL, deconjugates the tagged bile salts and releases radioactive CO_2 detected in breath.
- Test for protein-losing enteropathy: Tagged protein is administered intravenously and activity in the abdominal cavity is diagnostic of protein-losing enteropathy.
- ^{75}SeHCAT for bile salt malabsorption: Abnormal enterohepatic circulation leads to increased excretion of the bile salts. Normal retention is greater than 15% of the administered dose in 7 days; it is abnormal if the retention is less than 10%.

SUGGESTED READINGS

Mettler FA, Guiberteau MJ. Gastrointestinal tract. In Mettler FA, Guiberteau MJ (eds). Essentials of Nuclear Medicine Imaging, 5th ed. Philadelphia, Saunders, 2006, pp 203-242.

Skehan SJ, Mernagh JR, Nahmias C. Evaluation of the small intestine by nuclear medicine studies. In Gourtsoyiannis NC (ed). Radiological Imaging of the Small Intestine. Berlin, Springer, 2002, pp 131-155.

Ziessman HA, O'Malley JP, Thrall JH. Gastrointestinal system. In Ziessman HA, O'Malley JP, Thrall JH (eds). Nuclear Medicine: The Requisites, 3rd ed. St. Louis, Mosby, 2006, pp 346-383.

REFERENCES

1. Charron M, Di LC, Kocoshis S. CT and ^{99m}Tc-WBC vs. colonoscopy in the evaluation of inflammation and complications of inflammatory bowel diseases. J Gastroenterol 2002; 37:23-28.
2. Giaffer MH. Labeled leucocyte scintigraphy in inflammatory bowel disease: clinical applications. Gut 1996; 38:1-5.
3. Alberini JL, Badran A, Freneaux E, et al. Technetium-99m HMPAO–labeled leukocyte imaging compared with endoscopy, ultrasonography, and contrast radiology in children with inflammatory bowel disease. J Pediatr Gastroenterol Nutr 2001; 32:278-286.
4. Peters AM, Roddie ME, Danpure HJ, et al. ^{99m}Tc-HMPAO-labelled leucocytes: comparison with ^{111}In-tropolonate-labelled granulocytes. Nucl Med Commun 1988; 9:449-463.
5. Saverymuttu SH, Peters AM, Lavender JP. In-vivo assessment of granulocyte migration to diseased bowel in Crohn's disease. Gut 1985; 26:378-383.
6. Roddie ME, Peters AM, Danpure HJ, et al. Inflammation: imaging with Tc-99m HMPAO-labeled leukocytes. Radiology 1988; 166:767-772.
7. Mettler FA, Bhargavan M, Thomadsen BR, et al. Nuclear medicine exposure in the United States, 2005-2007: preliminary results. Semin Nucl Med 2008; 38(5):384-391.
8. Allan RA, Sladen GE, Bassingham S, et al. Comparison of simultaneous ^{99m}Tc-HMPAO and ^{111}In-oxime labeled white cell scans in the assessment of inflammatory bowel disease. Eur J Nucl Med 1993; 20:195-200.
9. Almer S, Granerus G, Ström M, et al. Leukocyte scintigraphy compared to intraoperative small bowel enteroscopy and laparotomy findings in Crohn's disease. Inflamm Bowel Dis 2007; 13:164-174.
10. Li DJ, Freeman A, Miles KA. Can ^{99m}Tc HMPAO leucocyte scintigraphy distinguish between Crohn's disease and ulcerative colitis? Br J Radiol 1994; 67:472-477.
11. Marsden DS, Alexander C, Yeung P, et al. Autoradiographic explanation for the uses of ^{99m}Tc in gastric scintigraphy. J Nucl Med 1973; 14:632.
12. Conway JJ. Radionuclide diagnosis of Meckel's diverticulum. Gastrointest Radiol 1980; 5:209-213.
13. Sfakianakis GN, Anderson GF, King DR. The effect of intestinal hormones of the Tc-99m pertechnetate imaging of ectopic gastric mucosa in experimental Meckel's diverticulum. J Nucl Med 1981; 22:678-683.
14. Schwartz MJ, Lewis JH. Meckel's diverticulum: pitfalls in the scintigraphic detection in the adult. Am J Gastroenterol 1984; 79:611-618.
15. Zuckier LS. Acute gastrointestinal bleeding. Semin Nucl Med 2003; 33:297-311.
16. Alavi A, Ring EJ. Localization of gastrointestinal bleeding: superiority of ^{99m}Tc sulfur colloid compared with angiography. AJR Am J Roentgenol 1981; 137:741-748.
17. Kwekkeboom DJ, Krenning EP. Somatostatin receptor imaging. Semin Nucl Med 2002; 32:84-91.
18. Maurer AH, Krevsky B, Whole-gut transit scintigraphy in the evaluation of small-bowel and colon transit disorders. Semin Nucl Med 1995; 25:326-338.

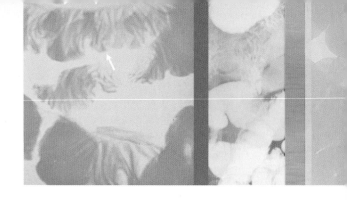

CHAPTER 45

Small Bowel Obstruction

Marie R. Koch, Zarine K. Shah, and William Bennett

SMALL BOWEL OBSTRUCTION: GENERAL CONSIDERATIONS

Etiology

Small bowel obstruction (SBO) is a common presentation for which safe and effective management depends on a rapid and accurate diagnosis. The morbidity and mortality associated with acute SBO continue to be significant, accounting for 12% to 16% of all surgical admissions in patients with acute abdominal conditions.[1] SBO can be caused by a variety of lesions, and the etiology can be broadly classified based on their location.

Intraluminal obstructions are relatively uncommon and can be caused by foreign bodies, bezoars, gallstones, parasites (e.g., *Ascaris lumbricoides*), and inspissated meconium in neonates or patients with cystic fibrosis.

Intramural causes are most commonly seen in patients with inflammatory bowel diseases, predominantly in Crohn's disease. Therapeutic irradiation or certain medications such as nonsteroidal anti-inflammatory drugs or potassium tablets can lead to ulcerations followed by strictures. Anticoagulants can cause intramural hematomas after trauma. In certain countries, tuberculosis of the small bowel is fairly common. Intramural tumors such as lipomas, leiomyomas, carcinoids, lymphoma, and, rarely, adenocarcinoma can lead to SBO, as well as metastatic tumors from sites such as the stomach, breast, colon, and ovaries. In children younger than 2 years of age, intussusception due to a polypoidal lesion within the bowel is a common abdominal emergency.

Extramural obstructions are the most common cause of SBO. These include adhesions due to prior surgery, congenital intraperitoneal bands, and congenital malrotation with short mesenteric attachment resulting in midgut torsion or volvulus. Bowel herniation is another cause of SBO. Bowel can get obstructed in any kind of hernia, but the most common types of hernias to cause SBO are femoral, indirect inguinal, or umbilical.[2,3] The causes of SBO by age are listed in Table 45-1.

Prevalence and Epidemiology

The leading cause of SBO in the United States is adhesions occurring after surgical procedures such as appendectomy, colorectal surgery, and gynecologic and upper gastrointestinal procedures. Other common causes are Crohn's disease, neoplasm, and hernia.

SBOs can be characterized as partial or complete and as nonstrangulated or strangulated. If left untreated, strangulated obstructions cause death in 100% of patients. Mortality decreases to 8% if surgery is performed within 36 hours and to 25% if the surgery is postponed beyond 36 hours.[2,3] The prevalence of SBO by cause is summarized in Box 45-1. Numbers vary between studies.[2,3]

Clinical Presentation

The diagnostic approach should focus on recognizing an obstruction, distinguishing partial from complete SBO, distinguishing simple from strangulated SBO, and identifying the underlying cause. Patients with SBO usually present with a variable period of abdominal pain, often accompanied by nausea and vomiting. Colicky pain is more often associated in patients with simple obstruction and increases in severity. It can be continuous or interspersed with pain-free intervals. Strangulated obstructions commonly present as constant pain. The presence of vomiting is another feature of SBO. In more proximal obstructions, vomiting is an early finding, with or without significant distention of the abdomen. In more distal obstruction, abdominal distention is marked, and vomiting is delayed as the bowel takes time to fill. Patients can have constipation or diarrhea, which is caused by secondary increased peristalsis distal to an obstruction. Whereas patients with partial obstruction might have diarrhea and can still pass flatus, patients with complete obstruction tend to have complete obstipation. Fever, hypotension, tachycardia, and leukocytosis are suggestive of strangulation.

TABLE 45-1 Causes of Small Bowel Obstruction by Age

Cause	Neonates and Infants < 2 Years	Children and Young Adults	Adults and the Elderly
Intraluminal	Meconium ileus Foreign bodies	Foreign bodies *Ascaris lumbricoides*	Foreign bodies Gallstones Food bolus
Intramural	Intussusception Congenital atresias and stenoses Henoch-Schönlein purpura	Crohn's disease Benign and malignant neoplasms Tuberculosis	Crohn's disease Benign and malignant neoplasm Radiation strictures Surgical anastomoses
Extramural	Midgut volvulus Inguinal hernia Congenital bands Postoperative adhesion	Inguinal hernia Adhesions Midgut volvulus	Adhesions (postoperative and inflammatory) Hernia Neoplasia

---

BOX 45-1 Prevalence of Small Bowel Obstruction by Cause

- Adhesions: 67% to 74%
- Neoplasms: 5% to 13%
- Inflammatory bowel disease: 4% to 7%
- Hernia: 2% to 8%
- Miscellaneous: 4% to 12%

BOX 45-2 Clinical Findings in Patients with Small Bowel Obstruction

- Abdominal pain
- Nausea and vomiting
- Abdominal distention
- Diarrhea or constipation; obstipation in complete small bowel obstruction
- Bowel sounds are hyperactive in early stages or hypoactive in late stages

---

On physical examination, patients will show abdominal distention. The degree of distention often depends on the level of obstruction. Bowel sounds can be hyperactive in an early stage of obstruction or hypoactive late in the course as well as with strangulated lesions. Strangulated SBO is also often associated with peritoneal signs. Peritonitis and perforation present as a silent tender abdomen and are late signs.[3,4] The most important clinical findings in patients with SBO are shown in Box 45-2.

Anatomy

The normal length of the entire small bowel is 3 to 6 meters, although this is quite variable. Loops of jejunum are mostly located in the left hypochondrium in an individual with normal gut rotation. The ileum is mostly in the midline of the pelvis. The terminal ileum is the narrowest part of the small bowel. The presence of valvulae conniventes differentiates small from large bowel on plain radiography, with valvulae being more prominent in the jejunum. Knowing the normal bowel gas pattern on abdominal radiographs is important because this determines the ability to detect deviation from the normal

pattern and classify this further.[3-5] The various bowel gas patterns are discussed in detail later in the section on radiographic imaging.

Pathology

Obstruction of the small bowel leads to proximal dilatation of the intestine due to accumulation of gastrointestinal secretions and swallowed air. This bowel dilatation stimulates cell secretory activity, resulting in more fluid accumulation. This leads to increased peristalsis both above and below the obstruction with frequent loose stools and flatus early in its course. Vomiting occurs if the level of obstruction is proximal. Increasing small bowel distention leads to increased intraluminal pressures. This can cause compression of mucosal lymphatics, leading to bowel wall lymphedema. With even higher intraluminal hydrostatic pressures, increased hydrostatic pressure in the capillary beds results in massive third spacing of fluid, electrolytes, and proteins into the intestinal lumen. The fluid loss and dehydration that ensue may be severe and contribute to increased morbidity and mortality.[3] Strangulated SBOs are most commonly associated with adhesions and occur when a loop of distended bowel twists on its mesenteric pedicle. The arterial occlusion leads to bowel ischemia and necrosis. If left untreated, this progresses to perforation, peritonitis, and death. Proximal to the obstruction, bacteria proliferate in the gut. Microvascular changes in the bowel wall allow translocation to the mesenteric lymph nodes. This is associated with an increase in incidence of bacteremia due to *Escherichia coli*.[6]

Imaging

SBO is a common clinical condition, and its diagnosis can be established if there is the classic triad of good clinical history, focused clinical examination, and targeted imaging and laboratory evaluation. The numerous causes of SBO result in a variety of clinical presentations for the condition based on the etiology; however, vomiting, abdominal distention, and colicky or constant abdominal pain (individually or as a combination) are often the presenting complaints. Imaging plays a very important role in making the diagnosis of this condition, and abdominal radiography, although not very sensitive or specific, is the first imaging test chosen because of its widespread availability and low cost. Depending on the imaging findings and the clinical condition of the patient, further imaging using either barium studies or cross-sectional imaging can be performed. With all methods, scanning should cover a field of view from the diaphragm to the pubic bone.

Radiography

Abdominal Radiography

Conventional abdominal radiography remains the preferred method of initial radiologic examination of symptomatic patients suspected of SBO.[7-12] The normal bowel gas pattern is either absence of small bowel gas or small amounts of gas within up to four variably shaped nondistended (<2.5 cm) loops of small bowel. A normal gas distribution and presence of stool in the large bowel should be recognized. A normal but nonspecific gas pattern describes a pattern of at least one loop of borderline or mildly distended small bowel (2.5 to 3 cm) with

three or more air-fluid levels on upright or lateral decubitus radiographs. The colonic gas and stool pattern is either normal or has a similar degree of borderline distention. This kind of pattern can result from many conditions such as low-grade obstruction, reactive ileus, and medication-induced hypoperistalsis. The probable SBO pattern consists of multiple gas or fluid-filled loops of dilated small bowel with a moderate amount of colonic gas. The presence of colonic gas can indicate early complete SBO, incomplete SBO, or a nonobstructive ileus. This diagnosis should prompt the radiologist to advise further imaging with CT. A definite SBO pattern shows dilated gas or fluid-filled loops of small bowel in the setting of a gasless colon (Fig. 45-1). These findings are diagnostic of SBO.[3,10,11] It is important to distinguish complete from partial SBO, because management is different. On plain films, the presence of residual colonic gas after 6 to 12 hours is suggestive of partial SBO (Fig. 45-2). Despite the description of the various gas patterns that can be seen on radiographs,

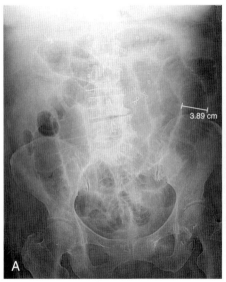
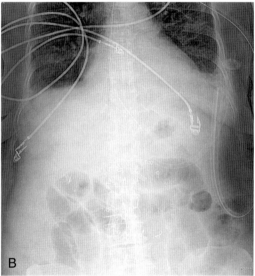

■ **FIGURE 45-1** Complete small bowel obstruction. **A,** Erect radiograph from an acute abdominal series of a 76-year-old woman shows multiple dilated loops of small bowel with air-fluid levels up to 3.9 cm in width. There is relative paucity of air in the colon, which suggests that the obstruction is complete. This patient has had multiple prior abdominal surgeries, as noted by the clips and mesh repair coils on the radiograph. **B,** Supine radiograph of the same patient confirms the findings. There is no free intraperitoneal air.

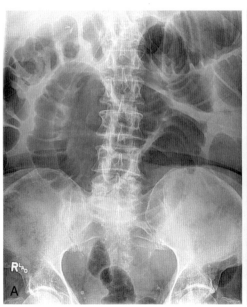
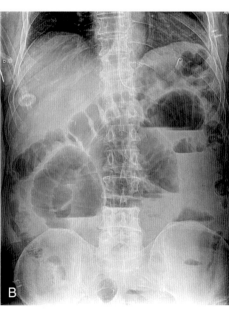

■ **FIGURE 45-2** Partial small bowel obstruction. Acute abdominal series in a 38-year-old woman with abdominal distention and vomiting. **A,** Supine radiograph shows multiple air-filled dilated loops of small bowel with gas in the colon. **B,** Erect radiograph shows multiple air-fluid levels wider than 3 cm each suggestive of small bowel obstruction. Presence of air in the colon suggests that the obstruction is not complete.

BOX 45-3 Manifestations of Small Bowel Obstruction on Plain Radiography

■ Loops of distended small bowel (>3 cm)
■ Dilated bowel loops proximal and collapsed bowel loops distal to obstruction
■ Gas and fluid levels (>3 air-fluid levels on an erect radiograph measuring > 3 cm)
■ Increased distance between valvulae conniventes ("stretch" sign)
■ Trapped gas between valvulae conniventes ("string-of-pearls" sign)

BOX 45-4 Most Common Manifestations of Small Bowel Obstruction on Barium Follow-through

■ Small amount of contrast agent through narrow lumen at the site of obstruction ("beak" sign)
■ Increased peristalsis to overcome obstruction leading to bulbous shape proximal to obstruction (snakehead appearance)
■ Stretched mucosal folds
■ Dilution of ingested barium in massively distended loops of small bowel (drawback of small bowel follow-through)

---

these are diagnostic in only 50% to 60% of cases.[1] Box 45-3 lists common manifestations of SBO on plain radiography.

Intraluminal Contrast Radiography

Barium can be safely used in the adynamic gut because it does not typically inspissate within it.[8] Evaluation of the small bowel using barium can be done by either nonintubation techniques or intubation and insufflations.[9] Nonintubation techniques include small bowel follow-through (SBFT) or per-enterostomy (colostomy or ileostomy) small bowel enemas. SBFT has limitations in the setting of SBO. The presence of significant bowel distention in patients with SBO can result in dilution of the ingested barium, resulting in incomplete opacification and poor mucosal detail. Also, in patients with bowel obstruction there is a prolonged transit time of the oral contrast agent that can be a limiting factor. The nonintubation techniques are unable to assess intestinal distensibility and fixity of bowel loops, which is another drawback. Despite these limitations, the SBFT technique is a viable alternative to enteroclysis in settings where intubation is not possible due to technical or patient-related factors.[10-13] Common manifestations of SBO on barium follow-through are listed in Box 45-4.

Barium Enteroclysis

Enteroclysis involves the intubation of small bowel to a point beyond the pylorus and often beyond the duodenojejunal flexure, enabling the infusion of nondiluted contrast medium into the jejunum. Based on findings of enteroclysis, SBO has been subdivided into three groups. This grading is, however, being used for the characterization of bowel obstruction on modalities such as CT. In Table 45-2 the causes of SBO are classified on the basis of the findings of enteroclysis.

Enteroclysis has a diagnostic value in patients in whom the diagnosis of low-grade SBO is clinically uncertain. Its ability to distinguish low-grade obstruction from normal bowel makes it important in assisting diagnosis.[14,15] Enteroclysis challenges the distensibility of small bowel and exaggerates the effect of mild or subclinical mechanical obstruction. The infusion technique promotes flow of contrast agent toward the site of obstruction despite diminished peristalsis. This distention facilitates evalua-

TABLE 45-2 Classification of Small Bowel Obstruction on the Basis of Enteroclysis Findings

Type of Obstruction	Description
Low grade	Sufficient contrast agent flow through obstruction to define mucosal folds distal to obstruction
High grade	Delayed passage of contrast agent leads to dilution by intestinal fluid. Minimal flow does not enable definition of mucosal folds.
Complete	No contrast agent passes the obstruction

tion of fixed and nondistensible bowel segments. Studies have shown that this technique can predict the presence of obstruction in 100%, the absence of obstruction in 88%, the level of obstruction in 89%, and the cause of obstruction in 86% of patients.[16] SBO is excluded when unimpeded flow of contrast agent is seen in normal-caliber loops from the duodenojejunal junction to the right colon. Mechanical SBO is confirmed when a transition point is demonstrated. By enteroclysis criteria, 3 cm is the upper limit of normal for jejunal caliber and 2.5 cm is the upper limit for the ileum.[14-17]

The level of obstruction is identified during the single-contrast phase of the study; the cause of obstruction is best evaluated during double-contrast evaluation in which mucosal detail is well appreciated. In partial SBO, enteroclysis has been almost 85% accurate in distinguishing adhesions from metastases, tumor recurrence, and radiation damage.[17]

Enteroclysis can also gauge the severity of intestinal obstruction, an advantage over other modalities. In low-grade partial SBO there is no delay in contrast medium arriving at the point of obstruction and adequate contrast medium passes distally such that the fold patterns of the distal bowel are well visualized. High-grade partial SBO is diagnosed when retained bowel fluid dilutes the barium and results in inadequate contrast density above the site of obstruction, allowing only small amounts of contrast medium to pass through the obstruction into the collapsed distal loops. Complete obstruction is diagnosed when there is no passage of contrast medium beyond the point of obstruction, as shown on delayed radiographs obtained up to 24 hours after the start of the examination.

Despite all its advantages, enteroclysis is not practiced widely because it requires conscious sedation, nasointestinal intubation, and constant radiologist involvement. It is often impractical to perform this as an outpatient procedure. In the acute setting when time is limited, CT is often the initial method of examination.

CT

CT is a valuable tool in the evaluation of patients with suspected SBO. The early diagnosis of SBO is critical in preventing complications such as ischemia or perforation. Reports on sensitivity and specificity vary between studies and seem to depend on the grade of obstruction. A low overall sensitivity (63%) of CT for all grades of SBO has been reported. Sensitivity increases with high-grade SBO (81% to 100%) and conversely worsens with low-grade SBO (48%).[17-19] CT can identify the location and severity of an SBO and detects the cause of the obstruction in 93% to 95% of cases. Closed-loop obstructions and strangulation are recognized, which is of great concern because clinical management and the decision for surgical intervention often depend on the exclusion of these complications.[17-19] Strangulation of bowel and ischemia occur as a complication of intussusception, volvulus (Fig. 45-3), torsion, or other types of closed-loop obstruction where there is compromise of the mesenteric vascular pedicle. The presence of pneumatosis intestinalis on CT is an indicator of strangulation and bowel ischemia (Fig. 45-4). Decreased enhancement of a segment of bowel wall in the arterial phase with increased enhancement in the venous phase seems to be highly specific for bowel ischemia.[1] Evaluation of the course of vascular arcades around the involved loops of bowel on CT helps identify patients who are at risk for the life-threatening complications of strangulation and ischemia. This is one of the major advantages of CT over other modalities for the diagnosis of this condition. CT is also useful in distinguishing high-grade obstruction from

an ileus pattern with reported sensitivities up to 100% as compared with 46% with plain radiographs.[18]

The speed of multidetector CT (MDCT) and the isotropic data available with the newer generation scanners have revolutionized abdominal imaging. The widespread use of 16-detector row scanners and the availability of 40- and 64-detector scanners enable rapid acquisition of scan data and have added significantly to CT diagnosis and evaluation of SBO.[20] MDCT allows multiplanar reformatted imaging to help identify the transition point of SBO more reliably and to assess adjacent structures as well as the mural and extramural extent of small bowel lesions. This aids planning for surgical resection.[21,22]

CT can be performed using barium and water as enteral contrast agents in combination with intravenous contrast agents. An intravenous contrast agent is used routinely in the absence of contraindications because it assists in the evaluation of bowel wall and mucosa, possible associated inflammatory or neoplastic processes, and mesenteric vasculature. In patients suspected of having ischemic bowel, scans should be performed in the arterial and venous phases to search for occluded arteries and veins, to depict vascular anatomy, and to assess bowel wall perfusion.[20]

Controversy exists about what oral contrast agent should be used in the setting of a suspected SBO, and practices vary by institution. Some authors use a positive oral contrast medium in this setting as tolerated by the patient because it is helpful in determining if an obstruction is complete.

Analysis of dilution effects on CT can be particularly helpful in patients whose plain radiographs did not show any gas-filled dilated loops (so-called gasless abdomen). It also can help in localizing the point of obstruction because the small bowel loops containing more dilute contrast medium are distal relative to those with more dense oral contrast.[20]

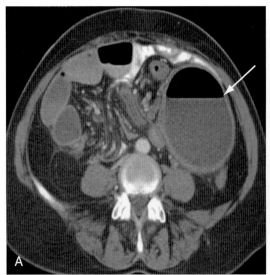 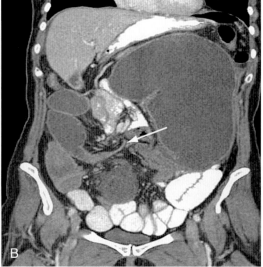

■ **FIGURE 45-3** Volvulus due to adhesions. **A,** Axial contrast-enhanced CT of a 53-year-old woman demonstrates a massively dilated loop of bowel in the left mid abdomen (*arrow*). Loops of small bowel proximal to this are dilated, confirming the diagnosis of small bowel obstruction. **B,** Coronal contrast-enhanced image shows the mesenteric "swirling" (*arrow*) and tapering of a small bowel loop at the transition point of the obstruction. Other images (not shown) showed the appendix next to the massively dilated loop of bowel, confirming that this was the cecum and aiding in the diagnosis of cecal volvulus. These findings were confirmed at surgery.

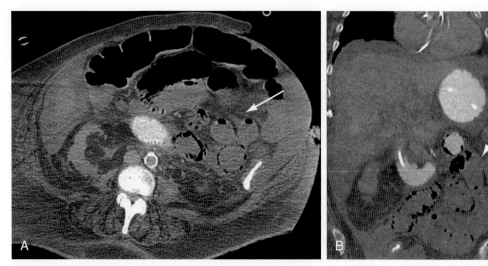

■ **FIGURE 45-4** Mesenteric ischemia. A 78-year-old woman presented with severe abdominal pain, hypotension, and tachycardia. **A,** Axial nonenhanced CT image of the abdomen reveals dilated small bowel loops with multiple air-fluid levels. A transition to normal small bowel was present in the right lower quadrant (*arrow*). Pneumatosis (air in the bowel wall) was seen, and mesenteric ischemia with involvement of the small bowel was suspected. Also noted is dense atherosclerotic calcification involving the visualized abdominal aorta. **B,** Coronal reconstructed image demonstrates the extent of the pneumatosis (*arrow*). The patient was taken to surgery, and extensive necrosed small bowel was resected. Extensive adhesions were present for which adhesiolysis was performed.

BOX 45-5 Most Common Manifestations of Small Bowel Obstruction on CT

- Dilated proximal bowel loop (>2.5 cm) and collapsed distal loop (<1 cm)
- Passage of contrast agent into collapsed segment indicating partial obstruction
- Accumulation of feces and gas proximal to obstruction (feces sign) indicating mechanical obstruction
- Bowel wall thickening, portal venous gas, and pneumatosis indicating strangulation

---

Other investigators have deemed oral contrast unnecessary if SBO is evident on plain radiographs because the contrast agent is unlikely to reach the obstruction and may make evaluation of bowel wall thickening difficult if it does reach the obstruction. If ischemia is suspected, water is used as the enteric contrast agent because positive contrast media interfere with vascular 3D reconstructions. In general, water is better tolerated than positive contrast media in patients with SBO.[1,23]

The most common manifestations of SBO on CT are shown in Box 45-5.

MRI

Although MRI can be used for evaluation of the small bowel, its role is not yet completely established. Advantages of MRI are the high soft tissue contrast and the acquisition of multiplanar images without exposing patients to ionizing radiation. This is especially important for young patients who are undergoing multiple evaluations (e.g., those with Crohn's disease) as well as for pregnant patients.

For imaging of SBO, the major advantage of MRI is the direct visualization of the small bowel wall. Fast sequences

enable acquisition of T1- and T2-weighted (T1W and T2W) images within a single breath-hold. For T2W images half-Fourier acquisition single-shot turbo spin-echo (HASTE) sequences with a fast acquisition time of approximately 1 second per image are used.[24] For T1W images, 2D or 3D spoiled gradient-recalled-echo (SPGR) before and after intravenous administration of a contrast agent are used. These ultra-fast sequences have the disadvantage of being prone to chemical shift artifacts but are especially useful in patients who are unable to hold their breath. The use of parallel imaging techniques is another option to minimize scan time, by reducing the number of phase encoding steps per repetition time. This allows even shorter scan times by maintaining spatial resolution or alternatively allowing higher spatial resolution by maintaining short acquisition time.

For both T1W and T2W sequences the addition of fat-saturated pulses has been shown to increase contrast between bowel and surrounding fat tissue.

The major problem of the just-mentioned MRI methods is flow artifacts that are generated by peristaltic motion that could imitate intraluminal lesions. This can be reduced by antiperistaltic medication.[25,26]

MRI of the small bowel is performed with oral contrast agents. Positive oral contrast agents, such as gadolinium chelates and ferrous and manganese ions are paramagnetic and reduce mainly T1 relaxation time. However, the use of positive contrast agents is limited because a hyperintense lumen often obscures pathologic processes of the bowel wall. Negative contrast agents, such as iron oxides, perfluoroocytl bromide, and barium sulfate produce low signal intensity on T1W as well as T2W images. T2 effects are predominant and caused by spin dephasing, which leads to a loss of signal intensity. One disadvantage of negative contrast agents are magnetic susceptibility artifacts by ferrous oxide on gradient-echo sequences.[25,26]

Biphasic contrast agents show different signal characteristics in different sequences. Manganese and gadolinium chelates at high concentrations lead to hyperintensity on T1W images and hypointensity on T2W images, whereas water, mannitol-based solutions, polyethylene glycol, and barium sulfate create hypointensity on T1W images and hyperintensity on T2W images. Disadvantages of these contrast agents are the intestinal absorption of water and unwanted intestinal side effects of mannitol solutions.[26,27]

MRI of the small bowel requires distention, because collapsed bowel loops can hide pathologic findings. There are two main approaches: imaging after administration of an oral contrast agent (MR follow-through) and imaging with distention by nasojejunal contrast application (MR enteroclysis).

For MR SBFT, image acquisition is preceded by oral ingestion of 600 to 1000 mL of contrast agent 20 minutes before the examination. A spasmolytic agent is added intravenously immediately before imaging is performed. T2W and T1/T2 hybrid sequences are acquired in axial and coronal planes, until the terminal ileum is completely distended.

With the MR enteroclysis technique a biphasic contrast agent is given through a nasojejunal tube. The volume of contrast agent depends on the subject and varies between 1500 and 2000 mL. It is preferably applied using a peristaltic pump with an infusion rate between 80 and 150 mL. The main advantages of MR enteroclysis are improved intestinal distention as well as real-time imaging with ultrafast sequences. In the evaluation of SBO, MRI can be especially useful for distinction of nonobstructive or partially obstructive lesions using real-time evaluation with MR enteroclysis.[28]

Ultrasonography

Ultrasonography is widely used in the assessment of acute abdominal pain. However, its use in the evaluation of SBO obstruction is limited. It is important to be aware of the findings of bowel obstruction on ultrasonography because this may be an incidental finding in a patient who is being evaluated for abdominal pain. In SBO, fluid accumulates in the bowel lumen. When there is no gas in the bowel lumen, as is often the case with mechanical obstruction or vascular compromise, fluid-filled bowel loops might be difficult to detect on plain radiographs. Contrast ultrasonography can be very useful to visualize SBO, because the intraluminal fluid is a natural contrast medium and helps demonstrating the origin of the obstruction. It can accurately detect the location of the obstruction. Characteristic features are rounded distended bowel loops with loss of definition and prominent valvulae conniventes. Ultrasonography is also able to assess the peristalsis and movements of intraluminal content.[29-31] Ultrasonography is less costly and less invasive than CT. Box 45-6 shows the most common manifestations of SBO seen on ultrasound evaluation.

Imaging Algorithm

There is no one generally accepted approach to evaluate patients with SBO. Plain radiography remains the initial modality of choice, because of its widespread availability,

---

BOX 45-6	**Most Common Manifestations of Small Bowel Obstruction on Ultrasonography**

- Luminal diameter greater than 2.0 to 2.5 in jejunum and greater than 1.5 to 2.0 in ileum
- Dilated segment longer than 10 cm
- Increased peristalsis in dilated loops
- Collapsed colon

---

accessibility, and low cost. However, plain films may be diagnostic in only 45% to 60% of cases.[15] The decision to use additional diagnostic imaging methods should be based on clinical presentation and findings on plain radiography. The definitive presence of SBO on plain radiograph confirms the diagnosis and is sufficient to decide if a patient is managed conservatively or if surgical exploration is necessary.

If conservative management is initiated or if there are doubts about the diagnosis, standard CT has emerged as the imaging modality of choice for further evaluation of SBO (Table 45-3). CT is helpful to exclude strangulation and enables better visualization of possible causes for the obstruction, especially if the lesion is extraluminal. CT enteroclysis should be performed only if conventional CT is nondiagnostic. Ultrasonography and MRI can occasionally be useful in the diagnosis of SBO and in the evaluation of possible causes. However, CT is superior to these imaging modalities because it is more comprehensive and not limited by intraluminal air. Nuclear medicine studies and PET/CT do not play a role in the diagnosis of acute SBO and are reserved for assessment of underlying causes of SBO. An imaging algorithm is provided in Figure 45-19.

Differential Diagnosis

A number of medical conditions can cause symptoms similar to those of SBO. Abdominal distention, vomiting, and constipation can be seen in patients with electrolyte disorders, uremia, diabetic ketoacidosis, and thyroid disorders as well as intoxication with anticholinergics or tricyclic antidepressants. Peritonitis of any cause can mimic the symptoms of SBO. The presence and characterization of pain is often the distinguishing feature from other pathologic processes. Imaging plays a critical role in the ultimate diagnosis of the condition.

Any condition resulting in small bowel dilatation or abdominal distention can be confused with SBO before clinical and radiographic investigations are completed and integrated. Obstruction typically results in distention that may include the colon in addition to small bowel. A concurrent inflammatory process, recent surgery, gastrointestinal infection, and electrolyte disturbances are predisposing factors for SBO, and appreciation of these comorbidities is important in scan interpretation. Cecal volvulus causes more proximal colonic obstruction and typically secondary small bowel dilatation as well. Recognition of the distended cecum is the key to differentiating volvulus from an isolated SBO. Shock bowel can present

TABLE 45-3 Accuracy, Limitations, and Pitfalls of the Modalities Used in Imaging of Small Bowel Obstruction (SBO)

Modality	Accuracy	Limitations	Pitfalls
Radiography	75% sensitivity 53% specificity	Barium studies cannot be performed in patients with perforation or complete SBO. Extended transit time in SBFT	Diagnosis might be missed if no gas present in the small bowel
CT	94% accuracy 92% sensitivity 96% specificity	Ionizing radiation Risk of contrast reaction	Low sensitivity for low-grade, partial or incomplete SBO
MRI	88% accuracy 90% sensitivity 86% specificity	Expensive Time consuming Not available everywhere	Patient factors: claustrophobia, pacemakers, metal implants
Ultrasonography	84% accuracy 83% sensitivity 100% specificity	Air can obscure the field of view Difficult in obese patients	Operator dependent
Nuclear medicine	79% sensitivity 98% specificity	Poor spatial resolution	Activity can be observed with other causes of inflammation.
PET/CT	Data not available	Ionizing radiation High cost	Differentiation of benign from borderline neoplasms can be difficult.

SBFT, small bowel follow-through.

as dilated loops of small bowel, but involvement of the colon and history should help differentiate the MDCT findings from SBO. Frank ischemia also can cause marked small bowel distention and simulate the appearance of obstruction. Ancillary findings of bowel wall thickening, segmental bowel perfusion abnormalities, and proof of arterial atherosclerotic disease provide evidence for an ischemic cause of the dilatation, however. Although Crohn's disease may cause SBO because of stricture formation, stenotic-phase disease, or superimposed acute disease, it also may result in areas of dilatation and narrowing without a true obstruction.[20]

Treatment

Medical Treatment

Initial nonsurgical management includes fluid administration, bowel decompression, analgesics, antiemetics, and antibiotics, which should cover gram-negative and anaerobic organisms. Initial decompression is achieved with a nasogastric tube for suctioning gastrointestinal contents and preventing aspiration. No clinical advantage for using a long tube (nasointestinal) instead of a short tube (nasogastric) has been observed. A nonoperative trial of as many as 3 days is warranted for partial or simple obstruction, given that adequate fluid resuscitation and nasogastric suctioning is provided. Resolution of the obstruction can occur in patients with these lesions in up to 72 hours.[4,5]

Surgical Treatment

A strangulated SBO is a surgical emergency. In patients in whom the SBO is complete, the risk of strangulation is high and early surgical intervention is necessary. Patients with simple complete obstructions in whom nonoperative trials fail also need surgical treatment but experience no apparent disadvantage from delayed surgery.[32]

> ### What the Referring Physician Needs to Know: General Considerations of Small Bowel Obstruction
>
> - Recognize SBO: clinical presentation and plain radiography (diagnostic in 45% to 60%).
> - Determine the site of obstruction.
> - Discriminate partial from complete obstruction.
> - Discriminate simple from strangulated obstruction.
> - Determine the cause (is there a cause that can be removed?).
> - Detect and treat associated complications.

BENIGN CAUSES OF SMALL BOWEL OBSTRUCTION

Etiology

The leading cause of benign SBO in the United States is adhesions occurring after surgical procedures such as appendectomy, colorectal surgery, and gynecologic and upper gastrointestinal procedures.[2] Single-band adhesions were most commonly found in cases with strangulating obstruction, whereas nonstrangulated obstructions were more commonly associated with multiple adhesions. Other common causes of SBO are inflammatory bowel diseases, hernias, gallstone ileus, Crohn's disease, hernia, and radiation injury or a combination of these findings.[1,31] Rare causes of nonmalignant SBO include phytobezoar after previous gastric surgery,[33] familial Mediterranean fever causing recurrent attacks of febrile inflammation of the peritoneum,[34] swallowed foreign bodies, parasites, tuberculosis, intra-abdominal abscess, and intramural hematoma. In pediatric patients, causes of SBO are intussusception, congenital intestinal atresia, malrotation of bowel with midgut volvulus, and necrotizing enterocolitis.

The varying incidence of etiologic factors in different studies can be attributed to the evaluation practices used as well as to referral patterns in institutions. There has also been a change in the etiology of SBO during this century, with hernia as the leading cause at the beginning of the 20th century. Elective treatment of groin hernias caused the decrease of strangulated hernia to only 2% to 5%.[2] Hernia is still the leading cause of SBO in developing countries, owing to a lack of access for elective repair.[35] Demographic factors also seem to play a role in the etiology of SBO, especially in diseases with a hereditary component such as Crohn's disease.

Prevalence and Epidemiology

Benign causes comprise 70% to 80% of all reasons for admission for SBO. Numbers vary in the literature, but the leading causes are adhesions (67% to 74%), inflammatory bowel diseases (7% to 10%), and hernia (2% to 8%).[2] Adhesions are due to previous surgery, most commonly appendectomy, colorectal resection, and gynecologic procedures. The terminology used in describing SBOs is presented in Box 45-7.

Clinical Presentation

Patients present with abdominal pain, accompanied by nausea and vomiting. SBO can be associated with consti-

---

BOX 45-7 Terminology in Bowel Obstruction

Simple obstruction: small bowel obstruction with intact blood supply
Strangulated obstruction: small bowel obstruction with bowel ischemia
Partial obstruction: narrowed lumen with conserved passage of gas and intestinal contents
Complete obstruction: total luminal occlusion with lack of gas and fecal material in colon or nondistended small bowel
Closed loop obstruction: bowel segment occluded at two points that are adjacent to each other

---

pation or diarrhea. Physical examination reveals abdominal distention and initially hyperactive bowel sounds, followed by hypoactive bowel sounds in later stages. The early diagnosis of SBO is crucial to prevent bowel ischemia or perforation.

Pathophysiology

Lower abdominal and pelvic operations are more likely to cause subsequent SBO than upper gastrointestinal procedures. The bowel is fixed at the root of the mesentery; therefore, the cranial part of the bowel is less mobile. In the pelvis, where the intestine is more mobile, it is more likely to undergo a torsion, leading to SBO.

Pathology

Postoperative adhesions can manifest as early SBO within 4 weeks of surgery (Fig. 45-5) or as delayed SBO years after a surgical procedure. Hernias account for 2% to 8% of all SBO cases in the United States.[2] They include inguinal, umbilical (Fig. 45-6), ventral wall (Fig. 45-7), femoral, obturator, and internal hernias (Fig. 45-8). A loop of small bowel can enter any form of hernia and become obstructed at the narrow neck of the hernia. This leads to a compromise of venous return of the entrapped bowel segment with congestion and edema, eventually resulting in ischemia, necrosis, and perforation in some cases. Inflammatory bowel diseases, such as Crohn's disease, are increasingly recognized as leading causes of SBO and account for approximately 10% of all cases. Patients most likely present with intermittent subacute or chronic forms of partial bowel obstruction. The obstruction can be caused by the primary inflammatory process itself or as a consequence of the formation of fibrotic strictures. Gallstone ileus is a rare complication of cholelithiasis; it has a high morbidity and mortality and most commonly presents in patients older than age 65.[2] It accounts for 1% to 4% of all mechanical SBO and is caused by impaction of a gallstone in the intestinal lumen.

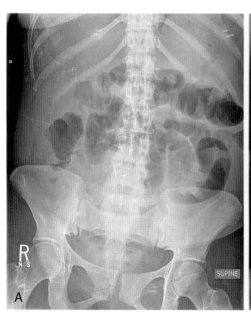
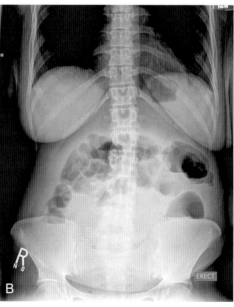

■ **FIGURE 45-5** Complete small bowel obstruction. **A,** A 25-year-old woman who is 5 days post cesarean section presented with vomiting and lower abdominal pain. **A,** Supine radiograph taken as a part of the acute abdominal series reveals multiple dilated air-filled loops of small bowel. The colon is gasless. **B,** Erect radiograph confirms small bowel obstruction. There is no free gas under the domes of the diaphragm. Presence of a smooth extrinsic mass effect on the small bowel loops due to the postpartum uterus is noted.

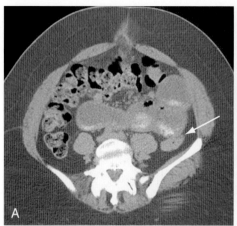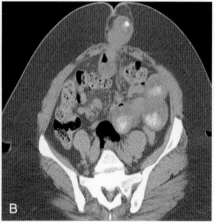

■ **FIGURE 45-6** Umbilical hernia. A 62-year-old woman presented with clinical symptoms consistent with small bowel obstruction. There was a vague fullness in the periumbilical region. **A,** Axial contrast-enhanced image demonstrates multiple dilated small bowel loops without dilatation of the colon (*arrow*), confirming the clinical suspicion of small bowel obstruction. **B,** Axial image at the level of the umbilicus is diagnostic for an umbilical hernia causing the bowel obstruction. The narrow neck of the hernial sac was compressing the loop of bowel reentering the peritoneal cavity. The hernia was surgically reduced.

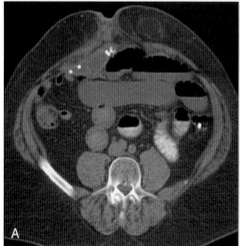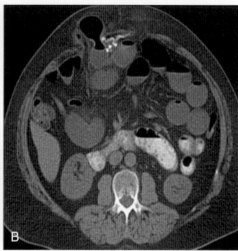

■ **FIGURE 45-7** Ventral wall hernia. **A,** Axial contrast-enhanced CT image in a 52-year-old woman shows multiple dilated loops of small bowel with air-fluid levels. There is a small amount of fluid in the colon with some air suggesting that the obstruction is not complete. This patient has a prior history of bowel surgery. **B,** Another axial contrast-enhanced image confirms that a ventral wall hernia through the surgical scar is the cause of the obstruction.

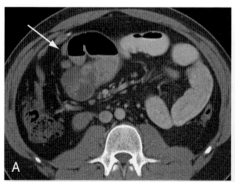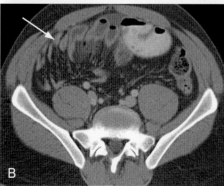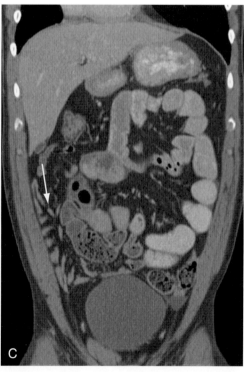

■ **FIGURE 45-8** Pericecal hernia. A 32-year-old man presented with acute abdominal pain and vomiting. **A,** Axial contrast-enhanced CT image shows multiple dilated loops of small bowel with a sudden abrupt change in caliber in the right lower quadrant (*arrow*). **B,** Nondilated loops of bowel are present in a nonanatomic location lateral to the cecum (*arrow*), which is confirmed by the coronal reformatted image (*arrow,* **C**). This was diagnosed as a case of pericecal hernia due to a congenital defect in the cecal mesentery. Internal hernias are uncommon, and recognizing the normal location of the bowel is very important for diagnosis.

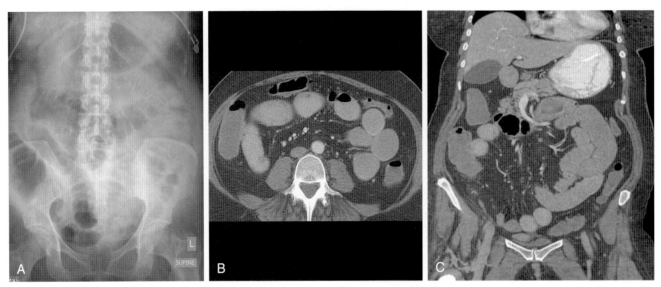

■ **FIGURE 45-9**   Ileus. **A,** Supine radiograph of the abdomen in a 52-year-old woman shows diffuse dilatation of small and large bowel loops. This patient had a history of constipation. The findings are diagnostic of functional ileus pattern of bowel. **B,** Axial CT image shows fluid-filled dilated small and large bowel loops. **C,** Coronal image confirms the findings of ileus. No transition point in the bowel and a proportionate dilatation of small and large bowel loops are diagnostic of ileus.

Imaging

Imaging is integral to the management of patients with SBO, and CT in particular has established its role for this indication, with a reported accuracy of 90% to 95%.[17,18] In most cases, management decisions are made regardless of the suspected cause of SBO. Some situations, however, warrant further investigation of the underlying cause, because patient management would differ from the general approach. These situations include incarcerated hernias, inflammatory bowel diseases, malignant tumors, intra-abdominal abscess, and recurrent SBOs.

Radiography

The most common general radiologic features of SBO that are seen on plain radiography were described earlier. Less common findings can be associated with specific circumstances or causes of SBO. It is not the role of plain radiography to detect the cause of intestinal obstruction in most cases. However, certain specific findings on plain radiographs can help in diagnosing the cause of SBO. Any cause of SBO can result in intramural gas secondary to ischemia, which can be appreciated on plain radiographs and is considered a poor prognostic sign. Another finding is closed-loop obstructions, which are most commonly caused by adhesions. A closed-loop obstruction develops when a bowel segment is not decompressed by the caudal passage of gas and fluid. It is important to distinguish paralytic ileus (Fig. 45-9A) from mechanical obstruction. Paralytic ileus can develop when an insult is not of the occlusive type or as expression of a worsening of a mechanical obstruction. Unlike in mechanical obstruction the patency of the intestinal lumen is maintained. Characteristic radiographic findings of paralytic ileus are multiple air-fluid levels with a reduced fluid component, increased diameter of bowel loops with decreased tone, thickened appearance of the intestinal wall, horizontal side by side

placement of distended bowel loops, and absence of gas in the colon.[36] On enteroclysis, the contrast medium should reach the cecum within 4 hours with paralytic ileus. If it remains stationary for longer than 4 hours, mechanical obstruction is suggested. If radiographic examination does not prove diagnostic, CT examination should be undertaken (see Fig. 45-9B, C). In cases of gallstone ileus, ectopic intraluminal calcified stones can be seen in addition to the classic findings of SBO. The cholecystoduodenal fistula causes accumulation of gas in the biliary tree (pneumobilia). Even though the triad of SBO, ectopic gallstones, and pneumobilia is considered pathognomonic of gallstone ileus, it is only seen in 30% to 35% of abdominal plain radiographs and is more easily demonstrated on CT.[37] However, these specific findings are not always present. The overall reported rate of diagnosed causes of SBO on plain radiography is only 2% to 7%.[30] In Crohn's disease, aphthoid ulcers develop into linear ulcers and fissures to produce an ulceronodular or "cobblestone" appearance. The bowel wall is thickened by a combination of fibrosis and inflammatory infiltrates.[38] SBFT (Fig. 45-10) is part of the standard radiologic approach to the investigation of Crohn's disease. It shows the entire small bowel but has limitations for Crohn's disease.

CT

Because of the very high resolution and the presence of intravenous contrast enhancement, CT can not only diagnose the presence of SBO but also possibly determine the cause and the complications of the condition. The presence or the amount of bowel dilatation is not a distinguishing factor between bowel obstruction and ileus. The identification of a site of transition in the small bowel and detection of change in caliber from dilated to nondilated bowel is important in diagnosing the condition and, in most cases, identifying the cause of obstruction.[30,31] Identification of the transition point often allows diagnosis of the cause of the bowel obstruction. Recent studies have found that in more complex cases off-axial (coronal and sagittal) reformatted images are of benefit in determining the site and cause of obstruction and that the presence of these images improves reader confidence in diagnosis.[21,22] There are, however, certain drawbacks for the coronal reformatted images, such as difficulties in determination of conditions involving the ventral abdominal wall because this is often not included when reformatted images are generated. There is also a learning curve for the interpreting radiologists when coronal images are being viewed.

The reformatted images should be used as an adjunct and not as a replacement for conventional axial imaging.[21,22]

The presence of intravenous contrast medium is especially useful in conditions in which an intramural pathologic process is causing SBO (e.g., Crohn's disease or infective or inflammatory enteritis). In patients with suspected Crohn's disease, cross-sectional images should be analyzed specifically for the presence and character of a pathologically altered bowel segment (wall thickness, pattern of attenuation, degree of enhancement, and length of involvement). CT of Crohn's disease shows bowel wall thickening and mural stratification as a target or double-halo appearance during acute inflammation. Inflamed mucosa and serosa enhance after contrast agent administration, and the intensity of contrast agent enhancement correlates with disease activity (Figs. 45-11 and 45-12). The stenosis and prestenotic dilatation as well as skip lesions can be identified. In chronic disease, mural stratification disappears and transmural fibrosis is seen. Mesenteric changes present as fibrofatty proliferation, lymphadenopathy, and hypervascularity of the vasa recta ("comb" sign). CT can also detect complications of Crohn's disease, such as fistulas, abscesses, strictures, and secondary tumors.[38,39]

It is also possible to determine complications such as vascular compromise resulting in bowel ischemia in the presence of intravenous contrast media. CT cannot identify a bowel adhesion itself. The diagnosis is made by the presence of an abruptly changing caliber of the small bowel lumen in the absence of another obstructing cause (Fig. 45-13). CT is superior to plain radiography in the diagnosis of a hernia, because anatomic relationships as well as complications can be determined. Especially in obturator hernias, which are difficult to detect clinically and are associated with bowel ischemia and high mortality, CT can establish a fast diagnosis followed by surgical intervention.[30,31] When SBO is caused by diverticulitis, CT findings consist of mural thickening, submucosal edema in small bowel adjacent to the diverticulitis, mesenteric inflammation, and typical signs of colonic diverticulitis, such as diverticula, colonic wall thickening, and abscess formation (Fig. 45-14).[40] Most adult intussusceptions in

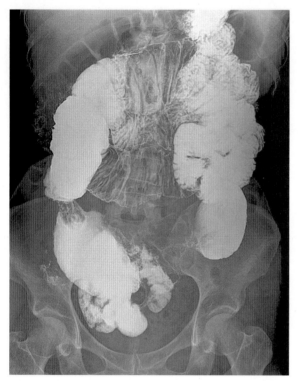

■ **FIGURE 45-10** Small bowel follow-through in Crohn's disease. Note the presence of massively dilated loops of small bowel filled with barium. There is a narrowed loop of small bowel in the left lower quadrant that is involved with Crohn's disease that was proven by CT.

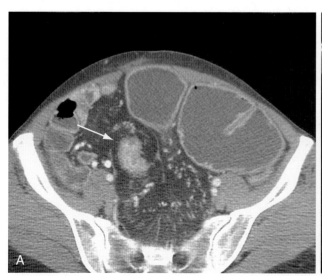

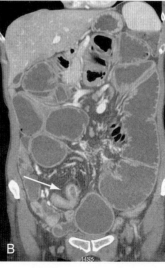

■ **FIGURE 45-11** Crohn's disease. **A,** Axial contrast-enhanced CT in a 68-year-old woman shows multiple significantly dilated loops of small bowel. There is a loop of ileum in the right lower quadrant that is thick walled and inflamed (*arrow*). The patient has symptoms of inflammatory bowel disease, and this appearance is consistent with Crohn's ileitis with small bowel obstruction. **B,** Coronal reconstructed image in the same patient clearly demonstrates the dilated fluid-filled loops of small bowel with the inflamed ileal loop in the right lower quadrant (*arrow*).

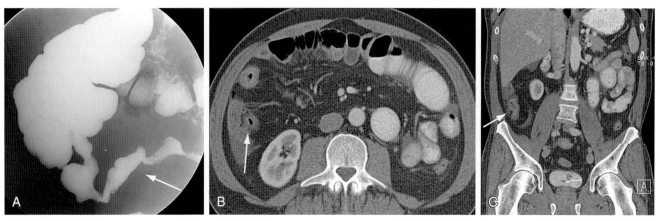

■ **FIGURE 45-12**   Crohn's disease small bowel follow-through (SBFT). A 36-year-old man presented with a known history of Crohn's disease. **A,** SBFT image at the level of the ileocecal junction shows nodularity of the terminal ileum. There were multiple dilated loops of small bowel proximal to the ileocecal junction (*arrow*). Delayed transit of barium to the ileocecal junction was noted. **B,** Axial contrast-enhanced CT image shows the dilated obstructed small bowel loops with a narrowed ileum at the ileocecal junction with inflammatory thickening of the wall of this loop of bowel (*arrow*). **C,** Coronal image at this level confirms the findings of Crohn's stricture with active inflammation (*arrow*). There were no complications of the disease diagnosed at this time.

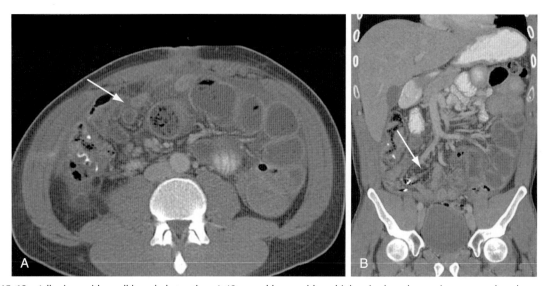

■ **FIGURE 45-13**   Adhesions with small bowel obstruction. A 48-year-old man with multiple prior bowel surgeries presented to the emergency department with a 3-day history of constipation and recent onset of vomiting. CT scan of the abdomen was performed with a high index of suspicion for bowel obstruction. **A,** Axial contrast-enhanced CT confirms small bowel obstruction up to the transition point at the right lower quadrant (*arrow*) very close to the site of prior bowel surgery. **B,** Coronal reformatted image shows the extent of the bowel obstruction and confirms the site of transition (*arrow*). Adhesions from prior bowel surgery were the cause for the obstruction. Conservative management was successfully performed in this patient.

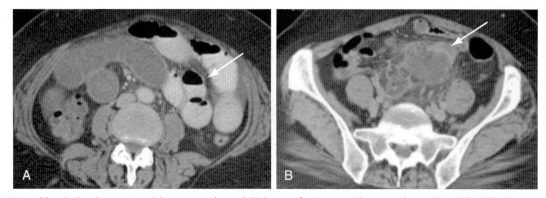

■ **FIGURE 45-14**   Diverticular abscess. **A,** Axial contrast-enhanced CT image of a 72-year-old woman shows dilated fluid-filled loops of small bowel with multiple air-fluid levels (*arrow*). There is the presence of air and some fluid in the colon. These features are suggestive of partial small bowel obstruction. **B,** Image in the pelvis demonstrates diverticulitis with a diverticular abscess (*arrow*). The small bowel obstruction is the result of the inflammation adjacent to the abscess.

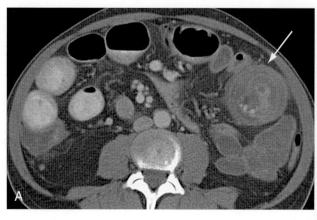
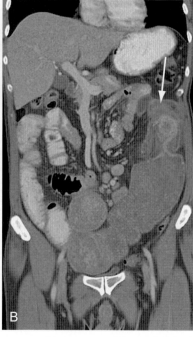

■ **FIGURE 45-15** Intussusception. A 62-year-old man presented to the emergency department with nausea, vomiting, and abdominal pain for 2 days. He had tenderness in the abdomen and hyperactive bowel sounds. **A,** Axial contrast-enhanced CT image demonstrates a whorled appearance of a loop of small bowel in the left mid abdomen (*arrow*) with dilated small bowel loops proximally. **B,** Coronal image clearly demonstrates the intussusceptions (*arrow*) and the proximal small bowel obstruction. This patient was taken to surgery, and a leiomyoma causing the intussusception was resected.

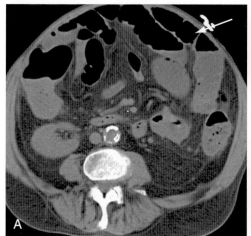
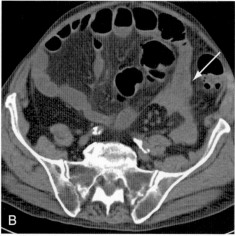

■ **FIGURE 45-16** Bowel wall hemorrhage. A 73-year-old man had a history of trauma. The patient was known to be on anticoagulants for the treatment of a prior pulmonary embolism. CT of the abdomen (**A**) and pelvis (**B**) was performed, and axial images displayed dilated loops of small bowel with obstruction at the site of bowel hematoma. This was seen as an area of bowel wall thickening and presence of stranding around the loops of small bowel (*arrows*).

the small bowel are transient and do not cause bowel obstruction. However, intussusceptions that lead to SBO are usually secondary to benign lesions, such as lipoma, leiomyoma, hemangioma, or neurofibroma. Fifteen percent of lesions causing small bowel intussusception are malignant and most often due to metastases. Adult intussusception appears as a complex soft tissue mass and can present as either a target-shaped lesion with concentric alternating layers of high and low attenuation when the CT beam is perpendicular to the longitudinal axis of the intussusceptions or as a sausage-shaped mass when the CT beam is parallel to the longitudinal axis (Fig.

45-15).[41] With intramural hematoma, CT findings are often nonspecific and depend on the age of the hematoma. In early stages the hemorrhage is hypodense, but it becomes hyperdense as time passes. Once lysis of the clot begins, the hemorrhage presents as decreased density (Fig. 45-16). The previously mentioned classic radiologic signs of gallstone ileus are not always present on initial plain radiographs. On CT, the gallstone is more reliably identified as is gas within the gallbladder due to biliary-enteric fistula.[37] CT also demonstrates a bezoar as a mass in the obstructed bowel segment. The mass may be mottled due to air trapped in the proximal bowel loop.

MRI

MRI with fast sequences (HASTE) uses the intrinsic intestinal fluid as contrast medium and avoids the time-consuming administration of oral contrast agents as needed for CT. Images are created rapidly during one breath-hold. The technique has been shown useful in finding the cause for SBO for some underlying pathologic processes.[24] Adhesions can manifest on MRI as sharply angled loops of dilated bowel and multiple transition points. With strictures, a focal narrowing of the bowel with abrupt change in caliber without a surrounding mass can be seen. Obstructing tumor masses cause increased signal intensity at the transition point, but further differentiation of the mass is not possible. The cause can be correctly identified in approximately 50% of the cases.[26]

MR enteroclysis is an emerging technique that combines the advantages of conventional enteroclysis with cross-sectional imaging. It can effectively determine the level and presence of SBO. Adequate small bowel distention is achieved by either duodenal intubation or oral contrast administration. MR enteroclysis shows a wide spectrum of imaging findings of Crohn's disease, including early nonspecific changes such as mucosal nodularity or aphthous-type ulcers, longitudinal or fissure ulcers, cobblestoning, intramural tracts, wall thickening, luminal narrowing and prestenotic dilatation, fibrofatty proliferation, mesenteric hypervascularity, the "comb" sign, associated mesenteric lymphadenopathy, and/or complications such as fistula formation, phlegmon, or abscess and can provide pictorial evidence of disease activity. In one study, MR enteroclysis showed 100% sensitivity in the diagnosis of lumen stenosis and demonstration of associated prestenotic dilatation.[42]

Ultrasonography

Ultrasonography can be used to locate dilated loops as well as to assess peristalsis and thus differentiate a mechanical obstruction from paralytic ileus. Its use is, however, limited owing to the inherent inability of sound waves to penetrate gaseous loops. The presence of free peritoneal fluid is a nonspecific finding of SBO. In some cases ultrasound can detect the cause of the obstruction such as gallstones, bezoars, foreign bodies, or mural thickening. Depiction of a calcified gallstone and gas in the biliary tree can be seen in SBO caused by gallstones. Intussusception can appear as a mass of concentric rings of alternating hyperechoic and hypoechoic layers, often referred to as a "target" or "doughnut" shape. Doppler ultrasonography is useful to assess the vascular flow to the intestine, with an absence of blood flow suggestive of necrosis. It is also used to demonstrate congenital abnormalities such as meconium ileus or jejunoileal atresia. In meconium ileus, bowel loops contain highly echogenic material.[29,30]

Nuclear Medicine

Nuclear medicine techniques do not play an important role in diagnosing benign SBO. One application is white blood cell scanning to localize inflammatory disease underlying the obstruction. ^{99m}Tc-hexamethylpropylene-amine oxime (HMPO) scanning has been shown useful in assessment of disease activity in patients with Crohn's disease and can distinguish it from other causes of mural thickening.[43]

Imaging Algorithm

An imaging algorithm is provided in Figure 45-19.

Classic Signs: Benign Causes of Small Bowel Obstruction

- Dilated small bowel loops with air-fluid levels
- Absent or minimal gas in the colon
- Localized transition zone
- Collapsed small bowel loops distal to the obstruction
- Small bowel feces sign

Treatment

Medical Treatment

General options for medical and surgical management were discussed earlier in this chapter. Management of specific causes depends on the etiology. Patients with SBO due to Crohn's disease can be managed nonsurgically in most cases with tube decompression in combination with treatment of the underlying inflammatory process. Parenteral nutrition should be provided for periods of prolonged bowel rest. Patients with partial SBO can be managed nonoperatively for up to several days. In 60% to 85% of these patients the obstruction will resolve without the need for surgical intervention. Parenteral nutrition should be provided for a prolonged period without oral nutritional intake.[4,5]

Surgical Treatment

Patients who present with SBO from adhesions usually benefit from early operative lysis by simple laparotomy or laparoscopy. Intraoperative measures such as minimizing serosal trauma, avoiding unnecessary dissection, and exclusion of foreign or nonabsorbable material should be taken to prevent formation of postoperative adhesions. When SBO is caused by a hernia, manual reduction of the obstruction can be tried for inguinal, umbilical, incisional,

---

What the Referring Physician Needs to Know: Small Bowel Obstruction from Benign Causes

- In patients with symptoms and nonspecific plain radiographs, CT after oral administration of a contrast agent is recommended.
- When CT is not diagnostic, CT or MR enteroclysis can be performed.
- When nonsurgical management is considered, CT can exclude strangulated obstruction.
- CT is the most comprehensive method to determine the cause of SBO.

and incarcerated hernias, followed by close observation of the patient. Elective repair of the hernia should be performed to prevent recurrence and strangulation. Irreducible hernias have to be managed by a primary operative approach.[32]

MALIGNANT CAUSES OF SMALL BOWEL OBSTRUCTION

Etiology

Primary tumors of the small bowel are uncommon and constitute only 2% to 3% of all tumors of the gastrointestinal tract. They are rarely suspected on a clinical basis, which can cause a delay in diagnosis, leading to significant morbidity and mortality. However, intestinal involvement from metastatic cancer is common. As cancer patients live longer with improved therapy, secondary tumors of the small bowel are becoming more likely.[44] The most common cause of SBO due to malignancy is secondary peritoneal implants, typically from intra-abdominal tumors of ovaries, pancreas, stomach, or colon. Lymphatic spread rarely causes masses large enough to obstruct the small bowel. Hematogenous spread from distant sites is rare and is mainly caused by breast and lung cancer. Obstruction by a tumor can be caused by either direct invasion or extrinsic compression.

Prevalence and Epidemiology

Although the small bowel comprises 75% of the total length and more than 90% of the mucosal surface of the gastrointestinal tract, less than 2% of malignant neoplasms of the entire tract are small bowel neoplasms.[45] Malignant tumors account for 7% to 25% of cases of SBO.[2] Any tumor of the small bowel can potentially cause obstruction, but few of these are primary tumors. Histologic evaluations of primary tumors showed lymphoma to be the most common tumor, followed by adenocarcinoma, carcinoid, and gastrointestinal stromal tumors (GISTs).[46] The incidence of metastatic cancer of the small bowel varies among different malignancies. Diffuse peritoneal carcinomatosis has been reported in up to 5% to 10% of patients with breast cancer and malignant melanoma. The majority of intestinal metastases are associated with primary lobular breast cancer.[44]

Clinical Presentation

Patients with SBO due to malignant neoplasm most frequently present with nonspecific symptoms of abdominal pain, associated with nausea and/or vomiting. Weight loss can be present due to the underlying malignancy. Clinical findings include abdominal distention with or without guarding and rigidity. A palpable abdominal mass can be present. Metastatic carcinoid tumors can present as flushing and diarrhea. GISTs are slow-growing tumors and are associated with a long period of symptoms. Patients are often anemic due to recurrent melena arising from ulcerated component. The time interval from diagnosis of the primary tumor to the development of SBO due to metastases varies widely and can be the initial presentation of the tumor. Symptoms are related to tumor size, location within the small bowel, blood supply, and tendency to undergo ulceration and necrosis. In a patient with a known history of malignancy, obstructive symptoms, or bleeding from the gastrointestinal tract, a metastatic lesion must be considered.[45]

Pathophysiology

Malignant tumors can be found in any part of the small bowel. Primary neoplasms are most often located in the jejunum (41%), followed be ileum (33%) and duodenum (22%). In 4%, tumors could be found in multiple sites of the small bowel.[47] The duodenum is the most frequent location of small bowel adenocarcinoma. Most carcinoid tumors of the small bowel occur in the appendix and distal ileum, which is also the most common site of clinically significant carcinoid tumors. Lymphoma occurs most commonly in the distal and terminal ileum, whereas GISTs are mostly found in ileum and jejunum.[45]

Pathology

Adenocarcinoma, carcinoid tumor, lymphoma, and GISTs are primary malignant tumors of the small bowel. Adenocarcinomas of the duodenum are either polypoid, ulcerated, or infiltrative. In the jejunum and ileum, adenocarcinomas are mostly annular, constricting, and particularly ulcerated; the remainder are polypoid and fungating.[45]

Most of the non-Hodgkin's lymphomas are of B cell type, except for the sprue-related T-cell lymphoma.[48] Hodgkin's disease accounts for only about 1% of all malignant lymphomas of the gastrointestinal tract. In adults, the most common lymphoma is histiocytic, whereas in children it is the well-differentiated lymphocytic type. A poor prognosis is associated with large tumor size, ulceration, multicentric origin, and presence of involved lymph nodes.

Small bowel carcinoids are usually submucosal-intramural tumors that bulge slightly into the lumen. They can become polypoid and cause intussusceptions or obstruction as they enlarge. More often, carcinoid-related obstructions are of lower grade and result from fibrosis rather than the mass effect of the tumor. GISTs arise from the muscular coats of the bowel wall and are most frequently subserosal and exoenteric. However, they may grow toward the bowel lumen and become polypoid. They assume a round or oval shape and frequently have a central area of mucosal ulceration that causes a high incidence of intestinal bleeding.[45,49]

Metastases may cause symptoms similar to primary intestinal neoplasms. Breast cancer is the leading cause of SBO due to metastases to the bowel wall. Metastases from breast cancer are usually associated with peritoneal carcinomatosis. The majority of metastatic SBO caused by breast cancer is due to the lobular variant. The characteristic subtype involved in SBO due to metastatic lung cancer is adenocarcinoma.[44] Other primary tumors that have been reported to metastasize to the small bowel are malignant.

Imaging

The diagnosis of malignant tumors as a cause of SBO is difficult. Because they are very rare, the index of suspicion is generally low. Symptoms are usually nonspecific and might be the same as symptoms caused by more common causes of SBO, such as adhesions. The workup should be the same as the general diagnostic workup for SBO, regardless of the underlying cause.[44]

Radiography

Contrast radiography remains the cornerstone of diagnosis for small bowel tumors. Enteroclysis has been considered a very useful diagnostic method for the detection of small bowel tumors. These examinations can provide accurate information on tumors in the bowel lumen but are limited in the evaluation of lesions of the intestinal wall and extraintestinal structures. The bowel obstruction due to malignant tumors presents with the same radiologic signs as do benign causes and was described previously. Additional findings are present on radiography and can be nonspecific, as in the form of diffuse thickening of mucosal folds with or without nodular filling. More specific findings depend on the underlying tumor.

Lymphoma is characterized by the presence of a narrowed segment of small bowel with nodular filling defects, aneurysmal dilatation of a bowel loop, and a polypoid or excavated mass. A large mass with necrosis and ulcerations, resulting in irregular cavities filled with barium as well as excavation and fistula formation, is suggestive of a GIST.[49] Primary adenocarcinomas of the small bowel most often present as solitary lesions located in the jejunum and are characterized on radiography by a polypoid mass with annular stricture and filling defects. On barium examination, the usual radiologic abnormality of a small bowel primary adenocarcinoma is the "apple core" lesion.[50] This is a short annular, circumferentially narrowed segment with features of mucosal destruction. It is frequently ulcerated and separated from the normal bowel wall above and below it by overhanging edges. The malignant stricture is usually central in position, rigid, and without change of shape during compression. The ulcerating form of adenocarcinoma appears as a short narrow lesion usually with an inconspicuous, mostly central ulcer. A polypoid mass that intussuscepts is also a rare manifestation of adenocarcinoma.[45]

Carcinoid tumors of the small bowel are commonly found in the distal ileum. They are associated with a broader spectrum of radiologic appearances, such as filling defects, strictures, kinking, stretching, thickening of the valvulae conniventes, and fixation of the bowel loops.[45,49]

In metastases the mechanism of tumor spread influences its radiographic appearance. Metastasis through intraperitoneal seeding is most commonly observed in pelvic small bowel loops and in the ileocecal region. When metastases are deposited on the serosal surface of a small bowel segment, rounded protrusions toward the lumen of lesions at least 1 cm in diameter can be demonstrated by a carefully performed contrast-enhanced examination. The folds may assume a curved appearance at the periphery of metastasis or may seem stretched. Metastatic infiltration and fixation of folds at the affected bowel edge are accentuated by a divergence of folds toward the unaffected side. An associated fibrous reaction may lead to angulation and tethering of folds.[49] The neoplastic implants (e.g., gastrointestinal, ovarian, and uterine) typically grow in relation to the concave or mesenteric border of bowel loops and can incite fibrosis. The early radiologic changes in hematogenous metastases to the small bowel are usually multiple nodules, seen mostly along the antimesenteric border, where the vasa rectae arborize into a rich submucosal plexus. Metastases can be seen generally as polypoid masses. Infiltrating ulcerative lesions may be seen as well. The polypoid lesions are more common and tend to be large and multiple and have a worse prognosis. Early melanoma metastases to the small bowel usually exhibit a smooth, rounded polypoid lesion of different sizes radiographically. The demonstration on barium examination of a nonobstructing, fairly large intraluminal mass favors the diagnosis of melanoma metastasis. This is due to the softness of the highly cellular mass, which contains little stroma. Metastases from lung cancer to the small bowel may be shown as single or multiple discrete intraluminal lesions, either flat or polypoid, which are frequently ulcerated.[45,49]

CT

CT has assumed an important role in the evaluation of SBO as well as in the detection of small bowel tumors. CT can directly depict tumors of the bowel wall as well as adjacent structures, such as mesentery, fibrofatty tissue, and lymph nodes, which can all be involved in malignant neoplastic processes and cause SBO by external compression. CT is useful for all malignant tumors to assess the local extent and to screen for distant metastases. Malignancy causing SBO can have various appearances on CT. Signs suggestive of malignancy are a mass larger than 2 cm with soft tissue density that is extending from the lumen to the serous surface. Other manifestations are eccentric or asymmetric mural thickening with compression of the lumen with proximally dilated and distally collapsed bowel and lobulated borders.

In their CT presentation adenocarcinomas are proximal solitary soft tissue masses causing lumen narrowing and obstruction. The lesions may be heterogeneous in attenuation and show moderate enhancement after intravenous contrast medium administration. Mesenteric extension should be suggested in cases with large mesenteric masses with heterogeneous attenuation and associated asymmetric narrowing of the small bowel wall. Regional lymph nodes, liver, peritoneal surfaces (Fig. 45-17), and ovaries may be involved by mesenteric spread.[49]

Lymphoma usually appears as a hypodense wall thickening that may be associated with nodal enlargement (Fig. 45-18). In contrast to adenocarcinoma and leiomyosarcoma, which tend to produce a focal or segmental lesion, lymphoma of the small bowel originates at multiple sites and extends along the axis of the small bowel. The principal radiologic presentation of small bowel lymphoma is circumferential segmental infiltration, endo-exoenteric disease with cavitation, aneurysmal dilatation, polypoid

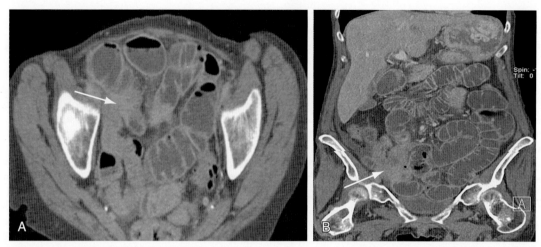

■ **FIGURE 45-17** Omental metastasis from endometrial cancer. A 67-year-old woman with a known history of endometrial cancer treated with total abdominal hysterectomy with bilateral salpingo-oophorectomy presented with signs of bowel obstruction. She had been followed for a period of nearly 5 years after surgery when she remained asymptomatic. **A,** Axial CT image demonstrates dilated fluid-filled small bowel with nodular deposits of enhancing tissue at the serosal surface in the pelvis. There is obstruction (*arrow*) to the loops due to these deposits, which is convincingly demonstrated on the coronal reformatted image (*arrow,* **B**). This patient had metastatic endometrial cancer with peritoneal and serosal implants causing bowel obstruction.

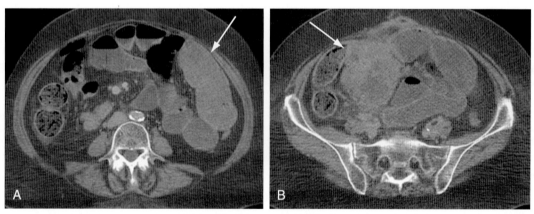

■ **FIGURE 45-18** Lymphoma. A 53-year-old woman presented with small bowel obstruction. There was a recent history of treated lymphoma. **A,** Axial contrast-enhanced CT image shows dilated loops of small bowel with air-fluid levels (*arrow*) up to a heterogeneously enhancing mass in the right lower quadrant (*arrow,* **B**). The loops of small bowel in close proximity to this mass are tethered to it, resulting in obstruction. This was diagnosed as a case of lymphomatous involvement of the small bowel.

lesions, mesenteric nodal lymphoma with secondary infiltration of the small bowel, and the possible transformation of diffuse nodular lymphoid hyperplasia into lymphoma (see Fig. 45-18). The infiltrating form generally displays moderate lumen widening and is the most common radiologic appearance, closely followed by the cavitary form.[45,49]

CT is extremely valuable in showing the extent of spread of a carcinoid tumor, which typically appears as a hypervascular mass with homogeneous attenuation in the root of the mesentery. Fibrous strands radiate from the mass in a characteristic pattern. More often, carcinoid-related obstructions are of lower grade and result from fibrosis rather than the mass effect of the tumor. Local serotonin output produces hypertrophy of the muscularis and fibrosis with crowding of folds and kinking of the lumen. This fibrosis is responsible for the fixation,

kinking, and angulation seen on the small bowel series and the stellate soft tissue density mass on CT scan examinations.[45]

The demonstration by enteroclysis of a smoothly rounded mucosa elevation of 5 to 10 mm in diameter located in the distal ileum should raise the suspicion for a carcinoid tumor. Carcinoid tumor lacks radiodiagnostic features characteristic for it, and it is indistinguishable from other lesions such as leiomyoma, lipoma, or adenoma. The presence of one or more additional polyps of similar appearance further supports the diagnosis of carcinoid. Fibrosis, as a result of serotonin's desmoplastic reaction, is responsible for the fixation, kinking, and angulation seen on small bowel series and the stellate soft tissue density mass on CT scan examinations.

Among all primary malignant tumors of the small bowel, GISTs account for 9% of the cases. Benign leiomyomas and

GISTs cannot be differentiated radiographically. Usually, smooth muscle cell tumors that are large or show significant ulceration are malignant. GISTs usually appear as an extrinsic mass displacing small bowel loops, owing to the predominant extraluminal growth pattern. Barium studies demonstrate a deformity of the small bowel segment from which the tumor originates. Flattening, stretching, and possible ulceration of the mucosa can be seen. Adjacent loops may adhere to the mass as a result of infiltration or tethering by the considerable saprophytic blood supply.[49] Because of the exoenteric growth type of GISTs, the manifestations on barium studies tend to be more subtle than the CT findings. The more characteristic CT pattern of a GIST is that of a bulky lesion, growing exoenterically. The soft tissue component of the tumor usually shows significant enhancement after intravenous contrast agent administration. Liposarcoma, angiosarcoma, and fibrosarcoma of the small bowel are rare tumors and are radiologically indistinguishable from GISTs.[45,49]

MRI

The role of MRI in small bowel tumors has not been fully evaluated; however, the technique is able to provide information of morphologic characteristics and internal constituents of tumors with benefits of direct multiplanar capability, excellent soft tissue contrast, and increased capability for assessing the biochemical changes.[26] Also, high contrast between a tumor and the adjacent bowel or surrounding fat enables MRI to depict the extent of lesions, especially with combined use of nonsuppressed T1W and of gadolinium-enhanced fat-suppressed T1W images. The latter sequence is considered most important for the characterization of small bowel tumors by their enhancement patterns, whereas most tumors show moderate signal intensity on T2W images (especially on true fast imaging with steady-state free precession [FISP] images). Small bowel adenocarcinoma may appear on MRI as either a focal rounded mass with extraluminal growth or as an annular constricting lesion narrowing the bowel lumen. Lymphoma typically demonstrates asymmetric but circumferential wall thickening, often associated with marked luminal dilatation and mesenteric lymphadenopathy, and a homogeneous, slightly increased signal intensity on T2W images combined with a moderate gadolinium enhancement. Carcinoid tumor typically appears as an ill-defined homogeneous mass that displaces bowel loops and may exhibit very low signal intensity on T2W images and strong gadolinium enhancement.[51]

Ultrasonography

Ultrasonography has also been used to diagnose neoplasms and can locate intraluminal, intramural, and extraluminal growth patterns, as well as those tumors with "dumbbell" shapes. It also detected metastases, particularly those with necrotic centers. In lymphomas of the small bowel a "sandwich" sign can be observed, caused by mural lymphomatous infiltrates and dilation of the bowel lumen. Lymphomatous infiltrates are usually anechoic.[52]

Nuclear Medicine

Scintigraphy with ^{111}In-octreotide or ^{99m}Tc-octreotate is the gold standard for the detection of somatostatin receptor–positive tumors such as carcinoid tumors of the small bowel that might be the cause of SBO. Despite the wide spectrum of imaging methods, carcinoid tumors can remain hidden before surgery. CT and MRI are efficient in the detection of larger primary tumors (>1 cm) and of liver and lymph node metastases. The efficiency of scintigraphy in the detection of carcinoids is 75% to 80%, and the efficiency of scintigraphy followed by radioguided surgery exceeds 90%.[53] Small intestine carcinoids with a relatively high malignant potential can cause serious difficulties in visualization. CT, MRI, and endoscopic capsules are insufficient, especially for the detection of small submucosal lesions.[54]

PET/CT

In SBO caused by primary tumors or metastatic disease, PET images can detect focal fluorodeoxyglucose (FDG) activity in the abdomen. CT alone is often not sensitive enough to detect intestinal metastases. However, co-registration of FDG-PET with CT images enables detection and localization of malignant lesions in the small bowel. The diagnosis of SBO by malignant tumor can be made by identification of an FDG-active point in combination with typical CT signs for SBO.[55] However, it can be difficult to differentiate nodal from intestinal disease based on the pattern of FDG uptake. The limited spatial resolution of FDG-PET precludes anatomic localization of areas of increased radiotracer accumulation. In addition, apparent accumulation of FDG in the small bowel may be a spurious finding resulting from a combination of normal peristaltic activity, gastrointestinal lymphoid tissue, and excreted radiotracer within the bowel lumen. Although such bowel activity can be intense, it tends to be diffuse rather than focal or multifocal.[56]

Imaging Algorithm

An imaging algorithm is provided in Figure 45-19.

Classic Signs: Malignant Causes of Small Bowel Obstruction

■ Lymphoma: aneurysmal dilation and polypoid mass
■ GIST: mass with necrosis and ulcerations with excavations and fistula
■ Adenocarcinoma: "apple core" lesion
■ Carcinoid tumor: mass with radiating fibrous strands

Treatment

Medical Treatment

Patients with SBO caused by a malignant tumor are initially managed like patients with SBO from adhesions

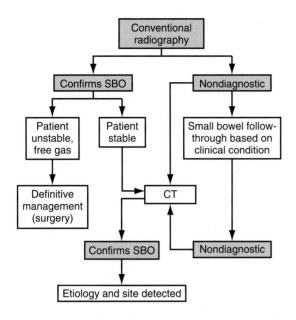

■ FIGURE 45-19 Imaging algorithm for suspected small bowel obstruction.

to remove the acute obstruction, followed by resection of the underlying malignancy. The most challenging situation is found in patients who have been treated for a malignant tumor or patients with peritoneal carcinomatosis.[4,5]

Surgical Treatment

The indication for laparotomy remains clinical, depending on the patient's symptoms. It also depends on the patient's ability to undergo surgery as well as on the extent of the primary tumor or metastatic spread. Retrospective analysis showed that about 35% of patients with cancer were diagnosed with complete SBO and that 96% of these patients required surgery. About half of the patients with partial SBO can be successfully managed without surgery. The entire bowel must be examined during surgery to exclude multiple lesions. Operative treatment has a better outcome than nonoperative management in terms of symptom-free interval and re-obstruction rates. However, it is marked by high postoperative morbidity. After a short

trial of nasogastric decompression, patients with obstruction secondary to malignant disease should be operated on if clinical factors indicate that they will survive the operation.[32,57]

What the Referring Physician Needs to Know: Malignant Causes of Small Bowel Obstruction

- Metastatic conditions causing SBO should be suspected in patients with known primary tumors.
- Clinical symptoms are nonspecific, and a high index of suspicion coupled with images is essential for diagnosis.
- CT is the mainstay in imaging evaluation because it is capable of identifying the cause and most often the site and severity of SBO and associated complications if present.
- Scintigraphy has a role in diagnosis of carcinoid tumors, which are often evasive.
- PET/CT can be used to detect the presence of malignant involvement of bowel if there is a diagnostic dilemma.

KEY POINTS

General Considerations

- Adhesions, Crohn's disease, neoplasia, and hernia are the most common causes of SBO.
- Conventional abdominal radiography is the method of choice for initial evaluation.
- Partial obstructions benefit from extended nonsurgical management.
- Most patients with complete SBO are managed after initial resuscitation because of risk of strangulation.

Benign Causes

- Benign causes comprise 70% to 80% of all cases of SBO.
- CT can reliably detect the severity and location of SBO as well as complications and causes.
- MRI, ultrasonography, and other methods are used for disease- or patient-specific indications.

Malignant Causes

- Primary tumors of the small bowel are rare and constitute only 2% to 3% of gastrointestinal tract tumors.
- The most common cause of malignant SBO is a peritoneal implant from an intra-abdominal tumor.
- Hematogenous spread from the small bowel is mainly from breast and lung carcinoma.
- Treatment is directed at removing the acute obstruction, followed by removal of the underlying tumor.

SUGGESTED READINGS

Elsayes KM, Menias CO, Smullen TL, Platt JF. Closed-loop small-bowel obstruction: diagnostic patterns by multidetector computed tomography. J Comput Assist Tomogr 2007; 31:697-701.

Fidler J. MR imaging of the small bowel. Radiol Clin North Am 2007; 45:317-331.

Maglinte DD. Small bowel imaging—a rapidly changing field and a challenge to radiology. Eur Radiol 2006; 16:967-971.

Maglinte DD, Howard TJ, Lillemoe KD, et al. Small-bowel obstruction: state-of-the-art imaging and its role in clinical management. Clin Gastroenterol Hepatol 2008; 6:130-139.

Mak SY, Roach SC, Sukumar SA. Small bowel obstruction: computed tomography features and pitfalls. Curr Probl Diagn Radiol 2006; 35:65-74.

Moran BJ. Adhesion-related small bowel obstruction. Colorectal Dis 2007; 9(Suppl 2):39-44.

Nicolaou S, Kai B, Ho S, et al. Imaging of acute small-bowel obstruction. AJR Am J Roentgenol 2005; 185:1036-1044.

Ros PR, Huprich JE. ACR Appropriateness Criteria on suspected small-bowel obstruction. J Am Coll Radiol 2006; 3:838-841.

Sandrasegaran K, Maglinte DD, Howard TJ, et al. The multifaceted role of radiology in small bowel obstruction. Semin Ultrasound CT MR 2003; 24:319-335.

Staunton M, Malone DE. Can diagnostic imaging reliably predict the need for surgery in small bowel obstruction? Critically appraised topic. Can Assoc Radiol J 2005; 56:79-81.

REFERENCES

1. Maglinte DD, Heitkamp DE, Howard TJ, et al. Current concepts in imaging of small bowel obstructions. Radiol Clin North Am 2003; 41:263-283.
2. Miller G, Boman J, Shrier I, Gordon PH. Etiology of small bowel obstruction. Am J Surg 2000; 180:33-36.
3. Herlinger H, Maglinte DDT. Small bowel obstruction. In Herlinger H, Maglinte DDT (eds). Clinical Radiology of the Small Intestine. Philadelphia, WB Saunders, 1989, pp 479-507.
4. Hayanga AJ, Bass-Wilkins K, Bulkley GB. Current management of small bowel obstruction. Adv Surg 2005; 39:1-33.
5. Bass KN, Jones B, Bulkley GB. Current management of small-bowel obstruction. Adv Surg 1997; 31:1-34.
6. Alexander JW, Boyce ST, Babcock GF, et al. The process of microbial translocation. Ann Surg 1990; 212:496-510.
7. Maglinte DD, Reyes BL, Harmon BH, et al. Reliability and role of plain film radiography and CT in the diagnosis of small bowel obstruction. AJR Am J Roentgenol 1996; 167:1451-1455.
8. Nolan DJ, Marks CG. The barium infusion in small intestinal obstruction. Clin Radiol 1981; 32:651-655.
9. Maglinte DDT, Miller RE. Intubation infusion method: reliability in diagnosis of mechanical partial small-bowel obstruction. Mt Sinai J Med 1984; 51:372-377.
10. Ericksen AS, Krasna MJ, Mast BA, et al. Use of gastrointestinal contrast studies in obstruction of the small and large bowel. Dis Colon Rectum 1990; 33:56-64.
11. Maglinte DD, Kelvin FM, O'Connor K, et al. Current status of small bowel radiography. Abdom Imaging 1996; 21:247-257.
12. Maglinte DDT, Lappas JC, Kelvin FM, et al. Small bowel radiography: how, when and why? Radiology 1987; 163:297-305.
13. Taverne PP, van der Jagt EJ. Small bowel radiography: a prospective comparative study of three techniques in 200 patients. Rofo 1985; 143:293-297.
14. Maglinte DDT, Peterson LA, Vahey TN, et al. Enteroclysis in partial small-bowel obstruction. Am J Surg 1984; 147:325-329.
15. Shrake PD, Rex DK, Lappas JC, Maglinte DD. Radiographic evaluation of suspected small-bowel obstruction. Am J Gastroenterol 1991; 86:175-178.
16. Maglinte DD, Balthazar EJ, Kelvin FM, Megibow AJ. The role of radiology in the diagnosis of small bowel obstruction. AJR Am J Roentgenol 1997; 168:1171-1180.
17. Megibow AJ, Balthazar EJ, Cho KC, et al. Bowel obstruction: evaluation with CT. Radiology 1991; 180:313-318.
18. Fukuya T, Hawes DR, Lu CC, et al. CT diagnosis of small-bowel obstruction: efficacy in 60 patients. AJR Am J Roentgenol 1992; 158:765-769.
19. Maglinte DDT, Gage SN, Harmon BH, et al. Obstruction of the small intestine: accuracy and role of CT in diagnosis. Radiology 1993; 186:61-64.
20. Qalbani A, Paushter D, Dachman AH. Multidetector row CT of small bowel obstruction. Radiol Clin North Am 2007; 45:499-512.
21. Jaffe TA, Martin LC, Miller CM, et al. Abdominal pain: coronal reformations from isotropic voxels with 16-section CT—reader lesion detection and interpretation time. Radiology 2007; 242:175-181.
22. Shah ZK, Uppot RN, Wargo JA, et al. Small bowel obstruction: the value of coronal reformatted images from 16-multidetector computed tomography—a clinicoradiological perspective. J Comput Assist Tomogr 2008; 32:23-31.
23. Gulati K, Shah ZK, Sainani N, et al. Gastrointestinal labeling for MDCT of abdomen: comparison of low density barium and low density barium in combination with water. Eur Radiol 2008; 18:868-873.
24. Lee JK, Marcos HB, Semelka RC. MR imaging of the small bowel using the HASTE sequence. AJR Am J Roentgenol 1998; 170:1457-1463.
25. Chou CK, Liu GC, Chen LT, Jaw TS. The use of MRI in bowel obstruction. Abdom Imaging 1993; 18:131-135.
26. Regan F, Beall DP, Bohlam ME, et al. Fast MR imaging and the detection of small-bowel obstruction. AJR Am J Roentgenol 1998; 170:1465-1469.
27. Laghi A, Carbone I, Paolantonio P, et al. Polyethylene glycol solution as an oral contrast agent for MR imaging of the small bowel. Acad Radiol 2002; 9:S355-S356.
28. Umschaden HW, Szolar D, Gasser J, et al. Small bowel disease: comparison of MR enteroclysis images with conventional enteroclysis and surgical findings. Radiology 2000; 215:717-725.
29. Schmutz GR, Benko A, Fournier L, et al. Small bowel obstruction: role and contribution of sonography. Eur Radiol 1997; 7: 1054-1058.
30. Suri S, Gupta S, Sudhakar PJ, et al. Comparative evaluation of plain films, ultrasound and CT in the diagnosis of intestinal obstruction. Acta Radiol 1999; 40:422-428.
31. Burkill G, Bell J, Healy J. Small bowel obstruction: the role of computed tomography in its diagnosis and management with reference to other imaging modalities. Clin Radiol 2001; 56:350-359.
32. Williams SB, Greenspon J, Young HA, Orkin BA. Small bowel obstruction: conservative vs. surgical management. Dis Colon Rectum 2005; 48:1140-1146.
33. Lo CY, Lau PWK. Small bowel phytobezoars: An uncommon cause of small bowel obstruction. Aust N Z J Med 1994; 64:187-189.
34. Ciftci AO, Tanyel FC, Buyukpamukcu N, et al. Adhesive small bowel obstruction caused by familial Mediterranean fever: the incidence and outcome. J Pediatr Surg 1995; 30:577-579.
35. Chiedozi LC, Aboh IO, Piserchia NE. Mechanical bowel obstruction: review of 316 cases in Benin City. Am J Surg 1980; 139:389-393.
36. Grassi R, Di Mizio R, Pinto A, et al. Serial plain abdominal film findings in the assessment of acute abdomen: spastic ileus, hypotonic ileus, mechanical ileus and paralytic ileus. Radiol Med 2004; 108:56-70.
37. Delabrousse E, Bartholomot B, Sohm O, et al. Gallstone ileus: CT findings. Eur Radiol 2000; 10:938-940.
38. Furukawa A, Saotome T, Yamasaki M, et al. Cross-sectional imaging in Crohn disease. RadioGraphics 2004; 24:689-702.
39. Gore RM, Balthazar EJ, Ghahremani GG, Miller FH. CT features of ulcerative colitis and Crohn's disease. AJR Am J Roentgenol 1996; 167:3-15.
40. Kim AY, Bennett GL, Bashist B, et al. Small bowel obstruction associated with sigmoid diverticulitis: CT evaluation in 16 patients. AJR Am J Roentgenol 1998; 170:1311-1313.
41. Gayer G, Zissin R, Apter S, et al. Adult intussusceptions—a CT diagnosis. Br J Radiol 2002; 75:185-190.
42. Gourtsoyiannis N, Papanikolaou N, Grammatikakis J, Prassopoulos P. MR enteroclysis: technical considerations and clinical applications. Eur Radiol 2002; 12:2651-2658.
43. Madsen SM, Thomsen HS, Munkholm P, et al. Inflammatory bowel disease evaluated by low-field magnetic resonance imaging: comparison with endoscopy, 99mTc-HMPAO leucocyte scintigraphy, conventional radiography and surgery. Scand J Gastroenterol 2002; 37:307-316.
44. Idelevich E, Kashtan H, Mavor E, Brenner B. Small bowel obstruction caused by secondary tumors. Surg Oncol 2006; 15:19-32.
45. Korman MU. Radiologic evaluation and staging of small intestine neoplasms. Eur J Radiol 2002; 42:193-205.

46. Nagi B, Verma V, Vaiphei K, et al. Primary small bowel tumors: a radiologic-pathologic correlation. Abdom Imaging 2001; 26: 474-480.

47. Garcia Marcilla JA, Sanchez Bueno F, Aguilar J, Parrilla Paricio P. Primary small bowel malignant tumors. Eur J Surg Oncol 1994; 20:630-634.

48. Kojima M, Nakamura S, Kurayabashi Y, et al. Primary malignant lymphoma of the intestine: clinicopathologic and immunohisto-chemical studies of 39 cases. Pathol Int 1995; 45:123-130.

49. Maglinte DDT, Herlinger H. Small bowel neoplasms. In Maglinte DDT, Herlinger H, Birnbaum BA (eds). Clinical Imaging of the Small Intestine, 2nd ed. New York, Springer, 1999, pp 377-438.

50. Maglinte DDT, Reyes BL. Small bowel cancer: radiologic diagnosis. Radiol Clin North Am 1997; 35:361-380.

51. Kim KW, Ha HK. MRI for small bowel diseases. Semin Ultrasound CT MR 2003; 24:387-404.

52. Miller JH, Hindman BW, Lam AH. Ultrasound in the evaluation of small bowel lymphoma in children. Radiology 1980; 135:409-414.

53. Benjegård SA, Forssell-Aronsson E, Wängberg B, et al. Intraoperative tumour detection using ^{111}In DTPA-D-Phe-octreotide and a scintillation detector. Eur J Nucl Med 2001; 28:1456-1462.

54. Caplin ME, Buscombe JR, Hilson AJ, et al. Carcinoid tumour. Lancet 1998; 352:799-805.

55. Strobel K, Skalsky J, Hany TF, et al. Small bowel invagination caused by intestinal melanoma metastasis: unsuspected diagnosis by FDG-PET/CT imaging. Clin Nucl Med 2007; 32:213-214.

56. Sam JW, Levine MS, Farner MC, et al. Detection of small bowel involvement by mantle cell lymphoma on F-18 FDG positron emission tomography. Clin Nucl Med 2002; 27:330-333.

57. Miller G, Boman J, Shrier I, Gordon PH. Small-bowel obstruction secondary to malignant disease: an 11-year audit. Can J Surg 2000; 43:353-358.

CHAPTER 46

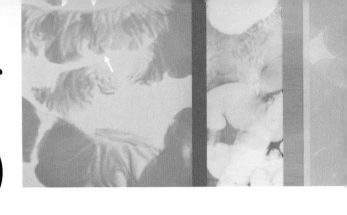

Acute Small Bowel Ischemia

Ashraf Thabet, T. Gregory Walker, and Sanjeeva P. Kalva

ETIOLOGY

Acute mesenteric ischemia of the small bowel has four major causes: (1) arterial embolism, (2) arterial thrombosis, (3) nonocclusive mesenteric ischemia, and (4) mesenteric venous thrombosis (Table 46-1). Less common causes include aortic dissection, spontaneous dissection of the celiac or superior mesenteric artery, and vasculitis.[1,2] Irrespective of cause, the common end result is an acute reduction in splanchnic blood flow that can lead to bowel necrosis.

PREVALENCE AND EPIDEMIOLOGY

Acute mesenteric ischemia affects approximately 1% of patients with acute abdomen and increases in incidence with age.[2-5] Mortality rates exceed 60%, exacerbated by delays in diagnosis.

Arterial embolism, the most frequent cause of acute mesenteric ischemia, is implicated in up to 50% of cases[6] and most often involves the superior mesenteric artery. The embolus is usually of cardiac origin; hence, myocardial infarction, arrhythmia, valvular disease, and ventricular aneurysm are important risk factors.[6]

Acute superior mesenteric artery thrombosis is the second most common cause of acute mesenteric ischemia, accounting for 25% of cases,[6] usually in the setting of severe atherosclerosis. Hypercoagulability is another important risk factor.

Nonocclusive mesenteric ischemia, implicated in 20% of patients with acute mesenteric ischemia, has a mortality rate as high as 70%.[7] It is most often seen in patients older than age 50 years with reduced cardiac output, hypovolemia, or hypotension. A low-flow state results in diffuse mesenteric vasoconstriction, which may be exacerbated in patients on vasopressor therapy.[6] The incidence of nonocclusive mesenteric ischemia is declining, presumably owing to advances in critical care medicine, including the use of vasodilator therapy.

Mesenteric venous thrombosis accounts for approximately 18% of cases of acute mesenteric ischemia.[6] It has a poor prognosis with a long-term survival of 30% to 40%.

Mesenteric venous thrombosis is considered acute when symptoms are present for less than 4 weeks. Risk factors include recent surgery, trauma, inflammatory disorders such as pancreatitis, and hypercoagulable states.

CLINICAL PRESENTATION

The clinical presentation of acute mesenteric ischemia is nonspecific and may mimic other common disease processes such as small bowel obstruction or pancreatitis. The presentation is also a function of the specific pathologic process that is compromising splanchnic blood flow—superior mesenteric artery embolism or thrombosis, nonocclusive mesenteric ischemia, or mesenteric venous thrombosis (see Table 46-1). Because of the nonspecificity of presentation, delays in diagnosis are common and many cases progress to bowel infarction.

Acute mesenteric ischemia classically presents as acute abdominal pain that is disproportional to the findings on physical examination.[1] Other findings may include dehydration, tachycardia, and altered mental status. Nonspecific laboratory findings such as an elevated serum lactate level and leukocytosis may be found with all major causes of acute mesenteric ischemia.

Both superior mesenteric artery occlusion and thrombosis may present acutely. Patients with superior mesenteric artery thrombosis, however, may report an antecedent history of postprandial pain, weight loss, and aversion to food. Because these symptoms are associated with chronic mesenteric ischemia due to atherosclerosis,[6] there may be an "acute on chronic" presentation, in which there may be a better developed collateral circulation than in patients with superior mesenteric artery embolism.[1]

Patients with nonocclusive mesenteric ischemia are usually older, critically ill, intubated, or on vasopressor or digitalis therapy and may be unable to communicate symptoms.[6] Clinicians must have a high index of suspicion, particularly in patients with unexplained failure to thrive.

Patients with acute mesenteric venous thrombosis are more typically symptomatic than patients with chronic mesenteric venous thrombosis and may present with slowly progressive diffuse abdominal pain and distention.[8,9]

TABLE 46-1 Clinical Features of Acute Small Bowel Ischemia

Cause	Onset of Presentation	Associated Features
SMA embolism	Acute	Myocardial infarction, arrhythmia, ventricular aneurysm, valvular disease, prior embolic event
SMA thrombosis	Acute or acute on chronic	Atherosclerotic disease, hypercoagulable state
Nonocclusive mesenteric ischemia	Acute, failure to thrive	Critical illness, hypotension, myocardial infarction, sepsis, disseminated intravascular coagulation, vasopressors
Mesenteric venous thrombosis	Acute (<4 wk) Chronic (≥4 wk)	Recent surgery, hypercoagulable state, oral contraceptive use

SMA, superior mesenteric artery.

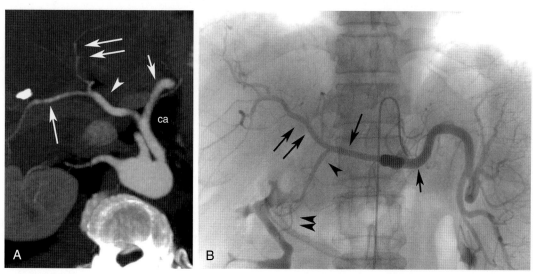

■ **FIGURE 46-1** **A,** Maximum intensity projection from CT angiogram of the abdomen demonstrates the celiac artery (ca), splenic artery (*short arrow*), common hepatic artery/hepatic artery proper (*arrowhead*), right hepatic artery (*single long arrow*), and left hepatic artery (*double long arrows*). The gastroduodenal artery is not shown. **B,** Selective contrast injection of the celiac artery demonstrates the splenic artery (*short arrow*), common hepatic artery (*single long arrow*), right hepatic artery (*double long arrows*), gastroduodenal artery (*single arrowhead*), and superior pancreaticoduodenal arcade (*double arrowheads*).

Bloody ascites, dehydration, Hemoccult-positive stool, and hypotension may be associated findings.[6]

ANATOMY AND PATHOPHYSIOLOGY

The arterial supply of the small bowel is predominantly from the celiac axis and the superior mesenteric artery. The inferior mesenteric artery and the internal iliac arteries may become important contributors in the setting of arterial disease.

The celiac artery gives origin to the left gastric artery and then it bifurcates into the splenic and common hepatic arteries (Fig. 46-1). The gastroduodenal artery is a branch of the common hepatic artery and gives off, among other vessels, the superior pancreaticoduodenal arteries.

The superior mesenteric artery arises from the anterior aspect of the aorta at the level of the L1 vertebral body (Fig. 46-2) and courses behind the body of the pancreas and then posterior and to the left of the superior mesenteric vein to supply the duodenum, small bowel, and colon proximal to the splenic flexure. The inferior pancreaticoduodenal artery arises from the superior mesenteric artery as the first branch and anastomoses with the

superior pancreaticoduodenal artery, forming the "pancreaticoduodenal arcades" (Fig. 46-3). The middle colic artery may arise from the right side of the superior mesenteric artery to supply the transverse colon. It bifurcates into a right branch, which anastomoses with the right colic artery, and a left branch, which anastomoses with the ascending branch of the left colic artery (Fig. 46-4). Multiple jejunal and ileal arteries as well as the right colic artery supplying the ascending colon arise from the superior mesenteric artery. More distally, the superior mesenteric artery terminates in the ileocolic artery, which supplies the terminal ileum, cecum, and ascending colon.

The inferior mesenteric artery arises from the left aspect of the aorta at the level of the L3 vertebral body (see Fig. 46-4). It divides into the left colic, sigmoid, and superior hemorrhoidal arteries, which supply the descending colon, sigmoid colon, and rectum, respectively. The ascending branch of the left colic artery anastomoses with the left branch of the middle colic artery, a branch of the superior mesenteric artery. The superior hemorrhoidal artery anastomoses with branches of the anterior division of the internal iliac arteries.

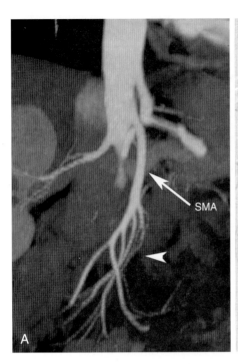
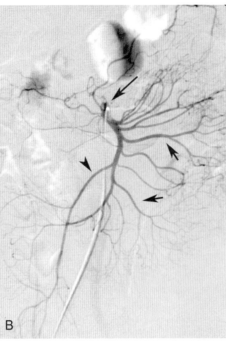

■ **FIGURE 46-2** **A,** Maximum intensity projection from CT angiogram of the abdomen demonstrates the superior mesenteric artery (SMA, *long arrow*) as well as jejunal and ileal branches (*arrowhead*). **B,** Selective contrast injection of the superior mesenteric artery (*long arrow*) demonstrates multiple jejunal and ileal branches (*short arrows*) as well as the ileocolic artery (*arrowhead*).

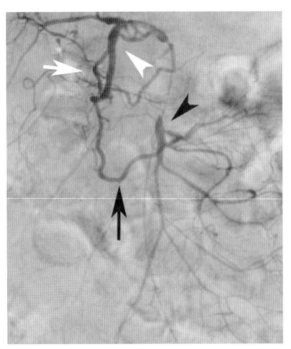

■ **FIGURE 46-3** Selective contrast injection of the gastroduodenal artery (*white arrowhead*) demonstrates the superior pancreaticoduodenal arteries (*white arrow*), which anastomose with the inferior pancreaticoduodenal arteries (*black arrow*) derived from the superior mesenteric artery (*black arrowhead*).

The marginal artery, defined as the artery closest to and parallel with the mesenteric margin of the intestine, gives off the vasa rectae, which are small vessels that supply the bowel wall.[10] In the colon, this artery is termed the *marginal artery of Drummond* (see Fig. 46-4). The middle colic artery may serve as the marginal artery for much of its distribution.[10]

The rich arterial supply of the bowel provides ample opportunity for collateral development in the setting of mesenteric arterial stenosis or occlusion (Fig. 46-5). The superior and inferior pancreaticoduodenal arteries can provide important collaterals between the celiac axis and the superior mesenteric artery (see Fig. 46-3). In addition, a persistent fetal arterial communication between the celiac axis and the superior mesenteric artery (often called the arc of Buehler) may exist in up to 2% of patients. Collateral pathways between the superior and inferior mesenteric arteries primarily involve communication between the left and middle colic arteries via the arc of Riolan (Fig. 46-6), located centrally in the mesentery, and the marginal artery of Drummond, located peripherally.[11] The internal iliac arteries may also provide collateral circulation to the principal mesenteric vessels.

The superior mesenteric vein is usually a single vessel that drains the small intestine and the ascending and transverse colon. Within the mesentery, the superior mesenteric vein courses anteriorly and to the right of the superior mesenteric artery (Fig. 46-7) and joins the splenic vein to form the main portal vein. The inferior mesenteric vein, which drains the left colic, sigmoid, and superior hemorrhoidal veins, usually terminates in the splenic vein or the superior mesenteric vein. Portal-to-portal collaterals may develop in the setting of chronic superior mesenteric vein occlusion; these are often submucosal and are prone to bleeding.[12] Portal-to-systemic collaterals (varices) may also develop in portal hypertension.

PATHOLOGY

Mesenteric blood flow is regulated by perfusion pressure, oxygen demand, α- and β-adrenergic stimulation, and humoral factors such as vasopressin.[6] At baseline, 20% to 25% of mesenteric capillaries may be open with considerable reserve against changes in blood flow.[11,13]

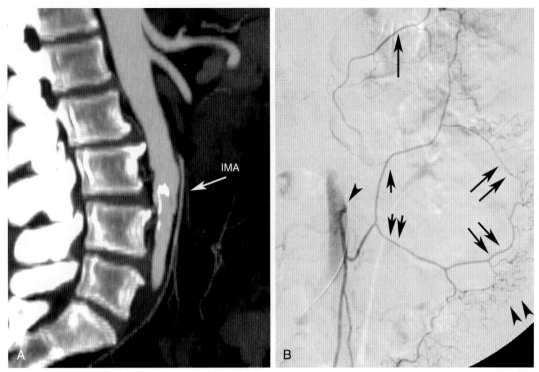

■ **FIGURE 46-4** **A,** Maximum intensity projection from a CT angiogram of the abdomen demonstrates the inferior mesenteric artery (IMA, *arrow*). **B,** Selective contrast injection of the inferior mesenteric artery (*single arrowhead*) demonstrates the ascending (*single short arrow*) and descending (*double short arrows*) branches of the left colic artery. The ascending branch anastomoses with the left branch of the middle colic artery (*single long arrow*), which is derived from the superior mesenteric artery. The marginal artery of Drummond (*double long arrows*) gives off arborizing vasa rectae (*double arrowheads*) to colon.

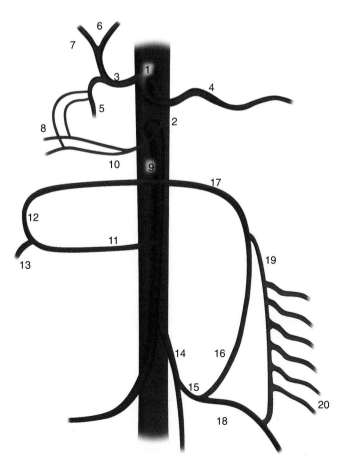

■ **FIGURE 46-5** Selected collateral pathways of the mesenteric circulation. The celiac artery (1) gives off the common hepatic artery (3), splenic artery (4), and ultimately the gastroduodenal artery (5), the left (6) and right (7) hepatic arteries, and superior pancreaticoduodenal arteries (8). The superior mesenteric artery (9) gives off the inferior pancreaticoduodenal arteries (10) as well as the middle colic (11) artery, which gives off left (12) and right (13) branches. Collateral circulation between the celiac axis and superior mesenteric artery may occur via a persistent direct fetal communication known as the arc of Buehler (2) or via the pancreaticoduodenal arcades, formed by communication of the superior (8) and inferior (10) pancreaticoduodenal arteries. The inferior mesenteric artery (14) gives off the left colic artery (15), which divides into ascending (16) and descending (18) branches. Collateral circulation between the superior and inferior mesenteric arteries may occur through the arc of Riolan (17) or the marginal artery of Drummond (19). Jejunal and ileal branches (20) are also demonstrated.

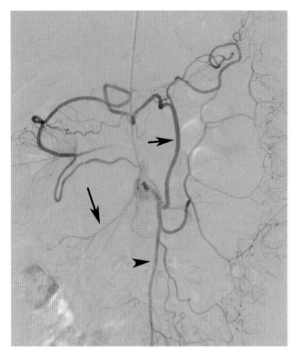

■ **FIGURE 46-6** Selective contrast injection of the inferior mesenteric artery (*arrowhead*) demonstrates a prominent arc of Riolan (*short arrow*). The arc of Riolan bridges the inferior and superior mesenteric arteries (*long arrow*).

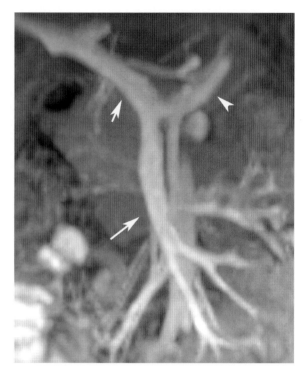

■ **FIGURE 46-7** MR angiogram demonstrates the superior mesenteric vein (*long arrow*) joining the splenic vein (*arrowhead*) to become the portal vein (*short arrow*).

Although the bowel can tolerate a considerable reduction in mesenteric perfusion, when there is a prolonged mismatch between demand and supply, ischemia will ensue. Prolonged ischemia may result in tissue damage due to reperfusion injury, resulting in increased microvascular permeability.[6,14] Ultimately, compromise of the intestinal mucosal barrier may occur, mediated by oxygen free radicals.[6,15]

Superior mesenteric artery emboli, as previously noted, are most often of cardiac origin, with approximately one third of patients having a history of prior embolic events.[6] Arterial emboli typically involve the superior mesenteric artery because of the oblique angle of its origin, with approximately 15% occluding the origin. A majority of emboli, however, will lodge distally in the superior mesenteric artery at branch points, and the distribution of ischemic bowel in many cases will therefore involve the distal jejunum and ileum, while sparing the proximal jejunum. Large emboli that initially occlude the superior mesenteric artery origin may propagate distally and potentially obstruct collateral flow from the celiac artery and inferior mesenteric artery. The clinical presentation is acute, with insufficient time to develop a collateral perfusion.

The most common site of arterial thrombosis is the origin of the superior mesenteric artery. Because of progressive atherosclerotic disease, collateral circulation may have developed and thus symptoms occur only when there is disease of multiple mesenteric arteries and major collateral vessels or when thrombosis occurs with insufficient collateral support. Acute hemodynamic compromise, dehydration, or hypercoagulability in the setting of visceral artery stenosis may prompt the thrombotic event.

In superior mesenteric artery thrombosis, a greater length of bowel may become ischemic or progress to infarction than with superior mesenteric artery embolus.

In nonocclusive mesenteric ischemia, diminished mesenteric arterial flow results from reduced perfusion pressure or vasoconstriction rather than from a physical impediment to blood flow. This reduced perfusion pressure resulting from various causes such as heart failure, hypotension, sepsis, disseminated intravascular coagulation, vasoconstrictive medications, and/or major surgery, eventually causes diffuse mesenteric vasoconstriction via autoregulatory mechanisms.

Mesenteric vein thrombosis, which is often associated with recent surgery, hypercoagulable state, or inflammatory disorders, usually begins in the venous arcades and can propagate to the superior mesenteric vein and portal vein; the inferior mesenteric vein is less frequently affected. Venous obstruction results in hypovolemia and hemoconcentration, arteriolar vasoconstriction, and reduced arterial inflow, ultimately leading to hemorrhagic bowel infarction. Infarcted bowel is segmental, and the transition between normal and ischemic bowel is typically more gradual compared with other causes of acute mesenteric ischemia.

IMAGING

Superior Mesenteric Artery Embolism

Because acute mesenteric ischemia may rapidly progress to bowel infarction, patients with peritoneal signs should proceed to emergent laparotomy. Nevertheless, imaging

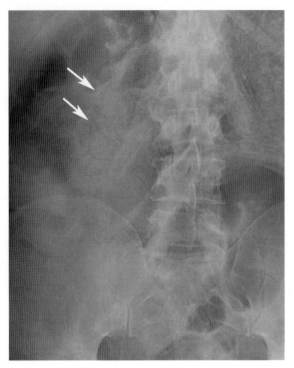

■ **FIGURE 46-8** Plain radiograph of the abdomen demonstrates curvilinear lucencies (*arrows*) within bowel wall, consistent with pneumatosis.

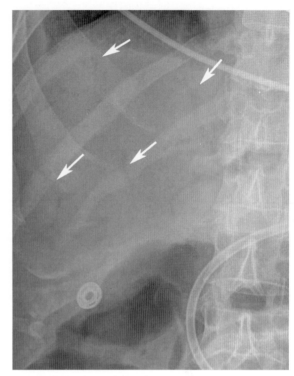

■ **FIGURE 46-9** Plain radiograph of the abdomen demonstrates branching linear lucencies (*arrows*) coursing to the periphery of the liver, consistent with portal venous gas.

can play an important role in the diagnosis of superior mesenteric artery embolism and operative planning.

Radiography

Plain radiography is nonspecific in all causes of acute mesenteric ischemia and may be normal in one fourth of cases. Plain radiographs may demonstrate dilated fluid-filled bowel loops, suggesting a nonspecific ileus, thumb-printing from focal submucosal hemorrhage, or separation of bowel loops due to mesenteric thickening. Pneumatosis (Fig. 46-8), mesenteric or portal venous gas (Fig. 46-9), and pneumoperitoneum indicate bowel infarction. Plain radiography may help to exclude some other causes of abdominal pain such as bowel obstruction.

CT

CT may demonstrate nonspecific fluid-filled dilated bowel with wall thickening, ascites, and mesenteric edema. CT may also demonstrate a water-halo sign, in which two concentric rings of different attenuation are seen in the bowel wall: either a high-attenuation outer ring with gray attenuation inner ring, or vice versa.[16] Similarly, a target sign (Fig. 46-10) may be seen, in which a central ring of gray attenuation is interposed between two rings of higher attenuation.[16] Inflammatory bowel disease may produce a similar appearance.

More specific findings include lack of bowel wall enhancement and infarcts of other visceral organs such as the kidney (Fig. 46-11). CT angiography (CTA) increases

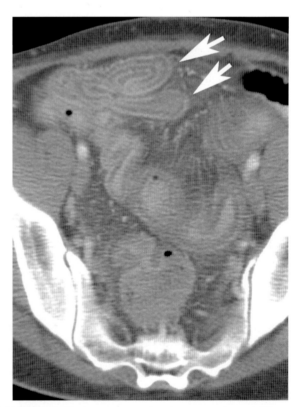

■ **FIGURE 46-10** Intravenous and oral contrast-enhanced CT scan of the abdomen and pelvis in a man with acute mesenteric ischemia of small bowel due to superior mesenteric artery embolism (not shown). A target sign (*arrows*) is characterized by an outer and inner hyperattenuating and middle hypoattenuating layer.

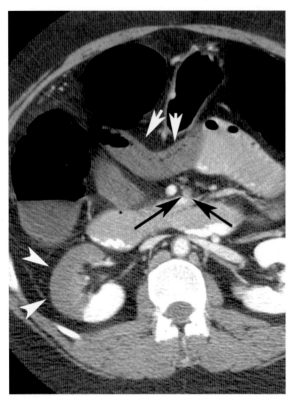

■ **FIGURE 46-11** Intravenous and oral contrast-enhanced CT scan of the abdomen and pelvis demonstrates wedge-shaped areas of nonenhancement in the right kidney (*arrowheads*) consistent with infarct in a patient with superior mesenteric artery embolism (*long black arrows*). Nonenhancement of bowel wall (*short white arrows*) is also a sign of ischemia.

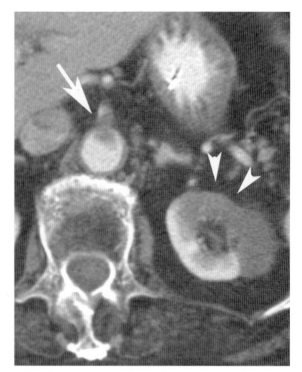

■ **FIGURE 46-12** Intravenous and oral contrast-enhanced CT scan of the abdomen and pelvis demonstrates a filling defect (*arrow*) within the origin of the superior mesenteric artery, consistent with embolus. Focal nonenhancement in the left kidney (*arrowheads*) is consistent with infarct and is further evidence of embolic phenomena.

the accuracy of the detection of a superior mesenteric artery embolus and should include initial noncontrast images for evaluation of vascular calcifications. CTA will demonstrate a filling defect within or nonopacification of the superior mesenteric artery (Figs. 46-11 to 46-13), although sensitivity diminishes with more distal emboli. Few to no collateral vessels are demonstrated. Image postprocessing, such as volume rendering and maximum intensity projections, facilitates diagnosis and operative planning.

Late-stage findings such as pneumatosis (Fig. 46-14), pneumoperitoneum, and mesenteric and portal venous gas (Fig. 46-15) are markers of bowel infarction and necrosis.[17] CT is helpful to evaluate other causes of abdominal pain as well.

MRI

Gadolinium-enhanced MR angiography (MRA) can be used to demonstrate superior mesenteric artery emboli[1] but is not the first-choice imaging modality in acute mesenteric ischemia, given long examination times that can delay treatment.

Ultrasonography

Although duplex sonography may detect occlusion at the origin of the superior mesenteric artery, more distal emboli may be missed. An occluded vessel will appear dilated and may contain echogenic debris with absent Doppler flow. Linear echogenic foci of intramural or portal venous gas may be detected and are signs of bowel infarction.[3] Ultrasonography is operator dependent and can be limited by bowel gas, body habitus, and patient noncooperation.

Nuclear Medicine

There is no role for scintigraphy in the evaluation of superior mesenteric artery embolism.

PET/CT

There is no role for PET/CT in the evaluation of superior mesenteric artery embolism.

Angiography

Angiography is the gold standard for the detection of superior mesenteric artery embolism, with sensitivity exceeding 90%.[18] Lateral aortography is used to evaluate the origins of the artery and celiac axis (Fig. 46-16). Anteroposterior aortography is useful to assess the aorta, renal arteries, and distal mesenteric vessels. The angiographic diagnosis of acute embolus is made when a filling defect is demonstrated that at least partially obstructs the artery,

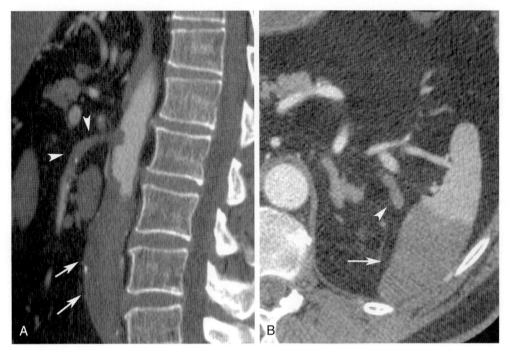

■ **FIGURE 46-13** **A,** Intravenous contrast-enhanced CT of the abdomen demonstrates embolic occlusion of the proximal superior mesenteric artery (*arrowheads*) as well as distal aorta (*arrows*). **B,** A wedge-shaped area of hypoattenuation in the spleen (*arrow*) is consistent with infarct from splenic artery embolism (*arrowhead*).

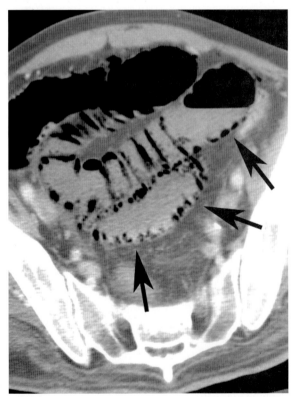

■ **FIGURE 46-14** Intravenous and oral contrast-enhanced CT of the abdomen and pelvis demonstrates linear foci of gas (*arrows*) within the wall of small bowel, consistent with pneumatosis intestinalis.

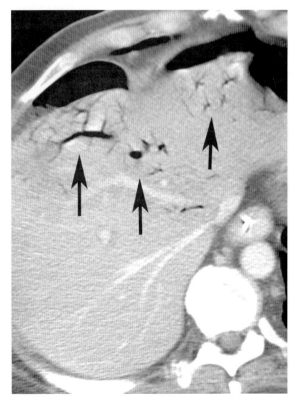

■ **FIGURE 46-15** Intravenous contrast-enhanced CT of the abdomen and pelvis demonstrates branching foci of air attenuation (*arrows*) extending into the periphery of the liver, consistent with portal venous gas.

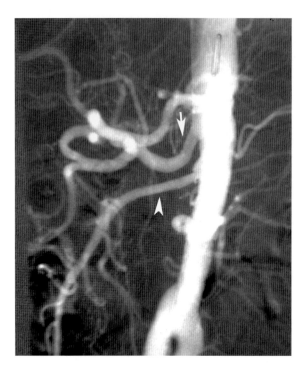

■ **FIGURE 46-16** Lateral aortogram demonstrates a normal celiac artery (*arrow*) as well as origin of the superior mesenteric artery (*arrowhead*).

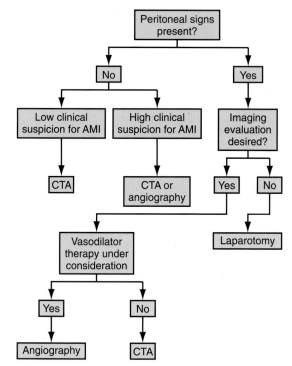

■ **FIGURE 46-17** Imaging algorithm for evaluation of clinically suspected occlusive acute mesenteric ischemia (AMI) of small bowel. The presence of peritoneal signs will prompt emergent laparotomy, although depending on the clinical situation, surgeon preference, and capacity to perform imaging quickly, imaging may be performed first. Patients with a high clinical suspicion for occlusive acute mesenteric ischemia who are not presenting with peritoneal signs may undergo imaging first to confirm the diagnosis; angiography may be preferred over CTA if transcatheter therapy is considered, although this may delay surgical therapy.

TABLE 46-2   Accuracy, Limitations, and Pitfalls of Modalities Used in Imaging of Superior Mesenteric Artery Embolism

Modality	Accuracy	Limitations	Pitfalls
Radiography	Poor	Sensitivity 30% Nonspecific	May not suggest disease until late stage of bowel infarction/perforation
CT	Sensitivity 64%-82% based on current literature, although expected to be higher with multidetector CT	Radiation	Distal emboli may be missed.
MRI	Although sufficient comparative data are lacking, sensitivity and specificity may be comparable to CT for vessel findings, but less accurate for bowel findings.	Long examination times High cost	Suboptimal evaluation of stented vessels Tailored examination less able to assess abdomen for other pathologic process compared with CT
Ultrasonography	Accuracy diminishes with more distal emboli and is operator dependent.	Patient body habitus Bowel gas Patient cooperation	Distal emboli may be missed.
Nuclear medicine	No role in the evaluation of acute mesenteric ischemia	Poor spatial resolution	
PET/CT	No role in the evaluation of acute mesenteric ischemia	Radiation High cost	
Angiography	Sensitivity 90%	Radiation Invasive	

with absence of collateral vessels.[12] Selective arteriography of the superior mesenteric artery can be performed in the absence of disease at its origin to assess for distal occlusion and may be accompanied by catheter-directed intervention, if appropriate.

Angiography, however, is invasive and time consuming and is associated with potential nephrotoxicity and other procedure-related morbidities.

Imaging Algorithm

An imaging algorithm is provided in Figure 46-17. See also Table 46-2.

Superior Mesenteric Artery Thrombosis

Superior mesenteric artery thrombosis may present as "acute on chronic" symptoms. Atherosclerotic disease

Classic Signs: Superior Mesenteric Artery Embolism

- Abdominal pain out of proportion to physical findings
- Filling defect within the superior mesenteric artery: branch points > origin
- Lack of bowel wall enhancement
- Infarcts of other visceral organs
- Late findings: Pneumatosis, portomesenteric venous gas, pneumoperitoneum

may affect several mesenteric vessels, with thrombotic occlusion of the superior mesenteric artery precipitating the acute clinical event.

Radiography

Plain radiography of the abdomen is nonspecific in all major causes of acute mesenteric ischemia.

CT

CT and CTA are useful in the evaluation of superior mesenteric artery thrombosis. Bowel findings overlap with that of superior mesenteric artery embolism. As previously noted, CTA should initially include noncontrast images so as to evaluate for vascular calcifications that may otherwise be obscured. Stenosis or occlusion may be demonstrated in the origin of the superior mesenteric, inferior mesenteric, or celiac arteries and collateral vessels may be identified. Thrombosis of a previously stented mesenteric artery may also cause acute mesenteric ischemia (Fig. 46-18). 3D image postprocessing can be useful in diagnosis and in planning revascularization.

MRI

Contrast-enhanced MRA may similarly demonstrate narrowing or cutoff of the superior mesenteric artery. Collateral vessels may be demonstrated. However, MRA is not advocated for the evaluation of acute mesenteric ischemia because long examination times can delay treatment.

Ultrasonography

Duplex sonography may demonstrate elevated peak systolic velocities in the proximal superior mesenteric artery, indicating stenosis, or lack of flow, suggesting occlusion. As with superior mesenteric artery embolism, ultrasonography is not advocated in the evaluation of acute mesenteric ischemia.

Nuclear Medicine

There is no role for scintigraphy in the evaluation of superior mesenteric artery thrombosis.

PET/CT

There is no role for PET/CT in the evaluation of superior mesenteric artery thrombosis.

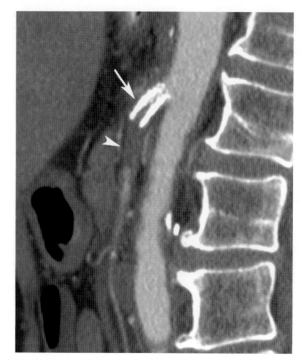

■ **FIGURE 46-18** CT angiogram in patient presenting with worsening abdominal pain demonstrates nonopacification of the superior mesenteric artery at the level of a stent (*arrow*) previously placed to treat chronic mesenteric ischemia. This is consistent with thrombosis that extends into the artery just distal (*arrowhead*) to the stent.

Angiography

Angiography can delineate important anatomic information, outline collateral vessels, and demonstrate visceral arterial stenoses and occlusions. The salient findings are nonopacification of the origin of the superior mesenteric artery and reduced bowel opacification. Although time consuming and invasive, it can enable therapeutic intervention through thromboaspiration, thrombolysis, and vasodilator therapy.

Imaging Algorithm

An imaging algorithm is provided in Figure 46-17. See also Table 46-3.

Classic Signs: Superior Mesenteric Artery Thrombosis

- Abdominal pain out of proportion to physical findings
- Nonopacification and/or narrowing of the origin of the superior mesenteric artery
- Severe atherosclerotic disease
- Late findings: Pneumatosis, portomesenteric venous gas, pneumoperitoneum

Nonocclusive Mesenteric Ischemia

Except for the absence of occlusive lesion within visceral arteries, the radiologic features of nonocclusive

TABLE 46-3   Accuracy, Limitations, and Pitfalls of Modalities Used in Imaging of Superior Mesenteric Artery Thrombosis

Modality	Accuracy	Limitations	Pitfalls
Radiography	Poor	Sensitivity 30% Nonspecific	May not suggest disease until late stage of bowel infarction/perforation
CT	Sensitivity 64%-82% based on current literature, although expected to be better with multidetector CT	Radiation	
MRI	Although sufficient comparative data are lacking, sensitivity and specificity may be comparable to CT for vessel findings but less accurate for bowel findings.	Long examination times High cost	Suboptimal evaluation of calcifications and stented vessels Tailored examination less able to assess abdomen for other pathology compared with CT
Ultrasonography	Accuracy dependent on ability to visualize proximal superior mesenteric artery	Patient body habitus Bowel gas Patient cooperation	Atherosclerotic disease burden may be underestimated due to incomplete visualization of mesenteric vessels.
Nuclear medicine	No role in the evaluation of acute mesenteric ischemia	Poor spatial resolution	
PET/CT	No role in the evaluation of acute mesenteric ischemia	Radiation High cost	
Angiography	Sensitivity 90%	Radiation Invasive	

mesenteric ischemia may be identical to other forms of acute mesenteric ischemia.

Radiography

Plain radiography of the abdomen is nonspecific in all major causes of acute mesenteric ischemia.

CT

CT may demonstrate bowel findings seen in other forms of acute mesenteric ischemia. Bowel wall which uniformly enhances greater than venous enhancement may be seen in shock bowel—a form of nonocclusive mesenteric ischemia seen in hypotensive and hypovolemic patients.[16] CTA may be used to exclude a lesion of the superior mesenteric artery. Late findings such as pneumatosis or pneumoperitoneum may be noted.

MRI

Although gadolinium-enhanced MRA may demonstrate absence of a lesion of the superior mesenteric artery, the long examination times should preclude the use of MRI in critically ill patients in whom nonocclusive mesenteric ischemia is suspected.

Ultrasonography

There is no role for ultrasonography in the assessment of nonocclusive mesenteric ischemia.

Nuclear Medicine

There is no role for scintigraphy in the evaluation of nonocclusive mesenteric ischemia.

PET/CT

There is no role for PET/CT in the evaluation of nonocclusive mesenteric ischemia.

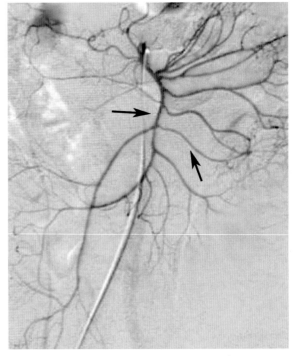

■ **FIGURE 46-19**   Superior mesenteric arteriogram demonstrates diffuse and segmental narrowing of the arterial branches (*arrows*) in a patient with nonocclusive mesenteric ischemia. Compare with Figure 46-2B.

Angiography

Patients suspected of having nonocclusive mesenteric ischemia should be promptly referred for angiography. There is diffuse constriction of vessels (Fig. 46-19) with reduced opacification of bowel parenchyma.[3] Major branches of the superior mesenteric artery may demonstrate segmental constrictions, producing a "string of sausages" sign.[6] Contrast material may reflux back into the aorta. The venous phase of mesenteric angiography is normal. Angiography also provides a tool for catheter

TABLE 46-4 Accuracy, Limitations, and Pitfalls of Modalities Used in Imaging of Nonocclusive Mesenteric Ischemia

Modality	Accuracy	Limitations	Pitfalls
Radiography	Poor	Insensitive Nonspecific	May not suggest disease until late stage of bowel infarction/perforation
CT	Poor Can help exclude occlusive disease	Radiation Diffuse mesenteric arterial narrowing not as well discerned as on angiography	
MRI	Poor Can help exclude occlusive disease	Long examination times High cost Diffuse mesenteric arterial narrowing not as well discerned as on angiography	Suboptimal evaluation of stented vessels Tailored examination less able to assess abdomen for other pathology compared with CT
Ultrasonography	Poor	Patient body habitus Bowel gas Patient cooperation	
Nuclear medicine	No role in the evaluation of acute mesenteric ischemia	Poor spatial resolution	
PET/CT	No role in the evaluation of acute mesenteric ischemia	Radiation High cost	
Angiography	Imaging test of choice as best demonstrates diffuse vessel narrowing	Radiation Invasive	

intervention through the infusion of vasodilators directly in the superior mesenteric artery.

Imaging Algorithm

Angiography is recommended in clinically suspected nonocclusive mesenteric ischemia (Table 46-4). CT may be performed first to exclude other pathologic processes.

Classic Signs: Nonocclusive Mesenteric Ischemia

- Critically ill patient, failure to thrive
- Vasopressor therapy, digitalis
- Lack of intraluminal filling defect within visceral vessels
- Diffuse narrowing of vessels with reduced opacification of bowel parenchyma on angiography
- "String of sausages" sign on angiography

Mesenteric Venous Thrombosis

Mesenteric venous thrombosis can be easily demonstrated on cross-sectional imaging with CT or MRI. It is not uncommon to identify incidental mesenteric venous thrombosis in asymptomatic patients undergoing CT and MRI for other reasons.

Radiography

Plain radiography of the abdomen is nonspecific in all major causes of acute mesenteric ischemia.

CT

CT/CTA is the test of choice for the evaluation of mesenteric thrombosis, with sensitivity exceeding 90%.[8,9] The most common CT finding is bowel wall thickening, typically associated with a target sign.[8,16] Small bowel dilata-tion, nonenhancement of the bowel wall, pneumatosis, portomesenteric gas, and pneumoperitoneum are findings that overlap with other forms of acute mesenteric ischemia. The most specific finding is a central focus of low attenuation within the venous lumen such as the superior mesenteric vein (Fig. 46-20) that is persistent on multiple phases of enhancement and may be surrounded by a rim-enhancing venous wall.[8] This finding, when coupled with bowel wall thickening and intraperitoneal fluid, is associated with a higher risk of bowel infarction compared with cases without intraperitoneal fluid.[8] Thrombus within multiple mesenteric veins is common.

MRI

Gadolinium-enhanced MR angiography is an excellent modality to evaluate mesenteric venous thrombosis. Lack of signal in the central superior mesenteric vein may be seen (Fig. 46-21). Image postprocessing can greatly facilitate the diagnosis. The lack of radiation is an advantage over CT, although images may be degraded due to turbulent flow. MRI examination times are significantly longer than those for CT and may be inappropriate in the evaluation of a patient with acute symptoms.

Ultrasonography

Duplex ultrasonography may be useful in assessing mesenteric venous thrombosis by demonstrating a lack of portomesenteric blood flow and intraluminal echogenic debris. However, evaluation is limited by bowel gas, patient body habitus, and patient noncooperation. Collateral vessels may be incompletely imaged or may be mistaken for patent central veins.[8]

Nuclear Medicine

There is no role for scintigraphy in the evaluation of mesenteric venous thrombosis.

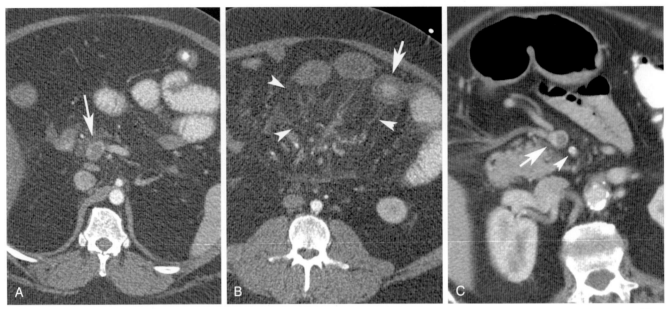

■ **FIGURE 46-20** **A,** Intravenous and oral contrast-enhanced CT of the abdomen and pelvis in a patient with abdominal pain demonstrates a filling defect within the superior mesenteric vein (*arrow*). **B,** Multiple loops of small bowel demonstrate wall thickening (*arrow*) with adjacent hazy attenuation of mesentery (*arrowheads*) consistent with venous congestion. **C,** In a different patient, CT demonstrates a filling defect within the superior mesenteric vein (*arrow*), which is located anterior and to the left of the superior mesenteric artery (*arrowhead*). The superior mesenteric artery demonstrates vascular calcifications, which are partially obscured by intraluminal contrast.

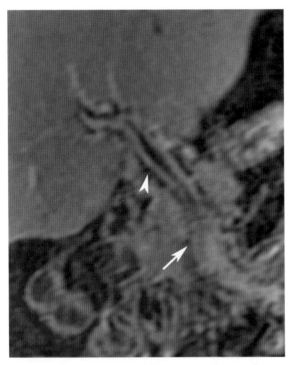

■ **FIGURE 46-21** MR angiogram demonstrates absence of enhancement of the superior mesenteric vein (*arrow*) and portal vein (*arrowhead*), consistent with thrombosis.

PET/CT

There is no role for scintigraphy in the evaluation of mesenteric venous thrombosis.

Angiography

Mesenteric venous thrombosis may be evaluated angiographically by direct portography, such as transhepatic or transjugular portography or splenoportography. Such techniques also provide an avenue for endovascular intervention such as angioplasty. Alternatively, mesenteric arteriography with delayed-phase imaging can be performed (so-called arterioportography). In addition to reduced arterial inflow and reflux of contrast back into the superior mesenteric artery, such indirect portography may demonstrate segments of nonopacified mesenteric and portal venous tributaries on delayed-phase images, signifying occlusions (Fig. 46-22). Portal-to-portal and portal-to-system collateral vessels may also be demonstrated.

Imaging Algorithm

An imaging algorithm is provided in Figure 46-17. See also Table 46-5.

Classic Signs: Mesenteric Venous Thrombosis

- Recent surgery, hypercoagulable state
- *CT or MRI:* Central well-defined filling defect within mesenteric vein; multiple veins may be affected
- *Angiography:* Segmental nonopacification of portomesenteric veins, slow arterial flow

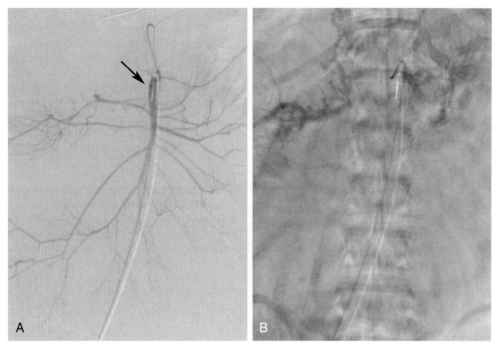

■ **FIGURE 46-22** **A,** Selective contrast injection of the superior mesenteric artery (*arrow*) demonstrates a normal arteriogram. **B,** Delayed venous phase of the arteriogram demonstrates nonopacification of the superior mesenteric vein and its tributaries, consistent with thrombosis.

TABLE 46-5 Accuracy, Limitations, and Pitfalls of Modalities Used in Imaging of Mesenteric Venous Thrombosis

Modality	Accuracy	Limitations	Pitfalls
Radiography	Poor	Insensitive Nonspecific	May not suggest disease until late stage of bowel infarction/perforation
CT	High accuracy with multiphasic imaging	Radiation	
MRI	Comparable to CT	Long examination times High cost	Suboptimal evaluation of calcifications and stented vessels
			Tailored examination less able to assess abdomen for other pathology compared to CT
Ultrasonography	Accuracy diminishes for evaluation of peripheral mesenteric veins	Patient body habitus Bowel gas	Collaterals may be missed or mistaken for patent mesenteric veins.
	Accuracy may be greater for portal compared to mesenteric vein thrombus	Patient cooperation	
Nuclear medicine	No role in the evaluation of acute mesenteric ischemia	Poor spatial resolution	
PET/CT	No role in the evaluation of acute mesenteric ischemia	Radiation High cost	
Angiography	High	Radiation Invasive	

DIFFERENTIAL DIAGNOSIS

The clinical presentation of acute mesenteric ischemia can be vague. A high index of suspicion is needed to facilitate early diagnosis and intervention and should be prompted when peritoneal signs are present. Clinicians may consider acute inflammatory disorders such as pancreatitis, cholecystitis, or inflammatory bowel disease, although pain may be more localized compared with acute mesenteric ischemia. Small bowel obstruction is also a consideration. Acute mesenteric ischemia should be considered strongly in patients with prior embolic events or cardiac disease or who are critically ill or are on vasopressor

therapy. Patients with a primary clotting disorder may prompt consideration of mesenteric venous thrombosis.

A bowel target sign on CT is nonspecific and may be attributed to mesenteric ischemia, inflammatory bowel disease, or infection. Pneumatosis intestinalis is more specific for ischemia, although infection and trauma are other possible causes.

A filling defect at a branch point of the superior mesenteric artery in the absence of prominent collateral vessels in a patient with a history of cardiac disease or prior embolic event favors embolism.

Nonopacification of the superior mesenteric artery particularly at its origin, severe atherosclerotic disease, presence of collateral vessels, and antecedent history of postprandial abdominal pain and weight loss favor thrombosis of the superior mesenteric artery.

Diffuse mesenteric arterial narrowing on angiography without evidence of occlusion suggests nonocclusive mesenteric ischemia, although vasculitis may also be considered.

Filling defects within mesenteric veins are diagnostic of mesenteric venous thrombosis and are often easily distinguished from extrinsic compression by tumor such as by pancreatic malignancy.

TREATMENT

Medical Treatment

Prompt treatment is imperative once the diagnosis of acute mesenteric ischemia is established. Medical therapy should begin with fluid resuscitation and, if there is no contraindication, anticoagulation. Broad-spectrum antibiotics should be administered early. Nasogastric tube decompression is indicated. When possible, vasoconstricting agents should be avoided.[18]

Therapy for nonocclusive mesenteric ischemia is primarily directed at reversing the offending stimulus (e.g., stopping digoxin). Catheter infusion of papaverine into the superior mesenteric artery may be helpful, but the primary stimulus must be addressed.

Similarly, mesenteric venous thrombosis may be treated medically unless there is evidence of bowel infarction, in which case laparotomy is mandated. Anticoagulation is the mainstay of therapy, and some patients recover spontaneously.[6] Long-term anticoagulation may be needed if a primary clotting disorder is discovered.

Surgical Treatment

Peritoneal signs should prompt laparotomy. Nonviable bowel is resected. Revascularization is pursued in superior mesenteric artery embolism and thrombosis and, in some cases, mesenteric venous thrombosis. Because vasospasm of otherwise unaffected mesenteric vessels may occur after revascularization, angiography and intra-arterial catheter infusion of a vasodilator such as papaverine may be performed before surgery unless reperfusion is established within 3 hours of onset.[18] Revascularization for superior mesenteric artery embolism may be performed via a transverse arteriotomy and embolectomy of the artery, which limits the potential iatrogenic reduction in arterial lumen diameter.[2,6]

Revascularization in the setting of superior mesenteric artery thrombosis may involve a longitudinal arteriotomy and thrombectomy of the artery, with subsequent patch angioplasty to preserve luminal diameter. If, however, a bypass graft is necessary to augment flow after thrombectomy, the arteriotomy site may serve as the distal anastomosis.[6] Bypass grafting is often necessary in severe atherosclerotic disease. Autologous vein grafts are mandated when there is intraperitoneal contamination from bowel perforation.

Thrombectomy is sometimes employed in cases of focal, acute mesenteric venous thrombosis within the proximal superior mesenteric vein.[8] Surgical thrombectomy is less feasible when there are numerous inaccessible thrombi. Intra-portomesenteric or intra–superior mesenteric arterial catheter infusion of thrombolytic agents is better suited in such cases.[8]

A second-look laparotomy is often needed within 48 hours after surgery for at least two reasons. First, many patients will suffer from post-treatment vasospasm of unaffected vessels, which may further compromise bowel viability. Second, intraoperative assessment of bowel viability is imperfect and a second look is needed to ensure all nonviable bowel is removed.

In select patients, percutaneous treatment of superior mesenteric artery obstruction such as by mechanical thrombectomy may be successful.[19,20] Many patients will require laparotomy, regardless, because of nonviable bowel. Further studies are required comparing percutaneous with surgical revascularization. Intra-arterial vasodilator therapy may be helpful in acute mesenteric ischemia to prevent or treat vasospasm.

What the Referring Physician Needs to Know

- CT and conventional angiography are the mainstays of imaging in acute presentations of mesenteric ischemia; MRI is the second choice owing to long examination times.
- Vessel anatomy and collateral mapping are helpful in operative planning.
- Angiography is extremely useful for both diagnosis and treatment; in some patients with peritoneal signs, emergent angiography before laparotomy may be performed to prevent post-treatment vasospasm.
- Bowel infarction and intraperitoneal contamination may prompt use of autologous veins for bypass grafting, if necessary.
- Surgery may not be necessary in nonocclusive mesenteric ischemia unless there is bowel infarction.
- Thrombosis of multiple mesenteric veins precludes surgical revascularization.

KEY POINTS

- Peritoneal signs should prompt emergent laparotomy.
- Bowel wall findings are more specific in late stages of acute mesenteric ischemia.
- Superior mesenteric artery emboli prefer to lodge at branch points.
- Infarcts in other visceral organs may suggest superior mesenteric artery embolism.
- Superior mesenteric artery thrombosis preferentially occurs at the origin of the artery.
- Collateral vessels are more typically seen in superior mesenteric artery thrombosis than embolism.
- Nonocclusive mesenteric ischemia typically occurs in critically ill patients or patients on vasopressors.
- Recent surgery or hypercoagulable state is associated with mesenteric venous thrombosis.

SUGGESTED READINGS

Bradbury MS, et al. Mesenteric venous thrombosis: diagnosis and noninvasive imaging. RadioGraphics 2002; 22:527-541.

Horton KM, Fishman EK. Volume-rendered 3D CT of the mesenteric vasculature: normal anatomy, anatomic variants, and pathologic conditions. RadioGraphics 2002; 22:161-172.

Kim AY, Ha HK. Evaluation of suspected mesenteric ischemia: efficacy of radiologic studies. Radiol Clin North Am 2003; 41:327-342.

Martinez JP, Hogan GJ. Mesenteric ischemia. Emerg Med Clin North Am 2004; 22:909-928.

Oldenburg WA, Lau LL, Rodenberg TJ, et al. Acute mesenteric ischemia: a clinical review. Arch Intern Med 2004; 164:1054-1062.

Shi MP, Hagspiel KD. CTA and MRA in mesenteric ischemia. I. Role in diagnosis and differential diagnosis. AJR Am J Roentgenol 2007; 188:452-461.

Shi MP, et al. CTA and MRA in mesenteric ischemia. II. Normal findings and complications after surgical and endovascular treatment. AJR Am J Roentgenol 2007; 188:462-471.

Wittenberg J, Harisinghani MG, Jhaveri K, et al. Algorithmic approach to CT diagnosis of the abnormal bowel wall. RadioGraphics 2002; 22:1093-1109.

REFERENCES

1. Shi MP, Hagspiel KD. CTA and MRA in mesenteric ischemia. I. Role in diagnosis and differential diagnosis. AJR Am J Roentgenol 2007; 188:452-461.

2. Milner R, Velazquez OC. Mesenteric ischemia and intestinal vascular disorders. In Lichtenstein GR, Wu GD. Requisites in Gastroenterology: Small and Large Intestine. St. Louis, Mosby, 2004, vol 2, pp 217-241.

3. Kim AY, Ha HK. Evaluation of suspected mesenteric ischemia: efficacy of radiologic studies. Radiol Clin North Am 2003; 41:327-342.

4. Kaleya RN, Sammartano RJ, Boley SJ. Aggressive approach to mesenteric ischemia. Surg Clin North Am 1992; 72:157-181.

5. Moore WM, Hollier LH. Mesenteric artery occlusive disease. Cardiol Clin 1991; 9:535-541.

6. Oldenburg WA, Lau LL, Rodenberg TJ, et al. Acute mesenteric ischemia: a clinical review. Arch Intern Med 2004; 164:1054-1062.

7. Bassiouny HS. Nonocclusive mesenteric ischemia. Surg Clin North Am 1997; 77:319-326.

8. Bradbury MS, et al. Mesenteric venous thrombosis: diagnosis and noninvasive imaging. RadioGraphics 2002; 22:527-541.

9. Rhee RY, Gloviczki P. Mesenteric venous thrombosis. Surg Clin North Am 1997; 77:327-338.

10. Horton KM, Fishman EK. Volume-rendered 3D CT of the mesenteric vasculature: normal anatomy, anatomic variants, and pathologic conditions. RadioGraphics 2002; 22:161-172.

11. Chow LC, Chan FP, Li KCP. A comprehensive approach to MR imaging of mesenteric ischemia. Abdom Imaging 2002; 27:507-516.

12. Kaufman JA, Lee MJ. Vascular and Interventional Radiology: The Requisites. St. Louis, Mosby, 2004.

13. Schneider TA, et al. Mesenteric ischemia: acute arterial syndromes. Dis Colon Rectum 1994; 37:1163-1174.

14. Schoenberg MH, Beger HG. Reperfusion injury after intestinal ischemia. Crit Care Med 1993; 21:1376-1386.

15. Zimmerman BJ, Grisham MB, Granger DN. Role of oxidants in ischemia/reperfusion-induced granulocyte infiltration. Am J Physiol 1990; 258:G185-G190.

16. Wittenberg J, Harisinghani MG, Jhaveri K, et al. Algorithmic approach to CT diagnosis of the abnormal bowel wall. RadioGraphics 2002; 22:1093-1109.

17. Sebastia C, et al. Portomesenteric vein gas: pathologic mechanisms, CT findings, and prognosis. RadioGraphics 2000; 20:1213-1224.

18. Martinez JP, Hogan GJ. Mesenteric ischemia. Emerg Med Clin North Am 2004; 22:909-928.

19. Hirsch AT, et al. ACC/AHA 2005 practice guidelines for the management of patients with peripheral arterial disease (lower extremity, renal, mesenteric, and abdominal aorta). Circulation 2006; 113:e463-e654.

20. Demirpolat G, Oran I, Tamsel S, et al. Acute mesenteric ischemia: endovascular therapy. Abdom Imaging 2007; 32:299-303.

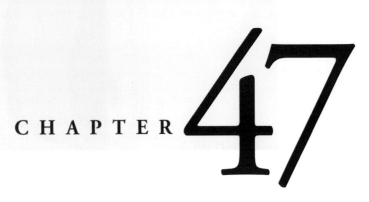
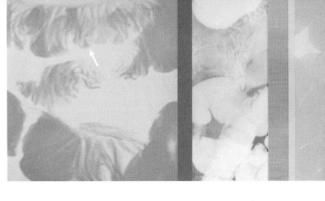

CHAPTER 47

Chronic Small Bowel Ischemia

Ashraf Thabet, T. Gregory Walker, and Sanjeeva P. Kalva

ETIOLOGY

Atherosclerotic disease is the primary cause of chronic mesenteric ischemia, accounting for more than 95% of cases.[1,2] Because of the rich arterial supply of the small bowel and the capability to develop collaterals, chronic mesenteric ischemia occurs only when there is disease of at least two of the three major mesenteric arteries: the celiac axis, superior mesenteric artery, and/or inferior mesenteric artery.

PREVALENCE AND EPIDEMIOLOGY

Chronic mesenteric ischemia occurs in patients older than age 50 years, and its prevalence increases with age.[2] Females are more commonly affected, with a female-to-male ratio of 3 : 1. Approximately 18% of people older than 65 years may have a mesenteric arterial stenosis exceeding 50%, but only a small percentage will have symptoms.[3,4] Up to 50% of patients with this disorder have had prior surgery for atherosclerotic disease.[5] Other risk factors include hypertension, smoking, and diabetes.

CLINICAL PRESENTATION

The classic presentation is intestinal angina, defined as recurrent postprandial abdominal pain subsiding in 1 to 2 hours with associated weight loss and aversion to food.[1] Because intestinal angina is rare, diagnosis is delayed and patients may have symptoms for months or years before presentation.

PATHOPHYSIOLOGY

An understanding of the anatomy and common collateral pathways of the mesenteric vasculature is critical to the imaging evaluation of patients with chronic mesenteric ischemia. Please refer to the discussion of mesenteric vessel anatomy in the previous chapter on acute small bowel ischemia.

PATHOLOGY

The predominant cause of chronic mesenteric ischemia is atherosclerotic disease affecting the proximal or ostial segments of the mesenteric arteries. As mentioned earlier, symptomatic patients have stenosis or occlusion of at least two mesenteric arteries (Figs. 47-1 and 47-2). In rare cases, only one vessel is involved and distal disease predominates, thus circumventing proximal collateral flow. The postprandial nature of the abdominal pain is consistent with an underlying mismatch between oxygen demand and supply that is exacerbated by food challenge.

Because most patients with mesenteric vascular disease are asymptomatic, its presence is not diagnostic of chronic mesenteric ischemia. In the setting of severe stenosis or occlusion of at least two mesenteric vessels, the diagnosis may be suggested by clinical findings in the absence of evidence of an alternative pathologic process.

IMAGING

Imaging is useful in the evaluation of chronic mesenteric ischemia because it can both accurately assess the atherosclerotic disease burden of the mesenteric vasculature and exclude other potential pathologic processes.

Radiography

Plain radiography is insensitive and nonspecific and is relegated to excluding other disorders, such as small bowel obstruction. A lateral abdominal radiograph may show calcified plaques at the origins of the mesenteric arteries.

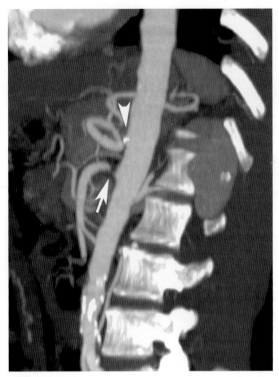

■ **FIGURE 47-1** Maximum intensity projection of a CT angiogram of the abdominal aorta demonstrates severe narrowing and calcification at the origin of the celiac artery (*arrowhead*). A severe stenosis is also demonstrated at the origin of the superior mesenteric artery (*arrow*).

CT

Contrast-enhanced CT and CT angiography (CTA) are the mainstays of evaluation. CT can evaluate inflammatory and neoplastic causes of abdominal pain. Findings of bowel wall thickening, target sign, pneumatosis, and portomesenteric gas indicate an acute process and are absent in chronic mesenteric ischemia. CTA is sensitive for detecting stenosis and/or occlusion (see Fig. 47-1) and may demonstrate collateral vessels; a noncontrast examination should be included, however, to assess for the presence of vascular calcifications.

MRI

Gadolinium-enhanced MR angiography (MRA) provides an accurate evaluation of the mesenteric vasculature (see Fig. 47-2)[6] but may not be as sensitive as CT in screening for other abdominal pathologic processes. 3D imaging techniques and postprocessing such as maximum intensity projections and volume rendering can facilitate diagnosis and operative planning. Limitations include susceptibility artifact from stents or poor demonstration of calcifications, with potential overestimation of severity of arterial stenoses.[1]

Other MR techniques to evaluate physiologic parameters of the mesenteric vasculature are performed before and after food challenge. Cine phase-contrast imaging assesses superior mesenteric vein flow, whereas MR

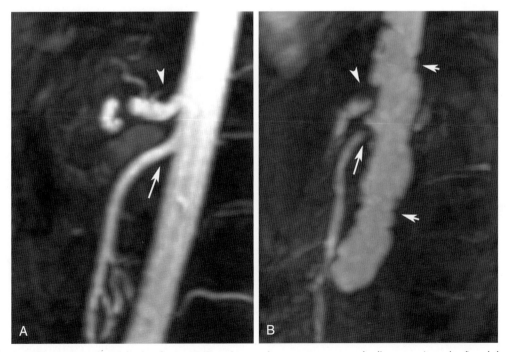

■ **FIGURE 47-2** **A,** Maximum intensity projection from an MR angiogram demonstrates a normal celiac artery (*arrowhead*) and the origin of the superior mesenteric artery (*arrow*). **B,** MR angiogram in a different patient with chronic mesenteric ischemia demonstrates diffuse wall irregularity (*short arrows*) of the aorta, consistent with atherosclerotic disease. Loss of signal at the celiac artery (*arrowhead*) and origin of the superior mesenteric artery (*long arrow*) is consistent with severe stenosis.

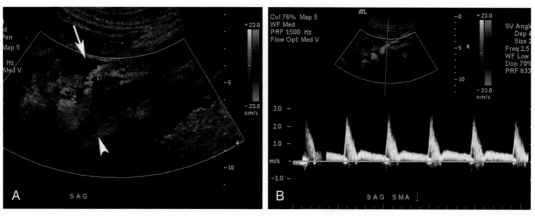

■ **FIGURE 47-3**   A, Color Doppler image of the abdominal aorta (*arrowhead*) demonstrates the takeoff of the superior mesenteric artery (*arrow*). B, Duplex ultrasonography of the proximal superior mesenteric artery demonstrates an elevated peak systolic velocity approaching 300 cm/s, suggestive of a stenosis greater than 70%.

oximetry evaluates the oxygenation of the blood of this vein.[7] Because mesenteric blood flow increases after food challenge,[7,8] a blunted superior mesenteric vein flow response implies chronic mesenteric ischemia on phase-contrast imaging.[7] MR oximetry takes advantage of the increased oxygen extraction of mesenteric blood in chronic mesenteric ischemia, given the inability to increase blood flow. Increased oxygen extraction reduces oxygen saturation and, consequently, the T2 value of the blood in the superior mesenteric vein.[7] Postprandial reduction of the T2 value of this blood has been demonstrated in patients with symptomatic chronic mesenteric ischemia, in contrast to a rise in T2 in asymptomatic patients.[7]

Ultrasonography

Duplex ultrasonography may be used to assess proximal superior mesenteric artery stenosis or occlusion (Fig. 47-3). A peak systolic velocity of greater than 275 cm/s correlates with a stenosis of at least 70%,[1,2] whereas lack of flow is consistent with occlusion. Ultrasonography, however, is limited by the patient's body habitus and overlying bowel gas. In addition, sonographic evidence of stenosis may suggest atherosclerotic disease but does not necessarily imply chronic mesenteric ischemia. Evaluation of the inferior mesenteric artery as well as more distal portions of the mesenteric vessels is limited.

Nuclear Medicine

There is no role for scintigraphy in the evaluation of chronic mesenteric ischemia.

PET/CT

There is no role for PET/CT in the evaluation of chronic mesenteric ischemia.

Angiography

Angiography is the gold standard in evaluating the mesenteric vasculature. Lateral aortography is used to assess the

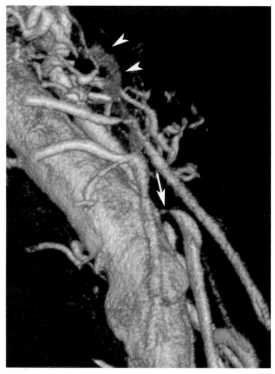

■ **FIGURE 47-4**   3D image obtained from a conventional aortogram demonstrates thrombosis of the superior mesenteric artery (*arrowheads*) and severe stenosis of the proximal inferior mesenteric artery (*arrow*).

origins of the celiac axis and superior mesenteric artery. The presence of collateral vessels such as the arc of Riolan (Figs. 47-4 and 47-5) may indicate a proximal mesenteric arterial stenosis or occlusion. Anteroposterior aortography and selective mesenteric angiography are used to assess distal disease as well as to demonstrate collateral vessels. Although invasive, costly, and associated with morbidities, angiography may be combined with interventions such as angioplasty and stenting (Fig. 47-6) to treat any identified pathologic process.

Imaging Algorithms

CT/CTA is the mainstay of evaluation of chronic mesenteric ischemia (Table 47-1). In addition to demonstrating the mesenteric arteries, CT can exclude other abdominal pathologic processes. Although MRA can assess the mesenteric arteries, it may overestimate stenoses and is limited when evaluating stented vessels. More specific physiologic parameters can be assessed with phase-contrast MR and MR oximetry, but these techniques are neither standardized nor widely available. Conventional angiography may be useful for problem solving and for intervention. Duplex ultrasonography avoids the radiation associated with CT or conventional angiography and is sensitive in evaluating the proximal superior mesenteric artery but is limited in evaluating other mesenteric vessels and collateral pathways.

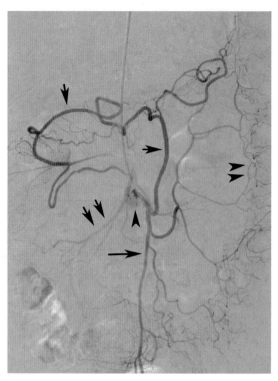

■ **FIGURE 47-5** Selective contrast injection of the inferior mesenteric artery (*single long arrow*) in the same patient as in Figure 47-4 demonstrates a prominent arc of Riolan (*single short arrow*), which reconstitutes the superior mesenteric artery (*double short arrows*). Severe stenosis of the origin of the inferior mesenteric artery as shown in Figure 47-4 results in reflux of contrast (*single arrowhead*) into the aorta. There is a poorly developed marginal artery of Drummond (*double arrowheads*).

Classic Signs: Chronic Small Bowel Ischemia

- Postprandial abdominal pain associated with food aversion and weight loss
- Narrowing of origin or proximal aspect of at least two of the following vessels: celiac artery, superior mesenteric artery, and inferior mesenteric artery
- Prominent collateral vessels
- Peak systolic velocity greater than 275 cm/s in the proximal superior mesenteric artery on ultrasonography

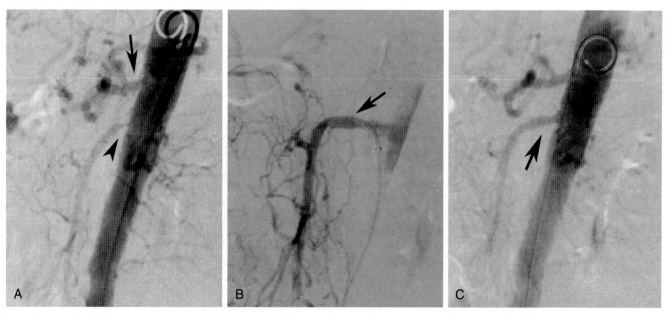

■ **FIGURE 47-6**   **A,** Lateral aortogram demonstrates a normal celiac origin (*arrow*) but severe stenosis of the origin of the superior mesenteric artery (*arrowhead*). **B,** Subsequently, angioplasty and stent placement (*arrow*) was performed. **C,** Repeat lateral aortogram demonstrates normal luminal diameter of the origin of the superior mesenteric artery (*arrow*).

TABLE 47-1 Accuracy, Limitations, and Pitfalls of the Modalities Used to Image the Major Mesenteric Arteries

Modality	Accuracy	Limitations	Pitfalls
Radiography	Poor	Insensitive Nonspecific	
CT	Highly accurate	Radiation	Presence of mesenteric arterial disease does not imply chronic mesenteric ischemia
MRI	100% sensitive, 95% specific for stenosis > 75%	Phase-contrast MR and MR oximetry are not widely available. High cost	Suboptimal evaluation of calcifications and stented vessels Tailored examination less able to assess abdomen for other pathology compared with CT
Ultrasonography	Accurate for evaluation of proximal superior mesenteric artery stenosis	Patient body habitus Bowel gas Patient cooperation	Distal mesenteric artery disease not well demonstrated Poor demonstration of collateral vessels
Nuclear medicine	No role in the evaluation of chronic mesenteric ischemia	Poor spatial resolution	
PET/CT	No role in the evaluation of chronic mesenteric ischemia	Radiation High cost	
Angiography	High	Radiation Invasive	

DIFFERENTIAL DIAGNOSIS

The clinical presentation of chronic mesenteric ischemia is nonspecific. New-onset or recent worsening of symptoms should prompt evaluation for acute mesenteric ischemia. Postprandial pain can be seen with gastroduodenal ulcers, which should be excluded by endoscopy. Weight loss is a nonspecific complaint that should prompt evaluation for malignancy.[2] Female patients in their third or fourth decade presenting with weight loss and epigastric pain that worsens with expiration suggests median arcuate ligament syndrome. Similarly, the finding in young female patients of abdominal pain and a history of hypertension may suggest fibromuscular dysplasia.

CT findings of target sign, bowel wall thickening, pneumatosis, or portomesenteric venous gas should prompt evaluation for acute ischemia. CT can assess numerous other causes of abdominal pain and/or weight loss, particularly malignancies such as pancreatic adenocarcinoma or lymphoma.

Angiographic demonstration of extrinsic narrowing of the celiac origin that worsens with expiration is compatible with median arcuate ligament syndrome.[2,9,10] Hemodynamically significant compression may cause enlargement of the gastroduodenal artery with superior mesenteric artery collateralization via the pancreaticoduodenal arcade.[9] Imaging that demonstrates beading of mesenteric arteries in a young female patient suggests fibromuscular dysplasia, whereas diffuse stenosis, aneurysms, vessel wall thickening, and enhancement may suggest vasculitis.[10,11]

TREATMENT

The traditional treatment for chronic mesenteric ischemia is surgical revascularization, which may consist of endarterectomy, reimplantation of the superior mesenteric artery, or bypass grafting.[12] Although multiple vessels may be diseased, in most instances revascularization of one vessel is needed, usually the superior mesenteric artery. Surgery has high long-term patency rates (70% to 93%) but may be associated with a morbidity of 29% and mortality of 7%,[13] with complication rates exacerbated by cardiovascular comorbidities, which are common in this patient population.

Endovascular therapies (e.g., angioplasty and/or stents) have been employed in treating stenotic mesenteric vessels since 1980,[14-16] but there are limited prospective trials comparing them with surgery. Although further studies are required, angioplasty and stenting have high technical success rates; restenoses may be re-treated percutaneously.[5] Although reported patency rates after percutaneous treatments are lower than surgery, new techniques and devices are expected to close these gaps. Percutaneous revascularization may be preferred in patients who are high-risk surgical candidates.

What the Referring Physician Needs to Know

- Atherosclerosis is responsible for over 95% of cases of chronic mesenteric ischemia.
- CT/CTA is the first step in imaging to assess the splanchnic arterial circulation as well as exclude other pathologic processes.
- 3D image postprocessing is useful in diagnosis and operative planning.
- Percutaneous therapies are an important alternative to surgical revascularization, particularly in high-risk surgical candidates.

KEY POINTS

- Chronic mesenteric ischemia is rare despite the high prevalence of atherosclerotic disease of mesenteric arteries.
- CT/CTA is the mainstay in evaluation of suspected chronic mesenteric ischemia.
- Stenosis or occlusion of the origin or proximal segments of at least two mesenteric arteries is typical.

- Chronic mesenteric ischemia suspected in young female patients should suggest fibromuscular dysplasia or median arcuate ligament syndrome.

SUGGESTED READINGS

Cademartiri F, et al. Multi-detector row CT angiography in patients with abdominal angina. RadioGraphics 2004; 24:969-984.

Chow LC, Chan FP, Li KCP. A comprehensive approach to MR imaging of mesenteric ischemia. Abdom Imaging 2002; 27:507-516.

Cognet F, et al. Chronic mesenteric ischemia: imaging and percutaneous treatment. RadioGraphics 2002; 22:863-880.

Horton KM, Fishman EK. Volume-rendered 3D CT of the mesenteric vasculature: normal anatomy, anatomic variants, and pathologic conditions. RadioGraphics 2002; 22:161-172.

Shi MP, Hagspiel KD. CTA and MRA in mesenteric ischemia. I. Role in diagnosis and differential diagnosis. AJR Am J Roentgenol 2007; 188:452-461.

Shi MP, et al. CTA and MRA in mesenteric ischemia. II. Normal findings and complications after surgical and endovascular treatment. AJR Am J Roentgenol 2007; 188:462-471.

REFERENCES

1. Kim AY, Ha HK. Evaluation of suspected mesenteric ischemia: efficacy of radiologic studies. Radiol Clin North Am 2003; 41:327-342.
2. Cognet F, et al. Chronic mesenteric ischemia: imaging and percutaneous treatment. RadioGraphics 2002; 22:863-880.
3. Cademartiri F, et al. Multi-detector row CT angiography in patients with abdominal angina. RadioGraphics 2004; 24:969-984.
4. Roobottom CA, Dubbins PA. Significant disease of the celiac and superior mesenteric arteries in asymptomatic patients: predictive value of Doppler sonography. AJR Am J Roentgenol 1993; 161: 985-988.
5. Hirsch AT, et al. ACC/AHA 2005 practice guidelines for the management of patients with peripheral arterial disease (lower extremity, renal, mesenteric, and abdominal aorta). Circulation 2006; 113: e463-e654.
6. Gilfeather M, et al. Gadolinium-enhanced ultrafast three-dimensional spoiled gradient-echo MR imaging of the abdominal aorta and visceral and iliac vessels. RadioGraphics 1997; 17:423-432.
7. Chow LC, Chan FP, Li KCP. A comprehensive approach to MR imaging of mesenteric ischemia. Abdom Imaging 2002; 27:507-516.
8. Burkart DJ, Johnson CD, Ehman RL. Correlation of arterial and venous blood flow in the mesenteric system based on MR findings. AJR Am J Roentgenol 1993; 161:1279-1282.
9. Horton KM, Talamini MA, Fishman EK. Median arcuate ligament syndrome: evaluation with CT angiography. RadioGraphics 2005; 25:1177-1182.
10. Shi MP, Hagspiel KD. CTA and MRA in mesenteric ischemia. I. Role in diagnosis and differential diagnosis. AJR Am J Roentgenol 2007; 188:452-461.
11. Ha HK, et al. Radiologic features of vasculitis involving the gastrointestinal tract. RadioGraphics 2000; 20:779-794.
12. Milner R, Velazquez OC. Mesenteric ischemia and intestinal vascular disorders. In Lichtenstein GR, Wu GD (eds): Requisites in Gastroenterology: Small and Large Intestine. St. Louis, Mosby, 2004, vol 2, pp 217-241.
13. Schaefer PJ, Schaefer FKW, Mueller-Huelsbeck S, Jahnke T. Chronic mesenteric ischemia: stenting of mesenteric arteries. Abdom Imaging 2007; 32:304-309.
14. Matsumoto AH, et al. Percutaneous transluminal angioplasty of visceral arterial stenosis: results and long-term clinical follow-up. J Vasc Interv Radiol 1995; 6:165-174.
15. Nyman O, Ivancey K, Lindle M, Uher P. Endovascular treatment of chronic mesenteric ischemia: report of five cases. Cardiovasc Intervent Radiol 1998; 21:305-313.
16. Maleux G, Wilms G, Stockx L, et al. Percutaneous recanalization and stent placement in chronic proximal superior mesenteric artery occlusion. Eur Radiol 1997; 7:1228-1230.

CHAPTER 48

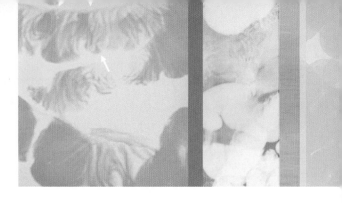

Benign Neoplasms and Wall Thickening of the Small Bowel

Aytekin Oto, Abraham H. Dachman, and Arunas E. Gasparaitis

Normal intestinal wall thickness depends on the degree of bowel distention and the imaging modality. The wall of the jejunum is slightly thicker than ileum. Individual wall thickness is about 2 mm in jejunum and 1 mm in the ileum on enteroclysis.[1] On CT, 3 mm is accepted as the upper limit of normal when the bowel is completely distended.[1]

The hallmark of benign wall thickening is homogeneous or stratified wall thickening. The stratified appearance is caused by submucosal decreased attenuation caused by edema, inflammation, and fat deposition and is also referred to as a "target" sign. In this chapter benign causes of small bowel wall thickening (Table 48-1) and benign small bowel neoplasms (Table 48-2) are discussed.

CROHN'S DISEASE

Etiology

Crohn's disease is an idiopathic, chronic, transmural disease affecting the entire gastrointestinal tract with a tendency toward segmental distribution. The etiology and pathogenesis remain unclear. Numerous environmental factors (e.g., smoking, diet, oral contraceptives, and non-steroidal anti-inflammatory agents), microbial influences along with immunologic dysregulation, and genetic factors have been suggested as the cause of this disease.[2] However, so far there is no compelling evidence that any of these factors alone can cause the disease. Today, it is believed that the combination and interaction of genetics, environmental influences, and immunologic abnormalities play the most important role.[2]

Prevalence and Epidemiology

Crohn's disease is seen more commonly in northern Europe and North America, and its incidence has increased in recent years and then reached a plateau.[3] The disease most commonly affects young adults between 15 and 25 years of age. A second peak in the elderly is thought to be caused by unrecognized ischemic colitis. Crohn's disease is seen two to four times greater in the Jewish population, especially in Ashkenazi Jews. The prevalence of disease is increased in the relatives of those who have the disease. For patients who have Crohn's disease, the occurrence of disease in their offspring is 9.2%.[4] However, classic mendelian inheritance patterns are not seen and Crohn's disease cannot be linked to a single gene locus.[2]

Clinical Presentation

Most patients present with recurrent episodes of abdominal pain, diarrhea, and low-grade fever. The pain is usually in the right lower quadrant and steady. Cramping abdominal pain may suggest intestinal obstruction. If there is colonic involvement, rectal bleeding and perianal fistulas may develop. A characteristic finding on physical examination is palpation of a tender mass, usually in the right lower quadrant, representing chronically inflamed terminal ileum. During the advanced stages of the disease, stricture formation and partial small bowel obstruction are common. Free perforation of the small bowel into the peritoneal cavity is rare, but small, sealed-off perforations are characteristic of the disease and may lead to fistula formation.

TABLE 48-1 Common Causes of Benign Small Bowel Wall Thickening

Inflammatory bowel disease (Crohn's disease, ulcerative colitis [backwash ileitis])
Infectious causes
Vascular causes
Miscellaneous causes (eosinophilic enteritis, Whipple's disease, amyloidosis, graft-versus-host disease, intestinal lymphangiectasia)
Benign neoplasms of small bowel

Extraintestinal manifestations are more common in Crohn's disease compared with ulcerative colitis. Biliary complications are the most common and include cholelithiasis and sclerosing cholangitis. Urolithiasis, sacroiliitis, peripheral arthritis, and ocular and skin manifestations are the other systemic complications, which can be seen in 20% to 30% of the patients.

The course of the disease is prolonged and unpredictable, characterized by acute exacerbations and remissions. It can be complicated by abscess/fistula formation, bowel obstruction, and development of bowel neoplasms. The risk of colorectal cancer is 4 to 20 times higher than that of the control population.[5]

Anatomy

Crohn's disease can involve the entire gastrointestinal tract in a discontinuous fashion. Terminal ileum and colon are the most frequently involved sites. Isolated small bowel involvement can occur in one third of the patients. The jejunum and ileum (sparing the terminal ileum) are affected by the disease in 3% to 10% of the patients.[6]

Pathology

The classic gross description of Crohn's disease is segmental, transmural inflammation of the bowel wall with skip lesions.[7] The mucosa shows multiple aphthous or linear ulcers, and the intervening normal mucosa has the appearance of pseudopolyps. Noncaseating granulomas are not pathognomonic but very suggestive of the disease but are found only in up to two thirds of biopsy specimens.[7] Fissures and fistula tracts are common, and the serosal surface may show transmural inflammation associated with a thickened layer of surrounding fat that is also referred to as "fibrofatty proliferation."

Imaging

Radiography

Plain radiographs of the abdomen are obtained in patients with acute presentation to evaluate for intestinal obstruction or perforation. Incidental findings may include gallstones and urinary stones. In cases of severe disease, wall thickening of the bowel segments also may be apparent on plain radiographs.

Despite advances in CT and MRI technology, barium studies remain the most sensitive radiologic test for detection of mucosal findings in the small bowel.

The literature comparing enteroclysis with small bowel follow-through (SBFT) is controversial. Enteroclysis certainly allows more accurate evaluation of the fold pattern, and carefully performed enteroclysis by an experienced radiologist can be definitive.[8] On the other hand, SBFT performed by intermittent fluoroscopy and spot films with adequate compression has been shown to approach the accuracy of enteroclysis.[9] The addition of peroral pneumocolon to the SBFT allows better evaluation of the terminal ileum.[10] In 2001, a wireless video capsule endoscope was approved by the U.S. Food and Drug Administration and has since been evaluated and found to be superior in the detection of early nonstricturing small bowel Crohn's disease.[11]

Coarsening of the villous pattern and thickening of the intestinal folds due to edema and inflammation can be seen in early disease. Ulcerations can be aphthous or linear. Aphthous ulcers are punctuate, shallow, discrete depressions surrounded by a halo. Linear ulcers can be long and run parallel to the mesenteric border (Fig. 48-1). Together with mesenteric border shortening and antimesenteric sacculations, these ulcers are very characteristic for Crohn's disease (Fig. 48-2). Linear ulcers may penetrate the entire wall of the bowel. Islands of intervening normal mucosa surrounded by denuded mucosa can give the appearance of "pseudopolyps," and multiple polypoid elevations can produce the "cobblestoning" appearance (Fig. 48-3).

Stenosis of the small intestine in Crohn's disease can be a combination of fibrosis, inflammation, and spasm. The "string" sign represents intense spasm of the bowel and indicates transmural inflammation (Fig. 48-4). This needs to be differentiated from strictures secondary to fibrosis that are not distensible and causing obstruction (Fig. 48-5). Asymmetric and discontinuous involvement of the bowel wall are the other hallmarks of Crohn's disease. Complications, such as sinus tracts, fistulas, and abscesses either ending blindly or penetrating the colon or another organ can be visualized by SBFT or enteroclysis (Figs. 48-6 and 48-7).

CT

CT has been traditionally used to evaluate patients with Crohn's disease when there is a clinical suspicion for a complication such as intestinal obstruction or fistula/abscess formation. With the advent of recent developments in CT technology and the recent introduction of novel oral contrast agents, new CT techniques (CT enterography and CT enteroclysis) dedicated to image the small bowel have emerged. These involve thin-slice, multidetector CT acquisition through the entire small bowel after administration of usually neutral oral (or nasoenteric) and intravenous contrast material. Classic CT features of active small bowel Crohn's disease are bowel wall thickening, mural hyperenhancement, and mural stratification (Fig. 48-8).[12] Narrowing of the lumen is another common finding, which can be fixed (due to fibrosis) or reversible (inflammation/spasm) (Fig. 48-9). CT can also give information about the mesentery, complications, and extraintestinal findings. Enlarged vasa recta and increased amount of fat surrounding the involved bowel segments

TABLE 48-2 Imaging Characteristics of Benign Neoplasms, Vascular Lesions, and Infectious Lesions of the Small Bowel and Inflammatory Bowel Disease

Lesion	Age	Sex	Distinguishing Clinical History	Distinguishing Clinical Presentation	Imaging Modality of Choice	Distinguishing Imaging Findings	Enhancement Pattern	Additional Findings
Benign neoplasms or neoplasm-like lesions	5th-6th decade	M = F	Could be incidental on imaging	Associated as a spectrum of polyposis syndromes *or* if large, can present as small bowel obstruction, intussusception, palpable mass. Rarely perforation is noted.	Enteroclysis, wireless capsule endoscopy, CT enterography	Lipomas are fat-containing lesions. GISTs are exophytic masses with hemorrhage, necrosis, and calcification.	Variable	If associated with syndromes
Inflammatory bowel disease	15-25 yr	M = F, four times more common in Ashkenazi Jews	Right lower quadrant pain, intermittent diarrhea, weight loss, rectal bleeding	Perianal fistula formation, extraintestinal manifestations	Enteroclysis and wireless capsule endoscopy for subtle mucosal involvement CT or MR enterography for extent of the disease and complications	Asymmetric and discontinuous involvement Coarsening of villous pattern and wall stratification Linear/aphthous ulcers Cobblestoning String sign due to inflammation and spasm Sinus tracts/fistulas and abscess formation	Fibrofatty proliferation, variable enhancement	Extraintestinal manifestations such as sclerosing cholangitis, joint involvement, etc.
Infectious diseases	Any age, more common in pediatric patients	M = F, endemic in some places	Immune suppression, recent history of travel or living in endemic places	Diarrhea, acute or chronic presentation, fever, abdominal pain	Usually none; in chronic cases or immune-compromised patients CT may be helpful.	Nonspecific findings; usually terminal ileum and right colon is involved	Variable, diffuse enhancement of the involved bowel segment	
Vascular diseases	More common in elderly patients	M = F	History of atherosclerotic disease, blood dyscrasia, abdominal surgery or infection	Abdominal pain, acute abdomen, gastrointestinal bleeding	CT; CT or MR angiography	Thrombus in the mesenteric vessels Intestinal wall thickening, "thumbprinting" Pneumatosis	Decreased or sometimes increased enhancement of the bowel wall	Atherosclerotic disease

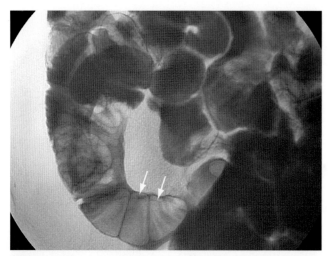

■ **FIGURE 48-1**   Linear ulceration (*arrows*) along the mesenteric border of a segment of ileum. These ulcers usually run parallel to the mesenteric border and can exceed 15 cm in length.

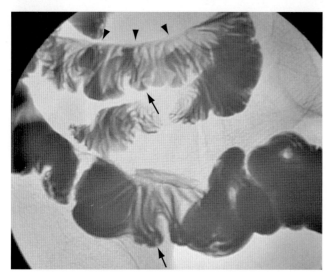

■ **FIGURE 48-2**   Asymmetric wall involvement in Crohn's disease. Mesenteric border of the small bowel segments is shortened and straightened (*arrowheads*) while there is redundancy and ulcerations (*arrows*) in the antimesenteric border. The combination of these findings is pathognomonic for Crohn's disease.

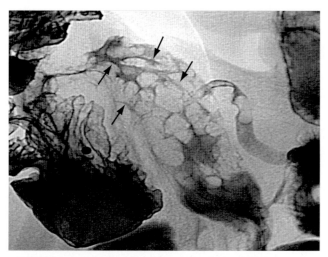

■ **FIGURE 48-3**   Classic cobblestone appearance. Multiple linear ulcerations (*arrows*) separating islands of normal mucosa.

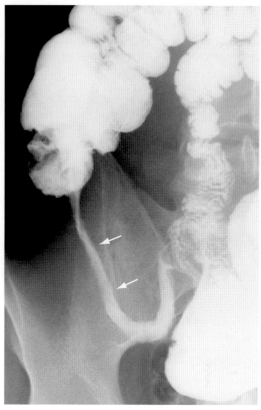

■ **FIGURE 48-4**   String sign (*arrows*). Decrease in the caliber is associated with spasm, and the most common site is the terminal ileum.

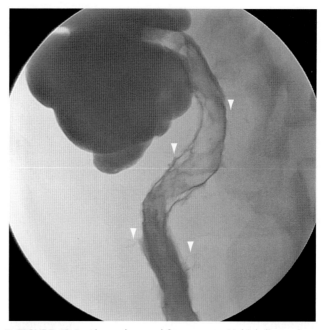

■ **FIGURE 48-5**   Linear ulcers and fissure tracts. Multiple linear ulcers are seen in the strictured terminal ileum. Linear extensions of barium outside the bowel wall (*arrowheads*) represent fissure tracts. Some of these may evolve into fistulas or abscesses.

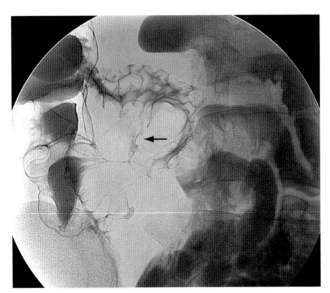

■ **FIGURE 48-6** Ileoileal fistula. Peroral pneumocolon study demonstrates the linear connection (*arrow*) between the terminal ileum and a distal segment of ileum representing the fistulous tract.

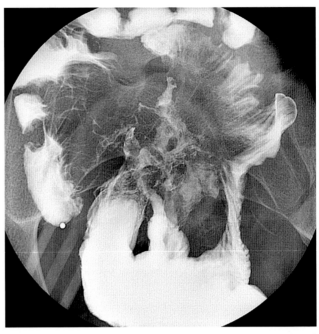

■ **FIGURE 48-7** Extensive fistula formation involving the small bowel and colon segments in Crohn's disease.

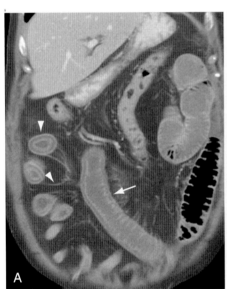

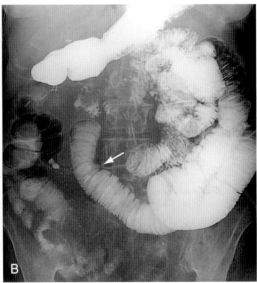

■ **FIGURE 48-8** CT enterography after administration of a neutral oral contrast agent (**A**) shows thick-walled jejunal (*arrow*) and ileal segments (*arrowheads*) with mural hyperenhancement and stratification. SBFT study (**B**) demonstrates the thickened, edematous folds in the involved jejunal segment (*arrow*).

are common findings (Fig. 48-10). Fistulas between the small bowel and colon or other organs can be seen as enhancing tracts (Fig. 48-11). Coronal and other multiplanar reformatted views may assist in better depiction of fistulous tracts. Positive oral contrast agents may be preferred if a fistula is clinically suspected.[12] In a prospective study by Hara and colleagues, Crohn's disease was depicted by CT enterography in 53%, ileoscopy in 65%, SBFT in 24%, and capsule endoscopy in 71% of the patients.[13] It is important to note that capsule endoscopy is contraindicated in patients with known strictures.

MRI

MR enterography and enteroclysis can provide a systematic evaluation of the entire small bowel and the mesentery without exposing the patients to ionizing radiation. In a study by Schreyer and colleagues, all pathologic findings seen on conventional enteroclysis were seen on MR enterography and MR enteroclysis.[14] Some reports have shown greater than 90% sensitivity and specificity with MRI in detection of Crohn's disease.[15] Increased enhancement and thickness of the bowel wall suggest active

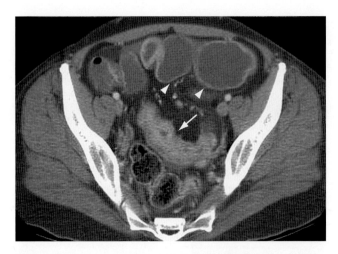

■ FIGURE 48-9 Axial CT image shows an inflamed, thick-walled distal ileum segment (*arrow*) causing dilatation of the proximal small bowel segments (*arrowheads*), representing bowel obstruction.

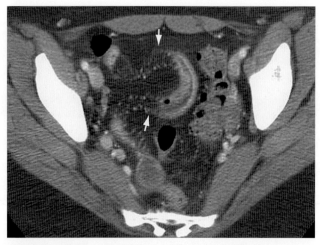

■ FIGURE 48-10 "Comb" sign and fibrofatty proliferation. Mesenteric vessels are prominent (*arrows*), and there is a focal increase in the amount of fat around the inflamed small bowel segment.

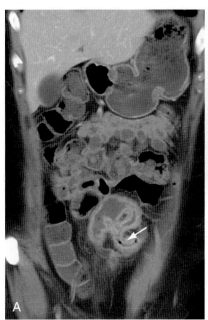

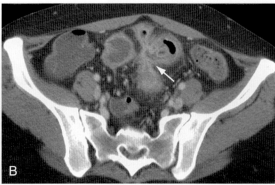

■ FIGURE 48-11 Ileosigmoid fistula. Coronal (**A**) and axial (**B**) CT enterography images demonstrate the fistulous communication (*arrows*) between the inflamed ileum and sigmoid colon segments. Exact localization of these fistulas is important for surgical planning.

inflammation (Fig. 48-12). High signal intensity in the bowel wall on T2-weighted (T2W) images also indicates active disease, and low signal on T2W images with lack of increased enhancement is suggestive of chronic Crohn's disease.[15]

Ultrasonography

During the past decade, advances in the resolution of ultrasound technology have led to better imaging of the bowel wall. Common ultrasonographic findings of Crohn's disease are thickened bowel wall and decreased peristalsis.[16] However, these changes are nonspecific. In some studies, the sensitivity of ultrasonography in the diagnosis of Crohn's disease was reported to be relatively high, but

it has also been shown that ultrasonography underestimates the extent of involvement.[16,17] Use of oral and intravenous contrast agents may further increase the diagnostic capability of ultrasonography.

Nuclear Medicine

Labeled white blood cell scans (indium-111 tropolone or technetium-99m hexamethyl propylene amine oxime [^{99m}Tc-HMPAO]) and granulocyte scintigraphy with labeled antibodies have been reported to detect the inflammation in Crohn's disease. Reported sensitivities vary between 5% and 70%, and they have been suggested to be more useful in reassessments rather than the initial diagnosis.[18]

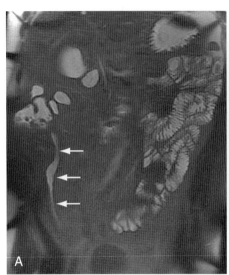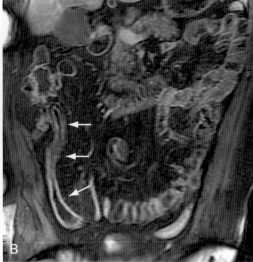

■ **FIGURE 48-12** MR enterography. Coronal fat-saturated T2W single-shot fast spin-echo (**A**) and contrast-enhanced T1W (**B**) MR images show the asymmetric stricture involving a long segment of the terminal ileum (*arrows*). Note the increased fat around the terminal ileum.

ity (85.4%) compared with the other imaging tools for the detection of inflamed bowel segments.[19]

Imaging Algorithm

In patients with suspected Crohn's disease, enteroclysis, SBFT, and CT or MR enterography (or enteroclysis) can be the initial test, depending on the experience of the radiologist. Capsule endoscopy is utilized as the initial diagnostic test for suspected nonstricturing small bowel Crohn's disease. Radiologic tests can also be helpful to exclude stenosis before the capsule endoscopy and provide more accurate localization of the pathology after the capsule endoscopy. Currently, CT enterography is the initial test for patients with acute presentation and suspected obstruction, fistula, or abscess (Table 48-3; see also Fig. 48-28 at the end of the chapter).

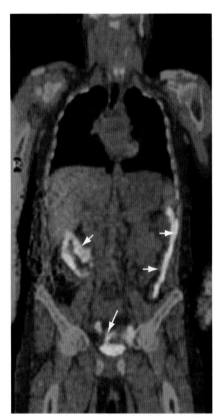

■ **FIGURE 48-13** Acute inflammation in PET/CT. Coronal PET/CT image shows increased FDG uptake in the small and large bowel segments (*arrows*). Acute inflammation was confirmed by colonoscopy in this patient.

Classic Signs: Crohn's Disease

- Cobblestoning: radiographic appearance caused by islands of normal mucosa (appearing as pseudopolyps) surrounded by denuded affected mucosa
- "String" sign: stenosis of the bowel caused by inflammation and spasm
- Fibrofatty proliferation: increased amount of fat around the involved bowel segments
- Wall stratification: low density between mucosal and serosal enhancement representing fat or inflammation

---

PET/CT

Recently, fluorodeoxyglucose (FDG)-labeled PET combined with CT (PET/CT) has been shown to be a reliable tool for detection of active disease in both the small and large bowel (Fig. 48-13). In a study comparing PET, MR enterography, and granulocyte scintigraphy with labeled antibodies, FDG-PET showed significantly higher sensitiv-

Differential Diagnosis

Infectious enteritis (*Yersinia, Mycobacterium tuberculosis, Campylobacter, Salmonella, Shigella, Entamoeba*) can be difficult to differentiate from Crohn's disease at the initial presentation. In patients presenting with acute abdomen or appendicitis, Meckel's diverticulitis needs to

TABLE 48-3 Limitations and Pitfalls of the Modalities Used in Imaging of Crohn's Disease

Modality	Limitations	Pitfalls
Radiography	Extraintestinal findings, detection of disease activity, radiation	
CT	Radiation, insensitive to early mucosal findings	Undistended bowel
MRI	Expensive, duration of the test	Undistended bowel
Ultrasonography	Unable to image the entire bowel	Nonspecific findings
Nuclear medicine	Radiation, poor spatial resolution	Normal bowel uptake
PET/CT	Expensive, radiation, relatively less data available	Normal bowel uptake

What the Referring Physician Needs to Know: Crohn's Disease

- Differentiation of Crohn's disease from other causes of enteritis
- Differentiation between active and chronic Crohn's disease
- Recognition of complications
- Monitoring of therapy

be differentiated from acute exacerbation or complications of Crohn's disease. In patients without small bowel involvement, differentiation from ulcerative colitis may be difficult. In elderly patients, ischemic enteritis should be differentiated from Crohn's disease.

Infectious enteritis can radiologically mimic Crohn's disease. Other differential diagnoses include ischemia, neoplasm (lymphoma and, rarely, adenocarcinoma), ulcerative colitis, radiation therapy, vasculitis, and, in children, lymphoid hyperplasia.

Treatment

Medical Treatment

Medical therapy is usually individualized and requires a combination of different drugs to achieve sustained response. The choice of drugs varies according to the severity of the disease, which is based on clinical, biochemical, endoscopic, and histologic findings. The Crohn's disease activity index (CDAI) score is commonly used to determine the severity of the disease. Different drugs used for Crohn's disease range from sulfasalazine, to antibiotics in mild cases, to oral corticosteroids, azathioprine, methotrexate, and tumor necrosis factor-α inhibitors in moderate and severe cases.[20] The use of tumor necrosis factor-α inhibitors has revolutionized the therapy of severe Crohn's disease.[20]

Surgical Treatment

Failure to respond to medical management and inability to tolerate effective therapy are the most common indications for surgical therapy.[5] Development of complications such as bowel obstruction and enterovesical fistulas and severe growth retardation in pediatric patients are the other surgical indications.[5]

INFECTIOUS CAUSES

Infectious diseases of the small bowel can be caused by various organisms, including bacteria, viruses, parasites, and fungi. Radiologic signs are often nonspecific, and bowel wall thickening is a common finding. Clinical information such as stool culture, the immune status, and geographic location of the patient is helpful for a specific diagnosis.

Etiology

Common bacterial causes of community-acquired infectious enterocolitis in the United States are *Campylobacter jejuni, Salmonella, Shigella, Escherichia coli,* and *Yersinia.*[21] Rotavirus and Norwalk virus are the most common pathogens in the children. Adenovirus and cytomegalovirus (CMV) should be considered in immunocompromised patients. *Giardia lamblia* is the most frequent cause of parasitic enteritis in the United States.[22] Other common parasitic infections that can affect the small intestine are *Ancylostoma, Ascaris, Cryptosporidium,* and *Taenia. Cryptosporidium* is a particularly common pathogen in the immunocompromised hosts. With the increasing population of immunocompromised patients (e.g., those with the acquired immunodeficiency syndrome), the incidence of *Mycobacterium tuberculosis* and *M. avium* complex (MAC) has increased during the past 2 decades.

Prevalence and Epidemiology

Acute diarrhea is one of the most common diagnoses in general practice. Immune status, clinical setting, and geographic location are important factors in disease expression and treatment.[23] Acute enteritis causes 3 to 6 million deaths (mostly of children) throughout the world.[21] Each year in the United States tens of millions of people acquire gastrointestinal infections with thousands of hospitalizations and deaths.[24] Chronic enteritis occurs less frequently and can be seen with parasites and, less commonly, with bacteria. Immunosuppressed individuals cannot clear pathogens effectively and can develop chronic diarrhea. *Campylobacter* and *Salmonella* can cause persistent diarrhea in patients with human immunodeficiency virus infection.[25]

Acute infectious diarrhea is acquired mostly through the fecal-oral route. Infection can also be transmitted via direct contact and ingestion of contaminated food and water. In developing countries, infectious enteritis can be endemic; and in most parts of the world a seasonality is recognized in the incidence of acute diarrhea.[23]

Clinical Presentation

Patients may present with abdominal pain, diarrhea (with or without blood), and fever. If the host is a child, elderly, or immunocompromised, dehydration may be frequently encountered. Growth retardation in children and weight loss in adults are the complications of chronic diarrhea. Enteropathogens may involve the entire small bowel, although certain pathogens are more likely to colonize at certain segments. For example, *M. tuberculosis* tends to involve the terminal ileum and ileocecal valve and *Giardia* primarily causes duodenal and proximal jejunal disease.

Pathology

In most cases, a pathogen enters and colonizes in an area of intestine. However, ingestion of the toxin alone can cause infection (*Staphylococcus aureus, Clostridium botulinum*). Most bacteria disrupt mucosal integrity through cytotoxic mediators. *Shigella* and enteroinvasive *Escherichia coli* can cause significant tissue invasion and destruction of the bowel mucosa. Rotavirus may disrupt the mucosa and produce villous atrophy. CMV produces characteristic nuclear and cytoplasmic inclusions that can be recognized on light microscopic examination. Whereas most infections elicit an inflammatory response, parasites such as *Giardia* or *Cryptosporidium* cause minimal mucosal response, and it may be difficult to localize these organisms in the villi.[26] A variety of parasitic worms also may be found in small bowel biopsy specimens.

MAC includes two related organisms. *M. avium* and *M. intracellulare* enter into the intestinal mucosa and are phagocytosed by histiocytes, which are unable to digest them. Acid-fast bacteria within the histiocytes or in the stool samples can be identified. The pathology resembles that of Whipple's disease, but the bacteria in Whipple's disease are not acid fast and histiocytes are typically foamy.[26] Pathology of infection with *M. tuberculosis* is similar to that of MAC with the addition of caseation granulomas in the wall or in the mesentery of the bowel.

Endoscopic findings in infectious enteritis range from normal intestine (mostly viral infections) to inflammation, atrophic/blunted villi, erosions, and ulcers.

Imaging

Radiography

Plain radiographic findings are often normal or nonspecific, showing mild ileus.

Barium studies are rarely indicated for acute disease. If the course is prolonged, it is important to differentiate an infectious cause from inflammatory, neoplastic, and vascular causes. The diagnosis depends on the findings of biopsy, stool examination, and culture.

Terminal ileum is most severely affected in infections with *Campylobacter, Yersinia,* and *Mycobacterium.* In infection with *Campylobacter* and *Yersinia,* the wall of the distal ileum demonstrates wall thickening with nodular folds and single or multiple, sometimes aphthous, ulcers.[27,28] In *Yersinia* infection, the bowel mostly retains its normal caliber. These changes can also extend to the cecum and ascending colon. In salmonellosis, barium studies are rarely indicated, and findings are nonspecific with aphthous ulcers and wall thickening most commonly in the region of the terminal ileum.[29] Shigellosis, on the

other hand, predominantly colonizes the colon and affects the small intestine by its enterotoxin.[29]

M. tuberculosis causes transaxial ulcerations, polyps, and thickening of the folds mostly in the ileocecal region in the early phase.[30,31] Involvement is more prominent in the cecum compared with the terminal ileum, and strictures may develop during the course of the disease. Strictures are usually short and have an hourglass configuration and sometimes cause small bowel obstruction. The cecum and ileocecal valve may be unrecognizable, with cephalad retraction of the cecum and straightening of the ileocecal angle.[31] Fistula formation and perforation are rare. Differentiation of ileocecal tuberculosis from Crohn's disease may be extremely difficult.

In the immunocompromised host, MAC, *Cryptosporidium,* and CMV are the most common infective agents causing enteritis. On barium studies, a diffuse granular pattern secondary to nodular thickening of mucosal folds is a common finding in MAC infection.[32] Ulcers are typical findings of CMV enterocolitis, and they can be large.[33] The ileocecal region is the most commonly involved area, and changes can extend into the cecum and the rest of the colon (Fig. 48-14). The barium study findings of cryptosporidiosis are nonspecific fold thickening and increase in intraluminal fluid.

CT

CT is usually not indicated in the evaluation of immunecompetent patients with acute enteritis, but it is important to know the CT findings to be able to consider acute enteritis in the differential diagnosis when these findings are incidentally encountered. Nonspecific wall thickening, mild ileus secondary to altered mobility of the involved small bowel segments, and mesenteric adenopathy are the common, nonspecific CT findings of acute enteritis.

CT can demonstrate the extent of the disease in patients with *M. tuberculosis* infection. CT findings include significant wall thickening mostly involving the ileocecal area, mesenteric adenopathy, and inflammatory mass-like lesions in the right lower quadrant.[34] CT can also show ascites and peritoneal and omental soft tissue densities representing peritonitis and may mimic peritoneal carcinomatosis (Fig. 48-15).

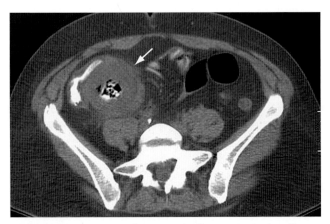

■ **FIGURE 48-14** CMV colitis. Note significant, concentric wall thickening of the terminal ileum (*arrow*).

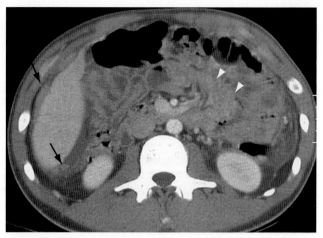

■ **FIGURE 48-15** Tuberculous peritonitis. Axial CT image shows peritoneal soft tissue nodules (*arrows*) with small amount of ascites. Small bowel wall thickening is also noted (*arrowheads*).

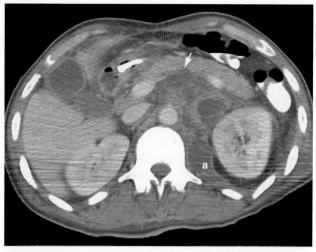

■ **FIGURE 48-17** MAC infection. Multiple enlarged retroperitoneal lymph nodes with central low densities (*arrow*) representing necrosis are typical for MAC infection in this patient with known HIV infection. There is also a retroperitoneal abscess on the left side (a).

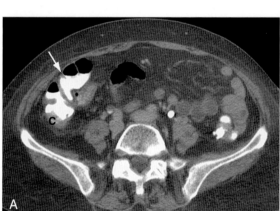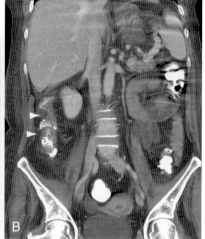

■ **FIGURE 48-16** Typhlitis in a neutropenic patient. Axial (**A**) and coronal (**B**) CT images demonstrate wall thickening of the terminal ileum (*arrow*, **A**), cecum (**C**), and ascending colon (*arrowheads*, **B**).

In the immune-compromised host, CT can help in differentiation of typhlitis (which requires medical treatment) from acute appendicitis and save the patient from unnecessary surgery.[35] CT features of typhlitis include segmental bowel wall thickening involving the terminal ileum, appendix, cecum and ascending colon, pneumatosis coli, and pericolonic fat stranding (Fig. 48-16). The extent of the colonic involvement is more substantial in typhlitis, and the presence of known risk factors favors the diagnosis of typhlitis (neutropenic colitis).[36] In patients with MAC infection, detection of mesenteric adenopathy with low attenuation centers indicating necrosis is very suggestive of the cause (Fig. 48-17). Similar lymph nodes can be seen in patients with Whipple's disease in the immune-competent host.

MRI

Limited experience is present about the MRI findings of infectious enteritis, and the role of MRI in the diagnosis of small bowel infections has not yet been established.

Ultrasonography

Acute infectious ileitis may show thickening of the ileal wall and mesenteric adenopathy.[26] An involved segment is usually aperistaltic, and the inflammation can also involve the cecum. Demonstration of the normal appendix on ultrasonography can rule out appendicitis.

Nuclear Medicine and PET/CT

The roles of nuclear medicine and PET/CT have not yet been established in the diagnosis of small bowel diseases.

Imaging Algorithm

Imaging is usually not indicated in immune-competent patients with acute enteritis (see Fig. 48-28). Clinical and laboratory evaluation with stool examination with or without cultures is usually enough to make the diagnosis or at least decide about the management. CT may be helpful to rule out a surgical diagnosis or complication of an infectious process. CT is also commonly utilized for the evaluation of immune-compromised patients with suspected enteritis to identify the etiology and the extent of the disease as well as to exclude complications or neoplastic etiology (Table 48-4). SBFT and enteroclysis can be obtained in chronic cases. Specific radiologic findings and location and extent of the disease can help in the accurate diagnosis when evaluated together with the clinical and laboratory information.

Differential Diagnosis

Most of the time, the clinical diagnosis of infectious enteritis is not difficult, although the specific pathogen cannot be determined in all of the cases. When the inflammation causes ileus, clinical presentation may mimic bowel obstruction. Sometimes, it may be difficult to exclude diseases causing acute abdomen. When the course of the infection is chronic, inflammatory, neoplastic, and vascular etiology should also be considered in the differential diagnosis.

When there is involvement of the ileocecal area, the differential diagnosis includes Crohn's disease, radiation enteritis, neoplasm (lymphoma, adenocarcinoma, carcinoid), or extrinsic inflammatory masses such as abscess/phlegmon from acute appendicitis. When the folds are thickened without narrowing and the history is more acute, then infection with *Yersinia, Salmonella,* or *Campylobacter* is the most likely cause. Luminal narrowing and mesenteric border ulcers are suggestive of Crohn's disease. Tuberculosis can mimic Crohn's disease with skip lesions but affects the right colon more than the terminal ileum. In tuberculosis, the ileocecal valve is patulous. Behçet's disease also has predilection for the terminal ileum, and the presence of other clinical manifestations helps to make the diagnosis.

When the involvement is more proximal (jejunum and proximal ileum), ulcerative jejunoileitis, eosinophilic enteritis, lymphoma, and abetalipoproteinemia can be considered in the differential diagnosis. Ulcerative jejunoileitis is a rare complication of celiac disease and may present as ulcer formation, which may eventually lead to stricture formation. Radiologically, it may be impossible to differentiate it from lymphoma. In the immunocompromised host, the main differential considerations are neoplasm (lymphoma, Kaposi's sarcoma) and graft-versus-host disease.

Treatment

Medical Treatment

The treatment of infectious enteritis depends on the infecting agent. Some organisms such as most viruses and non–*Salmonella typhi* usually cause self-limited disease in the immune-competent host and do not require antimicrobial therapy. In contrast, microorganisms such as most parasites, *M. tuberculosis,* and *Shigella* are treated with the appropriate antibiotic.[21] Because the management depends on the identity of the infecting agent, definitive microbiologic studies such as stool cultures, enzyme and toxin assays, and microscopic examination of stool should be performed. In patients with tuberculosis, long-term, triple-drug therapy with isoniazid, pyrazinamide, and rifampin is usually indicated. Agent-specific antimicrobial therapy is more aggressively pursued in the immune-compromised host. In all forms of infectious enteritis, supportive therapy to prevent dehydration and to maintain adequate nutrition is an essential part of the treatment. Further discussion of the specific medical therapy for specific infectious enteritis is beyond the scope of this chapter.

Surgical Treatment

Surgical therapy is rarely indicated. It is performed mostly for the complications of intestinal tuberculosis such as perforation, obstruction, or massive hemorrhage.[37]

TABLE 48-4 Accuracy and Limitations of the Modalities Used in Imaging of Infectious Causes of Small Bowel Disease

Modality	Accuracy	Limitations
Radiography		Nonspecific findings and cannot evaluate the extramural disease
CT	Very helpful in evaluation of acutely presenting immune compromised patients	Nonspecific findings and cannot evaluate the mucosal disease

---

What the Referring Physician Needs to Know: Infectious Causes of Small Bowel Disease

- CT can exclude abdominal acute inflammatory conditions that may mimic infectious enteritis and that will require surgery or drainage.
- When the clinical and laboratory information does not allow a definite diagnosis, radiologic information can help to exclude an ischemic, neoplastic, or inflammatory cause or in some cases suggest a specific infectious agent.

MISCELLANEOUS CAUSES OF BENIGN SMALL BOWEL WALL THICKENING

In this section, we will review the imaging findings of the relatively rare causes of benign small bowel wall thickening, including eosinophilic enteritis, graft-versus-host disease (GVHD), amyloidosis, Whipple's disease, and intestinal lymphangiectasia. Radiologic findings are mostly nonspecific in these diseases, and biopsy is usually required for definitive diagnosis.

Etiology

Eosinophilic enteritis is a rare inflammatory condition of unknown etiology characterized by focal or diffuse eosinophilic infiltration of the intestinal tract. GVHD occurs after bone marrow transplant when immunologically competent T lymphocytes are introduced into the immunocompromised host and may affect the skin, intestine, and liver. Amyloidosis is a rare systemic condition characterized by extracellular deposition of insoluble protein-mucopolysaccharide complex. The gastrointestinal tract can be involved in more than 70% of the cases with generalized amyloidosis. Primary amyloidosis is associated with multiple myeloma or Waldenström's macroglobulinemia, and secondary amyloidosis is associated with chronic inflammatory diseases such as rheumatoid arthritis or familial Mediterranean fever. Whipple's disease is a systemic disease caused by bacteria named *Tropheryma whippelii*. It can affect any system of the body, but the small intestine is frequently affected. Regional lymph nodes, heart, brain, and joints can also be involved. Lymphangiectasia can occur as a result of congenital hypoplasia of lymphatics in the bowel wall (primary) or obstruction of the lymphatics by retroperitoneal or mesenteric abnormalities (secondary). Primary lymphangiectasia is a rare disease, and patients are usually young adults.

Clinical Presentation

Eosinophilic enteritis is a disease of young adults and children. The symptoms vary depending on the location of eosinophilic infiltration within the digestive system and layers of the digestive system infiltrated with eosinophils.[38] Patients with predominantly mucosal disease may present with diarrhea, abdominal pain, and symptoms of malabsorption or protein-losing enteropathy. If the disease primarily affects the muscularis propria, partial obstruction can be seen. Ascites is common when serosa is the predominantly affected layer. Peripheral eosinophilia is present in most patients with eosinophilic enteritis.

Acute GVHD presents within the first 100 days of allogenic bone marrow transplantation. After marrow grafting, subacute disease can develop within 1 to 4 months and chronic GVHD may occur within 3 to 12 months. Severe diarrhea, abdominal pain, rash, dry mouth, and elevated liver enzymes are common findings.

Clinical presentation of small bowel amyloidosis depends on the involved bowel segment. Symptoms may include diarrhea, bleeding, malabsorption, hemorrhage, intestinal infarction, or even perforation. Biopsy of the small bowel is diagnostic.

Whipple's disease presents as abdominal pain, diarrhea, intestinal bleeding, loss of appetite, weight loss, fatigue, and weakness.[39] Arthritis and fever often occur several years before intestinal symptoms develop. Mesenteric adenopathy may cause intestinal lymphangiectasia, leading to protein-losing enteropathy. Neurologic changes may accompany the gastrointestinal findings. Definitive diagnosis requires small bowel biopsy.

Patients with primary lymphangiectasia present with protein-losing enteropathy, ascites, and pleural effusions. The disease is often associated with asymmetric edema of the extremities. Malabsorption, hypoalbuminemia, and lymphocytopenia can be seen secondary to development of lymphoenteric fistulas. Hypogammaglobulinemia, mainly affecting IgG and IgA, is also a common finding.

Pathology

Any segment of the gastrointestinal tract can be involved in eosinophilic enteritis. Most commonly involved areas are gastric antrum and proximal small bowel.[40] Eosinophilic infiltration of the submucosa is the hallmark of the disease. Infiltration may involve the mucosa, muscularis propria, and serosa.

Histologic analysis of GVHD shows varying degrees of epithelial cell apoptosis, crypt cell dropout, and mucosal inflammation.[41] Lymphocytic infiltration may be present in the thickened bowel wall.

Gastrointestinal system involvement is more common in primary amyloidosis. Primary amyloidosis is often referred to as light amyloidosis because the amyloid is made up of the light chains of immunoglobulins.[42] Amyloid is deposited in the submucosa and muscular layers of the bowel wall.

The mucosa and submucosa of the intestinal wall are diffusely infiltrated by foamy macrophages containing periodic acid–Schiff–positive material in Whipple's disease. The short, curved, rod-like Whipple bacillus can be identified within the cytoplasm.

In patients with intestinal lymphangiectasia, pathologic study shows dilated lacteals and lymphatics in the villi and edematous submucosa.[41] These findings can be focal or diffuse.

Imaging (Table 48-5; see also Fig. 48-28)

Radiography

In eosinophilic enteritis, barium studies of the small bowel show thickening of the small bowel folds and gastric

TABLE 48-5 Limitations and Pitfalls of the Modalities Used in Imaging for Miscellaneous Causes of Bowel Wall Thickening

Modality	Limitations	Pitfalls
Radiography	Nonspecific findings	Can be normal in mild disease
CT	Nonspecific findings, relatively insensitive to mucosal disease	Nondistended small bowel may mimic wall thickening

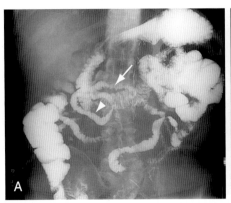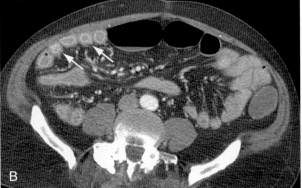

■ **FIGURE 48-18** Chronic graft-versus-host disease. **A,** SBFT shows thickened folds in the proximal jejunum (*arrow*) and fold effacement (*arrowhead*) and luminal narrowing in the ileum segments. Wide separation of the bowel segments is also noted. **B,** Axial CT image demonstrates the wall thickening involving the ileal segments with a mural stratification pattern and increased enhancement of the mucosa (*arrows*).

antrum. Nodularity may be present. When the disease predominantly affects the muscularis propria, narrowing of bowel lumen can be detected.[43]

In acute GVHD, barium studies may show thickened or effaced mucosal folds, decreased transit time, and shallow or deep ulcerations (Fig. 48-18).[44] Barium coating may persist over the mucosa for a few days. Rapid progression to luminal narrowing and to ribbon-like small bowel segments may be observed. Increased wall thickening, nodularity, and stenosis may be seen in subacute and chronic phases.

The radiologic findings in amyloidosis are not specific. Barium studies can be normal or demonstrate nonspecific fold thickening with or without nodular pattern (Fig. 48-19). Delayed contrast transit times have been reported owing to altered motility.[45]

In Whipple's disease, barium studies show diffuse thickening of the folds and sometimes a micronodular pattern with normal fold thickening.[46] Nodules measuring 1 to 2 mm may be diffuse or patchy in distribution.

In addition to nonspecific changes in barium studies, including mild fold thickening, dilatation, and increased fluid, enteroclysis can show a micronodular surface pattern produced by dilatation of the lacteals in the villi in patients with lymphangiectasia.[47]

CT

CT features of eosinophilic enteritis are nonspecific and have been recently described by Zheng and colleagues.[38] Small bowel wall thickening with or without a "halo" sign (specifying submucosal edema and benign etiology) and luminal narrowing can be demonstrated on CT.

Bowel wall thickening with or without proximal dilatation, engorgement of the vasa recta, mesenteric fat stranding, and mucosal and serosal enhancement are the described CT findings for GVHD (see Fig. 48-18).[48] Ascites, biliary abnormalities, and wall thickening involving other segments of the gastrointestinal tract can also be detected on CT.

CT findings of amyloidosis are normal or nonspecific in most cases. Bowel wall thickening is usually symmetric and may resemble ischemia.[45]

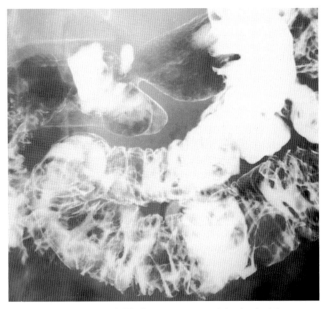

■ **FIGURE 48-19** Amyloidosis. Numerous nodules in the jejunum associated with thickening of the folds. Biopsy demonstrated amyloid deposition in the mucosa and submucosa.

The presence of enlarged low-density mesenteric lymph nodes associated with small bowel wall thickening is highly suggestive of Whipple's disease.[49] Hepatomegaly and ascites can also be present.

In patients with intestinal lymphangiectasia, CT shows diffuse wall thickening of the small bowel. The "halo" sign, characterized by an inner ring of low CT attenuation surrounded by a higher attenuation outer ring, was described for intestinal lymphangiectasia.[50] However, this sign is not specific and can also be seen in patients with Crohn's disease, ulcerative colitis, radiation enteritis, ischemic colitis, and pseudomembranous colitis.[45] CT can also demonstrate the etiology of secondary lymphangiectasia.

Nuclear Medicine

Lymphoscintigraphy using ^{99m}Tc-dextran can be used to localize the bowel segment with intestinal lymphangiectasia.[51] Protein-losing enteropathies can also be diagnosed by the rapid appearance of ^{99m}Tc-labeled albumin within the bowel after intravenous injection.

Classic Sign: Miscellaneous Causes of Bowel Wall Thickening

- "Halo" sign: nonspecific sign characterized by an inner ring of low CT attenuation surrounded by a higher attenuation outer ring in the small bowel wall. This sign may be seen in patients with intestinal lymphangiectasia as well as another colitis or enteritis.

Differential Diagnosis

Clinical presentation of these diseases is usually nonspecific and does not allow a definite diagnosis. GVHD is seen in a highly selective subgroup of patients, and the differential diagnosis for acute GVHD includes gastrointestinal infections, neutropenic enterocolitis, radiation changes, and chemotherapy side effects.

All of the other diseases discussed in this chapter can present as protein-losing enteropathy. Therefore, the differential diagnosis list is very long and includes inflammatory bowel disease, infectious enteritis, neoplasms, and connective tissue diseases. The diagnosis usually requires endoscopic biopsy of the duodenum or jejunum.

Common radiographic findings of these diseases are bowel wall thickening and micronodularity. Additional radiographic differential diagnosis includes infectious enteritis, Crohn's disease, radiation changes, intestinal ischemia, vasculitis, and submucosal hemorrhage (especially when the involvement is focal). The presence of micronodular pattern is more suggestive of Whipple's disease and lymphangiectasia. CT can help in the differential diagnosis in some cases by demonstrating extraintestinal findings such as low-density lymph nodes seen in patients with Whipple's disease.

Treatment

Medical Treatment

Medications are used for prevention of attacks or relief of acute symptoms in patients with eosinophilic enteritis. Corticosteroids are the most commonly used drugs. Azathioprine and other immunomodulators have also been used with some success.

Intensive prophylaxis with immunosuppressive drugs, selective depletion of T lymphocytes from the donor graft, using umbilical cord blood as the source of donor cells, and choosing more closely matched human leukocyte antigen donors have decreased the incidence and severity of GVHD.[52] Methylprednisolone or prednisone in combination with cyclosporine is usually administered in patients with acute GVHD. New drugs and new strategies such as sirolimus and monoclonal antibodies are available now or are in clinical trials that can supplement standard treat-

ment.[52] Primary therapy for chronic GVHD is administration of corticosteroids, usually cyclosporine and prednisone on alternating days.

Treatment of small intestine amyloidosis is supportive until the development of rare complications such as bleeding, ischemia, or obstruction. In secondary amyloidosis, treatment of the underlying cause (neoplasm or chronic infection) is the main focus.

Whipple's disease is treated with antibiotics, usually a combination of penicillin, streptomycin, and trimethoprim-sulfamethoxazole. Depending on the seriousness of the disease, treatment may also include fluid and electrolyte replacement, iron, folate, vitamin D, calcium, and magnesium. Relapses are common during the course of the disease.

Treatment of intestinal lymphangiectasia first starts with the treatment of the underlying cause, which can be inflammation or neoplasm. Supportive therapy includes a low-fat diet rich in medium-chain triglycerides and diuretics.

Surgical Treatment

Surgery is usually not indicated in the treatment of the diseases discussed in this section.

What the Referring Physician Needs to Know: Miscellaneous Causes of Bowel Wall Thickening

- The location and extent of the involved small bowel segments
- Any radiologic findings (intestinal or extraintestinal) that can help to make more specific diagnosis
- Development of complications such as strictures
- Exclusion of neoplasm and acute events requiring surgery

BENIGN NEOPLASMS OF THE SMALL BOWEL

Etiology

The etiology of most small bowel lesions is unknown. Most are thought to be acquired in adulthood, but there are some notable exceptions. There are lesions of congenital origin that may remain asymptomatic until adulthood. These include heterotopic pancreas, heterotopic gastric mucosa, duplication cysts, and myoepithelial hamartoma.

Prevalence and Epidemiology

Less than 2% to 5% of all gastrointestinal tumors originate in the small bowel.[53-57] The duodenum is more commonly involved than the remainder of the small bowel. Carcinoid, which can be benign or malignant, is probably the most common of the small bowel tumors, comprising 25% to 40% of the total. Gastrointestinal stromal tumors (GISTs) can also be either benign or malignant and comprise 9%

of small bowel tumors and are found in both the jejunum and ileum.[58] Of the benign-only tumors, lipomas are the second most common, and most are ileal in location. Excluding the malignant neuroendocrine tumors, benign tumors of neural origin are rare.[59] Most are gangliocytic paragangliomas found in patients with neurofibromatosis type 1 and, when present, are most commonly located in the duodenum. Other rare tumors include hemangiomas, lymphangiomas, hyperplastic polyps, inflammatory fibroid polyps,[60] and hamartomatous polyps associated with Peutz-Jeghers syndrome.[61]

Sporadic lesions have no strong gender or race predilection, although some series report a slight predilection in males. Some lesions are known to occur in association with syndromes, such as neural tumors in neurofibromatosis type 1, adenomas in association with polyposis syndromes (e.g., Gardner's syndrome), and hamartomas associated with Peutz-Jeghers syndrome or generalized juvenile polyposis.

Clinical Presentation

Excluding neurofibromatosis type 1 and congenital lesions that also present in childhood (e.g., duodenal duplications or ectopic pancreatic rests), the average age range at presentation is the 5th to 6th decades. Most benign tumors are clinically silent and may be discovered incidentally; however, large lesions or soft lesions may act as a lead point for an intussusception and cause symptoms of small bowel obstruction. This can occur in up to one third of benign tumors and cause symptoms such as early satiety, nausea, vomiting, constipation, abdominal distention, and a palpable mass. Large tumors may erode the overlying mucosa and cause bleeding (melena, gastrointestinal hemorrhage, pain, and, rarely, perforation). In fact, bleeding as a presenting sign is reported in almost 40% of benign small bowel tumors. Large hemangiomas for example can present with life-threatening hemorrhage. Other nonspecific symptoms may occur, such as anorexia and anemia. For patients with symptoms, diagnosis is usually made in 6 to 12 months from the onset of symptoms.

Peutz-Jeghers Syndrome

This syndrome occurs equally in men and women of all races and is usually diagnosed in the teens or early 20s. The incidence in the United States is 1 in 60,000 to 300,000 live births. There is often a family history of the syndrome. Melanotic macules can be found on the skin and, more importantly, to differentiate them from freckles, on the mucosa of the mouth and anus. The numerous polyps can cause acute intestinal obstruction due to intussusception in about 40% of patients. Other presentations include abdominal pain, gastrointestinal bleeding, and prolapse of a rectal polyp. Less common clinical findings include precocious puberty, gynecomastia in males when associated with a Sertoli cell testicular tumor, and irregular menses in females due to hyperestrogenism from a sex cord tumor). About half of the patients die in their 50s from cancer of the gastrointestinal tract or elsewhere (see Pathology).

Anatomy

The small intestine is divided into the duodenum, jejunum, and ileum. It is important to recognize the differences in the normal fold pattern in different parts of the small intestine, because some causes of benign small bowel disease can affect the fold pattern. The valvulae conniventes or small bowel folds are deeper and more prominent in the jejunum. In the ileum the folds are more shallow, farther apart, and more effaceable with distention or compression.

Pathology

Benign Neoplasms

Adenoma

As with the more well-known adenomas in the colon, small bowel adenomas are neoplastic growths from the mucosa that may be histologically tubular (most common), villous, or mixed tubulovillous with varying degrees of differentiation. Villous adenomas are rare in the small intestine and, when present, are most likely to occur in the duodenum (Fig. 48-20). About 85% of adenomas occur in the duodenum and 10% in the jejunum. Small bowel adenomas are usually solitary but can be multiple. They may occur in association with familial polyposis or Gardner's syndrome and are more likely than tubular adenomas to undergo malignant degeneration.[62] All adenomas of any variety are more likely to be malignant if they are large. Additionally, a unique adenoma occurring in the duodenal bulb (often near the apex of the bulb and always proximal to the ampulla of Vater) is the "Brunner gland adenoma," also classified by some as a "hamartoma," which may actually contain some ductal or stromal elements as well (Fig. 48-21).[63,64]

Lipoma

Lipomas are most common in the colon, and only 5% to 10% of gastrointestinal lipomas occur in the small intestine.[65,66] These are always benign submucosal lesions of mesenchymal origin that begin as sessile lesions but owing to their soft nature may become pedunculated when repeatedly stretched by peristalsis (Fig. 48-22). If that occurs, the lipoma can then serve as a lead point for intussusception. There is a variable amount of fibrous tissue in some lipomas; thus there is a spectrum from pure lipoma to fibrolipoma and fibroma.

Neural Tumors

Neural tumors originate in the submucosa, are usually solitary, and are varied in histologic category. Most are gangliocytic paragangliomas found in neurofibromatosis type 1 and, when present, are most commonly found in the duodenum, often near the ampulla of Vater. Malignant degeneration is rare.

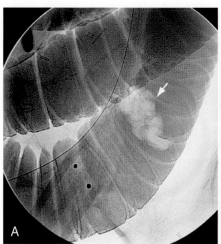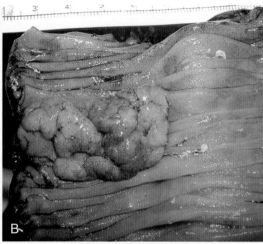

■ **FIGURE 48-20** Villous adenoma. **A,** Spot film from enteroclysis shows a lobulated polypoid mass projecting into the contrast-filled lumen (*arrow*). The surface features are well outlined by the graded compression of the loop, showing a frond-like appearance that corresponds well to the surgical specimen (**B**). This surface feature is characteristic of villous tumors.

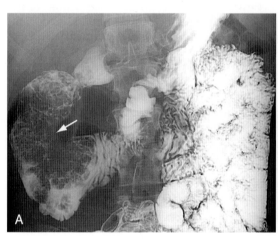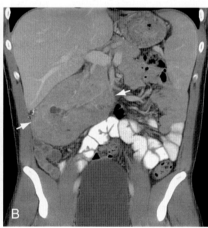

■ **FIGURE 48-21** Duodenal hamartoma. **A,** Spot film from SBFT demonstrates a large intraluminal polypoid mass (*arrow*) in the duodenum. **B,** Coronal CT image shows a large, well-defined, homogeneous, soft tissue mass (*arrows*) in the region of the duodenum. Histopathology revealed the diagnosis as hamartoma.

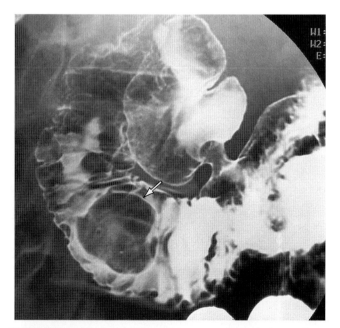

■ **FIGURE 48-22** Lipoma. Double-contrast radiograph shows a large, well-defined, compressible, polypoid mass (*arrow*) in the duodenum.

Vascular Tumors

These account for 5% to 10% of small bowel tumors and are submucosal lesions that come in three main types: capillary, cavernous (most common), and mixed.[67] They may be solitary or multiple and when multiple may rarely be part of a "systemic hemangiomatosis" involving multiple organs. The endoluminal shape may be that of a sessile polyp or a carpet lesion. When left untreated, the hemangiomas may develop phleboliths in venous-like channels and may undergo fibrosis. When not fibrotic, the gross appearance will be red and/or blue, suggesting the vascular nature of the lesions. However, when fibrosed, the lesion will be white and mimic other small bowel masses, in which case, if seen by endoscopy, it could be confused for a malignant mucosal lesion. If sampled, these lesions will bleed profusely.

Leiomyoma and Gastrointestinal Stromal Tumors

Stromal tumors are composed of nests of spindle-shaped cells usually located between the muscularis propria and muscularis mucosa. GISTs display immunochemical characteristics that are distinctive and express the CD117 and/

or CD34 antigen.[68] One third of GISTs occur in the small intestine. Because the overlying mucosa is grossly intact, these have radiologic and pathologic features of a submucosal lesion (Fig. 48-23). Malignant features are usually assessed by judging the number of mitotic cells per high power field, but clinical behavior as a benign or malignant lesion is variable. Nearly all lesions previously classified as leiomyomas and leiomyosarcomas now fall into the classification of GISTs. Rare variants such as leiomyoblastomas may occur.

The gross pattern of growth can be endoluminal or exophytic or both ("dumbbell"). They are often silent clinically and therefore can be large at the time of diagnosis. Large lesions often undergo necrosis and ulcerate.

Polyposis and Polyposis Syndromes

The most common polyposis syndrome to involve the small intestine is Peutz-Jeghers syndrome.[61] This is an inherited autosomal dominant disease (but some sporadic mutations occur). The disease is characterized by hamartomatous polyps with smooth muscle radiating within the polyp (in distinction from the hamartomas of Cronkite-Canada syndrome, which are characterized by cystic dilatation of glands). The polyps nearly always involve small intestine, but fewer polyps are commonly found in the stomach or colon. Mucocutaneous melanotic macules are seen on the hands, face, and lips that look like freckles but also involve buccal and sometimes anal mucosa. The presence of mucosal melanotic macules is essentially diagnostic. The hamartomas have no malignant potential, but sometimes a few adenomas or carcinomas may occur in the gastrointestinal tract (or elsewhere, including the esophagus, stomach, small intestine, colon, pancreas,

lung, breast, uterus, and ovary). There is an association with a mutation on the *STK11* and *CDK7* genes.

Tumor-like Benign Conditions

Heterotopic Pancreas

Congenital pancreatic tissue is known by several names: pancreatic rests, ectopic pancreas, accessory pancreas, and aberrant pancreas.[69] These tissues are distinct by location and vascular supply from the main body of the pancreas. They are surprisingly common in autopsy series but are asymptomatic. About 75% are located in the upper gastrointestinal tract, in which case they can become symptomatic. Symptoms include pain, gastrointestinal bleeding, and other obstructive symptoms. More commonly it is an incidental finding on endoscopy or upper gastrointestinal series in an infant or child. Small 2- to 5-mm submucosal nodule(s) are typically found on the greater curvature of the antrum or first portion of the duodenum, characterized by central umbilication. This characteristic central umbilication is thought to be an aborted form of a "pancreatic duct." Biopsy will reveal pancreatic tissue and confirm the diagnosis. If symptomatic, surgical resection is curative.

Hyperplasia of Brunner Gland

Brunner glands are mucosal and submucosal alkaline-secreting glands, most commonly found in the first and proximal second parts of the duodenum.[70] Brunner gland lesions have been classified as "hamartomas" or "hyperplasia" and by some as "adenomas." They are usually solitary and small but can be multiple (in which case the term *hyperplasia* is most appropriate) (Fig. 48-24). When multiple, they will produce a "cobblestone" pattern that should be distinguished from polyps due to Peutz-Jeghers

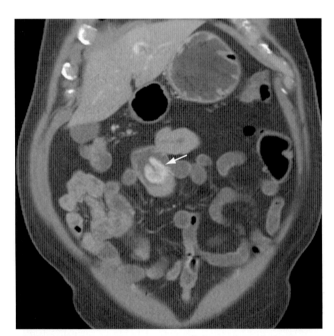

■ **FIGURE 48-23** Benign GIST. Coronal CT enterography image shows an enhancing small mass (*arrow*) within a midjejunal segment. No associated adenopathy, mass, or ascites is present. Surgery confirmed the diagnosis of a benign GIST.

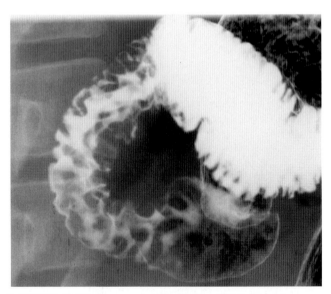

■ **FIGURE 48-24** Brunner gland hyperplasia. Thickening and nodularity of the duodenal folds. Most cases are associated with peptic duodenitis.

syndrome, lymphoid hyperplasia, carcinoid, or metastases. Solitary lesions can rarely be large or pedunculated and as such can cause gastric outlet or duodenal obstruction and gastrointestinal bleeding and be seen on upper gastrointestinal series or CT scans as a smooth intraluminal mass. They comprise 5% of all duodenal masses and are important to differentiate from other duodenal lesions.

Endometriosis

The association of gynecologic complaints and gastrointestinal symptoms in a premenopausal woman should raise the suspicion for endometriosis.[71] Endometriosis can implant on any peritoneal surface; although the cul-de-sac and sigmoid colon are the most commonly involved areas, the ileum and even jejunum or stomach also can be involved. When the small bowel is involved, the terminal ileum is the most common site (Fig. 48-25).[72] The endometrial implants behave similar to any process causing serosal implant on the surface of the bowel and mesentery (e.g., intraperitoneal spread of metastatic disease). They may cause distortion of loops, angulation, crenulation, or frank mechanical obstruction on small bowel series or CT.[72] Alternately, the lesions can present as submucosal masses and rarely act as a lead point for intussusception.

Inflammatory Fibroid Polyp

These are rare benign submucosal lesions that occur in the small intestine and are of unknown cause, although some familial cases have been reported.[73] More often, they are located in the stomach or terminal ileum, but they can occur anywhere in the gastrointestinal tract. About 70%

are pedunculated and therefore may act as a lead point for intussusception, causing pain, but other presentations, including bleeding, weight loss, diarrhea, or anemia, are reported. Most are found incidentally. When these polyps are symptomatic, polypectomy or resection is curative.

Heterotopic Gastric Mucosa

Heterotopic gastric mucosa can occur in a variety of locations, including the esophagus, duodenum, and colon, within a Meckel diverticulum, the gallbladder, and elsewhere.[74,75] The involved mucosa has an appearance similar to that of normal areae gastricae, as seen in the stomach on a double-contrast upper gastrointestinal series (Fig. 48-26). Unlike lymphoid hyperplasia, these lesions are usually angulated. The abnormality can often be seen to be contiguous with the pyloric channel, extending to involve the duodenal bulb for a variable distance. The appearance is essentially pathognomonic.

Lymphoid Hyperplasia

Lymphoid follicles are a normal feature in the small bowel mucosa. When prominent, the term *nodular lymphoid hyperplasia* applies. Nodular lymphoid hyperplasia can be a normal variant particularly in the terminal ileum in children. In adults, small bowel lymphoid follicles can become abnormally prominent due to inflammation or other reasons, such as common variable immunodeficiency, food hypersensitivity, bacterial overgrowth, lymphoma and other lymphoid malignancies, and near a carcinoma (Fig. 48-27). When symptomatic, this variant may be associated with diarrhea, weight loss, and pain.[76]

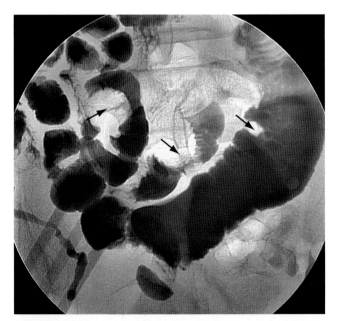

■ **FIGURE 48-25** Endometriosis. Spot film from a dedicated SBFT shows multifocal sites of angulation and tenting consistent with adhesions. At least three distinct sites of eccentric nodular luminal deformity (*arrows*) were present, each with a crenulated concave mural margin. These appeared to be caused by a discrete extraluminal soft tissue process.

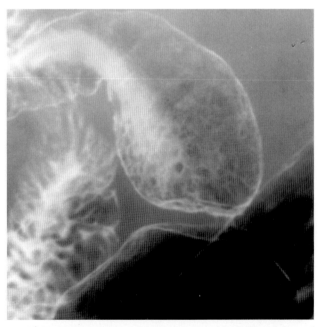

■ **FIGURE 48-26** Heterotopic gastric mucosa. Small filling defects of various sizes are shown on a double-contrast radiograph of the duodenal bulb.

In the duodenal bulb it can become prominent as well, for similar reasons.[74]

Mimics

An inverted Meckel diverticulum can appear as an elongated intraluminal "polyp" on fluoroscopic studies or CT, as can an inverted solitary diverticulum of any type.

Imaging

Solitary Benign Tumors

In addition to the radiographic studies listed below, gastroenterologists may use wireless capsule endoscopy (Fig. 48-28), which can show video images of the small bowel and demonstrate the shape and color of lesions.

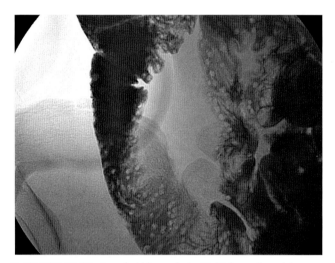

■ **FIGURE 48-27** Lymphoid hyperplasia. Multiple small, nodular filling defects are evenly distributed through several loops of small bowel.

This can be helpful in characterizing vascular lesions such as hemangiomas or varices, which will have a blue or reddish color or characteristic shape.

Radiography

If the lesions are large or cause intussusception, plain radiography may show dilated small bowel with a partial small bowel obstruction. Sometimes, complete mechanical obstruction may be present due to an intussusception.

Rarely, bowel gas may outline polyps or masses that project intraluminally, but this is more likely to be a retrospective observation than a prospective diagnostic feature. When the polyp contour is outlined by gas or on barium studies, the submucosal lesions have a smooth surface with acute angles except for lesions that are ulcerated. The adenomas have features of a mucosal lesion, irregular surface (especially for villous tumors), and acute angles.

Selective angiography of the gastroduodenal artery, superior mesenteric artery, or mesenteric branches can help to show sites of active bleeding and also help control bleeding by direct arterial embolization techniques.

CT

Partial or complete obstruction sites can be identified on CT and help with surgical planning. The size, shape, and density of the mass can be seen if the mass is large enough. CT is better than fluoroscopy in the accurate measurement of lesion size because there is some magnification factor associated with fluoroscopic measurements. The size of a GIST is an important factor in predicting its clinical behavior; larger lesions are more likely to be malignant. Lipomas are seen as fatty masses, which is a diagnostic factor. Most masses are hypodense and show some enhancement on portal venous phase imaging.

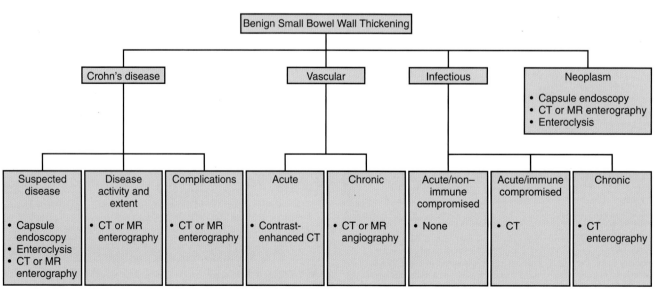

■ **FIGURE 48-28** Imaging algorithm for benign small bowel wall thickening.

Patients with active bleeding can undergo a three-phase CT angiographic technique to identify active extravasation of a contrast agent.

Necrosis of large masses such as GISTs can be seen as areas of heterogeneity and nonenhancement. Tumors with exophytic growth such as GISTs will also exert a mass effect on surrounding structures.

MRI

Similar to CT, MRI can show signs of bowel obstruction, mass size, and location and enhancement characteristics. Most soft tissue tumors, especially GISTs, tend to be isointense relative to skeletal muscle on T1-weighted (T1W) imaging and hyperintense on T2W imaging. Fatty tumors and those with hemorrhage can be best depicted on non-enhanced, non–fat-suppressed T1W spoiled gradient-recalled-echo images.

Ultrasonography

Except in children, ultrasonography is usually not performed in the evaluation of the small bowel.

Nuclear Medicine

In patients who present with signs of brisk gastrointestinal bleeding, a tagged red blood cell scan can help identify the site of bleeding.

PET/CT

PET/CT is not applicable unless malignancy or a neuroendocrine tumor is suspected.

Peutz-Jeghers Syndrome

Radiography

Barium studies show small bowel polyps that are too numerous to count and some gastric and colonic polyps. Both sessile and pedunculated lesions may be seen. Typically, some segments of the small bowel are spared but short segments with carpeting of polyps can be seen. Polyps may cause intussusception or obstruction.

CT

CT can show polyps and sites of intussusception or obstruction. Malignancies complicating the syndrome can be diagnosed and staged with CT.

MRI

Similar features to those of CT can be seen on MRI enteroclysis.

Ultrasonography

Ultrasonography can have a potential role for surveillance of the testes for males with the syndrome, surveillance of the pancreas for tumors, and surveillance of the ovaries for tumors.

PET/CT

Some rare malignancies, such as pancreatic cancer, can be staged with PET/CT.

Imaging Algorithm

Patients known to have Peutz-Jeghers syndrome should undergo surveillance for malignancy of the gastrointestinal tract, breasts, and testes. Imaging is used for initial diagnosis and for the evaluation of complications (Table 48-6).

Differential Diagnosis

The clinical differential diagnosis for partial or complete small bowel obstruction is extensive. In an adult with no prior surgery and no evidence of a primary malignancy, infection, or ischemia, a small bowel tumor should be included in the differential diagnosis.

TABLE 48-6 Accuracy, Limitations, and Pitfalls of the Modalities Used in Imaging for Benign Neoplasms of the Small Bowel

Modality	Accuracy	Limitations	Pitfalls
Radiography	Small bowel series or enteroclysis is best to detect small polyps and masses. Angiography can be done to detect bleeding sites or embolize active bleeding sites.	Limited evaluation of exophytic and extraluminal components of disease	Magnification factor will make lesion measurements less accurate than CT.
CT	Good for large masses, but if done as a "CT enterography" can be as good as a small bowel series or better	Not as good as barium studies in showing mucosal detail and small lesions or ulcerations within lesions	
MRI	Similar to CT	Spatial resolution not as good as CT	
Ultrasonography	Not generally done. May have a role in children		
Nuclear medicine	Not done for detection but can help localize bleeding		
PET/CT	Not applicable for benign lesions, except neuroendocrine lesions		

For patients with a gastrointestinal hemorrhage, the differential diagnosis is also vast. A small bowel tumor may be discovered if CT or a small bowel series or nuclear scintigraphy is used to search for a cause of the bleeding.

Treatment

Medical Treatment

Partial or complete small bowel obstruction is treated with decompression. Patients with anemia and active gastrointestinal bleeding are referred for diagnostic and therapeutic triage.

Surgical Treatment

High-grade obstruction (e.g., small bowel tumor causing intussusception) or a localized active bleeding site not amenable to minimally invasive angiographic embolization may require surgery. Large tumors causing symptoms that might also be malignant may be evaluated for elective resection.

What the Referring Physician Needs to Know: Benign Neoplasms of the Small Bowel

- Ninety percent of benign small bowel tumors are adenomas, GISTs, lipomas, or hemangiomas.
- Lesion location is important for suggesting some uncommon lesions: myoepithelial hamartoma occurs in the stomach or duodenum; Brunner gland polyps are in the first or second portion of the duodenum; inflammatory fibroid polyps occur in the terminal ileum (as can solitary carcinoid); gangliocytic paragangliomas are found near the ampulla of Vater.
- CT is the study of choice for the patient with a partial or complete small bowel obstruction.
- When there is strong indication of a small bowel lesion (e.g., a history of gastrointestinal bleeding in a patient with normal upper and lower bowel studies), consider wireless capsule endoscopy, dedicated small bowel series, or CT enterography (see Fig. 48-28).
- Incidental small lesions seen on CT should be evaluated in the clinical context. In most patients with no known underlying disease, a solitary soft tissue lesion is usually a GIST.
- Fatty lesions are "leave me alone" lesions consistent with lipoma.

KEY POINTS

Crohn's Disease

- Crohn's disease is a chronic disease affecting the entire gastrointestinal system.
- It causes transmural inflammation and presents as discontinuous involvement.
- The aims of imaging in Crohn's disease are early, noninvasive diagnosis, differentiation between active and chronic disease, determination of extent and activity of the disease, and recognition of complications.
- CT and MR enterography/enteroclysis have emerged as effective cross-sectional imaging methods, allowing the detection of intestinal and extraintestinal disease manifestations.

Infectious Causes of Small Bowel Disease

- Imaging is usually not indicated in immune-competent patients with acute enteritis. The diagnosis depends on the findings of biopsy, stool examination, and culture.
- Terminal ileum is most severely affected in *Campylobacter*, *Yersinia*, and *Mycobacterium* infections.
- *Mycobacterium tuberculosis* causes transaxial ulcerations, polyps, and thickening of the folds mostly in the ileocecal region in the early phase.
- In the immunocompromised host, *M. avium* complex, *Cryptosporidium*, and CMV are the most common infective agents causing enteritis.
- Ulcers are typical findings of CMV enterocolitis, and they can be large.
- CT features of typhlitis include segmental bowel wall thickening involving the terminal ileum, appendix, cecum, and ascending colon, pneumatosis coli, and pericolonic fat stranding.

Miscellaneous Causes of Bowel Wall Thickening

- Eosinophilic enteritis most commonly involves the stomach and proximal small bowel and is associated with peripheral eosinophilia.
- Acute GVHD develops within the first 100 days of allogenic bone marrow transplantation.
- CT can show low-density mesenteric lymph nodes in patients with Whipple's disease.
- Thrombocytopenia and low IgA levels are suggestive of intestinal lymphangiectasia in patients with diarrhea and steatorrhea.
- Gastrointestinal system involvement is more common in primary amyloidosis.
- Small bowel and/or rectal biopsy is required for the definitive diagnosis of the above diseases in most patients.

Benign Neoplasms of the Small Bowel

- Small bowel series and CT enterography are excellent studies to detect small bowel polyps and masses.
- The differential diagnosis can be tailored to the location of the lesions and their appearance.
- When numerous small bowel lesions are seen, consider polyposis syndromes or metastatic disease.
- If a lesion is soft enough to change size and shape, it is likely a lipoma, a diagnosis that can be made without biopsy based on CT features of gross fat content. Duplication cysts can also be soft and deformable.
- Demonstration of a phlebolith(s) in a lesion is diagnostic of a hemangioma.
- Tumor size is the best factor to predict benign versus malignant behavior of a GIST tumor, and the lesion is most accurately measured by CT rather than fluoroscopic studies.

SUGGESTED READINGS

Erturk SM, Mortele KJ, Oliva MR, Barish MA. State-of-the-art CT and MRI of the gastrointestinal system. Gastrointest Endosc Clin North Am 2005; 15:581-614.

Fidler J. MR imaging of the small bowel. Radiol Clin North Am 2007; 45:317-331.

Hoeffel C, Crema MD, Belkacem A, et al. MDCT spectrum of diseases involving the ileocecal area. RadioGraphics 2006; 26:1373-1390.

Macari M, Megibow AJ, Balthazar EJ. A pattern approach to the abnormal small bowel: observations at MDCT and CT enterography. AJR Am J Roentgenol 2007; 188:1344-1355.

Maglinte DD. Small bowel imaging—a rapidly changing field and a challenge to radiology. Eur Radiol 2006; 16:967-971.

Maglinte DD, Kelvin FM, O'Connor K, et al. Current status of small bowel radiography. Abdom Imaging 1996; 21:247-257.

Maglinte DD, Lappas JC, Heitkamp DE, et al. Technical refinements in enteroclysis. Radiol Clin North Am 2003; 41:213-229.

Maglinte DD, Sandrasegaran K, Lappas JC. CT enteroclysis: Techniques and applications. Radiol Clin North Am 2007; 45:289-301.

Rubesin SE. Simplified approach to differential diagnosis of small bowel abnormalities. Radiol Clin North Am 2003; 41:343-364.

Wittenberg J, Harisinghani MG, Jhaveri K, et al. Algorithmic approach to CT diagnosis of the abnormal bowel wall. RadioGraphics 2002; 22:1093-1109.

REFERENCES

1. Balthazar CJ. CT of the gastrointestinal tract: principles and interpretation. AJR Am J Roentgenol 1991; 156:23-32.
2. Thoreson T, Cullen JJ. Pathophysiology of inflammatory bowel disease: an overview. Surg Clin North Am 2007; 87:575-585.
3. Crohn DB, Ginzburg L, Oppenheimer GD. Regional ileitis: a pathologic and clinical entity. JAMA 1932; 99:1323-1329.
4. Orholm M, Fonager K, Sorensen HT. Risk of ulcerative colitis and Crohn's disease among offspring of patients with chronic inflammatory bowel disease. Am J Gastroenterol 1999; 94:3236-3238.
5. Fichera A, Michelassi F. Surgical treatment of Crohn's disease. J Gastrointest Surg 2007; 11:791-803.
6. Michelassi F, Balestracci T, Chappell R, Block GE. Primary and recurrent Crohn's disease: experience with 1,379 patients. Ann Surg 1991; 214:230-238.
7. Hamilton SR, Morson BC. Crohn's disease, pathology. In Berk JE (ed). Bockus Gastroenterology, 4th ed. Philadelphia, WB Saunders, 1985.
8. Fleckenstein P, Pederson G. The value of the duodenal intubation method (Sellink modification) for the radiological visualization of the small bowel. Scand J Gastroenterol 1975; 10:423-425.
9. Carlson HC. Perspective: the small bowel examination in the diagnosis of Crohn's disease. AJR Am J Roentgenol 1986; 147:63-65.
10. Kelvin FM, Gedgaudas RK, Thompson WM, et al. The peroral pneumocolon: its role in evaluating the terminal ileum. AJR Am J Roentgenol 1982; 139:115-121.
11. Triester SL, Leighton JA, Leontiadis GI, et al. A meta-analysis of the yield of capsule endoscopy compared to other diagnostic modalities in patients with non-stricturing small bowel Crohn's disease. Am J Gastroenterol 2006; 101:954-964.
12. Paulsen SR, Huprich JE, Hara AK. CT enterography: noninvasive evaluation of Crohn's disease and obscure gastrointestinal bleed. Radiol Clin North Am 2007; 45:303-315.
13. Hara AK, Leighton JA, Heigh RI, et al. Crohn's disease of the small bowel: preliminary comparison among CT enterography, capsule endoscopy, small-bowel follow-through, and ileoscopy. Radiology 2006; 238:128-134.
14. Schreyer AG, Geissler A, Albrich H, et al. Abdominal MRI after enteroclysis or with oral contrast in patients with suspected or proven Crohn's disease. Clin Gastroenterol Hepatol 2004; 2: 491-497.
15. Fidler J. MR imaging of the small bowel. Radiol Clin North Am 2007; 45:317-331.
16. Parente F, Greco S, Molteni M, et al. Imaging inflammatory bowel disease using bowel ultrasound. Eur J Gastroenterol Hepatol 2005; 17:283-291.
17. Pradel JA, David XR, Taourel P, et al. Sonographic assessment of the normal and abnormal bowel wall in nondiverticular ileitis and colitis. Abdom Imaging 1997; 22:167-172.
18. Sayfan J, Wilson DAL, Allan A, et al. Recurrence after strictureplasty for Crohn's disease: it is no more likely than after resection. Br J Surg 1989; 767:335-338.
19. Neurath MF, Vehling D, Schunk K, et al. Noninvasive assessment of Crohn's disease activity: a comparison of ^{18}F-fluorodeoxyglucose positron emission tomography, hydromagnetic resonance imaging, and granulocyte scintigraphy with labeled antibodies. Am J Gastroenterol 2002; 97:1978-1985.
20. Tamboli CP. Current medical therapy for chronic inflammatory bowel diseases. Surg Clin N Am 2007; 87:697-725.
21. Procop GW. Gastrointestinal infections. Infect Dis Clin North Am 2001; 15:1073-1108.
22. Addiss DG, Davis JP, Roberts JM, et al. Epidemiology of giardiasis in Wisconsin: increasing incidence of reported cases and unexplained seasonal trends. Am J Trop Med Hyg 1992; 47:13-19.
23. Ilnyckyj A. Clinical evaluation and management of acute infectious diarrhea in adults. Gastroenterol Clin North Am 2001; 30:599-609.
24. Altekruse SF, Cohen ML, Swerdlow DL. Emerging foodborne diseases. Emerg Infect Dis 1997; 3:285-293.
25. Lee SD, Surawicz CM. Infectious causes of chronic diarrhea. Gastroenterol Clin North Am 2001; 30:679-692.
26. Puylaert JB, Van der Zant FM, Mutsaers JA. Infectious ileocecitis caused by *Yersinia, Campylobacter* and *Salmonella:* clinical, radiological and US findings. Eur Radiol 1997; 7:3-9.
27. Ekberg O, Sjostrom B, Brahme F. Radiological findings in *Yersinia* ileitis. Radiology 1977; 123:15-19.
28. Brodey PA, Fertig S, Aron JM. *Campylobacter* enterocolitis: radiographic features. AJR Am J Roentgenol 1982; 139:1199-1201.
29. Speelman P, Kabir I, Islam M. Distribution and spread of colonic lesions in shigellosis: a colonoscopic study. J Infect Dis 1984; 150: 899.
30. Yao T, et al. Roentgenographic analysis of tuberculosis of the small intestine. Stom Intest 1977; 12:1467-1480.
31. Brombart M, Massion J, et al. Radiologic differences between ileocecal tuberculosis and Crohn's disease. Am J Dig Dis 1961; 6:589-612.
32. Poorman JC, Katon RM. Small bowel involvement by *Mycobacterium avium* complex in patients with AIDS: endoscopic histologic and radiographic similarities to Whipple disease. Gastrointest Endosc 1994; 40:753-759.
33. Barthazar EJ, Martino JM. Giant ulcers in the ileum and colon caused by cytomegalovirus in patients with AIDS. AJR Am J Roentgenol 1996; 166:1275-1276.
34. Ha HK, Ko GY, Yu ES, et al. Intestinal tuberculosis with abdominal complications: radiologic and pathologic features. Abdom Imaging 1999; 24:32-38.
35. Hoeffel C, Crema MD, Belkacem A, et al. Multi-detector row CT: spectrum of diseases involving the ileocecal area. RadioGraphics 2006; 26:1373-1390.
36. Yu J, Fulcher AS, Turner MA, Halvorsen RA. Helical CT evaluation of acute right lower quadrant pain: II. Uncommon mimics of appendicitis. AJR Am J Roentgenol 2005; 184:1143-1149.
37. Hassan I, Brilakis ES, Thompson RL, Que FG. Surgical management of abdominal tuberculosis. J Gastrointest Surg 2002; 6:862-867.
38. Zheng X, Cheng J, Pan K, et al. Eosinophilic enteritis: CT features. Abdom Imaging 2008; 33:191-195.

39. Maizel H, Ruffin JM, Dobbins WO III. Whipple's disease: a review of 19 patients from one hospital and review of the literature since 1950. Medicine 1970; 99:175-205.

40. Schulman A, Morton PCG, Dietrich PE. Eosinophilic gastroenteritis. Clin Radiol 1980; 31:101-104.

41. Baert AL, Sartor K. Radiological imaging of the small intestine. In Gourtsoyiannis NC, et al (eds). Pathology Pertinent to Radiology. Berlin, Springer-Verlag, 2002.

42. Kala Z, Valek V, Kysela P. Amyloidosis of the small intestine. Eur J Radiol 2007; 63:105-109.

43. Herlinger H, Malabsorption. In Gore RM, Levine MS (eds). Textbook of Gastrointestinal Radiology, 2nd ed. Philadelphia, WB Saunders, 2000.

44. Jones B, Kramer SS, Saral R, et al. Gastrointestinal inflammation after bone marrow transplantation: graft versus host disease or opportunistic infection? AJR Am J Roentgenol 1988; 150:277-281.

45. Horton KM, Corl FM, Fishman EK. CT of nonneoplastic diseases of the small bowel: spectrum of disease. J Comput Assist Tomogr 1999; 23:417-428.

46. Herlinger H. Radiology in malabsorption (editorial). Clin Radiol 1992; 45:73-78.

47. Aoyagi K, Iida M, Yao T, et al. Intestinal lymphagiectasia: value of double-contrast radiographic study. Clin Radiol 1994; 49:814-819.

48. Kalantari BN, Koenraad MJ, Cantisani V, et al. CT features with pathologic correlation of acute gastrointestinal graft-versus host disease after bone marrow transplantation in adults. AJR Am J Roentgenol 2003; 181:1621-1625.

49. Rijke AM, Falke TH, de Vries RR. Computed tomography in Whipple disease. J Comput Assist Tomogr 1983; 7:1101-1102.

50. Fakhri A, Fishman EK, Jones B, et al. Primary intestinal lymphangiectasia: clinical and CT findings. J Comput Assist Tomogr 1985; 9:767-770.

51. Puri AS, Aggarwal R, Gupta RK, et al. Intestinal lymphangiectasia: evaluation by CT and scintigraphy. Gastrointest Radiol 1992; 17:119-121.

52. Cutler C, Kim HT, Hochberg E, et al. Sirolimus and tacrolimus without methotrexate as graft-versus-host disease prophylaxis after matched related donor peripheral blood stem cell transplantation. Biol Blood Marrow Transplant 2004; 10:328-336.

53. Ramachandran I, Sinha R, Rajesh A, et al. Multidetector row CT of small bowel tumours. Clin Radiol 2007; 62:607-614.

54. Hoeffel C, Crema MD, Belkacem A, et al. Multi-detector row CT: spectrum of diseases involving the ileocecal area. RadioGraphics 2006; 26:1373-1390.

55. Horton KM, Fishman EK. MDCT of the duodenum: technique and clinical applications. Crit Rev Comput Tomogr 2004; 45:309-334.

56. Wittenberg J, Harisinghani MG, Jhaveri K, et al. Algorithmic approach to CT diagnosis of the abnormal bowel wall. RadioGraphics 2002; 22:1093-1107; discussion 1107-1109.

57. Blanchard DK, Budde JM, Hatch GF 3rd, et al. Tumors of the small intestine. World J Surg 2000; 24:421-429.

58. McGarrity TJ, Kulin HE, Zaino RJ. Peutz-Jeghers syndrome. Am J Gastroenterol 2000; 95:596-604.

59. Sathe PA, Kulkarni VM, Raut AA, et al. Ileal polyposis as manifestation of neurofibromatosis syndrome. Indian J Gastroenterol 2006; 25:159-160.

60. Hirasaki S, Matsubara M, Ikeda F, et al. Inflammatory fibroid polyp occurring in the transverse colon diagnosed by endoscopic biopsy. World J Gastroenterol 2007; 13:3765-3766.

61. Burton MJ, Seery JP, Taylor-Robinson SD, et al. Jejunal intussusception secondary to Peutz-Jeghers type hamartoma diagnosed on angiography. Clin Radiol 1999; 54:476-478.

62. Taylor SA, Halligan S, Moore L, et al. Multidetector-row CT duodenography in familial adenomatous polyposis: a pilot study. Clin Radiol 2004; 59:939-945.

63. Chappuis VS, Vernez M, Denys A, et al. Brunner gland hamartoma: a challenging diagnosis. Pancreas 2006; 33:202-203.

64. Merine D, Jones B, Ghahremani GG, et al. Hyperplasia of Brunner glands: the spectrum of its radiographic manifestations. Gastrointest Radiol 1991; 16:104-108.

65. Oyen TL, Wolthuis AM, Tollens T, et al. Ileo-ileal intussusception secondary to a lipoma: a literature review. Acta Chir Belg 2007; 107:60-63.

66. Metzger PP, Slappy AL, Chua HK. Ileal lipoma. Surg Rounds 2005; 28:84-86.

67. Boyle L, Lack EE. Solitary cavernous hemangioma of small intestine: case report and literature review. Arch Pathol Lab Med 1993; 117:939-941.

68. He LJ, Wang BS, Chen CC. Smooth muscle tumours of the digestive tract: report of 160 cases. Br J Surg 1988; 75:184-186.

69. Gurbulak B, Kabul E, Dural C, et al. Heterotopic pancreas as a leading point for small-bowel intussusception in a pregnant woman. JOP 2007; 8:584-587.

70. Patel ND, Levy AD, Mehrotra AK, Sobin LH. Brunner's gland hyperplasia and hamartoma: imaging features with clinicopathologic correlation. AJR Am J Roentgenol 2006; 187:715-722.

71. Scarmato VJ, Levine MS, Herlinger H, et al. Ileal endometriosis: radiographic findings in five cases. Radiology 2000; 214:509-512.

72. Attar A, Lagorce C. Small bowel obstruction caused by endometriosis. Clin Gastroenterol Hepatol 2007; 5:A30.

73. Wysocki AP, Taylor G, Windsor JA. Inflammatory fibroid polyps of the duodenum: a review of the literature. Dig Surg 2007; 24:162-168.

74. Glick SN, Gohel VK, Laufer I. Mucosal surface patterns of the duodenal bulb. Subject review. Radiology 1984; 150:317.

75. Langkemper R, Hoek AD, Dekker W, Op den Orth JO. Elevated lesions in the duodenal bulb caused by heterotopic gastric mucosa. Radiology 1980; 137:621.

76. Rubio-Tapia A, Hernández-Calleros J, Trinidad-Hernández S, Uscanga L. Clinical characteristics of a group of adults with nodular lymphoid hyperplasia: a single center experience. World J Gastroenterol 2006; 12:1945-1948.

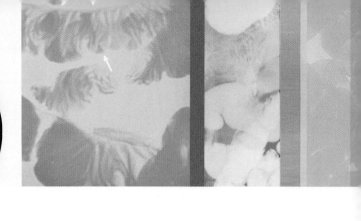

CHAPTER 49

Malignant Neoplasms and Wall Thickening of the Small Bowel

Aytekin Oto, Kirti Kulkarni, and Arunas E. Gasparaitis

Small bowel neoplasms remain a diagnostic challenge for radiologists and clinicians. The small bowel represents 75% of the total length of the gastrointestinal tract and more than 90% of the mucosal surface, but less than 2% of all gastrointestinal malignancies originate in the small bowel.[1] Malignant tumors of the small bowel may arise from the mucosal epithelium, lymphoid tissue, blood vessels, nerves, and muscle. Secondary involvement of the small bowel is more common than primary small intestinal malignancies. Considerable delay in the diagnosis of small bowel malignancies leads to low survival rates. Increased awareness of the small intestine as a potential source of nonspecific abdominal complaints or chronic anemia and the selection of the most accurate diagnostic tests would lead to improvement of a patient's prognosis.[2]

In this chapter both secondary and primary malignancies of the small bowel are reviewed with an emphasis on their imaging findings (Table 49-1).

SECONDARY MALIGNANCIES OF THE SMALL BOWEL

Etiology

Metastases are the most common secondary malignancies of the small bowel. Mechanisms of metastatic seeding to the small bowel include intraperitoneal seeding, direct extension along the fascia or mesenteric attachments, hematogenous spread, and lymphatic extension.[3] The mechanism of spread determines the radiologic appearance. Intraperitoneal spread is the most common mechanism and usually occurs as a result of spread via ascitic fluid. The primary neoplasms are usually gastrointestinal in men and ovarian in women.[4] Direct invasion of the

small intestine is seen from primary colon, pancreas, biliary, ovarian, renal, and adrenal malignancies. Hematogenous spread of primary neoplasms to the small bowel is rare. Melanoma, lung, breast, kidney, and gynecologic cancers are the most common tumors with embolic spread to the small bowel. Lymphatic dissemination to the small bowel plays a small role. A typical example is spread of cecal carcinoma to the terminal ileum by retrograde lymphatic flow after occlusion of the pericecal lymphatic vessels.[5] Melanoma is the extraintestinal malignancy with the greatest predilection to bowel metastasis, and the small bowel is the most common part of the gastrointestinal tract to be affected by metastatic melanoma.[6]

Clinical Presentation

The primary tumor is known in most cases. The complaints are commonly nonspecific, such as abdominal pain, weight loss, anemia, gastrointestinal bleeding, or obstruction. The interval between the diagnosis of malignancy and intestinal obstruction caused by the metastatic disease can vary widely.[7] Intermittent obstruction and anemia can be caused by intussusception, with metastatic lesions serving as a lead point. It is important to consider the possibility of metastatic small bowel lesions in the setting of nonspecific abdominal complaints or chronic unexplained iron deficiency anemia in patients with known malignancies.

Pathophysiology

When the mechanism of spread is direct invasion, the localization of an involved small bowel segment depends on the primary tumor. The infiltration involves a larger segment of small bowel in patients with ovarian cancer,

383

TABLE 49-1   Characteristics of Malignant Neoplasms of the Small Bowel

Lesion	Age	Sex	Distinguishing Clinical History	Distinguishing Clinical Presentation	Imaging Modality of Choice	Distinguishing Imaging Findings	Enhancement Pattern	Additional Findings
Adenocarcinoma	6th-7th decades	M = F	No specific symptoms, high level of suspicion is recommended in patients with long-standing disease, vague gastrointestinal symptoms, and weight loss	Abdominal pain (60%) Obstruction (40%) Gastrointestinal hemorrhage (24%)	Enteroclysis, CT enterography	Partial or complete small bowel obstruction or intussusception on plain film Barium studies: "apple core" lesion, asymmetric wall thickening or infiltrative pattern More in proximal small bowel	Heterogeneous enhancement (hemorrhage, necrosis, or ulceration in 40% of cases)	Local extension, regional abdominal lymphadenopathy, distant metastases
Carcinoid	6th-7th decades	M = F	Asymptomatic or present with carcinoid syndrome (cutaneous flushing, sweating, bronchospasm, abdominal pain, and diarrhea)	Classic carcinoid syndrome	Abdominal CT, CT enterography, nuclear scan	Intussusception on plain film Mesenteric mass on CT scan	Spiculated margins, low attenuation Mass with fat stranding and minimal enhancement Hypervascular liver metastases	Spokewheel or sunburst appearance on CT Encasement of mesenteric vessels leading to ischemia of affected bowel loops Octreoscan study is more sensitive in localizing carcinoids and metastatic disease compared with CT, MRI, or endoscopy.
Lymphoma	Bimodal, <10, >50	M > F	Chronic anemia, weight loss	Abdominal pain, diarrhea, steatorrhea	Abdominal CT or CT enterography	Four patterns of involvement: (1) multiple nodules at multiple sites; (2) single large mass, triggering point for intussusception; (3) infiltrative pattern, presents as asymmetric wall thickening or aneurysmal dilatation of bowel loop; (4) exophytic mass	Low-attenuation soft tissue mass with minimal enhancement	Enlarged lymph nodes in the chest, abdomen, or pelvis Aneurysmal dilatation of the involved bowel loop without obstruction
GIST	5th-6th decades	M > F	Incidental finding on imaging	Bleeding and abdominal pain; directly correlates with size of tumor	CT enterography or small bowel series	Intramural exophytic mass with or without internal calcifications and necrosis Submucosal lesion with smooth surface and acute angle	Circumscribed exophytic low-attenuation mass with heterogeneous enhancement depending on hemorrhage, necrosis	Liver metastases can be hypervascular.
Metastatic disease	After the 5th decade	M = F	History of a primary neoplasm, especially melanoma or gastrointestinal, pancreatic, or ovarian in origin	Gastrointestinal bleeding, increased abdominal pain, bowel obstruction in patients with known neoplasms	Abdominal CT	Diffuse or nodular peritoneal and intestinal wall thickening "Bull's eye" appearance on barium studies Intussusception	Variable	Primary tumor and other metastatic disease

but shorter segments in the case of primary colon carcinoma.[8] Pancreatic tumors and hepatic flexure tumors infiltrate the duodenum, whereas cecal tumors invade the terminal ileum.

Peritoneal fluid has a continuous flow within the anatomic pathways of peritoneal recesses and mesenteric reflections.[9] A primary neoplasm or metastatic lymph node can break into the peritoneal cavity and initiate the peritoneal spread.[10] The most common sites for the lodging and growth of peritoneal spread are the pouch of Douglas, right paracolic gutter, superior aspect of the sigmoid mesocolon, and the terminal portion of the mesentery in the right lower quadrant.[9] The negative pressure under the diaphragm and increased capillary forces make the dome of the liver a common spot for peritoneal deposits. Peritoneal deposits on serosal surfaces adhere through fibrinous exudation and may incite a desmoplastic response.

Pathology

Hematogenous metastases can be solitary or multiple and tend to be submucosal.[11] The masses are usually on the antimesenteric border where the vasa recta end in a rich submucosal plexus and can demonstrate central ulceration due to their limited blood supply.

Lymphatics parallel the arterial blood supply. When the local lymphatics are blocked by the primary tumor, retrograde lymphatic flow can cause the spread of tumor cells into the small bowel. Most commonly involved sites are the terminal ileum and proximal jejunum.

Imaging

Radiography

Direct invasion from another primary tumor usually produces mucosal destruction and narrowing of the lumen without the shouldering of the margins, which is a characteristic of a primary neoplasm (Fig. 49-1).[10] Chronic radiation changes need to be differentiated from secondary invasion. The duodenum is a common segment for secondary invasion and can be invaded by pancreatic, colon, renal, and adrenal tumors.

Peritoneal deposits may be seen as rounded protrusions toward the lumen of the small bowel. Discrete separation of ileal loops, often with a parallel configuration, angulated tethering of mucosal folds on their mesenteric border, and narrowing of loops are suggestive of peritoneal seeding associated with some desmoplastic reaction.[9] Striking angulation and marked fixation of small bowel loops can be seen in primary cancers, causing a significant desmoplastic reaction, such as pancreatic or gastric carcinoma.[9]

Multiple, round, polypoid nodules mostly seen along the antimesenteric border of the small bowel are the most common radiologic finding for hematogenous metastases, especially from a primary of malignant melanoma (Fig. 49-2). The metastatic nodules tend to ulcerate centrally, and, when the lesions are small, ulcerations appear as target lesions ("bull's eye" lesions) with collection of barium at the central ulcers.[12] These nodules can act as a lead point for intussusception. Larger masses may have

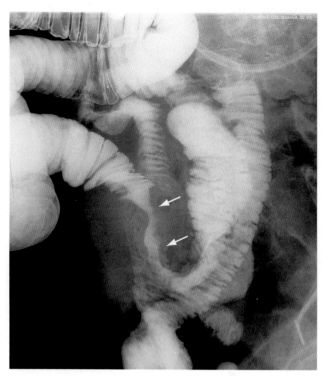

■ **FIGURE 49-1** Direct invasion by bladder cancer. Intramural masses with loop fixation and mucosal tethering of an ileum segment (*arrow*) are causing mild small bowel obstruction.

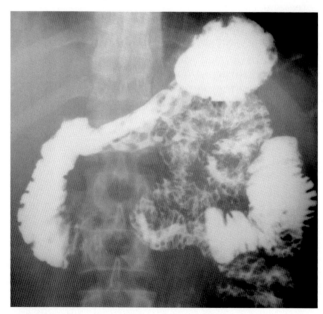

■ **FIGURE 49-2** Hematogenous metastasis from malignant melanoma. Multiple nodular filling defects throughout the stomach and jejunal segments are seen on SBFT. Some of these nodules demonstrate central ulcerations.

large ulcers or cavitations outlined with barium and may have a mass effect on the surrounding small bowel segments.[13] Breast cancer metastases are rare but described as spreading through the submucosa, causing multiple strictures and intestinal obstruction.[14] Metastases from carcinoma of the bronchus and renal cell carcinoma are usually seen as solid or multiple large mesenteric masses with frequent ulcerations.[15]

CT

CT can demonstrate the metastatic lesions in the small bowel wall, mesentery, peritoneal surfaces, and lymph nodes and therefore can give a better idea about the size and extent of the disease. CT can also depict the extension of disease to the surrounding organs. Another advantage of CT is its ability to identify the primary tumor (Fig. 49-3). Intestinal bowel wall or peritoneal thickening (either nodular or plaque-like), mesenteric or omental nodules, and/or fat stranding are the common CT findings in patients with metastases to small bowel segments (Fig. 49-4). Metastases from melanoma manifest as enhancing mural nodules or focal thickening of the intestinal wall (Fig. 49-5).[16]

MRI

MRI can provide a sensitive and accurate depiction of tumor involving the peritoneum and bowel serosa. Fat-suppressed, gadolinium-enhanced MRI is preferred for detection of small peritoneal or mesenteric tumors.[17] Peritoneal tumors are found to be more conspicuous on delayed MR images obtained 5 to 10 minutes after intravenous injection of gadolinium. Even small implants can be depicted on delayed, fat-suppressed, gadolinium-enhanced gradient-echo images.[17]

Ultrasonography

Ultrasonography can be sensitive for detection of serosal, neoplastic deposits along the anterior or lateral abdominal wall when performed with a high-frequency probe but is very limited in depiction of the deposits between the loops or along the posterior wall.[18] The focal thickened wall of the small bowel shows the nonspecific "pseudokidney" sign, which can be seen in both benign and malignant diseases.

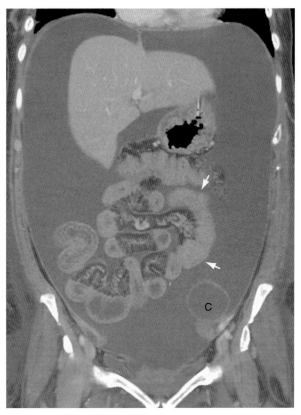

■ **FIGURE 49-4** Peritoneal carcinomatosis in a patient with ovarian cancer. Coronal CT image shows significant malignant ascites and diffuse wall thickening of the small bowel segments (*arrows*) secondary to peritoneal carcinomatosis. Additional cystic peritoneal metastatic mass (c) is seen in the left lower quadrant.

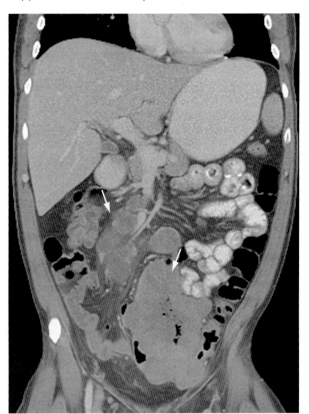

■ **FIGURE 49-5** Malignant melanoma metastasis. Coronal CT image shows multiple soft tissue masses in the small bowel wall and mesentery (*arrows*).

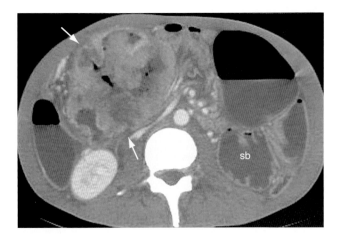

■ **FIGURE 49-3** Primary colon cancer arising from hepatic flexure invading small bowel segments. Axial CT image shows large, heterogeneous mass (*arrows*) invading the small bowel segments in the right upper quadrant. Small bowel segments in the left upper quadrant (sb) are dilated, representing obstruction.

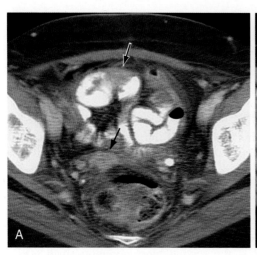 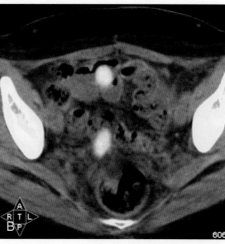

■ **FIGURE 49-6** Peritoneal metastasis from colon cancer on PET/CT. Subtle, peritoneal soft tissue deposits invading small bowel walls on axial CT image (*arrows,* **A**) are more obvious on the PET/CT image (**B**) demonstrating increased FDG uptake.

TABLE 49-2 Accuracy, Limitations, and Pitfalls of the Modalities Used in Imaging of Secondary Malignancies of the Small Bowel

Modality	Accuracy	Limitations	Pitfalls
Radiography	Enteroclysis is very accurate in detecting smaller lesions involving the small bowel wall.	Cannot show mesenteric, peritoneal disease or primary tumor	Radiation enteritis
CT	Very accurate in the detection of relatively larger intestinal lesions and extraintestinal disease	Limited sensitivity in detection of small mucosal or intramural lesions	Undistended bowel
MRI	Slightly more sensitive in depiction of small peritoneal lesions	Limited experience, longer study time, less spatial resolution compared with CT	

PET/CT

Peritoneal metastatic deposits can demonstrate uptake of fluorodeoxyglucose (FDG), and PET/CT may be a useful diagnostic tool when peritoneal biopsy is either unavailable or inappropriate (Fig. 49-6).[19] However, further studies are needed to better determine the role of FDG-PET for evaluation of peritoneal carcinomatosis.

Imaging Algorithm

Small bowel follow-through (SBFT) is noninvasive but relatively insensitive for detection of small intramural deposits and is completely blind to extraintestinal disease.

Enteroclysis can detect small intestinal metastases earlier than CT, but it is an invasive test. With the advances of CT technology, new techniques such as CT enterography or CT enteroclysis have emerged and can evaluate both intestinal and extraintestinal disease (Table 49-2).[20] Therefore, CT is often used as an initial tool for evaluation of abdominal symptoms in patients with known cancer. In cases complicated with bowel obstruction, CT should be the diagnostic test of choice (see Fig. 49-18).

Differential Diagnosis

Symptoms of metastatic disease to the small bowel are very nonspecific; therefore, the clinical differential diagnosis is very wide. Complications related to the treatment (irradiation or chemotherapy) of the primary cancer, bowel ischemia, infection, inflammation, paraneoplastic syndromes, primary gastrointestinal tumors, and other causes of abdominal pain must be considered.

The primary tumor is usually known and helps in determining the diagnosis. Adhesions, metastases, and radiation enteritis are considered in the differential diagnosis of small bowel obstruction in patients with known malignancies. Adhesions usually cause linear compression of the lumen with straight margins. Ileocecal metastatic disease may resemble Crohn's disease. Endometriosis can mimic multiple, small hematogenous metastases. Abdominal tuberculosis can cause peritoneal thickening, mesenteric fat stranding, bowel wall thickening, and adenopathy mimicking metastatic disease. Radiologic differentiation from neoplastic disease may be difficult.

Treatment

Medical Treatment

Medical treatment is aimed specifically against the primary tumor and may consist of hormone therapy, chemotherapy, and targeted biological therapy. There is a large variability in the expected effectiveness of the treatment as well as in the prognosis of patients.[6,7] Obstruction may be

---

Classic Sign: Secondary Malignancies of the Small Bowel

■ Target lesion (bull's eye): central ulceration of the hematogenous metastases, most common in the malignant melanoma metastases.

relieved and the symptoms may resolve after chemotherapy in patients with breast carcinoma.

Surgical Treatment

Surgical treatment of secondary intestinal malignancies aims to relieve the intestinal obstruction and/or to control the metastatic disease.[7] Radiologic demonstration of non-involved small bowel segments significantly contributes to the achievement of both of these targets. An accurate preoperative understanding of the extent of the disease is crucial for surgical planning. The specific anticancer therapy is almost always considered after surgery.

What the Referring Physician Needs to Know: Secondary Malignancies of the Small Bowel

- Knowing if small bowel metastases are present changes the staging, and their presence may cause complications such as intussusception, bleeding, or obstruction.
- Knowing the extent of disease is important for surgical planning and to decide between medical versus surgical treatment.
- Any complications related to metastatic disease should be considered.
- Abnormalities that may have a similar clinical presentation should be excluded.

PRIMARY MALIGNANCIES OF THE SMALL BOWEL

Etiology

The most common malignant primary small bowel neoplasms are small bowel adenocarcinoma, carcinoid, lymphoma, and gastrointestinal stromal tumors (GISTs). Small bowel adenocarcinoma is a rare neoplasm, and the most important risk factor in the development of adenocarcinoma is Crohn's disease. Higher incidence of small bowel adenocarcinoma is also associated with adenomatous polyps, villous adenomas, familial adenomatous polyposis, hereditary nonpolyposis colorectal cancer, celiac sprue, cystic fibrosis, and peptic ulcer disease.[21,22]

Carcinoid tumors originate from the diffuse endocrine system outside the pancreas and thyroid and most frequently occur in the gastrointestinal tract (66.9%), followed by the tracheobronchial system (24.5%).[21] They are frequently associated with specific syndromes such as Zollinger-Ellison syndrome, multiple endocrine neoplasia type 1, carcinoid syndrome, or neurofibromatosis type 1.

The exact etiology of small bowel lymphoma is unknown. Various predisposing factors have been postulated to be responsible for small bowel lymphoma. A few of the predisposing factors include celiac disease, previous extraintestinal lymphoma, immunosuppressed conditions such as human immunodeficiency virus (HIV) infection/AIDS, long-standing systemic lupus erythematosus, Crohn's disease, and post-chemotherapy conditions.

GISTs are CD117-positive mesenchymal tumors thought to originate from interstitial cells of Cajal that are normally part of the autonomic nervous system of the gastrointestinal tract.[23]

Prevalence and Epidemiology

Primary adenocarcinoma of the small intestine accounts for less than 1% of all primary gastrointestinal tumors, with an estimated annual incidence of 0.25 to 0.4 per 100,000 population.[21,22] It predominantly affects the duodenum and jejunum in 42% and 43% of cases, respectively. The ileum is involved in less than 15% of the patients, except in Crohn's disease.[21] The peak incidence is in the sixth and seventh decades of life.

Carcinoid is the second most common small bowel malignancy, representing approximately 25% of all primary small bowel tumors. It most commonly affects the ileum. The comprehensive epidemiologic data on gastrointestinal carcinoids in Western populations are derived from the analysis by Modlin and associates at the National Cancer Institute.[24] The data demonstrate an increase in the incidence of carcinoids over the past 30 years and that 41.8% of gastrointestinal carcinoids occur in the small intestine, followed in decreasing order of frequency by the rectum (27.4%), appendix (24.1%), and stomach (8.7%).[21] The appendix was thought to be the most common location for gastrointestinal carcinoids, but several authors have noted a decreased incidence of appendiceal carcinoids. This observation is probably due to the decreasing rate of appendectomies related to the increasing accuracy of diagnosing inflammatory appendicitis preoperatively.[24] The mean age at the time of diagnosis for all carcinoids is 61.4 years, and the disease occurs equally in men and women. Synchronous or metachronous malignancies occur in 29% of patients with small intestinal carcinoids.

Small bowel lymphoma is the third most common small bowel malignancy, representing 10% to 15% of small bowel malignancies. It can involve any portion of the gastrointestinal tract and predominantly targets the lymphoid follicles. It is most common in the ileum, and most present as intermediate- to high-grade non-Hodgkin's lymphoma; T-cell variants are more often associated with celiac disease. Mediterranean abdominal lymphoma is a variant associated with immunoproliferative small intestinal disease and consists of diffuse lymphomatous infiltration of mucosa and submucosa in long segments of the small intestine.

There is a slight male predominance with bimodal age distribution, with peaks in those younger than the age of 10 and older than the age of 50. Small bowel lymphoma is multifocal in 15% of cases. Increased incidence of small bowel lymphoma was reported among patients with celiac disease.[25]

GIST is the fourth common small bowel neoplasm. It comprises 9% of all small bowel malignant tumors.[26] GISTs rarely involve the duodenum. They occur in the fifth and sixth decades and are more common in males. It is difficult to distinguish benign from malignant GISTs based on radiographic appearance alone.

Clinical Presentation

There is a significant overlap among the clinical presentations of small bowel neoplasms. The clinical presentation and diagnosis of small bowel adenocarcinoma are usually delayed by 6 to 8 months primarily because small bowel carcinomas are not amenable to endoscopic examination when they are distal to the duodenum. Clinical presentation includes abdominal pain in 66%, obstruction in 40%, and gross intestinal hemorrhage in 24% of patients.[22] Especially in patients with long-standing bowel diseases, malignancy should be considered.

Patients with carcinoid tumor can be completely asymptomatic or may present with carcinoid syndrome (cutaneous flushing, sweating, bronchospasm, abdominal pain, and diarrhea) in less than 10% of cases.[27] The syndrome most commonly occurs in patients with ileal carcinoids and hepatic or retroperitoneal metastases.

Patients with small bowel lymphoma can present with chronic anemia, weight loss, fatigue, diarrhea, steatorrhea, or vague dull abdominal pain. A palpable mass can be present in one third of the cases. Acute gastrointestinal bleeding is less common than in small bowel adenocarcinoma, but the risk of perforation is higher.

When small, GISTs can be incidental on medical imaging. As they increase in size, the most common presenting symptom is gastrointestinal bleeding and abdominal pain. Less common symptoms are dysphagia, bowel obstruction, and a palpable mass.

Pathophysiology

Small bowel adenocarcinoma occurs most frequently in the duodenum. Carcinoid tumors are submucosal, are more common in the ileum, and produce a characteristic mesenteric mass through lymphatic spread. Lymphoma of the small bowel could be either a primary small bowel tumor or a manifestation of lymphomatous disease. In cases with primary small bowel lymphoma there is less evidence of mediastinal or peripheral lymphadenopathy or splenomegaly. The mesenteric lymph node involvement is limited to the region of involved bowel. Lymphoma can occur anywhere in the gastrointestinal tract but is more common in the distal small bowel. GISTs are more common in the jejunum and ileum and can be bulky, causing mass effect on adjacent organs with ulceration or necrosis.

Pathology

Grossly, small bowel adenocarcinomas present as solitary, infiltrative, polypoid, or annular obstructing lesions. Single or multiple ulcers can be associated with an infiltrative pattern. Histologically, they are most commonly mucin-secreting adenocarcinomas.

On gross pathologic study, carcinoids are white, yellow, or gray firm nodules that rarely exceed 3.5 cm in the intestinal wall. They can typically present as multiple nodules (30% of cases), exophytic masses, or intramural masses. They may protrude into the lumen as polypoid nodules or classically present as infiltrative fibrous lesions. These are typically slow-growing tumors that may cause

superficial ulcerations and hemorrhage. The metastatic deposits of carcinoid in the lymph nodes, mesentery, and liver vary in size and gross morphology. Extensive involvement of the subserosa and adjacent mesentery stimulates local release of serotonin, which is responsible for the development of desmoplastic reaction. Mesenteric arteries and veins located both near and far from the tumor may be thickened and may result in intestinal ischemia.[28,29]

Small bowel lymphoma is confined to a small bowel segment with regional lymphadenopathy. There is no evidence of hepatic or splenic involvement except by direct tumor extension and mediastinal lymphadenopathy. The peripheral blood smear and bone marrow biopsy could be normal. Small bowel lymphomas are usually diffuse and poorly differentiated and a common site of non-Hodgkin's lymphoma in children.

GISTs can present as exophytic large masses arising from the stromal layer with signs of central necrosis, hemorrhage, and ulceration. They can be characterized as benign, borderline, of low malignant potential, or malignant based on the pathologic appearance.

Imaging

The diagnosis of small bowel neoplasms can be challenging because these tumors are often small, infrequent, and difficult to detect radiographically. Currently, small bowel series and enteroclysis are used for evaluation of small bowel tumors in detecting small lesions. CT is now considered an important modality that helps in detection and staging of disease. Improvement in CT technology, including the introduction of multidetector-row scanners (MDCT) and advanced 3D imaging capabilities have improved interest in utilizing CT routinely to evaluate small bowel neoplasms and to evaluate a source of gastrointestinal bleeding or suspected obstruction, especially if the small bowel series or enteroclysis was negative. MDCT enteroclysis has an overall accuracy of 84.7% for depiction of small bowel neoplasms.[30] Gastroenterologists are routinely using wireless capsule endoscopy to capture video images of the small bowel, which is otherwise difficult to visualize by routine endoscopic procedures. These studies are gaining popularity in recent years and have complemented other radiographic modalities such as CT and MRI. It is routinely performed in patients with gastrointestinal hemorrhage of unknown etiology, anemia of chronic disease, and an obvious mass on CT scan.

Radiography

Plain films of the abdomen are helpful in evaluating partial or complete small bowel obstruction or intussusception as seen in cases of small bowel adenocarcinoma. Contrast radiographic studies are essential in the initial evaluation of small bowel diseases. Barium studies can demonstrate a wide spectrum of findings from "apple core" lesions, asymmetric wall thickening, to a more infiltrative process leading to a malignant stricture subsequently causing small bowel obstruction (Fig. 49-7).

Carcinoids can appear as trigger points leading to intussusception. Small bowel series are helpful in evaluating small polypoid and multifocal nodular appearances of carcinoid (Figs. 49-8 and 49-9). Ulcerations can be well appreciated on small bowel series as barium-filled craters on the surface of the lesion.[31]

In evaluating small bowel lymphoma, small bowel series can show luminal narrowing of the involved segment with loss of mucosal pattern, thickening of the folds, and intraluminal filling defects, possibly with dilatation of the involved segment (Figs. 49-10 and 49-11). Small bowel obstruction is seldom seen. Nodular lesions can vary in size and are irregularly distributed. Widening of the lumen rather than narrowing is noted from circumferential involvement and destruction of the myenteric plexus leading to aneurysmal dilatation (see Fig. 49-11).

SBFT and CT are commonly used to adequately make the diagnosis of GISTs. Small GISTs appear as intramural masses; and when they increase in size, they grow outward from the bowel. Internal calcifications and necrosis, creating a central hypodense cavity that can eventually ulcerate into the lumen of the bowel, may be seen (Fig. 49-12). GISTs can sometimes present with partial or complete small bowel obstruction. The submucosal lesions have a smooth surface with acute angles. The exophytic lesions

can cause significant mass effect on the adjacent bowel loops that can be evident on the plain film. The tumor can directly invade adjacent structures in the abdomen and, if metastatic, can spread to the liver and peritoneum.

CT

CT analysis of small bowel diseases requires meticulous bowel distention because specific attention should be made to the thickness of the intestinal wall, character of the wall, enhancement patterns, and alterations in the surrounding mesenteric fat and vasculature. Intravenous administration of a contrast agent is essential for a

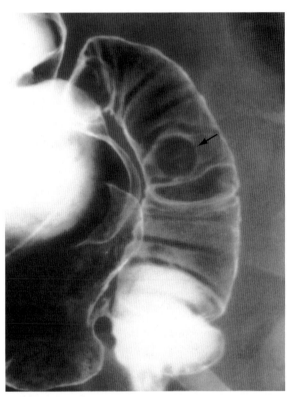

■ **FIGURE 49-9** Carcinoid tumor. Well-defined polypoid lesion in the terminal ileum (*arrow*) is incidentally noted on the peroral pneumocolon study. Surgery confirmed carcinoid tumor.

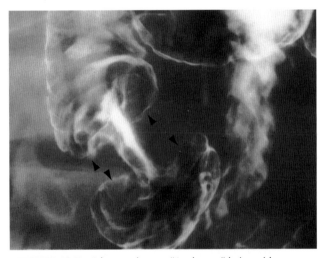

■ **FIGURE 49-7** Adenocarcinoma. "Apple core" lesion with concentric irregular narrowing of the lumen. *Arrowheads* indicate the overhanging edges (shouldering) at both ends of the lesion.

■ **FIGURE 49-8** Carcinoid tumor. **A,** Spot film from enteroclysis reveals irregular narrowing of an ileal segment (*arrow*) with kinking of the lumen and fixation of the loops. **B,** Mesenteric spiculated mass (*arrow*) and desmoplastic reaction in the small bowel mesentery (*arrowheads*) tethering adjacent small bowel loops are better demonstrated on the axial CT image.

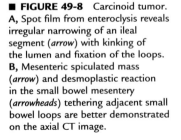
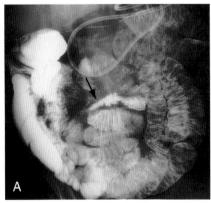
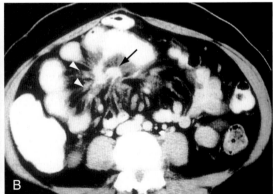

comprehensive CT examination of the small bowel and mesentery, especially when a small bowel neoplasm is suspected.

CT enterography with a negative contrast agent is routinely used to delineate detailed mucosal abnormalities. The high-density oral contrast agents can mix unevenly with gastric and intestinal fluid, resulting in pseudotumors, and also obscure the enhancing bowel wall or enhancing tumors such as carcinoid when the intravenous contrast agent is administered rapidly. Also, if 3D imaging of the small bowel or mesenteric vessels is planned, the use of high-density oral agents will hinder the postprocessing protocol. Therefore, the value of utilizing low-density agents as oral contrast for CT is gaining more popularity.

CT features of malignant small bowel neoplasms include a focal area of wall thickening causing malignant stricture, polypoid intraluminal masses, and "apple core" or infiltrative lesions (Fig. 49-13). Partial or complete small bowel obstruction may be noted. These tumors can demonstrate signs of necrosis, hemorrhage, and, occasionally, ulceration, as seen in 40% of cases.[21] CT staging of small bowel adenocarcinoma is extremely important and is determined by local extension beyond the bowel wall involving adjacent fat or structures, abdominal lymphadenopathy, or distant metastasis in the liver.

Small carcinoids frequently escape radiologic detection, but larger, polypoid lesions may be identified easily by CT. The submucosal carcinoid tumor is seldom identified on CT. Thirty percent of carcinoid tumors are multicentric and can present as multiple nodules and eventually extend into the adjacent mesentery.[32] The CT appearance is characteristically demonstrated as a soft tissue density mesenteric mass, with calcification seen in up to 70% of cases. The mass has spiculated margins, low attenuation, and adjacent fat stranding and occasionally causes encasement of mesenteric vessels, leading to ischemia of the affected bowel loops. Fibrosis in the mesentery may create

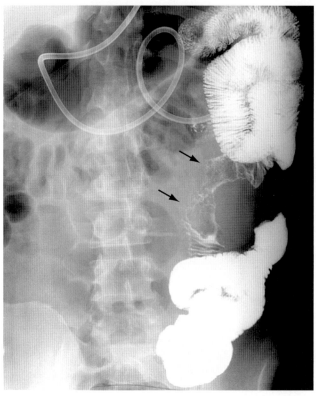

■ **FIGURE 49-10** Small bowel lymphoma. Circumferentially infiltrated lymphoma causing irregular narrowing of a jejunum segment (*arrows*).

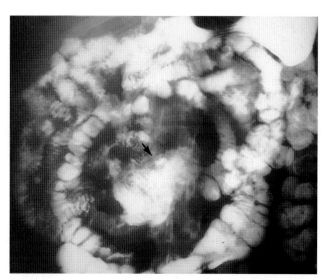

■ **FIGURE 49-11** Small bowel lymphoma. Dilated ileum segment with irregular contours (*arrow*), typical for lymphoma involvement.

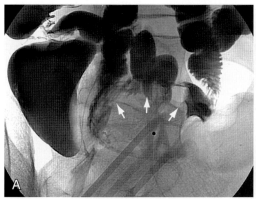

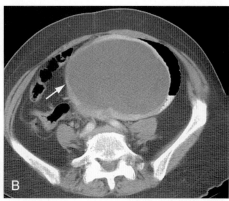

■ **FIGURE 49-12** Malignant GIST. **A,** Spot film from SBFT shows large excavated mass (*arrows*) displacing the adjacent small bowel loops. **B,** Axial CT image demonstrates the large mass (*arrow*) with homogeneously hypodense center.

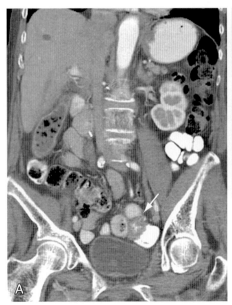

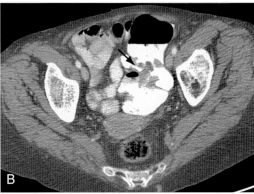

■ **FIGURE 49-13** Adenocarcinoma. Coronal (**A**) and axial (**B**) CT images reveal focal irregular narrowing and concentric wall thickening in an ileum segment (*arrows*) representing adenocarcinoma, which was later confirmed by surgery.

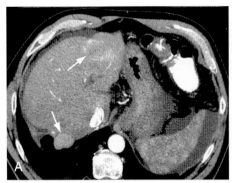

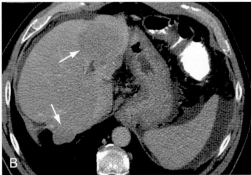

■ **FIGURE 49-14** Carcinoid metastasis in the liver. Focal lesions in the liver (*arrows*) enhancing on the arterial phase image (**A**) and washing out on the delayed phase image (**B**) with residual rim enhancement. These CT findings are consistent with metastatic disease in a patient with known carcinoid tumor.

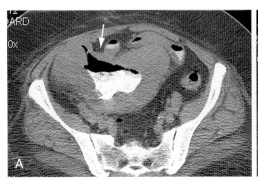

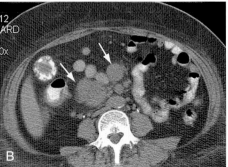

■ **FIGURE 49-15** Lymphoma. **A**, Axial CT image shows a dilated distal small bowel segment (*arrow*) with concentric wall thickening without causing any proximal bowel obstruction. **B**, Another axial image through the abdomen demonstrates multiple enlarged mesenteric lymph nodes (*arrows*).

a "spokewheel" or "sunburst" appearance of mesenteric vessels. Infiltrative tumors can present as asymmetric mural thickening, producing fibrosis and subsequent malignant stricture. At the time of diagnosis, 58% to 64% of patients with small intestinal carcinoids have disease that has spread beyond the intestine to regional lymph nodes or the liver.[21] Carcinoid metastasis to the liver is commonly hypervascular and best seen on the arterial phase imaging (Fig. 49-14).

CT appearance of intestinal lymphoma can be variable.[21] Multiple nodules may be seen within the small

bowel at multiple sites. This pattern is better appreciated on small bowel series.[22] A single large mass of varying size may act as a trigger point for intussusception but less likely is due to the soft nature of these tumors.[23] An infiltrative pattern may present as asymmetric small bowel wall thickening. The tumor infiltrates the muscular layer of the wall and may develop aneurysmal dilatation of bowel loops (50%).[33] An exophytic mass may cause a significant mass effect on the surrounding bowel and visceral structures based on its location. This pattern can simulate adenocarcinoma or GIST (Fig. 49-15). Small bowel lymphoma spreads through direct extension into adjacent organs or hematogenously to the liver. Non-Hodgkin's lymphoma can develop within the small bowel mesentery and encase the mesenteric vessels, seldom causing ischemia of the affected bowel loops owing to the soft nature of the mass. Peritoneal metastasis may also be seen.

Small GISTs (<2 cm) are rarely symptomatic and usually benign; they are often detected incidentally on imaging studies. Large GISTs (>2 cm) usually present as exophytic, well-defined tumors, with necrosis or hemorrhage causing a low-density center (Fig. 49-16).[34] Liver metastasis can appear of low-density or hypovascular on triple-phase imaging studies.

MRI

MRI is not commonly utilized for detection and staging of malignant small bowel neoplasms. However, MR enterography and MR enteroclysis are capable of detecting even small intraluminal neoplasms. MRI can also show peritoneal spread, liver metastasis, and metastatic lymph nodes (Fig. 49-17)

Ultrasonography

Ultrasonography is not routinely performed for small bowel lesions. It can be a good screening tool to look for liver metastases, abdominal lymphadenopathy, or ascites but is less sensitive than CT or MRI.

Nuclear Medicine

A tagged red blood cell scan is helpful in cases of acute gastrointestinal bleeding as a presenting symptom of small bowel adenocarcinoma. Localization of the primary tumor to facilitate surgery is better performed using Octreoscan in patients with carcinoid tumors. Data have shown that an Octreoscan study was positive in 94% of patients with metastatic disease as compared with CT, MRI, and endoscopic procedures.[28] Furthermore, primary carcinoid tumors and metastatic lesions of the small intestine were revealed in 16% and 33% of patients, respectively, and were missed on other imaging procedures (e.g., CT and MRI).[28]

PET/CT

PET may play a role in cases with widespread abdominal lymphadenopathy and liver metastases.

Imaging Algorithm

The current radiologic practice considers CT enterography to be the initial test in acute clinical settings such as

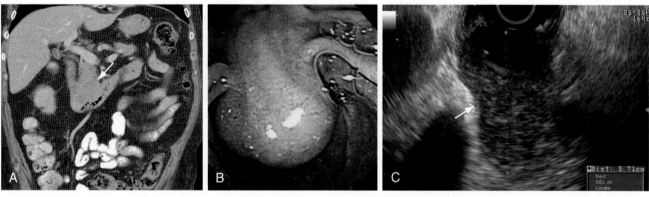

■ **FIGURE 49-16** Malignant GIST. Coronal CT (**A**), endoscopic (**B**), and endoscopic ultrasound (**C**) images show a well-defined, submucosal mass (*arrows*) in the second portion of the duodenum. Endoscopy confirms the normal mucosa. Surgery confirmed the diagnosis of a malignant GIST.

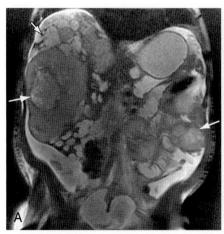
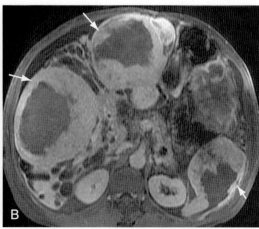

■ **FIGURE 49-17** Peritoneal spread from a malignant GIST. Coronal T2W (**A**) and contrast-enhanced axial T1W (**B**) MR images show multiple, large, peritoneal-based masses (*arrows*) and ascites. On the postcontrast images, the center of the mass lesions do not enhance, indicating necrosis.

TABLE 49-3   Accuracy, Limitations, and Pitfalls of the Modalities Used in Imaging of Primary Neoplasms of the Small Bowel

Modality	Accuracy	Limitations	Pitfalls
Radiography		Small lesion cannot be diagnosed. Metastatic disease cannot be evaluated.	Undistended bowel Uncooperative patient
CT		Small mucosal irregularities can be missed.	Acute setting; patient cannot drink oral contrast agent Compromised renal function; intravenous contrast agent cannot be administered
MRI	Better delineation of size, location, extent of disease; functionality of the bowel seen	Small mucosal irregularities can be missed.	Long scan time, cost, respiratory motion
Ultrasonography		Bowel lesions cannot be well demonstrated.	Low sensitivity and specificity
Nuclear medicine	Surgical planning in carcinoids; metastatic disease evaluation	Can be used in localization and confirmation for the diagnosis of carcinoid tumors	
PET/CT		Mostly used for metastatic disease	

suspected small bowel obstruction or gastrointestinal bleeding (Table 49-3). In patients with highly suspected small bowel neoplasm, SBFT and enteroclysis are reliable tools to come to a preliminary diagnosis (Fig. 49-18). Wireless capsule endoscopy is considered an adequate initial diagnostic test for suspected cases of small bowel neoplasm that cannot be evaluated by routine endoscopy. Radiologic tests can also be helpful to exclude stenosis before the capsule endoscopy and to assist in appropriate localization of the lesion after the procedure. MDCT is essential for disease staging. MR enterography is gaining attention because it is beneficial for surgical planning and ionizing radiation is not involved.

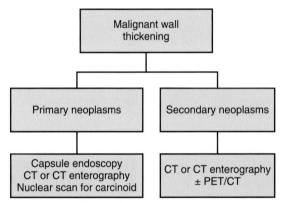

■ **FIGURE 49-18**   Imaging algorithm for malignant wall thickening of the small bowel.

Classic Signs: Primary Malignant Neoplasms of the Small Bowel

- Carcinoid tumors present with a fairly characteristic "mesenteric mass" on CT that can demonstrate spiculated margins, calcifications, hemorrhage, or necrosis (70%).
- Characteristic desmoplastic changes in the mesentery can cause a "spokewheel" appearance of the mesenteric vessels.
- Small bowel lymphoma can cause dilatation of the small bowel, resulting in "aneurysmal dilatation."
- The mesenteric lymph nodes in small bowel lymphoma encase the mesenteric vessels without invading them, leading to the "sandwich" sign.

Differential Diagnosis

Clinical symptoms of malignant small bowel neoplasms are nonspecific and include abdominal pain, gastrointestinal bleeding, and weight loss. It is important to consider small bowel malignancies as a potential cause of these symptoms and to have a high level of suspicion for catching them at an early stage. The clinical differential diagnosis is vast and includes ischemic, infectious, and inflammatory causes and other primary malignancies. Carcinoid tumors may have more specific clinical presentation at later stages when they are metastatic.

Small bowel lymphoma and adenocarcinoma can present as small bowel obstruction or intussusception. Both are difficult to differentiate based on radiologic findings. Focal amyloidomas of the small bowel may have the appearance of an ulcerated annular mass on CT and small bowel series and can mimic small bowel adenocarcinoma.[35] Bulky mesenteric lymphadenopathy favors lymphoma, whereas a metastatic liver lesion favors small bowel adenocarcinoma. The differential diagnosis of lymphoma can include tuberculosis and inflammatory small bowel disease. A mesenteric mass on CT is a characteristic feature of carcinoid tumor. The differential diagnosis includes lymphoma, desmoid tumor, metastases, and mesenteric lymphadenopathy. GISTs are typically extraluminal, causing a mass effect on adjacent structures. Size criteria greater than 2 cm can suggest a malignant GIST over a benign GIST. Frank invasion of mass into adjacent structures is more suggestive of malignant GIST.

Treatment

Surgical removal is the first line of treatment of small bowel adenocarcinoma. Five-year survival rates range from 10% to 60%, with a median around 30%.[36]

Factors associated with poor prognosis are age greater than 75 years, lack of surgical resection, advanced stage, and tumor arising in the duodenum.

Carcinoid tumors with metastatic disease have a positive Octreoscan study. This test is helpful in treatment planning and can predict the response to somatostatin analogs. Patients with positive Octreoscan are treated with somatostatin analogs, which results in control of symptoms (75%), stabilization of tumor growth (71%), or tumor shrinkage (9%).[28] Interferon-alfa can be added to the regimen in patients with no predictable response to maximum somatostatin analogs alone. Surgical excision is the treatment of choice in nonmetastatic carcinoid tumors. Transarterial chemoembolization is the procedure of choice for management of inoperable carcinoid liver metastases and shows promising results with partial response in at least 50% of patients and a mortality rate of 5%.[37]

Guidelines for the treatment of small bowel lymphoma are based on histology and staging of small bowel lymphoma. The treatment may range from resection followed by chemotherapy for local tumor to only chemotherapy in advanced tumors. The chemotherapy regimen depends on the histologic subtype of non-Hodgkin's lymphoma. Radiation therapy is the treatment of choice for initially bulky tumor sites, treatment of residual disease after chemotherapy, or serious local problems.

Current guidelines for the treatment of GISTs are surgery (first line), targeted therapy with imatinib mesylate (Gleevac), a tyrosine kinase inhibitor, or a combination of targeted therapy followed by surgery. The most important factors that decide mode of treatment are small bowel tumor size and cell division rate. Multiple clinical trials with imatinib have demonstrated significant shrinkage in the size of the tumor in more than 50% of cases with locally recurrent or metastatic GISTs. An additional 28% of cases demonstrated disease stabilization on imatinib.[38]

What the Referring Physician Needs to Know: Primary Malignant Neoplasms of the Small Bowel

- Acute presentation: Is there obstruction, perforation, or intussusception?
- Are the lesions synchronous or metachronous?
- After staging of the cancer, is the patient a surgical candidate?
- Is there association with Crohn's disease or a polyposis syndrome?
- What follow-up studies have been done?

KEY POINTS

Secondary Malignant Neoplasms

- There are four different ways of metastatic spread to small bowel: direct extension, peritoneal seeding, hematogenous spread, and lymphatic extension.
- The radiologic appearance changes with the mechanism of spread.
- Ovarian cancer in women and gastrointestinal cancer in men are the most common causes of peritoneal spread.
- Malignant melanoma commonly spreads hematogenously to the small bowel.
- Multiple round masses in the small bowel with central ulcerations are very suggestive of hematogenous metastatic spread.

Primary Malignant Neoplasms
Small Bowel Adenocarcinoma

- Predominantly affects the duodenum and jejunum
- More common in Crohn's disease
- Can present as small bowel obstruction, acute gastrointestinal bleeding, or intussusception

Carcinoid

- Appears more commonly in the ileum; 30% have multifocal disease
- Submucosal location, hypervascular tumor
- Synchronous or metachronous malignancies in 29% of patients with small intestinal carcinoids
- Mesenteric mass seen on CT
- "Spokewheel" appearance of mesenteric desmoplastic reaction caused by local release of serotonin

Small Bowel Lymphoma

- Second most frequent site of gastrointestinal tract involvement by lymphoma
- Most common in the ileum, rare in the duodenum
- Most cases due to non-Hodgkin's lymphoma
- Risk factors: celiac disease, immunocompromised state, chronic lymphocytic leukemia
- Polypoid lesions can cause intussusception.
- Infiltrative lesions can cause aneurysmal dilatation along the antimesenteric segment of the bowel.

GISTs

- Rarely involve the duodenum
- Extraluminal mass; size > 2 cm considered malignant
- Internal calcification; necrosis seen in 70% of cases
- Metastasize to peritoneum and liver but rarely to lymph nodes

SUGGESTED READINGS

Ashley SW, Wells SA Jr. Tumors of the small intestine. Semin Oncol 1988; 15:116-128.

Barclay THC, Schapira DV. Malignant tumors of the small intestine. Cancer 1983; 51:878-881.

Buckley JA, Jones B, Fishman EK. Small bowel cancer: imaging features and staging. Radiol Clin North Am 1997; 35:381-402.

Gourtsoyiannis N, Mako E. Imaging of primary small intestinal tumours by enteroclysis and CT with pathological correlation. Eur Radiol 1997; 7:625-642.

Levy AD, Sobin LH. From the archives of the AFIP: Gastrointestinal carcinoids: imaging features with clinicopathologic comparison. RadioGraphics 2007; 27:237-257.

Maglinte DD, Reyes BL. Small bowel cancer: radiological diagnosis. Radiol Clin North Am 1997; 35:361-380.

Ramachandran R, Sinha R, Rajesh A, et al. Multidetector row CT of small bowel tumours. Clin Radiol 2007; 62:607-614.

Rubesin SE, Gilchrost AM, Bronner M, et al. Non-Hodgkin lymphoma of the small intestine. RadioGraphics 1990; 10:985-998.

Sheth S, Horton KM, Garland MR, Fishman EK. Mesenteric neoplasms: CT appearances of primary and secondary tumors and differential diagnosis. RadioGraphics 2003; 23:457-473.

Wittenberg J, Harisinghani MG, Jhaveri K, et al. Algorithmic approach to CT diagnosis of the abnormal bowel wall. RadioGraphics 2002; 22:1093-1109.

REFERENCES

1. Barelay TH, Schapira DV. Malignant tumors of the small intestine. Cancer 1983; 51:878-881.
2. Fenoglio-Preiser C, Pascal RR, Perzin KH. Tumors of the Intestines. Washington, DC, Armed Forces Institute of Pathology, 1990, pp 175-250.
3. Meyers MA. Dynamic Radiology of the Abdomen: Normal and Pathologic Anatomy. New York, Springer, 1976, pp 37-80.
4. Meyers MA. Clinical involvement of mesenteric and antimesenteric borders of small bowel loops: II. Roentgen interpretation of pathologic alterations. Gastrointest Radiol 1976; 1:49-58.
5. Moffat RE, Gourley WK. Ileal lymph node metastases from cecal carcinoma. Radiology 1980; 135:55-58.
6. Gill SS, Heuman DM, Mihas AA: Small intestinal neoplasms. J Clin Gastroenterol 2001; 33:267-282.
7. Idelevich E, Kashtan H, Mavor E, Brenner B. Small bowel obstruction caused by secondary tumors. Surg Oncol 2006; 15:29-32.
8. Nolan D. Secondary neoplasms. In Gourtsoyiannis NC, Nolan DJ (eds). Imaging of Small Intestinal Tumours. Amsterdam, Elsevier, 1997, pp 193-211.
9. Meyers MA. Mesenteric seeding along the small bowel mesentery. AJR Am J Roentgenol 1975; 123:67-73.
10. Meyers MA. Intraperitoneal spread of malignancies and its effect on the bowel. Clin Radiol 1981; 32:129-146.
11. Walker MJ. Tumors that metastasise to the small intestine. In Nelson RL, Nyhus LM (eds). Surgery of the Small Intestine. Norwalk, CT, Appleton-Century-Crofts, 1987, pp 257-262.
12. Ollila DW, Essner R, Wanek LA, Morton DL. Surgical resection for melanoma metastatic to the gastrointestinal tract. Arch Surg 1996; 131:975-980.
13. Gourtsoyiannis NC, Nolan DJ. Imaging of Small Intestinal Tumours. Amsterdam, Elsevier, 1997.
14. Rees BI, Okwonga W, Jenkins IL. Ileal metastases from carcinoma of the breast. Clin Oncol 1976; 2:113-119.
15. McNeil PM, Wagman LD, Neifeld JP. Small bowel metastases from primary carcinoma of the lung. Cancer 1987; 59:1486-1489.
16. Kawashima A, Fishman EK, Kuhlman JE, Schuchter LM. CT of malignant melanoma: patterns of small bowel and mesenteric involvement. J Comput Assist Tomogr 1991; 15:570-574.
17. Low RN. MR imaging of the peritoneal spread of malignancy. Abdom Imaging 2007; 32:267-283.
18. Maccioni F, Rossi P, Gourtsoyiannis N, et al. US and CT findings of small bowel neoplasms. Eur Radiol 1997; 7:1398-1409.
19. Turlakow A, Yeung HW, Salmon AS, et al. Peritoneal carcinomatosis: role of (18)F-FDG-PET. J Nucl Med 2003; 44:1407-1412.
20. Paulsen SR, Huprich JE, Fletcher JG, et al. CT enterography as a diagnostic tool in evaluating small bowel disorders: review of clinical experience with over 700 cases. RadioGraphics 2006; 26:641-657.
21. Gourtsoyiannis NC, Nolan DJ. Imaging of Small Intestinal Tumours. Amsterdam, Elsevier, 1997.
22. Dabaji BS, et al. Adenocarcinoma of the small bowel: presentation, prognostic factors, and outcome of 217 patients. Cancer 2004; 101:518-526.
23. Sanders KM, Koh SD, Ward SM. Interstitial cells of Cajal as pacemakers in the gastrointestinal tract. Annu Rev Physiol 2006; 68:307-343.
24. Modlin IM, Latich I, Zikusoka M, et al. Gastrointestinal carcinoids: the evolution of diagnostic strategies. J Clin Gastroenterol 2006; 40:572-582.
25. Johnston SD, Watson RG. Small-bowel lymphoma associated with unrecognized celiac disease. Eur J Gastroenterol Hepatol 2000; 12:645-648.
26. Horton KM, et al. Multidetector-row computed tomography and 3-dimensional computed tomography imaging of small bowel neoplasms. J Comput Assist Tomogr 2004; 28:106-116.
27. Song T, Shen J, Guo HC, et al. Imaging and pathological features of gastrointestinal stromal tumors. Zhonghua Zhong Liu Za Zhi 2007; 29:386-390.
28. Nikou GC, Lygidakis NJ, et al. Current diagnosis and treatment of gastrointestinal carcinoids in a series of 101 patients: the significance of serum chromogranin-A, somatostatin receptor scintigraphy and somatostatin analogues. Hepatogastroenterology 2005; 52:731-741.
29. Oberg K. Neuroendocrine gastrointestinal tumours. Ann Oncol 1996; 7:453-463.
30. Pilleul F, Penigaud M. Possible small-bowel neoplasms: contrast-enhanced and water-enhanced multidetector CT enteroclysis. Radiology 2006; 241:796-801.
31. Levy AD, Sobin LH. Gastrointestinal carcinoids: imaging features with clinicopathologic comparison. RadioGraphics 2007; 27:237-257.
32. Modlin IM, Lye KD, Kidd A. Five-decade analysis of 13,715 carcinoid tumors. Cancer 2003; 97:934-959.
33. Gourtsoyiannis NC. Radiologic Imaging of the Small Intestine. New York, Springer, 2002.
34. Sandrasegaran K, Rajesh A. Gastrointestinal stromal tumors: CT and MRI findings. Eur Radiol 2005; 15:1407-1414.
35. Saidane AM, Losada M, Macari M. Focal amyloidoma of the small bowel mimicking adenocarcinoma on CT. AJR Am J Roentgenol 2005; 185:1187-1189.
36. Howe JR, Karnell LH, Menck HR, Scott-Conner C. The American College of Surgeons Commission on Cancer and the American Cancer Society. Adenocarcinoma of the small bowel: review of the National Cancer Data Base, 1985-1995. Cancer 1999; 86:2693-2706.
37. Wallace S, Ajani JA, Charsangavej C, et al. Carcinoid tumors: imaging procedures and interventional radiology. World J Surg 1996; 20:147-156.
38. Demetri GD, von Mehren M, Blanke CD, et al. Efficacy and safety of imatinib mesylate in advanced gastrointestinal stromal tumors. N Engl J Med 2002; 347:472-480.

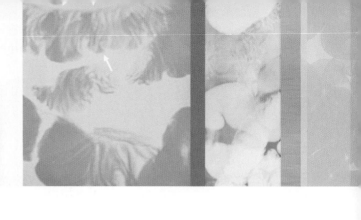

CHAPTER 50

Small Bowel Anomalies and Variants

Michael S. Gee and Sjirk J. Westra

TECHNICAL ASPECTS

Plain Radiography

Plain abdominal radiography is the traditional radiologic method for evaluating patients with abdominal symptoms. Supine and upright anteroposterior abdominal radiographs are obtained. Small bowel can be distinguished from colon in multiple ways radiographically, including smaller size, central location within the abdomen, and the presence of valvulae conniventes, which are thin mucosal folds that extend circumferentially to cross the entire bowel lumen (Fig. 50-1).

Fluoroscopic Methods: Small Bowel Series and Enteroclysis

In a small bowel series (SBS) a barium suspension is administered orally and followed by anteroposterior overhead films obtained every 15 to 20 minutes to monitor contrast transit until the contrast agent passes into the cecum. The patient continues to ingest barium during the course of the examination to maintain opacification of the entire small intestine. Compression views are then obtained once small bowel opacification has been achieved to evaluate individual bowel loops for a pathologic process (Fig. 50-2A).

In enteroclysis an enteral feeding tube is inserted via either an oral or nasal approach with focused instillation of barium solution into the small bowel via gravity drip, rapid injection, or use of a motorized pump.[1] The contrast agent is instilled at a relatively rapid rate to achieve adequate bowel distention. Double-contrast evaluation for mucosal abnormalities can be performed by subsequent administration of methylcellulose or air into the tube.

CT

CT evaluation of the small bowel is typically performed on a multislice helical scanner after administration of oral and intravenous contrast media. Most often, positive oral contrast agents are used to distend and opacify the small bowel lumen. Examples of neutral contrast agents are water, low-concentration barium, methylcellulose, and polyethylene glycol.[2] CT enterography (Fig. 50-3) makes use of large volumes of neutral oral contrast in combination with intravenous contrast and thin-section image acquisition for detection of small bowel disease.[3]

MRI

MRI has superior soft tissue contrast compared with CT and is routinely used in clinical practice for detection of perianal fistulas in patients with inflammatory bowel disease.[4] Historically, MRI evaluation of the small bowel has been limited by poor spatial resolution as well as motion artifacts from intestinal peristalsis and respiration. The recent development of rapid imaging sequences such as turbo spin-echo T2 and steady-state free precession, in combination with parallel imaging techniques, has shortened scan times and made high-resolution bowel MRI possible.[5] MR enterography is analogous to CT enterography and combines bowel distention with negative oral contrast and intravenous gadolinium to provide detailed images of the small bowel wall (Fig. 50-4). An additional advantage of MRI over CT is the lack of ionizing radiation exposure to the patient, which may pose a significant risk of malignancy for patients with chronic bowel diseases likely to require frequent imaging.[6]

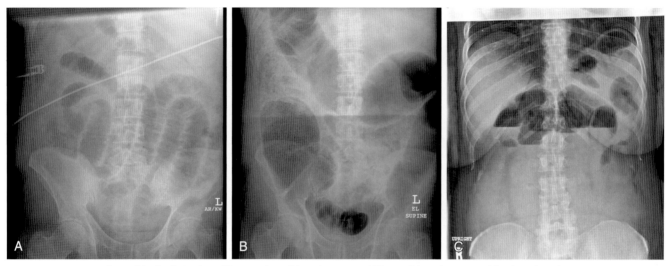

■ **FIGURE 50-1**   Radiographic discrimination of large and small bowel. **A,** Gas within small bowel. **B,** Gas within large bowel. **C,** Upright radiograph demonstrating dilated small bowel loops and air-fluid levels in patient with small bowel obstruction.

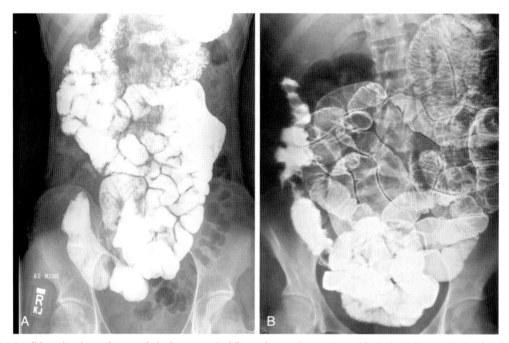

■ **FIGURE 50-2**   Small bowel series and enteroclysis detect terminal ileum changes in a patient with Crohn's disease. **A,** Overhead film from small bowel series shows barium passage to the cecum with strictures and dilation of terminal ileum. **B,** Enteroclysis shows two strictured areas on the terminal ileum.

PROS AND CONS

Pros and cons of commonly utilized small bowel imaging modalities are presented in Table 50-1.

CONTROVERSIES

There is some debate as to whether to use CT or barium fluoroscopy as the initial diagnostic study to detect small bowel pathology. One study compared barium enteroclysis to contrast-enhanced CT for evaluation of small bowel Crohn's disease.[7] Overall sensitivity and specificity were comparable for the two modalities (96%/98% for entero-

clysis vs. 94%/95% for CT). Given the widespread availability, rapid performance of CT relative to fluoroscopy, and lack of invasiveness, CT has become the most commonly used diagnostic modality. Another issue is whether MRI may be able to supplant CT for evaluation of small bowel disease in younger patients, in whom the ionizing radiation risk associated with CT may be significant. One study compared MRI and CT in patients with suspected gastrointestinal pathology and found that MRI was superior for demonstrating abnormal wall thickening and enhancement and worse for spatially resolving individual bowel loops.[8]

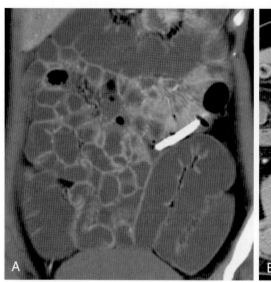

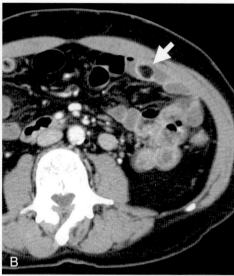

■ **FIGURE 50-3** CT enterography. **A,** Delineation of small bowel mucosa using neutral oral and intravenous contrast. **B,** Small bowel intramural lipoma (*arrow*) demonstrated by CT enterography.

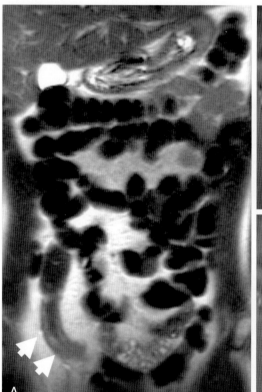

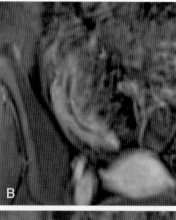

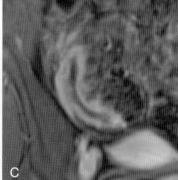

■ **FIGURE 50-4** MRI evaluation of the small bowel. **A,** T2-weighted image demonstrates distal ileal narrowing and wall thickening (*arrows*) in a patient with Crohn's disease. **B** and **C,** Dynamic T1-weighted postcontrast images obtained at 1 (**B**) and 5 (**C**) minutes demonstrate progressive transmural enhancement consistent with active inflammation.

NORMAL ANATOMY

The small bowel is primarily derived from the embryonic midgut, which is the portion of the abdominal gut tube that is supplied by the superior mesenteric artery.[9] The midgut extends from the duodenojejunal junction to the transverse colon. During the 6th week of gestation, the midgut herniates into the umbilicus and rotates 90 degrees counterclockwise about the superior mesenteric artery. During the 10th week of gestation, the midgut retracts into the abdomen and then rotates an additional 180 degrees. The cecum and terminal ileum then descend into the right lower abdomen, leading to the normal small bowel anatomic bowel configuration consisting of a long mesenteric root attached to the ligament of Treitz in the left upper quadrant and the cecum in the right lower quadrant (Fig. 50-5). The duodenum is derived from the foregut and assumes its normal C-shaped configuration in the upper abdomen after gastric rotation.

TABLE 50-1 Pros and Cons of Commonly Utilized Small Bowel Imaging Modalities

	PROS	CONS
Fluoroscopic small bowel series	Initial modality for small bowel evaluation Noninvasive Superior spatial resolution Relatively easy to perform	More operator and patient dependent
Fluoroscopic enteroclysis	Improved sensitivity for subtle disease due to bowel distention Superior spatial resolution	Invasive May require conscious sedation for patient compliance Time consuming
Ultrasonography	No ionizing radiation Ability to correlate imaging findings with area of clinical concern	Air within bowel lumen can confound evaluation Operator dependent Not good screening tool
CT	Noninvasive and widely available Can assess for extraintestinal pathology	Ionizing radiation Risk of reaction to IV contrast agents
MRI	No ionizing radiation Superior soft tissue contrast compared with CT	Long imaging times Expensive and not widely available Patient compliance issues (claustrophobia, respiratory motion)

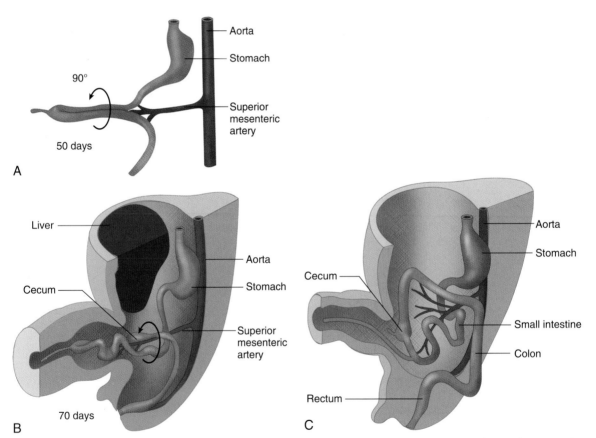

■ **FIGURE 50-5** Normal small bowel embryonic development. **A,** Midgut herniation into the umbilicus accompanied by 90-degree rotation. **B,** Retraction of small intestine into the abdominal cavity accompanied by additional 180-degree rotation. **C,** After inferior cecal migration, small bowel assumes final configuration. *(From Larsen WJ. Human Embryology. New York, Churchill Livingstone, 1993, Figure 9-9.)*

PATHOPHYSIOLOGY

Malrotation and Nonrotation

These intestinal rotational abnormalities are believed to arise during the 10th and 12th weeks of gestation, the time period in which the midgut reenters the abdominal cavity after previously herniating into the umbilical stalk. Malrotation refers to incomplete midgut rotation (<180 degrees) after it reenters the abdomen. This results in abnormal positioning of the duodenojejunal junction (ligament of Treitz) and a shorter than normal mesenteric base of attachment, which predisposes to volvulus.

Nonrotation results from excessive laxity of the umbilical ring that allows the midgut to retract into the abdomen with no additional rotation. The duodenum descends vertically to the right of the superior mesenteric artery, and the ligament of Treitz does not form, causing all of the small intestine to be located to the right of midline. The terminal ileum then crosses to the left of midline, and the entire colon is in the left abdomen. The overall incidence of symptomatic rotational abnormalities is estimated to be 1 in 6000 live births; however, in asymptomatic individuals the overall incidence is likely significantly higher.[10]

Intestinal Atresia

Two types of intestinal atresia occur most commonly. Duodenal atresia is an abnormality of foregut development, whereas ileal atresia arises from abnormal midgut development. Duodenal atresia is congenital obstruction of the second portion of the duodenum that is thought to arise from a defect in recanalization of the primitive gut tube that occurs during the 7th and 8th weeks of gestation.[9] It affects boys more than girls. Down syndrome is present in 30% of cases, and there is also an increased incidence of congenital heart disease, prenatal polyhydramnios, and premature birth.[11] Ileal atresia has been attributed to in-utero ischemia of the developing midgut[12] and is associated with maternal smoking and use of vasoconstricting medications. It is not uncommon for patients with intestinal atresia to have multiple atretic bowel segments.

Intussusception

Intussusception occurs when a portion of intestine becomes telescoped into an adjacent bowel segment. The portion of bowel that becomes prolapsed is termed the *intussusceptum,* whereas the portion of bowel that contains the intussusceptum is termed the *intussuscipiens.* Intussusception leads to venous congestion and bowel wall edema that, if left undiagnosed, leads to bowel ischemia and infarction. The large majority of cases are ileocolic, in which the distal ileum telescopes within the ascending colon. The typical age at presentation is between 6 months and 2 years of age, and in this age group the intussusception is usually idiopathic. In other cases, there is a pathologic small bowel mass that serves as a lead point for the intussusception. These cases usually present in children younger than age 6 months or older than 3 years of age. Causes of a pathologic lead point include Meckel's diverticulum, lymphoma, midgut duplication cyst, Henoch-Schönlein purpura, intestinal polyps, and cystic fibrosis.[13] Intussusception occurs less frequently in adults, comprising 5% of total cases. Adult intussusception is frequently transient, occurring more proximally in the small bowel compared with children (enteroenteric) and often discovered incidentally. Systemic conditions such as celiac disease and Crohn's disease are associated with transient nonobstructing intussusception.[14] In adults, intussusception with a pathologic lead point is most often due to a bowel mass that is either benign or malignant.

Internal Hernias

Internal hernias involve protrusion and trapping of small bowel loops through defects within the peritoneum or mesentery. Most commonly these hernias are congenital defects, although acquired hernias can occur as a result of surgery, trauma, or inflammation. The overall incidence of all abdominal internal hernias is 0.2% to 0.9% based on autopsy series.[15] The most common internal hernias are paraduodenal hernias, which comprise over 50% of all internal hernias.[16] Left paraduodenal hernias are caused by a defect in the descending colonic mesentery known as the fossa of Landzert, through which jejunal loops pass. Right paraduodenal hernias are caused by a defect in the ascending colonic mesentery known as the fossa of Waldeyer. Other types of hernias are more rare, including pericecal (13%), lesser sac (8%), and transmesenteric (8%). Lesser sac hernias enter the lesser peritoneal sac through the foramen of Winslow, which is normally protected by the transverse colon and greater omentum. Paracecal hernia occurs when a loop of ileum migrates posterior to the cecum during cecal descent after midgut rotation. Transmesenteric hernia occurs through a defect in the small bowel mesentery that can extend anywhere from the ligament of Treitz in the left upper quadrant to the cecum in the right lower quadrant.

Meckel's Diverticulum

Meckel's diverticulum is the most common congenital intestinal anomaly and is present in approximately 2% of the population.[17] The vitelline (omphalomesenteric) duct is a communication between the embryonic midgut and the yolk sac that normally involutes by week 9 of gestation. A Meckel diverticulum arises from incomplete obliteration of the ileal terminus of this duct. It is a true diverticulum arising from the antimesenteric border of the small bowel, usually within 100 cm of the ileocecal valve, and often can be several centimeters in length. The blood supply is via the vitelline artery, which arises from an ileal branch of the superior mesenteric artery. Sixty percent of Meckel's diverticula are lined by heterotopic tissue, most commonly gastric mucosa.[18]

IMAGING

Malrotation and Nonrotation

Although patients with midgut rotational abnormalities can become symptomatic at any age, the vast majority develop symptoms within the first month of life,[10] such as bilious vomiting. Both malrotation and nonrotation predispose to midgut volvulus due to reduction in length of the small bowel mesentery. The shortened mesenteric stalk can twist about itself more easily, leading to vascular compromise and intestinal ischemia. Intestinal obstruction in patients with malrotation can also be caused by Ladd's bands, which are fibrous stalks of peritoneum that extend between the cecum and abdominal wall. During malrotation, these bands can traverse and cause obstruction of the second portion of the duodenum. Volvulus typically presents clinically as acute severe abdominal pain associated with bilious vomiting. Other symptoms can include abdominal distention or lower gastrointestinal bleeding. Lesser degrees of mesenteric twisting that do not produce frank ischemia can produce episodic crampy abdominal pain and vomiting. Nonrotation is less commonly associated with obstruction and volvulus than malrotation because the mesenteric attachment is typically broader.[19] Most patients with nonrotation are identified incidentally in asymptomatic patients being evaluated for another pathologic process.

Radiography

Abdominal radiographs in asymptomatic patients typically appear normal but may show abnormal distribution of small and large bowel over the abdomen (Fig. 50-6B). In patients with volvulus, dilated proximal small bowel loops may be identified if bowel obstruction is significant.

Barium upper gastrointestinal series is the diagnostic study of choice to diagnose a rotational abnormality. Normally, the third and fourth portions of the duodenum cross to the left of midline and ascend to the level of the duodenal bulb. The position of the duodenojejunal junction (ligament of Treitz) is used to diagnose rotational anomalies based on these anatomic landmarks. In rotational abnormalities the distal duodenum does not reach these landmarks and instead crosses back toward the right (see Fig. 50-6A). A small bowel follow-through with contrast passage to the cecum is then able to discriminate between malrotation and nonrotation (see Fig. 50-6B). Midgut volvulus on small bowel series is manifest as a "corkscrew" appearance to the distal duodenum and proximal jejunum in the mid abdomen (see Fig. 50-6C). Bowel lumen proximal to this is usually dilated.

CT

CT is not typically required to diagnose rotational anomalies. Although not formally tested, CT may be comparable to an upper gastrointestinal series for diagnosis of malrotation, by combining the ability to assess bowel position with the ability to demonstrate reversal of the superior mesenteric vessel relationship.

Ultrasonography

Ultrasound can demonstrate reversal of the normal anatomic relationship of the superior mesenteric vessels, with the superior mesenteric vein located to the left of the superior mesenteric artery. The superior mesenteric artery is considered anatomically constant, whereas the position of the superior mesenteric vein reflects bowel positional anatomy.

Imaging Algorithms

1. An abdominal radiograph
2. Barium upper gastrointestinal series

Classic Signs: Malrotation and Nonrotation

- Reversal of superior mesenteric artery and vein on ultrasonography or CT
- Rotational abnormality on an upper gastrointestinal series: abnormal position of ligament of Treitz
- Corkscrew appearance of small bowel on small bowel series: midgut volvulus
- Bowel obstruction at level of the second portion of duodenum: obstructing Ladd band with malrotation

---

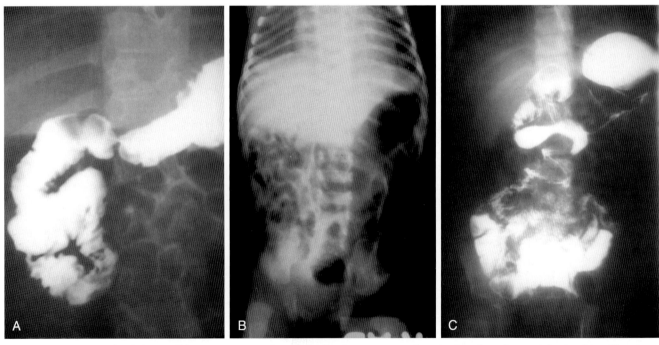

■ **FIGURE 50-6** Rotational abnormalities. **A,** Upper gastrointestinal series demonstrates malrotation based on abnormal duodenojejunal junction. **B,** Abdominal radiograph demonstrating nonrotation. **C,** "Corkscrew" appearance of small bowel volvulus.

Intestinal Atresia

Patients with intestinal atresia typically present with signs of obstruction in the first day of life. Symptoms include bilious vomiting, abdominal distention, and failure to pass meconium.

Radiography

Plain abdominal radiographs are helpful in a patient presenting with bowel obstruction to indicate the level of obstruction (high vs. low). Duodenal atresia will present as a high obstruction, with an air-filled, dilated stomach and proximal duodenum (Fig. 50-7A, the "double bubble" sign), and absence of distal bowel gas. Other causes of high intestinal obstruction in a neonate would include duodenal web, annular pancreas, and midgut volvulus. In contrast, ileal atresia will present as a low obstruction (see Fig. 50-7B), with multiple dilated, air-filled bowel loops in the abdomen. An upright or lateral decubitus film may demonstrate air/fluid levels within the distended bowel. Other causes of low intestinal obstruction would include Hirschsprung's disease, meconium ileus, and small left colon/meconium plug syndrome.

For duodenal atresia, a plain radiograph demonstrating the double bubble is sufficient for preoperative diagnosis. If bowel gas is seen distally, an upper gastrointestinal series can be considered to rule out a duodenal stenosis or web or, in rare cases, demonstrate duodenal atresia in which air and contrast can bypass the atretic bowel via the pancreaticobiliary system.

For ileal atresia, a contrast enema is typically the next step to exclude other causes of low intestinal obstruction. The colon will appear diffusely reduced in caliber (the so-called "microcolon" appearance) owing to lack of enteric contents passing through. However, long-segment Hirschsprung's disease and meconium ileus may also present as microcolon, and the critical finding for ileal atresia is a complete obstruction to the retrograde contrast passage in the collapsed small bowel that is distal to the atresia (see Fig. 50-7C).

Ultrasonography

A minority of cases of duodenal atresia are diagnosed prenatally with ultrasound. Polyhydramnios is observed from the fetal inability to swallow amniotic fluid. Prenatal ultrasonography can demonstrate a sonographic double-bubble sign of dilated, fluid-filled viscera in the upper abdomen corresponding to stomach and proximal duodenum, as well as paucity of bowel loops lower down in the abdomen.

Imaging Algorithms

1. Abdominal radiograph
2. Upper gastrointestinal series for upper gastrointestinal obstruction with bowel gas distally, to demonstrate causes other than duodenal atresia (duodenal stenosis/web, duplication cyst, malrotation/volvulus)
3. Contrast enema for lower obstruction to differentiate between ileal atresia and meconium ileus

---

Classic Signs: Intestinal Atresia

- Double bubble: dilated stomach and proximal duodenum on abdominal radiography or prenatal ultrasonography, indicative of duodenal atresia
- Microcolon and obstruction to retrograde contrast filling in the collapsed distal ileum on contrast enema: indicative of ileal atresia

---

Intussusception

The classic clinical triad of acute abdominal pain, hematochezia ("currant-jelly stool"), and palpable abdominal

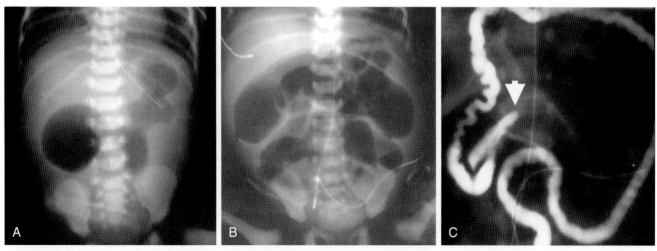

■ **FIGURE 50-7** Intestinal atresia. **A,** Abdominal radiograph demonstrating "double bubble" sign of duodenal atresia. **B,** Abdominal radiograph showing bowel gas pattern characteristic of a low intestinal obstruction such as ileal atresia. **C,** Contrast enema in patient with ileal atresia demonstrating "microcolon" as well as contrast cutoff at point of atretic ileum (*arrow*). Note dilated air-filled small bowel loops proximally to atresia.

mass is very specific for intussusception but only present in the minority of cases.[20] Other presenting symptoms include bilious vomiting, irritability, and intermittent crying.

Radiography

The most common radiographic sign of intussusception is a soft tissue mass in the right abdomen (Fig. 50-8A). Associated small bowel obstruction may also be present. A specific but infrequently observed radiographic finding is the "target sign."[21] The target sign is a soft tissue mass containing internal concentric areas of lucency corresponding to invaginated mesenteric fat or air within the intussusceptum. The use of abdominal radiography as a screening tool for intussusception is primarily to exclude other causes of abdominal pain such as adynamic ileus or lower lobe pneumonia. If there is a high clinical suspicion of intussusception, abdominal radiographs are also useful to evaluate for complications such as bowel obstruction and perforation.

Once the diagnosis of intussusception has been established, fluoroscopic reduction using air or water-soluble contrast is considered the primary therapeutic intervention.[22] It combines a high rate of technical success with avoidance of open surgery. Pneumatic reduction in particular has gained widespread acceptance recently because of ease and rapidity of performance, higher reduction rates compared with hydrostatic reduction, and avoidance of contrast contamination of the peritoneum in the rare case of iatrogenic perforation. Major contraindications to fluoroscopic reduction are free intraperitoneal air and signs of peritonitis. A catheter is introduced into the rectum, and air is insufflated under fluoroscopic guidance. Insufflation pressures are carefully monitored to minimize risk of bowel ischemia or perforation. Imaging during insufflation should demonstrate the "meniscus sign" corresponding to the interface between air-filled bowel and the soft tissue filling defect of the intussusception apex (see Fig. 50-8B). Successful reduction should result in resolution of this filling defect and vigorous retrograde reflux of air into the ileum. Published

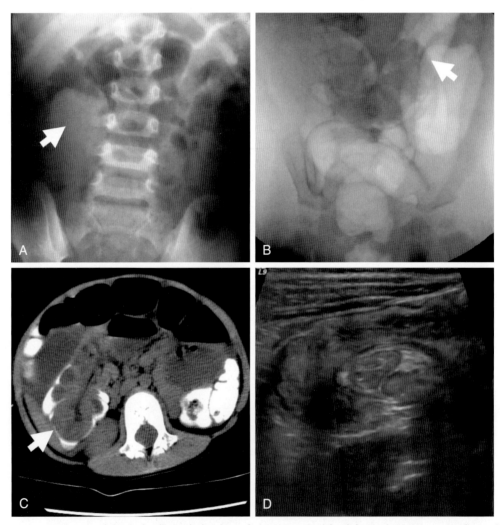

■ **FIGURE 50-8** Intussusception. **A,** Abdominal radiograph showing soft tissue mass in right abdomen (*arrow*) corresponding to intussusception. **B,** Pneumatic reduction showing "meniscus sign" (*arrow*) of interface between intussusceptum and adjacent air-filled colon and air dissecting around intussusceptum ("coiled spring sign"). **C,** CT with rectal contrast shows bowel-within-bowel appearance of intussusception. **D,** Ultrasound image shows "crescent-in-donut sign" of intussusception imaged transversely.

success rates for fluoroscopic reduction range from 80% to 95%.[22]

CT

CT is able to demonstrate a bowel-within-bowel appearance of intussusception with mesenteric prolapse (see Fig. 50-8C), as well as associated small bowel obstruction and free intraperitoneal air, with great accuracy.[23] Because of ionizing radiation exposure, CT is typically reserved for cases in which the plain radiograph and ultrasound image findings are indeterminate. CT may also be useful in cases of intussusception in older children, in which an underlying pathologic lead point is suspected.

Ultrasonography

Ultrasonography is a preferred modality for evaluation of intussusception, with multiple studies demonstrating a sensitivity and specificity of 88% to 100%.[21] Intussusception is seen sonographically in the transverse plane as bowel containing multiple concentric echogenic rings (sonographic target sign). The "crescent-within-donut" sign may be seen corresponding to prolapsed intussusceptum surrounded by its echogenic mesentery (see Fig, 50-8D).[21] Free intraperitoneal fluid in the paracolic gutter often accompanies intussusception. Sonographic signs, such as the presence of fluid within the intussusception or lack of color Doppler signal within the intussuscepted bowel wall, have been postulated to indicate bowel ischemia.[23] However, currently there is still debate concerning their significance.

Imaging Algorithms

1. Abdominal radiograph
2. Ultrasonography
3. Pneumatic reduction

Classic Signs: Intussusception

- Soft tissue mass on plain radiograph, with or without target appearance from trapped mesenteric fat
- Meniscus: abdominal radiograph or pneumatic reduction showing interface between intussusceptum and distal bowel gas
- Crescent-in-donut: ultrasound transverse plane showing intussusceptum surrounded by mesentery
- Coiled spring: air or contrast outlining of intussusceptum during fluoroscopic reduction

---

Internal Hernias

The most common clinical presentation of internal hernias is acute small bowel obstruction due to mechanical obstruction of herniated bowel loops. The severity of symptoms can be highly variable depending on the degree of spontaneous reducibility of the hernia and the presence or absence of incarceration. A typical clinical presentation is episodic periumbilical pain associated with recurrent

bowel obstruction (nausea, vomiting, abnormal bowel sounds, palpable abdominal mass).[16]

Radiography

Plain film radiography can demonstrate dilated small bowel loops if there is obstruction. The localized distribution of the abnormal bowel loops can be suggestive of an internal hernia.

Barium small bowel series can be used to better define the abnormal location of distended bowel loops. Other features seen on small bowel studies include crowding of small bowel loops within the hernia sac and absent or abnormal peristalsis.[24] Of note, barium studies are usually contraindicated in the emergent setting if there is a risk of bowel perforation.

CT

CT has emerged as the preferred imaging modality for evaluation of potential internal hernias.[16] Advantages include rapid image acquisition, 3D bowel evaluation, identification of secondary vascular and mesenteric anatomic alterations that accompany internal hernias, and assessment for ischemic changes in herniated bowel. In a right paraduodenal hernia, the normal duodenojejunal junction is absent and the herniated bowel loops cause anterior displacement of the superior mesenteric artery (Fig. 50-9A and 9D). In a left paraduodenal hernia, the herniated bowel loops typically are located between the stomach and pancreas and cause anterior displacement of the inferior mesenteric vein (see Fig. 50-9B and 9E). Lesser sac hernias are characterized by abnormal bowel loops in the left upper quadrant passing posterior to the gastrohepatic ligament and the stomach. Transmesenteric hernias are the most variable in appearance and can occur anywhere in the peritoneal cavity, although they tend to occur more often in the right mid abdomen (see Fig. 50-9C and F).[24]

Imaging Algorithms

1. Plain radiographs
2. CT

Classic Signs: Internal Hernias

- Focally dilated loops of small bowel localized to one side of abdomen
- Associated displacement of mesenteric vessels toward site of herniation

---

Meckel's Diverticulum

Although many people with Meckel's diverticula are asymptomatic, the majority of symptomatic patients present before age 2 with symptoms of small bowel obstruction. Inflammation or enterolith formation within the diverticulum can cause pain in the right lower quadrant and mimic appendicitis. Complications of Meckel's

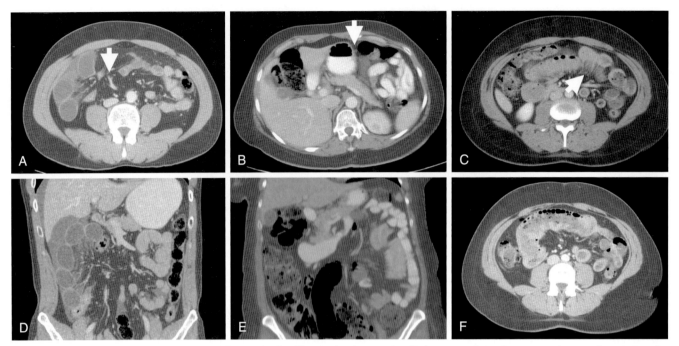

■ **FIGURE 50-9** Internal hernias. **A** and **D**, Right paraduodenal hernia showing anterior displacement of superior mesenteric artery (*arrow*). **B** and **E**, Left paraduodenal hernia showing anterior displacement of inferior mesenteric vein branches (*arrow*). **C** and **F**, Transmesenteric hernia showing anterior displacement of bowel and mesenteric vessels through mesenteric defect (**C**, *arrow*) with mechanical obstruction of small bowel upstream of the hernia (**F**).

diverticula include hemorrhage, diverticulitis, small bowel obstruction, intussusception, and diverticular herniation into the inguinal canal (Littre hernia). Diverticula are more often symptomatic if they contain ectopic gastric mucosa, possibly related to increased risk of hemorrhage and diverticulitis.

Radiography

Plain radiographic findings are often nonspecific. Dilated right lower quadrant small bowel loops can occasionally be identified if there is associated small bowel obstruction. Occasionally the diverticulum can be seen radiographically in the right lower quadrant if it contains either air or an enterolith.

Small bowel series or enteroclysis is rarely able to demonstrate a Meckel diverticulum due to its small size and rapid emptying of contrast. The diverticulum would appear as a blind-ending sac arising from the antimesenteric border of the ileum.

Angiography may be able to diagnose an occult Meckel diverticulum. The vascular supply to a Meckel diverticulum is a persistent vitelline artery, which can sometimes be seen angiographically as an elongated vessel originating from the main superior mesenteric artery or an ileal branch. It often is seen heading toward the right lower quadrant without sending branches to adjacent ileal arteries.[25] Additionally, Meckel's diverticula with gastric mucosa are more prone to hemorrhage, which can appear angiographically as a dense contrast blush at the end of the persistent vitelline artery (Fig. 50-10A).

CT

Meckel's diverticulum is difficult to distinguish from normal small bowel unless there is associated inflammation or bowel obstruction (see Fig. 50-10B). There are some data suggesting that CT enterography[3] may be more sensitive than conventional CT for diagnosing Meckel's diverticula owing to improved small bowel wall resolution.

Nuclear Medicine

Technetium pertechnetate scintigraphy can be used to detect Meckel's diverticula containing ectopic gastric mucosa. Nuclear scintigraphy with ^{99m}Tc-pertechnetate can be helpful for diagnosing Meckel's diverticula with gastric mucosa. Pertechnetate accumulates within mucin-secreting cells of the ectopic gastric mucosa. A Meckel diverticulum typically appears as a fixed focus of increased tracer activity in the right lower quadrant or mid abdomen that demonstrates progressive tracer accumulation and fading with a time course comparable to that of the stomach (see Fig. 50-10C).[26]

Imaging Algorithms

1. Abdominal radiograph
2. Technetium pertechnetate scintigraphy
3. CT
4. Angiography

See also Table 50-2.

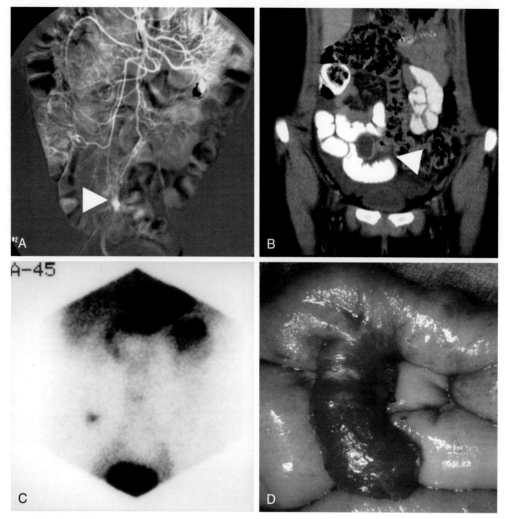

■ **FIGURE 50-10**   Meckel's diverticulum. **A,** Angiogram demonstrating focal contrast extravasation at the end of the vitelline artery (*arrow*) in a bleeding Meckel diverticulum. **B,** CT demonstrates a Meckel diverticulum containing fluid within its blind end (*arrowhead*). **C,** Technetium pertechnetate scintigraphy demonstrates a gastric mucosa–containing Meckel diverticulum in the right lower quadrant. **D,** Intraoperative photograph of Meckel's diverticulum shows an inflamed, hyperemic appearance.

TABLE 50-2   Accuracy, Limitations, and Pitfalls of the Modalities Used in Imaging of Small Bowel Anomalies and Variants

Modality	Accuracy	Limitations	Pitfalls
Radiography	Limited availability of studies directly comparing accuracy rates of different imaging modalities for detecting small bowel pathology	Poor soft tissue contrast	
CT		Ionizing radiation exposure	Risk of adverse reaction to iodinated contrast
MRI		Temporal and spatial resolution; expensive, long scan times	Inability to perform study in patients with claustrophobia or cardiac pacemakers
Ultrasonography		Operator dependence, air within bowel lumen limits evaluation	
Nuclear medicine		Limited utility for evaluating small bowel pathologic processes other than Meckel's diverticulum	May miss Meckel's diverticula without ectopic gastric mucosa
PET/CT		Not routinely used in small bowel diagnosis other than malignancy	Positive oral contrast can occasionally cause PET attenuation correction artifacts

Classic Signs: Meckel's Diverticulum

- Blind-ending sac on antimesenteric side of distal ileum
- Focus of increased tracer activity in right abdomen on technetium pertechnetate scintigraphy that accumulates tracer similar to stomach
- Vitelline artery on angiography: nonbranching vessel derived from the superior mesenteric artery heading to right lower quadrant

What the Referring Physician Needs to Know

- Evaluation of the small bowel typically is part of a general workup for causes of abdominal pain, with abdominal radiographs serving as the initial diagnostic examination.
- Barium studies (small bowel series and enteroclysis) have historically been the primary small bowel diagnostic examination but have mostly been replaced by CT in recent years.
- Advantages of multidetector CT include widespread availability, fast scan times, high spatial resolution in multiple imaging planes, and ability to assess for extraintestinal complications of disease.
- In children, ultrasonography and MRI are being increasingly utilized for small bowel evaluation due to the potential ionizing radiation risk associated with CT.

KEY POINTS

- Malrotation and nonrotation: abnormal embryonic midgut rotation predisposes to volvulus and small bowel ischemia. The upper gastrointestinal series is the diagnostic test of choice.
- Intestinal atresia: caused by embryonic bowel canalization defect or ischemia. Duodenal atresia causes a high obstructive pattern on radiographs, diagnosed by plain radiography or an upper gastrointestinal series. Ileal atresia causes a low obstructive pattern on radiographs, diagnosed by contrast enema.
- Intussusception: a portion of intestine becomes telescoped into an adjacent bowel segment, increasing the risk of bowel ischemia. Ultrasonography is the most reliable diagnostic test, followed by pneumatic reduction under fluoroscopic guidance.
- Internal hernia: bowel herniation through a defect in the mesentery can cause intermittent bowel ischemia. CT is the preferred modality for detection.
- Meckel's diverticulum: a remnant of persistent omphalomesenteric duct can become obstructed and inflamed. Nuclear scintigraphy and CT are primary diagnostic modalities.

SUGGESTED READINGS

Daneman A, Navarro O. Intussusception. I. A review of diagnostic approaches. Pediatr Radiol 2003; 33:79-85.

Martin LC, Merkle EM, Thompson WM. Review of internal hernias: radiographic and clinical findings. AJR Am J Roentgenol 2006; 186:703-717.

Gore RM, Levine MS. Textbook of Gastrointestinal Radiology, 2nd ed. London, WB Saunders, 2000.

Gosche JR, Vick L, Boulanger SC, Islam S. Midgut abnormalities. Surg Clin North Am 2006; 86:285-299.

REFERENCES

1. Maglinte DD, Lappas JC, Kelvin FM, et al. Small bowel radiography: how, when, and why? Radiology 1987; 163:297-305.
2. Young BM, Fletcher JG, Booya F, et al. Head-to-head comparison of oral contrast agents for cross-sectional enterography: small bowel distention, timing, and side effects. J Comput Assist Tomogr 2008; 32:32-38.
3. Paulsen SR, Huprich JE, Fletcher JG, et al. CT enterography as a diagnostic tool in evaluating small bowel disorders: review of clinical experience with over 700 cases. RadioGraphics 2006; 26:641-657; discussion 657-662.
4. Szurowska E, Wypych J, Izycka-Swieszewska E. Perianal fistulas in Crohn's disease: MRI diagnosis and surgical planning: MRI in fistulizing perianal Crohn's disease. Abdom Imaging 2007 Mar 3; Epub ahead of print.
5. Fidler J. MR imaging of the small bowel. Radiol Clin North Am 2007; 45:317-331.
6. Brenner DJ, Elliston CD, Hall EJ, Berdon WE. Estimates of the cancer risks from pediatric CT radiation are not merely theoretical: comment on "point/counterpoint: in x-ray computed tomography, technique factors should be selected appropriate to patient size. against the proposition." Med Phys 2001; 28:2387-2388.
7. Mako EK, Mester AR, Tarjan Z, et al. Enteroclysis and spiral CT examination in diagnosis and evaluation of small bowel Crohn's disease. Eur J Radiol 2000; 35:168-175.
8. Low RN, Francis IR. MR imaging of the gastrointestinal tract with i.v. gadolinium and diluted barium oral contrast media compared with unenhanced MR imaging and CT. AJR Am J Roentgenol 1997; 169:1051-1059.
9. Larsen WJ. Human Embryology. New York, Churchill Livingstone, 1993, p 479.
10. Gosche JR, Vick L, Boulanger SC, Islam S. Midgut abnormalities. Surg Clin North Am 2006; 86:285-299, viii.
11. Kimura K, Loening-Baucke V. Bilious vomiting in the newborn: rapid diagnosis of intestinal obstruction. Am Fam Physician 2000; 61:2791-2798.
12. Louw JH, Barnard CN. Congenital intestinal atresia; observations on its origin. Lancet 1955; 269:1065-1067.
13. Navarro O, Daneman A. Intussusception. III. Diagnosis and management of those with an identifiable or predisposing cause and those that reduce spontaneously. Pediatr Radiol 2004; 34:305-312; quiz 369.
14. Kim YH, Blake MA, Harisinghani MG, et al. Adult intestinal intussusception: CT appearances and identification of a causative lead point. RadioGraphics 2006; 26:733-744.
15. Ghahremani GG. Internal abdominal hernias. Surg Clin North Am 1984; 64:393-406.
16. Takeyama N, Gokan T, Ohgiya Y, et al. CT of internal hernias. RadioGraphics 2005; 25:997-1015.

17. Elsayes KM, Menias CO, Harvin HJ, Francis IR. Imaging manifestations of Meckel's diverticulum. AJR Am J Roentgenol 2007; 189:81-88.

18. Matsagas MI, Fatouros M, Koulouras B, Giannoukas AD. Incidence, complications, and management of Meckel's diverticulum. Arch Surg 1995; 130:143-146.

19. Filston HC, Kirks DR. Malrotation—the ubiquitous anomaly. J Pediatr Surg 1981; 16:614-620.

20. Daneman A, Alton DJ. Intussusception: issues and controversies related to diagnosis and reduction. Radiol Clin North Am 1996; 34:743-756.

21. del-Pozo G, Albillos JC, Tejedor D, et al. Intussusception in children: current concepts in diagnosis and enema reduction. RadioGraphics 1999; 19:299-319.

22. Daneman A, Navarro O. Intussusception. II. An update on the evolution of management. Pediatr Radiol 2004; 34:97-108; quiz 187.

23. Ko HS, Schenk JP, Troger J, Rohrschneider WK. Current radiological management of intussusception in children. Eur Radiol 2007: 17:2411-2421.

24. Martin LC, Merkle EM, Thompson WM. Review of internal hernias: radiographic and clinical findings. AJR Am J Roentgenol 2006; 186:703-717.

25. Brown RL, Azizkhan RG. Gastrointestinal bleeding in infants and children: Meckel's diverticulum and intestinal duplication. Semin Pediatr Surg 1999; 8:202-209.

26. Mettler FA, et al (eds). Essentials of Nuclear Medicine Imaging, 5th ed. Philadelphia, Saunders, 2006.

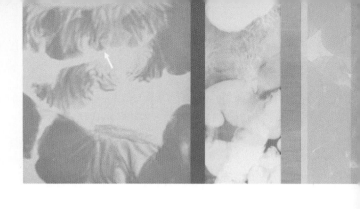

51

Conventional Imaging of the Colon and Rectum

Sunit Sebastian, Pardeep Mittal, Keerthana Kesavarapu, Todd Fibus, and William Small

TECHNICAL ASPECTS

Before the advent of cross-sectional imaging techniques, the double-contrast enema examination was the foremost radiologic method for the evaluation of the colon to detect mucosal lesions and precancerous polyps. The performance of a diagnostic high-quality double-contrast barium enema examination is an art form and requires skillful maneuvering of the patient and the barium pool with optimal use of fluoroscopy. In this chapter, we discuss the principles and techniques required for the performance of a safe and accurate double-contrast barium enema examination.

Single-Contrast Barium Enema Examination

A single-contrast examination can be performed very easily and quickly and is preferred in patients who are immobile, elderly, or incontinent.[1] The findings of single-contrast barium enema are less accurate than those of the double-contrast examination for detection of small polypoid lesions and for evaluation of inflammatory bowel disease (Fig. 51-1).[2]

Double-Contrast Barium Enema Examination

Attention to the clinical history of the patient is vital to tailor the examination according to the particular case in question. Barium enema examination should be performed 1 week after a recent polypectomy, mucosal cautery, or large forceps biopsy to avoid the risk of colonic perforation.[3,4]

Bowel Preparation

Rigorous colonic cleansing plays a vital role in the performance of an optimal diagnostic barium enema examination. Several colon cleansing regimens have been described.[5-7]

A standard bowel preparation is outlined in Table 51-1. The magnesium citrate keeps the feces semisolid, and the bisacodyl tablets stimulate colonic evacuation. Contraindications for the standard bowel preparation include bedridden patients, postoperative patients, patients with diabetes and hypothyroidism, and patients taking opiates.

Barium Suspension: Viscosity and Density

The barium suspension that is used to obtain adequate mucosal coating can be referred to as the radiologist's "paint."[8] A barium suspension of suitable viscosity will perform the following actions:

- Scrub colonic mucus and residual feces into the barium pool
- Adhere to mucosal surface for a sufficient amount of time to take radiographs
- Reabsorb residual water in the colon

Optimal density of the barium suspension ensures coating of the mucosal surface with a thin layer of barium and does not obscure lesions in the barium pool. Thus, a medium-viscosity and medium-density barium suspension is used.

Hypotonizing Agent

Glucagon, 1 mg, is administered intravenously and slowly over a 30- to 60-second period. Intestinal hypotony

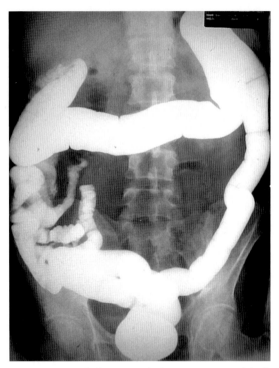

■ **FIGURE 51-1** Single-contrast barium enema: normal findings.

TABLE 51-1 Suggested Outline for Bowel Preparation

On the day before the study:

1. Twenty-four hours of clear liquids for breakfast, lunch, and dinner
2. Plenty of liquids or water between meals to maintain hydration
3. 16 oz of magnesium citrate at 5 PM
4. Four bisacodyl tablets at 8 PM

On the day of the examination: Nothing by mouth

facilitates colonic distention and reduces muscular tone to avoid spasms or peristaltic contractions.[9]

Procedure

Before starting the study the radiologist should confirm that the patients have complied with the preparation protocol. A preliminary abdominal radiograph is not usually necessary but may be obtained to ensure adequacy of the bowel preparation.[10] The procedure may need to be rescheduled with additional bowel cleansing if there is significant fecal residue in the colon. The radiologist should allay any apprehensions of the patient by explaining the study methodology and answering questions.

Digital Rectal Examination

A rectal examination before insertion of the enema tip is recommended to determine the course of the anal canal and check for inflammatory conditions or unsuspected rectal masses and rectal sphincter tone.[11] However, a rectal examination increases patient discomfort and prolongs examination time.

Rectal Catheter Insertion

The patient lies in a recumbent, left side down position. A thin layer of lubricant is applied on the external surface of the anus and the rectal catheter tip,[12] and the catheter is gently inserted into the anal canal. After the catheter tip passes the anal canal, it is directed posteriorly to parallel the course of the sacrum. If the rectal tone is good, the patient is encouraged to hold the barium. Balloon insufflation is performed only in patients who are leaking barium or air out of the anal canal.

Technique Tips:

● Rectal balloon inflation, if used, should be performed only after the rectum has been outlined by barium.
● Contraindications for inflating rectal balloons include suspected colitis, a history of pelvic radiation or colitis, suspected rectovaginal fistula, or Crohn's disease.[13]

Glucagon

Glucagon, 1 mg, can be administered intravenously to help prevent colonic spasm, enabling a more comfortable double-contrast examination of the colon. It also allows the radiologist to insufflate more air into the colon.[14]

Barium Instillation

The patient is placed in a prone position, and barium is slowly instilled into the colon by opening the tube only partially. Once a full column of barium has reached the descending colon, the tube is fully opened. The radiologist turns the patient 360 degrees at least once or twice to wash and coat the colon and displace barium pools from the colonic segments under evaluation. The patient is turned to the prone position to advance the barium into the midtransverse colon. The flow of barium across the mucosal surface must be carefully observed while the patient is turning to demonstrate superficial lesions. The distal rectum is then drained of the barium by dropping the barium bag to the floor and using gravity, to avoid creation of bubbles when air is insufflated into the rectum.

Technique Tip:

● Rapid distention and filling of the rectum will cause spasm of the physiologic sphincter at the rectosigmoid junction and increase the patient's urge to defecate.

Air Insufflation

Air is used to accelerate the movement of barium across the transverse colon and into the ascending colon. Air is insufflated by squeezing the bulb gently, thus insufflating air into the rectum. Rapid air insufflation is very uncomfortable and will cause rectosigmoid spasm with air or barium evacuation. Insufflation in one position only causes air to rise to the most nondependent area and causes patient discomfort. The patient is turned right side down to fill the proximal transverse colon and then turned into the supine position to fill the posteriorly located hepatic flexure.

The enema tip can be removed after an adequate amount of barium and air has been instilled into the colon, providing physical relief to the patient and allowing better evaluation of the distal rectum. The enema tip may need to be left in place in patients who are expelling gas and in patients who may need additional air to visualize the terminal ileum (e.g., patients with Crohn's disease).

Technique Tips:

- Air insufflation should be performed only after the barium has passed the splenic flexure of the colon.
- Avoid rapid air insufflations and always turn the patient in different obliquities to redistribute the air.

Radiographic Documentation: Spot Films and Overhead Views

Complementary radiologic projections are obtained to evaluate all colonic segments while continuously following the patient in different positions. Twelve to 14 spot films and 4 to 5 overhead films are obtained.[15] The routine sequence of images obtained in a double-contrast barium enema study is suggested in Table 51-2. However, a flexible approach is more practical for obtaining films depending on the position of the barium and comfort of the patient (Fig. 51-2).

Technique Tips:

- Spot films of the sigmoid colon are obtained before barium reaches the ascending colon. If barium refluxes through the ileocecal valve, the sigmoid colon may be partly obscured by barium in the distal ileum.
- Obtain views with the enema tip out of the rectum to avoid missing distal rectal lesions.
- Women should be instructed to manually elevate their left or right breast out of the radiation field during the evaluation of the splenic flexure or hepatic flexure, respectively. Breast elevation decreases radiation expo-

sure to the breast and prevents the breast shadow from overlying the splenic or hepatic flexure.
- Anterior cecal masses may need to be evaluated by spot films with the patient prone.
- Visualization of the appendix and terminal ileum can be facilitated by the examiner by applying compression with gloved fingers in either the erect or recumbent, left posterior oblique position.
- Postevacuation fluoroscopic spot films may be obtained with suspected fistulas or extraluminal collections associated with diverticulitis.

Erect Views

The erect position is useful for imaging the hepatic and splenic flexures and an elevated sigmoid colon. However,

TABLE 51-2 Sequence of Images Obtained in a Double-Contrast Barium Enema Evaluation

Spot Radiograph	Patient Position
Rectum (enema tip in)	Prone, left lateral
Rectum with air (enema tip out)	Supine, right lateral view
Proximal sigmoid colon	Left posterior oblique, prone
Distal sigmoid colon	Right posterior oblique, supine
Proximal descending colon	Erect
Distal descending colon	Recumbent right posterior oblique
Splenic flexure	Erect right posterior oblique
Hepatic flexure	Erect left posterior oblique
Proximal ascending colon	Prone or Trendelenburg left posterior oblique
Lateral wall of cecum	Supine, left posterior oblique
Medial wall of cecum	Supine, right posterior oblique
Remaining colonic segments	Supine

Overhead Radiograph	View
Rectosigmoid junction	Prone angled
Rectum	Left and right lateral decubitus cross-table view with horizontal beam
Rectum	Prone cross-table lateral views

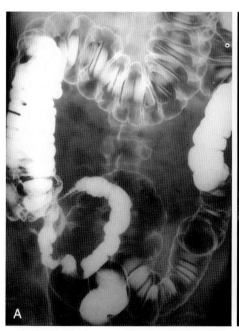
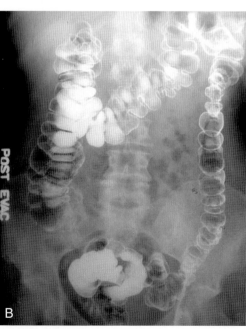

POST EVAC

■ **FIGURE 51-2** **A,** Upright radiograph of a double-contrast barium enema (normal study). **B,** Postevacuation film is important to detect lesions obscured by the barium pool.

TABLE 51-3 Technical Challenges during Double-Contrast Barium Enema Study

Problem	Implication	Solution
Poor bowel preparation	Simulates inflammatory bowel disease	Horizontal beam upright and lateral decubitus views; repeat study with preparation
Fecal residue	Simulates polyps	Found on dependent surface
Sigmoid diverticulosis	Difficult to detect polyps	Single-contrast examination of sigmoid
Patient incontinence	Leakage of air and barium	Intravenous glucagon prevents spasm; inflation of retention balloon
Nonfilling of right colon	Missed lesions	Postevacuation films; single-contrast study of right colon

because of the possibility of a vasovagal response, care must be taken while placing the patient in an erect position. The fluoroscopic table is slowly elevated into the erect position while assisting the patient to maintain equilibrium.

Technique Tips:

- Ensure that the patient's feet are always flat against the platform of the fluoroscopic table.
- Early removal of the rectal catheter helps prevent a vasovagal response.

The various technical challenges faced during the performance of a double-contrast barium enema examination and plausible solutions or methods to circumvent these issues are summarized in Table 51-3.

Technical Modifications

Peroral Pneumocolon

This is an excellent method to demonstrate terminal ileum and cecal pathologic processes. Glucagon, 1 mg, is administered intravenously and air is insufflated through the rectum after barium has reached the right colon to obtain double-contrast radiographs of the cecum and terminal ileum.[16]

Water-Soluble Contrast Enema

In patients with suspected colonic perforation or in postoperative patients, a water-soluble contrast agent such as diatrizoate meglumine and diatrizoate sodium is used to look for formation of fistulas and perforations (Fig. 51-3).[17]

In cystic fibrosis patients, a hyperosmolar water-soluble molar contrast agent can liquefy the viscous stool by drawing fluid into the bowel.

Colostomy Enema

Double-contrast examinations can be performed through a colostomy after resection of a previous rectal carcinoma to detect the presence of recurrence.

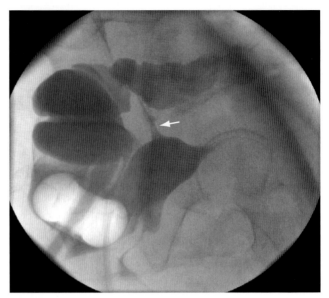

■ FIGURE 51-3 Barium enema with water-soluble contrast in a postoperative patient demonstrates a fistulous tract (*arrow*).

TABLE 51-4 Pros and Cons of a Barium Enema Study

Pros	Cons
Inexpensive	Replaced in larger centers by colonoscopy and cross-sectional studies
Very useful in small centers	
Adequate mucosal surface information	Lacks information of the mucosal, submucosal layers and the mesentery
	No extracolonic information
	Results depend on technical expertise of operator
	Residual barium in colon due to previous studies can pose difficulties in performance of future CT and MRI examinations

PROS AND CONS

The pros and cons of a barium enema study are outlined in Table 51-4.

COMPLICATIONS

The most serious complication is colonic perforation, which can be both intraperitoneal and extraperitoneal and is usually seen in a diseased rectum due to inflation of rectal balloon.[18] Air insufflations can cause abdominal discomfort and can be minimized by the use of carbon dioxide. Allergic reactions may be observed to barium, glucagon, or latex in gloves and rectal catheters. Transient bacteremia and septicemia are very rare complications of barium enema. Barium impaction can cause delayed complications several weeks after the barium enema with varying degrees of constipation and/or abdominal pain. Intramural leakage of barium may produce a granuloma, local inflammation, or ulceration.[19] Venous intravasation may result from barium breaching the colonic mucosa and is a feared complication because of its high mortality rate.[20]

CONTROVERSIES

The continued use of the double-contrast barium enema examination for detecting colorectal polyps has become an area of increasing controversy. It is reimbursed by Medicare for colon screening in asymptomatic individuals. However, two large prospective clinical trials show that the sensitivity of double-contrast barium enema examinations is about 50% for polyps measuring at least 10 mm in diameter.[21,22] At the same time, CT colonography shows far better performance with 55% to 96% sensitivity for patients with polyps 10 mm or larger.[23-25] Although the double-contrast barium enema procedure is an approved colon screening test, acceptance of CT colonography for colon screening is still delayed by critics who suggest the need for additional confirmatory data with large clinical trials.[26]

NORMAL ANATOMY

The goal of the double-contrast barium enema is to have a uniform coating of the mucosal surface with barium yet avoid the formation of barium pools, which can potentially obscure a pathologic process. It is important to be well versed with normal appearances and variations on a double-contrast study. The evaluation should always include the size, shape, position, and architecture of the colon.

Luminal Distention

When the lumen is optimally distended, the normal mucosal folds are just effaced. Inadequate distention may conceal lesions, but overdistention can also obscure lesions such as shallow ulcers. Adequate distention of the interhaustral sacculations will make the interhaustral folds appear as parallel lines perpendicular to the luminal axis of the bowel in the profile and en face views.

Luminal Contour

With adequate coating of barium, the contour of the lumen should appear in profile as a continuous white line.[27]

Mucosal Surface Variations

The normal mucosal surface usually has a smooth, featureless appearance. En face, the mucosal surface fades from the white line of the contour to a smooth, gray-white surface. Other potential anatomic features include the following:

● *Innominate grooves or areae colonicae:* seen as a fine network of lines and should not be mistaken for superficial ulceration
● *Transverse striations:* transient, secondary to contraction of the muscularis mucosa
● *Lymphoid follicles:* may appear as a pattern of fine 1- to 3-mm nodules on the mucosal surface. These follicles are more commonly seen in children, but enlargement of these lymphoid follicles may represent Crohn's disease, inflammation, and lymphoma.

IMAGING OF SPECIFIC LESIONS

Ulcerative Colitis

Confluent diffuse involvement affecting primarily the mucosa and submucosa of the colon is noted (Fig. 51-4).

Early Changes

● Fine granular pattern: early mucosal hyperemia and edema
● Mucosal stippling: due to barium adhering to the superficial ulcers
● "Collar button" ulcers: deeper ulcerations of thickened edematous mucosa with crypt abscesses extending in the submucosa
● Coarse granular pattern: due to replacement of diffusely ulcerated mucosa with granulation tissue

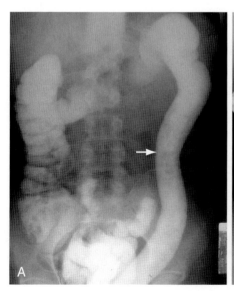
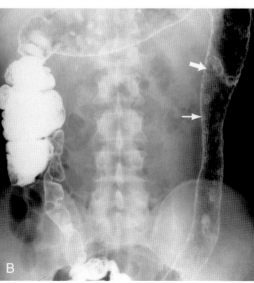

■ **FIGURE 51-4** Ulcerative colitis. **A,** The left hemicolon is diffusely mildly narrowed with loss of haustral markings (*arrow*). **B,** Double-contrast enema shows left-sided ulcerative colitis. Deep "collar stud" ulcers (*arrows*) are present on a background of abnormal mucosa.

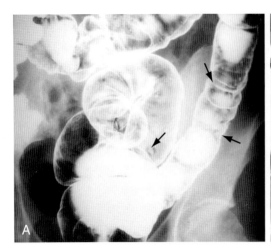

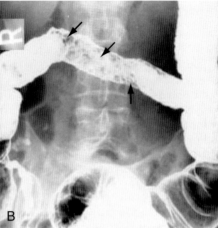

■ **FIGURE 51-5** Crohn's colitis. **A,** Discrete aphthoid ulcers are seen on double-contrast barium enema surrounded by normal mucosa (*arrows*). **B,** Note severe involvement of transverse colon with cobblestoning and ulceration (*arrows*).

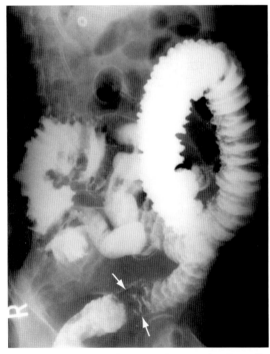

■ **FIGURE 51-6** Pseudomembranous colitis. Irregular plaque-like filling defect (*arrows*) seen in the sigmoid colon with slightly shaggy margins.

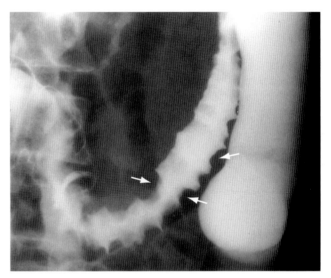

■ **FIGURE 51-7** Ischemic colitis. Double-contrast barium enema shows "thumbprinting" (*arrows*) in the descending colon due to submucosal edema or hemorrhage.

Late Changes

- Pseudo polyps: mucosal remnants in areas of extensive ulceration
- Inflammatory polyps: small islands of inflamed mucosa
- Postinflammatory polyps: mucosal tags seen in quiescent phases of the disease
- Filiform polyps: postinflammatory polyps having a worm-like appearance

Crohn's Disease

- Predominant right colon disease, discontinuous involvement with intervening regions of normal bowel, early aphthous ulcers (Fig. 51-5)
- Deep ulcerations in later stage
- Strictures, fistulas, and sinus formation

- Pseudodiverticula of the colon due to asymmetric fibrosis on one side of the lumen, causing saccular outpouching on the other side

Pseudomembranous Colitis

- Colitis that is patchy in distribution, with sparing of the rectum (Fig. 51-6)
- Irregular lumen with thumbprint indentations
- Superficial ulcers and plaque-like defects on the mucosal surface caused by the pseudomembranes

Ischemic Colitis

- The splenic flexure region and descending colon are watershed areas and most susceptible to ischemic colitis.
- *Early changes:* thickening of the colon wall, spasm, and spiculation
- *Late changes:* accumulation of blood and edema within the bowel wall, leading to multiple nodular defects in a pattern called "thumbprinting" (Fig. 51-7).

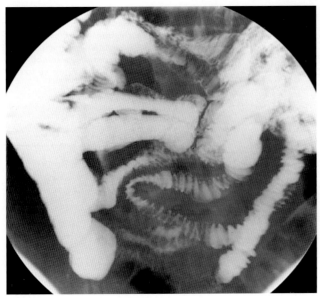

■ **FIGURE 51-8** Radiation colitis. Irregular mucosal thickening due to edema or intramural hemorrhage with separation of bowel loops is noted.

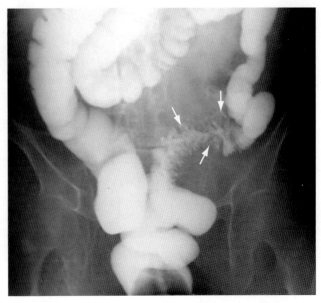

■ **FIGURE 51-9** Sigmoid diverticulitis. Multiple barium-filled outpouchings (*arrows*) are noted in the sigmoid colon with spasm, mural thickening, and lack of distensibility of a focal segment of sigmoid colon.

AIDS-Associated Colitis

● Right colon disease most common
● Wall thickening and ulceration noted

Radiation Colitis

● The rectosigmoid region is most commonly involved, owing to radiation of pelvic malignancy.
● Radiographic findings include thickened folds, spiculation, ulceration, stricture, and, occasionally, fistula formation (Fig. 51-8).
● Fibrosis results in a rigid, featureless bowel.
● Healing may include formation of pseudopolyps and postinflammatory polyps.

Diverticular Disease

Diverticulitis

● Barium enema examination is considered safe, except when signs of free intraperitoneal perforation or sepsis are present.
● Hallmarks of diverticulitis on barium enema include deformed diverticular sacs, demonstration of abscess, and extravasation of barium outside the colon lumen (Fig. 51-9).

Diverticular Abscess

● Extrinsic mass effect on the adjacent colon is shown when the colon lumen is narrowed but tapers at the margins of narrowing, in contrast to the abrupt narrowing of carcinoma.
● Barium leaks into the abscess cavities, or it may form tracks paralleling the colon lumen and often connecting multiple perforated sacs (the "double track" sign).

Lymphoid Hyperplasia

● The nodular lymphoid hyperplasia pattern of diffuse nodules larger than 4 mm is associated with allergic, infectious, and inflammatory disorders.

Lymphoma

● Non-Hodgkin's lymphoma is most common.
● Morphologic patterns include small to large nodules, which may ulcerate, cavitate, and perforate, and diffuse infiltration of the bowel wall, resulting in bulbous folds and a thickened bowel wall.

Lipoma

● The most common submucosal tumor of the colon; it is most frequent in the cecum and ascending colon.
● Barium studies demonstrate a smooth, well-defined, elliptical filling defect, usually 1 to 3 cm in diameter (Fig. 51-10).
● Tumors are soft and change shape with compression.

Extrinsic Masses

● Extrinsic masses commonly cause a mass effect on the colon that may simulate intrinsic disease (Fig. 51-11).
● Endometriosis commonly implants on the sigmoid colon and rectum.[8]
● Defects are sharply defined and can compress but do not usually encircle the lumen.
● Benign pelvic masses such as ovarian cysts, cystadenomas, teratomas, and uterine fibroids produce smooth extrinsic mass impressions on the colonic wall. The colon is displaced but not invaded.

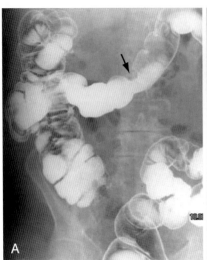

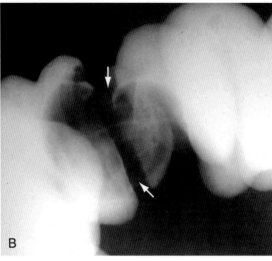

■ **FIGURE 51-10** Lipoma. **A,** A smooth-surfaced submucosal mass is seen in the transverse colon. **B,** Magnified spot image in another patient demonstrates a smooth-contoured lesion that proved to have fat density on CT.

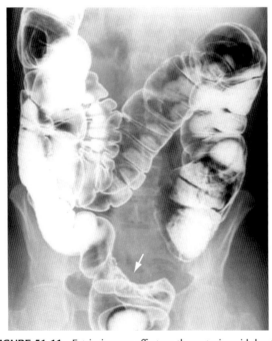

■ **FIGURE 51-11** Extrinsic mass effect on the rectosigmoid due to a large ovarian cyst. Note the smooth contour of the mass effect (*arrow*) without any signs of invasive disease.

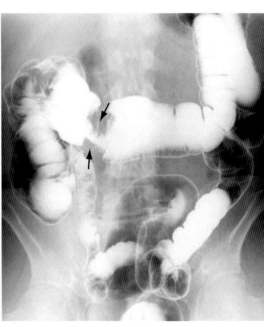

■ **FIGURE 51-12** Colon carcinoma. Annular constricting lesion seen as a short "apple core" segment (*arrows*) of narrowing with destruction of the mucosal pattern in the transverse colon.

Colorectal Carcinoma

● The rectum and sigmoid regions are the most common sites for carcinoma.
● Annular constricting lesions are the most common presentation and are seen as short "apple core" segments of narrowing with destruction of the mucosal pattern (Fig. 51-12).
● Other presentations include polypoid lesions, which are fungating and intraluminal, plaque-like lesions with submucosal spread and ulcerating tumors.
● Occasionally, colonic carcinoma may present as localized or free perforation or as ischemic colitis proximal to a chronically obstructing annular carcinoma.

Metastases

● Serosal involvement can cause a mass effect on the bowel or fixation, angulation, or traction changes with tethering and spiculation and narrowing.
● Common causes of direct spread of neoplasm to the bowel include primary tumors in the genital tract, kidney, and pancreas.

PATHOLOGY

The interpretation of double-contrast barium studies is a synthesis of excellent images and understanding of the basic tenets of pathology and pathophysiology of the underlying lesions.[27]

TABLE 51-5 Dependent and Nondependent Lesions

Lesion	Etiology	Dependent Surface	Nondependent Surface
Protrusions	Mucosal folds or polyps (Fig. 51-13)	Radiolucent filling defect since it displaces barium from the barium pool	Coated with barium, appears to be "etched in white"
Plaque-like lesions	Flat polyps	Best visualized in presence of a shallow barium pool	Difficult to visualize because it is faintly outlined with barium
Stalactite phenomenon	Barium droplet	Not seen	Transient, always seen on the nondependent surface as a protrusion
"Mexican hat" sign	Pedunculated polyp Associated with polyps only		Hanging from the nondependent surface Outer ring: head of the polyp Inner ring: stalk seen end-on through the head
"Bowler hat" sign	Polyp Diverticulum	Dome of the "hat" points inward toward the long axis of the bowel Dome of the "hat" points outward from the long axis of the bowel	
Depressed lesions	Ulcers or diverticula	Focal barium collections due to accumulation of barium	Devoid of barium or appear as a ring shadow if there is adequate coating of the sides
Barium pool	Any lesion	Best seen with a very shallow barium pool	Lesion seen if totally devoid of barium

The appearance of various lesions is based on their location on the dependent or nondependent surfaces, as summarized in Table 51-5.[28,29]

Artifacts

- Structures in front of or behind the bowel may be projected over the bowel and simulate lesions arising from the bowel.
- Flaking of barium suspensions produces an appearance suggestive of inflammatory bowel disease.
- Inadequate distention leads to apposition of the anterior and posterior colonic walls, causing a "kissing" artifact that may resemble a mass lesion.
- Air bubbles rise to the highest point of a column of contrast agent (the "carpenter's level" sign), but fecal material usually remains dependent. Plaques are flat lesions that barely rise above the mucosal surface.

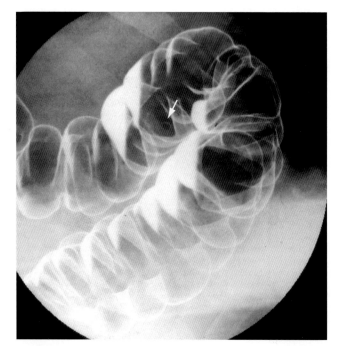

■ **FIGURE 51-13** Polyp seen as a well-defined radiolucent filling defect in the transverse colon.

Dependent and Nondependent Surfaces

- *Dependent surface:* The coating of barium is thicker, and a barium pool is formed in any depression.
- *Nondependent surface:* It has a thin coating of barium, since all the free barium moves onto the dependent surface.

Horizontal-beam radiographs clearly distinguish between these surfaces.

KEY POINTS

- Performance of a diagnostic high-quality double-contrast barium enema is an art form.
- Rigorous colonic cleansing plays a vital role in the performance of an optimal diagnostic barium enema examination.
- Technical tips can help circumvent potential challenges.
- Optical and virtual colonoscopies have resulted in the steady decline of the number of barium enema examinations performed.

SUGGESTED READINGS

Adam A, Dixon AK (eds). Grainger & Allison's Diagnostic Radiology, 5th ed. London, Elsevier, 2008.

Brant WE, Helms CA (eds). Fundamentals of Diagnostic Radiology, 3rd ed. Philadelphia, Lippincott Williams & Wilkins, 2006.

Eisenberg RL. Gastrointestinal Radiology: A Pattern Approach, 4th ed. Philadelphia, Lippincott Williams & Wilkins, 2003.

Gelfand D. The colon. Curr Opin Radiol 1990; 2:407-412.

Wolff BG, Fleshman JW, Beck DE, et al (eds). The ASCRS Textbook of Colon and Rectal Surgery. New York, Springer, 2007.

REFERENCES

1. Frederick MG, Ott DJ, Gelfand DW, et al. Gastrointestinal fluoroscopy in difficult patients. Appl Radiol 1997; 26:12-22.

2. Ott DJ. Accuracy of double-contrast barium enema in diagnosing colorectal polyps and cancer. Semin Roentgenol 2000; 35:333-341.

3. Harned RK, Consigny PM, Cooper NB. Barium enema examination following biopsy of the rectum or colon. Radiology 1982; 145:11-16.

4. Maglinte DDT, Strong RC, Strate RW, et al. Barium enema after colorectal biopsies: experimental data. AJR Am J Roentgenol 1982; 139:693-697.

5. Dodds WJ, Scanlon GT, Shaw DK, et al. An evaluation of colon cleansing regimens. AJR Am J Roentgenol 1977; 128:57-59.

6. Fork F-T, Ekberg O, Nilsson G, et al. Colon-cleansing regimens: a clinical study in 1200 patients. Gastrointest Radiol 1982; 7:383-389.

7. Gelfand DW, Chen YM, Ott DJ. Preparing the colon for the barium enema examination. Radiology 1991; 178:609-613.

8. Rubesin SE, Laufer I. Double contrast barium enema: technical aspects. In Levine MS, Rubesin SE, Laufer I (eds). Double Contrast Gastrointestinal Radiology. Philadelphia, WB Saunders, 2000, pp 331-356.

9. Ferrucci JT Jr. Hypotonic barium enema examination. Am J Roentgenol Radium Ther Nucl Med 1972; 116:304-308.

10. Eisenberg RL, Hedgcock MW. Preliminary radiograph for barium enema examination: is it necessary? AJR Am J Roentgenol 1981; 136:115-116.

11. Stewart ET, Dodds WJ, Nelson JA. The value of digital rectal examination before barium enema. Radiology 1980; 137:567.

12. Miller RE. A new enema tip. Radiology 1969; 92:1492.

13. Dodds WJ, Stewart ET, Nelson JA. Rectal balloon catheters and the barium enema examination. Gastrointest Radiol 1989; 5:227-234.

14. Skucas J. The use of antispasmodic drugs during barium enema. AJR Am J Roentgenol 1994; 162:1323-1325.

15. Rubesin SE, Maglinte DD. Double-contrast barium enema technique. Radiol Clin North Am 2003; 41:365-376.

16. Miller RE, Maglinte DDT. Barium pneumocolon: technologist-performed "7 pump" method. AJR Am J Roentgenol 1982; 139:1230-1232.

17. Shorthouse AJ, Bartram CI, Eyers AA, Thomson JP. The water-soluble contrast enema after rectal anastomosis. Br J Surg 1982; 69:714-717.

18. Blakeborough A, Sheridan MB, Chapman AH. Complications of barium enema examinations: a survey of UK consultant radiologists, 1992 to 1994. Clin Radiol 1997; 52:142-148.

19. Gelfand DW. Complications of gastrointestinal radiologic procedures: I. Complications of routine fluoroscopic studies. Gastrointest Radiol 1980; 5:293-315.

20. Rosenberg LS, Fine A. Fatal venous intravasation of barium during a barium enema. Radiology 1959; 73:771-773.

21. Winawer SJ, Stewart ET, Zauber AG, et al. A comparison of colonoscopy and double-contrast barium enema for surveillance after polypectomy. National Polyp Study Work Group. N Engl J Med 2000; 342:1766-1772.

22. Rockey DC, Paulson E, Niedzwiecki D, et al. Analysis of air contrast barium enema, computed tomographic colonography, and colonoscopy: prospective comparison. Lancet 2005; 365:305-311.

23. Chung DJ, Huh KC, Choi WJ, Kim JK. CT colonography using 16-MDCT in the evaluation of colorectal cancer. AJR Am J Roentgenol 2005; 184:89-103.

24. Pickhardt PJ, Choi JR, Hwang I, et al. CT virtual colonoscopy to screen for colorectal neoplasia in asymptomatic adults. N Engl J Med 2003; 349:2191-2200.

25. Cotton PB, Durkalski VL, Pineau BC, et al. Computed tomographic colonography (virtual colonoscopy): a multicenter comparison with standard colonoscopy for detection of colorectal neoplasia. JAMA 2004; 291:1713-1719.

26. van Dam J, Cotton P, Johnson CD, et al. AGA future trends report: CT colonography. Gastroenterology 2004; 127:970-984.

27. Laufer I. Barium studies: principles of double-contrast diagnosis. In Gore RM, Levine MS, Laufer I (eds). Textbook of Gastrointestinal Radiology. Philadelphia, WB Saunders, 1994, pp 38-49.

28. Laufer I, Kressel HY. Principles of double contrast diagnosis. In Laufer I, Levine MS (eds). Double Contrast Gastrointestinal Radiology. Philadelphia, WB Saunders, 1992, pp 9-54.

29. Ott DJ, Gelfand DW, Wu WC, Ablin DS. Colon polyp morphology on double-contrast barium enema: its pathologic predictive value. AJR Am J Roentgenol 1983; 141:965-970.

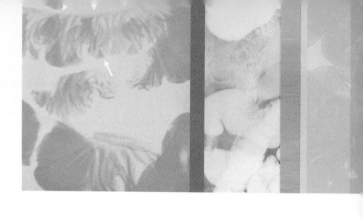

52

CT of the Colon and Rectum

Sunit Sebastian, Pardeep Mittal, and William Small

TECHNICAL ASPECTS

CT has the ability to accurately demonstrate intramural disease as well as extraluminal extension of colonic diseases. The use of a thin-section, high-volume, rapid-bolus scanning technique with state-of-the art multidetector CT (MDCT) technology is important in discriminating subtle intestinal abnormalities. In this chapter, we review technical considerations for the performance of colorectal CT with emphasis on distinctive CT patterns that may help distinguish specific diseases of the colon and rectum.

Imaging Protocol

The conventional CT technique consists of scanning the abdomen after the oral and intravenous administration of contrast material. A suggested protocol for scanning the colon and rectum is outlined in Table 52-1. Intravenous administration of contrast material should always be done to detect subtle bowel wall abnormalities. Delayed scans or decubitus views can help clarify subtle bowel findings, such as colonic leak or perforation, pneumatosis, fistulas, and sinus tracts. Administration of air or water through a rectal tube to distend the colon has also been reported to be helpful.[1]

Multiplanar reconstruction or 3D imaging can aid in visualizing tumor involvement of adjacent organs such as the bladder, vagina, and abdominal or pelvic musculature. This information is crucial for planning treatment and surgery. Thin sections and coronal and oblique reformatted images are helpful in outlining the course of fistulous tracts and bowel obstruction. They also provide detailed information on strictures and the exact location of large bowel obstruction (Fig. 52-1).[2]

Contrast Agents

Intravenous Contrast Agents

Intravenous contrast material is critical for enabling detection of subtle bowel wall abnormalities. The portal venous phase usually is sufficient for demonstrating mesenteric arteries and mesenteric veins. Administration of intravenous contrast material is also essential for complete staging of known colorectal cancer and for evaluation of recurrent or metastatic disease. At our institution, we routinely administer 130 to 150 mL of iohexol (Omnipaque 350) intravenously at a rate of 3 mL/s via a 20-gauge intravenous catheter after an 80-second delay. In patients with known Crohn's disease, it may be beneficial to scan the patient with a 45-second delay representing an "enteric" phase to optimize mural enhancement in the small and large bowel.[3]

Luminal Contrast Agents

Luminal distention with contrast material is essential for optimal assessment of the bowel wall. Both positive and neutral contrast material can be used for this purpose. However, nonopaque fluid distention may reveal luminally oriented features possibly obscured by positive oral contrast material.

Positive Contrast Opacification

Positive contrast opacification is accomplished by giving either 1% to 2% barium suspensions or 2% to 3% solutions of iodinated water-soluble agents. These commercial preparations with low percentages of barium are designed specifically for CT. The patient is instructed to ingest 1000 to 1250 mL of a 3% solution of oral diatrizoate sodium meglumine (Hypaque) 60 to 90 minutes before the CT study. In urgent cases, positive contrast agents can be administered via the rectum. Rectal contrast material distends the rectum and colon and helps differentiate between collapsed bowel wall and mural thickening due to inflammation. If necessary, a fistulous tract can be catheterized and rectal contrast material can be administered and a noncontrast CT is performed.

Neutral Contrast Opacification

Neutral agents such as water[4] or negative agents such as air or carbon dioxide[5] can also be easily administered via

TABLE 52-1 Suggested Protocol for Scanning the Colon and Rectum

Position/Landmark	Head first or feet first supine; xiphoid
Topogram Direction	Craniocaudal
Scan Type	Helical
Scan Start/End Locations	1 cm superior to diaphragm up to symphysis pubis
DFOV	38 cm
KVp	120 kV
mA	Smart mA (100-750) with noise index of 30
Rotation Time (s)	0.8
Pitch	1.375:1
Speed (mm/rotation)	55.00 mm
Detector Width x Rows	0.625 mm × 64
Slice Thickness/Spacing	Thin abdomen/pelvis: 0.6 mm × 0.6 mm for multiplanar reconstructions
Algorithm	Abdomen/pelvis: 5 mm × 5 mm for picture archiving and communications system
IV Contrast	130-150 mL at 3 mL/s
Scan Delay (s)	80

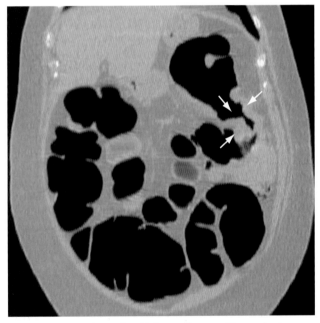

■ **FIGURE 52-1** Coronal multiplanar reformatted image demonstrates narrowing of the splenic flexure due to a stricture (*arrows*) with irregular nodular walls that was pathologically proven to be cancerous.

a rectal tube and provide excellent contrast for colonic imaging. Rectal water helps better demonstrate the colonic wall, depth of tumor invasion of the wall, and extension into the pericolic fat. However, it should not be used when a colonic perforation or postoperative leak is suspected.

Air or carbon dioxide can be used to distend the colon and is particularly helpful for detection of polyps and small masses, especially for CT colonography. Water or air is preferred over positive agents when performing 3D virtual colonoscopy or CT angiography because it does not interfere with data manipulation. Volumen is also an alternative that achieves the advantages of neutral-contrast

distention over a longer period of time owing to the rapid reabsorption of water.

Perfusion CT

Perfusion CT is a recent advancement that enables determination of tumor vascularity in rectal cancer and tumor response to chemotherapy and radiation therapy based on various perfusion parameters.[6] The CT perfusion software allows the simultaneous determination of blood flow, blood volume, vascular mean transit time, capillary permeability, and surface area product. High perfusion values suggest a high rate of angiogenesis and may indicate a high grade of tumor that could result in a poor response to therapy.

PROS AND CONS

CT has several advantages. It is widely available and easy to perform after protocol optimization. It accurately depicts the bowel wall, pericolonic soft tissues, and adjacent structures. CT can vividly assess inflammatory conditions and accurately stage abdominal neoplasms. 3D reconstruction images can identify the transition point in colonic obstruction, differentiating it from ileus. CT is also very sensitive in the detection of pneumoperitoneum and extravasation of oral contrast agent at the site of perforation. It also can be used to perform guided biopsies of suspicious lesions and percutaneous drainage of abscesses and intraluminal fluid collections.

However, CT also has a few limitations. It fails to depict early and superficial mucosal changes of inflammatory bowel disease. The depth of tumor invasion through the colonic wall cannot be accurately determined with CT.

The criteria for detection of metastatic lymphadenopathy on CT is based on size.[7] Lymph nodes larger than 1.0 to 1.5 cm in the short-axis diameter, although considered pathologic, may not contain any tumor, but smaller, presumably normal nodes may harbor tumor. Therefore, although CT has a high specificity for detection of larger metastatic lymph nodes, it has lower sensitivity for early disease.

CT colonography has proven to have a sensitivity and specificity similar to that of colonoscopy, but it still remains to be widely accepted as a cost-effective screening modality for colon cancer prevention.

NORMAL ANATOMY

Characteristic Features of the Colon

The colon is located in the periphery of the abdomen and is well outlined by fat. It can be distinguished from the small intestine on the basis of appearance, caliber, and location.

Taeniae coli are three longitudinal bands approximately 8 mm wide that run the length of the colon and are located on the dorsomedial, dorsolateral, and anterior walls. The taeniae merge where the appendix joins the cecum and at the rectosigmoid junction. Haustra are prominent sacculations formed in the spaces between the taeniae. The prominence of the haustra depends on the contraction of the taeniae. The appendices epiploicae are small packets of fat that run along the taeniae and vary in size.

The normal transverse diameter of the colon varies greatly. The cecum has the greatest diameter and is usually less than 9 cm in normal individuals. The transverse colon is usually less than 6 cm in diameter, and the descending colon and sigmoid colon are usually slightly smaller in caliber. The caliber of the rectum can vary significantly in normal individuals. The thickness of the colonic wall is best demonstrated if the colon is well distended and filled with air or water. In general, the normal colonic wall thickness is 1 to 2 mm[8] and is barely perceptible if the colon is well distended with contrast material or air. When the lumen is collapsed, the normal thickness can reach 3 to 4 mm.

Variations in Colon Anatomy

Redundancy of the sigmoid colon and cecum can lead to anomalous location and, at times, to volvulus or obstruction. If the colon is located between the anterior abdominal wall and the liver or between the diaphragm and the liver, this anatomic variant is called the Chilaiditi sign. It is usually asymptomatic, but, occasionally, the Chilaiditi syndrome develops and causes right upper quadrant pain, probably owing to colonic distention. However, colonic obstruction or volvulus as a complication of Chilaiditi syndrome is very rare.[9] The colon may occupy spaces in which normally other structures were or should have been present, as in renal agenesis, a pelvic kidney, or after hepatectomy and nephrectomy.

The appendix is found in the retrocecal area in about 66% of patients.[10]

DIAGNOSIS

Clinical Presentation

Although imaging is indispensable in the evaluation of diseases of the colon and rectum, a careful assessment of clinical features is beneficial in achieving a definitive diagnosis. The salient clinical features of different disease entities are summarized in Table 52-2.

The sites of involvement, as shown in Table 52-3, also provide clues for the diagnosis of the disease in question.

IMAGING OF SPECIFIC AREAS

There is considerable overlap in the imaging features of inflammatory and neoplastic conditions of the bowel. In addition to the algorithmic approach based on bowel wall attenuation proposed by Wittenberg and colleagues (see later), there are numerous other features that can serve as pathologic pointers on CT that can help to narrow the differential diagnosis.

Bowel Wall Thickening

The presence of bowel wall thickening, as an isolated finding, has limited value for analyzing a specific injury.

TABLE 52-2 Salient Clinical Features of Different Disease Entities of the Colon and Rectum

Disease Entity	Clinical Features
Ulcerative colitis and Crohn's disease	Abdominal pain, tenesmus (rectal urgency), bright red rectal bleeding, small-volume stools
Crohn's disease	Extraintestinal manifestations of erythema nodosum, large-joint nondestructive arthritis, and spondylitis
Amebic colitis	Colonic diarrhea with small volume of bloody stools
Pseudomembranous colitis	History of use of broad-spectrum antibiotics, watery diarrhea, and abdominal cramps
Neutropenic colitis	In patients with leukemia or AIDS and after transplantation or chemotherapy
Ischemic colitis	Age > 70, history of myocardial infarction, arrhythmia, embolus, thrombosis, shock, or trauma; abdominal pain and rectal bleeding
Radiation colitis	Sigmoid colon and rectum
Diverticulitis	Abdominal pain, cramping, diarrhea and constipation, rare gross bleeding or iron-deficiency anemia
Epiploic appendagitis	Right lower quadrant abdominal pain, low-grade fever, obstipation, and, rarely, elevated white blood cell count
Appendicitis	Right lower quadrant pain, obstipation, low-grade fever, and paraumbilical pain, diarrhea, and elevated white blood cell count

TABLE 52-3 Sites of Involvement of Diseases of the Colon and Rectum

Disease Entity	Sites of Involvement
Ulcerative colitis	Left-sided/diffuse, continuous; rectum always involved
	Backwash ileitis with dilated terminal ileum
Crohn's disease	Right-sided/diffuse, skip lesions; rectum may be spared
	Thick walled and narrowed terminal ileum ("string" sign)
Infectious colitis (*Schistosoma, Shigella,* cytomegalovirus, *Escherichia coli*)	Pancolitis
	Predominantly left-sided
	Diffuse
Amebic colitis	Right colon and rectum most severely affected
Pseudomembranous colitis	Pancolitis, skip lesions
Neutropenic colitis	Cecum and ascending colon
Ischemic colitis (Hypoperfusion, cocaine user)	Watershed areas: rectosigmoid junction, splenic flexure
	Left-sided
	Right-sided
Diverticulosis	Sigmoid
Epiploic appendagitis	Adjacent to the colon
Radiation colitis	Sigmoid colon and rectum
Colorectal cancers	Hepatic metastases

The assessment of bowel thickening must always take the degree of luminal distention into consideration.[11]

● The mean wall thickness in Crohn's disease is usually greater than that in ulcerative colitis.[12]

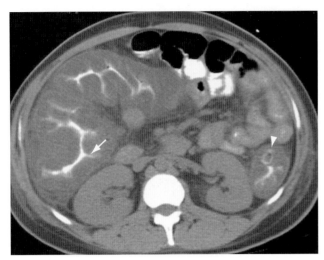

■ **FIGURE 52-2** Pseudomembranous colitis. Note marked mural thickening of the transverse and descending colon (*arrowhead*) with swollen haustra seen projecting into the bowel lumen between thin streaks of oral contrast medium (*arrow*).

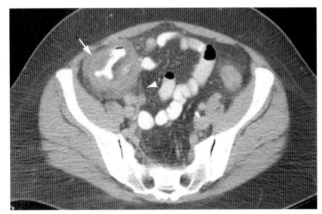

■ **FIGURE 52-3** Typhlitis/neutropenic colitis. The cecum is thickened due to submucosal edema (*arrow*). Note pericolonic stranding (*arrowhead*).

- In tuberculosis, the thickening of the wall of the colon and terminal ileum may be more prominent than in Crohn's disease.
- Coned-shaped cecum, without involvement of the terminal ileum, is unique to amebiasis.[13]
- Pseudomembranous colitis produces one of the most severe degrees of wall thickening among all types of colitis with the exception of Crohn's disease (Fig. 52-2). It also demonstrates skip areas, but the wall usually appears shaggier and more irregular than in Crohn's disease.
- In neutropenic colitis or typhlitis, the wall of the colon and small bowel is circumferentially thickened due to submucosal edema (Fig. 52-3). Pericolonic stranding, fluid, and pneumatosis may also be noted.
- Ischemic proctosigmoiditis should be considered when wall thickening associated with perirectal fat stranding is confined to the rectum and sigmoid colon in elderly patients.
- Long-segment involvement with pericolonic stranding, engorged mesenteric vessels, and fluid in the mesentery favors a diagnosis of diverticulitis (Fig. 52-4).

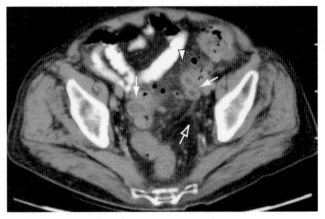

■ **FIGURE 52-4** Diverticulitis. Multiple inflamed diverticula are noted in the sigmoid colon with inflammatory infiltration into the pericolic fat (*arrowhead*). Multiple low-density intramural abscesses (*small white arrows*) are also seen with engorged vasa rectae (*lined arrow*).

- An inflamed appendix is enlarged, with a thickened wall that demonstrates increased enhancement. Pericecal inflammation in the absence of a visualized appendix is suggestive of appendicitis.
- The colon wall is usually not thickened in epiploic appendagitis.
- Features that indicate colon cancer are a focal concentric mass with overhanging shoulders and pericolonic nodes.

Morphology of Fat

In chronic ulcerative colitis, proliferation of perirectal fat is frequently present. This fat has a slightly increased attenuation (10 to 20 HU) compared with normal mesenteric fat (−55 to −75 HU).[14]

In Crohn's disease, mesenteric fat is increased and is called "creeping fat" or fibrofatty proliferation, which represents an attempt by the body to contain the inflammatory process. CT demonstrates an increase in fat in the mesentery that is of higher attenuation (20 to 60 HU) than subcutaneous fat because of edema and inflammatory cell infiltrates with loss of the sharp interface between the bowel wall and the mesentery.[15]

In epiploic appendagitis, CT reveals a well-defined oval or round pericolic area of fat with increased attenuation values with an enhancing rim located immediately adjacent to the colon (Fig. 52-5).[16] A central high attenuation dot within the inflamed appendage represents a thrombosed vein.[17] The fatty tissue in the epiploic appendix is not in direct continuity with the fecal stream, and so pyogenic abscess and sepsis are extremely rare in epiploic appendagitis.

Ascites

Ascites is not a specific sign and is associated with both benign and malignant conditions. It is often present in infectious types of colitis and is usually absent in inflammatory bowel disease. The presence of ascites in pseudomembranous colitis is one of the features that distinguishes it from Crohn's disease, in which ascites is very rare.[18] The

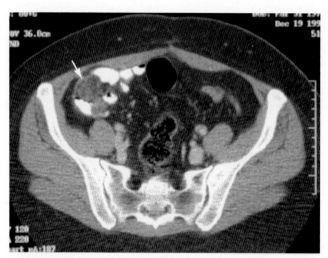

■ FIGURE 52-5 Right-sided epiploic appendagitis. Inflamed epiploic appendage (*arrow*) is seen as an ovoid fat density surrounded by a thickened rim of visceral peritoneum that shows as high attenuation and is in continuity with the ascending colon.

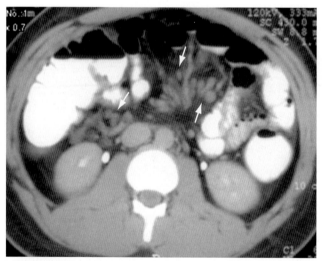

■ FIGURE 52-6 Mesenteric adenitis. Multiple enlarged mesenteric nodes (*arrows*) are noted in a patient with Crohn's disease.

presence of fluid in the root of the sigmoid mesentery and engorgement of adjacent sigmoid mesenteric vasculature favors the diagnosis of diverticulitis.

Lymphadenopathy

Enlarged mesenteric lymph nodes are seen in Crohn's disease (Fig. 52-6). However, the risk of lymphoma is increased in patients with Crohn's disease, and mesenteric lymph nodes larger than 1 cm should be investigated further and malignancy must be excluded.[19] The presence of pericolonic lymph nodes suggests the diagnosis of colon cancer rather than diverticulitis. In developing countries, if peritoneal thickening, ascites, abdominal lymphadenopathy, and thickened intestinal walls are seen on CT, a diagnosis of abdominal tuberculosis should be considered.[20]

Complications

CT is also useful in the identification of complications such as toxic megacolon, phlegmon, abscesses, fistula, and perforation; and timely management can prove to be vital in certain life-threatening conditions. In patients with Crohn's disease, the fistula is usually formed between the diseased terminal ileum and the bladder and is located on the right anterior surface of the bladder. Because diverticulitis typically involves the sigmoid colon, fistulas tend to occur in the left posterior portion of the bladder. In addition to demonstrating the presence and location of a fistula, CT can be helpful in planning subsequent surgery. CT is also useful for performing percutaneous CT-guided biopsies of suspicious lesions and appropriate planning of therapy, including the percutaneous drainage of these collections.

Distant metastasis of cancers of the colon and upper rectum occurs via the portal vein to the liver. However, the lower rectal cancers can drain into the pelvic veins and directly into the inferior vena cava to produce isolated pulmonary metastases without hepatic metastases.

Descriptive CT Signs

Some signs have been used to describe certain typical imaging features. However, these signs are not specific and are seen in several inflammatory conditions.

"Accordion" Sign

This sign is usually described in pseudomembranous colitis when the appearance of the colon may resemble that of an accordion owing to the trapping of positive contrast material between thickened haustral folds.[21] This sign lacks specificity and can be seen in patients with ischemia, cirrhosis, and infectious types of colitis caused by cytomegalovirus, *Cryptosporidium*, and *Salmonella*.

"Comb" Sign

When contrast-enhanced CT depicts hypervascularity of the mesentery with vascular dilatation, tortuosity, and wide spacing of the vasa recta, the "comb" sign is produced (Fig. 52-7).[22] This sign is not specific for active Crohn's disease; it can be seen in any moderate to severe acute inflammatory condition of the small or large bowel. The "comb" sign may be used to differentiate active inflammatory bowel disease from lymphoma and metastatic carcinoma, which tend to be hypovascular.

"Arrowhead" Sign

When inflammation from the appendix spreads to the cecum, cecal thickening is present and the contrast material in the cecal tip produces an arrowhead-shaped collection near the occluded appendiceal orifice.[23]

"Cecal Bar" Sign

The "cecal bar" sign occurs when a curved strip of cecal wall thickening is seen between the cecal lumen and an appendicolith.[24]

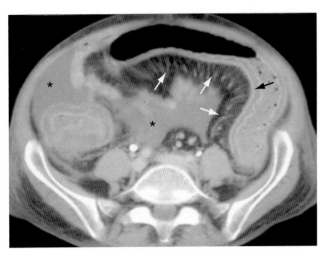

■ **FIGURE 52-7** "Comb" sign. Engorged vasa rectae (*small white arrows*) are seen supplying a thickened bowel segment (*black arrow*) in a patient with Crohn's disease. Ascites is also noted (*asterisks*).

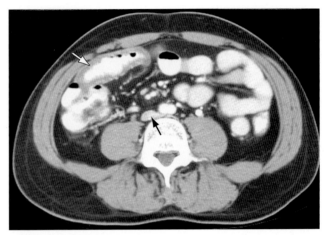

■ **FIGURE 52-8** White attenuation. Contrast enhancement in the diseased ileal loop (*white arrow*) is almost equal to inferior venal caval opacification (*black arrow*) in a patient with acute inflammatory Crohn's disease.

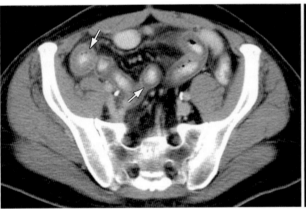

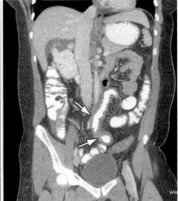

■ **FIGURE 52-9** "Water halo" pattern (*arrow*) due to angioedema seen in a patient on angiotensin-converting enzyme inhibitors, representing submucosal edema as a dominant component.

Imaging Algorithm

Wittenberg and associates[25] have proposed a practical algorithm that incorporates enhancement and attenuation values of the bowel wall after intravenous administration of a contrast agent to aid in the differentiation of benign from malignant disease. However, reliable clinical information must always be factored into the final diagnosis. The spectrum of these mural attenuation patterns includes white (avid contrast material enhancement), gray, "water halo" sign, "fat halo" sign, and black (pneumatosis). A single disease may simultaneously demonstrate multiple attenuation patterns in contiguous segments of bowel due to coexistent pathophysiologic events.

White Attenuation

White attenuation represents intense intravenous contrast enhancement of the thickened bowel wall. The relative attenuation is at least the same as, or greater than, venous opacification seen in the same scan. It is best discerned in bowel loops devoid of luminal contrast. Pericolonic vessels may usually appear prominent.

● *Pathophysiology:* vasodilation and/or injury to intramural vessels with accompanying interstitial leakage

● *Representative example:* shock bowel—diffuse ischemia of the small bowel in hypotensive adults due to blunt trauma[26]
● *Differential diagnosis:* acute inflammatory bowel diseases: acute ulcerative colitis and Crohn's disease (Fig. 52-8), vascular disorders; uncommon diagnosis: malignancy
● *Pitfalls:* Assessment is subjective, and there is no cutoff Hounsfield unit for designating white attenuation.

Gray Attenuation

Gray attenuation is the least specific of the five attenuation categories and is common in both benign and malignant diseases. A thickened bowel wall that shows little enhancement after administration of a contrast agent with its attenuation is comparable to that of enhanced muscle. A common cause of false-positive diagnosis in either the small intestine or colon is incomplete luminal distention.

"Water Halo" Pattern

The water halo sign is a strong indicator of acute bowel wall injury (Fig. 52-9).

● *Double halo:* A halo sign with two layers is composed of either a higher-attenuation outer annular ring (muscularis propria) surrounding a second, luminally oriented annular ring of gray attenuation or a higher-attenuation inner layer and an outer ring of gray attenuation.[27]

● *Target sign:* This is composed of three rings: outer high-attenuation muscularis propria, a middle ring of gray attenuation, and a luminally oriented ring of high attenuation.[28]

● *Pathophysiology:* The lower-attenuation (gray) layer of the "water halo" sign is believed to represent edema and is assumed to be located in the submucosa. The inner and outer rings of the target sign can conveniently be regarded as the mucosa and muscularis propria respectively, with the higher attenuation being the consequence of preferential enhancement.

● *Differential diagnosis:* Idiopathic inflammatory bowel diseases, vascular disorders, infectious diseases, radiation damage; uncommon diagnosis: malignancy

● *Pitfalls:* A positive Hounsfield unit value rather than the negative Hounsfield unit value of fat helps confirm the finding.

"Fat Halo" Pattern

The "fat halo" pattern refers to a three-layered target sign of thickened bowel in which the middle or "submucosal" layer has a darker attenuation of intramural fat (Fig. 52-10).

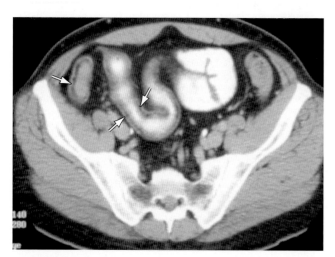

■ **FIGURE 52-10** "Fat halo" pattern in a patient with chronic ulcerative colitis demonstrating multiple thickened bowel segments with a central band of fat attenuation (*arrows*).

If the attenuation of the dark ring is measured in Hounsfield units, the numbers will largely be below −10 HU. However, the attenuation is seldom equal to that of pure mesenteric or retroperitoneal fat owing to either partial volume effect or coexistent edema.[29]

● *Differential diagnosis:* ulcerative colitis of colon, Crohn's disease in the colon; uncommon diagnoses: cytoreductive therapy exposure, chronic radiation enteritis

● *Pitfalls:* Intramural fat may exist in the colon as a "normal" variant in normal patients. The normal intramural fat layer is generally very thin with the muscularis propria also being uniformly thin, rarely exceeding 1 mm in thickness with no surrounding mesenteric abnormalities. The observation of the normal fat halo sign is most frequently made in undistended or poorly distended bowel loops. The clinical history must be considered in the final diagnosis.

Black Attenuation

Black attenuation is the equivalent of pneumatosis and usually represents an acute injury to the bowel, other than the rare, large cystic collections. Identifying gas within intramural or extramural vessels is also diagnostic of pneumatosis (Fig. 52-11).[30]

● *Pathophysiology:* represents acute injury to the bowel.
● *Representative example:* pneumatosis
● *Differential diagnosis:* ischemia, infection, and trauma; uncommon diagnosis: iatrogenic injury
● *Pitfalls:* Intraluminal gas collections that cling to the mucosa can be a source of false-positive findings. Differentiating dependently located gas bubbles in the cecum and ascending colonic wall from gas trapped between fecal debris and mucosa can be confirmed by rescanning the patient in a decubitus position.

Perfusion CT

The immediate or first-pass tumor enhancement after the administration of the intravenous iodinated contrast medium is largely due to the presence of the contrast medium within the intravascular space and its first-pass extraction into the extravascular space. As time progresses, leakage of the contrast medium into the extravascular space continues and the observed tumor enhancement

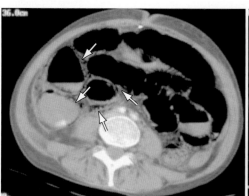
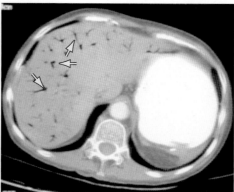

■ **FIGURE 52-11** Black attenuation pattern. The presence of intramural gas or pneumatosis (*white arrows*) is suggestive of acute injury to the bowel. CT of the liver shows gas in the portal vein (*yellow arrows*).

is due to the presence of the contrast medium in both the intravascular and the extravascular space. The intravascular component depends on the available volume of blood space (blood vessels within the tumor), and the extravascular component depends on vascular permeability. During the later phases, the contrast medium in the extravascular space of the tumor is cleared as the contrast medium reenters the vascular system and results in a return to baseline attenuation in the tumor.

KEY POINTS

- Multidetector CT is the initial diagnostic test for the evaluation of inflammatory and infectious diseases.
- CT can accurately depict the degree of bowel thickening, extent and location of the disease, and associated complications.
- Bowel attenuation and wall enhancement patterns can aid in narrowing the differential diagnosis.

SUGGESTED READINGS

Brant WE, Helms CA (eds). Fundamentals of Diagnostic Radiology, 3rd ed. Philadelphia, Lippincott Williams & Wilkins, 2006.

Messmann H. Atlas of Colonoscopy: Techniques, Diagnosis, Interventional Procedures. Stuttgart, George Thieme Verlag, 2005.

Ros PR, Mortele KJ, Lee S, Pelsser V (eds). CT and MRI of the Abdomen and Pelvis: A Teaching File, 2nd ed. Philadelphia, Lippincott Williams & Wilkins, 2006.

Rosenblum JD, Boyle CM, Schwartz LB. The Mesenteric Circulation—Anatomy and Physiology. Surg Clin North Am 1997; 77:289-306.

Wolff BG, Fleshman JW, Beck DE, et al (eds). The ASCRS Textbook of Colon and Rectal Surgery. New York, Springer, 2007.

REFERENCES

1. Amin Z, Boulos PB, Lees WR. Technical report: spiral CT pneumocolon for suspected colonic neoplasms. Clin Radiol 1996; 51:56-61.
2. Aufort S, Charra L, Lesnik A, et al. Multidetector CT of bowel obstruction: value of post-processing. Eur Radiol 2005; 15:2323-2329.
3. Booya F, Fletcher JG, Huprich JE, et al. Active Crohn disease: CT findings and interobserver agreement for enteric phase CT enterography. Radiology 2006; 241:787-795.
4. Angelelli G, Macarini L, Lupo L, et al. Rectal carcinoma: CT staging with water as contrast medium. Radiology 1990; 177:511-514.
5. Solomon A, Michowitz M, Papo J, Yust I. Computed tomographic air enema technique to demonstrate colonic neoplasms. Gastrointest Radiol 1986; 11:194-196.
6. Sahani DV, Kalva SP, Hamberg LM, et al. Assessing tumor perfusion and treatment response in rectal cancer with multisection CT: initial observations. Radiology 2005; 234:785-792.
7. Einstein DM, Singer AA, Chilcote WA, Desai RK. Abdominal lymphadenopathy: spectrum of CT findings. RadioGraphics 1991; 11:457-472.
8. Fisher JK. Abnormal colonic wall thickening on computed tomography. J Comput Assist Tomogr 1983; 7:90-97.
9. Plorde JJ, Raker EJ. Transverse colon volvulus and associated Chilaiditi's syndrome: case report and literature review. Am J Gastroenterol 1996; 91:2613-2616.
10. Kim S, Lim HK, Lee JY, et al. Ascending retrocecal appendicitis: clinical and computed tomographic findings. J Comput Assist Tomogr 2006; 30:772-776.
11. Thoeni RF, Cello JP. CT imaging of colitis. Radiology 2006; 240:623-638.
12. Fishman EK, Wolf EJ, Jones B, et al. CT evaluation of Crohn's disease: effect on patient management. AJR Am J Roentgenol 1987; 148:537-540.
13. Silva AC, Beaty SD, Hara AK, et al. Spectrum of normal and abnormal CT appearances of the ileocecal valve and cecum with endoscopic and surgical correlation. RadioGraphics 2007; 27:1039-1054.
14. Carucci LR, Levine MS. Radiographic imaging of inflammatory bowel disease. Gastroenterol Clin North Am 2002; 31:93-117.
15. Philpotts LE, Heiken JP, Westcott MA, Gore RM. Colitis: use of CT findings in differential diagnosis. Radiology 1994; 190:445-449.
16. Rao PM, Wittenberg J, Lawrason JN. Primary epiploic appendagitis: evolutionary changes in CT appearance. Radiology 1997; 204:713-717.
17. Rao PM, Novelline RA. Case 6: primary epiploic appendagitis. Radiology 1999; 210:145-148.
18. Markose G, Ng CS, Freeman AH. The impact of helical computed tomography on the diagnosis of unsuspected inflammatory bowel disease in the large bowel. Eur Radiol 2003; 13:107-113.
19. Friedman S. Cancer in Crohn's disease. Gastroenterol Clin North Am 2006; 35:621-639.
20. Pereira JM, Madureira AJ, Vieira A, Ramos I. Abdominal tuberculosis: imaging features. Eur J Radiol 2005; 55:173-180.
21. Macari M, Balthazar EJ, Megibow AJ. The accordion sign at CT: a nonspecific finding in patients with colonic edema. Radiology 1999; 211:743-746.
22. Madureira AJ. The comb sign. Radiology 2004; 230:783-784.
23. Rao PM, Wittenberg J, McDowell RK, et al. Appendicitis: use of arrowhead sign for diagnosis at CT. Radiology 1997; 202:363-366.
24. Rao PM, Rhea JT, Novelline RA. Sensitivity and specificity of the individual CT signs of appendicitis: experience with 200 helical appendiceal CT examinations. J Comput Assist Tomogr 1997; 21:686-692.
25. Wittenberg J, Harisinghani MG, Jhaveri K, et al. Algorithmic approach to CT diagnosis of the abnormal bowel wall. RadioGraphics 2002; 22:1093-1107.
26. Mirvis SE, Shanmuganathan K, Erb R. Diffuse small-bowel ischemia in hypotensive adults after blunt trauma (shock bowel): CT findings and clinical significance. AJR Am J Roentgenol 1994; 163:1375-1379.
27. Frager DH, Goldman M, Beneventano TC. Computed tomography in Crohn disease. J Comput Assist Tomogr 1983; 7:819-824.
28. Balthazar EJ, Hulnick D, Megibow AJ, Opulencia JF. Computed tomography of intramural intestinal hemorrhage and bowel ischemia. J Comput Assist Tomogr 1987; 11:67-72.
29. Jones B, Fishman EK, Hamilton SR, et al. Submucosal accumulation of fat in inflammatory bowel disease: CT/pathologic correlation. J Comput Assist Tomogr 1986; 10:759-763.
30. Connor R, Jones B, Fishman EK, Siegelman SS. Pneumatosis intestinalis: role of computed tomography in diagnosis and management. J Comput Assist Tomogr 1984; 8:269-275.

53

CT Colonography

Sunit Sebastian and William Small

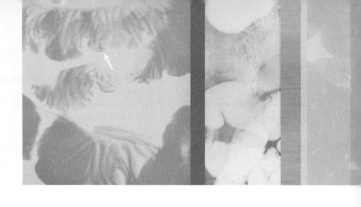

TECHNICAL ASPECTS

Colorectal cancer is one of the leading causes of cancer deaths in the United States,[1] second only to lung cancer in men and breast cancer in women. Colorectal cancer screening can be suitably employed in the early identification of precursor adenomatous polyps for screening symptomatic individuals to prevent colon cancer.[2] A simplified description of CT colonography would read as a highly sophisticated technique that employs rigorous bowel preparation (cleansing) followed by distention of the bowel with air or carbon dioxide and data acquisition using multidetector CT (MDCT). Specialized software is used for postprocessing the volumetric CT datasets to generate either 2D multiplanar images or 3D images of the colon. A detailed description of the various techniques and protocols essential for an optimal CT colonography is provided here. In addition, various methods of visualization, interpretation guidelines, and common pitfalls associated with the procedure are discussed.

Technique

A series of well-orchestrated, meticulous steps could yield a successful CT colonography examination. These steps include:

1. Colonic cleansing with residual stool and luminal fluid tagging
2. Colonic distention
3. Data acquisition
4. Visualization of CT colonography with 2D and/or 3D techniques

The examination can be entirely performed by a technologist after adequate training with minimal assistance from a radiologist. However, the presence of an onsite radiologist is preferred for consultation in difficult cases.

Colonic Cleansing

The presence of residual fluid or stool will result in a suboptimal CT colonographic study because it can obscure polyps or neoplasms or make differentiation between polyps and stool very difficult.[3] Hence, a robust colonic preparation is perhaps the most important step of the entire study. The objective of colonic cleansing is achieved by combining four basic components: dietary restriction, administration of a cathartic agent, tagging of residual stool, and tagging of residual luminal fluid.

The patient is instructed to consume a clear liquid diet the day before the examination. The main bowel cleansing agents include cathartics such as magnesium citrate and sodium phosphate and gut lavage solutions such as polyethylene glycol (PEG). The two popular commercial preparation kits are the 24-hour Fleet 1 Preparation (Fleet Pharmaceuticals, Lynchburg, VA) and the LoSo Preparation (EZ-EM, Westbury, NY). A time outline for bowel preparation is suggested in Table 53-1.

Sodium phosphate is an oral saline cathartic and is referred to as a "dry prep" because it leaves behind little residual fluid in the colon.[4] Magnesium citrate is also a saline cathartic that causes fluid to accumulate in the bowel because of its osmotic effects and promotes peristaltic activity and bowel emptying.

PEG is an effective agent for cleansing the bowel, but it often results in excessive fluid retention in the colon. It is considered a "wet prep" and is not the ideal bowel cleansing agent for virtual colonoscopy. The PEG preparation is associated with the poorest compliance because of its consistency and large volume of ingestion. In a study comparing PEG and sodium phosphate, the majority of the subjects were unable to complete the PEG regimen, whereas 84% of the patients found sodium phosphate to be tolerable as compared with only 33% of patients receiving PEG.[5] There is no significant difference between oral sodium phosphate and PEG electrolyte solution in the quality of bowel cleansing.[6] Magnesium citrate can be used in conjunction with a decreased volume (2 L) of PEG lavage solution to reduce preparation time and improve patient tolerance.[7] The advantages and disadvantages of using a dry or wet bowel cleansing agent are illustrated in Table 53-2.

TABLE 53-1 Suggested Protocol for Bowel Preparation

Preparation	Day before Examination	Morning of CT Colonography	Additional Instructions
Sodium phosphate	6 PM: 45 mL of sodium phosphate diluted in 4 oz of water orally 9 PM: four bisacodyl tablets (5-mg each) orally	10-mg bisacodyl suppository about 1 hr before the examination	Refrain from eating solids and maintain adequate hydration with clear liquids
Magnesium citrate	4 PM: 200-300 mL (10 oz) of magnesium citrate orally 6 PM: Four bisacodyl tablets are taken orally with 8 oz of water	10-mg bisacodyl suppository about 1 hr before the examination	

TABLE 53-2 Advantages and Disadvantages of Dry and Wet Preparation

Preparation	Advantages	Disadvantages
Dry prep: sodium phosphate or magnesium citrate	Less fluid to obscure colonic walls Better patient compliance More tolerable for consumption	More solid debris along the colonic wall makes 3D endoluminal view more time consuming
Wet prep: polyethylene glycol	Less debris along the wall Minimizes solid stool Preferred preparation for inpatients and elderly who cannot tolerate even moderate fluid or electrolyte shifts	More fluid can obscure colonic wall without stool subtraction Poor patient compliance due to large volume of ingestion Abdominal discomfort, bloating, and nausea and vomiting

Contraindications for Bowel Cleansing Agents

The use of a particular laxative is governed by the health status of the individual. Sodium phosphate can cause electrolyte disturbances leading to hyperphosphatemia, hypocalcemia, and hypernatremia. Hence it should not be used in patients with renal, cardiac, or hepatic insufficiency and preexisting electrolyte abnormalities.[8] Sodium phosphate also should be avoided in elderly hypertensive patients who are taking angiotensin-converting enzyme inhibitors. Although magnesium citrate also has been reported to cause electrolyte imbalances, these changes are less pronounced than those seen with sodium phosphate. Magnesium citrate should not be used in patients with renal failure.[9]

Residual Stool and Luminal Fluid Tagging

Dual-positive oral contrast agents are used for tagging of the residual stool and luminal fluid after catharsis.[10] Barium and/or iodine solution are ingested with meals, usually in conjunction with the oral cathartics, 24 to 48 hours before imaging to allow adequate incorporation of the positive contrast material with colonic contents. Tagged stool and residual fluid demonstrate higher attenuation and are easily discernible from the homogeneous soft tissue density of polyps and colonic folds. Either dilute 2% CT barium or 30% to 40% barium can be used for residual stool tagging; 30% to 40% barium can be very dense and cause artifacts and is also less well tolerated by patients.

Diatrizoate meglumine and diatrizoate sodium solution are used for uniform opacification of the residual luminal fluid and their added secondary cathartic effects eliminate a significant amount of adherent solid debris. The tagged residual stool and fluid are then eliminated by electronic subtraction of the high-density material. Pickhardt and colleagues[11] have demonstrated that patients who underwent residual stool and fluid tagging with electronic subtraction for a CT colonographic study demonstrated higher sensitivity for detection of adenomatous polyps measuring 8 mm or more than with conventional colonoscopy. The use of stool and fluid tagging provides a window of opportunity for possible elimination or significant decrease in the amount of laxative to be consumed by the patient. However, the American College of Radiology (ACR) practice guideline for performing virtual colonoscopy in adults currently does not recommend the routine use of oral contrast for labeling stool or fluid.[12]

Colonic Distention

Inadequately distended segments of the colon can make polyp and cancer detection difficult, compromising the sensitivity and specificity of the examination (Fig. 53-1). Room air or carbon dioxide may be used for colonic distention for the virtual colonoscopic examination. CT technologists after adequate training and experience could easily manage to perform the introduction of the rectal catheter. The need for radiologist intervention can be minimized for difficult situations or very apprehensive patients.

Room Air

Advantages of room air include ease of use, ready availability, and lack of additional cost and because it provides good colonic distention. However, because room air is

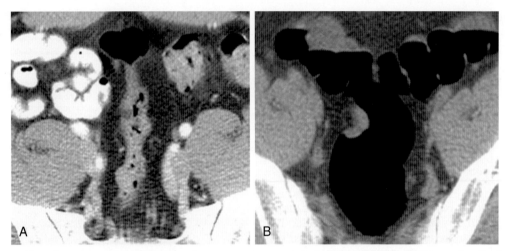

■ **FIGURE 53-1**   **A,** The collapsed segment of the rectum does not reveal any pathologic process even on careful inspection. **B,** Well-distended segment in the supine image revealed a 2-cm polyp within the rectum.

composed predominantly of nitrogen it is poorly absorbed through the colonic wall and patients can experience abdominal discomfort and pain after the CT colonography until the air is totally expelled distally by peristalsis. In addition, significant time may be required to teach patients to self-insufflate with room air, leading to increased operator dependence.

Carbon Dioxide

The patient is advised to evacuate just before the start of the study. Automatic carbon dioxide insufflation can be used as a useful alternative room air for colonic distention. A commercially available electronic insufflation device provides a constant flow of carbon dioxide into the colon per rectum at a relatively low level of preset pressure to reduce the risk of colonic perforation. Carbon dioxide is absorbed rapidly through the colonic wall and exhaled through the lungs. Shinners and associates[13] have observed decreased postprocedural discomfort and improved colonic distention using automated carbon dioxide as compared with patient-controlled room air. The automated CO_2 procedure is fairly easy to explain to the patient. Decreased operator dependence using the automated CO_2 technique can be attributed to a more definite determination of the end point of insufflation. The risk of perforation with automated CO_2 technique or patient-controlled distention methods probably approaches zero for screening CT colonography.[13]

Technique

Room Air

The patient is advised to evacuate just before the start of the study. With the patient in the left lateral decubitus position a small rubber catheter is used to insufflate the colon with a hand-held bulb syringe. Using an insufflation bulb, 50 to 70 puffs or 2 L of room air is administered until the patient experiences fullness or mild discomfort, which signals that the colon is well distended.

Automated CO_2 Technique

In the automated CO_2 technique a small-caliber, flexible rectal catheter is placed with the patient in the left lateral decubitus position and 1.0 to 1.5 L CO_2 is delivered by the automated device at equilibrium pressure of about 20 mm Hg. The patient is moved into the right lateral decubitus position until about 2.5 L of CO_2 has been introduced. The total volume of CO_2 used in the procedure can vary from 2 to 10 L owing to individual differences in colonic volume, colonic resorption, and reflux through the ileocecal valve. Finally, a scout image of the abdomen and pelvis is obtained with the patient in the supine position. The colonic distention can be checked on the CT scout image or on the review of the 2D transverse images during the examination. Adequate colonic distention will reveal an almost complete column of gas from the rectum to the cecum. However, additional CO_2 may be administered in the prone position if the colon is suboptimally distended. The virtual colonoscopy scan then is repeated in the prone position after a second scout localizing image. Scans performed in both the supine and prone positions provide improved colonic distention, particularly of the transverse and sigmoid colon as compared with supine or prone imaging alone.[14] Although dual-position scanning increases the radiation dose, it facilitates optimal bowel distention and differentiation of fecal material from polyps. Furthermore, persistent segments of focal collapse may need to be scanned with the patient in the right lateral decubitus position.

Use of Spasmolytic Agents

Glucagon

Glucagon causes relaxation of the smooth muscle in the gastrointestinal tract, including the colon, presumably improving patient comfort and colonic distention. One milligram of glucagon can be administered intravenously immediately before scanning. The ACR practice guidelines suggest that glucagon can be administered to relieve spasm or patient discomfort. However, mixed results are noted in the literature regarding the use of glucagon, with some groups claiming that it improves colonic distention[15] while other investigators report that it does not significantly improve colonic distention due to relaxation of the ileocecal valve allowing reflux of air into the small bowel.[16] Adverse reactions to glucagon are nausea, vomiting, and headache. A previous adverse reaction, insulinoma, pheochromocytoma, or poorly controlled diabetes are some of the contraindications for its use.

Hyoscine Butylbromide

This anticholinergic drug is administered intravenously and acts by blocking parasympathetic ganglia, causing relaxation of smooth muscle. Hyoscine butylbromide has been reported to be more effective than glucagon in distending the colon for barium enema examinations.[17] Adverse effects include blurring of vision, dry mouth, tachycardia, and acute urinary retention. Contraindications to the use of hyoscine butylbromide include glaucoma, obstructive uropathy, and myasthenia gravis. It is not approved for use in the United States but has been used widely in Europe and Asia.

Thus, the parenteral route of administration of spasmolytic agents accompanied by its own set of adverse reactions can create added patient anxiety, thereby increasing the duration and cost of the examination.

MDCT Protocol for CT Colonography

After air or CO_2 insufflation, CT colonography is performed first in the supine position in a cephalocaudad direction encompassing the entire colon and rectum. The patient is then placed in the prone position, and the scan is repeated over the same z-axis range. An optimal study can be performed using 4-, 8-, or 16-channel MDCT scanners with 1.25-mm collimation. The 16- and 64-slice MDCT scanners have considerably decreased scanning times, leading to virtual elimination of motion artifacts from peristalsis and respiration. The 64-slice scanners are generally not necessary because submillimeter collimation results in increased radiation dose. Screening CT colonography is a noncontrast study, and intravenous contrast material is not administered routinely. Oral contrast tagging and 3D polyp detection have a high diagnostic accuracy, making the use of intravenous contrast unnecessary for screening. Disadvantages of the use of intravenous contrast include the possibility of contrast reactions, higher radiation dose, increased interpretation times, and higher cost. Intravenous contrast could pose an added difficulty in differentiating an enhancing lesion from tagged material and should be avoided in patients with oral stool and fluid tagging. A suggested CT colonography MDCT protocol is illustrated in Table 53-3.

MDCT scanners generate volumetric datasets that can be used for traditional 2D axial images and multiplanar reformatted images as well as to produce 3D endoluminal views. A standard reconstruction kernel should be used for CT colonographic data reconstruction. State-of-the-art CT colonography also requires a sophisticated and specialized computer workstation with advanced graphic software that displays 2D and 3D views of the colon. The

TABLE 53-3 Suggested Protocol for CT Colonography Using 16-Slice MDCT

Technical Parameters	16-Slice MDCT
Scan position	Supine and prone
Scan area	Entire abdomen and pelvis
Scan direction	Craniocaudal
Respiratory phase	Inspiration
Detector configuration	16 × 0.625 mm
Pitch	1.375
Feed table (mm/rotation)	13.75
Gantry rotation time (s)	0.5
Kilovolt peak (kVp)	120
Milliampere (mA)	Smart mA (GE Medical Systems, Milwaukee, WI), with noise index of 50 or 35 to 75 mAs (effective) without automatic tube current modulation
Reconstruction	Standard/full
Thickness	1.25 mm
Interval	0.8 mm

thin-section source images are sent to a workstation for advanced modeling and interpretation and to the picture archiving and communications system for storage.

CT Colonography and Radiation Dose

CT colonography uses ionizing radiation; and because it is intended to be used as a screening test, optimization of scan parameters to minimize radiation exposure is necessary. The intrinsic high contrast between the intraluminal gas and the soft tissue of the colonic wall offers an opportunity to reduce the milliampere-second mAs to decrease the effective radiation dose. An automatic tube-current modulation system, which is routinely available nowadays with 16- and 64-slice CT scanners, can be set at a noise index of 50 to result in significant dose reduction. Macari and colleagues[18] have demonstrated effective radiation doses for CT colonography to be 5.0 mSv for men and 7.8 mSv for women. The radiation dose can be further reduced using ultra-low-dose CT colonography as demonstrated by Iannaccone and coworkers,[19] who employed an effective milliampere-second of 10 using a four-row MDCT to obtain an effective dose of 1.8 mSv in men and 2.4 mSv in women. Although there is a very small theoretical risk of cancer due to low-dose radiation exposure (0.14% for combined supine and prone virtual colonoscopy scans for a 50-year-old person),[20] the benefits of screening for colorectal cancer prevention clearly outweigh these risks.

CT Colonography Visualization

The CT colonography study can be interpreted using the conventional 2D multiplanar reconstruction (MPR) or 3D visualization using specialized software. The debate as to the relative value of 2D versus 3D for primary interpretation of CT colonography does not preclude the basic tenet of thorough colonic preparation and adequate reader training in CT colonography examinations. In practice, it is important to be comfortable in using both 2D and 3D methods. Depending on reader preference and training, either of the two methods could be used for primary reads

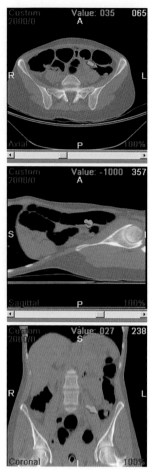

■ **FIGURE 53-2** Images can be viewed simultaneously with linked axial, coronal, sagittal, or oblique multiplanar reconstructed images.

and the other view could be used as a problem-solving tool. However, in practice use of both the 2D and 3D views provides better results in cohorts with low polyp prevalence as compared with using the 2D method alone.[21]

2D Visualization

Different images can be viewed simultaneously with linked axial, coronal, sagittal, or oblique multiplanar reformatted images (Fig. 53-2). Various window/level settings with presets for lung, soft tissue, and bone can be employed. Advantages of 2D visualization include familiarity of radiologists in the use of multiplanar reformatted images, detection of annular lesions, polyps submerged in fluid, and segments with partial or total luminal collapse. It is also excellent for confirming the soft tissue nature of polyps and recognizing the heterogeneous texture of stool. However, it can be a relatively ineffective and tedious method for detecting polyps in a cohort of low prevalence.

3D Visualization

3D visualization provides an endoluminal surface- or volume-rendered view of the colon that can be generated via a near-accurate automated center line (Fig. 53-3). The specialized software program eliminates gas-containing structures such as stomach, small intestines, and the lung bases and allows the user to bridge collapsed segments. The reader is able to fly through the colon at a set speed or manually with capabilities to manipulate the viewing direction and the viewing angle. Most software programs have the ability to compare the 3D images to

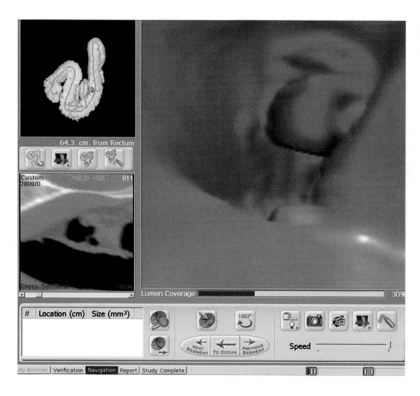

■ **FIGURE 53-3** 3D visualization provides an endoluminal surface- or volume-rendered view of the colon that can be generated via a near-accurate automated center line.

corresponding 2D images for immediate problem solving. To examine the entire colon, a fly-through should be performed in both antegrade and retrograde directions for both supine and prone positions, resulting in a total of four fly-throughs per CT colonographic study. Some of the disadvantages of 3D visualization include the possibility of solid stool to masquerade as a polyp; the ileocecal valve may appear rounded and elevated. However, correlation with 2D images can minimize these potential errors. Longer interpretation times for 3D endoluminal evaluation can be potentially fatiguing.

Newer Display Methods

To overcome problems posed by 2D and 3D methods, researchers have developed several interesting display methods. These include:

- *Virtual pathology/dissection:* The Virtual Dissection (VD) (GE Healthcare, Inc., Piscataway, NJ) program cuts the colon open and displays it either in segments or showing the entire colon in one screen.
- *Filet view:* It is similar to other cut-open views but additionally creates a movie loop of the cut-open colon displayed for a short segment at a time.
- *Panoramic views:* This 3D view enlarges the regular endoluminal view at its margins and depicts the colon in both the antegrade and retrograde directions in the same window.
- *Translucency rendering:* Color mapping is used in which a polyp has a red center and shifts to blue over green at its borders, while tagged stool appears white if the density of the tagged stool is 200 Hounsfield units or greater (Fig. 53-4).

CT Colonography Interpretation

The Working Group on Virtual Colonoscopy[22] has proposed a practical reporting scheme and categorization system for CT colonographic findings with follow-up

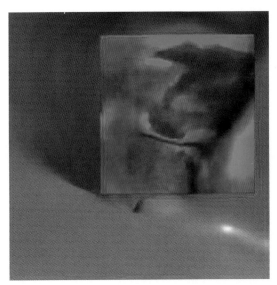

■ **FIGURE 53-4** Translucency rendering uses color mapping in which a polyp has a red center and shifts to blue over green at its borders.

recommendations. This report intends to facilitate uniformity and quality control in the performance of CT colonography. Although a detailed description is beyond the scope of this chapter, review and implementation of these recommendations are suggested. According to this report, for screening purposes the minimum size for reporting polyp lesions is 6 mm. Medium-sized lesions (6 to 9 mm) are rarely malignant, but these patients are offered sameday colonoscopy. Patients with lesions 1 cm or larger should be referred for colonoscopy.

PROS AND CONS

CT colonography could attract new patients who have previously refused colorectal screening, serving as a "compliance enhancer" owing to its relatively noninvasive nature and very low rate of complications.

Many young radiologists are better trained, and more interested, in cross-sectional scanning techniques than barium radiology. The latter is much more labor intensive and relatively poorly reimbursed, compared with virtual colonoscopy. The concern about insufficient number of gastroenterologists able to provide screening colonoscopy can be addressed with radiologists contributing to colorectal cancer screening with CT colonography.

CT colonography has potential disadvantages. The performance of an optimal CT colonographic study depends on adequate bowel preparation, reader training, and expertise. Virtual colonoscopy would have to be 54% less expensive than conventional colonoscopy to be as cost effective in a 10-year interval screening program.[23] In addition, significant abnormal findings have to be followed by colonoscopy for treatment (implying higher costs and a separate bowel preparation). The ability to detect extracolonic findings is a "double-edged sword." It can be a valuable tool for the identification of potentially life-threatening or significant extracolonic findings (e.g., lymphadenopathy, solid hepatic or renal masses, solid pancreatic mass, aortic aneurysm) that have the potential for positive effects on patient care.[24] However, this feature of virtual colonoscopy may also be a drawback: unnecessary workups for benign incidental findings could substantially add to the costs.[25] Moreover, a screening CT colonography is a noncontrast examination, which makes the evaluation of extracolonic solid organs suboptimal.

CONTROVERSIES

Two controversial large studies have been published in major journals regarding the efficacy of CT colonography. A large study by Pickhardt and coworkers[11] demonstrated outstanding results with virtual colonoscopy outperforming optical colonoscopy on a per polyp basis at both the 8-mm level (94% vs. 92%) and at the 10-mm level (94% vs. 88%). However, a subsequent study by Cotton and associates[26] found only a 52% sensitivity for 10-mm polyps and only 32% for polyps over 6 mm. This study was criticized by radiologist virtual colonoscopy researchers because of inadequate reader training, no documentation of examination quality, outdated scan techniques, and unorthodox reporting of results, which tended to bias the results in favor of optical colonoscopy.[27]

NORMAL ANATOMY

Knowledge of normal colonic anatomy and its variants, common pitfalls, and pseudolesions as demonstrated on CT colonography is essential to provide a confident and accurate report.[28] The common pitfalls of CT colonography are as follows:

Collapsed or underdistended segments are difficult to evaluate and significant pathologic processes may be missed. Furthermore, collapsed segments of colon may be misinterpreted as annular carcinomas or strictures. Supine and prone imaging and use of CO_2 for colonic distention may improve distention.

Fecal material can be a major source of false-positive findings on CT colonography and is misinterpreted as polyps or neoplasms. Fecal material may show the presence of a radiolucent area consistent with fat (Fig. 53-5). Use of both prone and supine imaging is helpful to differentiate mobile stool from a fixed lesion.

Intraluminal fluid may limit evaluation of the colonic mucosa and hide significant pathologic processes (Fig. 53-6). The use of phospho-soda colon preparations results in a drier colonic mucosa in addition to prone and supine imaging.

Haustral folds are poorly distended, thickened folds that may meet in the midline (kissing folds) and could mimic masses. Conversely, infiltrating tumors may appear as isolated haustral fold thickening.

Diverticula may become impacted with stool or inverted and may simulate polyps even on axial images. Stool-containing diverticula can usually be seen to project beyond the colonic lumen and have pockets of air or retained barium. Inverted diverticula need careful inspection of axial images that reveal the pericolic fat within them.

"Difficult" polyps include pedunculated polyps that may move with a change in patient position, thus being misinterpreted as stool (Fig. 53-7). Direct visualization of the stalk, homogeneous density of a polyp, and air trapped within the stool can aid in differentiation.

Flat or sessile polyps are only minimally raised from the colonic mucosa and can be missed (Fig. 53-8). Lung and soft tissue window settings with axial images supplemented with endoluminal views could be helpful.

A prominent ileocecal valve may mimic a mass lesion. The characteristic location of the valve on the medial wall of the cecum, its relationship to the terminal ileum, and the presence of fat within the valve are some of its signature features (Fig. 53-9). External compression or indentation of the air-distended colon by liver, loops of bowel, the psoas muscle, or aorta may simulate a mass on endoluminal images, especially in thin patients. Review of axial 2D images can overcome this misinterpretation.

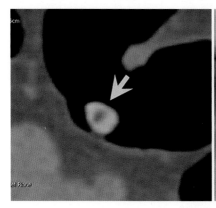
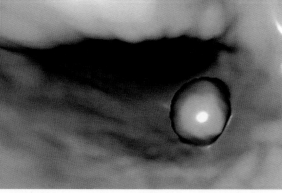

■ **FIGURE 53-5** Fecal material can be falsely interpreted as a polyp; it may show the presence of a radiolucent area consistent with fat and may change its position on supine and prone images.

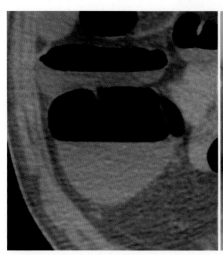
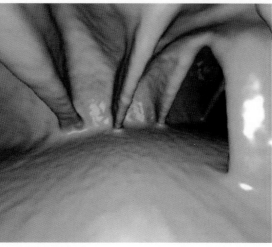

■ **FIGURE 53-6** Intraluminal fluid may limit evaluation of the colonic mucosa and hide a significant pathologic process.

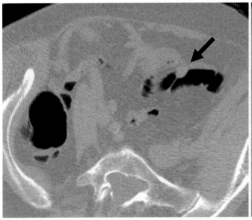
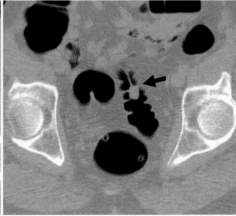

■ **FIGURE 53-7** Pedunculated polyps (*arrows*) may move with a change in patient position due to the presence of a long stalk and thus be misinterpreted as stool.

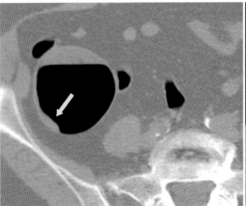
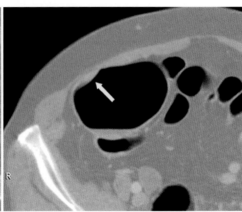

■ **FIGURE 53-8** Flat or sessile polyps (*arrows*) that are only minimally raised from the colonic mucosa can be missed. The apparent change in position of the lesion is due to movement of the cecum itself.

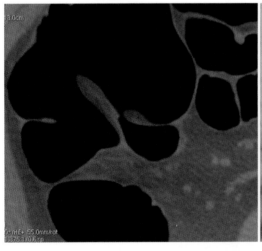
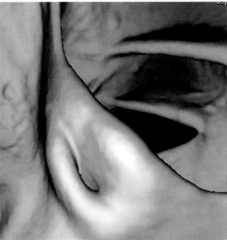

■ **FIGURE 53-9** A prominent ileocecal valve may mimic a mass lesion; characteristic location and the presence of fat aid in identification.

Breathing and peristalsis may cause misregistration artifacts on reconstructed images. Rapid image acquisition using multislice CT scanners has almost eliminated motion artifacts. Metallic artifact or beam hardening artifact may degrade both axial and endoluminal images particularly in the pelvis in patients with hip prostheses. Stair-step artifact is more prominent in the rectum and cecum on endoluminal images. They appear as multiple low-attenuation "rings" spiraling around the lumen of the distended colon but rarely interfere with interpretation.

FUTURE TRENDS AND DEVELOPMENTS

Computer-aided detection can be defined as a diagnosis made by utilizing the output of a computerized scheme for automated image analysis as a diagnostic aid. This second opinion has the potential to improve radiologists' detection performance and to reduce variability of the diagnostic accuracy among radiologists, without significantly increasing the reading time. However, computer-aided detection for CT colonography is still undergoing

TABLE 53-4 Pathologic and Molecular Pathways from Adenoma to Carcinoma

Pathway	Incidence	Molecular Genetic Pattern	Location
The APC, LOH, or MSS (microsatellite stable) pathway	60-80% of colorectal adenocarcinomas	*APC* mutation, loss of heterozygosity (LOH) of suppressor genes, chromosomal instability, and aneuploidy	Distal and left side of colon
The microsatellite instability (MSI) pathway	10-15% of colorectal adenomas—frequently mucin-producing carcinomas	Mutation in both alleles of a mismatch repair gene such as *hMLH1*, inactivation of the gene as a result of hypermethylation of its promoter region	Right sided
The MSI low pathway	5-10% of colorectal cancers More aggressive	Distinctive molecular profile of LOH without *APC* mutation but associated with low levels of MSI	Distal and left side of colon

active research and development and needs approval by the U.S. Food and Drug Administration. The future also promises that computer-aided detection software will be fully integrated with the visualization workstations like that for localizing polyps.[29]

PATHOPHYSIOLOGY

Advances in molecular genetics and new technologic approaches provide valuable insights into the evolution of colorectal cancer, enabling a more comprehensive understanding of the pathology and genetic basis of the disease process.[30]

Adenoma

Adenoma is considered to be the immediate precursor of colorectal cancer. The colonocytes that make up this minute neoplasm show an adenomatous phenotype or dysplasia; they are the progeny of crypt stem cells and typically exhibit *APC* gene mutations.

Adenoma Variants

The architectural pattern that the neoplastic glands of the adenoma assume as they grow can be described as tubular, villous, or tubulovillous:

● A tubular adenoma is composed of straight or branched J tubules (crypts) lined by adenomatous (dysplastic) epithelium.
● Villous growth (constituting greater than 75% of the polyp) consists of adjacent crypts that are elongated to give an appearance of hair-like or leaf-like extensions of adenomatous mucosa.
● Tubulovillous growth is composed of a villous component of 25% to 75% of the polyp, according to the standard nomenclature.

Adenoma Progression

By definition, all adenomas show at least low-grade dysplasia; the adenomatous phenotype represents transformed colonocytes that have enlarged elongated nuclei, mucus depletion of the cytoplasm, and disordered growth patterns of associated crypts or glands.

High-grade dysplasia represents the interface between benign adenoma and invasive cancer. There is increased nuclear atypia and extreme gland architectural abnormali-

ties, almost identical to the morphology of adenocarcinoma, devoid of invasion.

Advanced adenoma is usually an adenoma that has at least a 25% component of villous growth or is larger than 1 cm or shows high-grade dysplasia or invasive cancer on pathologic examination. It represents a biomarker for present and future colorectal cancer risk.

Classification of Adenoma Shape and Cancer Risk

Adenomas are classified according to their shape as flat or polypoid (protruding), the latter either sessile or pedunculated. The rate of invasive carcinoma in flat adenomas is slightly lower than but not remarkably different from those in protruded polyps. Depressed adenoma is an uncommon finding in a screening population but has a reported frequency of high-grade dysplasia or submucosal invasion up to 50%.

Adenoma Size and Cancer Risk

The most practical measure of high-grade dysplasia and malignant transformation risk in adenomas may be size. There is, however, no standard method for measuring adenoma size in current clinical practice.

Pathologic and Molecular Pathways from Adenoma to Carcinoma

Three distinctive pathways have been identified and are outlined in Table 53-4.

KEY POINTS

■ CT colonography can be suitably employed in the early identification of precursor adenomatous polyps for colorectal cancer.
■ A robust colonic preparation is the most important step of the CT colonography study.
■ CT colonography has proven to be as accurate as optical colonoscopy in the detection of significant polyps.
■ Knowledge of normal colonic anatomy and its variants, common pitfalls, and pseudolesions as demonstrated on CT colonography is essential to provide a confident and accurate report.
■ Future technologic advances such as computer-aided detection will further enhance the accuracy of CT colonography while decreasing interpretation time.

SUGGESTED READINGS

Dachman AH, Lefere P, Gryspeerdt S, Morin M. CT colonography: visualization methods, interpretation, and pitfalls. Radiol Clin North Am 2007; 45:347-359.

Hawes RH. Does virtual colonoscopy have a major role in population-based screening? Gastrointest Endosc Clin North Am 2002; 12:85-91.

Hofstad B. Colon polyps: prevalence rates, incidence rates, and growth rates. In Waye JD, Rex DK, Williams CB. Colonoscopy Principles and Practice. London, Blackwell, 2003, pp 358-376.

Kashida H, Kudo S. Magnifying colonoscopy, early colorectal cancer, and flat adenomas. In Waye JD, Rex DK, Williams CB. Colonoscopy Principles and Practice. London, Blackwell, 2003, pp 478-508.

Landeras LA, Aslam R, Yee J. Virtual colonoscopy: technique and accuracy. Radiol Clin North Am 2007; 45:333-345.

Mcahon PM, Gazelle GS. Colorectal cancer screening issues: a role for CT colonography? Abdom Imaging 2002; 27:235-243.

Mulhall BP, Veerappan GR, Jackson JL. Meta-analysis: computed tomographic colonography. Ann Intern Med 2005; 142:635-650.

Robinson C, Halligan S, Taylor SA, et al. CT colonography: a systematic review of standard of reporting for studies of computer-aided detection. Radiology 2008; 246:426-433.

REFERENCES

1. Jemal A, Thomas A, Murray T, Thun M. Cancer statistics, 2002. CA Cancer J Clin 2002; 52:23-47.
2. Rex DK, Johnson DA, Lieberman DA, et al. Colorectal cancer prevention 2000: screening recommendations of the American College of Gastroenterology. Am J Gastroenterol 2000; 95:868-877.
3. Fletcher JG, Johnson CD, Welch TJ, et al. Optimization of CT colonography technique: prospective trial in 180 patients. Radiology 2000; 216:704-711.
4. Gelfand DW, Chen MYM, Ott DJ. Preparing the colon for the barium enema examination. Radiology 1991; 178:609-613.
5. Hookey LC, Depew WT, Vanner SJ. A prospective randomized trial comparing low-dose oral sodium phosphate plus stimulant laxatives with large volume polyethylene glycol solution for colon cleansing. Am J Gastroenterol 2004; 99:2217-2222.
6. Arezzo A. Prospective randomized trial comparing bowel cleaning preparations for colonoscopy. Surg Laparosc Endosc Percutan Tech 2000; 10:215-217.
7. Sharma VK, Chockalingham SK, Ugheoke EA, et al. Prospective, randomized, controlled comparison of the use of polyethylene glycol electrolyte lavage solution in four-liter versus two-liter volumes and pretreatment with either magnesium citrate or bisacodyl for colonoscopy preparation. Gastrointest Endosc 1998; 47:167-171.
8. Wiberg JJ, Turner GG, Nuttall FQ. Effect of phosphate or magnesium cathartics on serum calcium: observations in normocalcemic patients. Arch Intern Med 1978; 138:1114-1116.
9. Ehrenpreis ED, Nogueras JJ, Botoman VA, et al. Serum electrolyte abnormalities secondary to Fleet's Phospho-Soda colonoscopy prep. Surg Endosc 1996; 10:1022-1024.
10. Zalis ME, Hahn PF. Digital subtraction bowel cleansing in CT colonography. AJR Am J Roentgenol 2002; 176:646-648.
11. Pickhardt PJ, Choi JR, Hwang I, et al. Computed tomographic virtual colonoscopy to screen for colorectal neoplasia in asymptomatic adults. N Engl J Med 2003; 349:2191-2200.
12. American College of Radiology. ACR practice guideline for the performance of computed tomography (CT) colonography in adults. Reston, VA, American College of Radiology, 2005, pp 295-299.
13. Shinners TJ, Pickhardt PJ, Taylor AJ, et al. Patient-controlled room air insufflation versus automated carbon dioxide delivery for CT colonography. AJR Am J Roentgenol 2006; 186:1491.
14. Yee J, Kumar NN, Hung RK, et al. Comparison of supine and prone scanning separately and in combination at CT colonography. Radiology 2003; 226:653-661.
15. Rogalla P, Lembcke A, Ruckert JC, et al. Spasmolysis at CT colonography: butyl scopolamine versus glucagon. Radiology 2005; 236:184-188.
16. Yee J, Hung RK, Akerkar GA, et al. The usefulness of glucagon hydrochloride for colonic distention in CT colonography. AJR Am J Roentgenol 1999; 173:169-172.
17. Goei R, Nix M, Kessels AH, et al. Use of antispasmodic drugs in double contrast barium enema examination: glucagon or Buscopan? Clin Radiol 1995; 50:553.
18. Macari M, Bini EJ, Xue X, et al. Colorectal neoplasms: prospective comparison of thin section low-dose multi-detector row CT colonography and conventional colonoscopy for detection. Radiology 2002; 224:383-392.
19. Iannaccone R, Laghi A, Catalano C, et al. Detection of colorectal lesions: lower-dose multi-detector row helical CT colonography compared with conventional colonoscopy. Radiology 2003; 229:775-781.
20. Brenner DJ, Georgsson MA. Mass screening with CT colonography: should the radiation exposure be of concern? Gastroenterology 2005; 129:328-337.
21. Macari M, Milano A, Lavelle M, et al. Comparison of time-efficient CT colonography with two- and three-dimensional colonic evaluation for detecting colorectal polyps. AJR Am J Roentgenol 2000; 174:1543-1549.
22. Zalis ME, Barish MA, Choi JR, et al. for the Working Group on Virtual Colonoscopy. CT colonography reporting and data system: a consensus proposal. Radiology 2005; 236:3-9.
23. Sonnenberg A, Delco F, Inadomi JM. Cost-effectiveness of colonoscopy in screening for colorectal cancer. Ann Intern Med 2000; 133:573-584.
24. Yee J, Kumar NN, Godara S, et al. Extracolonic abnormalities discovered incidentally at CT colonography in a male population. Radiology 2005; 236:519-526.
25. Hara AK, Johnson CD, MacCarty RL, Welch TJ. Incidental extracolonic findings at CT colonography. Radiology 2000; 215:353-357.
26. Cotton PB, Durkalski VL, Pineau BC, et al. Computed tomographic colonography (virtual colonoscopy): a multicenter comparison with standard colonoscopy for detection of colorectal neoplasia. JAMA 2004; 291:1713-1719.
27. Ferrucci JT. Colonoscopy: virtual and optical—another look, another view. Radiology 2005; 235:13-16.
28. Gryspeerdt S, Lefere P. How to avoid pitfalls in imaging: causes and solutions to overcome false negatives and false positives. In Lefere P, Gryspeerdt S (eds). Medical Radiology—Diagnostic Imaging. Virtual Colonoscopy: A Practical Guide. Berlin, Springer, 2006, pp 87-116.
29. Paik DS, Beaulieu CF, Mani A, et al. Evaluation of computer-aided detection in CT colonography: potential application to a screening population. Radiology 2001; 221:332.
30. Jass JR, Whitehall VLJ, Young J, Leggett BA. Emerging concepts in colorectal neoplasia. Gastroenterology 2002; 123:862-876.

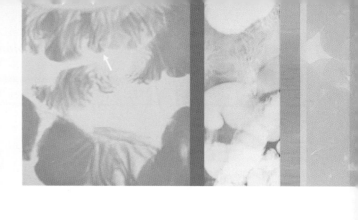

CHAPTER 54

Normal Anatomy and Variants of the Colon

Sunit Sebastian, Abhishek Rajendra Agarwal, Peter A. Harri, Pardeep Mittal, and William Small

TECHNICAL ASPECTS

The various methods of imaging the colon have continually evolved over time with conventional methods such as barium enema and transabdominal ultrasonography becoming less prevalent with increasing use of colonoscopy and CT. As elsewhere in the gastrointestinal tract, state of the art cross-sectional imaging methods such as multidetector CT (MDCT) and MRI provide exquisite details of inflammatory and neoplastic processes involving the colon. More recently, newer imaging techniques such as CT and MR colonography offer noninvasive methods for colonic evaluation. Although somewhat overshadowed by these imaging advancements, the plain abdominal radiograph still retains its significance, because it may be the initial investigation performed especially in acute settings.

In this chapter, we describe the normal gross and radiologic anatomy of the colon. Anatomic variants of the colon also are highlighted. The common theme underlining the imaging algorithm for most of the anomalies is discussed under appropriate headings.

PROS AND CONS

The pros and cons of various imaging modalities are outlined in Table 54-1.

NORMAL ANATOMY

Although a single organ, the colon is embryologically derived from two parts. The transverse colon and parts proximal to it are derived from the midgut being supplied by the superior mesenteric artery while the distal half of the colon is derived from the hindgut and is supplied by the inferior mesenteric artery.[1]

Embryology

The colon begins in the fourth week of gestation. It gets contribution from both the midgut and hindgut. The midgut gives rise to the small intestine and ascending and proximal transverse colon while the hindgut develops into the distal transverse, descending, and sigmoid colon, the rectum, and the proximal anus. Because the midgut grows considerably faster than does the rest of the embryonal body, it experiences various regular movements and rotations, which can be divided into three phases[2]:

Phase 1: Physiologic umbilical hernia (6th gestational week). The loop is located in the base of the umbilical cord (physiologic herniation) with the superior mesenteric artery as an axis. The intestinal loop rotates 90 degrees counterclockwise. As a result of this rotation, the proximal segment of the loop assumes a right-hand position, and the caudal segment, a left-hand position.

Phase 2: Closure of the physiologic umbilical hernia (10th gestational week). In the course of the repositioning of the umbilical hernia, an additional counterclockwise rotation of the midgut by 180 degrees occurs, resulting in a total rotation of 270 degrees. The cecal pouch becomes visible. The cecal pouch is located directly below the liver and grows out caudad. Finally, the cecum with the appendix is positioned in the right iliac fossa and the right flexure is formed.[3]

Phase 3: Peritoneal fixation of the midgut (12th gestational week). The mesenterium of the ascending and descending colon is pushed against the dorsal body wall and fuses completely with the parietal peritoneum. The ascending and the descending colon assume a secondary retroperitoneal position.

441

TABLE 54-1   Pros and Cons of Modalities Used in Imaging the Colon

Modality	Pros	Cons
Radiography	Used for initial evaluation Noninvasive Easily available	No functional evaluation Limited information
Barium enema	Provides information regarding mucosal surface Relatively inexpensive	Requires skill and technical expertise Ionizing radiation Time consuming No information regarding extracolonic findings
MDCT	Fairly easy to perform Exquisite anatomic detail Extracolonic information Multiplanar reconstruction and 3D postprocessing possible	Ionizing radiation Risk of intravenous contrast reactions
CT colonography[28]	Detection of precancerous adenomatous polyps Very low rate of complications Relatively noninvasive as compared with colonoscopy	Bowel preparation still required False-positive and false-negative findings Technical expertise and reader training Specialized software for 3D
MRI MR colonography	Exquisite information of the bowel wall No radiation Detection of precancerous adenomatous polyps	Expensive and not widely available Patient-limiting factors (e.g., claustrophobia, pacemaker) Technical expertise required

TABLE 54-2   Anomalies of Embryologic Development

Anomaly	Stage of Embryonal Development	Details of Anomaly
Nonrotation	Phase 2	Last step of the gut rotation of 180 degrees does not happen. Entire colon is in a double-folded position in the left part of the abdominal cavity (a so-called left colon), without any retroperitoneal fixation
Malrotation	Phase 2	Gut does not complete the last 90 degrees of the rotation. Cecum remains below the pylorus, becoming attached by Ladd's ligaments at the dorsal body wall.
Hyperrotation	Phase 2	Gut rotation of 450 degrees. Cecum lies directly at the left colic flexure.
Subhepatic cecum	Phase 2	Elongation of proximal colon and descensus of cecum does not occur. Cecum-appendix complex remains directly below the liver.
Inverse cecum	Phase 2	Early subhepatic fixation of the cecum below the liver directly after a normal gut rotation. During the elongation of the transverse colon, the cecum bends upward.
Retroperitoneal cecum	Phase 3	Peritoneal fixation of the midgut. Peritoneal membrane (Jackson's paracolic membrane) develops if the cecum is pushed under the laterodorsal peritoneal fixation and encloses the cecum-appendix complex and ascending colon.
Mobile cecum	Phase 3	Incomplete retroperitoneal fixation of ascending colon. Extreme cases completely lack retroperitoneal fixation; whole gut has a collective mesentery (commune mesenterium).

Table 54-2 provides a classification of anomalies of the colon based on alterations at different stages of embryologic development.

Normal Gross Anatomy

The large intestine is divided both anatomically and functionally into colon, rectum, and anus.[1] The colon begins with the cecum at the ileocolic junction and ends with the sigmoid colon at the rectosigmoid junction (Figs. 54-1 and 54-2).

The layered *wall architecture* of the colonic and rectal walls comprises the mucosa, submucosa, inner circular muscle, outer longitudinal muscle, and the serosa and is best seen on endoluminal ultrasound or MR images.[4] The outer longitudinal muscle layer in the colon is separated into three *teniae coli,* which traverse throughout its extent and shorten it to form *haustra,* the sacculations caused by puckering of the bowel wall. The haustral sacculations are fixed structures in the right and transverse colon; in the left colon the sacculations are transient outpouchings, created by the tone of the teniae coli.

The *cecum* is a wide, blind-ending pouch, having the widest diameter in the colon (7.5 to 8.5 cm) but the thinnest muscular wall. The cecum is mostly intraperitoneal and lies in the right iliac fossa. The cecum extends below the bi-lipped ileocecal valve with the appendix, a wormlike structure opening on its posteromedial wall, just inferior to the valve.

The *ileal orifice* is located at the ileal papilla within the lumen of the cecum and is lined by the ileocolic (superior) and ileocecal (inferior) lips. The ascending colon extends vertically in the right anterior pararenal space from the cecum superiorly up to the hepatic flexure near the right hepatic lobe.

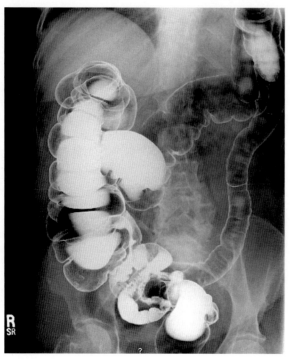

■ **FIGURE 54-1** Double-contrast barium enema depicting the normal mucosal pattern of the entire colon.

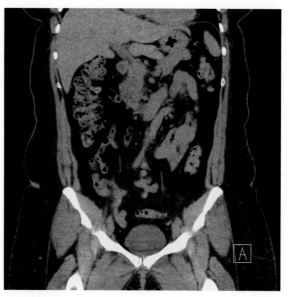

■ **FIGURE 54-3** Coronal CT reformatted image of the abdomen without oral or intravenous contrast enhancement demonstrating the ascending colon and cecum.

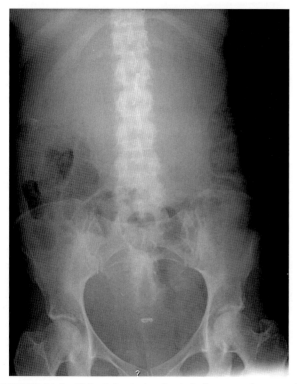

■ **FIGURE 54-2** Plain abdominal radiograph demonstrating normal gas pattern in the large bowel.

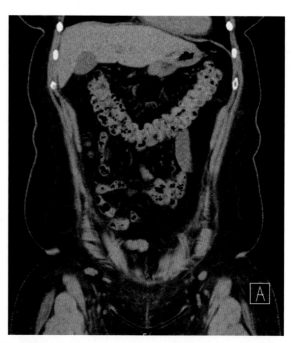

■ **FIGURE 54-4** Coronal CT reformatted image of the abdomen without oral or intravenous contrast enhancement demonstrating the transverse colon.

The *ascending colon* is fixed to the retroperitoneum and covered by peritoneum on its ventral surface only (Fig. 54-3).

The hepatic flexure extends intraperitoneally in a more horizontal course than the transverse colon with transi-

tion to the descending colon occurring at the splenic flexure near the splenic hilum.

The *transverse colon* is relatively mobile, suspended from the transverse mesocolon and tethered to the gastro-colic ligament. Both the hepatic and splenic flexures are supported by the left and right phrenicocolic ligaments, which are peritoneal folds connecting with the diaphragm. The greater omentum is attached to the anterosuperior surface of the transverse colon (Fig. 54-4).

The *descending colon,* like the ascending colon, is fixed to the retroperitoneum and oriented more vertically

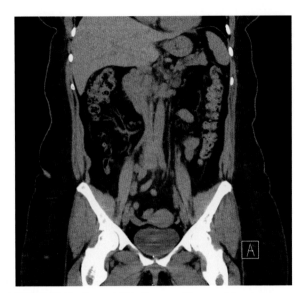

■ **FIGURE 54-5** Coronal CT reformatted image of the abdomen without oral or intravenous contrast enhancement demonstrating the descending colon.

TABLE 54-3 Gross Anatomic Distinguishing Features of Colon

Feature	Details
Omental appendices	Small fatty omentum-like projections on the antimesenteric surface
Teniae coli	Three in number: mesocolic, omental, and free
Haustra	Sacculations on the wall of the colon between the teniae
Caliber	Greater caliber than the small intestinal loops

on the left side of the abdomen. It extends into the left iliac fossa and continues as the sigmoid colon as it enters the brim of the true pelvis (Fig. 54-5).

The *sigmoid colon* is the narrowest and most mobile part of the colon. It is completely intraperitoneal with a sigmoid mesocolon responsible for its redundancy and mobility. The sigmoid colon is variable not only in its position but also in length,[5] and the mobility makes the sigmoid colon the most common site for a volvulus while its narrow diameter makes it most vulnerable to obstruction.

The sigmoid colon continues extraperitoneally at S2-S4 vertebral levels as the *rectum,* which follows the sacral promontory to the anal canal.

The gross anatomic characteristic features of the colon are outlined in Table 54-3.

Vascular Anatomy

The arterial and venous drainage of the colon is outlined in Table 54-4.[1,6]

Normal Radiologic Anatomy

Barium Enema

Both the single and double contrast techniques are used to evaluate the colon in a barium enema procedure. Luminal contour is demonstrated on double-contrast imaging as a continuous barium-etched white line and as a gently curved surface in the barium pool. The mucosal surface is normally smooth but may have a fine network of lines, the innominate grooves or areae colonicae, whereas an abnormal mucosal surface may have a granular, finely nodular, or an ulcerated appearance (see Fig. 54-1).

In some normal studies, lymphoid follicles can be seen as a pattern of fine 1- to 3-mm nodules on the mucosal surface. They are routinely seen in children but may also be occasionally appreciated in adults. Follicles larger than 3 mm may be considered abnormal.[7]

A lesion protruding into the lumen from the anterior surface (e.g., polyp) may appear as a ring shadow or barium-etched lines but may also be obscured by the barium pool on the opposing dependent surface. A lesion protruding from the posterior wall may appear as a radiolucent filling defect in the barium pool or may be obscured if the barium pool is deep. A lesion protruding outside from the posterior wall (e.g., ulcer or diverticulum) may appear as a focal barium collection if it is filled with barium. If the barium pool has been removed from the posterior wall, a depressed lesion may appear as a ring shadow on either the anterior or posterior wall.[8]

Ultrasonography

The normal colonic wall appears as five concentric, alternately echogenic and hypoechoic layers. These layers from lumen outward are as follows:

1. Thin hyperechoic: superficial mucosal surface
2. Hypoechoic: deep mucosa and muscularis mucosae
3. Hyperechoic: submucosa and muscularis propria interface
4. Hypoechoic: muscularis propria
5. Hyperechoic: marginal interface to serosa

The colonic wall is evaluated with graded compression with the thickness of the anterior wall of the colon measured as the distance between the innermost and outermost echogenic layers. The normal average thickness of the gut wall is 2 to 4 mm. The colonic wall is considered stratified when the mucosa, submucosa, and muscularis propria are visualized as separate layers.[9,10]

CT

On CT, the colon easily can be distinguished from small bowel by its location, size, and the presence of haustra. The colon is surrounded by homogeneous fat. The transverse diameter of the colon varies. The cecum, the widest portion of the colon, should measure less than 9 cm in diameter. The transverse colon measures less than 6 cm in diameter, and the descending/sigmoid colon is slightly

TABLE 54-4 Blood Supply of the Colon

Artery	Part of Colon Supplied	Branches
Superior mesenteric artery	Cecum	Right colic artery
	Ascending colon	Middle colic artery
	Proximal two thirds of transverse colon	Ileocolic artery
Inferior mesenteric artery	Distal third of transverse colon	Left colic
	Descending colon	Sigmoid
	Sigmoid colon	
	Rectum	
Venous Drainage of Colon		
Right colon	Superior mesenteric vein—joins splenic vein to form portal vein	
Left colon	Inferior mesenteric vein—joins splenic vein	
Watershed areas	Segmental ischemic colitis frequently affects these points, especially the one at the splenic flexure.	
Griffith's point	At the splenic flexure where branches of the middle colic and left colic meet	
Sudek's point	Where the last sigmoid branch and the superior hemorrhoidal artery meet	

smaller in caliber. The normal appendix can be identified on routine CT scan of the abdomen as a small thin-walled tubular structure arising from the posteromedial aspect of the cecum between the ileocecal valve and the cecal tip. The length of the appendix is quite variable, measuring up to 20 cm. The wall of the colon is very thin and barely perceptible if the colon is well distended with contrast medium. Gas, feces, and minimal fluid may normally be present within the colon.[11]

MRI

The normal colonic wall has a T1-weighted (T1W) signal intensity between that of water and muscle that is of a slightly higher signal intensity than the surrounding fat on fat-suppressed T1W sequences and has T2-weighted (T2W) signal intensity between that of fat and water. The wall appears as a thin-enhancing line after administration of gadolinium. Normal contrast enhancement is reported to be minimal. MRI with its superior soft tissue contrast enhancement enables the identification of the different layers of the bowel wall as well as identification of the peritoneal reflections.[12]

PATHOPHYSIOLOGY AND PATHOLOGIC CORRELATION

Nonrotation

The umbilical loop does not fulfill the last step of the gut rotation of 180 degrees, causing the entire colon to remain in a double-folded position in the left part of the abdominal cavity (a so-called left colon), without any retroperitoneal fixation.[2]

Barium, CT, and MRI findings include:

- Right-sided position of the entire small bowel
- Left-sided position of the large bowel loops
- Inverse relation of superior mesenteric vein to superior mesenteric artery
- Anomalous middle mesenteric artery in some cases[13]
- Volvulus complicating nonrotation

Subhepatic Cecum

The cecum fails to descend to its normal position in 6% of cases if the elongation of the proximal colon in the third phase of the gut rotation does not occur. The cecum/appendix complex remains directly below the liver. Many transitional forms exist between the normal position in the right iliac fossa and the subhepatic position. Appendicitis will be manifest as pain localized to the right upper quadrant.[14]

Barium and imaging findings include:

- Subhepatic location of the cecum/appendix complex
- Short length of ascending colon
- Appendix points downward

Mobile Cecum

A mobile cecum develops due to lack of retroperitoneal fixation of the beginning of the ascending colon. The colon may, in extreme cases, completely lack retroperitoneal fixation to the extent that the whole gut has a collective mesentery, called the commune mesenterium. The mobile cecum and common mesenterium predispose to a volvulus or to malposition of the appendix.

Barium and imaging studies show a change in position of cecum in sequential films or with patient movement.[15]

Hyperrotation

The cecum lies directly at the left colic flexure due to a gut rotation of 450 degrees. Another hypothesis is that an unlimited *descensus* of the cecum pushes the cecum at first into the pelvis and subsequently superiorly to the dorsal abdominal wall.[16]

Barium and imaging studies show the cecum in the left upper quadrant and excessive length of colon.

Inverse Cecum

Inverse cecum occurs due to an early subhepatic fixation of the cecum below the liver after a normal gut rotation. Elongation of the transverse colon causes the cecum to bend upward.

Barium and imaging studies show a high-placed cecum and an appendix pointing upward.

Retroperitoneal Cecum

A peritoneal membrane (Jackson's paracolic membrane) encloses the cecum/appendix complex and ascending colon. This membrane develops if the cecum is pushed under the laterodorsal peritoneal fixation.[17]

Retrogastric Colon

Three types have been described:

Type I: pancreaticogastric interposition of distal transverse colon and the splenic flexure with small bowel malrotation

Type II: pancreaticogastric interposition of distal transverse colon and the splenic flexure without obvious small bowel positional abnormality except for a caudal displacement of the duodenojejunal junction by the interposed colon

Type III: retrosplenic position of the radiologic splenic flexure without pancreaticogastric interposition

These anatomic variants in position may sometimes mimic lesser sac pathologic processes on imaging studies.

Plain radiographs and barium studies demonstrate a characteristic widening and a medial, paraspinal position of the splenic flexure, and lateral views on barium studies show a retrogastric location of the transverse colon.

Associated findings include:

● Shorter than average transverse colon
● Unusually low duodenojejunal junction (type II) *or*
● Frank small bowel malrotation (type I)

Cross-sectional imaging shows[18]:

● Transverse colon and splenic flexure posterior to the stomach and anterior to all or part of the pancreas (pancreaticogastric interposition)
● Transverse colon and splenic flexure posterior to the spleen and stomach (retrosplenic)[19]

Colonic Interpositions

Chilaiditi's Sign

Sometimes the hepatic flexure, a part of the transverse colon with or without part of small intestine, becomes interposed between the liver and diaphragm. This hepatodiaphragmatic interposition is known as Chilaiditi's sign and as Chilaiditi syndrome when symptoms are present. An increased prevalence has been reported with increasing age, cirrhosis, chronic obstructive pulmonary disease, near-term pregnancy, mental disorder, obesity, and primary lung cancer.

Plain radiographs and barium imaging show a gas-filled colon between the right dome of the diaphragm and liver shadow. The findings may mimic pneumoperitoneum.[20-22] Cross-sectional imaging shows the hepatic flexure portion of the transverse colon with or without part of small intestine is interposed between the liver and right dome of diaphragm. In splenodiaphragmatic interposition of the descending colon the left colic flexure and the beginning of descending colon are present behind the spleen just between the diaphragm and spleen.

Right Lower Quadrant Position of the Sigmoid Colon

The sigmoid colon is sometimes present in the right lower quadrant in infants and young children. Thus, care should be taken not to misinterpret air within a redundant right-sided sigmoid colon as air within the cecum in children being examined for a suspected abnormality such as volvulus, malrotation, appendicitis, or intussusception.[23]

Redundant Colon

A redundant colon results when extra loops of colon form, resulting in a longer than normal colon. It may predispose to constipation or a volvulus. It also can make colonoscopy difficult or even impossible.[24,25]

Imaging findings include:

● Normal rotation with excess length of colon, largest in distal colon
● Normal caliber and wall thickness of colon

ANATOMIC VARIANTS

Paucity of haustra is a normal phenomenon in the left colon. This knowledge is important when evaluating imaging studies for colitis, which can present on imaging studies as loss of normal haustra due to mucosal edema.

Barium may enter in innominate grooves simulating mucosal ulceration. These are distinguished from mucosal ulceration by their inconsistency.

Rectal ears are transitory protrusions of the rectum and are visible on barium films in young children.

Vascular Variants[1,26]

Vascular variants are outlined in Table 54-5.

Pseudolesions and Pathology Mimics

Pressure Effect and Displacements

Overdistended bladder may cause displacement of the colon, which disappears after catheterization. A large spleen may cause a pressure defect on the proximal descending colon. There may be pressure from the edge of the liver on the superior aspect of the hepatic flexure.

Pseudomass Lesions

Large ileocecal valves may simulate polypoid masses within the cecum.[27] Retrograde prolapse of an ileocecal valve may simulate a mass in the cecum. A prominent haustral pattern may give the appearance of diverticulosis. A physiologic colonic sphincter can mimic a colonic neoplasm. Sequential scans or postevacuation barium films may help in the differentiation.

TABLE 54-5 Variations in Vascular Anatomy

Artery/Area	Type	Details
Celiomesenteric trunk		Common origin of celiac plexus and superior mesenteric artery (SMA)
Middle mesenteric artery		Anomalous artery arising between the SMA and inferior mesenteric artery (IMA)
Right colic artery	Origin	Directly from SMA, middle colic artery, or ileocolic artery
	Absence	Ascending colon supplied by the middle colic and ileocolic arteries
Middle colic artery	Origin	From the celiac artery, IMA, common or right hepatic, right gastroepiploic, gastroduodenal, dorsal or transverse pancreatic and splenic artery
	Number	Complete absence
		Accessory or double middle colic artery
Blood supply to splenic flexure	If middle colic artery absent	From IMA via the left colic artery (~89%) and from SMA via the middle colic artery (~11%)
		Supplied by the right colic artery (originating from the SMA) and the left colic artery
	If left colic artery absent	Branches of the colosigmoid artery and the paracolic artery may form an anastomotic arcade (the meandering artery of Moskowitz or the marginal artery of Drummond).
Collateral circulation	Arc of Bühler	Direct communication between the celiac artery and SMA (~2%), a remnant of the embryonic ventral segmental arteries of the primitive intestinal vessels

Excessive fat in the pelvis (lipomatosis/obesity) can cause elongation, elevation, and narrowing of the pelvic colon. Lateral films may show an increased presacral space. Prominent lymphoid follicles in children simulating polyps cause confusion with polyposis coli.[7]

Appendiceal Variations

The position of the appendix varies among individuals. Five positions have been commonly identified:

1. Ascending appendix in the retrocecal recess (65.0%, most common type)
2. Descending appendix in the iliac fossa (31.0%)
3. Transverse appendix in the retrocecal recess (5%)
4. Paracecal and preilial ascending appendix (1.0%)
5. Paracecal and postilial ascending appendix (0.5%)

Nonfixed (appendix libera) and fixed (appendix fixa) appendices may occur. The position of a nonfixed appendix is changed permanently. The descending appendix is, most commonly, a nonfixed appendix.

KEY POINTS

- Knowledge of normal anatomy and variants is important to avoid misdiagnosis.
- CT and MR colonography represent newer noninvasive methods for colonic imaging.
- A working knowledge of embryology is necessary to understand congenital anomalies.

SUGGESTED READINGS

Gelfand D. The colon. Curr Opin Radiol 1990; 2:407-412.

Hamilton SR. Structure of the colon. Scand J Gastroenterol Suppl 1984; 93:13-23.

Kinner S, Lauenstein TC. MR colonography. Radiol Clin North Am 2007; 45:377-387.

Levine DS, Haggitt RC. Normal histology of the colon. Am J Surg Pathol 1989; 13:966-984.

Rosenblum JD, Boyle CM, Schwartz LB. The mesenteric circulation—anatomy and physiology. Surg Clin North Am 1997; 77:289-306.

Simpkins KC. Double-contrast examination: III. Colon. Clin Gastroenterol 1984; 13:99-121.

Summerton S, Little E, Cappell MS. CT colonography: current status and future promise. Gastroenterol Clin North Am 2008; 37:161-189.

REFERENCES

1. Hollinshead WH. Embryology and surgical anatomy of the colon. Dis Colon Rectum 1962; 5:23-27.
2. Strouse PJ. Disorders of intestinal rotation and fixation ("malrotation"). Pediatr Radiol 2004; 34:837-851.
3. Malas MA, Gokcimen A, Sulak O. The growing of the cecum and vermiform appendix during the fetal period. Fetal Diagn Ther 2001; 16:173-177.
4. Beynon J, Foy DM, Temple LN, et al. The endoscopic appearances of normal colon and rectum. Dis Colon Rectum 1986; 29:810-813.
5. Bhatnagar BNS, Sharma CLN, Gupta SN, et al. Study of the anatomical dimensions of the human sigmoid colon. Clin Anat 2004; 17:236-243.
6. Sunderland S. Blood supply of the distal colon. Aust NZ J Surg 1942; 11:253-263.
7. Kelvin FM, Max RJ, Norton GA, et al. Lymphoid follicular pattern of the colon in adults. AJR Am J Roentgenol 1979; 133:821-825.
8. Martel W, Robins JM. The barium enema: technique, value, and limitations. Cancer 1971; 28:137-143.

9. Bolondi L, Caletti G, Casanova P, et al. Problems and variations in the interpretation of the ultrasound feature of the normal upper and lower GI tract wall. Scand J Gastroenterol Suppl 1986; 123:16-26.

10. Ledermann HP, Börner N, Strunk H, et al. Bowel wall thickening on transabdominal sonography. Am J Radiol 2000; 74:107-115.

11. Desai RK, Tagliabue JR, Wegryn SA, Einstein DM. CT evaluation of wall thickening in the alimentary tract. RadioGraphics 1991; 11: 771-783.

12. Martin DR, Danrad R, Herrmann K, et al. Magnetic resonance imaging of the gastrointestinal tract. Topics Magn Reson Imaging 2005; 16:77-98.

13. Kawai K, Koizumi M, Honma S, et al. A case of nonrotation of the midgut with a middle mesenteric artery. Ann Anat 2006; 188: 13-17.

14. Silverstein IS. Subhepatic cecum and appendix. Mississippi Valley Med J 1950; 72:145-149.

15. Rogers RL, Harford FJ. Mobile cecum syndrome. Dis Colon Rectum 1984; 27:399-402.

16. Pellatt A, Evans A. A further case of hyperrotation of the colon. Anat Rec 1982; 204:289-293.

17. Reid DG. The genesis of Jackson's membrane: notes on the genito-mesenteric fold of peritoneum and the supra-adhesion foramen. J Anat Physiol 1914; 48:432-444.

18. Oldfield AL, Wilbur AC. Retrogastric colon: CT demonstration of anatomic variations. Radiology 1993; 186:557-561.

19. Oyar O, Yesildag A, Malas U, Gulsoy K. Splenodiaphragmatic interposition of the descending colon. Surg Radiol Anat 2003; 25:434-438.

20. Chilaiditi D. Zur Frage der hepatoptose und Ptose im Allgemeinen im anschlussan drei Falle von temporarer, partieller Leberverlagerung. Fortschr Geb Rontgenstr Nuklearmed Erganzungsband 1910-11; 16:173-208.

21. Vogel T, Berthel M. Chilaiditi's sign. Dig Liver Dis 2009; 41:71.

22. Nakagawa H, Toda N, Taniguchi M, et al. Prevalence and sonographic detection of Chilaiditi's sign in cirrhotic patients without ascites. AJR Am J Roentgenol 2006; 187:W589-W593.

23. Fiorella DJ, Donnelly LF. Right lower quadrant position of the sigmoid colon in infants and young children. Radiology 2001; 219:91-94.

24. Lichtenstein GR, Park PD, Long WB, et al. Use of a push enteroscope improves ability to perform total colonoscopy in previously unsuccessful attempts at colonoscopy in adult patients. Am J Gastroenterol 1999; 94:187-190.

25. Brummer P, Seppala P, Wegelius U. Redundant colon as a cause of constipation. Gut 1962; 3:140.

26. Sakorafas GH, Zouros E, Peros G. Applied vascular anatomy of the colon and rectum: clinical implications for the surgical oncologist. Surg Oncol 2006; 15:243-255.

27. Silva AC, Beaty SD, Hara AK, et al. Spectrum of normal and abnormal CT appearances of the ileocecal valve and cecum with endoscopic and surgical correlation. RadioGraphics 2007; 27:1039-1054.

28. Taylor SA, Halligan S, Bartram CI. CT colonography: methods, pathology and pitfalls. Clin Radiol 2003; 58:179-190.

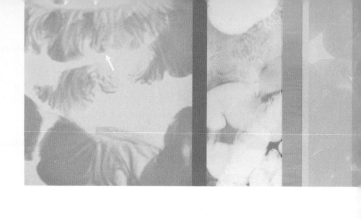

CHAPTER 55

Inflammatory and Infectious Colonic Lesions

Michael Macari

ETIOLOGY

Colonic inflammation may be caused by numerous processes.[1,2] It is typically thought of as colitis. Some inflammatory conditions of the colon such as diverticulitis and epiploic appendagitis are not typically thought of as colitis; however, they do represent inflammatory lesions of the colon and, on occasion, may be difficult to distinguish from each other and even from neoplastic conditions.

Colitis may be due to infection, autoimmune processes (Crohn's and ulcerative colitis), ischemia (of which there are numerous causes, including low flow, embolic, and vasculitis), irradiation, direct toxic insults, chronic abuse of cathartic agents, and intrinsic pathologic inflammatory conditions such as diverticulitis and epiploic appendagitis.[3-11]

In the case of ulcerative colitis and Crohn's colitis, ongoing activation of the mucosal immune system is thought to represent the underlying cause.[9,10] There are numerous stimulants to the activation of this abnormal autoimmune process in patients with Crohn's and ulcerative colitis, but both genetic and environmental factors are important.[9] Infectious colitis may be due to bacteria, parasites, or viruses. The patient's underlying immune status is important to know when considering the differential diagnosis of infectious colitis. In addition to typical infectious agents that may cause colitis, those persons with altered immunity are at risk for opportunistic infections. A history of recent travel and food ingestion can also be helpful when considering infectious causes. Although certain imaging findings are helpful in the differential diagnosis, they are often nonspecific in the case of infectious colitis, and culture of the stools is often necessary to determine the exact cause of infectious colitis.[1-3] A direct toxin or pathologic abnormality may be the cause of the colonic inflammation. In this chapter the focus is on the imaging findings and differential diagnosis of nonischemic causes of colonic inflammation.

PREVALENCE AND EPIDEMIOLOGY

The prevalence of colonic inflammation is related to the etiology of the process and the age of the patient.[8-10] Ulcerative colitis affects 10 to 12/100,000 individuals in the United States, with the peak incidence occurring between ages 15 and 25.[10] The prevalence of Crohn's disease is similar, affecting up to 20 to 40/100,000 individuals of Northern European descent.[11] Although most patients with these conditions are young, there is a bimodal age distribution with a second peak in older individuals.[9,10]

Diverticular disease affects up to 10% of the population older than the age of 50, and up to 20% of these patients will develop symptomatic diverticulitis.[12] Infectious colitis can affect anyone but is very common in immunocompromised individuals.[13-15] Other forms of colonic inflammation including stercoral colitis, epiploic appendagitis, cathartic colon, and glutaraldehyde colitis occur much less frequently.[2,5,6,16]

CLINICAL PRESENTATION

Most patients with colonic inflammation present with crampy abdominal pain, fever, leukocytosis, and some form of change in bowel habits.[1,2,9,10,12] The change in bowel habits is usually diarrhea. Diarrhea may be bloody or nonbloody and is related to the type of inflammation. Although the clinical presentation, nature and frequency of the diarrhea, age of the patient, and other epidemiologic factors may indicate a particular type of colonic inflammation, laboratory testing, cross-sectional imaging, endoscopy with biopsy, and culture of the stool are critical in establishing the correct diagnosis.

PATHOPHYSIOLOGY

By definition, colonic inflammation occurs in the colon. However, when considering the imaging findings that help to narrow the differential diagnosis of a pathologic

449

condition affecting the colon, several factors are important. These include the length of involvement, the location of involvement, the degree of thickening, and the extraintestinal manifestations of the disease. By carefully considering these anatomic considerations the differential diagnosis can be considerably narrowed.[4]

IMAGING

General Considerations

Because the clinical manifestations of patients with colonic inflammation are broad and overlap with other colonic diseases, an algorithm to help narrow the differential diagnosis is helpful. When evaluating colonic pathology on cross-sectional imaging, the differential diagnosis can be narrowed by determining several key observations. Even after using these critical imaging observations, uncertainty may still exist as to the specific etiology of the colonic inflammation. Nevertheless, this patterned approach is usually helpful when considering the cause of an abnormal segment of colon.

Length of Involvement

The length of diseased colon is important in narrowing the differential diagnosis. Certain entities tend to be focal, segmental, or diffuse.

Focal Disease (2 to 10 cm)

- Neoplasm
- Diverticulitis
- Epiploic appendagitis
- Infection (tuberculosis/amebiasis)

Segmental Disease (10 to 40 cm)

- Usually colitis
  - Crohn's colitis
  - Glutaraldehyde colitis
  - Ischemia
  - Infection
  - Ulcerative colitis (typically begins in the rectum and spreads proximally)
- Rarely neoplasm (especially lymphoma)

Diffuse Disease (Most of the Colon)

- Always benign
  - Infection
  - Ulcerative colitis
  - Vasculitis (almost always involves the small bowel as well)

Location of Involvement

Whereas almost any pathologic condition can affect any area of the colon, some pathologic entities have a propensity to localize to certain areas of the colon. Certain entities tend to occur in the cecum or rectum.

Cecal Region

- Amebiasis
- Typhlitis (neutropenic colitis)
- Tuberculosis

Isolated Splenic Flexure/Proximal Descending Colon

- Watershed area for low-flow intestinal ischemia

Rectum

- Early stages of ulcerative colitis
- Stercoral colitis

Multiple Skip Regions

- Crohn's disease

Degree of Thickening

There is quite a bit of overlap in the degree of colonic wall thickening among different colonic pathologic processes. Mild thickening may be seen in plaque-like tumors and mild colonic inflammation. Marked colonic thickening greater than 1.0 to 1.5 cm may be seen in pseudomembranous, tuberculous, and cytomegaloviral colitis as well as colonic neoplasms and vasculitis.[4] Occasionally, the degree of thickening and the imaging appearance of colon cancer and diverticulitis may overlap (Figs. 55-1 and 55-2).[17-19] In both cases the disease is usually focal or involves a short segment of colon and may be associated with marked thickening of the bowel wall. Inflammatory changes in the mesentery have been shown to favor the diagnosis of diverticulitis, and adjacent lymphadenopathy has been shown to favor colon cancer.[17,19] Quantitative CT perfusion measurements may enable differentiation of cancer from diverticulitis. A recent study showed increased blood volume, blood flow, and permeability in patients with colon cancer when compared with those with diverticulitis.[18] However, because there is considerable overlap in the degree of thickening of different colonic pathologic processes, overall the degree of thickening has limited value in itself for narrowing the differential diagnosis.

Pattern of Enhancement

The pattern of enhancement has been shown to be important in discriminating different forms of intestinal pathology.[4]

Target/Double Halo

- Edema
  - Infection, inflammation (ulcerative and Crohn's colitis), ischemia, vasculitis
- Submucosal fat
  - Chronic inflammation
  - Normal variant
- Neoplasm
  - Rarely scirrhous carcinoma of rectum

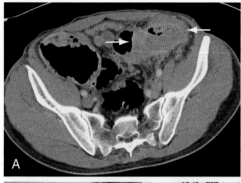

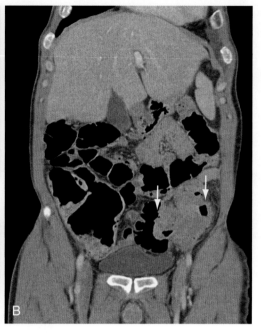

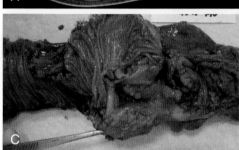

■ **FIGURE 55-1** **A,** Axial contrast-enhanced CT image shows marked thickening of the sigmoid colon (*arrows*). **B,** Coronal reformatted CT from same examination better demonstrates segmental (approximately 10 cm) distribution of disease (*arrows*). **C,** Resected specimen reveals florid diverticulitis.

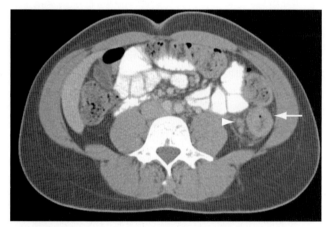

■ **FIGURE 55-2** Axial CT scan shows focal thickening of the descending colon (*arrow*) with adjacent adenopathy (*arrowhead*). Resected specimen revealed adenocarcinoma. Lymphadenopathy adjacent to focal colon thickening favors the diagnosis of colon cancer over diverticulitis.

Homogeneous

● Neoplasm, chronic inflammation

Heterogeneous

● Neoplasm

Diminished

● Ischemia

Extraintestinal Manifestations

When an abnormal segment of colon is evaluated the adjacent mesentery, presence and attenuation of abdomi-

nal lymph nodes, and status of the vasculature all need to be assessed.[4,8,14] Abnormalities pertaining to these structures can be helpful in narrowing the differential diagnosis. Low-attenuated lymph nodes are often associated with tuberculosis. Mesenteric changes including fibrofatty proliferation, sinus formation, and hyperemia in the vessels subtending an abnormal segment suggest Crohn's disease. Filling defects in the vessels suggest colonic ischemia.

Radiography

The hallmark of acute colonic inflammation on radiographs of the abdomen is the "thumbprinting" sign (Fig. 55-3). This finding represents thickened haustral folds (in general due to edema) with intracolonic gas outlining the thickened haustral folds. This is a nonspecific finding and is related to edema in the colonic submucosa. This finding correlates with the "double halo" or "target" sign that is seen on CT.[1,2,4] Thumbprinting on radiographs and the double halo sign on CT may be seen in any form of acute colonic inflammation, including infection, ischemia, ulcerative colitis, Crohn's disease, and vasculitis.

Another finding that may be present on plain radiographs and may suggest a specific diagnosis is an ahaustral colon. On imaging, this manifests as a featureless tubular appearance of the colon. This is usually seen in the descending colon and represents chronic scarring that may occasionally be seen in ulcerative colitis and rarely in cathartic colon (Fig. 55-4).

Finally, plain radiographs of the abdomen may show small filling defects in the colon (Fig. 55-5). The differential diagnosis when this is seen includes a polyposis syndrome such as familial adenomatous polyposis and postinflammatory pseudopolyps in the colon, which may be seen in ulcerative colitis and Crohn's disease. Other than these imaging findings, radiographs of the abdomen

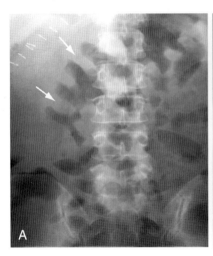
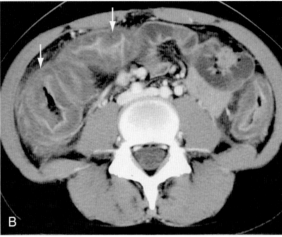

■ **FIGURE 55-3**   **A,** Radiograph of the abdomen shows "thumbprinting" in the transverse colon (*arrows*). **B,** Contrast-enhanced CT in the same patient shows marked colonic wall thickening (*arrows*) with mural stratification. The patient had had a cholecystectomy and had *Clostridium difficile* colitis.

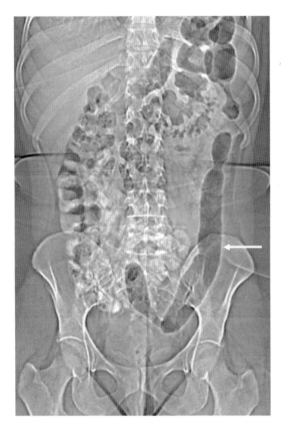

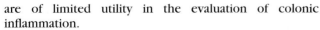

■ **FIGURE 55-4**   Scout radiograph for CT shows ahaustral left colon (*arrows*). Differential diagnosis includes cathartic colon (melanosis coli) and chronic ulcerative colitis. The patient had chronic ulcerative colitis.

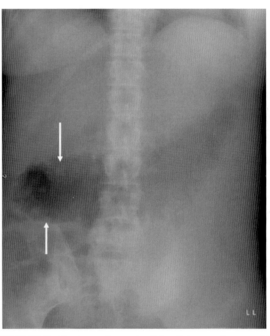

■ **FIGURE 55-5**   Supine radiograph of the abdomen shows multiple small filling defects in the transverse colon (*arrows*). The differential diagnosis includes polyposis syndrome and postinflammatory polyps. There were postinflammatory polyps in this patient with ulcerative colitis.

are of limited utility in the evaluation of colonic inflammation.

Barium studies of the colon used to be the primary noninvasive imaging technique to evaluate the colon in case of colonic inflammation. However, CT and endoscopy are now the primary imaging techniques to evaluate the patient with colonic inflammation.

CT

Normal Colon

CT is the primary imaging tool used to evaluate patients with abdominal pain and suspected colonic disease. There are three main findings on CT that correlate with colonic inflammation. These are colonic wall thickening, mural stratification ("target" sign) after the intravenous administration of a contrast agent, and pericolonic fat stranding.

The normal colonic wall is thin, measuring between 1 and 2 mm when the lumen is well distended. However, there is considerable variation in the thickness of the normal colonic wall depending on the degree of luminal distention. As a result, different criteria have been used to diagnose colonic wall thickening.[1,2,4,20,21]

The variability in colonic wall thickness related to the degree of distention is well known based on observations at CT colonography. It is not unusual for the wall of the normal colon to measure up to 5 mm in the supine position and 1 mm in the prone position and vice versa. This is directly related to the amount of gas in the segment of colon.

Frequently, because of internal fecal contents, fluid, or colonic redundancy the true thickness is difficult to ascertain. This is most true for the sigmoid colon and is a location where bowel wall thickening is often "over-called" on CT. In these cases, carefully following the colonic wall to a region where the colon is well distended with gas will often demonstrate the true thickness of the wall (Fig. 55-6). Observing the enhancement pattern and changes in the pericolonic fat are also helpful in determining whether the bowel is truly abnormal.

Typically, no specific colonic preparation is utilized when performing routine abdominal and pelvic CT. That is, neither gas nor fluid is administered per rectum before data acquisition. However, if there is a concern regarding the true thickness of the colonic wall, insufflation of the colon with room air via a small rectal catheter can be very helpful in revealing the true thickness.

The normal colonic wall enhances after an adequate intravenous bolus of contrast agent has been administered. When abdominal CT is performed, a 20- to 22-gauge catheter should be inserted into an arm vein and 1.5 to 2.0 mL/kg of iodinated contrast agent should be injected at a rate of at least 2.5 to 3.0 mL/s. Enhancement is usually greater on the mucosal aspect of the bowel wall. This enhancement should not be mistaken as a pathologic process. Recognizing that the wall is not thickened and that no perienteric inflammation is present will allow one to differentiate normal enhancement from a pathologic process. If an intravenous contrast agent is not administered, significant colonic pathologic processes may be overlooked (Fig. 55-7).

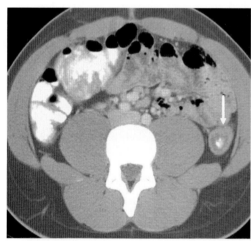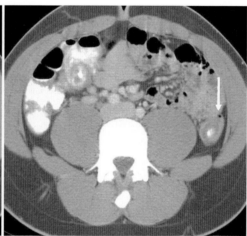

■ **FIGURE 55-6** Oral and intravenous contrast-enhanced CT (*left*) shows apparent thickening of the descending colon (*arrow*). Image obtained 1 cm caudal (*right*) shows small bubble of gas adjacent to nondependent wall (*arrow*). The true thickness of the colon wall is 1 to 2 mm. Note there is no pericolonic stranding to suggest a pathologic process.

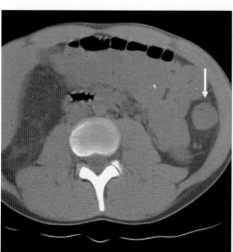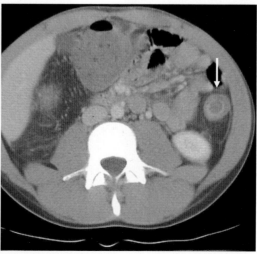

■ **FIGURE 55-7** Axial unenhanced CT image (*left*) shows no obvious abnormality in the descending colon (*arrow*). Two hours later the scan was repeated after intravenous contrast agent administration (*right*). Note target appearance (*arrow*) to the enhancement of the descending colon consistent with acute inflammation. Biopsy revealed Crohn's disease.

Multidetector CT of the colon should be performed on at least a 4-detector row scanner, but optimal evaluation is obtained on a 16-detector row or higher scanner. These scanners can acquire submillimeter isotropic data that are necessary for 3D displays. At our institution we utilize either a 16 × 0.75-mm or 64 × 0.6-mm detector configuration depending on whether a 16- or 64-row detector scanner is used to reconstruct either 1.0- or 0.8-mm slices. From this dataset, the technologist will generate a set of axial 4.0-mm sections and a set of 3.0-mm thick coronal multiplanar reconstructed images at 3.0-mm intervals encompassing the entire bowel. Coronal images can be extremely helpful when evaluating the bowel because of the redundant nature of both the small bowel and colon.

Specific Pathologic Causes of Colonic Inflammation

The hallmark of inflammation at CT is the "double halo" or "target" sign (Fig. 55-8).[1,2,4] The target sign was first described as a specific sign for Crohn's disease, but it is now recognized that any non-neoplastic condition may lead to a target appearance in the small bowel or colon (Figs. 55-9 to 55-12).[21] Rarely, infiltrating scirrhous

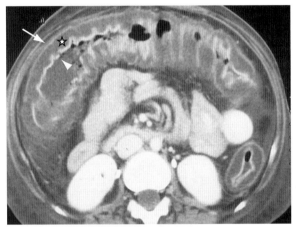

■ **FIGURE 55-8** Axial contrast-enhanced CT image shows target appearance to the enhancement of the abnormal colon. Enhancement of serosa and muscularis (*arrow*), enhancement of the mucosa (*arrowhead*), and low attenuation of the submucosa (*star*) represent the target appearance.

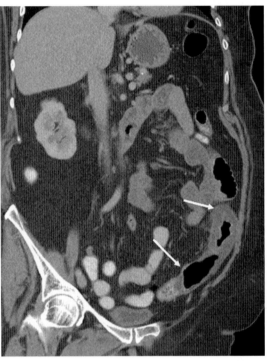

■ **FIGURE 55-10** Oblique coronal reformatted image shows 12-cm segment of thickening of the descending colon (*arrows*). The patient had a colonoscopy the previous day with random biopsies in the region. The findings are consistent with glutaraldehyde colitis.

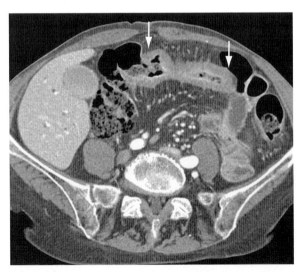

■ **FIGURE 55-9** Axial contrast-enhanced CT shows 15-cm segment of colonic wall thickening with target appearance and irregularity to the mucosa (*arrows*). There is prominence of the vasa recta adjacent to this segment and fibrofatty proliferation consistent with Crohn's colitis.

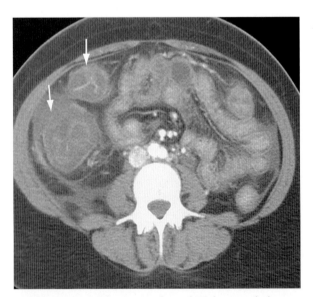

■ **FIGURE 55-11** Axial contrast-enhanced CT shows marked thickening of ascending colon and transverse colon with target appearance (*arrows*). The patient had lupus vasculitis, and this inflammation/ischemia in the colon improved after corticosteroid therapy.

carcinomas of the stomach or colon may display a target or double-halo appearance at CT. It may be difficult to distinguish rectosigmoid inflammation from an infiltrating neoplasm (Fig. 55-13). Although infiltrating scirrhous type neoplasms frequently show marked thickening, adjacent adenopathy, and an abrupt transition, a high index of suspicion is necessary to consider this in the differential diagnosis.

As discussed earlier, the extraintestinal manifestations of colonic inflammation and the clinical history can be very useful in narrowing the differential diagnosis.

Focal colonic inflammation in the cecum may be caused by ischemia, infection, fecal impaction, Crohn's disease, and typhlitis.[22,23] The imaging appearance of these entities may be similar, but there are usually imaging findings that aid in distinguishing these processes.

Focal inflammation in the cecum with an associated liver abscess should raise the possibility of amebiasis (Fig. 55-14).[2,23] Amebiasis is caused by the protozoa *Entamoeba histolytica,* which is endemic in various parts of the tropics. The disease manifests clinically as bloody diarrhea;

and, although any area of the colon may be involved, it has a propensity for the right colon and especially the cecal region. The terminal ileum is usually spared, and with chronic disease the cecum may obtain a cone-like configuration. Amebic liver abscess is the most important complication and is present in approximately 94% of fatal cases.[23]

Intestinal tuberculosis is typically acquired by ingesting contaminated milk or swallowing tracheobronchial secretions in patients with pulmonary tuberculosis.[2] However, intestinal and peritoneal tuberculosis may be present with no pulmonary findings. Intestinal tuberculosis typically affects the ileocecal region (Fig. 55-15). The imaging appearance of the tuberculosis in the colon resembles Crohn's disease.[24,25] There are typically focal or short segments of colonic wall thickening with associated mesenteric changes, including fistula and abscess. On barium examinations, linear ulcers that mimic Crohn's disease may be seen. A distinguishing feature often present with intestinal tuberculosis is the associated low-attenuated mesenteric lymphadenopathy (see Fig. 55-15). This is likely due to the caseating necrosis seen with tuberculosis.

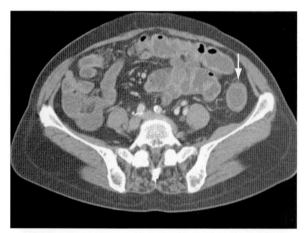

■ **FIGURE 55-12** Axial contrast-enhanced CT shows mild wall thickening in the descending colon (*arrow*). The finding is nonspecific. At colonoscopy, melanotic changes were present and biopsy revealed "melanosis coli," indicative of chronic laxative abuse.

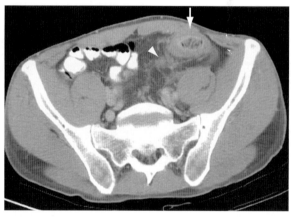

■ **FIGURE 55-13** Axial contrast-enhanced CT shows mural stratification in the sigmoid colon extending from the rectum (*arrow*). Note lymphadenopathy (*arrowhead*). Biopsy revealed infiltrating scirrhous carcinoma. A "double halo" appearance is almost always indicative of inflammation or ischemia. Rarely, infiltrating adenocarcinomas of the rectum and stomach may show a "double halo" appearance on contrast-enhanced CT.

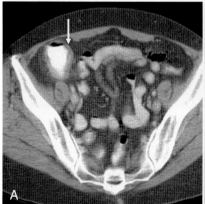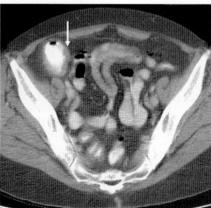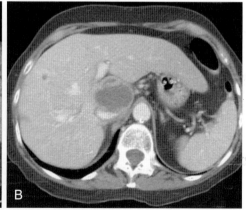

■ **FIGURE 55-14** **A,** Axial contrast-enhanced CT scans (*left* and *right*) several millimeters apart show focal thickening of the cecum (*arrows*) with irregularity to the mucosa and minimal stranding of the adjacent fat. The remainder of the bowel was normal. **B,** Axial contrast-enhanced CT image in the same patient shows a hepatic abscess in the caudate lobe. Amebiasis was confirmed at histologic evaluation.

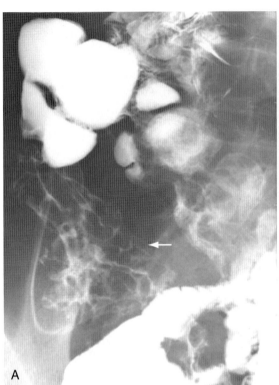

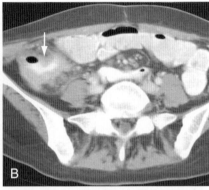

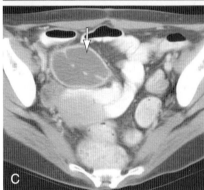

■ **FIGURE 55-15   A,** Spot radiograph of the cecum from a barium enema shows multiple linear ulcerations (*arrow*). The finding suggests Crohn's disease. **B,** Axial contrast-enhanced CT image in same patient shows nonspecific thickening of ileocecal region (*arrow*). **C,** Axial contrast-enhanced CT several centimeters caudal shows large, low-attenuated lymph node (*arrow*). Tuberculosis was confirmed at biopsy and culture.

Typhlitis, also known as neutropenic colitis, primarily affects the cecal region, but any region of the small bowel or colon may be involved, including the appendix (Fig. 55-16).[22] The condition is seen most frequently in patients being treated for acute leukemia. The colonic inflammation is usually multifactorial and is often due to a combination of fungal and bacterial infections as well as to ischemia and hemorrhage. CT is the modality of choice in the evaluation of patients with suspected neutropenic colitis, and colonoscopic evaluation is often contraindicated because these patients are usually quite sick, the colon is very friable and at risk for perforation, and, in addition to the neutropenia, thrombocytopenia is often present. Therefore, these patients are at risk for bleeding. Therapy is usually antimicrobial and supportive.

Stercoral colitis is an inflammatory colitis related to increased intraluminal pressure from impacted fecal material in the colon (Fig. 55-17).[5] This rare condition, first reported in 1894, has been primarily described in the surgical and gastrointestinal literature. As a result of the fecal impaction a focal pressure colitis may occur with ulceration, resulting in colonic perforation. When stercoral colitis is associated with colonic perforation, a 35% mortality rate has been reported.[5]

Radiation-induced colitis is less frequent than radiation-induced enteritis but does occur.[1,2] It tends to be segmental and corresponds to the radiation port. Whenever a localized inflammatory process is noted in the small bowel or colon that does not seem to localize to any specific vascular territory, radiation injury should be suspected. In the acute stages, nonspecific bowel wall thickening may be present with a target appearance and perienteric fat stranding. In the chronic stages, fibrosis and stricture with obstruction may occur.

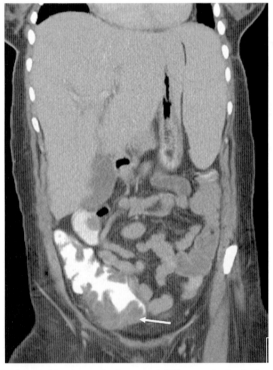

■ **FIGURE 55-16**   Coronal reformatted CT image obtained after oral contrast administration shows only marked thickening of the cecum (*arrow*). The patient had acute myelogenous leukemia and was neutropenic. Note hepatosplenomegaly.

Glutaraldehyde colitis is a direct toxic response to the colon due to inadequate removal of the disinfectant glutaraldehyde from the colonoscope before an endoscopic procedure (see Fig. 55-10).[16] The condition typically occurs 24 to 48 hours after colonoscopy. Patients will

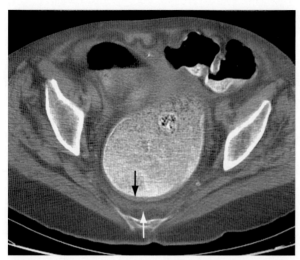

■ **FIGURE 55-17** Axial contrast-enhanced CT image of the rectum shows fecal impaction with wall thickening (*black arrow*) and perirectal fat stranding (*white arrow*). Findings are indicative of stercoral colitis.

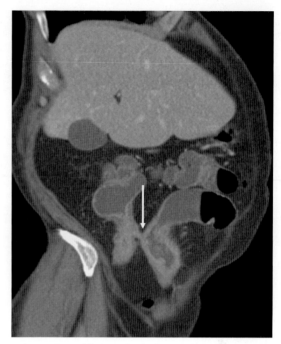

■ **FIGURE 55-18** Oblique coronal reformatted CT image shows tethering and probable fistulization (*arrow*) of the right colon and small bowel in this patient with known Crohn's disease.

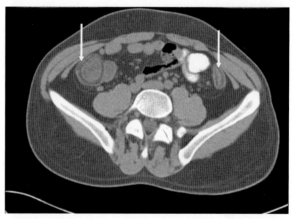

■ **FIGURE 55-19** Axial CT performed after oral administration of a contrast agent shows only target appearance to the right and left colon (*arrows*). Region of interest cursor placed in the submucosa measured −50 HU. Findings are consistent with chronic inflammation in this patient with a 2-year history of ulcerative colitis.

present with severe crampy abdominal pain, bloody diarrhea, and occasionally mild leukocytosis.[16] At CT the colon usually shows segmental, circumferential, mural stratification with moderate to marked wall thickening. Often the location is proximal to the rectum and is at the site of a mucosal biopsy. The proximal location is thought to be related to the disinfectant being trapped in the chamber of the biopsy forceps. As the biopsy device is utilized, the glutaraldehyde acts as a toxin to the colonic mucosa, causing intramural hemorrhage. The condition is self-limiting, and conservative management leads to improvement.

Although Crohn's disease may be focal, it is usually segmental, involving anywhere between 10 and 30 cm of intestine.[8,26-28] Crohn's disease is often associated with numerous skip lesions. Extraintestinal manifestations of the disease include sinus formation, fistula, abscess, the "comb" sign, and fibrofatty proliferation. These imaging features help to distinguish Crohn's disease from other entities (Fig. 55-18).[26,27]

Irregularity of the mucosa with ulceration may be seen on CT and suggests the diagnosis of Crohn's disease.[28] This may enable differentiation of Crohn's disease and other entities such as amebiasis and tuberculosis from other conditions such as vasculitis and low-flow ischemia, which typically show a submucosal pattern of bowel thickening (compare Figs. 55-9 and 55-14 with 55-11).[28,29] Although the mucosal changes may be assessed at CT, they are usually better evaluated at endoscopy.

In cases of chronic colitis, whether it be Crohn's or ulcerative colitis, submucosal fat deposition may occur (Fig. 55-19).[8] Recognition of the fat attenuation within the submucosa will allow differentiation from edema. However, a recent study has shown that submucosal fat deposition may be a normal variant and not necessarily associated with chronic bowel inflammation.[30] In a study of 100 patients undergoing noncontrast CT to evaluate for kidney stones, 21 patients were shown to have submucosal adipose tissue in the bowel and in 4% it was in the terminal ileum. These patients had no history of chronic

bowel inflammation. Therefore, if this finding is seen at CT, correlation with the clinical history is essential.

As discussed earlier, ulcerative colitis is an autoimmune condition associated with mucosal ulceration, edema in the wall, and occasionally extraintestinal manifestations such as bony ankylosis and primary sclerosing cholangitis (Fig. 55-20).[8] Typically, the bowel wall thickening in ulcerative colitis shows mural stratification and the degree of thickening is mild; however, occasionally bowel wall thickening can exceed 1 cm in patients with severe ulcerative colitis.[3] Ulcerative colitis begins in the rectum; and as the inflammation progresses, the disease continues into the more proximal colon without skip areas.[8]

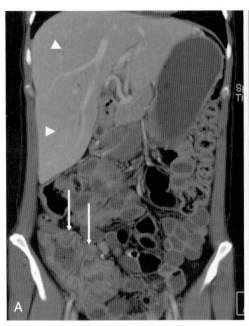

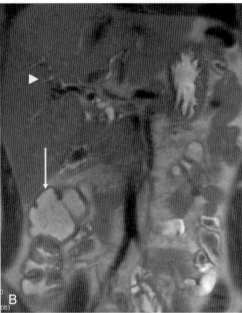

■ **FIGURE 55-20** **A,** Coronal reformatted CT image in this patient with chronic ulcerative colitis shows mural stratification in the right colon (*arrows*). Note mild biliary dilatation (*arrowheads*) in this patient with known sclerosing cholangitis. **B,** Coronal MR image in same patient shows mural stratification in the right colon (*arrow*). Note mild biliary dilatation (*arrowhead*). MRI can often show similar findings to those of CT without the need for ionizing radiation.

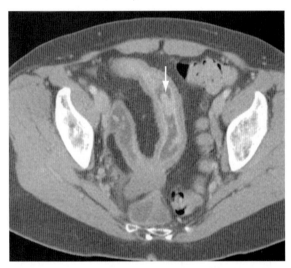

■ **FIGURE 55-21** Axial contrast-enhanced CT of the ileum shows segmental wall thickening, a target appearance, and an enhancing intraluminal filling defect (*white arrow*) consistent with a postinflammatory pseudopolyp in this patient with long-standing Crohn's disease.

In both Crohn's disease and ulcerative colitis postinflammatory pseudopolyps may be seen on CT (Figs. 55-21 and 55-22).[8,31] These lesions represent an abnormal proliferation of the inflamed colonic mucosa. They can get quite large and morphologically may be difficult to distinguish and make detection of carcinoma in the colon challenging. This is a major problem because in both chronic ulcerative colitis and Crohn's colitis the risk of colon cancer is increased over the general population.

When colonic inflammation affects the entire colon a "pancolitis" is present. The differential diagnosis of pancolitis is infection and ulcerative colitis.[4] Rarely, vasculitis may affect the entire colon, but the small bowel usually also is associated.[29]

Pseudomembranous colitis, also known as antibiotic-related colitis, is due to *Clostridium difficile* overgrowth and is a major cause of hospital-acquired morbidity in the United States today. *C. difficile* is a gram-positive anaerobic bacillus that can cause a spectrum of enteric disease ranging from mild diarrhea to fulminant life-threatening colitis.[3] Almost all cases of pseudomembranous colitis are associated with recent antibiotic therapy.[3] Infrequently, a prior history of antibiotic use may not be elicited in documented cases of *C. difficile* colitis. Almost all antibiotics and some antineoplastic agents have been implicated as a factor leading to *C. difficile* colitis. By altering the normal colonic flora, antibiotic use allows *C. difficile* to proliferate, resulting in the clinical disease. Earlier recognition and treatment of *C. difficile*–related colitis with appropriate antibiotics decreases the incidence of fulminant colitis that may develop in these patients. Previously the most common cause of toxic megacolon was ulcerative colitis; however, pseudomembranous colitis is currently the most common cause of this life-threatening condition.[32,33]

Pseudomembranous colitis is clinically suggested when a patient has had a recent history of antibiotic use, concurrent diarrhea, and positive stool assay for *C. difficile.* On CT, the colon may look normal or show marked wall thickening.[3,34,35] The "accordion" sign is defined as alternating edematous haustral folds separated by transverse mucosal ridges filled with oral contrast material, simulating the appearance of an accordion (Fig. 55-23).[34,35] This CT finding was originally reported to be a specific sign of severe *C. difficile*–related colitis. In cases of *C. difficile* colitis, the high attenuation oral contrast agent is trapped between thickened edematous folds and pseudomembranes on the colonic mucosa. The degree of colonic wall thickening caused by the pseudomembranes and edematous tissues that develops in this condition has been suggested as the reason for the sign's specificity.[34] However, a number of other conditions may cause an appearance of an accordion at CT, including lupus, ischemia, edema

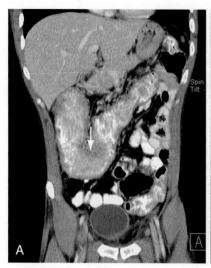
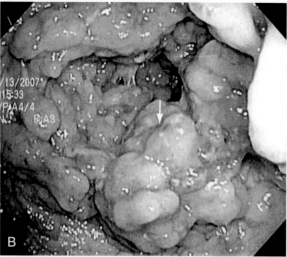

■ **FIGURE 55-22** **A,** Coronal reformatted CT image obtained after oral and intravenous administration of contrast agents in a patient with chronic ulcerative colitis shows irregular frond-like filling defects (*arrow*). **B,** Endoscopic image from same patient shows multiple irregular filling defects (*arrow*). Biopsy revealed postinflammatory pseudopolyps.

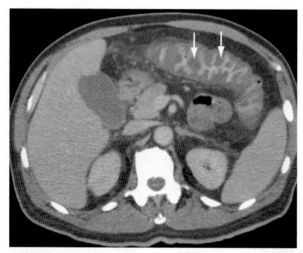

■ **FIGURE 55-23** Axial contrast-enhanced CT image shows marked thickening of the wall of the colon (*arrows*) with barium trapped between the folds. The finding is consistent with the "accordion" sign in this patient with pseudomembranous colitis.

associated with portal hypertension, and many other infectious causes, including cytomegaloviral colitis in immunocompromised patients.[3,36,37]

In patients with cirrhosis the finding of bowel edema has been reported at both barium enema studies and on CT.[37,38] Intestinal wall thickening is common on contrast-enhanced images and is seen in up to 64% of patients. The bowel edema may be mild or marked when due to portal hypertension (Fig. 55-24). When edema from portal hypertension is present in the colon, it can look like any other form of intestinal inflammation and may mimic infection or even ischemia. The edema typically occurs in the ascending colon. Observation that the patient has cirrhosis and correlation with clinical findings will usually suggest the correct diagnosis.

As demonstrated earlier, the differential diagnosis of colonic inflammation is broad. CT is the primary noninvasive imaging modality used to evaluate the patient with colonic inflammation. This is often supplemented with endoscopic evaluation. In addition to all of the previously

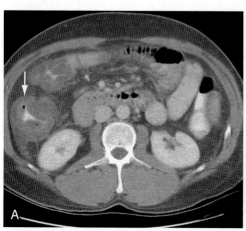
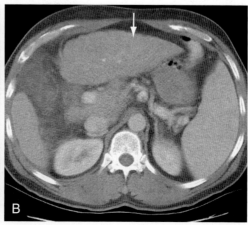

■ **FIGURE 55-24** **A,** Axial contrast-enhanced CT image shows marked thickening of the right colon (*arrow*). The patient had no intestinal symptoms. **B,** Axial contrast-enhanced CT image in the same patient shows cirrhosis (*arrow*). The findings in the colon are consistent with edema related to portal hypertension.

listed causes of colonic inflammation, colonic ischemia should always be considered in the differential diagnosis of a thickened colon.[39] Careful inspection of the mesenteric vasculature should always be performed; and if there is concern because of the results of the imaging study, correlation with serum lactic acid level should be performed; the lactic acid level will usually be elevated in cases of colonic ischemia.

MRI

The concern for radiation-induced carcinogenesis has recently increased.[40,41] This is primarily related to the increased number of CT examinations that are being performed and the increased number of acquisitions that are being obtained with each examination. There is a definite role of MRI in the evaluation of colonic inflammation.[41,42] Although CT is still the primary imaging modality that is used to evaluate colonic inflammation, MRI allows detection of the same findings as CT. In particular, MRI is useful in observing patients with Crohn's disease (see Fig. 55-20). These patients are young and typically receive multiple CT examinations over their lifetime. It is likely that, in the future, MRI will play a greater role in the evaluation of patients with colonic inflammation.

Classic Signs

■ Thumbprinting: indicates colonic edema on plain films.
■ Ahaustral colon: indicates chronic colonic inflammation on plain radiograph or CT.
■ "Target" sign: indicates colonic edema; very rarely can be seen in scirrhous carcinomas of the colon.
■ "Comb" sign: prominent vasa recta subtending an inflamed segment of bowel seen commonly in Crohn's disease.
■ Fibrofatty proliferation: proliferation of adipose tissue around a segment of chronic Crohn's disease.
■ Low-attenuated caseating adenopathy: seen commonly in tuberculosis.

DIFFERENTIAL DIAGNOSIS

The conditions listed below can all be a cause of either focal, segmental, or diffuse colonic disease:

● Crohn's disease
● Ulcerative colitis
● Diverticulitis
● Infectious colitis
● Ischemic colitis
● Epiploic appendagitis
● Vasculitis
● Colon cancer

Imaging, especially with CT and endoscopy, can help narrow the differential diagnosis of these conditions:

● Crohn's disease
● Ulcerative colitis
● Diverticulitis
● Infectious colitis
● Ischemic colitis
● Epiploic appendagitis
● Vasculitis
● Colon cancer

TREATMENT

Most cases of colonic inflammation are treated conservatively with anti-inflammatory medications, antibiotics, and/or supportive care depending on the etiology of the inflammation.

If medical management fails, the bowel perforates, or toxic megacolon develops, surgical intervention is warranted in cases of colonic inflammation.

What the Referring Physician Needs to Know

■ Although radiographs of the abdomen may suggest the diagnosis, plain radiographs have limited use in the evaluation of colonic inflammation.
■ Barium studies (barium enema) used to be the primary noninvasive imaging technique to evaluate colonic inflammation.
■ CT and endoscopy are now the primary imaging techniques to evaluate the patient with colonic inflammation.
■ CT is the primary noninvasive imaging modality to evaluate colon inflammation.
■ The differential diagnosis of colonic inflammation is broad, and by using a patterned approach on CT the differential diagnosis can usually be narrowed.
■ MRI, because of its similar sensitivity to CT and lack of ionizing radiation, may play an important role in the future in the evaluation of patients with colonic inflammation.

KEY POINTS

■ Many different inflammatory and infectious conditions can affect the colon.
■ The location in the colon, length of involvement, and enhancement pattern are helpful in narrowing the differential diagnosis.

■ Diverticular disease and colon cancer may have a similar imaging appearance at MDCT.
■ When a confident diagnosis cannot be made, endoscopic correlation is indicated.

SUGGESTED READINGS

Balthazar EJ. CT of the gastrointestinal tract: principles and interpretation. AJR Am J Roentgenol 1991; 156:23-32.

Gore RM, Balthazar EJ, Ghahremani GG, Miller FH. CT features of ulcerative colitis and Crohn's disease. AJR Am J Roentgenol 1996; 167:3-15.

Horton KM, Corl FM, Fishman EK. CT evaluation of the colon: inflammatory disease. RadioGraphics 2000; 20:399-418.

Macari M, Balthazar EJ. Review: computed tomography of bowel wall thickening: significance and pitfalls of interpretation. AJR Am J Roentgenol 2001; 176:1105-1116.

Thoeni RF, Cello JP. CT imaging of colitis. Radiology 2006; 240: 623-638.

REFERENCES

1. Horton KM, Corl FM, Fishman EK. CT evaluation of the colon: Inflammatory disease. RadioGraphics 2000; 20:399-418.
2. Thoeni RF, Cello JP. CT imaging of colitis. Radiology 2006; 240:623-638.
3. Macari M, Balthazar EJ, Megibow AJ. The accordion sign on CT: a nonspecific finding in patients with colonic edema. Radiology 1999; 211:734-746.
4. Macari M, Balthazar EJ. Review: computed tomography of bowel wall thickening: significance and pitfalls of interpretation. AJR Am J Roentgenol 2001; 176:1105-1116.
5. Heffernan C, Pachter HL, Megibow AJ, Macari M. Original report: Stercoral colitis leading to fatal peritonitis: CT findings. AJR Am J Roentgenol 2005; 184:189-193.
6. Singh AK, Gervais DA, Hahn PF, et al. CT appearance of acute epiploic appendagitis. AJR Am J Roentgenol 2004; 183:1303-1307.
7. Balthazar EJ. CT of the gastrointestinal tract: principles and interpretation. AJR Am J Roentgenol 1991; 156:23-32.
8. Gore RM, Balthazar EJ, Ghahremani GG, Miller FH. CT features of ulcerative colitis and Crohn's disease. AJR Am J Roentgenol 1996; 167:3-15.
9. Podolsky DK. Inflammatory bowel disease. N Engl J Med 2002; 347:417-429.
10. Hanauer SB. Inflammatory bowel disease. N Engl J Med 1996; 334:841-848.
11. Bernstein CN. The epidemiology of inflammatory bowel disease in Canada: a population-based study. Am J Gastroenterol 2006; 101:1559-1568.
12. Ferzoco LB, Raptopoulos V, Silen W. Acute diverticulitis. N Engl J Med 1998; 338:1521-1526.
13. Radin R. HIV infection: analysis in 259 consecutive patients with abnormal abdominal CT findings. Radiology 1995; 197:712-717.
14. Bini EJ, Cohen J. Diagnostic yield and cost-effectiveness of endoscopy in chronic human immunodeficiency virus–related diarrhea. Gastrointest Endosc 1998; 48:354-361.
15. Lew EA, Poles MA, Dietrich DT. Diarrheal diseases associated with HIV infection. Gastroenterol Clin North Am 1997; 26:259-290.
16. Birnbaum BA, Gordon RB, Jacobs JE. Glutaraldehyde colitis: radiologic features. Radiology 1995; 195:131-134.
17. Padidar AM, Jeffrey RB, Mindelzun RE, Dolph JF. Differentiating sigmoid diverticulitis from carcinoma on CT scans: mesenteric inflammation suggests diverticulitis. AJR Am J Roentgenol 1994; 163:81-83.
18. Goh V, Halligan S, Taylor SA, et al. Differentiation between diverticulitis and colorectal cancer: quantitative CT perfusion measurements versus morphologic criteria. Radiology 2007; 242:456-462.
19. Chintapalli KN, Esola CC, Chopra S, et al. Pericolic mesenteric lymph nodes: an aid to distinguishing diverticulitis from cancer in the colon. AJR Am J Roentgenol 1997; 19:1253-1255.
20. Karahan OI, Dodd GD III, Chintapalli KN, et al. Gastrointestinal wall thickening in patients with cirrhosis: frequency and patterns at contrast-enhanced CT. Radiology 2000; 215:103-107.
21. Frager DH, Goldman M, Beneventano TC. Computed tomography in Crohn disease. J Comput Assist Tomogr 1983; 7:819-824.
22. Kirkpatrick ID, Greenberg HM. Gastrointestinal complications in the neutropenic patient: characterization and differentiation with abdominal CT. Radiology 2003; 226:668-674.
23. Elizondo G, Weissleder R, Stark DD, et al. Amebic liver abscess: diagnosis and treatment with MR imaging. Radiology 1987; 165:795-800.
24. Baoudiaf M, Zidi SH, Soyer P, et al. Tuberculous colitis mimicking Crohn's disease: utility of computed tomography in the differentiation. Eur Radiol 1998; 8:1221-1223.
25. Makanjuola D. Is it Crohn's disease or intestinal tuberculosis? CT analysis. Eur J Radiol 1998; 1:55-61.
26. Madureira AJ. The comb sign. Radiology 2004; 230:783-784.
27. Herlinger H, Furth EE, Rubesin SE. Fibrofatty proliferation of the mesentery in Crohn disease. Abdom Imaging 1998; 23:446-448.
28. Macari M, Megibow AJ, Balthazar EJ. A pattern approach to the abnormal small bowel: Observations at MDCT and CT enterography. AJR Am J Roentgenol 2007; 188:1344-1355.
29. Lalani TA, Kanne JP, Hatfield GA, Chen P. Imaging findings in systemic lupus erythematosus. RadioGraphics 2004; 24:1069-1086.
30. Harisinghani MG, Wittenberg J, Lee W, et al. Bowel wall fat halo sign in patients without intestinal disease. AJR Am J Roentgenol 2003; 181:781-784.
31. Zegel H, Laufer I. Filliform polyposis. Radiology 1978; 127:615-619.
32. Bartlett JG, Perl TM. The new *Clostridium difficile*—what does it mean? N Engl J Med 2005; 355:2503-2504.
33. McDonald LC, Killgore GE, Thompson A, et al. An epidemic, toxin gene-variant strain of *Clostridium difficile*. N Engl J Med 2005; 355:2433-2441.
34. O'Sullivan SG. The accordion sign. Radiology 1998; 206:177-178.
35. Fishman EK, Kavuru M, Jones B, et al. Pseudomembranous colitis: CT evaluation of 26 cases. Radiology 1991; 180:57-60.
36. Wall SD, Jones B. Gastrointestinal tract in the immunocompromised host: opportunistic infections and other complications. Radiology 1992; 18:327-335.
37. Karahan OI, Dodd GD, Chintapalli KN, et al. Gastrointestinal wall thickening in patients with cirrhosis: frequency and patterns at contrast enhanced CT. Radiology 2000; 215:103-107.
38. Balthazar EJ, Gade MF. Gastrointestinal edema in cirrhotics. Gastrointest Radiol 1976; 1:215-223.
39. Balthazar EJ, Yen BC, Gordon RB. Ischemic colitis: CT evaluation of 54 cases. Radiology 1999; 211:381-388.
40. Jaffe TA, Gaca AM, Delaney S, et al. Radiation doses from small-bowel follow-through and abdominopelvic MDCT in Crohn's disease. AJR Am J Roentgenol 2007; 189:1015-1022.
41. Brenner DJ, Hall EJ. Computed tomography—an increasing source of radiation exposure. N Engl J Med 2007; 357:2277-2284.
42. Gourtsoyiannis N, Papanikolaou N, Grammatikakis J, et al. Assessment of Crohn's disease activity in the small bowel with MR and conventional enteroclysis: preliminary results. Eur Radiol 2004; 14:1017-1024.

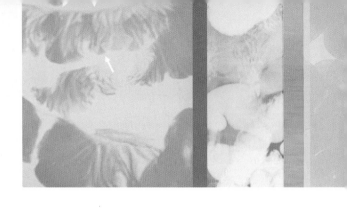

CHAPTER 56

Colonic Vascular Lesions

Naveen M. Kulkarni and Ozden Narin

ETIOLOGY

Vascular lesions of colon are an important medical problem and have now been recognized as a significant cause of gastrointestinal bleeding.[1] They can be solitary or multifocal, benign or malignant, or they can be associated with a syndrome or systemic disorder. There are three main groups: vascular malformations, neoplastic lesions, and non-neoplastic lesions (Fig. 56-1). Vascular malformations can be broadly classified into arterial, venous, and arteriovenous types. Neoplastic lesions include hemangiomas, hemangioendotheliomas, and angiosarcomas. Non-neoplastic lesions can be further divided into inflammatory lesions (e.g., vasculitis) and obstructive lesions (e.g., ischemic colitis). Few systemic conditions and syndromes present with vascular lesions, such as colonic varices in portal hypertension or vasculitis in systemic lupus erythematosus and polyarteritis nodosa, Ehlers-Danlos syndrome, Osler-Weber-Rendu disease, Marfan syndrome, and systemic sclerosis. This chapter focuses on the important vascular lesions that cause gastrointestinal bleeding and that are representative of the spectrum of vascular lesions of the gastrointestinal tract.

PREVALENCE AND EPIDEMIOLOGY

The prevalence is related to the etiology and age of the patient. The prevalence of angiodysplasia is 0.8% in healthy patients older than 50 years who are undergoing screening colonoscopy.[2] These lesions characteristically appear in the right colon and cecum in older patients, although they may be found anywhere in the lower gastrointestinal tract, may be multiple, and can occur in younger patients.[1,3] Dieulafoy's lesion involving the colon is rare and more frequently affects the stomach. It is twice as common in men as in women and presents at a mean age of 52 years.[4] Hemangiomas are benign vascular tumors that can be found throughout the gastrointestinal tract, often in the rectum or colon. The incidence of gastrointestinal hemangioma is reported as 0.3%, and these tumors account for

5% to 10% of all benign intestinal tumors.[5] In some populations these lesions are multiple and associated with skin lesions, such as the blue rubber bleb nevus syndrome with purple-blue cutaneous hemangiomas or the Klippel-Trenaunay syndrome with port-wine–colored cutaneous hemangiomas, hemihypertrophy, and varicose veins.[6-8] Rare vascular malignant neoplasms of the gastrointestinal tract include angiosarcomas, hemangiopericytomas, and hemangioendotheliomas.[6,9,10] The incidence of these lesions is highly variable. Telangiectases are similar to angiodysplasias but occur in all the layers of the bowel wall, are usually congenital, and often occur in other organ systems.[1] Hereditary hemorrhagic telangiectasia (Osler-Weber-Rendu disease) is an autosomal dominant disorder with telangiectases involving the lips; mucous membranes, especially in the mouth and nose; gastrointestinal tract, especially the stomach and small bowel; liver; lung; retina; and central nervous system.[11,12]

CLINICAL PRESENTATION

Although many vascular lesions are asymptomatic, those that present with bleeding require expeditious localization and control. These lesions may be responsible for different types of gastrointestinal bleeding: severe, acute, and overt, on the one hand, and chronic or occult, on the other.[1,13] Some of these lesions are difficult to localize on cross-sectional imaging and colonoscopy and necessitate use of more invasive modalities such as angiography. Although the clinical presentation, age of the patient, and other epidemiologic factors may indicate a particular type of colonic vascular lesion, endoscopy with biopsy and visceral angiography are critical in establishing the correct diagnosis.

PATHOPHYSIOLOGY AND PATHOLOGY

Pathology of vascular lesions involving the colon depends on the underlying etiology, which can be vascular, neoplastic, or non-neoplastic in origin.

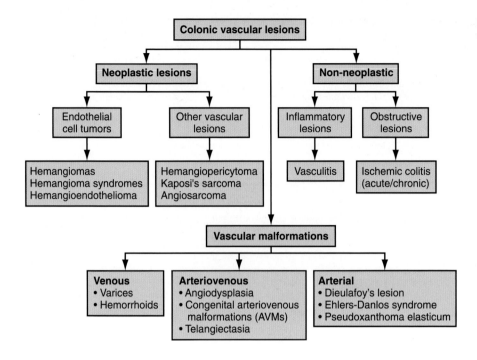

Angiodysplasia

These lesions are acquired vascular ectasias, possibly caused by chronic, low-grade colonic obstruction. Histologic identification is difficult unless special techniques are used.[14,15] Microscopically, angiodysplasias are composed of clusters of dilated, tortuous, thin-walled veins, venules, and capillaries localized in the colonic mucosa and submucosa.

Dieulafoy's Lesion

Dieulafoy's lesion belongs to an arterial type of vascular abnormality with abnormally large (caliber-persistent) submucosal end-arteries; and, in some instances, there is a small, overlying mucosal defect.[16-18]

Congenital Arteriovenous Malformations

Histologically, arteriovenous malformations are persistent congenital communication between arteries and veins located in the submucosa. Characteristically, arterialization of the veins is seen. The veins are tortuous and dilated, having thick walls with smooth muscle hypertrophy and intimal thickening.[19,20]

Hemangioma

Hemangioma is the second most common vascular lesion of colon and may be solitary or may be multiple in patients with multisystem involvement.[6,9,21] Histologically, hemangiomas can be divided into cavernous, capillary, and mixed. Cavernous hemangiomas are composed of large, dilated spaces filled with blood and are covered with a thin wall of abnormal vessels. Capillary hemangiomas consist of conglomerates of small, thin-walled vessels.[6,9]

TABLE 56-1 Clinical Factors in Differentiating Colonic Vascular Lesions

Age

Elderly
Angiodysplasia
Dieulafoy's lesion
Ischemic colitis

Children
Hemangiomas
Hereditary hemorrhagic telangiectasia

Location of Involvement
Angiodysplasia—cecum and proximal ascending colon
Hemangiomas—predilection for rectosigmoid region

Multifocal Involvement
Hemangioma

IMAGING

Because the clinical presentation and manifestations of patients with colonic vascular lesions in the form of lower gastrointestinal bleeding overlaps with other colonic diseases, a precise identification of etiology is only possible by using different imaging modalities. A high degree of suspicion is necessary when considering a patient with a lower gastrointestinal hemorrhage. A precise knowledge of clinical background with imaging findings can help narrow the differential diagnosis. Although there is no specific algorithm the information presented in Tables 56-1 and 56-2 should be kept in mind when there is a high index of suspicion of a vascular lesion.

Angiodysplasia

Angiodysplasia or vascular ectasia is the most common vascular malformations of the gastrointestinal tract in the

TABLE 56-2 General Information and Diagnostic Modalities

	Angiodysplasia	Hemangioma	Dieulafoy's Lesion
Age	Older than 50 years	Younger age group	No specific age distribution
Diagnostic Modalities	Endoscopy, catheter angiography or CT angiography	CT and endoscopy	Endoscopy and angiography
Radiographs	N/A	Phleboliths can be seen on radiographs.	N/A
CT/CTA Findings	Ectatic, dilated vessels in the wall of colon, an early filling vein, and an enlarged ileocolic artery	Enhancing lesion with phleboliths	N/A
MRI Findings	N/A	Thickened colon wall with high signal intensity on T2-weighted imaging	N/A
Colonoscopy	Lesions are flat, 2-5 mm in diameter, and red.	Elevated blue nodular lesions or dilated vessels	Caliber-persistent artery protruding from the mucosa

N/A, not applicable.

elderly and one of the major causes of lower gastrointestinal bleeding. Accurate diagnosis may require a combination of diagnostic techniques, such as angiography, nuclear scanning, and colonoscopy.[15,22-24]

Barium Studies

Because the lesions of angiodysplasia are small in diameter and do not distort the mucosa, double-contrast barium enema studies are of no value in the diagnosis of angiodysplasia. This technique is useful, however, to rule out other causes of gastrointestinal bleeding, such as neoplastic lesions.[22]

CT

The role of CT is still evolving, and at present there is limited literature on its role in evaluating angiodysplasia. Recently, there have been some reports of being able to detect these lesions by multidetector CT (MDCT) scans and CT angiographic (CTA) techniques. In a study of 30 patients with clinical suspicion of angiodysplasia, CTA had a sensitivity of 78% and a specificity of 100% when compared with colonoscopy, which had a sensitivity of 68% to 80% and a specificity of 90%. Accumulation of ectatic, dilated vessels in the wall of colon, an early filling vein, and an enlarged ileocolic artery (Fig. 56-2) can be observed in CTA images.[25]

MRI

The role of MRI is still investigational and evolving.

Nuclear Medicine

Nuclear scintigraphy is a sensitive method of detecting gastrointestinal bleeding at a rate of 0.1 mL/min. It is more sensitive than angiography but less specific than a positive endoscopic or angiographic examination (Fig. 56-3). A major disadvantage of nuclear imaging is that it localizes bleeding only to an area of the abdomen. Nuclear scintigraphy has proven more useful as an adjunct

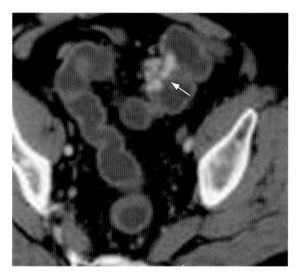

■ **FIGURE 56-2** Axial, contrast-enhanced CT at the level of the pelvis shows a tangle of vessels in the sigmoid colon (*arrow*) caused by angiodysplasia. (*Reprinted from Miller FH. Case 185. In Miller FH, Rubesin SE [eds]. The Teaching Files: Gastrointestinal. Philadelphia, Elsevier Saunders, 2009; Courtesy of Richard M. Gore, MD, Evanston, IL.*)

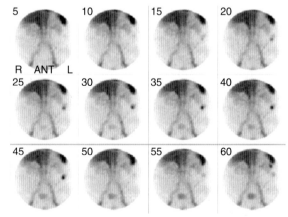

■ **FIGURE 56-3** Serial images from ^{99m}Tc red blood cell scintigram show radionuclide tracer uptake in the descending colon caused by bleeding angiodysplasia.

to angiography by localizing and confirming the presence of bleeding, minimizing the number of angiograms that do not yield meaningful diagnostic information, and allowing rapid selection of the artery to be injected by angiography.[15,26,27]

Colonoscopy

Three main ideas underlying colonoscopy are:

● Determination of the location of lesion and type of bleeding
● Identification of patients with ongoing hemorrhage or at high risk for rebleeding
● Potential for endoscopic intervention

Angiodysplastic lesions are often described as discrete and small, with scalloped or frond-like edges and a visible draining vein (Fig. 56-4). They can be flat or slightly

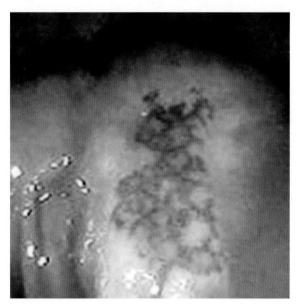

■ **FIGURE 56-4** Angiodysplasia identified on cecal wall during colonoscopy.

raised and can be hidden within mucosal folds.[22,24] The endoscopist's ability to diagnose the specific nature of a vascular lesion is limited by the similar appearance of different types of lesions. The following lesions should be considered in the differential diagnosis:

● Hereditary hemorrhagic telangiectasia
● Angiomas
● Focal hypervascularity of radiation colitis
● Ulcerative colitis
● Crohn's disease
● Ischemic colitis

Because the appearance of vascular lesions is influenced by a patient's blood pressure, blood volume, and state of hydration, such lesions may not be evident in those with severely reduced blood volume or shock; thus, accurate evaluation may not be possible until red cell and volume deficits are corrected.[27]

Angiography

Angiography is used to determine the site and nature of lesion during active bleeding. Three reliable angiographic signs of angiodysplasia are a densely opacified, slowly emptying, dilated, tortuous vein; a vascular tuft; and an early-filling vein. The slowly emptying vein persists late into the venous phase, after the other mesenteric veins have emptied (Fig. 56-5). When the lesion is bleeding, intraluminal extravasation of contrast material usually appears during the arterial phase of angiography and persists throughout the study.[20,27] Extravasation identifies the site of active bleeding, but in the absence of other signs of angiodysplasia it suggests another cause for the bleeding.

Hemangiomas

Hemangiomas are the second most common vascular lesion of the colon and may occur as solitary or multiple lesions limited to the colon or as part of diffuse gastrointestinal or multisystem angiomatoses.[5,8] Hemangiomas may be classified as cavernous, capillary, or mixed types.

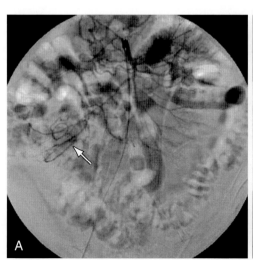
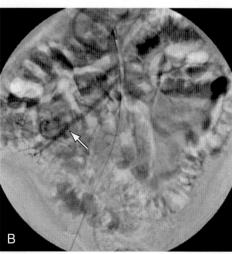

■ **FIGURE 56-5** **A,** Early angiogram shows focal arterial enlargement (*arrow*). **B,** On a subsequent angiogram, accompanying enlarged draining vein is seen (*arrow*) consistent with cecal angiodysplasia.

The capillary hemangiomas are usually incidental findings at autopsy. Diffuse cavernous hemangioma of the rectosigmoid colon is the most common type (75% to 80%).[8,28-30] Most are small, ranging from a few millimeters to 2 cm, but larger lesions occur, especially in the rectum. Patients with the blue rubber bleb nevus and Klippel-Trenaunay syndrome can have lesions anywhere in the gastrointestinal tract.[6,9] The diagnosis is best established by CT and endoscopy, including enteroscopy, because radiographic studies, including angiography, are frequently normal.

Radiography

The diagnosis of cavernous hemangioma of the rectum often can be suggested on plain films of the abdomen by the presence of phleboliths and displacement or distortion of the rectal air column.[3,31] However, absence of phleboliths does not rule out the diagnosis.

Barium Studies

Like plain abdominal radiographs, barium studies are too nonspecific and insensitive in evaluating the vascular lesion. A barium contrast examination shows only poorly specific signs such as large polypoid or obstructing lesions that may change configuration after compression or distention. The affected bowel lumen may show narrowing and rigidity, scalloping of the wall, and widening of the presacral space when the rectum is involved.[3,8,28,31] Furthermore, dense barium interferes with subsequent MDCT examinations, colonoscopy, and transcatheter interventions.

CT

On CT, hemangiomas present as an enhancing lesion or clusters of intraluminal polypoid lesions that may diffusely infiltrate the submucosa with extraserosal extension into the mesentery and adjacent organs.[8,32] Presence of a phlebolith can confirm the diagnosis (Fig. 56-6). CT helps in localization, assessment of the extent of the lesion, and pericolonic involvement to guide surgical management. When the extent of the lesion is limited, with no phleboliths, thickening of colon or rectosigmoid wall might not be specific enough for CT to be diagnostic.[6,9] Moreover, CT may not be preferred when repeated examinations might be necessary for follow-up in young patients because it involves radiation exposure and requires injection of iodinated contrast material.

MRI

The colon wall will be markedly thickened with high signal intensity on T2-weighted images. This feature appears to be related to slow flow in vascular malformation. Sometimes serpiginous structures that are thought to represent small vessels supplying the diffuse cavernous hemangioma may be seen.[7,33,34] MRI allows correct evaluation of the extent of bowel wall involvement and visualization of extracolonic extension.[28,35] Depiction of phleboliths by MRI again can help in confirming the diagnosis.

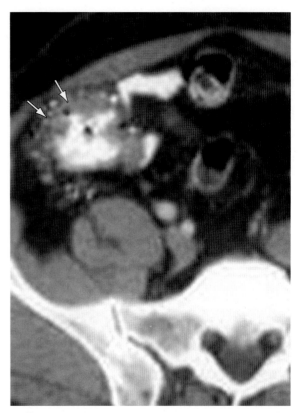

■ **FIGURE 56-6** Axial contrast-enhanced CT scan shows cecum wall thickening with avid enhancement and calcified phleboliths (*arrows*). (*Reprinted from Rubesin SE, Furth EE. Other tumors of the colon. In Gore RM, Levine MS [eds]. Textbook of Gastrointestinal Radiology, 3rd ed. Philadelphia, Elsevier Saunders, 2007, p 1171.*)

Endoscopy

Endoscopically, one sees elevated plum-red nodules or vascular congestion; ulcers and proctitis also may be present. Hemangiomas may also present as sessile polypoid lesions, appearing bluish. The entire colon needs screening to look for multiple lesions, especially in patients with systemic disorders in which pancolonic involvement is common. Endoscopic biopsy should be avoided due to bleeding risk.[6,36-39]

Angiography

Angiography can demonstrate these lesions but seldom is necessary to establish the diagnosis.

Dieulafoy's Lesion

This vascular lesion is an unusual cause of massive gastrointestinal hemorrhage, usually from the stomach but sometimes from the small or large bowel. The vascular abnormality is the presence of arteries of persistently large caliber in the submucosa and, in some instances, the mucosa, typically with a small, overlying mucosal defect.[4] It may be difficult to find a Dieulafoy lesion in a patient with lower gastrointestinal bleeding because the overlying mucosal defect may be small and hidden between the mucosal folds and the caliber-persistent vessel may constrict and retract after the bleeding episode.[18,40]

Nuclear Scintigraphy

The approach for Dieulafoy's lesion is similar to that mentioned in the discussion on angiodysplasia.

Endoscopy

Endoscopy reveals a reddish-brown protruding spot with small erosion and no ulcer.[26] Because the lesion is so small it can easily be missed, especially when the colon is full of blood. It can be noticed more easily when pulsating or oozing blood or a longitudinal clot with small area of adhesion to the colon wall can be seen.[16,17,41-43]

Angiography

In difficult cases angiography may be useful when endoscopy fails to identify the lesion, especially in nongastric sites. On angiography, abnormal blush with extravasation of contrast agent is appreciated.[16,17,41-44]

Congenital Arteriovenous Malformations

Arteriovenous malformations (AVMs) are embryonic growth defects and are considered to be developmental anomalies. Although AVMs are found mainly in the extremities, they may occur anywhere in the vascular tree. In the colon, they may be small and resemble angiodysplasia or they may involve a long segment of bowel. The most extensive lesions typically are in the rectum and sigmoid.[45] AVMs of the bowel are characterized by thick-walled blood vessels that extend through the mucosa and submucosa into the muscle. Conversely, vascular ectasia (angiodysplasia) is characterized by thin or normal-sized blood vessels that proliferate in the submucosa.[45,46] True AVMs tend to occur in younger patients, whereas vascular ectasia is a disease of the elderly that predominates in the right colon. Unlike vascular ectasia, which may be subtle on pathologic examination, AVMs represent substantial lesions that may actually distort adjacent tissues.[43,45,47] Although AVMs may be detected by endoscopy or exceptionally by barium studies, only the visible mucosal component of the AVMs is assessable by these means. Definitive diagnosis and determination of the site and extension of intestinal AVMs is still best achieved by selective mesenteric angiography. Involved vessels and flow pattern, as depicted by angiography, are used to classify AVMs into low- and high-flow AVMs.

CT

CT appears to be able to reveal AVMs of bowel and can be performed in patients who are hemodynamically stable and do not require emergency vascular or surgical intervention. Rapid scanning techniques and administration of contrast material at rates typically used in CT angiography are essential for an accurate diagnosis. Use of water as oral contrast media is also critical to distend the bowel and highlight enhancing vessels within the bowel wall. Use of oral contrast media can obscure identification of blood within the bowel lumen and interfere with diagnosis of an AVM.

On unenhanced CT, blood may be evident within the lumen or bowel wall. On enhanced CT, during the arterial phase, dilated vessels in the bowel wall enhance similar to that of aorta. Active contrast agent extravasation may also be appreciated. These enhancing vessels will tend to become less conspicuous in the venous phase.

Effort should be made to screen other parts of bowel because AVMs are known to be multiple.

Endoscopy

Flat or elevated, bright red lesions can be seen.

Angiography

The constant angiographic sign of an arteriovenous malformation is the enlargement and increase in the number of arteries, small vessels, and veins. The feeding artery is dilated, and an early venous return is observed.[20,48] Patients with significant bleeding from large AVMs should undergo resection of the involved segment; transendoscopic therapy may be beneficial for smaller lesions.

TREATMENT
Medical Treatment

Management of incidentally detected vascular lesion is expectant, and in such cases no therapy is warranted. Hormonal therapy, using estrogens in combination with progestins, has been used to treat patients with a variety of vascular lesions of the gastrointestinal tract, in an attempt to reduce or terminate bleeding. It is likely that hormonal therapy affects different vascular lesions differently and that vascular lesions in the small intestine may respond differently to such treatment than the same lesions in the colon. Bleeding can also be controlled endoscopically or angiographically in most patients, thereby avoiding the morbidity and mortality of emergency operation (Table 56-3). Argon and neodymium:yttrium-aluminum-garnet (Nd:YAG) laser, endoscopic sclerosis, monopolar and bipolar electrocoagulation, hemoclips in combination with cautery, and endoscopic band ligation have been used to ablate vascular lesions throughout the gastrointestinal tract and can be used to control active bleeding. Angiography with superselective microcoil embolization is largely used to control bleeding and has replaced intraarterial vasopressin infusion. Vasopressin is still recommended, however, when intestinal lesions are diffuse throughout the bowel or when superselective catheterization is not possible.

Surgical Treatment

Surgical management either in the form of segmental or hemicolectomy depending on the site and multiplicity of

TABLE 56-3 Treatment Options for Colonic Lesions

	Angiodysplasia	Hemangioma	Dieulafoy's Lesion
Medical Treatment	Systemic hormonal therapy with estrogen	N/A	N/A
Interventional Therapy			
Colonoscopy	Endoscopic thermocoagulation, electrocoagulation, or photocoagulation	Endoscopic polypectomy if the lesion is pedunculated, polypoid, and ≤ 2.5 cm	Bipolar cautery, laser photocoagulation, and hemoclipping
Angiography	Superselective arterial embolization or direct vasopressin infusion	Not useful	Embolization with absorbable sponges
Surgical Therapy	Reserved for severe bleeding	Surgical resection of hemangioma	Reserved for intractable bleeding

lesion is indicated when a vascular lesion has been identified by either colonoscopy or angiography and when therapy by either or both of these two modalities is unsuccessful, cannot be performed, or is unavailable (see Table 56-3).

What the Referring Physician Needs to Know

■ Vascular lesions should be considered in both acute and chronic gastrointestinal bleeding, especially when initial endoscopic examination reveals no abnormalities.

■ Multiplicity of vascular lesions should always be considered when initial endoscopic or vascular therapy is unsuccessful and bleeding seems to continue based on clinical evidence.

■ Argon plasma coagulation is a preferred method of therapy in several vascular abnormalities.

■ The roles of CT- and MRI-based diagnostic imaging techniques for vascular lesions of all types are evolving, and conventional angiography at present is more important for therapy than for diagnosis.

SUGGESTED READINGS

Bounds BC, Kelsey PB. Lower gastrointestinal bleeding. Gastrointest Endoscopy Clin North Am 2007; 17:273-288.

Cappell MS. Gastrointestinal vascular malformations or neoplasms: arterial, venous, arteriovenous, and capillary. In Yamada T, Alpers DH, Kaplowitz N, et al (eds). Textbook of Gastroenterology, 4th ed. Philadelphia, Lippincott Williams & Wilkins, 2003, pp 2722-2741.

Gore RM, Yaghmai V, Thakra KH, et al. Imaging in intestinal ischemic disorders. Radiol Clin North Am 2008; 46:845-875.

Paterno F, Longo WE. The etiology and pathogenesis of vascular disorders of the intestine. Radiol Clin North Am 2008; 46:877-885.

Regula J, Wronska E, Pachlewski J. Vascular lesions of gastrointestinal tract. Best Pract Res Clin Gastroenterol 2008; 22:313-328.

Richardson JD. Vascular lesions of the intestines. Am J Surg 1991; 161:283-293.

REFERENCES

1. Farman J. Vascular lesions of the colon. Br J Radiol 1966; 39: 575-582.

2. Foutch PG, Rex DK, Lieberman DA. Prevalence and natural history of colonic angiodysplasia among healthy asymptomatic people. Am J Gastroenterol 1995; 90:564-567.

3. Boley SJ, Brandt LJ, Mitsudo SM. Vascular lesions of the colon. Adv Intern Med 1984; 29:301-326.

4. Fockens P, Tytgat GN. Dieulafoy's disease. Gastrointest Endosc Clin North Am 1996; 6:739-752.

5. Yorozuya K, Watanabe M, Hasegawa H, et al. Diffuse cavernous hemangioma of the rectum: report of a case. Surg Today 2003; 33:309-311.

6. Vilallonga R, Espin Basany E, Armengol M. Cavernous hemangioma: unusual benign tumor of the transverse colon. Turk J Gastroenterol 2009; 20:146-149.

7. Kandpal H, Sharma R, Srivastava DN, et al. Diffuse cavernous haemangioma of colon: magnetic resonance imaging features: report of two cases. Australas Radiol 2007; 51(Spec No):B147-B151.

8. Wang AY, Ahmad NA. Diffuse cavernous hemangioma of the colon and rectum. Clin Gastroenterol Hepatol 2007; 5:A25.

9. Sylla P, Deutsch G, Luo J, et al. Cavernous, arteriovenous, and mixed hemangioma-lymphangioma of the rectosigmoid: rare causes of rectal bleeding—case series and review of the literature. Int J Colorectal Dis 2008; 23:653-658.

10. Genter B, Mir R, Strauss R, et al. Hemangiopericytoma of the colon: report of a case and review of literature. Dis Colon Rectum 1982; 25:149-156.
11. Byrne ST, McDonald MJ, Poonnoose SI. Ten-year follow-up of a patient with Osler-Weber-Rendu syndrome and recurrent cerebral abscess secondary to pulmonary arteriovenous fistula. J Clin Neurosci 2009; 16:1095-1096.
12. Giordano P, Nigro A, Lenato GM, et al. Screening for children from families with Rendu-Osler-Weber disease: from geneticist to clinician. J Thromb Haemost 2006; 4:1237-1245.
13. Zuccaro G. Epidemiology of lower gastrointestinal bleeding. Best Pract Res Clin Gastroenterol 2008; 22:225-232.
14. Boley SJ, Sammartano R, Adams A, et al. On the nature and etiology of vascular ectasias of the colon: degenerative lesions of aging. Gastroenterology 1977; 72:650-660.
15. Sharma R, Gorbien MJ. Angiodysplasia and lower gastrointestinal tract bleeding in elderly patients. Arch Intern Med 1995; 155: 807-812.
16. Jain R, Chetty R. Dieulafoy disease of the colon. Arch Pathol Lab Med 2009; 133:1865-1867.
17. Njeru M, Seifi A, Salam Z, Ognibene L. Dieulafoy lesion: a rare cause of gastrointestinal bleeding. South Med J 2009; 102:336-337.
18. Schmulewitz N, Baillie J. Dieulafoy lesions: a review of 6 years of experience at a tertiary referral center. Am J Gastroenterol 2001; 96:1688-1694.
19. Cooperman AM, Kelly KA, Bernatz PE, Huizenga KA. Arteriovenous malformation of the intestine: an uncommon cause of gastrointestinal bleeding. Arch Surg 1972; 104:284-287.
20. Moore JD, Thompson NW, Appelman HD, Foley D. Arteriovenous malformations of the gastrointestinal tract. Arch Surg 1976; 111: 381-389.
21. Ng EK, Cheung FK, Chiu PW. Blue rubber bleb nevus syndrome: treatment of multiple gastrointestinal hemangiomas with argon plasma coagulator. Dig Endosc 2009; 21:40-42.
22. Foutch PG. Angiodysplasia of the gastrointestinal tract. Am J Gastroenterol 1993; 88:807-818.
23. Dodda G, Trotman BW. Gastrointestinal angiodysplasia. J Assoc Acad Minor Phys 1997; 8:16-19.
24. Accordino R, Paties C, Inzani E, et al. [Angiodysplasia of the right colon]. Minerva Chir 1995; 50:703-706.
25. Junquera F, Quiroga S, Saperas E, et al. Accuracy of helical computed tomographic angiography for the diagnosis of colonic angiodysplasia. Gastroenterology 2000; 119:293-299.
26. Regula J, Wronska E, Pachlewski J. Vascular lesions of the gastrointestinal tract. Best Pract Res Clin Gastroenterol 2008; 22:313-328.
27. Wolff WI, Grossman MB, Shinya H. Angiodysplasia of the colon: diagnosis and treatment. Gastroenterology 1977; 72:329-333.
28. Holman CC. Haemangioma of the sigmoid colon: report of a case. Br J Surg 1948; 36:210.
29. Olnick HM, Woodhall JP Jr, Clay CB Jr. Hemangioma of the colon. J Med Assoc Ga 1957; 46:383-384; passim.
30. Clark HH, McKay ER. Mixed cavernous and capillary hemangiomatosis involving the large bowel. J Int Coll Surg 1957; 27:218-225.
31. Camilleri M, Chadwick VS, Hodgson HJ. Vascular anomalies of the gastrointestinal tract. Hepatogastroenterology 1984; 31:149-153.
32. Hervias D, Turrion JP, Herrera M, et al. Diffuse cavernous hemangioma of the rectum: an atypical cause of rectal bleeding. Rev Esp Enferm Dig 2004; 96:346-352.
33. Eadie DG. Cavernous haemangioma of the descending colon. Br J Surg 1958; 46:223-224.
34. Ichikawa T, Koyama A, Fujimoto H, et al. Diffuse arteriovenous malformation involving jejunum and total colon with mesenteric varices: case report. Clin Imaging 1994; 18:221-223.
35. Bailey JJ, Barrick CW, Jenkinson EL. Hemangioma of colon. JAMA 1956; 160:658-659.
36. Czekajska-Chehab E, Borowiec D, Drop A, et al. Diffuse hemangioma of the rectum detected on multi-slice CT in an 18-year-old woman with Klippel-Trenaunay syndrome. Ann Univ Mariae Curie Sklodowska Med 2004; 59:356-360.
37. Machicado GA, Jensen DM. Endoscopic diagnosis and treatment of severe lower gastrointestinal bleeding. Indian J Gastroenterol 2006; 25(Suppl 1):S43-S51.
38. Matsuhashi N, Nakagama H, Moriya K, et al. Multiple diffuse hemangiomas of the large intestine. Gastroenterol Jpn 1991; 26:654-660.
39. Scopinaro F, Signori C, Massa R, et al. Right colonic hemangioma diagnosed by scintigraphy with ^{99m}Tc sucralfate: a case report. Ital J Surg Sci 1989; 19:89-92.
40. Katsinelos P, Pilpilidis I, Paroutoglou G, et al. Dieulafoy-like lesion of the colon presenting with massive lower gastrointestinal bleeding. Surg Endosc 2004; 18:346.
41. Bou Jaoude J, Hobeika E, Yaghi C, et al. [Endoscopic treatment of Dieulafoy's lesion: a case report and review of the literature]. J Med Liban 2003; 51:55-58.
42. Golubovic G, Kiurski M, Spica V, et al. [Vascular gastric anomalies as a cause of relapsing bleeding]. Vojnosanit Pregl 2008; 65: 710-713.
43. Yano T, Yamamoto H. [Vascular lesions of the small intestine]. Nippon Rinsho 2008; 66:1335-1341.
44. Labenz J, Borsch G. [Vascular anomalies as the cause of recurrent intestinal hemorrhages]. Dtsch Med Wochenschr 1990; 115: 575-579.
45. Lesur G, Julie C, Romdhane N, Bruneval P. Vascular malformation of the colon and lower gastrointestinal tract. Gastroenterol Clin Biol 2006; 30:483-484.
46. Marescaux J, Petit B, Pavis d'Escurac X, et al. [Vascular malformations of the colon: a frequently undetected etiology of lower digestive hemorrhage]. Presse Med 1986; 15:2204-2207.
47. de la Torre L, Carrasco D, Mora MA, et al. Vascular malformations of the colon in children. J Pediatr Surg 2002; 37:1754-1757.
48. Pariente D, Cauquil P, Gallaire C, Roche A. Vascular malformations of the cecum: treatment by embolization: apropos of 2 cases. Gastroenterol Clin Biol 1988; 12:61-65.

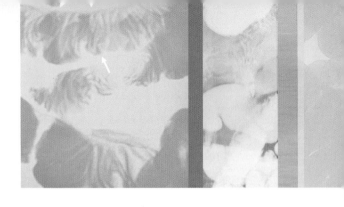

57

Colon Cancer and Screening Strategies

David A. Rosman, Dipti K. Lenhart, and Dushyant V. Sahani

ETIOLOGY

The etiologic factors in the development of colorectal carcinoma and its precursor lesion, the colonic adenoma, are multifactorial and include both genetic predisposition as well as environmental insults. Some of the risk factors for colorectal carcinoma include familial polyposis syndrome, ulcerative colitis, family history of colorectal cancer, age, male gender, smoking, alcohol intake, and obesity.[1]

PREVALENCE AND EPIDEMIOLOGY

Colon cancer is the third most commonly diagnosed cancer and third most common cause of cancer-related death in both men and women. It is responsible for 10% of new cancer cases and 9% of cancer-related deaths annually in the United States, representing an estimated 146,970 new cases and 24,680 deaths each year. The lifetime risk of developing colorectal carcinoma is 5.5% in men and 5.1% in women.[2] Winawer and associates demonstrated a marked reduction in colorectal carcinoma incidence after colonoscopic polypectomy, indicating that screening techniques are essential in the prevention and early detection of colorectal carcinoma.[3]

CLINICAL PRESENTATION

The clinical presentation of colorectal cancer includes blood in stool, change in bowel habits, bowel obstruction, bowel perforation, abdominal pain, diminished appetite, or systemic symptoms such as generalized fatigue and weight loss. However, colorectal carcinoma is often detected in asymptomatic patients during a screening examination.

The late presentation of colon cancer includes symptoms related to metastatic disease. Colon cancer spreads hematogenously most commonly to the liver and lungs and via lymphatics to regional lymph nodes.

Laboratory findings can include microcytic anemia related to blood loss and elevation of the carcinoembryonic antigen tumor marker.

PATHOPHYSIOLOGY AND PATHOLOGY

Histology of Colonic Polyps

Colonic polyps are growths into the bowel lumen and can develop as isolated polyps or in the setting of polyposis syndromes. Isolated colonic polyps of all sizes are seen in approximately 37.6% of the screening population,[4] whereas potentially clinically significant polyps greater than or equal to 6 mm have a prevalence of 14%.[5] Polyps are histologically characterized as adenomatous, hyperplastic, and other. The "other" category includes juvenile/hamartomatous polyps, inflammatory polyps, lymphoid aggregates, mucosal tags, and submucosal lipomas.

Of all the types of polyps, only adenomatous polyps are of concern with respect to colon cancer. The adenoma is a precursor lesion that can potentially harbor dysplasia and develop into colon cancer; this prevailing view on the pathogenesis of colon cancer is called the "adenoma-carcinoma sequence" (see later).

Adenomas are further characterized into three subtypes based on their histologic architecture: tubular, tubulovillous, and villous. Adenomas containing less than 25% villous features are classified as tubular adenomas; those with 25% to 75% villous features are tubulovillous adenomas; and those with more than 75% villous features are villous adenomas.

Adenomas can also be characterized based on the degree of cellular atypia seen on pathology (mild, moderate, or severe dysplasia), depending on the amount of nuclear changes and number of mitotic figures.[6]

With imaging studies and/or colonoscopy as screening tools, the radiologist and gastroenterologist cannot visually distinguish between the different types of polyps (with the exception of lipomas), nor can they determine the histology or degree of cellular atypia of an adenoma. Thus, generally all encountered polyps seen on colonoscopy and those meeting a certain size threshold on noninvasive studies such as CT colonography are removed.[7]

Location of Adenomas

Adenomas can develop anywhere in the colon or rectum but are seen with the greatest frequency in the sigmoid colon. In a recent colonoscopy/CT colonography series, the distribution of adenomas and carcinomas was as follows: rectal, 13.4%; sigmoid colon, 25.1%; descending colon, 10.7%; transverse colon, 18.4%; ascending colon, 19.8%; and cecum, 12.6%.[8]

Adenoma-Carcinoma Sequence

The currently accepted evolution of colon cancer is via the "adenoma-carcinoma sequence," a name first coined by Jackman and Mayo in 1951[9] and further developed and refined by pathologists, including Morson, Muto, and Bussey.[6,10]

The model for progression from normal epithelium to adenoma to carcinoma is a series of genetic mutations.[11] Colonic neoplasms are thought to arise as a result of mutational activation of oncogenes (*RAS* gene on chromosome 12p) coupled with the mutational inactivation or loss of tumor suppression genes (familial adenomatous polyposis gene on chromosome 5q, *TP53* gene on chromosome 17p, and *DCC* gene on chromosome 18q). These mutations act at a number of steps in the progression from normal epithelium to hyperproliferative epithelium to early, intermediate, and late adenoma and, finally, to carcinoma.

The degree of dysplasia is highly correlated with the risk of malignancy because on a genetic and cellular level increasing atypia leads to a stepwise progression toward carcinoma. The presence of high-grade dysplasia is therefore the best predictor of which adenomas will go on to become carcinomas.

There is a close relationship between the size of an adenoma and its propensity to harbor malignancy. In a colonoscopy series of a nonscreening population, the rate of carcinoma in adenomas greater than 2 cm was 19.4%, whereas that in adenomas less than 1 cm was 0.07%.[12] In an older surgical series, the rate of carcinoma in adenomas more than 2 cm was 46%, whereas that in adenomas less than 1 cm was 1.3%.[10]

Accordingly, adenoma size is correlated with the degree of cellular dysplasia. Some authors have also proposed a direct relationship between increasing villous component seen on histology and the degree of dysplasia.[13] As a result, the degree of dysplasia, adenoma size, and histologic characteristics are used as markers for malignancy risk in removed polyps.

Advanced Adenoma

Screening studies should be targeted toward the removal of adenomas that have the highest potential of developing into colorectal carcinoma. These "advanced adenomas" have traditionally been defined by any of the following three criteria: high-grade dysplasia, size greater than or equal to 1 cm, or a substantial (>25%) villous component (i.e., tubulovillous or villous adenomas). These lesions are at high risk of developing into colorectal carcinomas compared with their less-advanced counterparts. In an asymptomatic screening population, the overall prevalence of an advanced adenoma or carcinoma (collectively termed *advanced neoplasia*) is 3.3%.[4]

Multiple Adenomas

Patients who have an adenoma, advanced or otherwise, detected on a screening study are more likely to have additional adenomas detected on the same examination (synchronous) or on future examinations (metachronous). The presence of multiple adenomas (two or more) has also been shown to confer an increased risk of an individual's risk of developing an advanced adenoma on subsequent follow-up studies.[14] Therefore, the factors that inform our current screening guidelines include adenoma size, histology (i.e., presence of villous component), cellular features (i.e. degree of dysplasia), and total number.

SCREENING

Theory of Screening and Cost-Benefit Analysis

The goal of any cancer screening, including colon cancer screening, is to achieve a reduction in mortality by identifying disease at earlier stages and thus reducing the incidence of advanced disease.

Five-year survival is 90% for disease confined to the wall of the bowel; however, it falls to 68% for regional disease and plummets to 10% for metastatic disease.[15] It thus becomes clear that if cancer can be caught at earlier stages, mortality from the disease will be drastically reduced. In fact, prospective randomized trials and observational studies have demonstrated a reduction in mortality by detection of invasive disease and subsequent therapy.[16-19]

The American Cancer Society first issued formal guidelines for colorectal screening in 1980,[20] followed by guidelines from the U.S. Preventive Services Task Force,[21,22] the American College of Radiology,[23] and the U.S. Multi-Society Task Force on Colorectal Cancer.[24,25] Although there are differences between the guidelines, there is growing consensus, with the latest iteration being a collaborative effort by all of these groups.[26] The recommendations include continued support of the fecal occult blood test (FOBT) as well as the fecal immunohistochemical test (FIT) and stool DNA testing, assuming a patient is willing to undergo an invasive procedure in the instance of a positive test. The recommendations prefer tests that detect lesions earlier, including optical colonoscopy (OC) every 10 years or flexible sigmoidoscopy (FSIG), CT colonography (CTC), or double-contrast barium enema (DCBE) every 5 years.

The clinical effectiveness of screening is often assessed in terms of life-years gained. A measure of this is the incremental cost-effectiveness ratio (ICER), defined as the difference in cost between strategies divided by the difference in life expectancy between those strategies. Although controversial, an ICER threshold of $50,000 per life-year gained is often used to differentiate a relatively efficient procedure from an inefficient procedure.[27,28] Pickhardt and colleagues compared CTC and optical colonoscopy screening strategies for a population of 100,000 and found a nonscreening cumulative loss of 29,925 life-years due to colorectal cancer. Five-year CTC demonstrated a gain of 6250 life-years due to colorectal cancer prevention and early treatment, and 10-year optical colonoscopy demonstrated a gain of 6032 life years. If CTC is reduced to a 10-year interval, the life-years gained is 5518. CTC also identified aortic aneurysms, saving an additional 1536 life-years for a total of 7786 years of life saved. Compared with no screening, 10-year screening protocols cost just over $1000 per year of life saved, yielding a remarkable cost-benefit ratio.[28]

Screening Modalities

Fecal Occult Blood Test and Other Stool-Based Examinations

Theory

The principle behind the FOBT and other stool-based examinations is that invasive carcinoma will cause bleeding, which can then be detected using a variety of methodologies, including guaiac staining, immunohistochemistry, and DNA. Small polyps tend not to bleed, and larger lesions tend to bleed intermittently. As a result, these tests are subject to sampling error and are also more likely to detect cancer rather than precancerous lesions.[29,30]

Benefit

FOBT is supported by randomized controlled studies, which have demonstrated that its use leads to cancers being detected at an earlier and more curable stage compared with no screening, leading to reductions in colorectal cancer mortality of 15% to 33%.[31-33]

Limitations

The limitations of stool testing include the necessity for annual testing, low individual test sensitivity, and the need to follow up any positive test with an invasive test.[26] Furthermore, the sensitivity is highly variable and dependent on hydration status of the feces, brand and style of the test, as well as chosen target lesion (i.e., adenoma versus carcinoma). As mentioned earlier, small polyps are unlikely to bleed; thus sensitivity for these tests is very low, and FOBT is useful only for detecting advanced adenomas and cancers, with a sensitivity ranging from 37.1% to 79.4% when used correctly.[29] A large number of physicians use an in-office FOBT examination that has been demonstrated to have only a sensitivity of 4.9% for advanced adenoma and only 9% for cancer.[34]

Recommendation

Given the limited availability of all screening modalities for the entire population, the Multi-Society Task Force continues to recommend properly performed stool testing as one alternative screening methodology.

Flexible Sigmoidoscopy

Theory

FSIG is an optical endoscopic procedure that examines the most distal portion of the colon lumen. It is most often performed with a 60-cm endoscope but can also be performed with a variety of alternative scopes.

Benefits

FSIG was associated with a 60% to 80% reduction in colorectal cancer mortality for the area of colon within its reach. Overall decreased incidence compared with an unscreened group has also been demonstrated.[35-38] Its principal advantages over colonoscopy are that it requires a less extensive bowel preparation than a full colonic examination, and because it is less invasive than colonoscopy, sedation is not required. It also allows for concurrent sampling and/or removal of detected lesions.

Limitations

Like colonoscopy, FSIG can be complicated by patient discomfort and, more importantly, bowel perforation. Its greatest limitation, however, is its failure to evaluate the entire colon. Defenders of FSIG note that many people who have a proximal lesion will also have a distal lesion that would be detected on FSIG; thus, the incremental benefit of colonoscopy or colonography over FSIG is less pronounced. Lastly, there is substantial variation in the depth of insertion of the scope given the lack of sedation, and insufficient insertion leads to inadequate examination.[39,40]

Recommendation

The Multisociety Task Force continues to recommend FSIG every 5 years up to a distance of 40 cm within the colon.

Double-Contrast Barium Enema

Theory

DCBE is a fluoroscopic examination executed by coating the mucosa with barium and distending the colon with air insufflated through a tube inserted in the rectum. Multiple images are obtained both fluoroscopically as well as overheads.

Benefits

DCBE evaluates the entire colon and detects most cancers and the majority of significant polyps. Sensitivity for cancer has been shown to vary from 85% to 97%.[41] In a meta-analysis, DCBE was 70% sensitive and 71% specific for polyps greater than or equal to 10 mm.[42] When performed properly, the examination can be completed with minimal discomfort.[43]

Limitations

Because it is an imaging examination, DCBE does not permit tissue biopsy. No randomized controlled studies have been performed to evaluate its efficacy, and the studies that have been done are predominately retrospective. The differential in results highlights the operator dependency of the examination. With the advent of CT colonography and increased use of colonoscopy, fewer DCBE examinations are performed annually and, consequently, radiologists currently in training will have less experience with DCBE than their predecessors.

Recommendation

Although there remains controversy, DCBE, every 5 years, continues to be recommended by some as an acceptable screening methodology in asymptomatic, average risk populations aged 50 and older.[26]

Colonoscopy

Theory

Colonoscopy is an optical procedure that evaluates the entire colon. It is one of the most commonly performed medical procedures with 14.2 million performed in 2002.[44] Patients require an extensive colonic cleansing preparation, and the procedure is performed under sedation. Because it allows for direct optical visualization, biopsies are often performed.

Benefits

The greatest advantage to colonoscopy is that usually the entire colon can be screened and suspicious lesions sampled in a single visit. The seminal paper by Winawer and colleagues demonstrated a reduction in incidence of colon cancer of 76% to 90%.[21] Although no prospective randomized controlled trial has been performed to evaluate colonoscopy,[26] its health benefits are undisputed. A Veteran's Affairs study demonstrated a 50% reduction in mortality when colonoscopy was performed on a symptomatic population.[45] Numerous additional cohort studies have demonstrated reductions in colorectal carcinoma incidence and mortality.[46] Multiple additional studies by Winawer and his colleagues have reinforced these benefits.[14,24,25,47]

Limitations

The limitations of colonoscopy include the need for colon cleansing and patient sedation. Because of sedation, a patient chaperone is needed. Controlled studies have shown the colonoscopy miss rate for large adenomas 10 mm or larger to be 6% to 12%.[48,49] The additional risks

of colonoscopy related to sedation and biopsy include cardiopulmonary events such as arrhythmia and hypotension as well as postpolypectomy bleeding and perforation.[48,50]

Recommendation

Colonoscopy every 10 years beginning at age 50 is recommended as a screening option for colorectal cancer.[26]

CT Colonography

Theory

CT colonography (CTC) is a minimally invasive examination that uses CT to acquire images of the colon and 2D and 3D displays for interpretation. The mechanism and technique are explained in detail elsewhere in this book.

Benefits

CTC evaluates the entire colon, including those segments that are particularly redundant and difficult to evaluate with colonoscopy. Additionally the examination can be performed without sedation. The examination can also detect extracolonic findings. In one study, 9% of the total patients had clinically important extracolonic findings.[51] Meta-analysis of 33 studies on nearly 6400 patients demonstrated an 85% to 93% sensitivity and 97% specificity for polyps 10 mm and larger. The 96% sensitivity of CTC for invasive cancer was comparable to that of optical colonoscopy.[49,52-54]

Limitations

One of the greatest limitations of CTC is its availability. Because funding is not widely available for screening CTC, the professional capacity is markedly limited.[26] CTC requires a cathartic bowel preparation, although studies are underway to eliminate this need. The most notable limitation is that CTC is an imaging study only, and patients must be referred to optical colonoscopy for biopsy and/or removal if a significant colonic lesion is encountered. However, Pickhardt and colleagues have demonstrated a coordinated approach with gastroenterology that allows for same-day colonoscopy and biopsy in instances of positive CTC findings.[59]

Recommendation

CTC every 5 years for patients older than 50 years of age is an acceptable screening option for colorectal cancer.[26]

Recommendation

An overall recommendation given the multiple methodologies of screening is challenging. The U.S. Multisociety Task Force leaned heavily toward screening tests that could prevent cancer rather than simply detect it at a later stage and thus implied a preference away from stool testing and toward direct mucosal evaluation. At this time there is insufficient capacity to screen the entire population using any one modality. Given this, and the fact that

TABLE 57-1　Accuracy, Limitations, and Pitfalls of the Modalities Used in Screening for Colon Cancer

Modality	Accuracy	Limitations	Pitfalls
FOBT	37-79% cancer[29]	Positive result requires invasive test; does not detect small lesions	Single test is insufficient.
FSIG	60-70% advanced adenoma and cancer[26]	Does not detect proximal disease	Less accurate in older patients because proximal disease is more common after age 65
DCBE	85-97% cancer[26] 70% advanced adenoma[60]	Positive result requires invasive test.	Operator dependent
CTC	85-93% sensitive; 97% specific for 10-mm polyp[49,52-54]	Positive result requires invasive test; limited availability	Training dependent
OC	88-94% sensitive for 10-mm polyp[48,49]	Tortuous colon can lead to incomplete studies. Invasive test with risks of bleeding, perforation	

patients have shown varied preferences for the screening tests, the goal is to encourage screening using any modality with which a patient is willing to comply, with preference for those modalities that evaluate the entire colonic mucosa (Table 57-1).[55-58]

IMAGING

Early-Stage Adenocarcinoma and the Adenomatous Polyp

The primary target of colon cancer screening is the early adenocarcinoma or the adenomatous polyp.[26] It has been estimated that 35% to 50% of the adult population older than 50 years of age will have at least one polyp; however, the majority of these will be diminutive lesions.[59] The prevalence using a 6-mm threshold is approximately 14%.[59] Using a 10-mm threshold, the prevalence falls to 5% to 6%.[59] It thus becomes a critical question as to the appropriate polyp size as the target for screening examinations and the actions to be taken on discovery of the target lesion.

The Diminutive Lesion (<6 mm)

The American Gastroenterological Association Future Trends Report from 2004 claimed that such diminutive polyps are not a compelling reason for colonoscopy and polypectomy. Approximately a third of such polyps are adenomatous, with the majority presenting as mucosal tags or hyperplasia.[59] Lieberman and associates noted that despite the increased number of diminutive polyps compared with small polyps, the prevalence of advanced histology in diminutive polyps is lower.[60] Although some continue to argue for colonoscopy in diminutive lesions, there is near consensus that these lesions do not require intervention.

The Small Lesion (6-9 mm)

Two thirds of small polyps are adenomatous, and approximately 4% will have advanced histology.[8,59,61] With an 8% screening prevalence of small adenomas and 4% advanced histology, the overall prevalence of the advanced, small adenoma is 0.3%. In Pickhardt and colleagues' screening

experience of over 1000 small polyps, they did not find any invasive cancers.[59] Without any intervention, the 5-year colorectal cancer death rate in patients with 6- to 9-mm polyps is 0.08%, a sevenfold decrease from that of the *a priori* screening population.[59] Pickhardt and colleagues recommend a 3-year CTC surveillance for 6- to 9-mm lesions discovered on CTC but agreed with the American Gastroenterological Association that there remains a need to define the natural history of such polyps with a large longitudinal study.[61]

The Large Polyp (≥10 mm)

This group is the least controversial, and there is near unanimity that these lesions merit tissue sampling. Studies have shown a 30.6% prevalence of advanced histology in large polyps.[60] If these are detected on CTC, these patients should be referred to colonoscopy for biopsy.

What the Referring Physician Needs to Know

- There is a 90% 5-year survival rate for cancer limited to the colon; it is 68% for regional disease and 10% for metastatic disease.
- Screening has a definite benefit in the prevention of colorectal carcinoma.
- Both CTC and optical colonoscopy are cost effective in colorectal cancer screening.

KEY POINTS

- CTC is comparable to optical colonoscopy in detection of clinically significant (≥10 mm) lesions.
- Acceptable screening options include:
  - CTC every 5 years
  - Optical colonoscopy every 10 years
  - FSIG every 5 years
- Less preferred but acceptable screening options:
  - Stool-based examinations conducted as a full program
  - DCBE every 5 years
- Different patients have different preferences. The key goal is to screen as many people as possible!

REFERENCES

1. American Cancer Society. Colorectal Cancer Facts & Figures 2008-2010; 1-32. Available at http://www.cancer.org/downloads/STT/F861708_finalforweb.pdf.

2. Jemal A, et al. Cancer statistics, 2009. CA Cancer J Clin 2009; 59: 225-249.

3. Winawer SJ, et al. Prevention of colorectal cancer by colonoscopic polypectomy. The National Polyp Study Workgroup. N Engl J Med 1993; 329:1977-1981.

4. Kim DH, et al. CT colonography versus colonoscopy for the detection of advanced neoplasia. N Engl J Med 2007; 357: 1403-1412.

5. Pickhardt PJ, Kim DH. Colorectal cancer screening with CT colonography: key concepts regarding polyp prevalence, size, histology, morphology, and natural history. AJR Am J Roentgenol 2009; 193: 40-46.

6. Morson B. President's address: the polyp-cancer sequence in the large bowel. Proc R Soc Med 1974; 67:451-457.

7. Zalis ME, et al. CT colonography reporting and data system: a consensus proposal. Radiology 2005; 236:3-9.

8. Johnson CD, Chen MH, et al. Accuracy of CT colonography for detection of large adenomas and cancers. N Engl J Med 2008; 359: 1207-1217.

9. Jackman RJ, Mayo CW. The adenoma-carcinoma sequence in cancer of the colon. Surg Gynecol Obstet 1951; 93:327-330.

10. Muto T, Bussey HJ, Morson BC. The evolution of cancer of the colon and rectum. Cancer 1975; 36:2251-2270.

11. Fearon ER, Vogelstein B. A genetic model for colorectal tumorigenesis. Cell 1990; 61:759-767.

12. Odom SR, et al. The rate of adenocarcinoma in endoscopically removed colorectal polyps. Am Surg 2005; 71:1024-1026.

13. O'Brien MJ, et al. The National Polyp Study: patient and polyp characteristics associated with high-grade dysplasia in colorectal adenomas. Gastroenterology 1990; 98:371-379.

14. Winawer SJ, et al. Randomized comparison of surveillance intervals after colonoscopic removal of newly diagnosed adenomatous polyps. The National Polyp Study Workgroup. N Engl J Med 1993; 328:901-906.

15. Ries L, Melbert D, Krapcho M, et al (eds). SEER Cancer Statistics Review 1975-2004. Bethesda, MD, National Cancer Institute, 2007.

16. Smith RA, Cokkinides V, Eyre HJ. Cancer screening in the United States, 2007: a review of current guidelines, practices and prospects. CA Cancer J Clin 2007; 57:90-104.

17. Selby JV, Friedman GD, Quesenberry CP Jr, Weiss NS. A case control study of screening sigmoidoscopy and mortality from colorectal cancer. N Engl J Med 1992; 326:653-657.

18. Kronborg O, Fenger C, Olsen J, et al. Randomised study of screening for colorectal cancer with faecal occult blood test. Lancet 1996; 348:1467-1471.

19. Mandel JS, Church TR, Bond JH, et al. The effect of fecal occult-blood screening on the incidence of colorectal cancer. N Engl J Med 2000; 343:1603-1607.

20. Eddy D. ACS report on the cancer-related health checkup. CA Cancer J Clin 1980;30:193-240.

21. U.S. Preventive Services Task Force. Guide to Clinical Preventive Services, 2nd ed. Baltimore, Williams & Wilkins, 1996.

22. U.S. Preventive Services Task Force. Screening for colorectal cancer: recommendation and rationale. Ann Intern Med 2002; 137:129-131.

23. Heiken JP, Bree RL, Foley WD, et al. Colorectal cancer screening. American College of Radiology (ACR) Appropriateness Criteria. Reston, VA, American College of Radiology, 2006.

24. Winawer SJ, Fletcher RH, Miller L, et al. Colorectal cancer screening: clinical guidelines and rationale. Gastroenterology 1997; 112: 594-642.

25. Winawer SJ, Fletcher RH, Rex D, et al. Colorectal cancer screening: clinical guidelines and surveillance: clinical guidelines and rationale—update based on new evidence. Gastroenterology 2003; 124:544-560.

26. Levin B, Lieberman DA, McFarland B, et al. Screening and surveillance for the early detection of colorectal cancer and adenomatous polyps, 2008: A joint guideline from the American Cancer Society, the U.S. Multi-Society Task Force on Colorectal Cancer, and the American College of Radiology. CA Cancer J Clin 2008; 58: 130-160.

27. Tengs TO, Wallace A. One thousand health related quality-of-life estimates. Med Care 2000; 38:583-637.

28. Pickhardt PJ, Hassan C, Laghi A, Kim DH. CT colonography to screen for colorectal cancer and aortic aneurysm in the Medicare population: cost-effectiveness analysis. AJR Am J Roentgenol 2009; 192: 1332-1340.

29. Allison JE, Tekawa IS, Ransom LJ, Adrain AL. A comparison of fecal occult blood tests for colorectal cancer screening. N Engl J Med 1996; 334:155-159.

30. Simon JB. Occult blood screening for colorectal carcinoma: a critical review. Gastroenterology 1985; 88:820-837.

31. Hardcastle JD, Chamberlain JO, Robinson MH, et al. Randomised controlled trial of faecal-occult-blood screening for colorectal cancer. Lancet 1996; 348:1472-1477.

32. Kronborg O, Fenger C, Olsen J, et al. Randomised study of screening for colorectal cancer with faecal-occult-blood test. Lancet 1996; 348:1467-1471.

33. Young GP, St John DJ. Selecting an occult blood test for use as a screening tool for large bowel cancer. In Rozen P, Reich CB, Winawer SJ (eds). Frontiers of Gastrointestinal Research. Advances in Large Bowel Cancer: Policy, Prevention, Research and Treatment. Basel, Karger, 1991, pp 135-156.

34. Collins JF, Lieberman DA, Durbin TE, Weiss DG. Accuracy of screening for fecal occult blood on a single stool sample obtained by digital rectal examination: a comparison with recommended sampling practice. Ann Intern Med 2005; 142:81-85.

35. Selby JV, Friedman GD, Quesenberry CP Jr, Weiss NS. A case control study of screening sigmoidoscopy and mortality from colorectal cancer. N Engl J Med 1992; 326:653-657.

36. Newcomb PA, Norfleet RG, Storer BE, et al. Screening sigmoidoscopy and colorectal cancer mortality. J Natl Cancer Inst 1992; 84:1572-1575.

37. Thiis-Evensen E, Hoff GS, Sauar J, et al. Population-based surveillance by colonoscopy: effect on the incidence of colorectal cancer. Telemark Polyp Study I. Scand J Gastroenterol 1999; 34:414-420.

38. Newcomb PA, Storer BE, Morimoto LM, et al. Long-term efficacy of sigmoidoscopy in the reduction of colorectal cancer incidence. J Natl Cancer Inst 2003; 95:622-625.

39. Schoen RE, Pinsky PF, Weissfeld JL, et al. Results of repeat sigmoidoscopy 3 years after a negative examination. JAMA 2003; 290: 41-48.

40. Doria-Rose VP, Newcomb PA, Levin TR. Incomplete screening flexible sigmoidoscopy associated with female sex, age, and increased risk of colorectal cancer. Gut 2005; 54:1273-1278.

41. Johnson CD, Carlson HC, Taylor WF, Weiland LP. Barium enemas of carcinoma of the colon: sensitivity of double- and single-contrast studies. AJR Am J Roentgenol 1983; 140:1143-1149.

42. Sosna J, Sella T, Sy O, et al. Critical analysis of the performance of double-contrast barium enema for detecting colorectal polyps > or = 6 mm in the era of CT colonography. AJR Am J Roentgenol 2008; 190:374-385.

43. Scholz FJ. Tips for the comfortable double-contrast barium enema: the open tube technique with active drainage. Semin Roentgenol 2000; 35:342-356.

44. Seeff LC, Richards TB, Shapiro JA, et al. How many endoscopies are performed for colorectal cancer screening? Results from CDC's survey of endoscopic capacity. Gastroenterology 2004; 127: 1670-1677.

45. Muller AD, Sonnenberg A. Prevention of colorectal cancer by flexible endoscopy and polypectomy: a case control study of 32,702 veterans. Ann Intern Med 1995; 123:904-910.

46. Kahi CJ, et al. Effects of screening colonoscopy on colorectal cancer incidence and mortality. Clin Gastroenterol Hepatol 2009; 7: 770-775.

47. Rex DK, Bond JH, Winawer S, et al. Quality in the technical performance of colonoscopy and the continuous quality improvement process for colonoscopy; recommendations of the U.S. Multisociety Task Force on Colorectal Cancer. Am J Gastroenterol 2002; 97: 1296-1308.

48. Rex DK, Cutler CS, Lemmel GT, et al. Colonoscopic miss rates of adenomas determined by back to back colonoscopies. Gastroenterology 1997; 112:24-28.

49. Pickhardt PJ, Nugent PA, Mysliwiec PA, et al. Location of adenomas missed by optical colonoscopy. Ann Intern Med 2004; 141:352-359.

50. Gatto NM, Frucht H, Sundararajan V, et al. Risk of perforation after colonoscopy: a population-based study. J Natl Cancer Inst 2003; 95:230-236.

51. Yee J, Kumar NN, Godara SS, et al. Extracolonic abnormalities discovered incidentally at CT colonography in a male population. Radiology 2005; 236:519-526.

52. Farrar WD, Sawhney MS, Nelson DB, et al. Colorectal cancers found after a complete colonoscopy. Clin Gastroenterol Hepatol 2006; 4:1259-1264.

53. Halligan S, Altman DG, Taylor SA, et al. CT colonography in the detection of colorectal polyps and cancer; systematic review, meta-analysis, and proposed minimum data set for study level reporting. Radiology 2005; 237:893-904.

54. Mulhall BP, Veerappan GR, Jackson JL. Meta-analysis: computed tomographic colonography. Ann Intern Med 2005; 142:635-650.

55. Vernon SW. Participation in colorectal cancer screening; a review. J Natl Cancer Inst 1997; 89:1406-1433.

56. Schroy PC 3rd, Heeren TC. Patient perceptions of stool based DNA testing for colorectal cancer screening. Am J Prev Med 2005; 28:208-214.

57. Tangka FK, Molinari NA, Chattopadhyay SK, Seeff LC. Market for colorectal cancer screening by endoscopy in the United States. Am J Prev Med 2005; 29:54-60.

58. Lafata JE, Divine G, Moon C, Williams LK. Patient-physician colorectal cancer screening discussions and screening use. Am J Prev Med 2006; 31:202-209.

59. Pickhardt PJ, Kim DH. Colorectal cancer screening with CT colonography: key concepts regarding polyp prevalence, size, histology, morphology and natural history. AJR Am J Roentgenol 2009; 193:40-46.

60. Lieberman D, Morave M, Holub J, et al. Polyp size and advanced histology in patients undergoing colonoscopy screening: implications for CT colonography. Gastroenterology 2008; 135:1100-1105.

61. Pickhardt PJ, Choi JR, Hwang I, et al. Nonadenomatous polyps at CT colonography: prevalence, size distribution, and detection rates. Radiology 2004; 232:784-790.

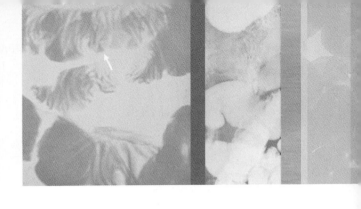

58

Imaging of the Postoperative Bowel

Efrén J. Flores and Dushyant V. Sahani

During daily radiology practice many cases are encountered that demonstrate postoperative changes related to different types of bowel surgery. Considering how extensive the bowel is as an organ (i.e., from the esophagus to the rectum), the surgical procedures performed on different sections of the bowel are innumerable and their detailed discussion is beyond the scope of this chapter. To have a better understanding of the imaging findings related to these procedures, it is important to be familiar with the anatomy of the performed surgical technique. Taking this into consideration, our purpose in this chapter is to present some tools to approach the postoperative bowel by briefly discussing the commonly performed surgical procedures of the bowel, their appearance on imaging, and the common complications to look for on imaging.

PROCEDURES

Esophageal Resection

In light of various surgical procedures that can be performed in the esophagus and the possible approach to surgery (e.g., transthoracic, transhiatal), the planned procedure will be selected based on the location of esophageal disease. All the surgical techniques utilized for esophageal resection have a characteristic in common: a segment of the esophagus will be resected and reconstructed. Among those techniques the most frequently performed are the transthoracic esophagectomy (either right-sided or left-sided approach), transhiatal esophagectomy, the Ivor-Lewis technique, and esophagectomy with aperistaltic colonic interposition.

Indications, Contraindications, Purpose, and Underlying Mechanisms

Esophageal resection is the treatment of choice for several benign and neoplastic conditions. Benign causes include conditions such as esophageal perforation, refractory peptic stricture that does not resolve with stenting, and large leiomyomas (>5 cm). The most common neoplastic causes include adenocarcinoma and squamous cell carcinoma of the esophagus.

Once the medical reason for surgery is established and the affected part of the esophagus is localized, the surgeon will determine the technique to utilize. For example, right-sided transthoracic esophagectomy (Fig. 58-1) is preferred in cases involving the upper two thirds of the esophagus because the aorta does not limit access to the esophagus, whereas the left-sided approach is used in cases involving the distal esophagus. The Ivor-Lewis procedure is an excellent procedure for patients with midesophageal carcinomas, Barrett's esophagus, and esophageal destruction (e.g., perforation, caustic injury, persistent esophageal ulcer).[1] This procedure combines a laparotomy with right thoracotomy and intrathoracic anastomosis. This technique permits direct visualization of the thoracic esophagus and a full lymphadenectomy. Disadvantages of this technique include a limited proximal resection margin, intrathoracic location of the anastomosis, and the complexity associated with an above-and-below the diaphragm procedure.

Transhiatal esophagectomy was developed due to the multiple complications involved with the thoracotomy approach, and decreased morbidities associated with the transhiatal technique have made this procedure a more popular approach. This technique involves mobilization of the esophagus through the esophageal hiatus; then the entire thoracic esophagus is transected, and finally the esophagus is reconstructed with the stomach by an anastomosis with the remaining cervical esophagus (Fig. 58-2).

Esophagectomy with aperistaltic colonic interposition (Fig. 58-3) is a procedure in which a segment of the colon is used to reconstruct the esophagus. This technique is performed in cases of neoplastic disease in which tumor extension to the stomach precludes a 5-cm resection margin or if the patient has previously undergone a gastrectomy.[2,3]

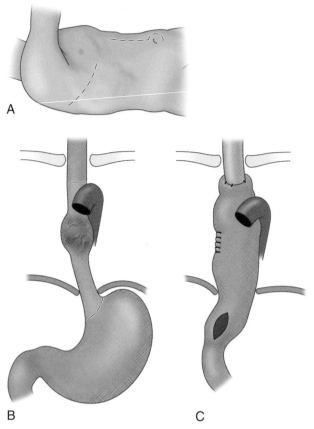

■ **FIGURE 58-1**   Overview of right thoracotomy (**A**) with esophageal resection, (**B**) gastric mobilization, and (**C**) intrathoracic anastomosis. (*Redrawn from Townsend CM. Sabiston Textbook of Surgery, 17th ed. Philadelphia, Elsevier Saunders, 2004, p 1134.*)

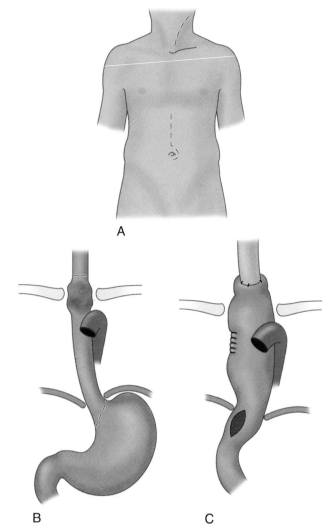

■ **FIGURE 58-2**   A to C, Overview of transhiatal esophagectomy with gastric mobilization and gastric pull-up for cervical-esophagogastric anastomosis. (*Adapted from Ellis FH Jr: Esophagogastrectomy for carcinoma: technical considerations based on anatomic location of lesion. Surg Clin North Am 1980; 60:275.*)

Expected Appearance on Relevant Modalities

As previously mentioned, the common denominator for all these techniques is an esophageal resection, reconstruction, and creation of an anastomosis. It is important to know the location of the anastomosis to optimally evaluate the patient. At our institution, the operative report is reviewed before evaluating the patient in the fluoroscopy suite. In the preoperative or postoperative setting the radiologic imaging modality of choice is barium esophagography. Preoperatively it allows for evaluation of the lesion in question, the location (Figs. 58-4 and 58-5) of this lesion in the esophagus (upper, middle or lower third), which is important in terms of deciding right versus left thoracotomy, and the preoperative functionality of the esophagus. Postoperatively, it allows evaluation of patency of the anastomosis, functionality of the reconstructed esophagus, and possible recurrent disease. In cases in which there is a concern of perforation, water-soluble contrast media should be used initially to exclude this possibility and prevent complications such as a chemical mediastinitis.

Considering that most complications occur at the anastomosis site, when reviewing these cases this area should be thoroughly evaluated. In cases of transhiatal esopha-

gectomy and gastric pull-through, images on barium esophagography will demonstrate a narrowing within the cervical esophagus that represents the anastomotic site and a reconstructed esophagus demonstrating the folds that are typical of stomach mucosa (Figs. 58-6 and 58-7). In the cases in which an Ivor-Lewis or a left/right thoracotomy and esophagectomy techniques were performed the images on the barium esophagogram will show that the anastomotic site is located within the chest (Figs. 58-8 and 58-9).

Potential Complications and Radiologic Appearance

Possible complications in cases of patients with esophagectomy can be divided into intraoperative and

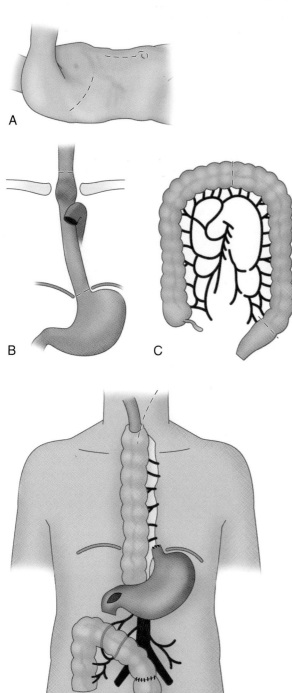

A

B

C

D

■ **FIGURE 58-3** Overview of esophagectomy with interposition of an antiperistaltic segment of left colon. **A,** Incisions. **B,** Extent of esophageal resection (*between dashed lines*). **C,** Preparation of segment of left colon (*between dashed lines*). **D,** Completed operation. (*Redrawn from Townsend CM. Sabiston Textbook of Surgery, 17th ed. Philadelphia, Elsevier Saunders, 2004, p 1140.*)

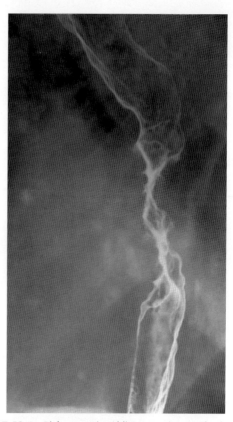

■ **FIGURE 58-4** Right posterior oblique spot image of a double-contrast esophagogram demonstrates an irregular "apple core" lesion within the middle third of the esophagus.

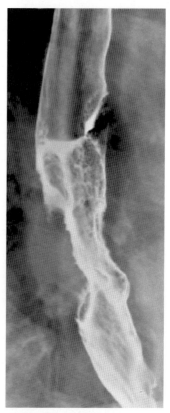

■ **FIGURE 58-5** Left posterior oblique image of a double-contrast esophagogram demonstrates an irregular narrowing secondary to an esophageal adenocarcinoma affecting the lower third of the esophagus.

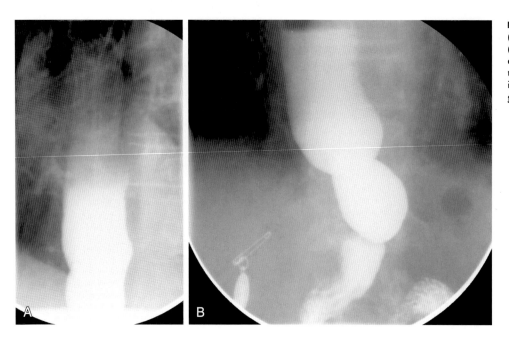

■ **FIGURE 58-6** Anteroposterior (**A**) and right posterior oblique (**B**) images of a barium esophagogram demonstrating the typical appearance of a patient who is status post esophagectomy and gastric pull-through.

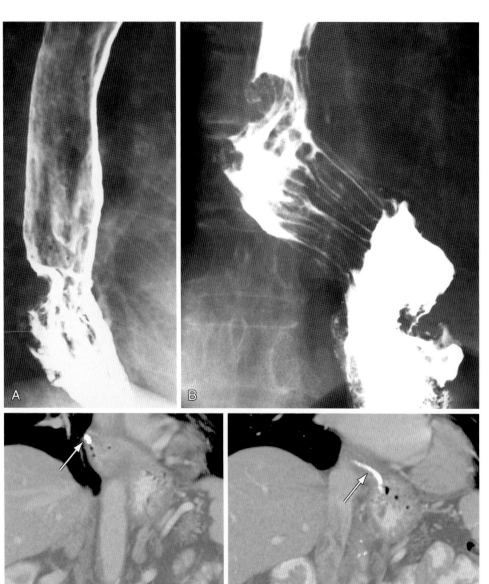

■ **FIGURE 58-7** Spot right posterior oblique images of a barium esophagogram at the level of the distal esophagus (**A**) and proximal stomach (**B**) in a patient who underwent partial distal esophagectomy and reanastomosis. Coronal CT images (**C** and **D**) demonstrate a linear hyperdensity near the gastroesophageal junction (*arrows*) representing the new gastroesophageal anastomosis.

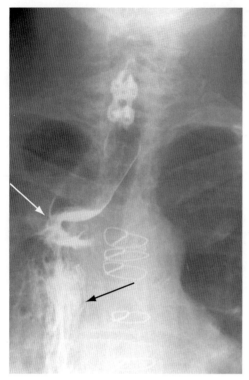

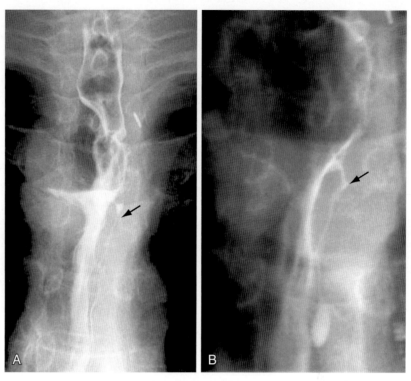

■ **FIGURE 58-8** Frontal image of a barium esophagogram of a patient who underwent an Ivor-Lewis procedure shows a narrowing within the cervical esophagus (*white arrow*) with the distal reconstructed esophagus demonstrating mucosal folds typical of stomach mucosa (*black arrow*).

■ **FIGURE 58-10** Spot anteroposterior (**A**) and right posterior oblique (**B**) images of a barium esophagogram from a patient with recent esophagectomy and gastric pull-through with anastomosis demonstrate a small linear area of extraluminal contrast medium (*arrows*) consistent with an anastomotic leak.

postoperative complications.[4] Laryngeal nerve injury, tracheobronchial tree injury, arrhythmias, and hemorrhage are among the most common intraoperative complications. Postoperative complications include pulmonary (atelectasis, pleural effusions), anastomotic leak/ stricture, and the two most feared complications of anastomosis failure and leak (Fig. 58-10) and of recurrent disease in patients with esophageal cancer. At our institution, those patients who are within the recent postopera-

tive period (first 24 hours) are first evaluated with water-soluble contrast medium to rule out the possibility of anastomotic leak. If extraluminal contrast agent is seen, images at other angles (e.g., right posterior oblique, anteroposterior, left posterior oblique) and with magnification should be obtained because this is important for documentation and a true leak may be managed surgically. If an anastomotic leak is excluded, the examination can be continued with barium for improved detail.

■ **FIGURE 58-9** **A,** Coronal CT image of the same patient as in Figure 58-8 demonstrates stomach replacing the distal esophagus. **B,** Axial CT image at the level of the upper thorax demonstrates a linear high-density material (*arrowheads*) adjacent to the reconstructed esophagus, representing the suture material used for the thoracic anastomosis.

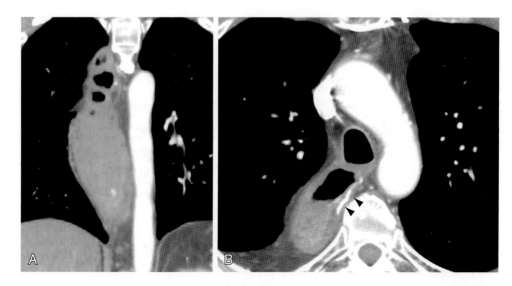

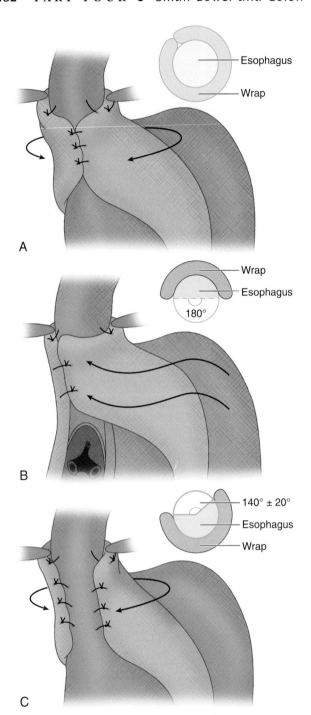

■ FIGURE 58-11 Overview of the most common fundoplications. **A,** Nissen fundoplication. Most surgeons perform a "floppy" wrap and add sutures posteriorly to approximate the crura of the diaphragm. **B,** The Belsey Mark IV repair is performed transthoracically, whereas the Hill procedure (**C**) is performed via the abdominal route. (*Redrawn from Townsend CM. Sabiston Textbook of Surgery, 17th ed. Philadelphia, Elsevier Saunders, 2004, p 1160.*)

Antireflux Surgery

Gastroesophageal reflux disease is a common occurrence among patients and is usually manifested as heartburn and dysphagia. There are many medications available for treatment of this condition; however, in cases in which the

TABLE 58-1 Types of Antireflux Surgery and Indications

Esophageal Length and Preoperative Motility	Recommended Antireflux Surgery
Normal length and motility	Nissen fundoplication
Normal length but abnormal motility	Hill or Belsey operation
Normal length and motility but prior stomach surgery	Hill operation

symptoms are refractory to medical management or in which there is evidence of severe esophageal injury then surgical intervention is an option for more permanent relief of symptoms.

Indications, Contraindications, Purpose, and Underlying Mechanisms

The purpose of antireflux surgery is to construct a valve mechanism that reestablishes the gastroesophageal junction competence. Among surgical techniques available for treatment, the three most popular are the Nissen fundoplication, the Belsey Mark IV repair, and the Hill posterior gastropexy (Fig. 58-11). These procedures can be performed through laparotomy (Nissen, Hill), thoracotomy (Belsey), or laparoscopy (Nissen, Hill).

As described in Table 58-1, the surgical technique of choice depends on the patient's preoperative esophageal length and motility. The Nissen fundoplication is the most common and popular technique owing to improvement in symptoms and decreased morbidity related to the laparoscopic approach. This procedure is recommended in patients with normal esophageal length and normal motility. In patients with normal esophageal length and decreased motility, a complete fundoplication is discouraged and a Hill or Belsey technique is recommended. For those patients with a small stomach due to prior surgery, the Hill procedure is the procedure of choice.[3]

Expected Appearance on Relevant Modalities

The esophagus is the main organ evaluated for this procedure, and barium esophagography remains the optimal study for evaluation of these patients. In the preoperative setting it provides information regarding

- Esophageal motility
- Presence of sliding or paraesophageal hernia (>5 cm)
- Significant esophageal stricture or Barrett's esophagus (segment > 3 cm)

If a hernia is present it is important to document if it is present when the patient is upright and if there is a stricture that is more than 3 cm. This will determine the surgical procedure to be performed. In the postoperative setting, this study will provide information about patency of the procedure and functionality of the esophagus. The typical appearance of a fundoplication on barium esophagography is a smooth circumferential narrowing of the distal esophagus that extends for 2 to 3 cm and is associated with a filling defect within the stomach fundus

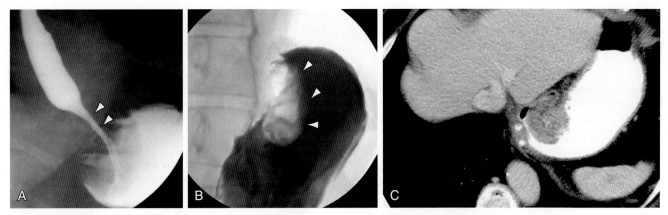

■ **FIGURE 58-12** Spot radiographs from barium esophagography at the level of the distal esophagus (**A**) and proximal stomach (**B**) reveal a typical fundoplication defect (*arrowheads*). Note the circumferential narrowing of the distal esophagus and gastroesophageal junction, extending for 2 to 3 cm. The wrap is subdiaphragmatic. CT image (**C**) from a patient who is status post Nissen fundoplication demonstrates a curved apparent gastric wall thickening that represents the stomach fundus wrapped around the distal esophagus at the gastroesophageal junction.

representing the portion used for the wraparound (Fig. 58-12).[5]

Potential Complications and Radiologic Appearance

In the postoperative setting, those patients who present with symptoms such as dysphagia, epigastric pain, or recurrent reflux warrant an evaluation to assess the status of the fundoplication. These symptoms may be secondary to one of the following complications: (1) a tight fundo-

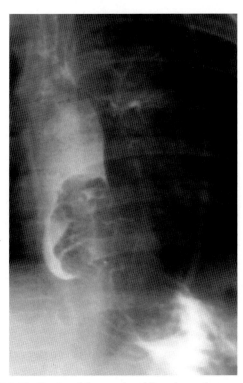

■ **FIGURE 58-13** Spot left posterior oblique image from a patient status post Nissen fundoplication who complained of dysphagia shows the filling defect at the stomach fundus typical of a fundoplication. However, the stomach fundus and proximal body have herniated above the diaphragm.

plication or a long fundoplication that prevents adequate passage of a food bolus, (2) partially or completely herniated fundoplication (Fig. 58-13) and acquired paraesophageal hernia, or (3) partially or completely disrupted fundoplication.[6]

Gastric Bypass

Obesity has become an increasing problem, with some calling it an epidemic. As part of the solutions offered for this problem, gastric bypass or bariatric surgery is a procedure that has become more commonly used with patients as an alternative to improve long-term outcome. The weight loss that results from this procedure not only improves the quality of life of these patients[7] but also makes them less likely to require medications for cardiovascular disease or diabetes.[8]

Indications, Contraindications, Purpose, and Underlying Mechanisms

This type of surgery is indicated in patients who have a body mass index (BMI) of more than 40 kg/m^2 or a BMI of 35 kg/m^2 associated with other comorbidities, such as sleep apnea, diabetes, and obesity-related cardiomyopathy.

Bariatric procedures are divided into two main categories: restrictive and malabsorptive techniques (Table 58-2). The main purpose of restrictive procedures is to reduce the caloric intake by limiting the stomach's capacity.

TABLE 58-2 Types of Gastric Bypass Surgery
Restrictive
Vertical banded gastroplasty
Gastric banding
Malabsorptive
Jejunoileal bypass
Biliopancreatic diversion with duodenal switch
Combined
Roux-en-Y gastric bypass

Vertical banded gastroplasty (Fig. 58-14A) and laparoscopic adjustable gastric banding (Fig. 58-14B) are among these procedures. The malabsorptive procedures aim to reduce the absorption of calories by reduction of the length of the small intestine. These procedures include the biliopancreatic diversion with duodenal switch and the jejunoileal bypass (Fig. 58-15). However, the Roux-en-Y gastric bypass is a combination of both, in which the gastric pouch serves as the restrictive component and the gastrojejunal anastomosis represents the malabsorptive component (Fig. 58-16). The laparoscopic Roux-en-Y gastric bypass has become the preferred method owing to decreased hospital stays and faster recovery.[9,10]

To perform these types of surgeries, the anatomy of the upper gastrointestinal system has to be intact. The possibility of underlying malignancy or an inflammatory process

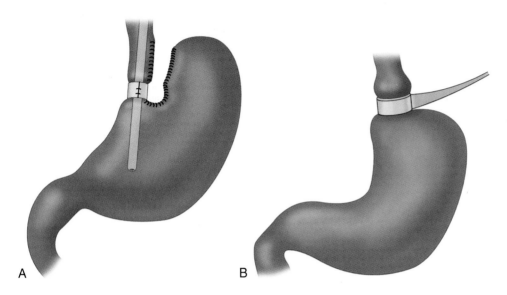

A   B

■ **FIGURE 58-14** **A,** Vertical banded gastroplasty. Vertical staple line is used to exclude part of the stomach. **B,** Lap-band adjustable banding. This adjustable band is placed laparoscopically to decrease the size of the stomach, and it can be adjusted. (*Redrawn from Cameron JL. Current Surgical Therapy, 7th ed. St. Louis, Elsevier Mosby, 2005.*)

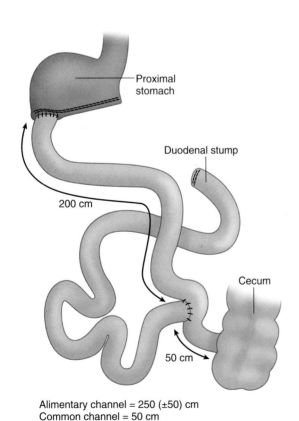

Alimentary channel = 250 (±50) cm
Common channel = 50 cm

■ **FIGURE 58-15** Anatomic configuration of the biliopancreatic diversion. (*Redrawn from Townsend CM. Sabiston Textbook of Surgery, 17th ed. Philadelphia, Elsevier Saunders, 2004, p 377.*)

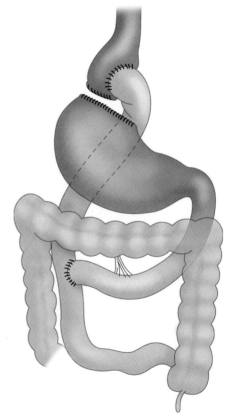

■ **FIGURE 58-16** Roux-en-Y gastric bypass. Illustration includes exclusion of part of the stomach and a gastrojejunostomy. (*Redrawn from Cameron JL. Current Surgical Therapy, 7th ed. St. Louis, Elsevier Mosby, 2005, p 99.*)

affecting this system needs to be excluded before performance of the surgery.

Expected Appearance on Relevant Modalities

First, because of the body habitus and morbid obesity of these patients, imaging is challenging. Fluoroscopy and CT need to be adjusted to acquire adequate images on these patients, because proper evaluation is extremely important, especially in the recent postoperative setting. The two main imaging modalities used to evaluate these patients are barium esophagography and CT. The esophagography will allow evaluation of the anatomy, patency of the anastomosis in cases of Roux-en-Y gastric bypass, and functionality of the gastric bypass (Fig. 58-17). CT

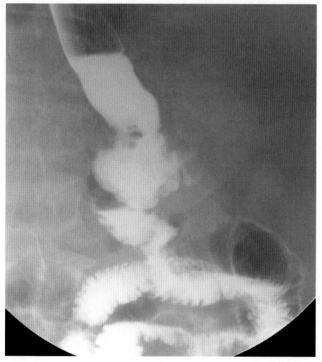

■ **FIGURE 58-17** Spot anteroposterior image from a patient after Roux-en-Y gastric bypass demonstrates a stomach pouch filled with contrast medium and passage of the medium into the gastrojejunal anastomosis without evidence of obstruction or extraluminal filling.

allows for evaluation of possible complications related to the surgery such as free fluid in the abdomen from anastomotic leak and abscess (Fig. 58-18) or secondary complications related to the altered anatomy such as afferent loop syndrome. At our institution, the day after Roux-en-Y gastric bypass surgery, all patients are evaluated with modified barium esophagography to verify that the anastomosis is intact and no contrast medium is seen within the excluded stomach or located outside the bowel lumen. Water-soluble contrast agent is used first in case there is extraluminal contrast filling. Once this possibility is excluded, we continue the examination with barium for improved detail (Fig. 58-19). At the end of the examination, we take an overhead image to evaluate that contrast medium is moving distally into the small bowel without evidence of obstruction. In some cases in which the transit time is slow, the patient should be evaluated again several hours later with a plain radiograph of the abdomen to confirm that contrast agent is seen in the distal small bowel without evidence of obstruction. At the gastrojejunal anastomosis of patients who have undergone Roux-en-Y gastric bypass it is typical to encounter a narrowing within the first 24 hours after surgery due to postoperative edema.

In patients with laparoscopic adjustable gastric banding, the bands in the left upper quadrant where the stomach is located can be seen on plain radiographs. These are connected to the device that adjusts the band (Fig. 58-20). On CT, basically the same findings can be seen (Fig. 58-21). The most important part of each evaluation is to comment if the components of the laparoscopic adjustable gastric banding are intact and that there is no contrast opacification within the excluded stomach.

Potential Complications and Radiologic Appearance

There are many possible complications in the postoperative setting that can be divided into those that occur within the first days after surgery or those that present later after surgery. These complications include bleeding, infection, anastomotic ulcer, stricture, and internal hernia, among others (Table 58-3). In these patients, fluoroscopy and CT are key in evaluating these complications and both studies are complementary. Although fluoroscopy will

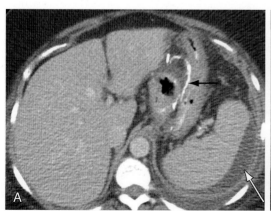

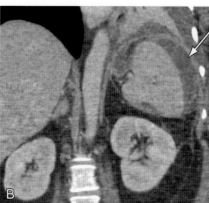

■ **FIGURE 58-18** Axial (**A**) and coronal (**B**) CT images from a patient after Roux-en-Y gastric bypass surgery who had an anastomotic leak and now presented with left upper quadrant pain secondary to a rim-enhancing fluid collection in the left subphrenic space consistent with an abscess (*white arrow*). Note the linear hyperdensity along the stomach that represents suture material from surgery (*black arrow*).

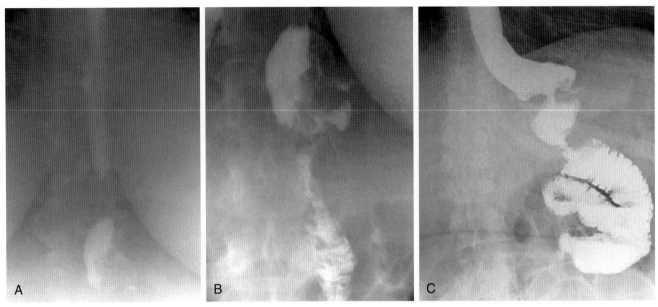

■ FIGURE 58-19 Anteroposterior (**A**) and left posterior oblique (**B**) images of esophagography performed with water-soluble contrast medium in a patient who is post Roux-en-Y gastric bypass demonstrate that the gastrojejunostomy and jejunojejunostomy anastomosis are intact without evidence of extraluminal contrast filling or contrast agent within the excluded stomach. **C,** Spot anteroposterior image of a barium esophagogram demonstrates intact anastomosis and also improved detail with barium as compared with a water-soluble contrast agent.

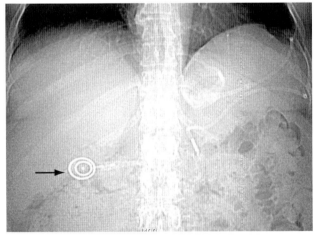

■ FIGURE 58-20 Scout image from CT scan from a patient after laparoscopic adjustable gastric banding demonstrates intact bands in the left upper quadrant. These are connected to the device that adjusts the size that is located in the right side of the abdomen (*arrow*).

TABLE 58-3 Potential Complications in Gastric Bypass Patients

First 24 Hours
Anastomotic leak
Anastomotic stricture
Small bowel obstruction
Stricture at mesocolic window

Late Complications
Gastrogastric fistula
Internal hernia
Ulcer at anastomosis

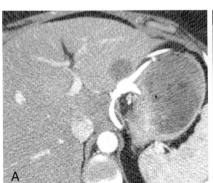
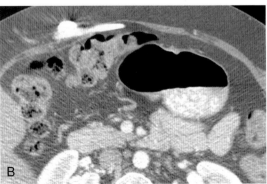

■ FIGURE 58-21 Axial CT images of a patient after laparoscopic adjustable gastric banding demonstrate the intact bands adjacent to the stomach (**A**) and the device that adjusts the bands located in the soft tissues of the anterior abdominal wall (**B**).

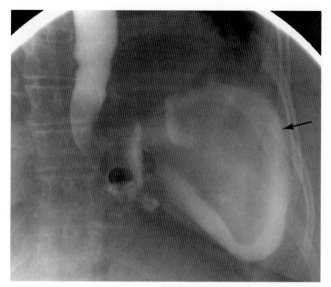

■ **FIGURE 58-22** Spot image of an esophagogram performed with water-soluble contrast agent from a patient after Roux-en-Y gastric bypass demonstrates contrast agent within the peritoneal cavity in the left upper quadrant (*arrow*).

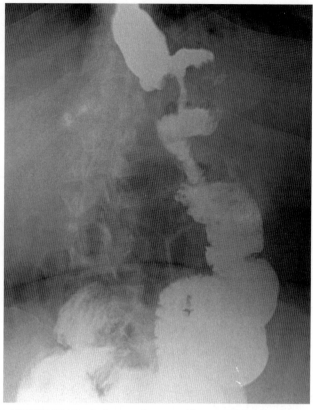

■ **FIGURE 58-23** Barium esophagogram from a patient after Roux-en-Y gastric bypass demonstrates a long-segment narrowing at the jejuno-jejunostomy (distal anastomosis) that caused this patient to have obstructive symptoms. During surgery it was found this was caused by a narrowing at the mesocolon.

provide details and functionality of the anastomosis, CT is central in evaluating patients whose condition is unstable and those who present with life-threatening complications such as pneumoperitoneum and closed-loop bowel obstruction.

Within the first day, the most feared complication that a radiologist should be aware of in patients who underwent a malabsorptive technique or Roux-en-Y gastric bypass procedure is a leak at the anastomotic site because this complication could be life threatening and needs immediate attention (Fig. 58-22). Narrowing of the anastomosis in the postoperative setting may be secondary to postoperative edema; however, if this narrowing is symptomatic and prevents passage of contrast agent, this is significant and has to be documented. This could be secondary to tight sutures; or, in cases of Roux-en-Y gastric bypass, if a retrocolic approach was used, there could be a stricture at the site where the Roux limb goes through the mesocolon (Fig. 58-23).

In patients in whom a gastric pouch is created, degradation of the suture line or a gastrogastric fistula is another complication that could present with a patient complaining of decreased satiety or weight gain (Fig. 58-24). Small bowel obstruction could be secondary to postoperative edema. However, if this condition develops later, this could be secondary to an internal hernia, intussusception (Fig. 58-25), or adhesions.[11] An internal hernia can occur through defects in the small bowel mesentery or transverse mesocolon or through a potential space posterior to the Roux limb termed the *Peterson space.*[12] In these cases, it is important to be confident about the diagnosis; if a possible transition point can be located, this would be helpful for the surgeon because these patients will need surgical exploration. Prompt diagnosis is important because perforation or anastomotic leak are possibilities secondary to tension caused by severe small bowel obstruction. In this case, CT plays an important role for displaying the anatomy of the abdomen and because of

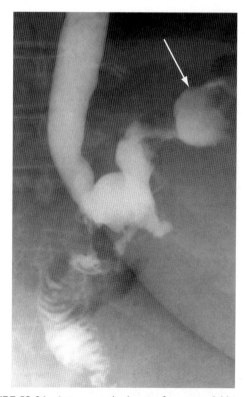

■ **FIGURE 58-24** Anteroposterior image of a water-soluble esophagogram shows contrast agent within the excluded stomach segment (*arrow*) in this patient who had a Roux-en-Y gastric bypass.

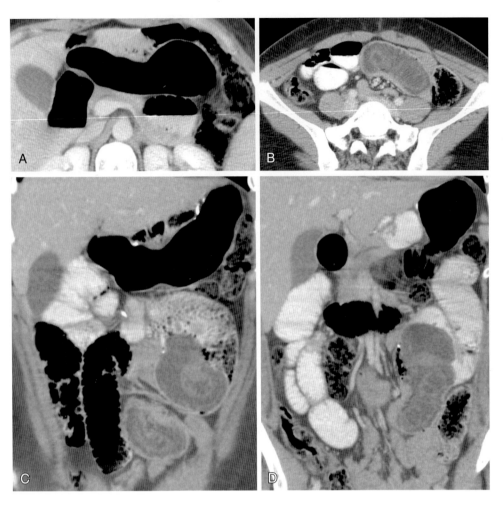

■ **FIGURE 58-25** CT images from a patient with intussusception after Roux-en-Y gastric bypass. **A,** Axial CT image at the level of the stomach and duodenum; the excluded stomach and duodenum are markedly distended with gas. Axial (**B**) and coronal (**C** and **D**) CT images of the same patient demonstrate an intussusception at the level of the distal anastomosis that is causing the obstructive symptoms in this patient.

its role in locating an exact or approximate location for a transition point.

Ulcers can develop in these patients; however, because of altered anatomy, diagnosis by radiology may be difficult and the patient may be better evaluated with endoscopy.

Gastrectomy, Billroth I and II Procedures, and Esophagojejunostomy

The incidence of gastric cancer has decreased in the United States since 1930; however, approximately 21,260 new cases are diagnosed yearly.[13] Although surgical resection of a gastric tumor and adjacent lymph nodes is the best option for patients in terms of managing this disease, the choice of either total or subtotal gastrectomy depends on the tumor location. If the tumor is located in the upper third of the stomach, is infiltrative, or is a large midgastric mass, total gastrectomy is the preferred surgical option. If the tumor is located in the distal two thirds of the stomach, subtotal gastrectomy may be an option in these patients. In cases in which a gastric tumor is known or suspected, the precise location should be described on imaging because this is key in surgical planning. Gastrectomy is used not only for the treatment of neoplastic disease but also for the treatment of severe peptic ulcer disease and complications related to this disease (e.g., severe perfora-

tion and ulceration, stricture causing gastric outlet obstruction).

After a partial or total gastrectomy, the most common types of anastomosis are Billroth I gastroduodenostomy, Billroth II gastrojejunostomy, or a Roux-en-Y loop or total gastrectomy with esophagojejunostomy.

Indications, Contraindications, Purpose, and Underlying Mechanisms

The main indication to perform a gastrectomy is for the treatment of gastric cancer. When a partial gastrectomy is performed, a Billroth I or II reanastomosis is commonly used to restore part of the anatomy. The Billroth I procedure involves an antrectomy and an end-to-end anastomosis between the remnant of the stomach and the duodenum. In the Billroth II operation, after the antrectomy is performed, the duodenal stump is closed and a gastrojejunal anastomosis is created. Also, a side-to-side duodenojejunal anastomosis may be created and the anastomotic loop may be placed in a retrocolic or antecolic position, depending on the surgeon's preference (Fig. 58-26). The retrocolic gastrojejunostomy creates a shorter afferent loop compared with the antecolic, resulting in better nutritional status and less postoperative herniation.[14] Conversely, because the anastomotic site is where the recurrence of gastric cancer first occurs, the antecolic

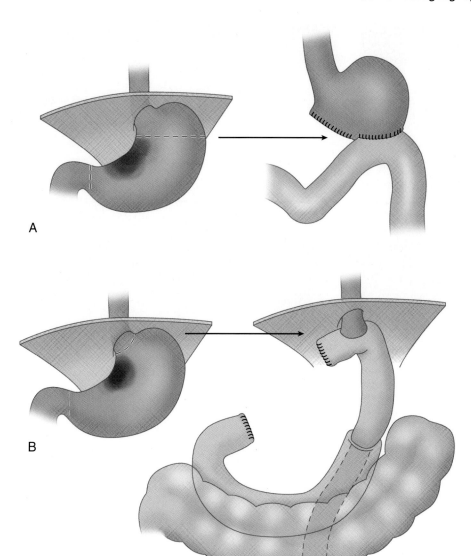

■ **FIGURE 58-26** **A,** Total gastrectomy with a Roux-en-Y anastomosis. **B,** Subtotal gastrectomy with a Billroth II anastomosis. (*Redrawn from Townsend CM. Sabiston Textbook of Surgery, 17th ed. Philadelphia, Elsevier Saunders, 2004, p 1310.*)

gastrojejunostomy is performed in patients with advanced gastric cancer to maintain the anastomosis out of the lesser sac.[15]

In cases in which a total gastrectomy is performed, a Roux-en-Y esophagojejunostomy with end-to-side anastomosis is created.

Expected Appearance on Relevant Modalities

Radiology is crucial in the evaluation of patients with symptoms after gastrectomy and proximal small bowel surgeries.[16] For adequate radiologic interpretation, reviewing the surgical note or knowing the type of procedure the patient underwent should be the first step. Single- and double-contrast fluoroscopic imaging is excellent to follow to the anastomosis, searching for anastomotic leaks and strictures, and to evaluate functionality after surgery (Fig. 58-27).

Nowadays CT has become the primary means for evaluating patients, especially if they are complaining of acute symptoms or if there is a suspicion for recurrent disease. On CT, surgical staples or sutures indicate where an anastomosis has been created and they serve as guidelines for the anatomy after surgery (Fig. 58-28). Particular attention should be given to the anastomotic site because this is where complications and recurrent disease in the cases of neoplasm frequently occur. Multiplanar reconstructions of multidetector CT images (MDCT) assist in delineation of the anatomy after surgery. MRI still has a limited role in evaluation of the small bowel, especially in postsurgical cases with acute complications.

After Billroth I surgery, initially the duodenum is seen anterior to the gastroduodenal anastomosis; however, afterward the duodenum returns to the normal position at the subhepatic and peripancreatic space (Fig. 58-29).[14]

In cases of patients with Billroth II gastrojejunostomy, the anastomosis can be located on CT by following the remnant stomach and the duodenal stump is usually located in its anatomic location (subhepatic, peripancreatic spaces).

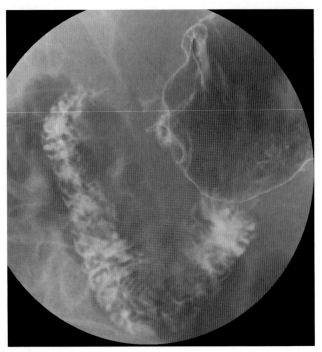

■ **FIGURE 58-27** Spot image of double-contrast small bowel series from a patient after a Billroth II operation shows the changes related to antrectomy and end-to-end anastomosis between the remnant stomach and duodenum.

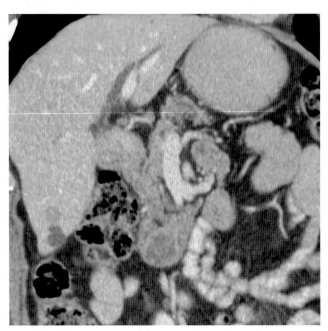

■ **FIGURE 58-29** Coronal MDCT image several months after Billroth I surgery shows the duodenum to be in the typical anatomic location in the subhepatic, peripancreatic space.

■ **FIGURE 58-28** MDCT images on patient after Billroth I surgery: axial (**A**) and coronal (**B**) MDCT images demonstrate the changes related to antrectomy and gastroduodenal anastomosis. Linear high-density material at the distal stomach is the suture material used for the anastomosis (*arrow*, **B**).

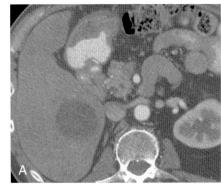

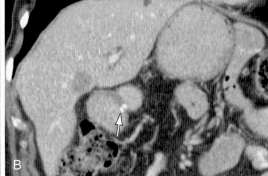

Potential Complications and Radiologic Appearance

MDCT is useful in identifying postoperative anatomic changes, complications, and tumor recurrence.[14] There is a vast constellation of postsurgical complications after a partial or total gastrectomy that includes the following:

● Early or late dumping syndrome
● Postvagotomy diarrhea
● Roux stasis syndrome
● Alkaline reflux gastritis
● Duodenal stump leakage
● Intra-abdominal bleeding
● Afferent or efferent loop syndrome

Afferent loop syndrome, duodenal stump leakage (Fig. 58-30), and postoperative hemorrhage are complications that require prompt recognition because they can be life-threatening and management is surgical.

Among these complications, afferent loop syndrome is a life-threatening condition that is underdiagnosed. It can be further divided into acute and chronic afferent loop syndrome. The acute syndrome presents as complete obstruction of the afferent loop (Fig. 58-31) and is a surgical emergency with a reported mortality up to 57%. Afferent loop syndrome can be caused by several conditions (Fig. 58-32), including:

● Entrapment of the afferent loop by adhesions
● Internal hernia through mesocolic defect[16]
● Volvulus of the intestinal segment
● Recurrence of cancer at the anastomosis
● Scarring due to marginal ulceration

The afferent loop is composed by the duodenal stump. Patients with a jejunal portion of the afferent limb longer than 10 to 15 cm, with an antecolic position of the gastrojejunostomy, or with a mesocolic defect not

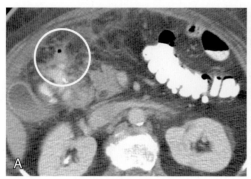
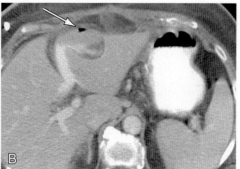

■ **FIGURE 58-30** Axial MDCT images from a patient after Billroth II surgery demonstrate (**A**) perforation at the duodenal stump (*circle*) with (**B**) extraluminal oral contrast filling, a small pocket of gas, and a fluid collection anterior to the liver (*arrow*).

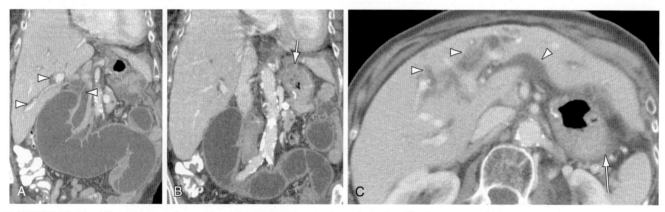

■ **FIGURE 58-31** Afferent loop syndrome. Coronal (**A**) MDCT image of a patient after Billroth II surgery who is now presenting with acute obstruction of the afferent limb. Note the dilatation of the common bile duct and the proximal intrahepatic biliary tree (*arrowheads,* **A** and **C**). Coronal (**B**) and axial (**C**) MDCT images on the same patient demonstrate the obstructed afferent limb and increased thickening, nodularity, and heterogeneous enhancement (*arrows*) of the stomach that was secondary to recurrent gastric carcinoma.

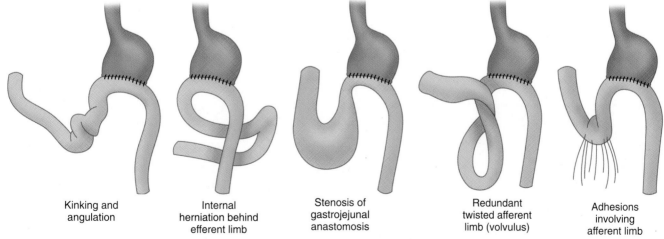

Kinking and angulation

Internal herniation behind efferent limb

Stenosis of gastrojejunal anastomosis

Redundant twisted afferent limb (volvulus)

Adhesions involving afferent limb

■ **FIGURE 58-32** Causes of afferent loop syndrome. (*Redrawn from Townsend CM. Sabiston Textbook of Surgery, 17th ed. Philadelphia, Elsevier Saunders, 2004, p 1297.*)

TABLE 58-4 Predisposing Conditions for Development of Afferent Loop Syndrome

- Jejunal portion of the afferent limb is longer than 10-15 cm.
- Gastrojejunostomy is placed in antecolic position instead of retrocolic position.
- Mesocolic defects are not properly closed after construction of retrocolic anastomosis.

properly closed after surgery have an increased chance of developing afferent loop syndrome (Table 58-4). When the afferent loop is partially or completely obstructed, pooling of enteric secretions from the pancreas and bile result in overdistention of the afferent limb, causing a blowout of the duodenal stump. Other complications that may result from this entity include ascending cholangitis and pancreatitis.

In addition, postgastrectomy patients suffer from metabolic conditions that include dumping syndrome, either early or late, as well as other metabolic disturbances related to the altered anatomy and absorption of nutrients.

Early dumping syndrome symptoms occur 20 to 30 minutes after ingestion of a meal and are accompanied by symptoms that include nausea, dizziness, tachycardia, and fainting. The symptoms are related to the rapid passage of food of high osmolarity into the stomach and the subsequent release of several humoral agents. Late dumping syndrome appears within 2 to 3 hours; and although this condition is related to rapid transit time, it is more related to carbohydrates being delivered to the small intestine, which results in hyperglycemia that causes a release of large amounts of insulin. This results in overcorrection of hyperglycemia, and hypoglycemia occurs. In most cases, both dumping syndromes can be managed conservatively by lifestyle changes that include eating smaller but more frequent meals that are low in carbohydrates. Other measures, such as surgery, are reserved for the small percentage of patients who fail conservative management.

Surgery of Small Bowel, Colon, and Rectum

Previously we discussed surgical procedures that involved the proximal small bowel. However, the complexity of

the small bowel, colon, and rectum prevents us from a detailed description of each possible procedure that may be performed, and the purpose of this section is to provide some of the indications for surgery and their respective radiologic appearances.

Indications, Contraindications, Purpose, and Underlying Mechanisms

Small bowel surgery is the treatment option in cases of refractory inflammatory bowel disease with stricture (Fig. 58-33), small bowel perforation, carcinoma (Fig. 58-34), closed-loop obstruction (Fig. 58-35), severe/strangulating small bowel obstruction, pneumatosis intestinalis, and small bowel fistula, among others. Most of these cases

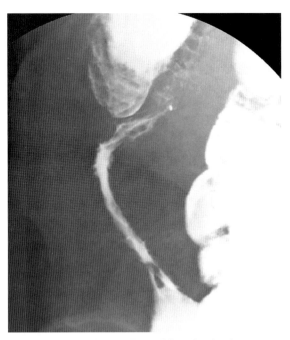

■ **FIGURE 58-33** Spot image of a small bowel series demonstrates a long-segment stricture at the terminal ileum in a patient with Crohn's disease.

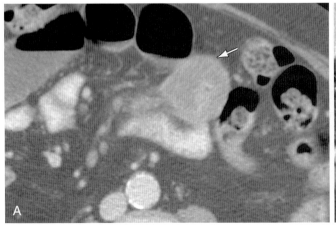

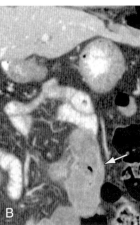

■ **FIGURE 58-34** Axial (**A**) and coronal (**B**) MDCT images demonstrate circumferential small bowel wall thickening (*arrows*) in a short segment of the small bowel in a patient diagnosed with lymphoma of the small bowel.

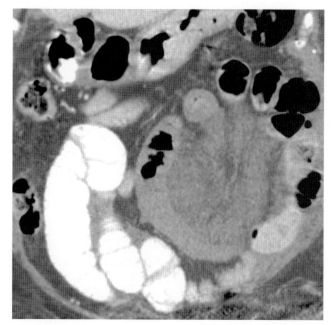

■ **FIGURE 58-35** Coronal MDCT image demonstrates a focal dilatation and twisting of the small bowel with mesenteric edema in a patient with closed-loop obstruction.

involve a partial resection of the affected segment with anastomosis of the remaining small bowel.

Partial or complete colonic resection (Fig. 58-36) is the treatment option for conditions such as colon cancer (Fig. 58-37) and acute conditions such as perforated diverticulitis (Fig. 58-38), toxic megacolon, severe colitis (Fig. 58-39), severe colonic obstruction, or refractory lower gastrointestinal bleeding. The colon can also be resected partially or completely and used for anastomosis in cases of complete esophagectomy and colonic interposition (Fig. 58-40). In cases in which the entire colon needs to be removed, a total colectomy is performed. A total

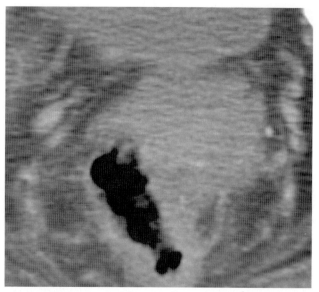

■ **FIGURE 58-37** Axial MDCT image demonstrates focal asymmetric thickening of the distal sigmoid colon in a patient diagnosed with adenocarcinoma of the colon.

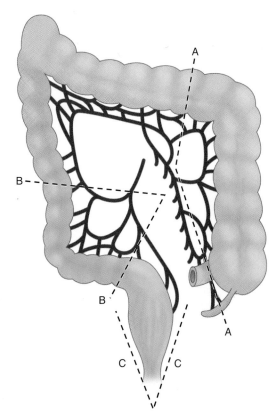

■ **FIGURE 58-36** Operative procedures for right-sided colon cancer, sigmoid diverticulitis, and low-lying rectal cancer. Right hemicolectomy involves resection of the terminal ileum and colon up to the division of the middle colic vessels (A). Sigmoidectomy consists of removing colon between the partially retroperitoneal descending colon and the rectum (B). Abdominoperineal resection of the rectum is a combined approach through the abdomen and perineum with resection of the entire rectum (C). (*Redrawn from Townsend CM. Sabiston Textbook of Surgery, 17th ed. Philadelphia, Elsevier Saunders, 2004, p 1459.*)

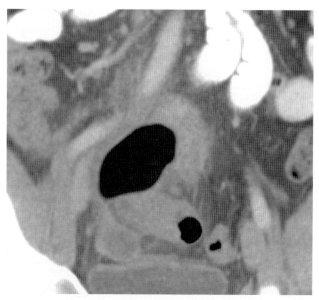

■ **FIGURE 58-38** Coronal MDCT image shows a fluid collection with an air-fluid level and adjacent fat stranding in a patient diagnosed with perforated diverticulitis.

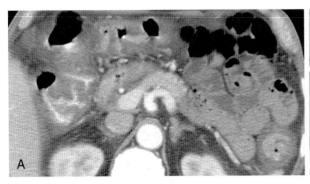
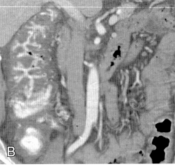

■ **FIGURE 58-39** Axial (**A**) and coronal (**B**) MDCT images demonstrate diffuse circumferential colon wall thickening consistent with pancolitis.

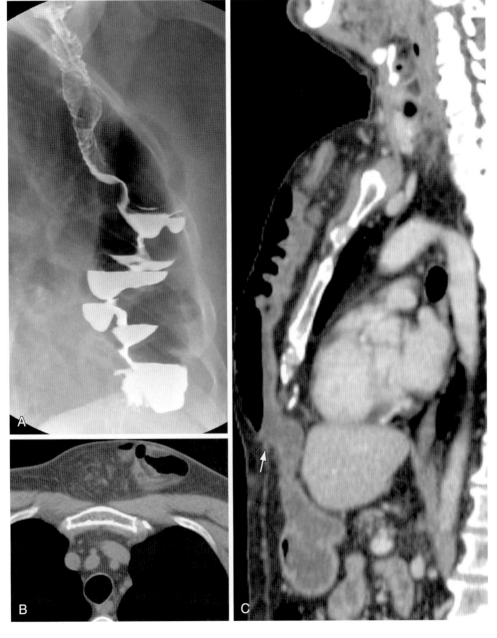

■ **FIGURE 58-40** Spot image from a barium swallow study (**A**) from a patient after total esophageal resection and colonic interposition. Note the haustrae typical of colonic tissue. Axial (**B**) and coronal (**C**) MDCT images on the same patient demonstrate the loop of colon located in the anterior chest wall with an anastomosis to the stomach (*arrow*).

proctocolectomy removes all of the colon, rectum, and anus; and a ileal pouch/anal anastomosis or end ileostomy with permanent ileal stoma can be performed. A colostomy is performed when part of the colon needs to be bypassed temporarily or permanently. If the distal rectum and anal sphincter are preserved, the colostomy can be reversed (colostomy takedown), whereas in cases in which rectum and anal sphincter have been removed, the colostomy is permanent.

Surgery involving the rectum is primarily for treatment of rectal carcinoma (Figs. 58-41 and 58-42). In the United States, approximately 8500 people die of rectal cancer each year.[17] Surgery is the primary therapy, with a 5-year survival after potential curative resection for stage I, II, and III disease of 80% to 90%, 50% to 60%, and 30% to 40%, respectively.[18,19] For rectal carcinoma, high-resolution MRI is applied as part of the initial evaluation because it provides excellent visualization of the tumor and can define tumor infiltration of the mesorectal fascia and perirectal lymph nodes.[20,21] PET and PET/CT may also be included as part of the evaluation for local invasion and distal metastasis. These findings are important for presurgical planning because they will determine which of the three major curative options for rectal cancer can be utilized: local excision, sphincter-preserving abdominal surgery (low anterior resection), or abdominal perineal resection.

Expected Appearance on Relevant Modalities

In addition to Billroth I or Billroth II cases, which involve the proximal small bowel and have a specific appearance, radiology of the postoperative small bowel is incredibly variable and depends on the section of the small bowel involved. In cases in which a routine postoperative evaluation is warranted, a small bowel series should be performed to delineate the postoperative anatomy and functionality of the anastomosis created (Fig. 58-43). If the surgery is recent and there is a concern of leak or breakdown of the anastomosis, water-soluble contrast media may be used in those cases to exclude this possibility. When reviewing postsurgical MDCT images of patients who have small bowel resection, searching for the sutures will point to the anastomosis (Fig. 58-44). Multiplanar MDCT reconstructions also assist in evaluation of the postoperative anatomy. As previously mentioned, the anastomotic site requires special attention because most complications or recurrent disease occur at this site.

Patients who had colon surgery will present with either partial or complete resection of the large bowel. In patients in whom a partial resection has been performed,

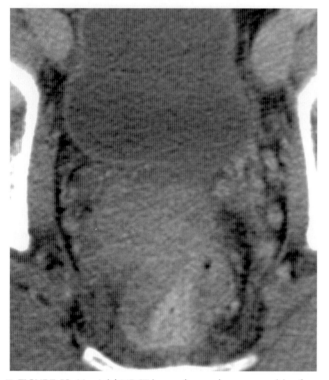

■ **FIGURE 58-41** Axial MDCT image shows a large mass arising from the rectum consistent with the patient's diagnosed rectal carcinoma.

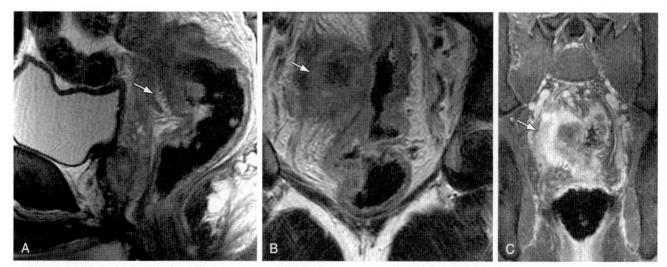

■ **FIGURE 58-42** Sagittal (**A**) and coronal (**B**) T2-weighted MR images of the pelvis from the same patient as in Figure 58-41 demonstrate a large rectal mass (*arrows*). **C,** Coronal post-gadolinium image shows avid enhancement within the rectal mass (*arrow*). Note the improved anatomic detail of the rectum and perirectal region, which is key in presurgical planning.

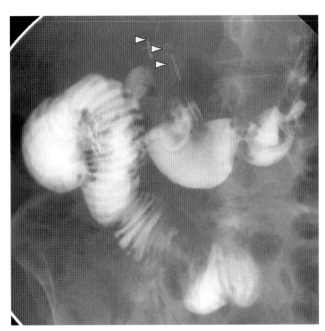

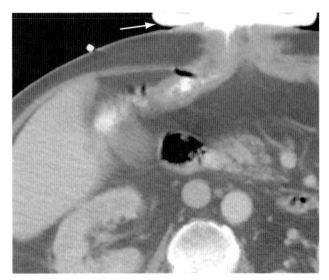

■ **FIGURE 58-45** Axial MDCT image from a patient after partial colon resection and colostomy shows part of the colonic lumen projecting outside the patient where the colostomy bag is located. Note oral contrast medium collecting in the bag (*arrow*).

■ **FIGURE 58-43** Spot image of a small bowel series shows surgical staples (*arrowheads*) in the right upper quadrant near the duodenal anastomosis in this patient who underwent partial resection of the duodenum.

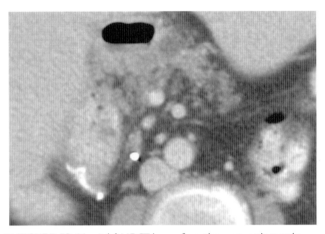

■ **FIGURE 58-44** Axial MDCT image from the same patient as in Figure 58-43. Note the linear high-density material in the duodenum representing the suture material used for anastomosis after partial resection of the duodenum.

a diverting colostomy may be a temporary or permanent solution. On MDCT images part of the colonic lumen can be identified outside the patient where the colostomy bag is located (Fig. 58-45). For those patients who have a temporary colostomy, referring physicians may require a preoperative evaluation of the colon before reversal or takedown of the colostomy. For this evaluation, fluoroscopy plays an important role. A barium enema (Fig. 58-46) is used for evaluation of the caliber of the colonic segment that has been excluded owing to the diverting colostomy. This is important to verify there is no extraluminal contrast agent and the caliber of the colon is adequate before reanastomosis at surgery. For evaluation of the colostomy site, a small catheter (e.g., Foley catheter) may be intro-

duced into the colostomy and contrast agent may be instilled. This allows for evaluation of possible extraluminal contrast filling and anatomy of the colostomy site and contiguous large bowel (Fig. 58-47).

Patients who undergo a total colectomy with sparing of the rectal sphincter may have a Hartmann closure or an ileal pouch/anal anastomosis (Fig. 58-48) as options to avoid a permanent stoma, thus allowing patients to have bowel movements per rectum. The ileal pouch/anal anastomosis is a procedure in which a distal ileal loop reservoir and a diverting ileostomy are created initially. Several months later an anastomosis between the ileostomy and the ileal loop is created. Radiology evaluation of these patients is central in patient care and may be performed with a barium enema using a No. 14-Fr Foley catheter. This may be secured in position by inflating the balloon, not to exceed the diameter of the pouch. Barium is instilled through the catheter in a retrograde fashion to evaluate the patency and anatomy of the pouch (Fig. 58-49) and the possibility of any leaks.[22] MDCT is used when there is a suspicion of acute symptoms related to surgery. The normal appearance of the ileal pouch/anal anastomosis on MDCT demonstrates two rows of sutures delineating where the pouch was created (Fig. 58-50).

Surgery of the rectum may be complicated because many cases involve rectal cancer or a fistula. These can complicate the postoperative course, and careful follow-up evaluation is recommended. For cases of rectal cancer, the primary goal of surgery is removal of the primary tumor along with the adjacent mesorectal tissue and regional lymph nodes. Reestablishment of bowel continuity at the time of surgery has become the rule rather than the exception in modern rectal cancer surgery. Nevertheless, it is a secondary objective and cancer removal should not be compromised in an attempt to avoid a temporary or permanent colostomy.[23] In the postoperative setting of patients with continued bowel after rectal surgery, the anastomosis site should be the focus of the evaluation

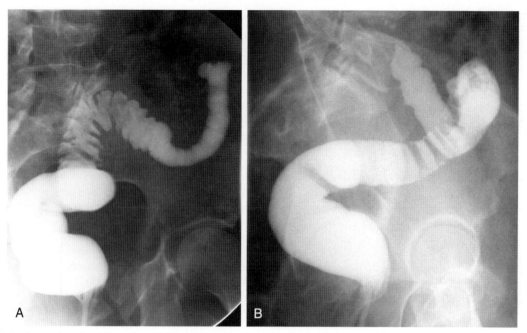

■ **FIGURE 58-46** Anteroposterior (**A**) and lateral (**B**) spot images of a barium enema from a patient after partial colonic resection and colostomy show that the excluded colon appears intact with no extraluminal contrast agent or severe stricture.

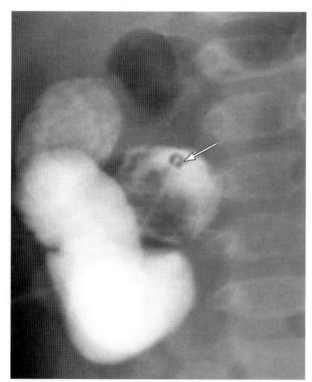

■ **FIGURE 58-47** Oblique spot image from a patient after a colostomy shows opacification of the colon without evidence of extraluminal contrast medium. Note the catheter (*arrow*) located within the colon that was used to instill the contrast agent into the ostomy.

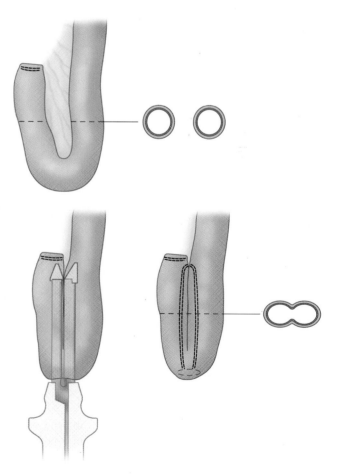

■ **FIGURE 58-48** Creation of an ileal J-pouch with a linear stapler. (*Redrawn from Townsend CM. Sabiston Textbook of Surgery, 17th ed. Philadelphia, Elsevier Saunders, 2004, p 1433.*)

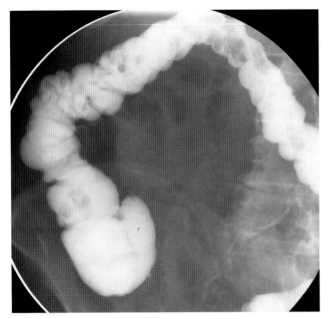

■ **FIGURE 58-49** Oblique spot fluoroscopy image demonstrates the typical appearance of an ileal pouch/anal anastomosis with an ileal loop reservoir and rectal anastomosis.

Potential Complications and Radiologic Appearance

With any surgical procedure involving the bowel and the creation of a new anastomosis, the most dreaded complication is breakdown of this site and leakage. Awareness of this possibility should always be increased, in particular for those postoperative patients presenting with acute symptoms.

In cases in which a surgical procedure involving the large bowel has been performed, complications may vary depending if the patient has a colostomy or reanastomosis of the colon to the rectum. Special care of the colostomy is important because there is a concern for infection or fistula. If a patient presents with acute symptoms after recent surgery, one must be aware of severe complications, for instance, a fluid collection or perforation (Fig. 58-51). When a Hartmann pouch or an ileal pouch/anal anastomosis has been created, other possible complications can arise that include (Table 58-5) portal vein thrombosis,[23] small bowel obstruction, pouch fistula, pouchitis (Fig. 58-52), anastomotic leakage, and pelvic abscess (Fig. 58-53), among others.[22]

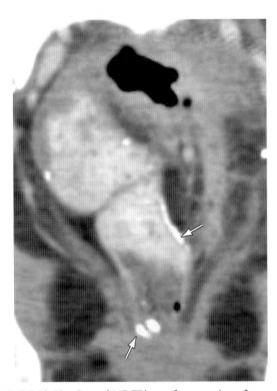

■ **FIGURE 58-50** Coronal MDCT image from a patient after total colectomy and ileal pouch/anal anastomosis demonstrates two rows of sutures delineating the ileal pouch (*arrows*).

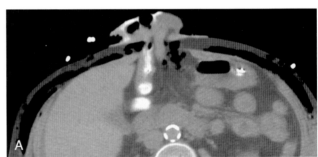

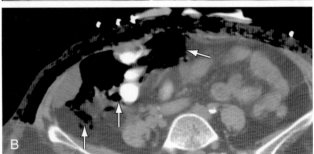

■ **FIGURE 58-51** **A,** Axial image at the level of the colostomy shows subcutaneous emphysema in the anterior abdominal wall. **B,** Axial image at a lower level demonstrates subcutaneous emphysema and free intraperitoneal air (*arrows*). During surgery it was discovered that this patient had a perforation of the colon adjacent to where the colostomy was created.

to assess for patency, recurrent disease, or other possible complications. Although MDCT plays an important role for evaluation in the postoperative setting, MRI and PET or PET/CT have become key in those patients who have been diagnosed with rectal cancer, owing to the increased sensitivity of these studies in discovering recurrent disease.

TABLE 58-5 Possible Complications after Ileal Pouch Creation

• Portal vein thrombosis	• Pelvic infection
• Pouch fistula	• Anastomosis leakage
• Stricture	• Pouchitis
• Pelvic abscess	• Anastomotic separation

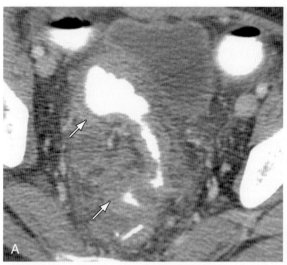
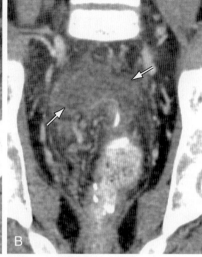

■ **FIGURE 58-52** Axial (**A**) and coronal (**B**) MDCT images from a patient after total colectomy and creation of an ileal pouch demonstrate bowel wall thickening (*arrows*) at the pouch in this patient diagnosed with pouchitis.

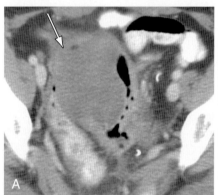
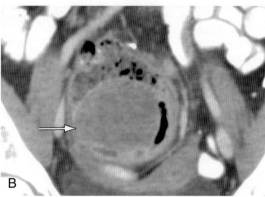

■ **FIGURE 58-53** Axial (**A**) and coronal (**B**) MDCT images from a patient after total colectomy and creation of an ileal pouch demonstrate a fluid collection (*arrows*) adjacent to the ileal pouch consistent with an abscess.

What the Referring Physician Needs to Know

ESOPHAGEAL RESECTION

■ Preoperatively and postoperatively, barium esophagography remains the imaging choice for esophagus.

■ For optimal preoperative planning, report the exact location of the lesion in the preoperative setting.

■ The most common site of complications is at the anastomosis site.

■ In cases of esophageal neoplasms, recurrence commonly occurs at the anastomosis.

ANTIREFLUX SURGERY

■ Antireflux surgery is an option for refractory cases.

■ Preoperative functionality and esophageal length are key in choosing a surgical technique.

■ Fundoplication patency and esophageal functionality should be evaluated in the postoperative setting.

■ If the fundoplication is longer than 3 cm, the patient may complain of dysphagia.

GASTRIC BYPASS

■ Perform an evaluation with water-soluble contrast within the first 24 hours.

■ An anastomotic leak is a life-threatening complication on the first day.

■ Most patients are obese, and image quality could be suboptimal.

■ Always look at the site of the anastomosis during evaluation.

■ If closed-loop obstruction or an internal hernia is suspected, CT is more helpful.

GASTRECTOMY, BILLROTH I AND II PROCEDURES, AND ESOPHAGOJEJUNOSTOMY

■ Be able to recognize the most common procedures.

■ If available, review the type of surgical procedure the patient had before imaging.

■ Be aware of the most frequent complications seen on imaging and provide proper recommendations to expedite patient management.

■ Multiplanar MDCT reconstructions are very useful for discerning the anatomy after surgery.

■ Acute afferent loop syndrome, duodenal stump leak, and intra-abdominal hemorrhage are emergencies, and prompt recognition is key for appropriate patient care.

SURGERY OF SMALL BOWEL, COLON, AND RECTUM

■ Fluoroscopy and MDCT are key in evaluating the postoperative small bowel.

■ MRI has taken an important role in the preoperative planning of rectal cancer.

■ Radiology plays a critical role in the routine postoperative evaluation of patients with ileal pouch/anal anastomosis.

KEY POINTS

Esophageal Resection

■ Barium esophagography is the study of choice.
■ Carefully examine the site of anastomosis.
■ If a leak is seen, obtain images at different angles to clearly document this finding.
■ In the postoperative setting, CT can be an alternative for initial evaluation of patients with acute symptoms.

Antireflux Surgery

■ Be aware of complications, because some of them may require urgent surgery.
■ If symptoms of dysphagia or recurrent reflux occur, look carefully for a tight or disrupted fundoplication.

Gastric Bypass

■ Imaging may be challenging in these patients due to body habitus, and radiology equipment needs to be adjusted to acquire adequate images.
■ CT and fluoroscopy are complementary evaluations for these patients.
■ Before evaluating each patient, review what type of bypass surgery was performed on the patient.

■ CT is the best study for patients whose condition is unstable.

Gastrectomy, Billroth I and II Procedures, and Esophagojejunostomy

■ Gastrectomy is a treatment option for esophageal cancer and intractable ulcers.
■ MDCT is essential in evaluating patients after gastrectomy who present with acute symptoms.
■ MRI and ultrasonography have a limited role in evaluation of the postoperative small bowel.
■ Communicate urgent findings of complications related to surgery to expedite patient care.

Surgery of Small Bowel, Colon, and Rectum

■ Fluoroscopy is useful for depicting anatomy and functionality of the postoperative bowel.
■ Suture lines seen on MDCT are useful for guidance to identify the anastomosis and for evaluation of this particular area.
■ MRI and PET/CT play a key role as part of the initial preoperative evaluation of rectal carcinoma and in follow-up studies for evaluation of recurrent disease.

SUGGESTED READINGS

Baker ME, Einstein DM, Herts BR, et al. Gastroesophageal reflux disease: integrating the barium esophagram before and after antireflux surgery. Radiology 2007; 243:329-339.

Beets-Tan RGH, Geerard L, Beets GL. Rectal cancer: review with emphasis on MR imaging. Radiology 2004; 232:335-346.

Canon CL, Morgan DE, Einstein DM, et al. Surgical approach to gastroesophageal reflux disease: what the radiologist needs to know. RadioGraphics 2005; 25:1485-1499.

Kim KW, Choi BI, Han JK, et al. Postoperative anatomic and pathologic findings at CT following gastrectomy. RadioGraphics 2002; 22: 323-336.

Kim SY, Lee KS, Shim YM, et al. Esophageal resection: indications, techniques, and radiologic assessment. RadioGraphics 2001; 21: 1119-1137.

Kim TJ, Lee HK, et al. Postoperative imaging of esophageal cancer: what chest radiologists need to know. RadioGraphics 2007; 27:409-429.

MERCURY Study Group. Extramural depth of tumor invasion at thin-section MR in patients with rectal cancer: results of the MERCURY study. Radiology 2007; 243:132-139.

REFERENCES

1. Kim SY, Lee KS, Shim YM, et al. Esophageal resection: indications, techniques, and radiologic assessment. RadioGraphics 2001; 21: 1119-1137.

2. Baba M, Aikou T, Natsugoe S, et al. Appraisal of ten-year survival following esophagectomy for carcinoma of the esophagus with emphasis on quality of life. World J Surg 1997; 21:282.

3. Orlando RC. Reflux esophagitis. In Yamada T (ed). Textbook of Gastroenterology. Philadephia, JB Lippincott, 1995, p 1214.

4. Kim TJ, Lee HK, et al. Postoperative imaging of esophageal cancer: what chest radiologists need to know. RadioGraphics 2007; 27: 409-429.

5. Canon CL, Morgan DE, Einstein DM, et al. Surgical approach to gastroesophageal reflux disease: what the radiologist needs to know. RadioGraphics 2005; 25:1485-1499.

6. Baker ME, Einstein DM, Herts BR, et al. Gastroesophageal reflux disease: integrating the barium esophagram before and after antireflux surgery. Radiology 2007; 243:329-339.

7. Karlsson J, Sjostrom L, Sullivan M. Swedish obese subjects (SOS)—an intervention study of obesity: two-year follow-up of health-related quality of life (HRQL) and eating behavior after gastric surgery for severe obesity. Int J Obes Relat Metab Disord 1998; 22:113.

8. Narbro K, Nagren G, Jonsson E, et al. Pharmaceutical costs in obese individuals: comparison with a randomly selected population sample and long-term changes after conventional and surgical treatment: the SOS intervention study. Arch Intern Med 2002; 162:2061.

9. Nguyen NT, Goldman C, Rosenquist CJ, et al. Laparoscopic versus open gastric bypass: a randomized study of outcomes, quality of life, and costs. Ann Surg 2001; 234:279-289.

10. Lujan JA, Frutos MD, Hernandez Q, et al. Laparoscopic versus open gastric bypass in the treatment of morbid obesity: a randomized prospective study. Ann Surg 2004; 239:433-437.

11. Fleser PS, Villalba M. Afferent limb volvulus and perforation of the bypassed stomach as a complication of Roux-en-Y gastric bypass. Obes Surg 2003; 13:453-456.

12. Scheirey CD, Scholz FJ, Shah PC, et al. Radiology of the laparoscopic Roux-en-Y gastric bypass procedure: conceptualization and precise interpretation of results. RadioGraphics 2006; 26:1355-1371.

13. Jemal A, Siegel R, Ward E, et al. Cancer statistics, 2007. CA Cancer J Clin 2007; 57:43.

14. Kim KW, Choi BI, Han JK, et al. Postoperative anatomic and pathologic findings at CT following gastrectomy. RadioGraphics 2002; 22:323-336.

15. Greenfield LJ. Complications of gastric surgery. In Greenfield LJ (ed). Complications in Surgery and Trauma. Philadelphia, JB Lippincott, 1990, pp 457-467.
16. Smith C, Dezie DJl, Kubicka RA. Evaluation of the postoperative stomach and duodenum. RadioGraphics 1994; 14:67-86.
17. Nour S, Beck J, Stringer MD. Colostomy complications in infants and children. Ann R Coll Surg Engl 1996; 78:526-530.
18. Jemal A, Murray T, Samuels A, et al. Cancer statistics, 2003. CA Cancer J Clin 2003; 53:5.
19. Willett CG, Lewandrowski K, Donnelly S, et al. Are there patients with stage I rectal carcinoma at risk for failure after abdominoperineal resection? Cancer 1992; 69:1651.
20. Beets-Tan RGH, Beets GL. Rectal cancer: review with emphasis on MR imaging. Radiology 2004; 232:335-346.
21. Vliegen RFA, Beets GL, Lammering G, et al. Mesorectal fascia invasion after neoadjuvant chemotherapy and radiation therapy for locally advanced rectal cancer: accuracy of MR imaging for prediction. Radiology 2008; 246:454-462.
22. Alfisher MM, Scholz FJ, Roberts PL, Counihan T. Radiology of ileal pouch-anal anastomosis: normal findings, examination pitfalls, and complications. RadioGraphics 1997; 17:81-98.
23. Stocchi L, Nelson H, Sargent D, et al. Impact of surgical and pathologic variables in rectal cancer: a United States community and cooperative group report. J Clin Oncol 2001; 19:3895.

PART

FIVE

Liver and Pancreas

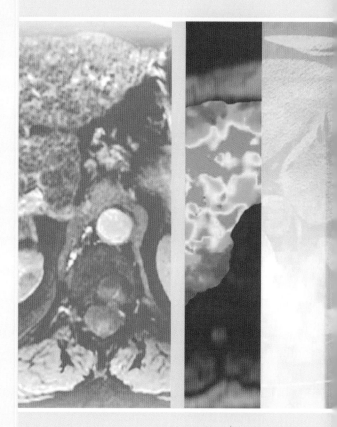

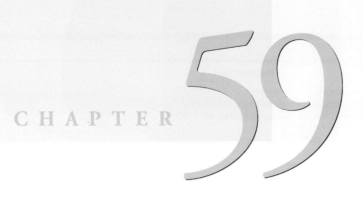
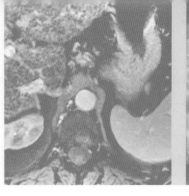
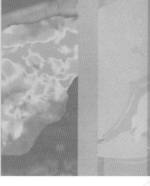

CHAPTER 59

Ultrasonography of the Liver

Rocio Perez Johnston, Anna Galluzzo, and Dushyant V. Sahani

TECHNICAL ASPECTS

Ultrasonography is a widely accessible, noninvasive imaging method that has many advantages over other imaging methods. It is portable, is relatively inexpensive, has high spatial and temporal resolution, does not involve ionizing radiation, and can be repeated frequently. Despite increased utilization of other imaging modalities such as CT and MRI, ultrasonography remains, in many settings, the first-line imaging techniques for the liver and bile ducts. There are multiple indications for liver ultrasonography that include screening for pathologic processes, diagnosis, and guidance for interventional procedures (Table 59-1).[1-3]

Technique

Patient Preparation and Positioning

Whenever possible, 4- to 6-hour fasting is desirable, not only to allow the gallbladder to distend but also to reduce the artifacts from bowel gas that interfere in the visualization of the left hepatic lobe. However, in the acute setting or in patients with unstable clinical status such as in admitted patients, preparation is not a prerequisite.

A curvilinear probe of 3 to 5 MHz is generally effective for optimal evaluation of the liver. However, in small adults or children when body penetration is not an issue, a linear probe of higher frequency such as 7.5 to 10 MHz is preferred.

Generally, a supine or right anterior supine position allows assessment of the entire liver. However, if excessive overlying bowel gas from the colon or stomach is present, changing the patient's position to the right anterior oblique or left anterior oblique might help to displace bowel gas.

In an effort to image the superior segments of the liver, scanning in full inspiration is preferred in cooperative patients. In patients who are unable to breath-hold or are uncooperative, other modified scanning approaches (see later) can help overcome these limitations.

Scanning Approach and Anatomic Overview

To adequately scan the parenchyma of the liver, and adequately localize a lesion, one needs to acknowledge the hepatic segmental nomenclature as well as the separating landmarks (Table 59-2).

The majority of the liver parenchyma lies above the costal margin. A subcostal approach with superior angulation allows a good overview of the parenchyma. Intercostal scanning can be helpful to visualize the subphrenic space.

The approaches generally used are those in the longitudinal and transverse planes (Tables 59-3 and 59-4, Figs. 59-1 and 59-2).

When the lower segments of the right lower lobe have not been adequately visualized on the previously mentioned scanning orientations, the patient can be placed slightly on the left, for a left anterior oblique approach. In this setting, the transverse colon and the duodenum are displaced to the midline of the abdomen, allowing better visualization of the right lobe. If the described scans still do not allow good visualization of the parenchyma and vascular structures, the patient can be placed in the left lateral decubitus position.

Advanced Techniques and Applications

Harmonic Imaging

Patients with certain types of body composition (e.g., obesity) can be difficult to scan, and acoustic noise such as grating lobes can be easily generated. Therefore, the image quality can be improved with harmonic imaging. This technique can also improve the image quality of cystic structures (simple cysts, gallbladder, and abscesses)

TABLE 59-1   General Indications for Liver Ultrasonography

Type of Examination	Indications
Screening ultrasonography	Metastases in patients with known primary neoplasm
	Hepatocellular carcinoma in patients with cirrhosis
	Diffuse liver disease in patients with family history and steatosis
	Complications in asymptomatic post-transplant patients
Diagnostic ultrasonography	*Parenchyma:* diffuse or focal lesions, diffuse liver disease
	Bile ducts: Chronic cholecystitis, cholangitis, sclerosing cholangitis, bile duct cysts
	Vascular: portal vein thrombosis, Budd-Chiari syndrome
Emergency ultrasonography for right upper quadrant pain	Acute cholecystitis, choledocholithiasis, infectious hepatitis, hepatic trauma, abscesses, hemorrhagic lesions, metastatic disease
Emergency ultrasonography for hepatic transplant	*Parenchyma:* infarct, abscess, preexisting donor disease, biloma, metastatic disease, and post-transplantation lymphoproliferative disorder
	Bile ducts: leaks, strictures, stones, sludge, recurrent disease (sclerosing cholangitis)
	Vascular:
	Hepatic artery: thrombosis, stenosis, and pseudoaneurysms
	Portal vein: thrombosis and stenosis
	Inferior vena cava: thrombosis
	Perihepatic complications: fluid collections, ascites
Guidance for interventional procedures	*Ultrasound-guided biopsy*
	Grading and staging chronic liver disease
	Hepatitis C and B, nonalcoholic fatty liver disease, alcoholic liver, autoimmune hepatitis, storage disease (iron overload, Wilson's disease)
	Evaluation of hepatomegaly
	Evaluation of liver mass
	Evaluation after liver transplantation
	Evaluation of fever of unknown cause
	Radiofrequency ablation: hepatocellular carcinoma, liver metastases
	Liver abscess drainage

TABLE 59-2   Anatomic Landmarks

Segments	Landmarks
Caudate and left lobe	Ligamentum venosum
Left lateral and medial	Ligamentum teres, left hepatic vein, umbilical segment of left portal vein
Left medial and right anterior	Interlobar fissure, middle hepatic vein, gallbladder
Right anterior and posterior	Right hepatic veins
Superior and inferior segments of right and left lobes	Portal vein and respective branches

as well as vascular structures as in the hepatic hilum (Fig. 59-3).

Doppler Imaging

Doppler ultrasonography is a noninvasive technique that provides information about the condition of blood vessels and the flow direction. It is commonly used to detect flow in focal lesions as well as to determine any vascular abnormality of the major hepatic vessels, especially in post-transplant patients. The main indications for Doppler imaging of the liver are listed in Table 59-5.

Contrast-Enhanced Ultrasonography

Contrast-enhanced ultrasonography is a dynamic technique that uses a microbubble contrast agent that acts as a blood pool tracer and enables tissue perfusion and vascular enhancement. The contrast agent facilitates real-time

TABLE 59-3   Longitudinal Planes of Scanning

	Sweep transducer in sagittal orientation along the costal margin starting at the midline toward the right lateral abdominal wall.
Left Hepatic Lobe	Longitudinal view with the probe positioned slightly to the left of midline: left lobe (LL), abdominal aorta (Ao), left hepatic and portal vein (see Fig. 59-1A)
	Longitudinal view with the probe positioned slightly right to midline: left lobe, inferior vena cava (IVC), left or middle hepatic vein (LHV and MHV), porta hepatis anterior to IVC (see Fig. 59-1B)
Caudate Lobe	Longitudinal view, with the probe located lateral of midline: caudate lobe (CL), left lobe (LL), ligamentum venosum (LV), right portal vein (see Fig. 59-1C)
Right Lobe	Longitudinal view, with the probe positioned in the right subcostal margin: medial and lateral segments of right lobe (RL), right portal vein (RPV), right kidney (RK), and hepatorenal recess (HRR) (see Fig. 59-1D, E)

assessment of tissue dynamics in various phases of contrast enhancement to facilitate lesion detection and characterization. Indications for this method are summarized in Table 59-6.[4,5]

When compared with B-mode ultrasonography, contrast-enhanced ultrasonography markedly improves sensitivity (75% vs. 95%) and specificity (60% vs. 75%) for differentiating between benign and malignant focal liver lesions.[6]

However, this technique is operator dependent and there is a limited field of view for deeply located or very small lesions. The body habitus of some patients represents a major obstacle to the utilization of contrast-enhanced ultrasonography.

Before injection of the contrast agent, baseline gray-scale and Doppler images are acquired. After identification of the target lesion, the transducer (2 to 5 MHz) is kept in a stable position while the imaging mode is changed to a low mechanical index, contrast-specific setting.[4] This low setting leads to effective tissue signal suppression but provides an adequate depth penetration for visualization of the lesion and identification of other anatomic landmarks, such as the diaphragm.

The intravenous contrast agent is administered as a bolus injection, followed by a 5- to 10-mL saline flush. Simultaneous display of B-mode and low mechanical index, contrast-specific ultrasound modes can be performed for real-time assessment. Constant scanning for 60 to 90 seconds is recommended to continuously assess dynamics of tissue perfusion in arterial, portovenous, and sinusoidal phases (Table 59-7). For assessment of a delayed phase, scanning may be used intermittently until the clearance of the microbubbles from the liver microvasculature has been observed. The real-time scanning should be documented on video or digital media.

NORMAL ANATOMY
Relevant Morphologic Features

As mentioned earlier, for assessing broad overview of the parenchyma each segment should be carefully evaluated in sagittal and transverse projections. The operator should assess for liver size, contours, echogenicity, and focal masses.

The normal liver size is difficult to determine on ultrasonography. It has been estimated that a longitudinal diameter of 16 cm at the midclavicular line can indicate hepatomegaly. However, consideration is important of certain anatomic variants such as Riedel's lobe, which can simulate hepatomegaly.[7]

TABLE 59-4 Transverse Planes of Scanning

	Place transducer under costal margin and angulate it in the cephalic direction as parallel to the diaphragm as possible. Sweep transducer from cephalic to caudal direction.
Hepatic Veins	Transverse view with the probe sharply angulated in cephalic direction: superior aspect of segments VII and VIII and IVC and three hepatic veins as they drain into the IVC; "playboy bunny" sign (see Fig. 59-2A)
Left Lobe, Caudate Lobe	Transverse view with the probe angulated in cephalic direction: left lobe and left portal vein, ligamentum venosum, caudate lobe (see Fig. 59-2B, C)
Right Lobe, Left and Caudate Lobes	Transverse view with slight angulation: porta hepatis (PH) and left and right portal veins can be identified. Caudate lobe is seen anterior to IVC; or, if probe is inferiorly angled, porta hepatis is seen anterior to IVC (see Fig. 59-2D, E)
Right Lobe	Transverse view with minimal angulation: right hepatic lobe, right portal vein with branches, and IVC (see Fig. 59-2F)
Right Lobe and Right Kidney	Transverse view, with probe slightly directed caudad: lower segments of the right lobe and right kidney located in the posterior border (see Fig. 59-2G)

IVC, inferior vena cava.

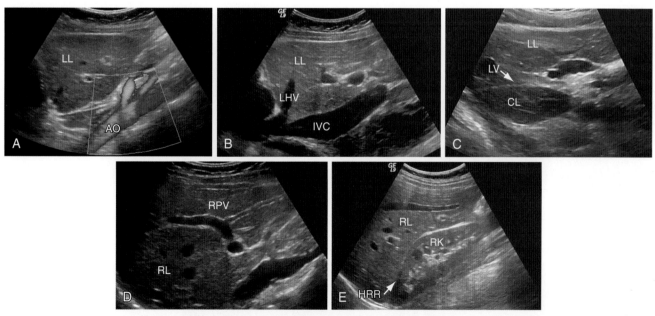

■ **FIGURE 59-1** A to E, Longitudinal planes of scanning and anatomic landmarks (see Table 59-3 for abbreviations and further description).

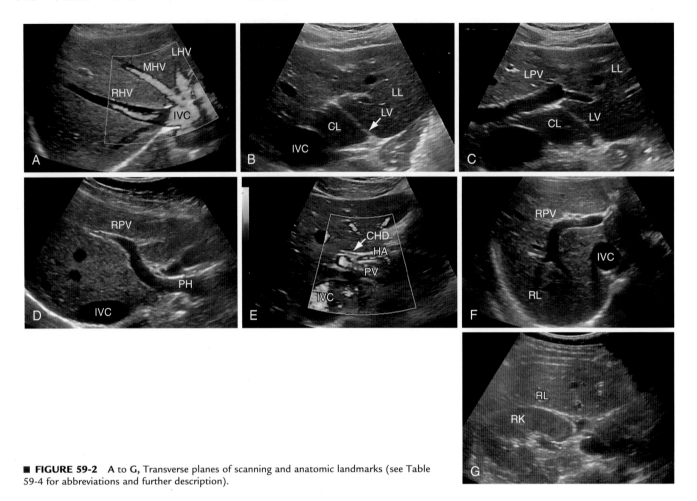

■ **FIGURE 59-2**   A to G, Transverse planes of scanning and anatomic landmarks (see Table 59-4 for abbreviations and further description).

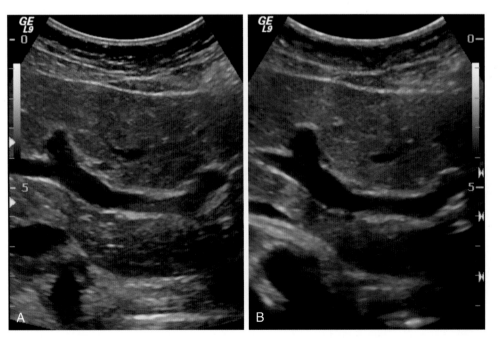

■ **FIGURE 59-3** Harmonic imaging. Subcostal view of the liver at the level of the bifurcation of the left and right portal veins. **A,** Gray-scale B-mode image is used to assess the vessels. **B,** The same image with harmonic settings allows a better visualization of the lumen and wall of the portal vessel.

TABLE 59-5 Major Indications for Doppler Ultrasonography in the Liver

Underlying Condition	Pathology
Cirrhotic liver	Portal vein thrombosis, portal hypertension, transjugular intrahepatic portosystemic shunt malfunction, portal vein aneurismal ectasia, and assessment of vascularity of single lesions
Noncirrhotic liver	Post-biopsy complications, portal vein thrombosis, hepatic trauma, and assessment of vascularity of single lesions
Transplant liver	Hepatic artery stenosis and pseudoaneurysm, portal vein thrombosis, hepatic veins and inferior vena cava thrombosis

TABLE 59-6 Recommended Uses and Indication of Contrast-Enhanced Ultrasonography

Diagnostic Imaging	Incidental findings on routine ultrasound
	Lesions or suspected lesion in chronic hepatitis or liver cirrhosis
	Lesions or suspected lesion in patient with known history of malignancy
	Characterization of portal vein thrombosis in malignant lesions
Interventional Application	Assessment of the vascularity of a target lesion
	Ablation needle/probe positioning into lesions not well delineated in B-mode ultrasonography
	Immediate assessment of therapeutic result to detect residual viable tumor areas
	Postablation follow-up to assess treatment response and tumor recurrence
Therapeutic Follow-up	Pretreatment staging and assessment of target lesion vascularity
	Depiction of margins of the lesion including relationship with adjacent and intralesional vessels
	Differentiation of necrosis from residual viable tumor after treatment

TABLE 59-7 Assessment of the Different Vascular Phases through Contrast-enhanced Ultrasonography

Phase	Post-injection Time (s) Start	Post-injection Time (s) End
Arterial	10-20	25-35
Portovenous	30-45	120
Sinusoidal	> 120	240-360 (bubbles disappear)

The normal echogenicity of the liver parenchyma is homogeneously mid-echogenic, slightly hypoechoic when compared with the spleen, and hyperechoic to isoechoic with respect to the renal cortex. When diffuse abnormal parenchymal echogenicity is encountered, diffuse pathologic processes are suggested.

The border of the liver should be smooth. If nodular or irregular borders are present, cirrhosis or diffuse

metastatic infiltration is suggested. It is important to look for small or focal outpouchings of the liver contour and to dismiss the presence of any focal isoechoic subcapsular lesion, such as focal nodular hyperplasia, some metastases, and small hepatocellular carcinomas. Therefore, to detect poorly conspicuous lesions, it is important to look for secondary signs, such as deformation of the liver contour, compression of vascular structures, and displacement of the bile ducts and gallbladder.

The portal vein, as well as both of its branches, the hepatic veins, and the hepatic artery should all be assessed for thrombosis with color Doppler imaging. Differentiating portal veins and hepatic veins can be difficult. The portal triad contains a branch of the portal vein, hepatic artery, and bile duct, contained within connective tissue, giving the portal veins a more echogenic wall, which hepatic veins do not have.[7,8]

Normal Hemodynamics

The liver receives a dual blood supply from the portal vein and the hepatic artery. The portal vein supplies around 75% of the blood flow, carrying partially oxygenated venous blood from the bowel and spleen. Its intrahepatic portion can be identified within the porta hepatis adjacent to the hepatic artery and common hepatic duct. It is relatively unaffected by the systemic pressure changes from the cardiac cycle, and therefore the portal flow has little or no pulsatility, presenting a monophasic pattern, with an approximate flow velocity of 15 to 20 cm/s. The flow within the portal vein should always be directed toward the liver (hepatopetal) (Fig. 59-4). With the usual intercostal or subcostal approach, blood flow in the main and left portal veins is directed toward the transducer, whereas the flow in the right portal veins moves away from it.[7,9]

Reversal of blood flow within the main portal vein or its branches, from the normal hepatopetal to hepatofugal direction away from the liver parenchyma, can be a sign of portal hypertension and is more often present in patients with advanced hepatic disease. The hepatic veins

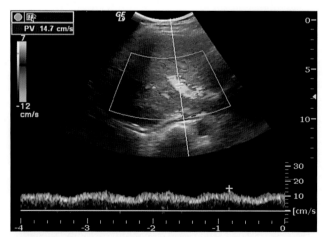

■ **FIGURE 59-4** Normal portal vein in a healthy 27-year-old woman. Color and duplex Doppler image demonstrates normal hepatopetal portal flow with venous monophasic waveform and minimal respiratory cycling.

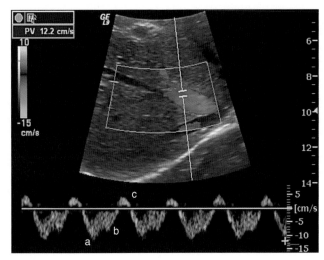

■ FIGURE 59-5   Normal middle hepatic vein in a 29-year-old woman. Color and duplex Doppler image demonstrates normal triphasic flow: a, atrial diastole; b, ventricular systole; c, atrial systole.

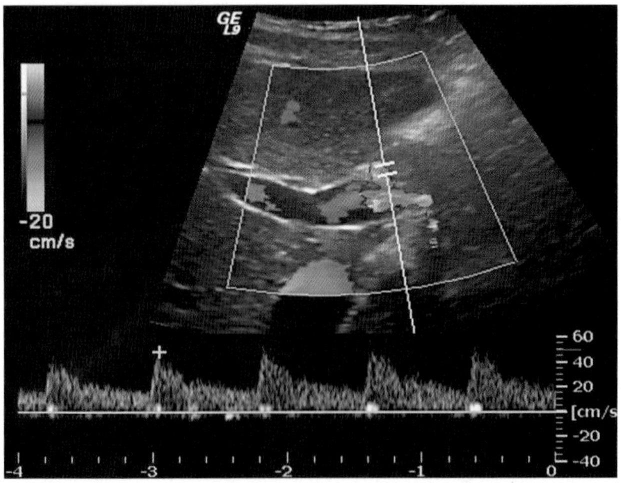

■ FIGURE 59-6   Normal hepatic artery in an asymptomatic 30-year-old woman. Color and duplex Doppler image of the porta hepatis shows a normal low-resistance arterial spectral pattern.

TABLE 59-8	**Morphologic Findings to Be Assessed in a Focal Lesion**
Location	For a solitary mass or a cluster of small masses, their location should be specified (segment).
Distribution	Disseminated or focal (periportal, perivenous, parahilar, or subcapsular)
Size	Useful for follow-up studies. Ideally all three dimensions should be reported (longitudinal, transverse, anteroposterior).
Shape	Round, oval, irregular
Margin	Well-defined margins: sharp or blurred; smooth or irregular
Center/Edge	Center may be hyperechoic, hypoechoic, or anechoic; edge can have hypoechoic or hyperechoic rim.
Flow	Present or absent; arterial or venous; distribution: diffuse, central, or peripheral
Surrounding tissue	Normal, hypoechoic, or hyperechoic secondary to edema or chronic inflammation

TABLE 59-9	**Examples of Focal Lesions According to Their Echogenicity**
Anechoic	Simple cysts, polycystic liver disease, biloma, abscess, hematoma, hydatid cyst, hepatic peliosis, lymphoma, metastasis, biliary cyst
Hypoechoic	Metastasis, lymphoma, abscess, hematoma, complicated cyst, adenoma, FNH, HCC, atypical hemangioma
Isoechoic	FNH, adenoma, HCC, metastasis, atypical hemangioma
Hyperechoic	Hemangioma, bile duct hamartoma, regenerative nodules, porphyria, HCC, FNH, metastasis, abscess, focal fatty changes
Irregular/Heterogeneous	HCC, metastasis, alveolar hydatid disease, Thorotrastosis
Calcified/Echodense	Granulomatous calcifications, periportal "comet tail," calculus, foreign body

HCC, hepatocellular carcinoma; FNH, focal nodular hyperplasia.

drain into the inferior vena cava near the right atrium, and the flow is dependent on the right-sided heart cycle. The flow pattern is triphasic, consisting of two anterograde waveforms corresponding to the atrial diastole and ventricular systole as well as one retrograde pulse secondary to the right-sided heart contraction of the atrial systole (Fig. 59-5). The main hepatic artery runs anterior to the main portal vein within the porta hepatis. It provides only 20% to 30% of the liver parenchyma circulation, but it is the main supplier to the biliary tree. The normal hepatic flow pattern is a low-resistance arterial waveform with continuous well-maintained anterograde diastolic flow (Fig. 59-6). The normal systolic velocity measures 30 to 40 cm/s with a diastolic velocity of 10 to 15 cm/s. The resistive index in the hepatic artery varies from 0.55 to 0.8.[10,11]

ASSESSING FOCAL LESIONS OF THE LIVER

To determine the presence or absence of focal masses, careful scanning of all segments in various planes should be performed. If a mass has been detected, several criteria have to be accounted for in their analysis (Tables 59-8 and 59-9).

Focal Liver Lesions

The typical enhancement patterns of the common benign and malignant liver lesions are summarized in Figures 59-7 to 59-11 and 59-12 to 59-14, respectively, in various phases of contrast enhancement (A = early arterial phase; B = arterial phase; C = portal venous phase; and D = sinusoidal phase; the white color depicts the contrast-enhanced areas).[6,12]

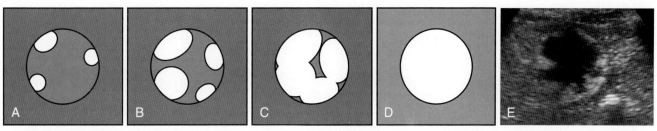

■ **FIGURE 59-7**   Cavernous hemangioma. A common pattern of a liver hemangioma is one of peripheral nodular enhancement on the arterial phase (**A** and **B**) with progressive, centripetal filling in the portovenous phase (**C**) and sinusoidal phase (**D**). **E,** Late arterial phase of contrast-enhanced ultrasound evaluation in an asymptomatic 50-year-old patient shows peripheral nodular enhancement of a hemangioma.

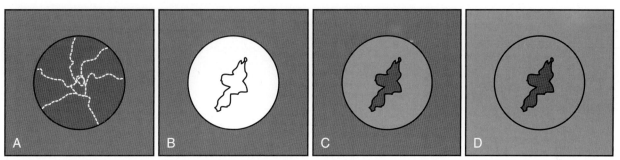

■ **FIGURE 59-8**   Focal nodular hyperplasia. **A,** The classic appearance is an early and centrifugal enhancement from the central feeding artery with spread to the periphery, giving a spokewheel pattern. **B,** On the late arterial phase, homogeneous enhancement persists. **C** and **D,** However, in the later phases, the lesion turns slightly hyperechoic or isoechoic to the parenchyma. The enhancement of central scar is generally not seen.

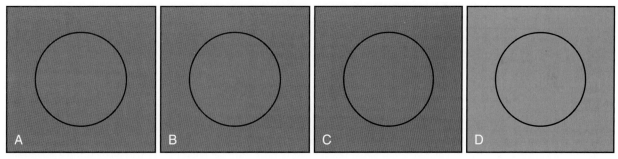

■ **FIGURE 59-9**   Focal fatty sparing. **A** to **D,** Demonstration of homogeneous enhancement similar to the liver parenchyma in all the phases of contrast enhancement.

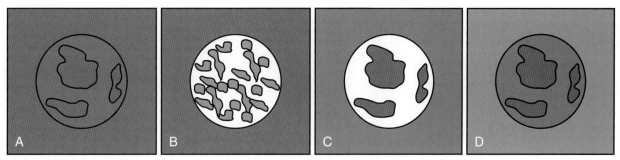

■ **FIGURE 59-10**   Adenoma. **A** and **B,** The common enhancement pattern shows a hypervascular lesion with centripetal enhancement on the arterial phases. **C** and **D,** In the portal venous and sinusoidal phases the lesion can be heterogeneous owing to the presence of fat, necrosis, or hemorrhagic areas.

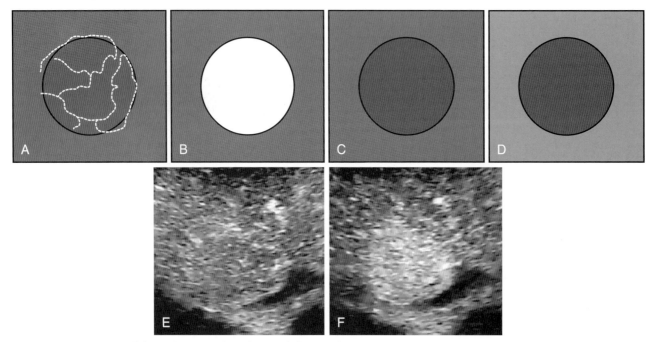

■ **FIGURE 59-11** Abscess. **A,** No enhancement is seen in the early arterial phase. **B,** Typically, peripheral rim enhancement in the late arterial phase surrounds an inner hypovascular area. **C and D,** There is a gradual wash-out of contrast medium from the rim in portal and sinusoidal phases. Central necrosis, a common feature of abscess, appears hypoechoic and shows lack of enhancement in all dynamic phases.

■ **FIGURE 59-12** Hepatocellular carcinoma. In the early arterial phase (**A**) heterogeneous enhancement is present; subsequently there is an intensive and homogeneous enhancement in the late arterial phase (**B**). Because of rapid wash-out in the portovenous phase (**C**), the lesion remains hypoechoic in the subsequent sinusoidal phase (**D**). **E and F,** Contrast-enhanced ultrasound images of a 63-year-old patient with cirrhosis being evaluated for a 4-cm suspicious solid lesion. Heterogeneous peripheral enhancement in the early arterial phase (**E**) and intense homogeneous enhancement in the late arterial phase (**F**) are observed, characteristic of hepatocellular carcinoma. Percutaneous biopsy confirmed the diagnosis.

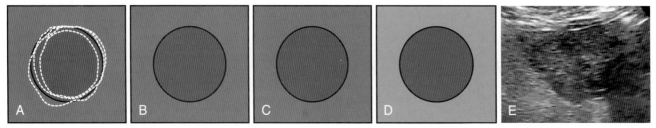

■ **FIGURE 59-13** Hypovascular metastasis. **A to D,** Note the peripheral enhancement in the arterial phase with wash-out of the contrast material and hypoechoic appearance in the remaining vascular phases. **E,** Contrast-enhanced ultrasound image of a 68-year-old patient with a history of colon cancer shows a predominantly hypoechoic lesion, with mild heterogeneous enhancement in the early arterial phase.

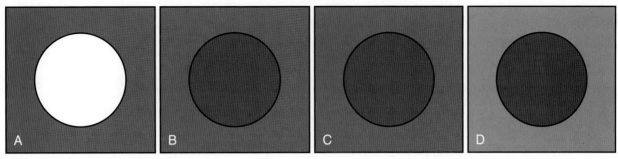

■ **FIGURE 59-14** Hypervascular metastasis. **A** to **D,** Typically, a homogeneous enhancement in the arterial phase with wash-out and classic hypoechoic pattern on the subsequent phases is evident.

TABLE 59-10 Etiology of Diffuse Liver Disease

Type of Disease	Possible Cause
Inflammation/fibrosis	Cirrhosis
Metabolic storage disorders	Steatosis, iron overload, Wilson's disease, amyloidosis, Gaucher's disease
Diffuse neoplastic disease	Metastatic disease, lymphoma, hepatocellular carcinoma
Diffuse vascular disease	Budd-Chiari syndrome, passive hepatic congestion
Granulomatous	
Noninfectious	Sarcoidosis, primary biliary cirrhosis, autoimmune cholangitis, idiopathic granulomatous hepatitis
Infectious	*Bacterial:* mycobacterial, brucellosis, listeriosis, melioidosis, tularemia, bartonellosis
	Viral: cytomegalovirus, Epstein-Barr virus, hepatitis C and B
	Fungal: histoplasmosis, coccidioidomycosis, blastomycosis, nocardiosis, candidiasis
	Parasitic: schistosomiasis, ascariasis
	Protozoal: visceral leishmaniasis, toxoplasmosis

TABLE 59-11 Possible Causes of Diffuse Liver Disease According to the Echogenicity of the Parenchyma

Predominantly Hypoechoic
Acute hepatitis
Acute liver congestions
Amyloidosis
Lymphoma

Predominantly Hyperechoic
Steatosis
Hemochromatosis
Fibrosis

Heterogeneous Texture
Cirrhosis
Diffuse tumor growth

echogenicity and reduced penetration of the sound beam with relatively decreased definitions of portal venues. In the second pattern, in which the parenchyma presents decreased echogenicity, there is accentuation of the portal venous structures. This is often seen in the setting of acute hepatitis, leukemia, and a few other diseases (Table 59-11). According to the findings, the severity of the disease can be categorized into mild, moderate, or severe.[14]

Diffuse Liver Disease

In many instances, imaging is used to determine the etiology of diffuse liver disease, which can be caused by diverse pathologic processes (Table 59-10). Ultrasonography, although nonspecific, generally is the first-line modality for assessment of the liver parenchyma, with a reported sensitivity ranging from 56% to 89% in detecting abnormalities.[13]

Two patterns of diffuse liver abnormalities have been reported. The most common pattern, the "bright liver," has been reported in fatty infiltration, chronic hepatitis, and cirrhosis. In this setting the liver exhibits increased

---

KEY POINTS

■ Ultrasonography of the liver is a sensitive imaging technique to evaluate the liver parenchyma and bile ducts.
■ Doppler imaging is useful to establish the presence or absence of a vascular pathologic process.
■ Contrast-enhanced ultrasonography is a promising technique and will aid in evaluating liver pathologic processes and liver vasculature.

SUGGESTED READINGS

Kono Y, Mattrey R. Ultrasound of the liver. Radiol Clin North Am 2005; 43:815-826.

Swart J, Sheth S. Role of vascular ultrasound in the evaluation of liver disease. Ultrasound Clin 2007; 2:355-375.

REFERENCES

1. Chong W, Shah M. Sonography of right upper quadrant pain. Ultrasound Clin 2008; 3:121-138.
2. Chalasani N, Horlander J, Said A, et al. Screening for hepatocellular carcinoma in patients with advanced cirrhosis. Am J Gastroenterol 1999; 94:2988-2993.
3. Douglas B, Charboneau W, Reading C. Ultrasound-guided intervention. Radiol Clin North Am 2001; 39:415-428.
4. Claudon M, Cosgrove D, Albrecht T, et al. Guidelines and good clinical practice recommendations for contrast enhanced ultrasound (CEUS)—update 2008. Ultraschall Med 2008; 29:28-44.
5. Hohmann J, Albrecht T, Hoffmann CW, et al. Ultrasonographic detection of focal liver lesions: increased sensitivity and specificity with microbubble contrast agents. Eur J Radiol 2003; 46:147-159.
6. Bartolotta TV, Midir M, Quaia E, et al. Benign focal liver lesions: spectrum of findings on SonoVue-enhanced pulse-inversion ultrasonography. Eur Radiol 2005; 15:1643-1649.
7. Rumack CM, Wilson SR, Charboneau JW. Diagnostic Ultrasound, 3rd ed. St. Louis, Elsevier Mosby, 2005.
8. Schmidt G. Differential Diagnosis in Ultrasound Imaging: A Teaching Atlas. Stuttgart, Georg Thieme, 2005.
9. Swart J, Sheth S. Role of vascular ultrasound in the evaluation of liver disease. Ultrasound Clin 2007; 2:355-375.
10. Ackermand S, Irshad A. The role of sonography in the liver transplantation. Ultrasound Clin 2007; 2:377-390.
11. McNamara M, Lockhart M, Robbin M. Emergency Doppler evaluation of the liver and kidneys. Radiol Clin North Am 2004; 42: 397-415.
12. Konopke R, Bunk A, Kersting S. The role of contrast-enhanced ultrasound for focal liver lesion detection: an overview. Ultrasound Med Biol 2007; 33:1515-1526.
13. Needleman L, Kurtz A, Rifkin M, et al. Sonography of diffuse benign liver disease: accuracy of patterns recognition and grading. AJR Am J Roentgenol 1985; 146:1011-1015.
14. Mergo P, Ros P, Buetow P, Buck J. Diffuse disease of the liver: radiologic-pathologic correlation. RadioGraphics 1994; 14: 1291-1307.

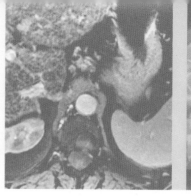
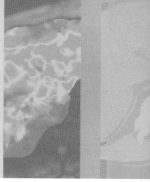

CHAPTER 60

CT of the Liver

Anand Singh, Gordon J. Harris, Hiroyuki Yoshida, and Dushyant V. Sahani

TECHNICAL ASPECTS

The advent of multidetector computed tomography (MDCT) scanners has led to alteration and improvement of various CT applications and protocols. The scanners are now capable of producing images as thin as 0.625 mm of isotropic voxel resolution, which improves the detection of liver lesion conspicuity and, more importantly, the detection and characterization of small malignant tumors with better characterization of the benign pathologic processes and the details of vascular flow.[1,2]

Because of reduction in the hepatic arterial phase acquisition time and thin collimation provided from MDCT, image postprocessing and CT angiography are much better, with a significant reduction in volume averaging artifacts.[3,4]

The enhancement pattern of the arterial phase is dependent on various factors, such as the iodine administration rate, which is further dependent on the flow rate or the concentration of the contrast agent administered. For arterial phase imaging, it is crucial to ensure that the injection duration is longer than the scan duration to obtain good vascular enhancement due to contrast recirculation. However, parenchymal enhancement is independent of the injection flow rate and depends on the total volume (dose) of contrast agent administered, which should be 120 to 150 mL of 300 mgI/mL to obtain an optimal liver parenchymal enhancement. However, with higher-concentration contrast media this volume can be lowered to 80 to 120 mL (370 mgI/mL). For example, for vascular mapping of the liver (CT angiography), the arterial phase imaging is of paramount importance and administration of a smaller volume of high-concentration contrast media at a higher rate proves more efficient. Contrast media then enter the extracellular space by diffusion, which reduces the conspicuity and contrast of the liver lesion, causing its relative obscuration, which is called the equilibrium phase. Ensuring scan completion before the setting in of the equilibrium phase is therefore important.

Dual-Phase Imaging

Normally, 75% of liver blood supply comes from the portal venous system and the remaining 25% comes from the hepatic arterial system.[5] When the iodinated contrast media is injected rapidly (3 to 5 mL/s), the hepatic arterial system is usually the first to opacify, that is, 20 to 30 seconds followed by the portal venous system (50 to 60 seconds); and lastly the hepatic venous opacification occurs at 65 to 75 seconds. Depending on the scan delay used to acquire the hepatic arterial phase, the images can either show mere opacification of hepatic arterial anatomy without parenchymal enhancement (early arterial phase) or with parenchymal enhancement (late [dominant] arterial phase). This is a vital consideration in tailoring MDCT protocols because hypervascular lesions are best visualized in the dominant arterial phase. In other words, better hepatic parenchymal contrast in the hepatic arterial phase is produced as a consequence of better enhancement of only the hypervascular lesions in relation to the rest of the hepatic parenchyma (Fig. 60-1). On the other hand, hypovascular lesions are more evident on the portal venous phase, and usually appear hypodense compared with the contrast enhancement of background liver parenchyma.[6] Hence the dual-phase CT of the liver is performed in the late hepatic arterial phases and the portal venous phases. The use of triple-phase scanning (early and late hepatic arterial and portal venous phase acquisitions) has been discouraged because there is no significant identified benefit to obtaining early arterial phase scans. Moreover, there is the disadvantage of increased radiation dose to the patient (Fig. 60-2).[7]

Role of High-Concentrated Iodinated Contrast Media

With old scanners (conventional, helical, and dynamic), liver CTs were usually performed during the pre-equilibrium phase because of factors such as decreased scan

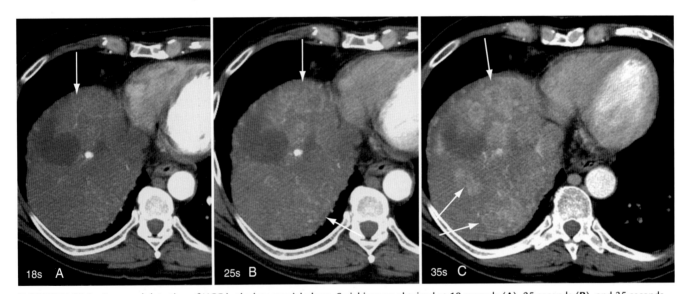

■ **FIGURE 60-1** Hepatocellular carcinoma. Coronal reformatted CT images of the liver showing intensely enhancing HCC (*arrow*) in the arterial phase (**A**). Note better lesion to parenchymal contrast in this phase in comparison to portal venous phase image (**B**) where the lesion is not appreciated (*arrow*). *(From Sahani DV, Singh AH. Dual-phase liver MDCT. In Mannudeep K, Saini S, Rubin G (eds). MDCT from Protocols to Practice. Berlin, Springer-Verlag, 2006, pp 83-92. Reprinted with permission.)*

■ **FIGURE 60-2** Improved detection of HCC in the late arterial phase. Serial images obtained at 18 seconds (**A**), 25 seconds (**B**), and 35 seconds (**C**) after initiation of contrast injection. Although arterially enhancing lesions are seen on images **A** and **B**, better enhancement and more lesions (*arrows*) are evident on the late arterial phase image (**C**). *(From Sahani DV, Singh AH. Dual-phase liver MDCT. In Mannudeep K, Saini S, Rubin G (eds). MDCT from Protocols to Practice. Berlin, Springer-Verlag, 2006, pp 83-92. Reprinted with permission.)*

speed and lengthened time of contrast delivery. MDCT has provided definitive advantages, including reduction in scanning time, which can be further complemented by increasing the injection speed.

In patients with decreased cardiac output, obesity, cirrhosis of the liver, or portal vein thrombosis in whom there is decreased liver perfusion, the role of high-concentration iodinated contrast media is important. The maximum hepatic enhancement in obese patients is significantly lower than in normal individuals, and this can be attributed to the decreased liver perfusion in obese patients, whereas in cirrhosis it is the decreased portal perfusion that delays and reduces the peak contrast enhancement, with the plateau occurring late in the portal phase.[8,9] This can increase the odds of missing a hypovas-cular metastatic lesion during the late phase if a standard concentration of iodinated contrast media is used.

The use of high-concentration iodine improves visualization of the characteristic heterogeneous enhancement pattern of liver seen in cirrhotic patients. In addition, the lesion to liver contrast can be improved when high iodine concentration contrast media are used, which also results in higher mean attenuation of liver substance in the portal venous phase (Fig. 60-3).[10,11]

Other Technical Factors

In addition to the previously mentioned factors, various other technical and physiologic factors affect the MDCT contrast enhancement for the liver.[12,13]

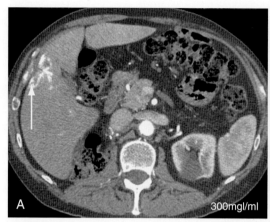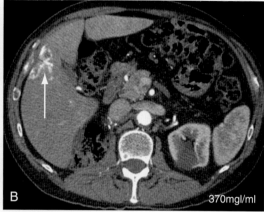

■ **FIGURE 60-3** Comparison of low- and high-concentration contrast for characterization of a hemangioma (*arrows*). Arterial phase axial CT images of the liver performed with 300 mgI/mL (**A**) and 370 mgI/mL (**B**) concentration contrast media in a patient with a liver lesion. There is slightly improved enhancement of the aorta and the liver hemangioma on the image in **B** obtained with the use of higher-concentration contrast media. (*From Sahani DV, Singh AH. Dual-phase liver MDCT. In Mannudeep K, Saini S, Rubin G (eds). MDCT from Protocols to Practice. Berlin, Springer-Verlag, 2006, pp 83-92. Reprinted with permission.*)

Scan Delay and Contrast Delivery

If the contrast volume is kept constant and the rate is increased, then the delay for peak aortic enhancement decreases.[12] However, optimal enhancement in larger patients can be achieved by increasing the injection rate. Thus the time required for each of the phase acquisitions varies from patient to patient depending on the medical condition, body size, and various other physical factors.

Because the fixed time delays do not take into account the patient-to-patient variability in cardiac output or the contrast circulating time, almost all recent scanners are now equipped with automated scanning trigger software. A region of interest is selected usually in the aorta above the celiac origin, the threshold enhancement of which serves as an indicator of scan commencement after injection of the contrast agent. The scans can be initiated either manually or automatically. Alternatively, a test bolus of 10 to 15 mL/4 s of contrast is injected and serial cuts are obtained through the upper aorta to judge the maximal opacification and determine the appropriate scan delay time. A test bolus is accurate but does entail additional contrast and time for scan.

However, for venous phase imaging, delays of 65 to 70 seconds, 60 seconds, and lesser time from start of injection are usually planned in 4-slice, 16-slice, and 64-slice scanners, respectively, and are usually dependent on the performance of the automated triggering system or test bolus method.

Contrast Volume

For liver imaging due to concerns about the image quality, 120 to 150 mL of contrast media of 300 mgI or 100 to 120 mL of 370 mgI is recommended.[14] Patients with cirrhosis particularly require a higher volume of contrast agent to achieve optimal parenchymal enhancement owing to decreased liver perfusion, but authorities have discouraged the use of any iodinated contrast above 150 mL.

The injection rate is a crucial factor while considering the amount of contrast volume that needs to be injected. Although an injection rate of 3 to 4 mL/s may be used for injection of 300 mgcI/mL, it is advisable to increase the injection rate 4 to 5 mL/s to ensure optimal opacification and contrast volume in desired structures. Increasing the injection rate of less volume of high concentration of iodinated contrast media, in other words, compensates for the volume compromise. Thus, with use of higher or lower iodine concentration contrast media, appropriate adjustments in injection rate and contrast volume are needed.

Pitch and Scan Collimation

It has been proven that the use of 2.5-mm collimation markedly improves the detection of liver lesions compared with the imaging by scanners with higher collimation such as 10 mm, 7.5 mm, and 5 mm.[3] For hepatic parenchymal imaging, 2.5-mm collimation is typically selected with 4-slice MDCT, but with increasing detector rows in the CT scanners, such as 16- and 64-slice CT, collimations as thin as 1.25 mm and 0.625 mm can be obtained, with a resultant increase in radiation dose to the patient. In light of such adversity, 2.5-mm collimation is usually adequate to provide optimal images of liver lesions except in cases of CT angiography protocols in which collimation of as low as 0.625 is chosen to ensure good postprocessing quality of the 3D images (Fig. 60-4). Table speed is the most important determinant of the pitch that is used for the scan. Higher scan speed results in higher pitch and better image quality. Because the newer MDCT scanners are now equipped to provide thin axial slices owing to their respective detector configuration and presence of more data elements, they also reduce the noise in the images. A pitch above 1.00 ensures optimal image quality of axial slices and the reconstructions.

CT protocols for some common liver indications are given in Table 60-1.

Technical Aspects for Image Postprocessing

The advent and advances in MDCT technology have immensely helped in exploring dimensions of image

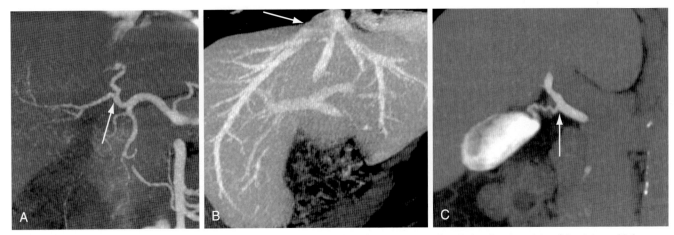

■ FIGURE 60-4 Thick volume MIP-CT images from a 34-year-old female liver donor. **A,** Coronal MIP showing the origin of the right and left hepatic arteries from the proper hepatic artery (*arrow*). **B,** Coronal MIP showing hepatic venous confluence (*arrow*) on venous phase acquisition. **C,** Thick coronal MIP reformatted image of a CT cholangiogram showing the site of insertion of the cystic duct into the bile duct (*arrow*). (*B from Sahani DV, Singh AH. Dual-phase liver MDCT. In Mannudeep K, Saini S, Rubin G (eds). MDCT from Protocols to Practice. Berlin, Springer, 2006, pp 83-92. Reprinted with permission.*)

TABLE 60-1 MDCT Protocols for the Liver

Parameters	4-Channel	16-Channel	64-Channel
Detector collimation (mm)	1.25	1.25	0.625
Table speed (mm/s)	15	13.75	55
Pitch		1.0-1.5	
Slice arterial (mm) (CTA)	1.25	1.0	1.0
Slice arterial (mm) (liver)	2.5-5.0	2.5	2.5
Slice venous (mm) (CTA)	2.5	2.0	2.0
Slice venous (mm) (liver)	5.0	5.0	5.0
Delay arterial bolus tracking/automated trigger (s)		Empirical delay: 25-30 s	
Delay venous (s)	65-70 s	60 s	50-60 s
120-150 mL of 300 mgI/mL nonionic contrast at 4 mL/s or 80-100 mL of 370 mgI/mL at 5 mL/s			

postprocessing. It is now possible to get raw axial datasets that are conducive for postprocessing. Higher scan speed of newer MDCT scanners can provide artifact-free images of isotropic voxel resolution. However, the fact of most concern is balancing the dataset requirements for postprocessing with appropriate parameters of CT protocols such that the radiation dose to the patient is kept under control. The dual-phase acquisition, as low as 0.625 mm for arterial phase on a 64-slice MDCT scanner, is justified for CT angiography of the liver, but it is advisable to increase the thickness of scan acquisitions wherever possible. Plain scan acquisitions can be avoided in cases of CT angiography for preoperative evaluation of liver donors but become essential to acquire in cases of preoperative planning of patients with liver tumors, in which case arterial phase acquisitions can be attained at thicker scan collimation such as 2.5 mm (Fig. 60-5). The thinner the axial sections, the better the image quality; a scan thickness of 2.5 mm is just about appropriate for ensuring optimal 3D postprocessing, even for advanced applications such as liver and tumor volume estimations and performance of computer-assisted techniques (Fig. 60-6). A reduction in scan length wherever possible should be employed and appropriate calibration of kilovoltage and milliampere setting should be chosen to reduce radiation dose delivery to the patient while simultaneously ensuring absence of image noise.

For patients during follow-up and those who need frequent CT scans with postprocessing for monitoring disease progression, axial sections as thick as 10 mm can be acquired for the delayed phase if vascular phase acquisitions have been kept thin to ensure good quality of postprocessed images.

Postprocessing Techniques for CT Angiography

The advances in MDCT scanners have propelled the benefits of image postprocessing and extended its applicability to the clinical scenario.[15,16] The most frequently employed postprocessing applications are common algorithms such as maximum intensity projection (MIP) and volume rendering (VR), which provide justification to the thin acquisitions if liver CT angiograms are performed for purposes of preoperative planning of tumor and donor surgeries and placement of intra-arterial chemotherapy pumps. Certain advanced applications such as volumetry and computer-assisted detection have recently gained importance owing to technical advances in liver and tumor segmentation techniques, which are complementing a busy work flow.

Preoperative knowledge of the arterial variants can avoid complications such as inadvertent ligation or injury of various hepatic arteries, hepatic ischemia, and hemor-

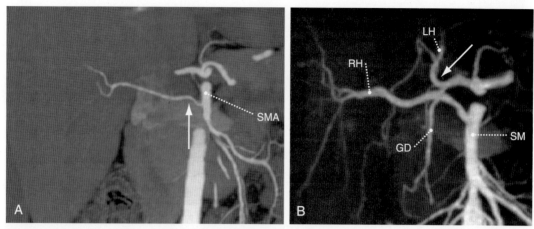

■ **FIGURE 60-5** MDCT-MIP images from a 43-year-old man showing hepatic arterial anatomy. **A,** Accessory origin of right hepatic artery (*arrow*) is seen from the superior mesenteric artery (SMA). **B,** A background-subtracted MIP highlighting the gastroduodenal (GD), the right hepatic (RH), the left hepatic (LH) origin from the proper hepatic (*arrow*), and the superior mesenteric (SM) arteries. (*A from Sahani DV, Singh AH. Dual-phase liver MDCT. In Mannudeep K, Saini S, Rubin G (eds). MDCT from Protocols to Practice. Berlin, Springer-Verlag, 2006, pp 83-92. Reprinted with permission.*)

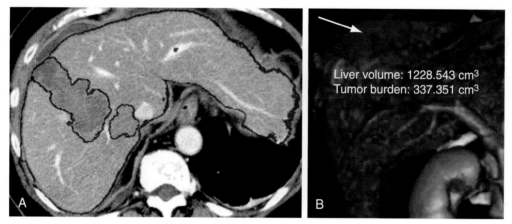

■ **FIGURE 60-6** Computer-assisted generation of liver and tumor volumes using MDCT dataset from a 42-year-old male patient with hepatocellular carcinoma. **A,** Segmentation of liver (*red*) and tumor (*blue*) by detection of their margins. **B,** Automated generation of liver and tumor volumes based on segmentation of structures. The area of tumor is displayed in red (*arrow*).

rhage and biliary leak. The variations in the celiac axis anatomy with respect to liver supply are common, and preoperative knowledge is especially important in obese patients who have large amounts of lymphatic and fatty tissue in the duodenal hepatic ligament and the porta hepatis.[17] The techniques usually used for CT angiography of liver are VR and MIP.[18] Optimal delay time, contrast concentration, and opacification are important. MIP is the most frequently employed postprocessing algorithm for liver because it provides an optimum contrast for highlighting the liver vascular anatomy and its variants, which is crucial for preoperative planning (Figs. 60-7 and 60-8). It is essential to visualize subtle vascular details in relation to the liver's segmental anatomy, such as the arterial branch to segment 4 of the liver, or if any variation exists to such details. Such considerations in the reports have to be emphasized because this helps surgeons to plan their resections accordingly. In addition, 3D vascular maps also help surgeons to increase their preoperative confidence with localization of such small-diameter vessels, which is essential for prevention of torrential bleeding complica-

tions. Volume rendering has an additive effect to the MIP images, but at times visualization of very thin diameter vessels may pose a problem. However, as a routine practice, it is advisable for the radiologists to view CT angiographic liver studies by reviewing axial datasets followed by MIPs acquired in axial and coronal planes and eventually the 3D vascular maps to counterconfirm their findings, while for clinicians 3D image maps of MIPs and VR are optimal for providing semblance to the intraoperative picture (Fig. 60-9).[19] Minimum intensity projections (MinIP) can be good for visualization of biliary ductal anatomy in case of dilatation but are usually not favored as a standard of practice in imaging because dilatation of the biliary ductal system is clearly evident on routine axial images.

The quality of the 3D images is largely dependent on the source images for reconstruction. As with other forms of visualization, such as multiplanar reconstruction (MPR), VR, and MIP, the source images should be of thin collimation and have a greater longitudinal coverage with about 50% overlap and a sufficient signal-to-noise ratio.

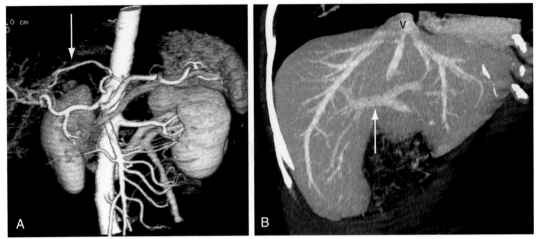

■ **FIGURE 60-7**   Preoperative planning for living related liver transplantation: color-coded volume-rendered CTA image (**A**) demonstrates an anomalous origin of the left hepatic artery from the left gastric artery (*arrow*). A venous phase, subvolume MIP image in the coronal oblique plane (**B**) demonstrates normal portal and hepatic venous anatomy (*arrow*). *(From Sahani DV, Singh AH. Dual-phase liver MDCT. In Mannudeep K, Saini S, Rubin G (eds). MDCT from Protocols to Practice. Berlin, Springer-Verlag, 2006, pp 83-92. Reprinted with permission.)*

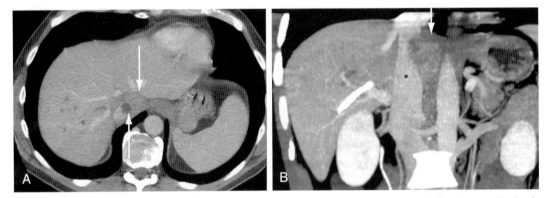

■ **FIGURE 60-8**   Preoperative planning of cholangiocarcinoma. **A,** Contrast-enhanced axial image shows an infiltrative mass in the dome of the liver with suspicion of inferior vena cava invasion (*arrow*) seen as a filling defect. **B,** However, the corresponding coronal subvolume MIP image confirmed only extrinsic compression and not invasion of the inferior vena cava (*asterisk*) by the tumor (*arrow*) and therefore surgery was feasible. *(From Sahani DV, Singh AH. Dual-phase liver MDCT. In Mannudeep K, Saini S, Rubin G (eds). MDCT from Protocols to Practice. Berlin, Springer-Verlag, 2006, pp 83-92. Reprinted with permission.)*

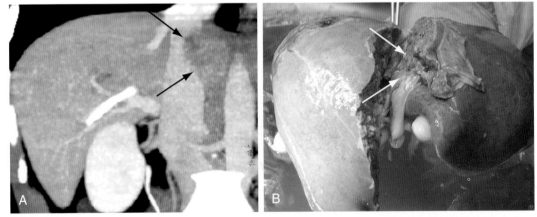

■ **FIGURE 60-9**   Images from a 49-year-old male patient with cholangiocarcinoma. **A,** Coronal MDCT reformatted image shows invasion of the intrahepatic inferior vena cava by the tumor (*arrows*). **B,** An intraoperative picture of partially resected liver tumor confirming the same finding (*arrows*).

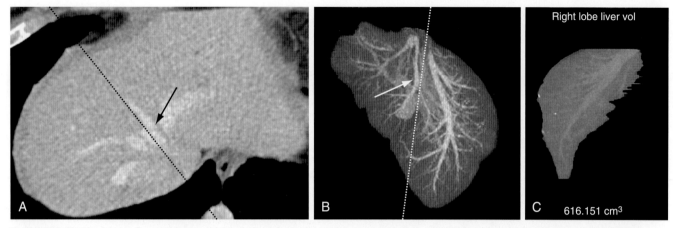

■ FIGURE 60-10 Images from a 38-year-old female liver donor illustrating the technique for generation of partial liver volumes. Axial MDCT image (**A**) and a coronal volume-rendered MDCT posterior reconstruction (**B**) show the manually computer-generated intervening plane that divides the liver into two parts and is parallel to the right side of the middle hepatic vein (*arrow*). This corresponds to the median fissure, which extends from the gallbladder fossa to the inferior vena cava (Cantlie's line). **C,** Subsequent generation of right lobe liver volume is shown.

TABLE 60-2 Recommended CT Postprocessing Applications for Some Common Liver CT Protocols

CT Protocols	Reformatted—*MIPs: Coronal + Axial	Volume MIP + †VR-Manually Created	Advanced Applications
Liver donor	+	+ (Hepatic vasculature)	Segmentation and volumetry (total and partial liver)
CTA of liver (other indications)	+	+ (Hepatic vasculature)	–
Tumor: pretreatment evaluation	+	+ (Hepatic vasculature)	Segmentation + tumor volume
Tumor treatment follow-up	+	–	Volumetry†
CT cholangiography	+	+ (biliary ductal details and gallbladder)	–

*CT acquisitions needed at 2.5-mm or less collimation.
†VR, volume rendered.

Advanced Postprocessing Applications

Most of the workstations are now equipped to provide advanced postprocessing application tools for segmentation, volume estimations, and virtual endoscopy. Segmentation of the liver on CT to estimate total liver volume, partial liver lobe volume, and tumor volumes is an advanced application, the automation of which is being actively investigated (Fig. 60-10).[20] Knowledge of total and partial liver volumes is important for planning liver transplants, whereas estimation of liver tumor volumes is a vital indicator for assessing response to chemotherapy and for planning for irradiation.[21] Considering the volume of CT cases of such patients, recent work is more focused on automating these advanced postprocessing applications by computer-aided techniques. Virtual CT cholangioscopy refers to navigation through the common bile duct for assessment of calculi and stenosis, but feasibility of this application for its merger with current work flow is still under investigation.[22]

Postprocessing applications for commonly requested MDCT protocols are given in Table 60-2.

Liver Tumors

The two most important factors that influence the detection of a lesion are the size of the lesion and its intrinsic vascularity. A minimum of a 10-HU difference between lesion and normal liver parenchyma is required for the lesion to be detected.

Most hypervascular tumors such as hepatocellular carcinomas and metastases from melanoma, breast cancer, carcinoid, thyroid medullary carcinomas, islet cell tumors, and renal cell carcinomas derive their blood supply from the hepatic artery and its branches and thus show increased enhancement on the hepatic arterial phase of the scan. Certain benign lesions also show increased vascularity in the hepatic arterial phase of the scan, such as focal nodular hyperplasia and hemangiomas. MDCT can detect the peripheral rim enhancement in the hypovascular lesions and subtle enhancement pattern of tiny hypodense liver lesions in the hepatic arterial phase (Fig. 60-11).[23] An important consideration while imaging liver tumors is to look for arterioportal shunting, which is frequently seen in certain malignant lesions owing to the development of hepatic artery to portal venous collaterals secondary to vessel compression by the tumor. Because of such capabilities of the MDCT scanners, to outline smaller and subtle lesions much earlier in the disease process, routine screening for hepatitis B patients is performed to detect early development of neoplasia in the liver where small tumors of less than 5-cm diameter can be detected, leading to early consideration of liver transplantation for such patients.

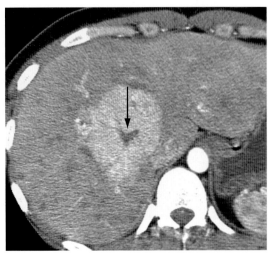

■ **FIGURE 60-11** Focal nodular hyperplasia. A dynamic late arterial phase axial image shows a well-defined, heterogeneously enhancing liver lesion with central scar (*arrow*) that appears as a hypoattenuating area. *(From Sahani DV, Singh AH. Dual-phase liver MDCT. In Mannudeep K, Saini S, Rubin G (eds). MDCT from Protocols to Practice. Berlin, Springer-Verlag, 2006, pp 83-92. Reprinted with permission.)*

Characterization of focal nodular hyperplasia (FNH) has also been improved by MDCT where features such as its intense enhancement pattern with a low-attenuation central area on the arterial phase and its rapid wash out on the venous phase are more clearly evident.[24,25]

The only factor that helps in differentiating a tiny benign lesion from a malignant one is the pattern of enhancement after administration of a contrast agent. For example, attenuation values in small hemangiomas are similar to those of the aorta on arterial phase images and of the hepatic veins on the venous phase, which is not the case with hypervascular malignant lesions, which may differ in their enhancement attenuation values when compared with the aorta and hepatic veins.

Liver Cirrhosis

It is important to detect the subtle changes in the liver parenchyma in terms of density and heterogeneity for a confident diagnosis of liver cirrhosis. This heterogeneous enhancement pattern in cirrhosis is mainly due to regenerative nodules, periportal fibrosis, and microcirculatory shunts between the portal venous and hepatic venous systems. With appropriate calibration of the automated bolus tracking technique on the newer-generation MDCT scanners, better accuracy in timing of the arterial phase and the venous phases can be achieved, which is important in cirrhotic patients who have decreased liver perfusion. More so, the use of high-concentration contrast further improves the visualization of the heterogeneity of the liver substance. Such technical upgrades also improve depiction of other features, such as collateral circulation and varices in the case of portal hypertension. MDCT images of better resolution have helped to highlight small lesions, which may represent a focus or foci of hepatocellular carcinoma that are interspersed within the substance of a cirrhotic liver, which are otherwise difficult to visualize.

Vascular Pathologic Processes

Any obstruction to the hepatic venous outflow is called the Budd-Chiari syndrome. Acute obstruction is usually caused by a blood clot that occurs in hypercoagulable states due to malignancies, genetic disorders such as protein C and antithrombin III deficiency, and physiologic alterations in blood clotting mechanisms during pregnancy. Chronic conditions may result owing to fibrotic changes in hepatic vasculature, which may occur in cirrhosis.[26] Any obstruction to hepatic outflow results in generalized liver enlargement as a compensatory mechanism, which is more markedly prominent in the caudate lobe component of the parenchymal substance due to a compensatory mechanism. A characteristic mottled enhancement pattern is observed on MDCT with a delay in peripheral contrast enhancement. Marked enlargement of the hepatic veins compared with the rest of the surrounding venous vasculature differentiates this condition from right-sided or congestive heart failure, which usually results in dilatation and generalized increase in venous blood volume.

Similarly, portal vein thrombosis can result from tumor invasion, external compression by tumors, or coagulation abnormalities (Fig. 60-12). The hallmark of portal vein thrombosis is the presence of a filling defect inside the vein due to the clot. This is usually well depicted if the scan is acquired at the peak of the venous enhancement. A long-standing thrombus in a portal vein can give rise to chronic conditions such as portal cavernoma, in which numerous collateral veins form around the thrombosed portal vein to compensate for compromised circulation.[27,28]

Dynamic CT perfusion is a relatively new technique for assessing neoangiogenesis in the liver and the response to therapy for liver tumors that estimates the blood flow, blood volume, mean transit time, and capillary permeability surface area of the tumor and the normal liver substance. A noncontrast CT scan of the liver is obtained to localize the tumor for further investigation by dynamic scanning. A region of interest is selected, and dynamic scanning of this area is performed 8 to 10 seconds after initiation of intravenous administration of a contrast medium injected at a rate of 6 to 9 mL/s. About four sections are obtained through the same region every 12 seconds for 4 to 5 minutes. The representative parameters are then averaged across all the sections and values compared with the average of normal liver parenchyma (Fig. 60-13).[29]

Imaging of the Biliary System

Visualization of common bile duct and gallbladder pathologic processes such as calculi can be easily seen on the regular axial images due to their hyperdensity. However, on CT the bile duct is very thin and of low attenuation, which makes its satisfactory visualization difficult. MR cholangiopancreatography images provide a much better contrast in visualization of biliary ductal details and are thus preferred. Diagnostic confidence in assessing biliary ductal details given its fluid hypodensity is always a problem on CT. However, the reliability of CT cholangiography has been recently confirmed for evaluation of the

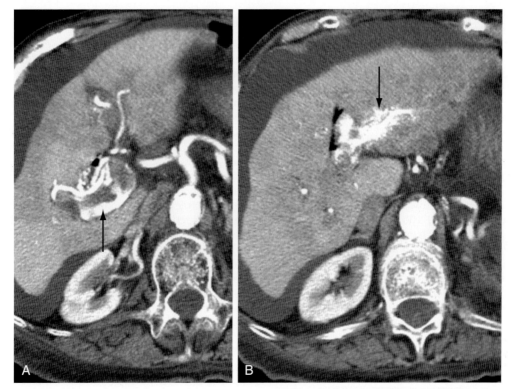

■ **FIGURE 60-12** Tumor invasion in the portal vein from HCC. Two arterial phase axial images of the liver are shown. **A,** Tumor thrombus is seen in the right portal vein (*arrow*). Also note the enhancement/contrast in the portal vein in the arterial phase. **B,** Intensely enhancing arterioportal shunts from the tumor (*arrow*) around the left portal vein. Also seen is evidence of liver cirrhosis and ascites. *(From Sahani DV, Singh AH. Dual-phase liver MDCT. In Mannudeep K, Saini S, Rubin G (eds). MDCT from Protocols to Practice. Berlin, Springer-Verlag, 2006, pp 83-92. Reprinted with permission.)*

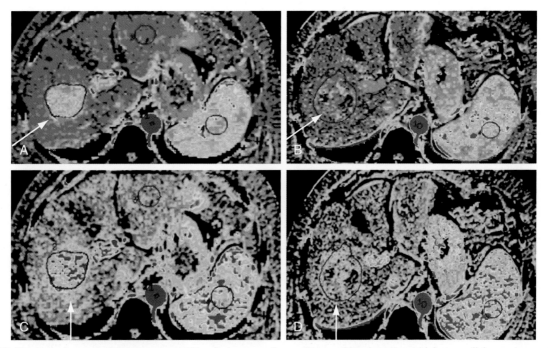

■ **FIGURE 60-13** Pretreatment and post-treatment CT perfusion maps from a 52-year-old male patient with hepatocellular carcinoma. Note the increased blood flow (*arrow,* **A**) and increased blood volume (*arrow,* **C**) in the pretreatment images compared with the post-treatment appearances (*arrows,* **B** and **D**).

intrahepatic biliary anatomy of patients who are candidates for liver surgery, who have nondilated biliary ducts and bilirubin levels no higher than 2 mg/dL.[30] Iodipamide meglumine injection 52% (Cholografin Meglumine) is a radiopaque contrast agent for rapid intravenous cholangiography. After intravenous administration, iodipamide is metabolized by the liver and rapidly secreted within 10 to 15 minutes, thus permitting visualization of the hepatic and common bile ducts (Table 60-3). The contrast outlines the gallbladder within an hour. It is important to premedicate the patient before injection to reduce the chances of adverse reactions, which are slightly more than that of the regular intravenous contrast medium that is presently used. For similar reasons, slow intravenous infusion of this agent mixed with 80 to 100 mL of normal saline is advised, which reduces the chances of adverse reactions. Scanning after a delay of 45 to 60 minutes from start of injection is usually enough for obtaining delineation of the biliary system. CT cholangiography has especially proved more beneficial for preoperative imaging of liver donors because it provides better resolution in delineation of subtle details, such as biliary drainage of segment 4 of the liver (Fig. 60-14).[31]

TABLE 60-3 Protocol for CT Cholangiography*

Parameters	16-Channel	64-Channel
Premedication	Prednisolone, 50 mg orally, given at 13 hr, 7 hr, and 1 hr before contrast injection. Last dose to be given along with diphenhydramine, 50 mg.	
Contrast injection	Slow IV drip: 20 mL of meglumine iodipamide mixed with 80 mL of normal saline and infused over 45 minutes	
Scan delay	45-60 min after start of contrast injection	
Extent	Dome of diaphragm to umbilicus	
Slice thickness	2.5	2.5
Table speed (mm/s)	13.75	55

*In cases of assessing liver donors, contrast injection is to be initiated after the CT angiography.

PROS AND CONS

MDCT ensures availability of thin-section datasets of isotropic voxel resolution, which has immensely improved the depiction of liver lesion conspicuity and its characterization. However, appropriate tailoring of MDCT liver protocols is crucial for ensuring optimal scan quality while keeping a check on the radiation dose.

Triple-phase imaging, namely, scan acquisition in early arterial, late arterial, and portal venous phases, has therefore become unpopular; and more realistic and dose-saving protocols with dual-phase imaging of the liver on MDCT have been followed. With advances in CT scanners, the role of high iodine concentration contrast media has also been highlighted in cirrhotic patients to achieve a higher mean attenuation in the liver substance. However, certain factors such as cardiac output, body weight, and pathologic conditions including cirrhosis and portal vein thrombosis can alter blood flow, which is an important consideration for planning scan acquisitions and assigning delay time for contrast injection. Certain software upgrades have enabled the advent of automated scanning trigger software that allows scan acquisitions only when a particular attenuation value is achieved in the aorta after injection of a contrast agent. Contrast volume and rate of injection are other important factors to be considered and altered while using media of different iodine concentrations.

Ensuring a pitch above 1.00 and scan collimation of less than 2.00 mm provides a dataset that is conducive for postprocessing and thus ensures a better display of vascular maps and variants in hepatic vasculature by simple postprocessing algorithms such as MIP and volume renderings. The role of MDCT and image resolution provided by thin scan acquisition has also propelled the importance of advanced postprocessing applications such as liver segmentation, segmentation of hepatic vasculature for preoperative planning, volume estimation of total and partial liver volumes, along with estimation of tumor burden. Such advances have opened doors for developments of computer-aided techniques, and automated tumor segmentation and volume estimation are becoming increasingly popular at certain centers and research platforms.

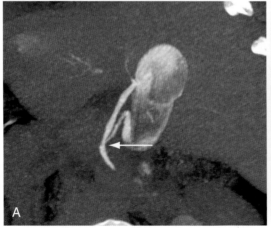 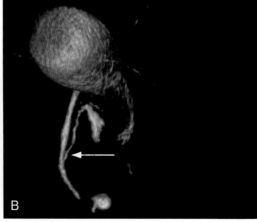

■ **FIGURE 60-14** CT cholangiogram MIP (**A**) and volume-rendered (**B**) images from a 36-year-old male liver donor with situs inversus totalis. Note the low insertion of the cystic duct into the bile duct (*arrows*).

MDCT has also improved detection of hidden liver lesions that appear to be masked by the heterogeneous appearance and enhancement patterns of liver cirrhosis. Thin-section datasets and optimal postprocessing also lead to better depiction of vascular pathologic processes such as Budd-Chiari syndrome and portal vein thrombosis. Scan quality, accuracy in contrast injection rate and, timing and

software upgrades at MDCT scanners and newer workstations provide diverse options for assessing perfusion in tumors and monitoring response to therapies.

CT cholangiography has been found to be more useful and cost effective than MRI in preoperative evaluation of liver donors, and its further clinical applicability and feasibility is being actively investigated.

KEY POINTS

- The advanced MDCT scanners are capable of producing images as thin as 0.625 mm of isotropic voxel resolution, which improves the detection of liver lesion conspicuity and, more importantly, detection and characterization of small liver malignancies with better characterization of the benign pathologic processes and the vascular flow details.
- In patients with decreased cardiac output, obesity, cirrhosis of the liver, or portal vein thrombosis in whom there is decreased liver perfusion, adjustment of volume and rate of injection of contrast media and use of high-concentration iodinated contrast media are particularly important.
- A scan acquired at 2.5-mm collimation is usually adequate for optimal imaging of liver lesions except for CT angiography protocols, in which collimation of as low as 0.625 mm should be chosen to ensure optimal postprocessing quality of the 3D images.
- 3D vascular maps help the surgeons to increase their diagnostic and preoperative confidence with such small-diameter

vessels, which is essential before surgery to prevent torrential bleeding complications.
- Certain advanced applications such as volumetry and computer-assisted diagnosis have recently gained importance, along with advances in liver and tumor segmentation techniques.
- Certain benign lesions also show increased vascularity in the hepatic arterial phase of the scan (e.g., focal nodular hyperplasia and hemangiomas). MDCT can detect the peripheral rim enhancement in the hypovascular lesions and subtle enhancement pattern of tiny hypodense liver lesions in the hepatic arterial phase.
- Dynamic CT perfusion is a relatively new technique for assessing neoangiogenesis and response to therapy in liver tumors. It estimates the blood flow, blood volume, mean transit time, and capillary permeability surface area of the tumor.

SUGGESTED READINGS

Atasoy C, Akyar S. Multidetector CT: contributions in liver imaging. Eur J Radiol 2004; 52:2-17.

Brink JA. Contrast optimization and scan timing for single and multidetector-row computed tomography. J Comput Assist Tomogr 2003; 27(Suppl 1):S3-S8.

Catalano OA, Singh AH, Uppot RN, et al. Vascular and biliary variants in the liver: implications for liver surgery. RadioGraphics 2008; 28:359-378.

Gletsos M, Mougiakakou SG, Matsopoulos GK, et al. A computer-aided diagnostic system to characterize CT focal liver lesions: design and optimization of a neural network classifier. IEEE Trans Inf Technol Biomed 2003; 7:153-162.

Kopp AF, Heuschmid M, Claussen CD. Multidetector helical CT of the liver for tumor detection and characterization. Eur Radiol 2002; 12:745-752.

Laghi A. Multidetector CT (64 slices) of the liver: examination techniques. Eur Radiol 2007; 17:675-683.

Lu R, Marziliano P, Hua Thng C. Liver tumor volume estimation by semi-automatic segmentation method. Conf Proc IEEE Eng Med Biol Soc 2005; 3:3296-3299.

Ong KO, Leen E. Radiological staging of colorectal liver metastases. Surg Oncol 2007; 16:7-14.

Oto A, Tamm EP, Szklaruk J. Multidetector row CT of the liver. Radiol Clin North Am 2005; 43:827-848, vii.

Spielmann AL. Liver imaging with MDCT and high concentration contrast media. Eur J Radiol 2003; 45(Suppl 1):S50-S52.

REFERENCES

1. Tsurusaki M, Sugimoto K, Fujii M, Sugimura K. Multi-detector row helical CT of the liver: quantitative assessment of iodine concentration of intravenous contrast material on multiphasic CT—a prospective randomized study. Radiat Med 2004; 22:239-245.

2. Abdelmoumene A, Chevallier P, Chalaron M, et al. Detection of liver metastases under 2 cm: comparison of different acquisition protocols in four row multidetector-CT (MDCT). Eur Radiol 2005; May 3. Epub ahead of print.

3. Weg N, Scheer MR, Gabor MP. Liver lesions: improved detection with dual-detector-array CT and routine 2.5-mm thin collimation. Radiology 1998; 209:417-426.

4. Spielmann AL: Liver imaging with MDCT and high concentration contrast media. Eur J Radiol 2003; 45(Suppl 1):S50-S52.

5. Bader TR, Prokesch RW, Grabenwoger F. Timing of the hepatic arterial phase during contrast-enhanced computed tomography of the liver: assessment of normal values in 25 volunteers. Invest Radiol 2000; 35:486-492.

6. Hollett MD, Jeffrey RB Jr, Nino-Murcia M, et al. Dual-phase helical CT of the liver: value of arterial phase scans in the detection of small (< or =1.5 cm) malignant hepatic neoplasms. AJR Am J Roentgenol 1995; 164:879-884.

7. Ichikawa T, Kitamura T, Nakajima H, et al. Hypervascular hepatocellular carcinoma: can double arterial phase imaging with multidetector CT improve tumor depiction in the cirrhotic liver? AJR Am J Roentgenol 2002; 179:751-758.

8. Furuta A, Ito K, Fujita T, et al. Hepatic enhancement in multiphasic contrast-enhanced MDCT: comparison of high- and low-iodine-

concentration contrast medium in same patients with chronic liver disease. AJR Am J Roentgenol 2004; 183:157-162.

9. Vignaux O, Legmann P, Coste J, et al. Cirrhotic liver enhancement on dual-phase helical CT: comparison with non-cirrhotic livers in 146 patients. AJR Am J Roentgenol 1999; 173:1193-1197.

10. Murakami T, Kim T, Takamura M, et al: Hypervascular hepatocellular carcinoma: detection with double arterial phase multi-detector row helical CT. Radiology 2001; 218:763-767.

11. Awai K, Takada K, Onishi H, Hori S: Aortic and hepatic enhancement and tumor-to-liver contrast: analysis of the effect of different concentrations of contrast material at multi-detector row helical CT. Radiology 2002; 224:757-763.

12. Saini S: Multi-detector row CT: principles and practice for abdominal applications. Radiology 2004; 233:323-327.

13. Kalra MK, Maher MM, Toth TL, et al. Techniques and applications of automatic tube current modulation for CT. Radiology 2004; 233:649-657.

14. Choi BI, Han JK, Cho JM, et al. Characterization of focal hepatic tumors: value of two-phase scanning with spiral computed tomography. Cancer 1995; 76:2434-2442.

15. Singh AK, Sahani DV, Blake MA, et al. Assessment of pancreatic tumor resectability with multidetector computed tomography semi-automated console-generated images versus dedicated workstation-generated images. Acad Radiol 2008; 15:1058-1068.

16. Singh AK, Sahani DV, Kagay CR, et al. Semiautomated MIP images created directly on 16-section multidetector CT console for evaluation of living renal donors. Radiology 2007; 244:583-590.

17. Stemmler BJ, Paulson EK, Thornton FJ, et al. Dual-phase 3D MDCT angiography for evaluation of the liver before hepatic resection. AJR Am J Roentgenol 2004; 183:1551-1557.

18. Johnson PT, Halpern EJ, Kuszyk BS, et al. Renal artery stenosis: CT angiography comparison of real-time volume rendering and maximum intensity projection algorithms. Radiology 1999; 211: 337-343.

19. Lee WJ. [Applications of multidetector-row CT for the imaging diagnosis of liver disease.] Korean J Gastroenterol 2006; 48:241-246. Korean.

20. Carrascosa PM, Capuñay CM, Sisco P, et al. [Liver evaluation with multidetector CT: angiotomography, volume determination and virtual hepatectomy.] Acta Gastroenterol Latinoam 2006; 36:131-138. Spanish.

21. Duran C, Aydinli B, Tokat Y, et al. Stereological evaluation of liver volume in living donor liver transplantation using MDCT via the Cavalieri method. Liver Transpl 2007; 13:693-698.

22. Koito K, Namieno T, Hirokawa N, et al. Virtual CT cholangioscopy: comparison with fiberoptic cholangioscopy. Endoscopy 2001; 33:676-681.

23. Schwartz LH, Gandras EJ, Colangelo SM, et al. Prevalence and importance of small hepatic lesions found at CT in patients with cancer. Radiology 1999; 210:71-74.

24. Mortele KJ, Praet M, Van Vlierberghe H, et al. CT and MR imaging findings in focal nodular hyperplasia of the liver: radiologic-pathologic correlation. AJR Am J Roentgenol 2000; 175:687-692.

25. Carlson SK, Johnson CD, Bender CE, Welch TJ: CT of focal nodular hyperplasia of the liver. AJR Am J Roentgenol 2000; 174:705-712.

26. Mergo PJ, Ros PR. Imaging of diffuse liver disease. Radiol Clin North Am 1998; 36:365-375.

27. Bluemke DA, Soyer P, Fishman EK. Helical (spiral) CT of the liver. Radiol Clin North Am 1995; 33:863-886.

28. Bradbury MS, Kavanagh PV, Chen MY, et al. Noninvasive assessment of portomesenteric venous thrombosis: current concepts and imaging strategies. J Comput Assist Tomogr 2002; 26:392-404.

29. Sahani DV, Holalkere NS, Mueller PR, Zhu AX. Advanced hepatocellular carcinoma: CT perfusion of liver and tumor tissue—initial experience. Radiology 2007; 243:736-743.

30. Morosi C, Civelli E, Battiston C, et al. CT cholangiography: assessment of feasibility and diagnostic reliability. Eur J Radiol 2008; Jul 3. Epub ahead of print.

31. Wang ZJ, Yeh BM, Roberts JP, et al. Living donor candidates for right hepatic lobe transplantation: evaluation at CT cholangiography—initial experience. Radiology 2005; 235:899-904.

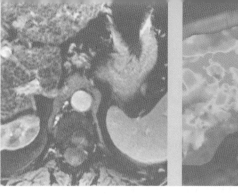
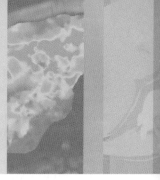

61

MRI of the Liver: From Sequences to Protocol

Danny Kim and Bachir Taouli

INDICATIONS

There are many indications for performing MRI of the liver. The American College of Radiology (ACR) practice guideline highlights the most common recommended indications (Table 61-1).[1] MRI of the liver is a clinically proven and valuable tool in the detection, evaluation, and monitoring of focal and diffuse liver disease.

TECHNICAL ASPECTS

MRI of the liver can be performed using different hardware and software configurations that are available to the radiologist. Recommendations for performing an optimal examination include using magnets with field strengths of 1.5 T or higher (3.0-T magnets are now commercially available), gradient rise times of at least 600 ms, torso phased-array coils, MR-compatible power injector, oxygen availability for patients with breath-holding difficulty, and a dedicated 3D workstation to review the images and perform advanced postprocessing techniques. In the past few years there has been tremendous progress in the development of hardware and sequence design, high-performance gradients, parallel imaging technique, and advanced torso phased-array coils, enabling faster scanning and improved image quality.

Faster scanning has many benefits. The primary benefit is the reduction of scan times to fit within a breath-hold (<25 seconds). By acquiring images during a breath-hold, respiratory motion artifact is greatly reduced. Technologists should practice breath holding with the patient before the examination to familiarize him or her with the technique and improve compliance. Suspending respiration at end-expiration results in more reproducible levels of lung volume and permits accurate slab selection and ability to perform subtraction imaging with better registration of pre- and post-contrast images.

A combination of T1-weighted, T2-weighted, and contrast-enhanced sequences are classically used to perform a routine MRI examination. In Table 61-2, a standard liver MRI protocol as used in our institution is outlined. Each of these sequences will be discussed in the sections that follow.

T1-Weighted Imaging

Normal hepatic parenchyma has a relatively short T1 relaxation time of approximately 575 ms at 1.5 T and demonstrates signal intensity that is isointense or hyperintense to muscle and hyperintense to spleen.[2] Most focal hepatic lesions, including cysts, hemangiomas, hepatocellular carcinomas, and metastases, possess longer T1 relaxation times and consequently appear hypointense relative to hepatic parenchyma on T1-weighted images. Other lesions, such as fat-containing lesions (adenomas and some hepatocellular carcinomas), hemorrhagic lesions, melanin-containing lesions, and proteinaceous lesions possess shorter T1 relaxation times and appear hyperintense relative to hepatic parenchyma. T1-weighted turbo spin-echo (TSE) or spin-echo (SE) imaging is almost never used for liver imaging owing to a longer acquisition time compared with gradient-recalled-echo (GRE) sequences. The T1-weighted in- and opposed-phase GRE sequence provides T1-weighted images. Short repetition time (TR) and short echo time (TE) are used to obtain T1 weighting. This sequence, also known as chemical shift imaging, is valuable in determining the T1-weighted signal properties of lesions and to detect the presence of microscopic or intravoxel fat within focal and diffuse liver diseases.[3] The difference in the local molecular environment between protons in fat and protons in water results in different precessional frequencies of these protons when they are placed in a uniform magnetic field. At 1.5 T, fat protons will precess approximately 220 Hz slower than water protons. At 3.0 T, fat protons will precess approximately 440 Hz slower than water protons.[4] Although this difference is small when compared with the Larmor frequency of protons of approximately 64 MHz at 1.5 T, it is easily exploited to detect the presence of a mixture of fat and water protons within an imaging voxel. At 1.5 T, this difference in precessional frequencies results in fat and water protons being out-of-phase and in-phase at approximately 2.2 and 4.4 ms, respectively. At 6.6 ms, the protons will be out-of-phase again. Consequently, obtaining dual echoes at these strategic times will enable discrimination of the proton population in an imaging voxel. And, by collecting dual echoes during one acquisition, the registration of images between out-of-phase and in-phase images is optimized.

A voxel containing pure fat protons or pure water protons will not demonstrate loss of signal on the opposed-phase sequence because all the protons will precess at the same frequency. However, if there is a mixed population of fat and water protons there will be loss of signal on the opposed-phase sequence because the number of fat protons will cancel an equal number of water protons (Fig. 61-1). The resultant signal will arise from the absolute value of the difference in number between fat protons and water protons. This means a voxel containing 70% fat protons and 30% water protons will demonstrate an equal amount of signal loss on the opposed-phase sequence as a voxel containing 30% fat protons and 70% water protons (fat/water ambiguity). Consequently, a small degree of signal loss may not necessarily translate into "mild" fatty infiltration; in these cases MR spectroscopy has a role in determining the dominant species.[5] For a voxel containing an equal number of fat and water protons, there will be cancellation of all the protons, resulting in no signal from that voxel. This phenomenon is also responsible for the India ink artifact that occurs at interfaces between water-and fat-containing structures, as commonly seen at the surfaces of abdominal organs (Fig. 61-2).

MRI is also effective in detecting the presence of iron deposition because of the paramagnetic properties of iron. In the dual-echo sequence, the presence of iron will result in $T2^*$ effects that decrease the signal intensity as the TE is increased. This occurs because of increased dephasing in the region containing iron. Consequently, the second echo will yield lower signal intensity of iron-containing structures. This phenomenon is the reason why the out-of-phase images must be obtained before the in-phase images. If the out-of-phase images are obtained after the in-phase images and there is signal loss on the out-of-phase images, it is unclear whether the signal loss occurred secondary to the cancellation of fat and water protons of fatty infiltration or whether there is signal loss from the $T2^*$ effects of iron deposition on this longer TE sequence. By acquiring the out-of-phase images first, fatty infiltration will demonstrate lower signal on the out-of-phase, shorter TE images while iron deposition will demonstrate lower signal on the in-phase, longer TE images (Fig. 61-3). Chemical shift imaging also allows characterization of focal liver lesions. For example, intracellular lipid may be seen within hepatocellular carcinoma, regenerative nodules, hepatic adenoma, focal nodular hyperplasia, and focal fatty infiltration.[6]

T2-Weighted Imaging

The echo-train turbo spin-echo T2-weighted sequence is a fat-suppression sequence that provides T2-weighted images. Echo-train imaging acquires multiple echoes to spatially encode an image after a single excitation pulse.[2] The echo train length (ETL), or number of echoes acquired, is a measure of the efficiency of the echo-train pulse sequence compared with conventional spin-echo sequences. The higher the echo-train length, the shorter the acquisition time. The ETL can be adjusted so that the acquisition times are decreased sufficiently to fit during a breath-hold. Breath-hold imaging results in fewer motion-related artifacts. Frequency-selective fat suppression is performed to improve image contrast and conspicuity of lesions and pathologic processes. The drawback of this sequence compared with conventional spin-echo sequences is decreased image contrast owing to the combined T1- and T2-weighted imaging effects of using a range of echo times. Using longer ETLs will result in a longer effective TE and in greater T2 weighting. The T2-weighted sequence is valuable for detecting lesions and pathologic processes. Most normal tissues possess

---

TABLE 61-1 ACR Practice Guideline Indications for MRI of the Liver

Primary Indications
Detection of focal hepatic lesions
Hepatic lesion characterization
Evaluation for known or suspected metastasis
Evaluation of hepatic vascular patency
Evaluation of diffuse liver disease
Evaluation of cirrhotic liver
Clarification of findings from other imaging studies or laboratory abnormalities

Extended Indications
Potential living donor evaluation
Evaluation of tumor response to treatment
Evaluation of known or suspected congenital abnormalities

TABLE 61-2 New York University Liver MRI Protocol

Sequence	Plane	TR/TE	Slice/Gap	Matrix
T1-Weighted Gradient-Recalled-Echo In- and Out-of-Phase	Axial	188/2.2-4.4	8/1	256×118
T2-Weighted Turbo Spin-Echo Fat-Suppressed	Axial	5300/93/TI 180	8/1	256×98
Half-Fourier Acquisition Single-Shot Turbo Spin-Echo (HASTE)	Coronal	900-Infinity/65	4/1	256×256
Time of Flight	Axial oblique	26/9-10	5	138×256
Diffusion-Weighted MRI	Axial	2000/67-82	7/1.4	144×192
3D T1-Weighted Fat-Suppressed Gradient-Recalled-Echo Volumetric Interpolated Breath-hold Examination [VIBE] (precontrast, arterial, portal, equilibrium)	Axial	3.5/1.6	2.1-2.5	98×256

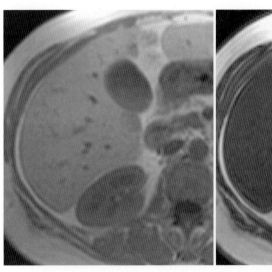
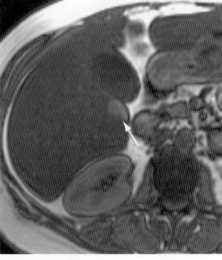

■ **FIGURE 61-1** Axial T1-weighted in-phase (*left*) and out-of-phase (*right*) images of the liver demonstrate signal loss of the hepatic parenchyma on the out-of-phase image consistent with hepatic steatosis. There is an area of fatty sparing adjacent to the gallbladder fossa (*arrow*).

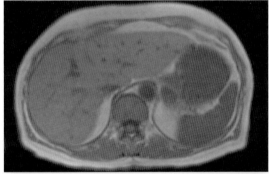
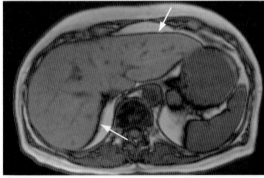

■ **FIGURE 61-2** Axial T1-weighted in-phase (*top*) and out-of-phase (*bottom*) images of normal liver demonstrate no signal loss of the hepatic parenchyma on the out-of-phase image. There is a dark line at the fat/water interfaces (India ink artifact, *arrows*) on the out-of-phase image.

short T1 and T2 values (Fig. 61-4). Benign liver lesions such as cysts and hemangiomas (Fig. 61-5), malignant lesions such as hepatocellular carcinoma and hepatic metastases (Fig. 61-6), and fluid such as edema and ascites possess long T1 and T2 values, which increase their conspicuity.

HASTE Sequence

The half-Fourier acquisition single-shot turbo spin-echo sequence (HASTE) is a long echo train imaging technique that enables acquisition of T2-weighted images in less time than conventional spin-echo imaging. HASTE is a single-shot technique that fills just over half of k-space in one echo train.[2] The remainder of k-space is mathematically filled based on the symmetric properties of k-space. The acquisition times are generally less than 1 second, permitting essentially motion-free T2-weighted images. This technique is useful in uncooperative patients or patients who cannot adequately hold their breath. The main drawback, however, is the low signal-to-noise ratio. Consequently, the sensitivity for liver lesion detection is diminished. In this protocol, the HASTE images are mainly used for assessment of the biliary tree (Fig. 61-7).

Contrast-Enhanced Imaging

The 3D T1-weighted fat-suppressed GRE sequence, performed before and after contrast administration, is the workhorse of the liver MR examination secondary to its high spatial and temporal resolution.[7-9] This volumetric acquisition allows accurate detection and characterization of focal and diffuse liver diseases and accurate depiction of the segmental, vascular, and biliary anatomy with high precision to guide further therapeutic management.[8,10] The advantages over 2D imaging include thinner sections; no gaps between slices, thereby minimizing partial volume effects; higher signal-to-noise ratios; and nearly isotropic voxels, enabling advanced 3D image postprocessing. Contrast-to-noise ratios may be improved by implementing fat-suppression techniques. The complete volume of the liver may be imaged within a single breath-hold to minimize respiratory and other motion artifacts and allow advanced 3D image postprocessing. At our institution, the volumetric interpolated breath-hold examination (VIBE) was developed on the Siemens platform to serve this purpose.[7] Contrast-enhanced images are essential in detecting and characterizing focal and diffuse liver diseases. Image acquisition during the hepatic arterial, portal venous, and equilibrium phases (Fig. 61-8), and a delayed phase for certain lesions, can demonstrate enhancement patterns that are characteristic of particular liver lesions,

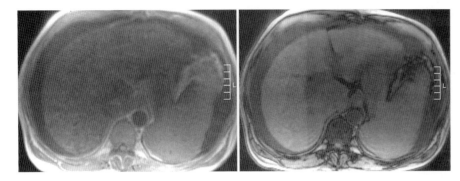

■ **FIGURE 61-3**   Axial T1-weighted in-phase (*left*) and out-of-phase (*right*) images of the liver in a patient with cirrhosis demonstrate signal loss of the hepatic parenchyma on the in-phase image consistent with diffuse iron deposition. There is associated perihepatic and perisplenic ascites.

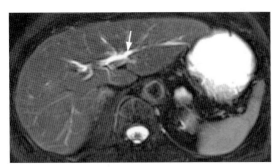

■ **FIGURE 61-4**   Axial fat-suppressed T2-weighted image through the normal liver and spleen. Note the relative low signal intensity of the liver parenchyma compared with the spleen. Most focal liver lesions have higher signal intensity than normal liver parenchyma, which increases their conspicuity on this sequence. There is minimal intrahepatic biliary distention in this patient after cholecystectomy.

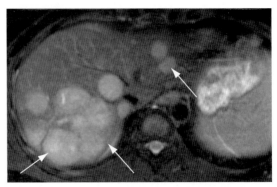

■ **FIGURE 61-6**   Axial T2-weighted image demonstrating multiple hyperintense hepatic metastases of both hepatic lobes (*arrows*).

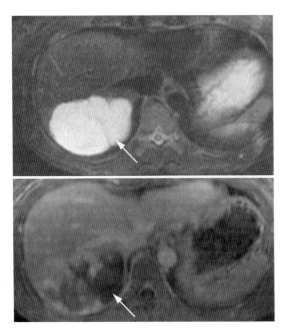

■ **FIGURE 61-5**   Hepatic hemangioma. Axial fat-suppressed T2-weighted image (*top*) demonstrates a large hyperintense lesion in the right hepatic lobe (*arrow*). Axial post-contrast fat-suppressed T1-weighted image (*bottom*) obtained during the portal venous phase demonstrates the characteristic nodular peripheral enhancement of the hepatic hemangioma (*arrow*).

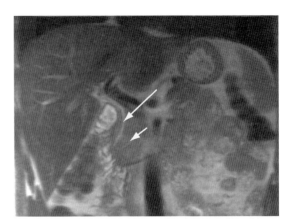

■ **FIGURE 61-7**   Coronal half-Fourier acquisition single-shot turbo spin echo sequence (HASTE) image demonstrates the normal common bile duct (*long arrow*) and distal pancreatic duct (*short arrow*).

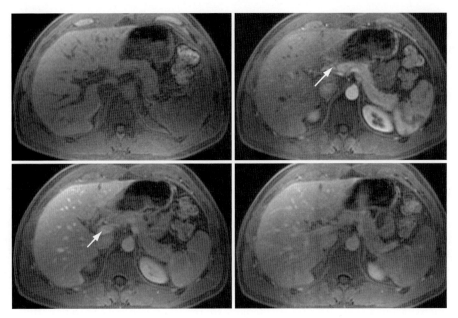

■ **FIGURE 61-8** Axial post-contrast 3D gradient-echo fat-suppressed T1-weighted images of the normal liver obtained before (*left upper image*) and after intravenous contrast administration, during the arterial (*right upper image*), portal venous (*left lower image*), and equilibrium phases (*right lower image*). Note the hepatic artery opacification (*long arrow*) during the arterial phase and the portal vein opacification (*short arrow*) during the portal venous phase.

allowing for their accurate diagnosis or, at least, narrowing of the differential diagnosis.[9] Hypervascular liver lesions include hepatocellular carcinoma, focal nodular hyperplasia, hepatic adenoma, hypervascular metastases, and cavernous hemangioma. In the case of cavernous hemangioma, the arterial phase images may demonstrate the characteristic discontinuous nodular peripheral enhancement to confirm the diagnosis (see Fig. 61-5). Delayed-phase–enhancing liver lesions include cholangiocarcinoma, the central scar of focal nodular hyperplasia, hepatic fibrosis, and peliosis hepatis. The enhancement pattern of different liver lesions is discussed in further detail elsewhere in this text.

To accurately image the liver during the hepatic arterial, portal venous, and equilibrium phases, the circulation time must be determined for the individual patient because the circulation time can vary significantly from patient to patient. Different methods can be used to accomplish this task. In our institution, we use a timing bolus scan.[11] In this protocol, a 1-mL test dose of gadolinium contrast may be infused, followed by a 20-mL saline flush, both infused at a rate of 2 mL/s with a power injector. At the same time, axial images may be acquired at the level of the upper abdominal aorta at 2-second intervals. From these images, the time for peak enhancement of the aorta may be determined. For a sequential MR acquisition, where the center of k-space is filled during the middle of the acquisition time, the following formula may be used to calculate the scan delay:

$$T \text{ (scan delay)} = T \text{ (circulation time)} + \frac{1}{2}T \text{ (contrast infusion)} - \frac{1}{2}T \text{ (acquisition time)}$$

The circulation time is the time for peak enhancement of the aorta. Contrast infusion time is the duration of the contrast infusion (10 seconds for 20 mL of contrast infused at 2 mL/s). Acquisition time is approximately 20 seconds. For liver MRI, a simplification of this formula where T

(scan delay) = T (circulation time) may be used. For the portal venous phase images, 45 seconds is added to the arterial phase scan delay. For the equilibrium phase images, 120 seconds is added to the arterial phase scan delay. Additional delayed phase images may be acquired if delayed enhancing lesions are suspected.

Time-of-Flight (TOF) Sequence

The oblique axial time-of-flight gradient-echo sequence is obtained at the level of the porta hepatis with the saturation band placed craniad to the selected slice. This sequence is used to determine patency and flow direction of the portal vein (Fig. 61-9). If no flow is detected in the

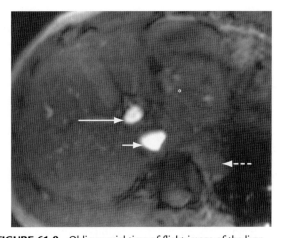

■ **FIGURE 61-9** Oblique axial time-of-flight image of the liver obtained through the porta hepatis with the saturation band positioned cranial to the slice. High signal intensity within the portal vein (*long arrow*) indicates portal vein patency with hepatopetal flow. High signal intensity within the inferior vena cava (*short arrow*) indicates cranial directed flow. Note the low signal intensity within the aorta (*dashed arrow*) secondary to saturation of flow from the cranial positioned saturation band.

portal vein, the portal vein may be thrombosed or possess hepatofugal flow. To differentiate between these two possibilities, the saturation band may be placed caudad to the selected slice. If flow is still not seen, the vessel is thrombosed. If flow is identified, then hepatofugal flow is present.

Gadolinium Contrast Agents

At the present time there are five U.S. Food and Drug Administration (FDA)-approved gadolinium-containing contrast agents (Magnevist, MultiHance, Omniscan, Opti-MARK, and ProHance). Gadolinium is a toxic, paramagnetic, heavy metal ion. Through a chelating process, the gadolinium is surrounded by an organic molecule to form a stable complex, enabling its use in clinical MR examinations. The chelating process reduces the risk of toxicity from free gadolinium exposure. Contrast material is useful in detecting and characterizing lesions, evaluating perfusional properties of tissues, and demonstrating vascular anatomy. The mechanism of action is a shortening of the T1 relaxation time, resulting in increased signal intensity on T1-weighted images. The FDA-approved dose for gadolinium contrast material in MRI examinations is 0.1 mmol/kg. It is cleared from the body through glomerular filtration with only a minimal amount excreted in breast milk.

Recently, a rare and potentially life-threatening condition called nephrogenic systemic fibrosis/nephrogenic fibrosing dermopathy (NSF/NFD) has been reported in patients with advanced renal failure receiving gadolinium-containing contrast material.[12-15] This disease causes fibrosis of the skin and connective tissues throughout the body. Patients may develop skin thickening to such an extent that it results in decreased joint mobility. Fibrosis may also occur in other parts of the body, including the diaphragm, musculature of the lower abdomen and extremities, and the pulmonary vasculature. The clinical course of NSF/NFD is progressive and may be fatal. No treatment has been identified. Consequently, extreme caution is advised in administering gadolinium-based contrast material in those patients with impaired renal function. In our institution, we do not recommend the use of gadolinium in patients with a glomerular filtration rate less than 30 mL/min/1.73 m^2.

SPIO (Superparamagnetic Iron Oxide) Particles (Ferumoxides)

SPIO particles distribute specifically in the hepatic Kupffer cells, with superparamagnetic properties, producing magnetic susceptibility effect and subsequent darkening of the liver parenchyma and spleen, increasing lesion-liver contrast and lesion detection on T2-weighted images. SPIO-enhanced MRI has been shown to be superior to dual-phase CT in the depiction of colorectal metastases.[16] SPIO particles have been used sequentially with gadolinium chelates within one study session with a benefit for screening for hepatocellular carcinoma[17] and for diagnosis of hepatic fibrosis.[18]

TECHNIQUE OPTIMIZATION AND NEW DEVELOPMENTS

Parallel Imaging and Multichannel Systems

Parallel imaging with multichannel systems offers the potential to decrease imaging times without sacrificing spatial resolution. More than one receiver coil is required with each coil having its own receiver channel. This technique utilizes the difference in signal detected by receiver coils positioned over different parts of the body. By incorporating the differences in sensitivity of multiple coils to detect signal from the same source, information regarding spatial localization may be obtained and reduce the number of phase-encoding steps required to produce an image. Consequently, imaging times will be decreased. Two main techniques of parallel imaging are known as simultaneous acquisition of spatial harmonics (SMASH) and sensitivity encoding (SENSE). There are several challenges to realize when incorporating these techniques. First, special coils must be designed with independent coil elements having their own receiver channels. Second, accuracy of coil sensitivity measurements may be difficult to determine. Third, extensive computational time is required to integrate the independent data from multiple channels. Finally, the signal-to-noise ratio will be decreased because of the undersampling of k-space.

3.0-T Considerations

High field strength imaging at 3.0 T offers several potential advantages but presents a new set of challenges.[4] The potential advantages include higher signal-to-noise ratio, higher spatial resolution, faster imaging, and improved MR spectroscopy secondary to increased spectral separation. Pulse sequence parameters used on lower field strength systems cannot be simply transferred to the 3.0-T systems. For example, the T1 and T2* relaxation times will differ at this higher field strength and necessitate modification of the echo times, particularly for chemical shift imaging. Another challenge is the increased specific absorption rate (SAR) at 3.0 T. Because SAR is proportional to the square of the main magnetic field, radiofrequency deposition is four times greater at 3.0 T than at 1.5 T. Strategies to limit SAR that have gained interest include modifications of the pulse sequence design using variable-rate selective excitation methods and variable flip angle sequences and implementing parallel imaging techniques.[4] Other challenges with less straightforward solutions include the heterogeneities in the main magnetic field (B0) and the magnetic field associated with the radio-frequency excitation pulse (B1). Ongoing research efforts will undoubtedly present new strategies to tackle these challenges.

Diffusion-Weighted MRI

Diffusion-weighted MRI (DWI)—by means of apparent diffusion coefficient (ADC) calculation—can be used for in-vivo quantification of the combined effects of capillary

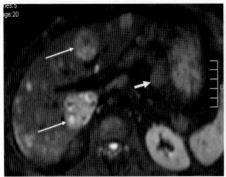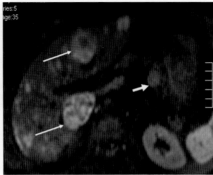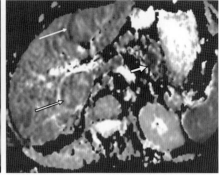

■ **FIGURE 61-10** Single-shot echoplanar imaging diffusion-weighted images in a patient with metastatic neuroendocrine tumor of the pancreas. Diffusion images show the pancreatic body lesion (*short arrow*) and multiple liver metastases (*long arrows*), which are hyperintense at b = 0 (*left image*) and remain hyperintense at b = 500 s/mm² (*middle image*) compared with the normal pancreatic/liver parenchyma, consistent with malignant lesions. ADC map (*right image*) shows a low ADC of the pancreatic and liver lesions.

perfusion and diffusion. DWI has the unique capability of tissue characterization without the need for intravenous contrast, which makes it a potential alternate or adjunct technique to gadolinium-enhanced sequences, owing to the recently recognized risk of nephrogenic systemic fibrosis in patients with renal insufficiency.

We use a breath-hold or respiratory-triggered single-shot epiplanar sequence to obtain diffusion-weighted images on 1.5-T or 3.0-T scanners with phased-array coils and parallel imaging. We typically use b-values of 0, 50, and 500 s/mm²; 50 is used for detection and 500 for characterization. DWI has mostly been used for focal liver lesion detection and characterization.[19-22] DWI images with low b-values are similar to T2-weighted black blood images whereby background signal of vessels in the liver parenchyma is suppressed and better lesion conspicuity could be obtained,[23] whereas higher b-values give diffusion information that helps lesion characterization.[21] In our experience, DWI performs better than T2-weighted imaging for liver lesion detection using DWI with a b-value of 50 s/mm² (sensitivity of detection of lesions was 87.7% for DWI vs. 70.1% for T2 [$P < .0001$]).[24] In addition, it has been shown that ADC values are higher in benign lesions, compared with malignant lesions (Fig. 61-10). In our experience, the use of a threshold ADC value less than 1.5×10^{-3} mm²/s for diagnosis of malignant liver lesions would result in a sensitivity and specificity of 84% and 89%.[21]

Dynamic Contrast-Enhanced MRI

DCE MRI involves the use of continuous high temporal imaging after the injection of gadolinium chelates. Data on DCE MRI of the liver are limited, with promising results for the estimation of diffuse liver disease and focal liver lesions.[25-28]

PROS AND CONS

The advantages of MRI compared with other imaging modalities include its superior soft tissue contrast, avoidance of ionizing radiation, and avoidance of iodinated contrast media. The disadvantages include its high cost, long length of examination, recently described risks of NSF/NFD associated with gadolinium-based contrast media in renal failure patients (see earlier),[12-15] and the presence of multiple contraindications. These contraindications include cardiac pacemakers, the presence of metallic elements in the body (e.g., cerebral aneurysm clips, shrapnel in critical locations of the body), inability to lie flat for the duration of the examination, claustrophobia, first-trimester pregnancy, and known allergy to gadolinium-based contrast media. The likelihood of obtaining valuable clinical information will be increased by screening for appropriate patients, integrating the results of prior imaging examinations and clinical findings, and selecting an appropriate imaging protocol.

KEY POINTS

- ■ MRI of the liver is a valuable tool in the detection, evaluation, and monitoring of focal and diffuse liver diseases.
- ■ The advantages of MRI compared with other imaging modalities include superior soft tissue contrast, avoidance of ionizing radiation, and avoidance of iodinated contrast media.
- ■ The disadvantages of MRI include high cost, long length of examination, recently described risks of nephrogenic systemic fibrosis/nephrogenic fibrosing dermopathy associated with gadolinium-based contrast media in renal failure patients, and the presence of multiple contraindications.

SUGGESTED READINGS

Elsayes KM, Narra VR, Yin Y, et al. Focal hepatic lesions: diagnostic value of enhancement pattern approach with contrast-enhanced 3D gradient-echo MR imaging. RadioGraphics 2005; 25:1299-1320.

Lee VS, Hecht EM, Taouli B, et al. Body and cardiovascular MR imaging at 3.0 T. Radiology 2007; 244:692-705.

Prasad SR, Wang H, Rosas H, et al. Fat-containing lesions of the liver: radiologic-pathologic correlation. RadioGraphics 2005; 25:321-331.

REFERENCES

1. American College of Radiology: Practice guideline for the performance of magnetic resonance imaging (MRI) of the liver. In ACR Practice Guideline, 2005, pp 427-430.
2. Lee VS. Cardiovascular MRI. Physical Principles to Practical Protocols. Philadelphia, Lippincott Williams & Wilkins, 2005, p 402.
3. Merkle EM, Nelson RC. Dual gradient-echo in-phase and opposed-phase hepatic MR imaging: a useful tool for evaluating more than fatty infiltration or fatty sparing. RadioGraphics 2006; 26:1409-1418.
4. Lee VS, Hecht EM, Taouli B, et al. Body and cardiovascular MR imaging at 3.0 T. Radiology 2007; 244:692-705.
5. Chang JS, Taouli B, Salibi N, et al. Opposed-phase MRI for fat quantification in fat-water phantoms with 1H MR spectroscopy to resolve ambiguity of fat or water dominance. AJR Am J Roentgenol 2006; 187:103-106.
6. Prasad SR, Wang H, Rosas H, et al. Fat-containing lesions of the liver: radiologic-pathologic correlation. RadioGraphics 2005; 25:321-331.
7. Rofsky NM, Lee VS, Laub G, et al. Abdominal MR imaging with a volumetric interpolated breath-hold examination. Radiology 1999; 212:876-884.
8. Lee VS, Lavelle MT, Krinsky GA, Rofsky NM. Volumetric MR imaging of the liver and applications. Magn Reson Imaging Clin North Am 2001; 9:697-716, v-vi.
9. Elsayes KM, Narra VR, Yin Y, et al. Focal hepatic lesions: diagnostic value of enhancement pattern approach with contrast-enhanced 3D gradient-echo MR imaging. RadioGraphics 2005; 25:1299-1320.
10. Lavelle MT, Lee VS, Rofsky NM, et al. Dynamic contrast-enhanced three-dimensional MR imaging of liver parenchyma: Source images and angiographic reconstructions to define hepatic arterial anatomy. Radiology 2001; 218:389-394.
11. Earls J, Rofsky N, DeCorato D, et al. Hepatic arterial-phase dynamic gadolinium-enhanced MR imaging: optimization with a test examination and a power injector. Radiology 1997; 202:268-273.
12. Thomsen HS. Nephrogenic systemic fibrosis: a serious late adverse reaction to gadodiamide. Eur Radiol 2006; 16:2619-2621.
13. Grobner T. Gadolinium—a specific trigger for the development of nephrogenic fibrosing dermopathy and nephrogenic systemic fibrosis? Nephrol Dial Transplant 2006; 21:1104-1108.
14. Boyd AS, Zic JA, Abraham JL. Gadolinium deposition in nephrogenic fibrosing dermopathy. J Am Acad Dermatol 2007; 56:27-30.
15. Sadowski EA, Bennett LK, Chan MR, et al. Nephrogenic systemic fibrosis: risk factors and incidence estimation. Radiology 2007; 243:148-157.
16. Ward J, Naik KS, Guthrie JA, et al. Hepatic lesion detection: comparison of MR imaging after the administration of superparamagnetic iron oxide with dual-phase CT by using alternative-free response receiver operating characteristic analysis. Radiology 1999; 210:459-466.
17. Imai Y, Murakami T, Yoshida S, et al. Superparamagnetic iron oxide-enhanced magnetic resonance images of hepatocellular carcinoma: correlation with histological grading. Hepatology 2000; 32:205-212.
18. Aguirre DA, Behling CA, Alpert E, et al. Liver fibrosis: noninvasive diagnosis with double contrast material-enhanced MR imaging. Radiology 2006; 239:425-437.
19. Kim T, Murakami T, Takahashi S, et al. Diffusion-weighted single-shot echoplanar MR imaging for liver disease. AJR Am J Roentgenol 1999; 173:393-398.
20. Nasu K, Kuroki Y, Nawano S, et al. Hepatic metastases: diffusion-weighted sensitivity-encoding versus SPIO-enhanced MR imaging. Radiology 2006; 239:122-130.
21. Taouli B, Vilgrain V, Dumont E, et al. Evaluation of liver diffusion isotropy and characterization of focal hepatic lesions with two single-shot echo-planar MR imaging sequences: prospective study in 66 patients. Radiology 2003; 226:71-78.
22. Yoshikawa T, Kawamitsu H, Mitchell DG, et al. ADC measurement of abdominal organs and lesions using parallel imaging technique. AJR Am J Roentgenol 2006; 187:1521-1530.
23. Hussain SM, De Becker J, Hop WC, et al. Can a single-shot black-blood T2-weighted spin-echo echo-planar imaging sequence with sensitivity encoding replace the respiratory-triggered turbo spin-echo sequence for the liver? An optimization and feasibility study. J Magn Reson Imaging 2005; 21:219-229.
24. Parikh T, Drew S, Lee V, et al. Focal liver lesion detection and characterization with diffusion-weighted MR imaging: comparison with standard breath-hold T2-weighted imaging. Radiology 2008; 246:812-822.
25. Jackson A, Haroon H, Zhu XP, et al. Breath-hold perfusion and permeability mapping of hepatic malignancies using magnetic resonance imaging and a first-pass leakage profile model. NMR Biomed 2002; 15:164-173.
26. Materne R, Smith AM, Peeters F, et al. Assessment of hepatic perfusion parameters with dynamic MRI. Magn Reson Med 2002; 47:135-142.
27. Annet L, Materne R, Danse E, et al. Hepatic flow parameters measured with MR imaging and Doppler US: correlations with degree of cirrhosis and portal hypertension. Radiology 2003; 229:409-414.
28. Hagiwara M, Rusinek H, Lee VS, et al. Advanced liver fibrosis: diagnosis with 3D whole-liver perfusion MR imaging initial experience. Radiology 2008; 246:926-934.

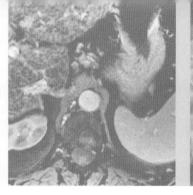
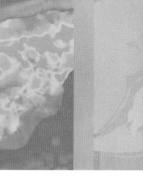

CHAPTER 62

Nuclear Imaging of the Liver

Miguel Hernandez Pampaloni, Saurabh Jha, and Daniel A. Pryma

TECHNICAL ASPECTS

Radiopharmaceuticals

Various technetium-99m (^{99m}Tc)-labeled hepatobiliary radiopharmaceuticals have been used over the years. ^{99m}Tc-disofenin (DISIDA, 2,6-diisopropylacetanilidoiminodiacetic acid) or ^{99m}Tc-mebrofenin (BRIDA, bromo-2,4,6-trimethylacetanilidoiminodiacetic acid) are administered intravenously in doses of 1.5 to 5.0 mCi (50 to 200 MBq) for adults, with 3 to 10 mCi (100 to 370 MBq) used for hyperbilirubinemia. ^{99m}Tc-mebrofenin may be selected instead of ^{99m}Tc-disofenin in moderate-to-severe hyperbilirubinemia owing to its somewhat higher hepatic extraction. For infants and children, the administered dose is 0.05 to 0.2 mCi/kg (2 to 7 MBq/kg) with a minimum of 0.4 to 0.5 mCi (15 to 20 MBq).

CHOLESCINTIGRAPHY

A gamma camera with a large field of view and equipped with a low-energy, all-purpose, or high-resolution collimator is typically used. A diverging collimator may be needed for a camera with a smaller field of view. Whenever possible, continuous computer acquisition should be performed (1 minute per frame) (Fig. 62-1). Imaging should begin at injection and continue serially for 60 minutes or until activity is seen in both the gallbladder (which confirms patency of the cystic duct) and the small bowel (which confirms patency of the common bile duct). Additional views (e.g., right lateral, left, or right anterior oblique) may be obtained as needed to clarify anatomy. Standing and ingestion of water help move duodenal activity distally. When acute cholecystitis is suspected and the gallbladder is not seen within 60 minutes, 3- to 4-hour delayed images should be obtained or morphine augmentation may be used in lieu of delayed imaging. Delayed imaging at 18 to 24 hours may be necessary in some patients (e.g., severely ill patients or those with suggested common bile duct obstruction, suggested leak, or suggested biliary atresia).[1-3]

Several studies have reported an overall sensitivity of 98% and specificity of 90%.[4,5] The false-positive rate is as low as 0.6% and as high as 27%.[6,7] Although reports have suggested high accuracy for ultrasonography, cholescintigraphy has consistent, superior accuracy in direct comparison studies.[6,8] Cases of acute cholecystitis superimposed on chronic cholecystitis can be misinterpreted as chronic cholecystitis. The criterion of complete cystic duct obstruction and/or gallbladder wall edema is most appropriate because it recognizes the natural history of acute cholecystitis.

Patient Preparation

Fasting for 3 to 4 hours before cholescintigraphy has become standard protocol. Half the normal subjects who eat within 1 hour of cholescintigraphy will have gallbladder nonvisualization.[9] Postprandially, the gallbladder is contracted owing to endogenous stimulation by cholecystokinin (CCK). Gallbladder nonvisualization often occurs in patients fasting for more than 24 hours.[10] Without stimulus to contraction, the gallbladder fills to capacity but water reabsorption allows further inflow of bile. The increasingly concentrated viscous bile may prevent ^{99m}Tc-iminodiacetic acid (^{99m}Tc-IDA) entry into the gallbladder. A meal containing fat would be required to contract the gallbladder. Total parenteral nutrition (TPN) is associated with a high incidence of hepatobiliary disease; up to 40% of patients require emergency cholecystectomy.[11]

Cholecystokinin and Morphine Sulfate

Cholecystokinin has been used for many years in conjunction with cholescintigraphy to empty concentrated bile from the gallbladder, to shorten the length of the procedure, and to reduce the number of false-positive studies for acute cholecystitis.[12] In 1978, Paré and colleagues

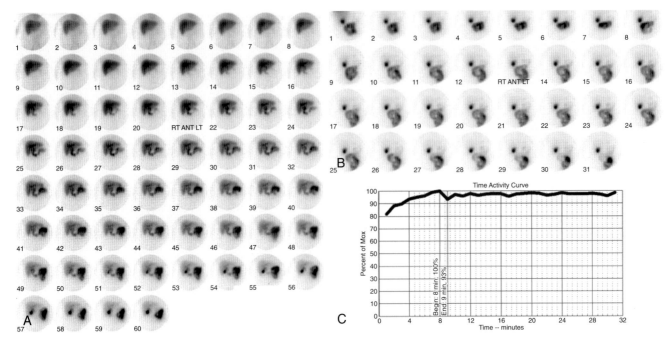

■ **FIGURE 62-1**   A, Dynamic images at 1 minute per frame after injection of 5 mCi ⁹⁹ᵐTc-mebrofenin. There is appropriate tracer concentration by the liver with gallbladder filling and excretion into the small bowel during the initial 60 minutes, excluding cholecystitis. The patient was subsequently given 0.02 μg/kg CCK as a slow intravenous infusion over 30 minutes during imaging at 1 minute per frame (**B**), which demonstrates little gallbladder contraction during the CCK infusion. The time activity curve (**C**) confirms an abnormal gallbladder ejection fraction.

administered CCK to patients who had nonvisualization of the gallbladder at 2 hours and then readministered the radiopharmaceutical.[13] In patients with acute cholecystitis, nonvisualization persisted. In 8 of 16 patients with chronic cholecystitis, the gallbladder did not initially visualize. Delayed biliary-to-bowel transit raises the question of partial common duct obstruction. Delayed imaging or repeat sincalide administration can differentiate obstruction from functional causes. Sincalide pretreatment does not preclude good gallbladder contraction with repeat administration at 60 minutes because the serum half-life of CCK is 2.5 minutes. Proper methodology is critical when administering sincalide to ensure adequate gallbladder contraction. Sincalide, a synthetic C-terminal octapeptide of CCK, in doses of 0.01 to 0.02 μg/kg, may be given intravenously 30 to 60 minutes before the hepatobiliary tracer injection to minimize the potential for a false-positive study. This may occur in patients who have fasted longer than 24 hours, are on parenteral hyperalimentation (especially TPN), or have a severe intercurrent illness.

To assess gallbladder contraction the study involves a 30-minute intravenous infusion of 0.01 to 0.02 μg/kg sincalide after the gallbladder is maximally filled with radiopharmaceutical (usually 60 minutes after the injection) and there is minimal activity in the liver. Dynamic acquisition then continues for 30 minutes (see Fig. 62-1). When performing and interpreting this procedure, the physician must adhere to a specific technique (i.e., dosage and duration of infusion) and normal values must be validated for that technique preferably at each local institution.[14,15]

A shorter sincalide infusion produces a supraphysiologic serum level that may cause gallbladder spasm and a false-positive result. Sincalide infusion does not guarantee

gallbladder contraction. Patients with chronic cholecystitis or diabetes or who are on therapeutic drugs known to inhibit gallbladder contraction (e.g., narcotics, octreotide, calcium blockers, progesterone) may not respond to CCK. Recent administration of morphine sulfate can inhibit the effect of CCK on gallbladder contraction.

Intravenous morphine sulfate contracts the sphincter of Oddi.[16] With 2.5 mg of morphine sulfate, biliary flow resistance doubles and intraductal pressure increases by 60%.[17] Peak effect occurs at 5 minutes. In 1984, Choy and coworkers reported on the use of morphine sulfate as an alternative to delayed imaging.[18] The theory was that morphine would increase bile duct pressure enough to overcome a partial or functional cystic obstruction and, thus, reduce the incidence of false-positive studies and the length of the study. Multiple studies have confirmed a high accuracy of morphine-augmented cholescintigraphy.[19] The sensitivity of morphine-augmented cholescintigraphy for the diagnosis of acute cholecystitis has been uniformly high, between 92% to 100%. False-negative studies are uncommon. Specificity has had a wider range: 69% to 100%.[20] Similar to the delayed imaging method, an increased false-positive rate occurs in patients with prolonged fasting, TPN, severe intercurrent illness, chronic cholecystitis, and hepatic insufficiency. Delayed imaging beyond the 30 minutes after morphine rarely converts a false-positive finding to a true negative finding.[21]

Morphine should not be given if there is a suggestion of partial biliary obstruction (e.g., delayed common duct or biliary-to-bowel clearance). Morphine would make it impossible to differentiate a partial biliary obstruction from a functional obstruction secondary to the drug. There are no absolute contraindications to morphine administration except allergy. Relative contraindications might include hyperamylasemia and narcotic addiction. Re-injection of the radiopharmaceutical has been recommended at morphine administration if the tracer has completely cleared from the liver. The advantage of earlier administration is to further shorten the study. If the morphine is given at 30 minutes, the study can be completed by 60 minutes.[19]

Most investigators have used a standard morphine dose of 0.04 mg/kg. A few have given a standard dose of 2 mg,[19] and one investigation used a variable dose ranging from 0.05 to 0.2 mg/kg. The dose is infused over 1 to 3 minutes. After morphine is administered, gallbladder filling begins within 5 to 10 minutes and is diagnostic by 20 to 30 minutes. Choy and colleagues showed that the second portion of the duodenum cleared within 5 to 10 minutes after morphine administration, accompanied by a slight widening of the common bile duct, presumably caused by cessation of bile flow caused by contraction of the sphincter of Oddi.[18] Kim and associates, using quantitative analysis, also noted a transient decrease in bile flow in half the patients.[22]

It has been suggested that pretreating all patients with CCK before radiopharmaceutical injection could shorten the study and make delayed imaging unnecessary. A retrospective review investigated 155 patients pretreated with sincalide; and if there was gallbladder nonvisualization at 90 minutes, morphine was administered. Morphine decreased nonvisualization from 28% to 12%, with a concomitant decrease in the false-positive rate and increase in the positive predictive value.[23]

Hemangioma Scintigraphy

Hemangiomas are the most common hepatic benign lesion. They are typical incidental findings and may occur in up to 7% of the population.[24] They are usually less than 3 cm in diameter, and they do not require any medical intervention. For the proper identification, 20 mCi (740 MBq) of ^{99m}Tc-labeled autologous red blood cells is routinely used. Imaging normally consists of three phases—arterial perfusion (blood flow), immediate blood pool, and delayed blood pool—often preceded by a structural modality such as CT, MRI, or ultrasonography to identify the lesion location. The arterial perfusion phase is commonly obtained at a rate of 1 frame per second during the injection of the radiopharmaceutical, and it is helpful for revealing the regional distribution of the hepatic arterial blood flow. Immediate blood pool images are acquired during the next 5 minutes or up to 1 to 2 million counts. Delayed blood pool images are normally acquired 2 to 3 hours after the injection and are used to characterize the maximal wash-in of the radiotracer into the hemangioma. Anterior and oblique planar projections are typically used along with single-photon emission computed tomography (SPECT) to identify small lesions.

Pros and Cons

Cholescintigraphy has proven to be the best, single non-invasive test for the diagnosis of acute cholecystitis because it can directly show cystic duct obstruction.

Failure of gallbladder filling in the presence of normal hepatic uptake and biliary excretion reliably indicates acute cholecystitis, whereas normal gallbladder visualization excludes the diagnosis. Cholescintigraphy can also diagnose low-grade or early biliary obstruction before ultrasonography shows biliary dilatation. The adjunctive use of CCK can be used to identify chronic cholecystitis or biliary dyskinesia as a cause of pain.

Controversies

Hepatocellular disease is seen on cholescintigraphy as delayed uptake and excretion of ^{99m}Tc-IDA. The altered pharmacokinetics may result in nonvisualization of the gallbladder at the expected intervals. A 40% to 60% false-positive rate was reported in early studies.[25] However, with delayed imaging, 83% of patients have gallbladder visualization.[3] Severe intercurrent illness (e.g., massive trauma, sepsis, life-threatening postoperative complications, acute respiratory diseases) has been associated with false-positive cholescintigraphy results.[2,26]

Acute pancreatitis is a reported cause of false-positive cholescintigraphy. Zeman and colleagues reported four of seven false-positive studies in patients with acute pancreatitis.[1] Common causes for acute pancreatitis are alcoholism and biliary tract disease. The pathophysiology of biliary pancreatitis is uncertain, but precipitating factors include pancreatic duct obstruction by an impacted stone in the ampulla of Vater or by inflammatory spasm of the ampullary sphincter. The mortality rate of pancreatitis associated with gallstone disease is high (20% to 50%), compared with that associated with alcoholism (2% to 5%).

Chronic cholecystitis is a frequent cause for false-positive cholescintigraphy. More than 90% of patients with chronic cholecystitis have normal findings on 60-minute cholescintigraphy.[27] However, of those patients with delayed gallbladder filling, more than 70% have chronic cholecystitis.[28] Delayed filling is caused by a functional resistance to flow through the cystic duct caused by viscous bile, sludge, and stones within the gallbladder or by chronic mucosal thickening and, rarely, fibrosis.

NORMAL HEPATOBILIARY SCINTIGRAPHY IN ADULTS

A normal hepatobiliary scintigram is characterized by immediate demonstration of hepatic parenchyma, followed by activity in the intrahepatic and extrahepatic biliary ductal system, gallbladder, and upper small bowel. All these structures should be visualized within 1 hour. Gallbladder visualization implies a patent cystic duct and excludes acute cholecystitis with a high degree of certainty. Normal excretion of a small percentage of the tracer by the kidneys may mimic gallbladder or small bowel on occasion but may be clarified by a lateral image.

NORMAL HEPATOBILIARY SCINTIGRAPHY IN INFANTS

In neonates, extraction of tracer by the liver is prompt and has a uniform distribution, which reaches a maximum tracer accumulation within 5 minutes. The gallbladder may be visualized as early as 10 minutes, but occasionally it is not seen in the neonatal period. The significance of a nonfunctioning gallbladder in the neonatal period is uncertain but most likely represents biliary stasis and reduced bile flow. Bowel activity is seen usually by 30 to 40 minutes. The hepatic, cystic, and common bile ducts are not normally visualized in the neonatal period. From 12 months of age the hepatic, cystic, and common bile ducts become more obvious.

PATHOPHYSIOLOGY

Acute Cholecystitis

Cystic duct obstruction is the initial pathophysiologic landmark of acute cholecystitis. If patency is not promptly reestablished after the obstruction to the venous and lymphatic outflow has occurred, neutrophils infiltrate the gallbladder wall, followed by mucosal hemorrhage and necrosis. Gangrenous cholecystitis occurs in up to 20% of patients, and perforation occurs in up to 10% of patients. A severely inflamed gallbladder may become adherent to contiguous structures. The pain of biliary colic lasts minutes to hours and is followed by a diminution in intensity. The pain of acute cholecystitis is unremitting for days and accompanied by fever and leukocytosis.

Complications of acute cholecystitis include hydrops, emphysematous cholecystitis, and empyema. Perforation is the most serious complication and has a high mortality rate. In subacute or chronic perforations with fistula formation, repeated bouts of cholecystitis lead to fibrosis with adherence to adjacent structures. Inflammation and pressure necrosis can develop around gallstones impacted in the gallbladder wall, with erosion into contiguous organs.

Acute acalculous cholecystitis occurs in 5% to 15% of patients with acute cholecystitis. There are no stones in the gallbladder or cystic duct. These patients are critically ill, often are postoperative, and have had severe trauma, extensive burns, or other serious illnesses. Diagnosis is difficult and delayed owing to the patient's multiple medical problems, resulting in high morbidity and mortality.

Cholecystectomy has been the definitive therapy for acute cholecystitis for many decades. In recent years, laparoscopic cholecystectomy has become the treatment of choice for patients with symptomatic gallstone disease, acute cholecystitis, and more complicated problems, including common bile duct stone disease.[29] Although delayed surgery is considered safer, increased adhesions make the gallbladder more difficult to remove laparoscopically. The open approach is still often used for patients with gallbladder perforation, pericholecystic abscess, or empyema.

Early diagnosis of acute cholecystitis is essential for prompt, therapeutic decisions and prevention of complications. When the etiology of abdominal pain is uncertain, ultrasonography is often performed first because nonbiliary disease and bile duct dilatation can be detected. CT is used as an alternative to ultrasonography in the setting of an acute abdomen or when gastrointestinal symptoms predominate over signs or symptoms of biliary disease. When the clinical index of suspicion for acute cholecystitis is high, cholescintigraphy should be the initial imaging study (Fig. 62-2).

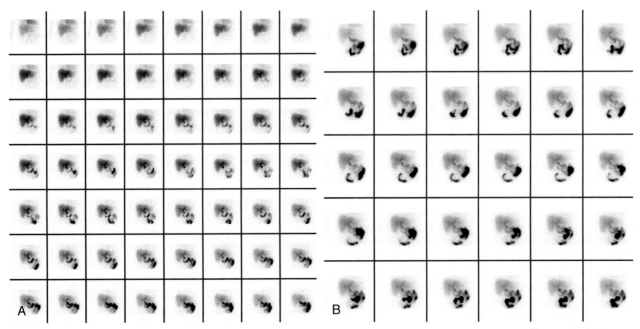

■ **FIGURE 62-2** Acute cholecystitis. The initial 56 frames (**A**) at 1 minute per frame after intravenous injection of 5 mCi ^{99m}Tc-mebrofenin demonstrate appropriate tracer concentration by the liver and a patent common bile duct. The gallbladder was not visualized. Therefore, 0.04 mg/kg of morphine sulfate was given intravenously and imaging continued at 1 minute per frame for 30 minutes (**B**), during which the gallbladder was persistently nonvisualized. Cholecystectomy confirmed acute cholecystitis.

The hallmark of acute cholecystitis (acalculous as well as calculous) is persistent gallbladder nonvisualization after morphine administration or on 3- to 4-hour delayed images. A pericholecystic hepatic band of increased activity (the "rim sign")[30] is often associated with severe phlegmonous/gangrenous acute cholecystitis. The rim sign has been variously reported to occur in 18% to 61% of patients with acute cholecystitis.[31,32] Several studies also found that the rim sign had a strong association with gangrene and perforation. Although the overall sensitivity of the rim sign for acute cholecystitis is not high, it has a high positive predictive value for complicated acute cholecystitis. Possible pathophysiologic mechanisms that have been postulated for the rim sign include (1) inflammation and edema of hepatic parenchyma adjacent to the inflamed gallbladder, causing obstruction and impaired drainage of bile canaliculi; (2) injury of local hepatocytes in the inflamed region, resulting in reduced ability to excrete the tracer; (3) increased blood flow to the region surrounding the gallbladder due to inflammatory hyperemia; (4) extravasation of a small amount of tracer into the gallbladder fossa via a gangrenous, perforated gallbladder; and (5) incomplete obstruction with faint gallbladder visualization.[33]

Increased blood flow to the gallbladder fossa is another secondary sign of acute cholecystitis. All patients with a rim sign had increased flow, although only 46% with increased flow had a rim sign. Other investigators reported that increased flow was seen in 53% of patients with acute cholecystitis and 47% had a rim sign.[34,35] Scintigraphic evidence for perforation is present in approximately half the cases. The rim sign and increased flow are indirect, insensitive, and nonspecific cholescintigraphic findings of gangrene and perforation.[36]

The high accuracy for acute calculous cholecystitis is due to detection of the pathophysiologic abnormality cystic duct obstruction, which is reported as nonfilling of the gallbladder. However, with the acalculous form of the disease, patients may not have cystic duct obstruction.[37] The cystic duct may be partially obstructed by edema, cellular debris, or inspissated bile, and other patients may have direct inflammation of the gallbladder wall from sepsis, toxemia, or ischemia, without cystic duct obstruction. Several publications reported sensitivities higher than 90%.[38,39]

It would not be surprising to discover that cholescintigraphy has a high false-positive rate for acute acalculous cholecystitis. These patients are often affected with serious illnesses, have fasted for a prolonged period, and are receiving TPN. However, studies with a limited number of patients have reported specificities close to 100%.[40]

Biliary Obstruction

Common causes for biliary obstruction include malignancy, choledocholithiasis, and inflammatory stricture. Much less common causes are sclerosing cholangitis, choledochal cyst, hemobilia, duodenal diverticulum, echinococcosis, and ascariasis. Stone formation is related to the secretion of lithogenic bile. Approximately 90% of calculi form in the gallbladder and pass into the biliary duct via the cyst duct. The clinical presentation of biliary obstruction varies, depending on the duration, the degree, and the site of obstruction. Painless jaundice, a common presentation, is gradual in onset and is usually caused by malignancy. Sudden, severe abdominal pain occurs with acute, complete biliary obstruction, usually due to cholelithiasis. Persistence of obstruction beyond 2 to 3 days may result in cholangitis, with symptoms of biliary colic and fever, chills, and jaundice (i.e., Charcot's triad). Intermittent colicky pain is most commonly due to benign causes of partial obstruction (e.g., stones or biliary stricture). Stones often incompletely obstruct, producing fluctuating symptoms and often normal or low levels of hyperbilirubinemia. Small stones may pass into the duodenum with transient symptoms. The serum alkaline phosphatase value increases early in the natural history of obstruction. Released from the biliary ductal epithelium, it is the most sensitive indicator. After complete biliary obstruction, hepatic bile secretion decreases as biliary pressure increases. Secretion ceases when the back-pressure equals or exceeds the secretory pressure of hepatocytes, usually after 1 to 2 days. By 24 to 48 hours, bile duct dilatation of extrahepatic and intrahepatic ducts occurs proximal to the site where obstruction occurs.

Noninvasive imaging is critical for the prompt workup and diagnosis of patients with suspected biliary obstruction, whether it presents as painless jaundice or abdominal pain. Real-time ultrasonography is commonly used to screen patients with suspected biliary obstruction. Detection of extrahepatic and intrahepatic biliary dilatation is often diagnostic. In early obstruction, ducts may not be dilated. Dilatation is most prevalent in high-grade obstruction of several days' duration and in those patients with malignant causes. Cholescintigraphy plays an important role in the differential diagnosis of biliary obstruction despite advances of other anatomic imaging modalities that rely on detecting biliary dilatation. Both bilirubin and ^{99m}Tc-IDA radiopharmaceuticals share a common organic anion receptor–mediated endocytosis mechanism for uptake by the hepatocyte. When serum bilirubin levels are high, bilirubin occupies available receptor sites and blocks ^{99m}Tc-IDA uptake. ^{99m}Tc-IDA radiopharmaceuticals used in the early days of cholescintigraphy had only moderate sensitivity for detection of obstruction (i.e., 78% to 85%), which is slightly lower than that reported for ultrasonography. However, modern-day radiopharmaceuticals (e.g., ^{99m}Tc-disofenin and ^{99m}Tc-mebrofenin) have high hepatic extraction and permit visualization of bile flow at serum bilirubin levels of 20 mg/dL or higher. Here, the higher hepatic extraction of ^{99m}Tc-mebrofenin (98% vs. 88%, respectively) is advantageous.

Patients with early, low-grade, or intermittent biliary obstruction may not have dilated ducts. Physiologic abnormalities precede morphologically evident disease, and discordance in favor of cholescintigraphy, compared with morphologic imaging modalities, can be as high as 23%.[41] Cholescintigraphy can be diagnostic for patients whose symptoms are suggestive of biliary obstruction but who are not clearly jaundiced, have only mild liver function abnormalities, and have normal results of ultrasonography. It can also distinguish cholecystitis from biliary obstruction or suggest concomitant disease. The patient with prior bouts of obstruction and common duct exploration, in whom a dilated, atonic, but nonobstructed duct is suspected, can benefit from cholescintigraphy as well. Normal scintigraphic drainage can avert needless additional evaluation.

Some patients may have postoperative stones that formed in the biliary tree since the time of surgery. Choledocholithiasis causes serious complications of ductal stricture, cholangitis, biliary cirrhosis, biliary fistulas, and hepatic abscess. Common duct stones sometimes act in a ball valve fashion, causing mild, intermittent obstruction. Cholescintigraphy with ^{99m}Tc-IDA derivatives has been used to diagnose biliary obstruction since 1978.[42] Delayed imaging was recommended to differentiate complete from partial obstruction, although partial obstruction was defined as biliary clearance by 24 hours.[43] Morphine-like drugs may cause the scintigraphic pattern of partial obstruction.[44,45]

The sensitivity and specificity of cholescintigraphy to differentiate biliary tract obstruction from other causes were 97% and 90%, respectively, in a 1986 study of 96 jaundiced patients.[46] The cholescintigraphic findings of partial biliary obstruction included segmental biliary narrowing, abrupt biliary cutoff, intraluminal filling defects, and persistent pooling in major ducts after CCK administration.[47]

Quantitative methods have been used to improve the accuracy for cholescintigraphic diagnosis of partial biliary obstruction. Regions of interest were selected for the liver and biliary structures, and various quantitative parameters were calculated.[48,49] When image analysis and a semiquantitative scoring method were combined for diagnosing partial obstruction, it was diagnosed with 100% accuracy after cholecystectomy.[50]

The pattern of high-grade biliary obstruction is easily recognized as prompt hepatic uptake with no gallbladder or biliary duct visualization or biliary-to-bowel transit. The diagnosis can be made in most patients at 60 minutes in those with good hepatic function. Delayed imaging beyond 1 hour may detect transit into biliary ducts at 2 to 24 hours in some patients. Although they have an incomplete obstruction, it is still high grade. The term *high grade* for this pattern is probably more correct than the term *complete obstruction*. The term *partial obstruction* should be reserved for the pattern of clearance into the biliary tract during the first hour but little or no clearance from biliary ducts, regardless of whether there is some biliary-to-bowel transit. CCK administration at 1 hour can obviate the need for delayed images. In the setting of hepatic insufficiency, delayed imaging is always indicated.

The pattern of delayed bile duct clearance and biliary-to-bowel transit has causes other than obstruction (e.g., morphine-like drugs, CCK given before cholescintigraphy, chronic cholecystitis) and normal variation.[51] Morphine-like drugs should not be given for 4 to 6 hours before the study. Delayed imaging can usually differentiate functional from obstructive causes.

Bile Leaks

Bile leaks after cholecystectomy are common. Small quantities of leakage after cholecystectomy do not usually lead to serious medical complications. Gilsdorf and associates performed cholescintigraphy routinely 2 to 4 hours after open cholecystectomy.[52] Bile leaks were detected in 44% of patients. The cause of bile leakage after cholecystectomy is often caused by surgical transection of small biliary radicles entering directly into the gallbladder bed (i.e., bile ducts of Luschka). Less frequently, biliary extravasation occurs from direct injury to the biliary tree at surgery.

Laparoscopic cholecystectomy has replaced the open procedure in all but complicated cases. The procedure is associated with less discomfort, shorter postoperative recovery and hospital stay, and better cosmetic result. The incidence of bile duct injuries and significant bile leakage is only slightly higher than that with open cholecystectomy, from 0.5% to 2.0%.[53]

Symptoms of bile leakage are often mild and nonspecific in the early postoperative period. Most perihepatic, postoperative fluid collections are small and asymptomatic and resolve spontaneously. Symptomatic leakage is usually caused by local inflammatory or compressive effects of bile collection or infection. Large leaks with bile ascites are indicative of significant biliary tract or small intestine injury and require prompt repair. Bile salts are the toxic component of bile and produce a chemical peritonitis and associated cytokine release, resulting in serious alterations in fluid transport across peritoneal membranes.

CT and ultrasonography have high sensitivities for detection of perihepatic fluid collections and free peritoneal fluid. However, they often cannot determine the type of fluid present. Postoperative collections other than bile include seroma, hematoma, lymphocele, and abscess. Cholescintigraphy can confirm that a fluid collection is derived from the biliary system, identify active biliary leakage, and estimate the rate of leakage (Fig. 62-3). Negative cholescintigraphy should lead to a search for other causes of the patient's symptoms. Even if a leak is confirmed by paracentesis, negative cholescintigraphy indicates that the leak has either ceased or is slow enough that it will likely resolve spontaneously, and aggressive therapy is not warranted.

Published reports of the use of cholescintigraphy for diagnosis of biliary leakage date back to 1974, using ^{131}I-rose bengal.[54,55] Since 1978, ^{99m}Tc-IDA radiotracers have been used.[56] Numerous studies have defined the clinical role for cholescintigraphy for detection of different presentations of bile leakage[57] after cholecystectomy or laparoscopic cholecystectomy.[58] Several studies have emphasized its use for detection of various manifestations of biliary leakage, including intrahepatic leaks,[59] bilomas,[60] fistula to gastrointestinal organs,[61] and leakage from a perforated duodenal ulcer.[62,63]

Rapid leaks can often be detected and localized during the first 30 to 60 minutes after radiopharmaceutical injection. This process is seen as rapidly increasing activity outside the normal hepatobiliary structures. After cholecystectomy, biliary leakage often collects in the gallbladder fossa and then extravasates either down the right paracolic gutter, spreads over the dome of the liver, and/or localizes to the left upper quadrant. Biliary leaks may accumulate in a loculated collection or biloma or diffusely throughout the abdomen (i.e., bile ascites). With

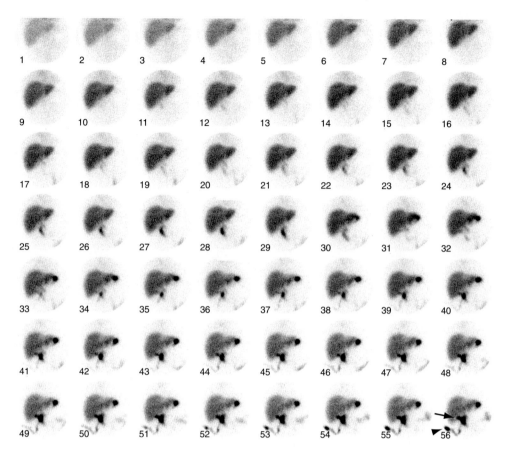

■ **FIGURE 62-3** Anterior images of the abdomen at 1 minute per frame after injection of 5 mCi ^{99m}Tc-mebrofenin in a patient with pain after cholecystectomy demonstrate concentration of tracer by the liver with excretion into the small bowel. However, a significant portion of the excreted tracer is seen leaking into the gallbladder fossa (*arrow*) and into a drain (*arrowhead*).

peritoneal free leakage, the intestines will often be outlined with small bowel loops, giving a cold "stepladder" appearance. Leakage exits via a fistula to another organ (e.g., bronchi, stomach, bowel, or skin). Activity exiting a surgical drain may be the only evidence of a leak. Careful attention to drains, tubing, and collection bags is critical for proper diagnosis. It is common for patients to have multiple drains, some placed free within the peritoneum and others placed within a biliary structure. The specific anatomy of biliary-enteric anastomoses is also essential to understand the biliary and bowel drainage pattern.

Delayed imaging and multiple views are often helpful for detection and correct localization of biliary leakage. This process is particularly useful when the diagnosis is suspected but initial images appear normal. Delayed imaging can often confirm slow extravasation and/or small collections. The decreasing adjacent liver activity and progress of bowel clearance can facilitate diagnosis. Lateral decubitus images can sometimes confirm fluid collections.

Scintigraphy is more sensitive than CT or ultrasonography for the detection of biliary leaks. CT and ultrasonography may demonstrate the presence of a fluid collection; however, scintigraphy is better able to establish an active hepatobiliary component associated with the fluid collection. In the setting of a clinically high suspicion of biliary leak, endoscopic retrograde cholangiopancreatography is often performed to identify the leak and in some cases also to repair the leak. If the clinical suspicion for an active biliary leak is low, then scintigraphy is preferred because it is a sensitive, noninvasive, and inexpensive test.

Hemangioma

The classic scintigraphic appearance of the hemangioma is absent visualization during the arterial perfusion phase imaging, whereas the activity becomes more intense than in surrounding liver during the immediate blood pool phase. At 2 to 3 hours, imaging activity greater than in the adjacent liver is often observed. The overall imaging accuracy for detecting hemangiomas has been reported to be 90%, especially when SPECT is used to detect small and peripheral lesions.[64] False-positive results have been described in a very small number of cases of patients with hemangiosarcoma or hepatocellular carcinoma.[65,66]

HEPATOBILIARY SCINTIGRAPHY IN CHILDREN

Assessment of the hepatobiliary system by nuclear medicine techniques in the infant younger than 1 year of age is usually performed to help determine the cause of jaundice. The majority of cases occur in children in the first 3 months of life. Hyperbilirubinemia in the neonatal period is common and most often due to benign physiologic jaundice, a self-limiting condition. Persistent jaundice beyond 2 weeks of age in full-term infants and 3 weeks in

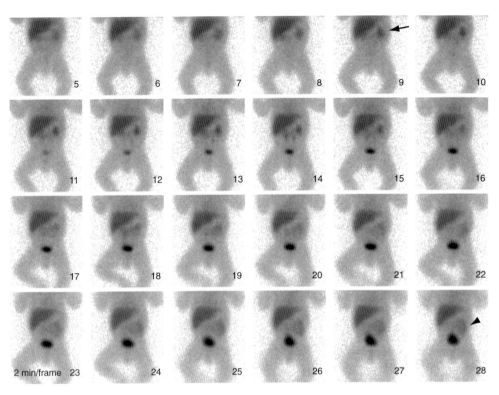

■ **FIGURE 62-4** Anterior images at 2 minutes per frame in a 27-day-old male neonate with hyperbilirubinemia. Initially, excreted activity in the kidneys (*arrow*) can mimic bowel activity. However, at the end of the first hour of imaging, small bowel activity can be visualized (*arrowhead*), excluding biliary atresia.

preterm infants is not physiologic, however, and evaluation of these patients must be undertaken.[67,68] Cholestasis or prolonged elevation of the serum conjugated bilirubin level is always pathologic. Cholestasis can be attributed to either intrahepatic causes of an infectious, metabolic, or genetic nature or extrahepatic abnormalities causing mechanical obstruction to bile flow.

Biliary Atresia

The pathogenesis of biliary atresia remains unknown.[67-69] In the majority of infants, obstructive obliteration of the biliary tree occurs perinatally or postnatally.[70] Histopathology shows both chronic and acute inflammatory changes, and the process may be progressive, because the pathologic process has been reported to continue after surgical relief of the obstruction.[71] The diagnosis of biliary atresia in the neonatal period is often difficult. Its early diagnosis and the distinction of biliary atresia from other causes of jaundice are vital, because early intervention is paramount for the successful surgical correction of biliary atresia.[72] Ultrasonography is used as one of the first imaging modalities to visualize the anatomy of the hepatobiliary system and exclude congenital abnormalities of the liver and biliary system. The abnormality most commonly diagnosed by ultrasonography is congenital bile duct dilatation or choledochal cyst.

Hepatobiliary scintigraphy is based on the fact that radiotracers are transported to the liver bound to albumin and are actively taken up by the hepatocytes. Excretion into the bile ducts is by both active and passive transport mechanisms. Depending on the agent, 2% to 15% is excreted by the kidneys. With increasing hepatocellular dysfunction, a higher percentage of tracer is excreted through the renal pathway.[73]

In neonates being investigated to differentiate between intrahepatic and extrahepatic causes of cholestasis, pretreatment with phenobarbital, 5 mg/kg/day, is usually given orally in two divided doses daily for a minimum of 3 to 5 days before the hepatobiliary imaging study to enhance the biliary excretion of the radiotracer and increase the specificity of the test. ^{99m}Tc-mebrofenin may be preferred over ^{99m}Tc-disofenin in suspected biliary atresia (Fig. 62-4).[73,74] Care should be taken if the patient has fasted for more than 24 hours or has been on total parenteral nutrition for extended periods. This may cause failure of visualization of the gallbladder. Prolonged fasting results in gallbladder atony and increased intraluminal gallbladder pressure from retained bile and sludge, secondary to the absence of endogenous CCK.[75] Fasting, however, should not cause absent or reduced flow into the duodenum.

Gallbladder function is assessed with a fatty meal or CCK. In neonates, if the gallbladder has been visualized, a normal feeding is given to assess gallbladder function and quantitate gallbladder ejection fraction. In older infants, a fatty meal or CCK also may be given.[76] CCK should be infused over a 30-minute period and data collected for 30 minutes. Infusion of CCK over a shorter period (1 to 3 minutes) may cause side effects of cramping and abdominal pain.

Hepatic extraction fraction (HEF) is defined by the extraction of tracer by the liver and reflects hepatocyte function and may be assessed visually and quantitatively. Visual inspection usually gives the diagnostic information required to differentiate conditions causing reduced hepatocyte function (e.g., neonatal hepatitis) and those with preserved hepatocyte function (e.g., biliary atresia). In some equivocal cases quantitation by HEF will add information to help differentiate biliary atresia, and it is useful for determining the degree of liver dysfunction semiquantitatively. The HEF is calculated from the hepatic phase of the study and is a measure of the efficiency of the hepatocyte in extracting the radiopharmaceutical from the blood. The normal HEF in a pediatric population is 92%.[74,77] Hepatic half-lives are defined as hepatic parenchymal clearance/excretion and can be quantitatively assessed by determining the half-life from a peripheral region of liver parenchyma. The region of interest should exclude major bile ducts when possible. The excretion half-life is calculated by a least squares fit to the clearance curve.

Patients with biliary atresia who present within the first 2 months of life show prompt hepatic extraction with an HEF greater than 92%, nonvisualization of the gallbladder, prolonged retention of tracer in the liver, and no excretion of tracer into the bowel at 1, 4, and 24 hours. Patients presenting when older than 3 months of age usually have compromised hepatocyte function and show reduced hepatic extraction, reflected by a reduction in HEF, and no biliary excretion. In this situation, differentiation from severe neonatal hepatitis or cholestasis is more difficult. In cases in which there is good extraction of tracer by the liver and only minimal biliary excretion seen on hepatobiliary scan findings, close follow-up is recommended. The hepatobiliary scan should be repeated if jaundice remains and acholic stools are seen.

The sensitivity of scintigraphy for the diagnosis of biliary atresia was reported by Gerhold and colleagues as 91% accuracy, 97% sensitivity, and 92% specificity.[78] Specificity was increased by premedication with phenobarbital (5 mg/kg/day for 5 days).

Neonatal Hepatitis

Neonatal hepatitis more commonly affects male patients and is associated with infection (cytomegalovirus, rubella, toxoplasmosis, herpes simplex virus, and viral hepatitis), α_1-antitrypsin deficiency, and idiopathic onset. In patients with neonatal hepatitis, the HEF is generally reduced, reflecting the reduced hepatocyte extraction of tracer.[79] There is persisting and delayed clearance of tracer from the blood pool that is particularly evident by prolonged cardiac blood pool activity. If the hepatocellular dysfunction is severe, some of these patients will also show absent excretion of tracer into the biliary tree over 24 hours. The presence of any bowel activity rules out biliary atresia. Occasionally, 24-hour images are required and may show activity in the gut or rectum. Lateral views are useful to separate the pelvic activity of rectum and bladder. As the degree of liver dysfunction increases, there is a concurrent increase in renal excretion.

Other Causes of Congenital Hepatobiliary Dysfunction

Many patients present during the first months of life with cholestatic jaundice and acholic stools. Choledochal cysts have been reported in association with biliary atresia. Choledochal cysts can be associated with simple hepatic cysts, stone formation, cholangitis, pancreatitis, portal hypertension, and biliary atresia. The ultrasonographic appearance of choledochal cysts ranges from mild dilatation of the common bile duct to cystic dilatation, which may involve major intrahepatic ducts and the cystic duct. Extremely large cystic structures may obstruct biliary flow completely. Hepatobiliary scan appearance may show good extraction and excretion of tracer, a photopenic area in the porta hepatis depending on the size of the anatomic abnormality, and accumulation of tracer in the dilated ducts or cysts. There might be complete obstruction with negligible biliary flow and nonfilling of the cystic mass. In addition, choledochal cysts may contract with a stimulus of a fatty meal or CCK. The presence of activity in the peritoneal cavity is a rare complication owing to rupture of the choledochal cyst.

In patients with congenital cystic abnormalities the liver shows good perfusion and function with excretion of tracer into the biliary system. If there is connection of the cyst to the biliary system there initially may be a photon-deficient area seen in the early parenchymal phase of the study and delayed filling of the cyst with tracer. Idiopathic perforation of the extrahepatic biliary system is the second most common cause of surgical jaundice in infants. Perforation usually occurs at the junction of the common duct and cystic duct. Presentation with jaundice and abdominal distention usually occurs in the first 1 to 2 weeks of life. Scintigraphy may show a photopenic area caused by the pseudocyst with slow accumulation into the cyst or dispersion of tracer into the peritoneal cavity. The pseudocyst may enlarge to a size that causes compression of the extrahepatic bile ducts. The pseudocyst may also mimic a choledochal cyst on ultrasonography.

The bile plug syndrome is characterized by a partial or complete obstruction of the extrahepatic biliary system by inspissated bile plugs. Patients with increased bile viscosity are at risk, particularly infants with dehydration, cystic fibrosis, and hemolytic disorders, those on total parenteral nutrition, and those after extensive ileal resections. Scintigraphy shows a variable pattern. However, it usually shows good extraction of tracer by the liver with poor excretion into the gut, typical of severe cholestasis. Occasionally, however, there is reduced extraction similar to patients with hepatocellular dysfunction from neonatal hepatitis.

Arteriohepatic dysplasia, or Alagille syndrome, is characterized by paucity of interlobular bile ducts associated with congenital abnormalities.[80] These include typical facial features, pulmonary artery stenosis, complex congenital heart disease, and vertebral anomalies. There is also a nonsyndromic form of paucity of the interlobular bile ducts. Scintigraphy shows good extraction of the tracer but marked holdup in liver parenchyma similar to severe cholestasis with usually minimal excretion into the gut. Occasionally no excretion is seen, and in these patients scintigraphy cannot distinguish Alagille syndrome from biliary atresia.

Hepatobiliary involvement in neonates with cystic fibrosis ranges from hepatomegaly or mild cholestatic jaundice to severe cholestasis with acholic stools. Biliary obstruction in neonates with cystic fibrosis is due mainly to inspissation of biliary secretions and generally resolves by 3 to 4 months of age. Biliary atresia must be excluded if there are acholic stools. Scintigraphy of cystic fibrosis patients in the neonatal period usually shows moderately good extraction of tracer with poor excretion. However, cholestasis may be severe and show no excretion into the gut. Premedication with phenobarbital is highly recommended for this group of patients.[79]

Cholecystitis is presumed to occur less frequently in children than in adults, but its incidence in children has probably been underestimated.[81,82] Cholecystitis with underlying cholelithiasis is more common in children with hemolytic anemias. Acute calculous cholecystitis occurs when the cystic duct becomes obstructed by gallstones, leading to gallbladder distention and edema. Bile stasis may then lead to bacterial overgrowth. Acalculous cholecystitis occurs infrequently in the adult population but proportionately is a more common cause of cholecystitis in children. Acalculous cholecystitis can occur in prolonged illness, sepsis, or trauma. These conditions (and their treatment) predispose to increasing cholesterol saturation, biliary stasis, and cholestatic hypofunction. Biliary sludge may then form with resultant cystic duct obstruction. The associated inflammation and edema may compromise blood flow and promote bacterial infection. Infections such as scarlet fever and other streptococcal infections as well as vasculitis from Kawasaki disease and polyarteritis nodosa can lead to acalculous cholecystitis in children. Chronic cholecystitis most often is related to gallstone formation; however, cases of chronic acalculous cholecystitis (biliary dyskinesia) are believed to be related to gallbladder dysfunction, causing chronic bile stasis and sphincter of Oddi dysfunction.[83]

Acute cholecystitis is associated with nonvisualization of the gallbladder on hepatobiliary scintigraphy with a diagnostic accuracy of 98% and a specificity of 100% in adults. However, in children, visualization of the gall-bladder does not exclude cholecystitis because gallbladder visualization, although infrequent, is possible in acalculous cholecystitis. In acalculous cholecystitis, the cystic duct may be partially obstructed and associated edema of the cystic duct may result in gallbladder nonvisualization. If the gallbladder is visualized, infusion of 0.02 mg/kg sincalide permits further assessment. Poor contraction of the gallbladder after infusion of sincalide may occur in partial cystic duct obstruction, acalculous cholecystitis, or chronic cholecystitis. Chronic cholecystitis is associated with a gallbladder ejection fraction of less than 35%. No normal values for gallbladder ejection fraction have been established in children, and it is expected that there is significant overlap between the normal and abnormal range. Additionally, chronic cholecystitis may be accompanied by a delay in gallbladder filling in the absence of hepatic dysfunction. As in adults, morphine augmentation of hepatobiliary scintigraphy of acute cholecystitis may help reduce the number of false-positive studies in children and reduce scanning time; however, in acute acalculous cholecystitis, it may overcome functional obstruction of the cystic duct, resulting in a false-negative result.[84]

KEY POINTS

■ The most common indications for imaging evaluation of the hepatobiliary system and functional assessment of the integrity of the hepatobiliary tree include the following:
  ● Suspected acute cholecystitis
  ● Suspected chronic biliary tract disorders
  ● Common bile duct obstruction
  ● Detection of bile leak
  ● Evaluation of congenital abnormalities of the biliary tree

---

REFERENCES

1. Eikman EA, Cameron JL, Colman M, et al. A test for patency of the cystic duct in acute cholecysitis. Ann Intern Med 1975; 82:318-322.
2. Zeman RK, Burrell MI, Cahow CE, et al. Diagnostic utility of cholescintigraphy and ultrasonography in acute cholecystitis. Am J Surg 1981; 141:446-451.
3. Mauro MA, McCartney WH, Melmed JR. Hepatobiliary scanning with [99m]TcPIPIDA in acute cholecystitis. Radiology 1982;142:193-197.
4. Samuels BI, Freitas JE, Bree RL, et al. A comparison of radionuclide hepatobiliary imaging and real-time ultrasonography for detection of acute cholecystitis. Radiology 1983; 147:2017-2020.
5. Ralls PW, Colletti PM, Halls JM, et al. Prospective evaluation of ^{99m}Tc-IDA cholescintigraphy and gray-scale ultrasound in the diagnosis of acute cholecystitis. Radiology 1982; 144:369-371.
6. Worthen NJ, Usler JM, Funamura JL. Cholecystitis: prospective evaluation of sonography and ^{99m}Tc-HIDA cholescintigraphy. AJR Am J Roentgenol 1981; 137:973-978.
7. Shuman WP, Mack LA, Rudd TG, et al. Evaluation of acute right upper quadrant pain: sonography and ^{99m}Tc-PIPIDA cholescintigraphy. AJR Am J Roentgenol 1982; 139:61-64.
8. Chatziioannou SN, Moore WH, Ford PV, Dhekne RD. Hepatobiliary scintigraphy is superior to abdominal ultrasonography in suspected acute cholecystitis. Surgery 2000; 127:609-613.
9. Baker RJ, Marion MA. Biliary scanning with Tc-99, pyridoxylideneglutamate—the effect of food in normal subjects: concise communication. J Nucl Med 1977; 18:793-795.
10. Larson MJ, Klingensmith WC, Kuni CC. Radionuclide hepatobiliary imaging: non-visualization of the gallbladder secondary to prolonged fasting. J Nucl Med 1982; 23:1003-1005.
11. Warner BW, Hamilton FN, Silberstein EB, et al. The value of hepatobiliary scans in fasted patients receiving total parenteral nutrition. Surgery 1987; 102:595-599.
12. Nicholson RW, Hastings DL, Testa HF, et al. HIDA scanning in gallbladder disease. Br J Radiol 1980; 53:878-882.
13. Paré P, Shaffer EA, Rosenthall L. Nonvisualization of the gallbladder by ^{99m}Tc-HIDA cholescintigraphy as evidence of cholecystitis. Can Med Assoc J 1978; 118:384-386.
14. Ziessman HA, Muenz LR, Agarwal AK, et al. Normal values for sincalide cholescintigraphy: comparison of two methods. Radiology 2001; 221:404-410.

15. Ziessman HA. Cholescintigraphy: clinical indications and proper methodology. Radiol Clin North Am 2001; 39:997-1006.

16. Murphy P, Salomon J, Roseman D: Narcotic anesthetic drugs: their effects on biliary dynamics. Arch Surg 1980; 115:710-711.

17. Dedrick FD, Tanner WW, Bushkin FL. Common bile duct pressure during enflurane anesthesia: effects of morphine and subsequent naloxone. Arch Surg 1980; 115:820-822.

18. Choy D, Shi EC, McLean RG, et al. Cholescintigraphy in acute cholecystitis: use of intravenous morphine. Radiology 1984; 151:203-207.

19. Fink-Bennett D, Balon H, Robbins T, Tsai D. Morphine-augmented cholescintigraphy: its efficacy in detecting acute cholecystitis. J Nucl Med 1991; 32:1231-1233.

20. Fig LM, Wahl RL, Stewart RE, Shapiro B. Morphine-augmented hepatobiliary scintigraphy in the severely ill: caution is in order. Radiology 1990; 175:467-473.

21. Flancbaum L, Choban PS. Use of morphine cholescintigraphy in the diagnosis of acute cholecystitis in critically ill patients. Intensive Care Med 1995; 21:120-124.

22. Kim CK, Palestro CJ, Solomon RW, et al. Delayed biliary-to-bowel transit in cholescintigraphy after cholecystokinin treatment. Radiology 1990; 176:553-556.

23. Chen CC, Holder LE, Maunoury C, et al. Morphine-augmentation increases gallbladder visualization in patients pretreated with cholecystokinin. J Nucl Med 1997; 38:644-647.

24. Iskak KG, Rabin L. Benign tumors of the liver. Med Clin North Am 1975;59:995-1013.

25. Kalf V, Froelich JW, Lloyd R, et al. Predictive value of an abnormal hepatobiliary scan in patients with severe intercurrent illness. Radiology 1983; 146:191-194.

26. Pitt HA, King W III, Man LL, et al. Increased risk of cholelithiasis with prolonged total parenteral nutrition. Am J Surg 1983; 146:106-112.

27. Shuman WP, Gibbs P, Rudd TG, et al. PIPIDA scintigraphy for cholecystitis: false positive in alcoholism and total parenteral nutrition. AJR Am J Roentgenol 1982; 138:1-5.

28. Drane WE, Nelp WB, Rudd TG. The need for routine delayed radionuclide hepatobiliary imaging in patients with intercurrent disease. Radiology 1984; 151:763-769.

29. Meyers WC, Branum GD, Farouk M, et al. A prospective analysis of 1518 laparoscopic cholecystectomies. N Engl J Med 1991; 324:1075-1078.

30. Swayne LC, Ginsberg HN. Diagnosis of acute cholecystitis by cholescintigraphy: significance of pericholecystic hepatic uptake. AJR Am Roentgenol 1989; 152:1211-1213.

31. Greer P, Lacayo L, Reiner DK, et al. The rim sign: the ghostly portender of acute cholecystitis. Am J Gastroenterol 1992; 87:627-629.

32. Bushnell DL, Perlman SB, Wilson MA, et al. The rim sign: association with acute cholecystitis. J Nucl Med 1986; 27:353-356.

33. Bohdiewicz PJ. The diagnostic value of grading hyperperfusion and the rim sign in cholescintigraphy. Clin Nucl Med 1993; 18:867-871.

34. Brachman MB, Tanasescu DE, Ramanna L, et al. Acute gangrenous cholecystitis: radionuclide diagnosis. Radiology 1984; 151:209-211.

35. Jacobson AF. False-negative morphine-augmented hepatobiliary scintigraphy with a rim sign. Clin Nucl Med 1995; 20:579-581.

36. Shih WJ, Domstad PA, Kenady D, et al. Scintigraphic findings in acute gangrenous cholecystitis. Clin Nucl Med 1987; 12:717-720.

37. Shuman WP, Rogers JV, Rudd TG, et al. Low sensitivity of sonography and cholescintigraphy in acalculous cholecystitis. AJR Am J Roentgenol 1984; 142:531-534.

38. Swayne LC. Acute acalculous cholecystitis: sensitivity in detection using technetium-99m iminodiacetic acid cholescintigraphy. Radiology 1986; 160:33-38.

39. Prevot N, Mariat G, Mahul P, et al. Contribution of cholescintigraphy to the early diagnosis of acute acalculous cholecystitis in intensive-care-unit patients. Eur J Nucl Med 1999; 26:1317-1325.

40. Mariat G, Mahul P, Prevot N, et al. Contribution of ultrasonography and cholescintigraphy to the diagnosis of acute acalculous cholecystitis in intensive care unit patients. Intensive Care Med 2000; 26:1658-1663.

41. Zeman RK, Lee C, Jaffe MH, et al. Hepatobiliary scintigraphy and sonography in early biliary obstruction. Radiology 1984; 153:793-794.

42. Nielsen SP. Hepatobiliary scintigraphy and hepatography with Tc-99m diethyl-acetanilido-iminodiacetate in obstructive jaundice. J Nucl Med 1978; 19:452-457.

43. Klingensmith WC, Kuni CC, Fritzberg AR. Cholescintigraphy in extrahepatobiliary obstruction. AJR Am J Roentgenol 1982; 139:65-70.

44. Taylor A, Kiper MS, Witztum K, et al. Abnormal ^{99m}Tc-PIPIDA scans mistaken for common duct obstruction. Radiology 1982; 144:373-375.

45. Egbert RN, Braunstein P, Lyos K, et al. Total bile duct obstruction. Arch Surg 1983; 118:709-712.

46. Lee AW, Ram MD, Shih WJ, et al. Technetium-99m BIDA biliary scintigraphy in the evaluation of the jaundiced patient. J Nucl Med 1986; 27:1407-1412.

47. Pitluk HC, Beal JM. Choledocholithiasis associated with acute cholecystitis. Arch Surg 1979; 114:887-888.

48. Darweesh RMA, Dodds WJ, Hogan WJ, et al. Efficacy of quantitative hepatobiliary scintigraphy and fatty-meal sonography for evaluating patients with suspected partial common duct obstruction. Gastroenterology 1988; 94:779-786.

49. Kloiber R, AuCoin R, Hershfield NB, et al. Biliary obstruction after cholecystectomy: diagnosis with quantitative cholescintigraphy. Radiology 1988; 169:643-647.

50. Sostre S, Kaloo AN, Spiegler EJ, et al. A noninvasive test of sphincter of Oddi dysfunction in postcholecystectomy patients: the scintigraphic score. J Nucl Med 1992; 33:1216-1222.

51. Ziessman HA. Cholecystokinin cholescintigraphy: clinical indications and proper methodology. Radiol Clin North Am 2001; 39:997-1006.

52. Gilsdorf JR, Phillips M, McLeod MK, et al. Radionuclide evaluation of bile leakage and the use of subhepatic drains after cholecystectomy. Am J Surg 1986; 151:259-262.

53. The Southern Surgeons Club: a prospective analysis of 1518 laparoscopic cholecystectomies. N Engl J Med 1991; 324:1073-1078.

54. Silverberg M, Rosenthall L, Freeman LM. Rose bengal excretion studies as an aid in the differential diagnosis of neonatal jaundice. Semin Nucl Med 1973; 3:69-80.

55. Wiener SN, Vyas M. The scintigraphic demonstration of bile leakage utilizing I-131 rose bengal. J Nucl Med 1974; 15:1074-1075.

56. Rosenthall L, Fonesceca C, Arzoumanian A, et al. Tc-99m IDA hepatobiliary imaging following upper abdominal surgery. Radiology 1979; 130:735-738.

57. Weissmann H, Chun K, Frank M, et al. Demonstration of traumatic bile leakage with cholescintigraphic and ultrasonography. AJR Am J Roentgenol 1979; 133:843-847.

58. Rosenthal L. An update on radionuclide imaging in hepatobiliary disease. JAMA 1981; 245:2065-2068.

59. Scott-Smith W, Raftery AT, Wraight EP, et al. Tc-99m labeled HIDA imaging in suspected biliary leaks after liver transplantation. Clin Nucl Med 1983; 10:478-479.

60. Walker AT, Shapiro AW, Brooks DC, et al. Bile duct disruption and biloma after laparoscopic cholecystectomy: imaging evaluation. AJR Am J Roentgenol 1992; 158:785-789.

61. Kuni CC, Klingensmith WC, Koep LJ, et al. Communication of intrahepatic cavities with bile ducts: demonstration with Tc-99m diethyl IDA imaging. Clin Nucl Med 1980; 5:349-351.

62. Lee CM, Stewart L, Way LW. Postcholecystectomy abdominal bile collections. Arch Surg 2000; 135:538-542.

63. Ramachandran A, Gupta SM, Johns WD. Various presentations of postcholecystectomy bile leak diagnosed by scintigraphy. Clin Nucl Med 2001; 26:495-498.

64. Kudo M, Ikekubo K, Yamamoto K, et al. Distinction between hemangioma of the liver and hepatocellular carcinoma: value of labeled RBC-SPECT scanning. AJR Am J Roentgenol 1989; 152:977-983.

65. Ginsberg F, Slavin JD, Spencer RP. Hepatic angiosarcoma: mimicking of angioma on three-phase technetium 99m red blood cell scintigraphy. J Nucl Med 1986; 27:1861-1863.

66. Middleton ML, Milstein DM, Freeman LM. Hepatic mass lesions: Scintigraphic uptake with emphasis on hemangioma detection. In Freeman LM (ed). Nuclear Medicine Annual. New York, Raven Press, 1994, pp 55-90.

67. McEvoy C, Suchy FJ. Biliary tract disease in children. Pediatr Clin North Am 1996; 43:75-97.

68. Hicks BA, Altman RP. The jaundiced newborn. Pediatr Clin North Am 1993; 40:1161-1175.

69. Balistreri W. Liver and biliary system. In Behrman RE, Kliegman RM, Nelson WE, Vaughan VC (eds). Nelson Textbook of Pediatrics, 14th ed. Philadelphia, WB Saunders, 1992, pp 1001-1015.

70. Kasai M, Suzuki K, Ohashi E, et al. Technique and results of operative management of biliary atresia. World J Surg 1978; 2:571-580.

71. Miyano T, Fujimoto T, Ohya T, Shimomura H. Current concept of the treatment of biliary atresia. World J Surg 1993; 17:332-336.

72. Whitington PF. Chronic cholestasis of infancy. Pediatr Clin North Am 1996; 43:1-26.

73. Nadel H. Hepatobiliary scintigraphy in children. Semin Nucl Med 1996:26:25-42.

74. Krishnamurphy S, Krishnamurphy K. Quantitative assessment of hepatobiliary diseases with 99mTc-IDA scintigraphy. In Freeman LM, Weissmann HS (eds). Nuclear Medicine Annual. New York, Raven Press, 1988, pp 309-313.

75. Fink-Bennett D. Gallbladder and bile ducts. In Wagner HN, Szabo Z, Buchanan JW (eds). Principles of Nuclear Medicine, 2nd ed. Philadelphia, WB Saunders, 1995, pp 946-958.

76. Howman-Giles R, Moase A, Gaskin K, Uren R. Hepatobiliary scintigraphy in a pediatric population: determination of hepatic extraction by deconvolution analysis. J Nucl Med 1993; 34:214-221.

77. Landing BH. Considerations of the pathogenesis of neonatal hepatitis, biliary atresia and choledochal cyst: the concept of infantile obstructive cholangiopathy. Prog Pediatr Surg 1974; 6:113-139.

78. Gerhold JP, Klingensmith WC, Kuni CC, et al. Diagnosis of biliary atresia with radionuclide hepatobiliary imaging. Radiology 1983; 146:499-504.

79. Gaskin KJ, Waters DL, Howman-Giles R, et al. Liver disease and common bile duct stenosis in cystic fibrosis. N Engl J Med 1988; 318:340-346.

80. Alagille D, Odievre M, Gautier M, Dommergues JP. Hepatic ductular hypoplasia associated with characteristic facies, vertebral malformations, retarded physical, mental and sexual development, and cardiac murmur. J Pediatr 1975; 86:63-71.

81. Shaffer EA. Gallbladder disease. In Walker WA, Durie PR, Hamilton JR, et al (eds). Pediatric Gastrointestinal Disease, 3rd ed. Hamilton, Ontario, Canada, BC Decker, 2000, pp 1291-1311.

82. Wessmann HS, Frank MS, Bernstein LH, et al. Rapid and accurate diagnosis of acute cholecystitis with ^{99m}Tc-HIDA cholescintigraphy. AJR Am J Roentgenol 1979; 132:523-528.

83. Gilger MA. Diseases of the gallbladder. In Wyllie R, Hyams JS (eds). Pediatric Gastrointestinal Disease, 2nd ed. Philadelphia, WB Saunders, 1999, pp 651-662.

84. Freitas JE. Cholescintigraphy. In Ell PJ, Gambhir SS (eds). Nuclear Medicine in Clinical Diagnosis and Treatment, 3rd ed. Edinburgh, Churchill Livingstone, 2004, pp 919-926.

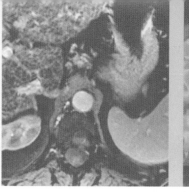
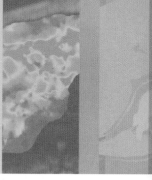

CHAPTER 63

Benign Focal Lesions

Daniele Marin and Giuseppe Brancatelli

ETIOLOGY

Although benign hepatic tumors have been classified into several histiotypes according to their cell of origin (i.e., hepatocytes, biliary epithelium, or mesenchymal cells), our focus in this discussion is on those lesions most frequently encountered in clinical practice, including simple (nonparasitic) hepatic cyst, hemangioma, hepatocellular adenoma (HCA), focal nodular hyperplasia (FNH), large benign regenerative nodules, and hepatic abscess (Table 63-1).

PREVALENCE AND EPIDEMIOLOGY

With the widespread use of sensitive imaging studies, benign hepatic tumors are increasingly reported. Notably, even in patients with a known primary malignancy, about 50% of small hepatic lesions (<1.5 cm) are benign.[1]

CLINICAL PRESENTATION

Most benign hepatic tumors are an incidental finding in asymptomatic patients during imaging workup for an unrelated medical problem. Larger lesions may occasionally produce signs and symptoms related to mass effect, such as abdominal discomfort and pain.

Hepatocellular adenoma can manifest as acute onset of abdominal pain after intratumoral hemorrhage, whereas hepatic abscess is often accompanied with fever and leukocytosis.

PATHOPHYSIOLOGY

Although benign tumors can occur in every portion of the liver, the right and left hepatic lobes are unequally affected by some histiotypes.

PATHOLOGY

Pathologic findings vary greatly according to the specific tumor type, and their appearance will be described in the sections on specific lesions.

IMAGING

Although combining multiple imaging studies allows a confident diagnosis in the majority of cases, atypical lesions may still represent a diagnostic challenge.

Radiography

Because of poor soft tissue resolution, a plain abdominal radiograph does not provide any clinical information in the investigation of patients with benign hepatic tumors, although in some cases larger lesions may be suspected owing to deformation of a visible liver border, mass effect on adjacent structures, or calcification.

CT

With the advent of multidetector CT (MDCT), remarkable improvements have been accomplished with scanning speed, scan volumes, and image quality. As a result, CT currently represents the main imaging modality for evaluating the liver.

Besides lesion detection, the main goal of CT is to firmly establish a diagnosis of benign hepatic tumors. Indeed, mistaking an incidental benign lesion for a malignant tumor may lead to unnecessary, aggressive management, or possibly preclude surgery when benign and malignant lesions coexist within the same liver. Although simple cysts can be confidently characterized based only on their appearance at precontrast and single-phase contrast-enhanced CT during the portal venous phase, reliable diagnosis of other benign hepatic tumors generally requires assessment of lesion enhancement pattern with multiphasic contrast-enhanced CT (i.e., hepatic arterial phase, portal venous phase, and delayed phase).

MRI

MRI represents a powerful technique for the detection and characterization of either benign or malignant liver tumors. A comprehensive MRI protocol includes pulse sequences that assess different tissue characteristics such

TABLE 63-1 Clinical and Radiologic Features of Benign Hepatic Neoplasms

Neoplasm	Sex	Age	Capsule	Size	Number	Calcifications	Fat	Scar	Bleed	Associated Signs and Predisposing Factors
Hepatic cyst	F > M	5-6th decade	No	Variable	One or few	Rare (peripheral)	No	No	Rare	Congenital
Cavernous hemangioma	F > M	2-5th decade	No	Variable (3-20 cm)	One or few	Sometimes in large ones	No	Rare (larger lesions)	No	Congenital
Capillary hemangioma	F > M	2-5th decade	No	Usually smaller than 2 cm	One or few	No	No	No	No	Congenital
Focal nodular hyperplasia	F >> M	3-4th decade	No	3 cm (1-14 cm)	One or few	1%	Very rare	Present in 50% Hyperintense on T2-weighted images and on delayed post-gadolinium T1-weighted images	No	Vascular abnormality
Hepatic adenoma	F >> M	3-4th decade	25%	5.5 cm	One or few	5%	Often	No	Yes	Oral contraceptives assumption
Large benign regenerative nodules	F > M	3-4th decade	No	0.5-4 cm	Multiple	No	No	Larger lesions	No	Budd-Chiari syndrome and other vascular disorders
Pyogenic abscess	F = M	5-7th decade	Yes	Variable	One or few	No	No	No	No	Bacterial

as T1 and T2 contrast of liver tumors, as well as assessment of tumor-specific enhancement patterns after intravenous administration of gadolinium-based extracellular contrast agents. Liver-specific MR contrast media, which include reticuloendothelial system–specific and hepatocyte-selective contrast agents, have the potential to further increase the conspicuity and characterization of focal hepatic lesions by providing both anatomic and functional information.

Ultrasonography

Because of its high contrast resolution, low cost, and wide availability, ultrasonography frequently represents the primary modality for the study of the liver. However, operator dependency, substantial image degradation in either obese or meteoric patients, and a limited field of view, represent major limitations that explain the low appeal of ultrasonography among referring physicians and surgeons.

Some benign liver tumors, such as simple cysts or hemangiomas, typically demonstrate a classic, virtually diagnostic appearance at ultrasonography. Some other lesions (e.g., FNH, small hepatic adenoma, or large benign regenerative nodules) may, however, be difficult to distinguish from normal liver owing to their hepatocellular nature.

Recent development of microbubble contrast agents has substantially enhanced the diagnostic information available.[2] Besides the evaluation of tumor enhancement pattern during both arterial and portal venous phases, contrast-enhanced images can also be acquired during a late parenchymal phase with potential improvement of lesion detection.

Nuclear Medicine

Although nuclear medicine can provide important information for the diagnosis of either FNH and hemangioma, its role has been almost entirely supplanted by contrast-enhanced CT and MRI in daily clinical practice.

PET/CT

The role of PET/CT in the diagnosis of benign tumors of the liver has not been explored.

SPECIFIC LESIONS
Simple (Bile Duct) Cyst
Etiology

Simple (nonparasitic) cysts likely result from a congenital defective development of the intrahepatic biliary ducts.

Prevalence and Epidemiology

Simple hepatic cysts are among the most common liver lesions, with an estimated incidence of 2.5% in the general population.[3] Although cysts can occur in both sexes at all ages, middle-aged women are more frequently affected (male-to-female ratio, 1:5).

Clinical Presentation

Typically, cysts are incidental imaging findings in asymptomatic patients. Occasionally, larger lesions may produce signs and symptoms related to mass effect, such as abdominal discomfort, chronic pain, nausea and vomiting, or early satiety due to compression of the stomach. Rarely, acute pain can develop after intralesional hemorrhage, spontaneous or traumatic rupture, torsion of an exophytic cyst, or secondary infection.[3]

Pathophysiology

Simple cysts originate twice as frequently within the right lobe of the liver than the left lobe.

Pathology

Typically, simple cysts manifest as either solitary or multiple, well-defined lesions, varying in size from a few millimeters to several centimeters. Cysts do not communicate with the biliary tree and typically contain clear fluid. Occasionally, cystic content may, however, be mucoid, purulent (if the cyst is infected), or hemorrhagic.[3]

At histology, the cyst lining consists of a single layer of columnar or cuboid epithelium, which is identical to bile duct epithelium. Epithelial cells rest on a basement membrane surrounded by a thin fibrous stroma.[3]

Liver Function

Liver function test results are generally unremarkable, although larger cysts may produce mild increase of alkaline phosphatase and bilirubin levels.

Imaging

Because of the high incidence in the general population, simple hepatic cysts are frequently discovered at either ultrasonography, CT, or MRI of the liver.

Radiography

Although larger lesions may deform one of the visible borders of the liver or cause mass effect on adjacent structure, a plain abdominal radiograph does not usually detect simple hepatic cysts.

CT

At precontrast CT, cysts manifest as rounded or oval, thin-walled, well-defined, water-attenuating (from −10 to +10 HU) lesions.[4] Although cysts are almost invariably unicameral in shape, multiple lesions can manifest as a multicameral appearance when clustered together.

At contrast-enhanced CT, neither the cystic content nor the peripheral wall shows perceptible enhancement (Fig. 63-1).[4] Rarely, complicated cysts may show atypical appearances, such as parietal calcifications, mural nodularity, or fluid levels that may resemble a cystic liver tumor or hepatic abscess.

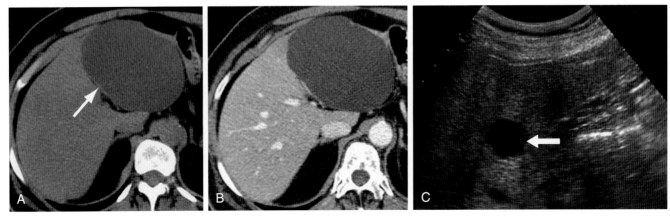

■ **FIGURE 63-1** Typical presentation of hepatic (bile duct) simple cyst. **A,** Transverse precontrast CT image shows a large, sharply defined lesion (*arrow*) in the left lobe of the liver that is hypoattenuating compared with the surrounding hepatic parenchyma and aorta. Hypoattenuation to aorta on precontrast images is the single most important finding to diagnose cystic lesions at CT. **B,** Corresponding contrast-enhanced CT scan during portal venous phase demonstrates absence of lesion enhancement. **C,** Ultrasound image in a different patient shows a round, well-circumscribed mass (*arrow*) with imperceptible wall and increased through-transmission of sound waves.

MRI

Because cysts are composed almost entirely of fluid, their T1 and T2 values are extremely long, thus explaining the very low signal intensity on T1-weighted images and markedly high signal intensity on T2-weighted images. Characteristically, cysts further increase their signal on T2-weighted images at longer echo times (e.g., >120 ms) because of signal suppression from most abdominal parenchymal tissues. Hemorrhagic cysts can show variable signal intensity on T1- and T2-weighted images according to the age of hemorrhage as well as a fluid/fluid level due to mixed blood product.[4]

As in the case of contrast-enhanced CT, simple cysts do not enhance on gadolinium-enhanced MRI.

The lack of communication between cysts and the biliary tree can be demonstrated with T2-weighted MR cholangiopancreatography (MRCP). This finding can be further corroborated on T1-weighted MRCP after administration of hepatobiliary excretion of liver-specific MR contrast agents, which demonstrate markedly increased signal intensity of the biliary tree and gallbladder but not of the noncommunicating liver cyst.

Ultrasonography

Typically, hepatic cysts manifest as well-defined, anechoic lesions with well-defined margins and posterior acoustic enhancement on gray-scale ultrasonography (see Fig. 63-1). Complicated cysts may show atypical appearances, such as internal septations, debris, and a thickened wall with or without calcification.

Nuclear Medicine

Findings at radionuclide scintigraphy are rarely diagnostic for hepatic cysts.

PET/CT

Findings at PET/CT are rarely diagnostic for hepatic cysts.

Imaging Algorithm

An ideal algorithm is presented in Figure 63-15 at the end of this discussion.

Classic Signs: Simple Cysts

- Thin wall
- Anechoic cystic content and posterior echo enhancement
- No contrast enhancement after intravenous injection of a contrast agent
- Fluid filled
- Homogeneous

Differential Diagnosis

Clinical findings usually do not contribute to the diagnosis of simple hepatic cysts. Strong hyperintensity on heavily T2-weighted MR images allows differentiation from most hepatic metastases, with the exception of those originating from neuroendocrine tumors. Unlike hepatic abscesses or cystic neoplasms, hepatic cysts present with a very thin, almost imperceptible nonenhancing wall, as well as lack of intralesional septa and mural nodules. Polycystic liver disease will usually consist of numerous cystic lesions, with size varying from a few millimeters to several centimeters, and is associated with adult recessive polycystic kidney disease. Hydatid cyst usually contains several daughter cysts and is surrounded by calcified walls. Biliary hamartomas are usually numerous and smaller than 15-mm cystic lesions, whereas Caroli's disease will consist of multiple segmental biliary dilatation, typically showing the "central dot sign," owing to a portal venous branch surrounded by a cystic lesion secondary to arrested development of the intrahepatic biliary tree (Fig. 63-2; Table 63-2).

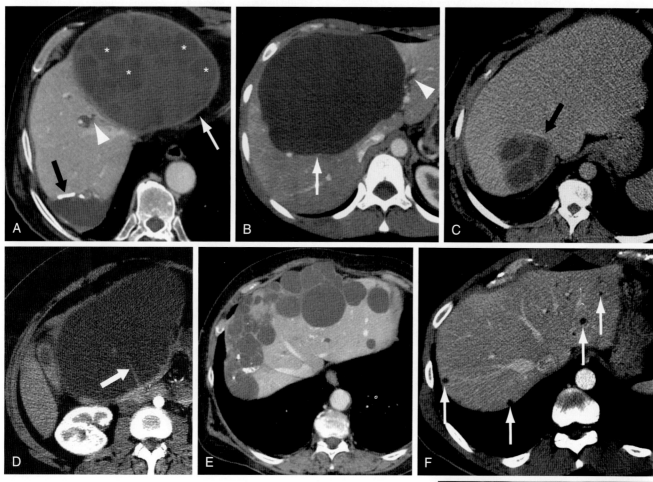

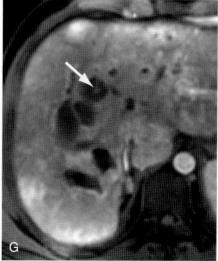

■ **FIGURE 63-2** Imaging findings and differential diagnosis among different cystic lesions of the liver, including hydatid cyst, simple cyst, pyogenic abscess, biliary cystadenoma, polycystic liver disease, biliary hamartomas, and Caroli's disease. **A** to **F**, Portal venous phase CT. **G,** Gadolinium-enhanced T1-weighted gradient-recalled-echo MR image. **A,** Calcified wall (*black arrow*), thick enhancing wall (*white arrow*), and daughter cysts (*asterisks*) are typical of hydatid cyst. **B,** A simple hepatic cyst has no visible wall (*arrow*). Note the mild intrahepatic biliary dilatation (*arrowhead*) due to mass effect in both cases. Other findings that may help in narrowing differential diagnosis when facing cystic liver lesions are (**C, D**) thick enhancing walls (*arrow, C*) and internal septa (*arrow, D*) in pyogenic liver abscess and biliary cystadenoma, (**E**) multiplicity and partially calcified walls in polycystic liver disease, (**F**) small size (<15 mm) and multiplicity (*arrows*) in biliary hamartomas, and (**G**) demonstration of a "dot sign" (*arrow*) due to a centrolesional portal venous branch in Caroli's disease.

TABLE 63-2 Demographics and Pathologic and Clinical Features of Hydatid Cyst, Simple Cyst, Pyogenic Abscess, Biliary Cystadenoma, Polycystic Liver Disease, Biliary Hamartomas, and Caroli's Disease

	Hydatid Cyst	Simple Cyst	Pyogenic Abscess	Biliary Cystadenoma	Polycystic Liver Disease	Biliary Hamartomas	Caroli's Disease
Sex	F = M	F > M	F = M	F > M	F > M	M > F	F > M
Age	3-4th decade	5-6th decade	5-7th decade	2-5th decade	5-6th decade	Any age	2-3rd decade
Frequency	Depend on geographic area	Very common	Common	Rare	Rare	Common	Very rare
Clinical Features	Asymptomatic	Asymptomatic	Fever, pain	Asymptomatic	Mass effect	Asymptomatic	Fever (cholangitis)
Location	Right lobe > left	All liver segments	Right lobe > left	Right lobe > left	All liver segments	All liver segments	All liver segments
Number	Multiple (60%)	Solitary > Multiple	Multiple	Solitary	Multiple	Multiple	Multiple
Size	3-30 cm	0.5-30 cm	0.5-10 cm	1-20 cm	1-10 cm	<15 mm	0.5-5 cm
Wall Calcification	Yes	Rare, peripheral	No	Rare	Rare	No	No
Septations	Present	Absent	Present	Present	Absent	Absent	Absent
Gas	No	No	Present (20%)	No	No	No	No
Inflammatory Changes	Absent	Absent	Present	Absent	No	No	No
Multiplicity	Possible	Absent	Present	No	No	No	Yes
Signs at Imaging and Associated Conditions	Intralesional daughter cysts and wall calcifications	Increased through-transmission at ultrasonography, hypoattenuation to blood pool at unenhanced CT	Cluster sign		Adult recessive polycystic kidney disease	Multiplicity and small (<15 mm) size, congenital hepatic fibrosis, Caroli's disease	Dot sign, congenital hepatic fibrosis, biliary hamartomas

Treatment

Medical Treatment

Because simple cysts are rarely complicated, they should be treated conservatively.

What the Referring Physician Needs to Know: Simple Cysts

- Simple cysts are among the most common liver lesions.
- They occur most often in middle-aged women.
- Conservative management is warranted.
- Ultrasonography is usually sufficient to confirm or rule out the diagnosis.

Surgical Treatment

Percutaneous catheter drainage with alcohol sclerosis may be an effective therapy for larger, symptomatic cysts. Rarely, hepatic cysts are treated surgically.

Hepatic Hemangioma

Etiology

Hemangiomas are probably congenital in origin, and no definite predisposing factors have been identified. Because they increase with multiparity, female sex hormones have been suggested as a cause.

Prevalence and Epidemiology

Hemangioma is the most common benign hepatic tumor with an estimated incidence of 5% to 20% in the general population.[5] Although hemangiomas can occur in both sexes at all ages, middle-aged women are more frequently affected, perhaps reflecting the causative effect of female sex hormones.[5]

Clinical Presentation

Typically, hemangiomas are incidental imaging findings in asymptomatic patients. Occasionally, larger lesions may produce signs and symptoms related to mass effect, such as upper abdominal mass, abdominal discomfort, and pain. Rarely, sudden onset with acute pain can develop after either spontaneous or traumatic rupture of larger lesions. Giant hemangiomas can also manifest as thrombo-cytopenia and consumptive coagulopathy.

Pathophysiology

Hemangiomas can occur on all liver segments with equal frequency.

Pathology

Characteristically, hemangiomas manifest as either solitary or multiple, well-defined masses, varying in size from few millimeters to several centimeters.[5] Hemangiomas are infrequently detected or are generally smaller when occurring within a cirrhotic liver, probably owing to progressive tumor shrinkage by liver fibrosis.[6] On sectioning, hemangiomas show a typical red-blue appearance with a spongy or honeycombing surface.[5] Organized thrombi, fibrosis, and calcification may be noted grossly, particularly in the central area of larger lesions. Occasionally, sclerosis may involve the entire lesion, which manifests as a firm, gray-white nodule of fibrous tissue (the so-called sclerosed hemangioma).

Association of hemangioma with other benign liver lesions, such as FNH and hepatic adenoma, has been described.[7]

At histology, hemangioma consists of several communicating blood-filled spaces, lined by a single layer of flat endothelial cells, which are supported by a thin basement membrane.[5]

Liver Function

Liver function test results are generally unremarkable, although patients with giant hemangiomas can occasionally have a mild increase in alkaline phosphatase level.

Imaging

Because of the high incidence in the general population, hemangiomas are frequently discovered incidentally at either ultrasonography, CT, or MRI of the liver.

Radiography

Although larger lesions may deform one of the visible borders of the liver or cause mass effect on adjacent structures, more often a plain abdominal radiograph does not provide any clinical information in patients with hemangiomas.

CT

At precontrast CT, hemangiomas manifest as hypoattenuating lesions relative to the liver. However, because lesions may be hyperattenuating if occurring in the setting of diffuse fatty liver disease due to uniformly decreased attenuation of the hepatic parenchyma,[8] a more reliable criterion for the diagnosis of hemangioma is isoattenuation to aorta and intrahepatic vessels. Central calcifications may occur in giant hemangiomas.

At contrast-enhanced CT, hemangiomas classically show early, peripheral, nodular enhancement, with centripetal progression. The enhancing areas of hemangiomas are isoattenuating to aorta during the hepatic arterial phase and to blood pool during the portal venous phase and delayed phase (Fig. 63-3).[9,10] When all typical criteria are observed, lack of complete lesion enhancement on the delayed phase should not dissuade from the diagnosis of hemangioma. Giant hemangiomas usually lack complete enhancement on delayed phase imaging owing to thrombosis or sclerosis of the central portion of the tumor.

Small hemangiomas (<2.0 cm)—also known as "capillary hemangiomas" or "flash filling hemangiomas"—may enhance rapidly and homogeneously during the hepatic arterial phase (Fig. 63-4), thus mimicking other benign or malignant hypervascular liver tumors (Tables 63-3 and 63-4). Transient peritumoral enhancement during the hepatic arterial phase is frequently observed owing to associated arteriovenous shunt.

A sclerosed hemangioma usually lacks any contrast enhancement at different vascular phases.

MRI

Because hemangiomas are composed almost entirely of blood, their T1 and T2 values are very long, thus explaining the very low signal intensity on T1-weighted images and markedly high signal intensity on T2-weighted images, even at longer echo times (e.g., >120 ms).[11] The complex internal architecture of giant hemangiomas can be better depicted on T2-weighted images as low-signal strands of fibrous stroma, which gives the lesion a characteristic appearance.

On gadolinium-enhanced MRI, the tumor enhancement pattern is substantially comparable to that at CT (Fig. 63-5).

Ultrasonography

Typically, hemangioma manifests as a homogeneous, hyperechoic mass with well-defined margins on gray-scale ultrasonography (see Fig. 63-3). Occasionally, lesions appear iso- or hypoechoic relative to the liver, surrounded by a peripheral hyperechoic rim.

With microbubble contrast agents, a contrast enhancement pattern closely resembles that found on CT and MRI (Fig. 63-6).

Nuclear Medicine

Technetium-99m pertechnetate–labeled red blood cell scintigraphy has been regarded as a reference standard for the diagnosis of hemangiomas. Because hemangiomas have increased blood volume relative to the liver, they manifest as a hot spot on blood pool scanning (30 to 50 minutes after injection of the radiotracer).

PET/CT

PET/CT has no role in the diagnosis of hemangiomas.

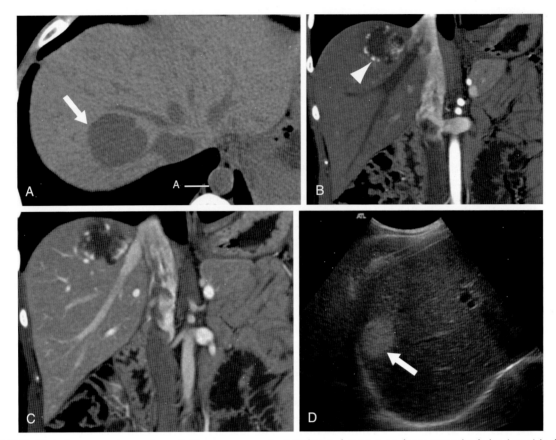

■ **FIGURE 63-3** Typical cavernous hemangioma. **A,** Transverse precontrast CT image shows a 4-cm, hypoattenuating lesion (*arrow*) in the right lobe of the liver. Note the equal attenuation of the lesion with both aorta (A) and intrahepatic vessels. **B** and **C,** Coronally reformatted images of the same patient demonstrate nodular, peripheral, discontinuous enhancement (*arrowhead,* **B**) on both (**B**) hepatic arterial phase and (**C**) portal venous phase, which is comparable to vessels on all vascular phases. **D,** Ultrasound image in a different patient shows a homogeneous, well-defined, hyperechoic lesion (*arrow*) of the right hepatic lobe.

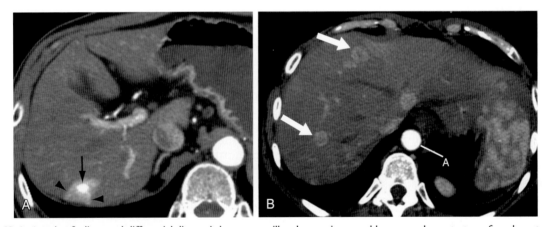

■ **FIGURE 63-4** Imaging findings and differential diagnosis between capillary hemangioma and hypervascular metastases from breast carcinoma on transverse contrast-enhanced CT during hepatic arterial phase. **A,** Capillary hemangioma (*arrow*) manifests as an isoattenuating lesion compared with the aorta, surrounded by a wedge-shaped, homogeneous, moderately hyperattenuating area (*arrowheads*) due to arteriovenous shunt. **B,** Hypervascular metastases (*arrows*) are multiple and demonstrate more heterogeneous enhancement, which is not as strong as aorta (A). Enhancement characteristics along with a history of primary tumor allow the correct diagnosis.

TABLE 63-3 Differential Features between Capillary Hemangioma, Cavernous Hemangioma, Metastases, Focal Nodular Hyperplasia, and Large Benign Regenerative Nodules

	Capillary Hemangioma	Cavernous Hemangioma	Metastases	Focal Nodular Hyperplasia	Large Benign Regenerative Nodules
Sex	F > M	F > M	M = F	F >> M	F > M
Age	2-5th decade	2-5th decade	6-7th decade	3-4th decade	3-4th decade
Ultrasound Findings	Hypointense with hyperechoic border	Hyperechoic	Hypoechoic	Isoechoic	Variable
Sustained Enhancement on Portal Venous and Delayed Phases	Yes	Yes	No	Yes	Yes
Isoattenuating to Vessels at CT	Yes	Yes	No	No	No
Hyperintensity on T2	Strong	Strong	Mild*	Mild	No
Homogeneous Enhancement on Hepatic Arterial Phase	Yes	No	No	Yes	Yes
Enhancement	Homogeneous	Peripheral, discontinuous	Peripheral, ring-like	Homogeneous	Homogeneous
Calcifications	No	Central if present	No†	1%	No
Scar	No	Rare (larger lesions)	No	Yes	Larger lesions
Necrosis	No	No	Yes	No	No
Number	Single > multiple	Single > multiple	Multiple	Single (75%)	Multiple
History of Malignancy	No	No	Yes	No	No

*Except for neuroendocrine tumors, mucinous colon cancer, and breast cancer that may be strongly hyperintense.
†Except for mucinous colon cancer metastases that may have scattered calcifications.

TABLE 63-4 Differential Features between Focal Nodular Hyperplasia, Large Benign Regenerative Nodules, Hepatocellular Adenoma, Hepatocellular Carcinoma, Hypervascular Metastases, and Cavernous Hemangioma

	FNH	LBRN	HCA/ Adenomatosis	HCC	Hypervascular Metastases	Cavernous Hemangioma
Sex	F >> M	F > M	F >> M	M > F	M = F	F > M
Age	3-4th decade	3-4th decade	3-4th decade	6-7th decade	6-7th decade	2-5th decade
History of Cirrhosis	No	No	No	Yes	No	No
Association with Use of Oral Contraceptives	No	No	Yes	No	No	No
Liver Morphology	Normal	Normal	Normal	Abnormal	Normal	Normal
Ultrasound Findings	Isoechoic	Variable	Variable	Hypoechoic	Hypoechoic	Hyperechoic
Hypervascularity on Hepatic Arterial Phase	Strong	Strong	Mild	Mild	Mild	Nodular, peripheral
Homogeneity	Yes	Yes	No	No	No	No
Calcifications	1%	No	Rare	Rare	No	Rare (larger lesions)
Signal Drop on Out-of-Phase MRI	No	No	Yes	Rare	No	No
Signal Intensity on T2	Hyperintense (mild)	Hypointense	Hyperintense (mild)	Hyperintense (mild)	Hyperintense (mild*)	Hyperintense (strong)
Wash Out on Portal Venous and Delayed Phases	No	No	Yes	Yes	Yes	No
Delayed Enhancement on Hepatobiliary Phase at MRI	Yes	Yes	No	No	No	No
Ferromagnetic Agent Uptake at MRI	Yes	No	No	No	No	No

*Except for neuroendocrine tumors, mucinous colon cancer, and breast cancer that may be strongly hyperintense.

Imaging Algorithm

An ideal algorithm is presented in Figure 63-15.

Classic Signs: Hemangiomas

- Isoattenuation to blood pool on all phases
- Peripheral, nodular enhancement
- Centripetal enhancement
- Marked hyperintensity on T2-weighted MR images

Differential Diagnosis

Clinical findings usually do not contribute to the diagnosis of hepatic hemangiomas. Unlike most primary or secondary hypervascular malignant liver tumors, hemangiomas invariably show sustained enhancement comparable to blood pool during the portal venous and delayed phases of CT (see Fig. 63-4) or MRI. In addition, unlike most malignant liver tumors, marked hyperintensity of hemangiomas on T2-weighted MR images (see Fig. 63-5) typically persists with longer echo times (see Table 63-3).

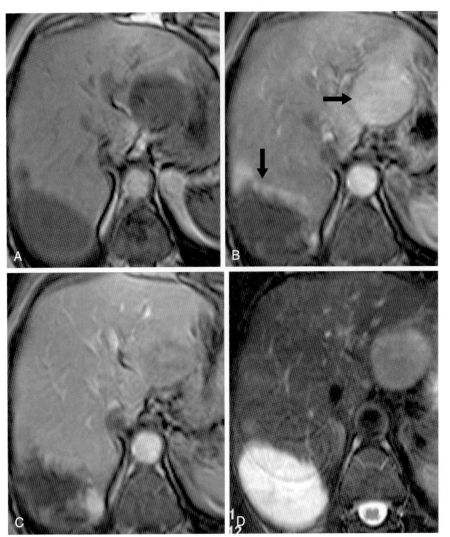

■ **FIGURE 63-5** Imaging findings and differential diagnosis at MRI between cavernous hemangioma and hypervascular sarcoma metastasis coexisting in the same liver. **A,** Although both lesions are hypointense to surrounding liver parenchyma on T1-weighted gradient-recalled echo MRI, metastasis (*horizontal arrow,* **B**) shows moderate hypervascularity and rapid wash out on gadolinium-enhanced T1-weighted gradient-recalled-echo MR image during hepatic arterial phase (**B**) and portal venous phase (**C**), respectively. **B** and **C,** On the same imaging phases, cavernous hemangioma (*vertical arrow,* **B**) typically shows nodular, peripheral, discontinuous enhancement, which progresses centripetally. **D,** Fat-suppressed T2-weighted fast-spin-echo MR image shows strong hyperintensity of hemangioma while only moderate hyperintensity of metastasis.

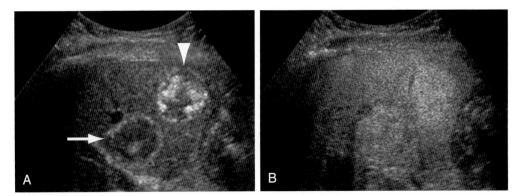

■ **FIGURE 63-6** Typical ultrasound images of two hepatic hemangiomas. **A,** During hepatic arterial phase, lesions show either minimal, peripheral enhancement (*arrow*) or prominent, peripheral, globular enhancement (*arrowhead*). **B,** During portal venous phase, both lesions show centripetal progression of enhancement to complete fill. (*Courtesy of Dr. Tommaso V. Bartolotta, University of Palermo.*)

Metastases from neuroendocrine tumors, mucinous cancer of the colon, and breast cancer may show strong hyperintensity on T2-weighted images that may mimic hemangiomas (see Table 63-3). Biopsy may be necessary in doubtful cases.

Treatment

Medical Treatment

Because hemangiomas virtually never cause complications, they should be treated conservatively.

Surgical Treatment

Larger lesions can be treated surgically (i.e., enucleation or resection) when clinically symptomatic.

What the Referring Physician Needs to Know: Hemangiomas

- Hemangiomas occur most often in middle-aged women.
- If the appearance is classic for hemangioma at ultrasonography, no further evaluation should be required in patients without a history of underlying malignancy.
- Conservative management is warranted, unless large symptomatic lesions are present.
- Lesions may occasionally enlarge.
- Biopsy can be safely performed in the case of atypical lesions.

Hepatocellular Adenoma

Etiology

Although the etiology of hepatocellular adenoma (HCA) is unknown, steroid medications (i.e., estrogen-containing or androgen-containing) represent the main promoters of lesion growth. The incidence of HCA is increased in the setting of type I glycogen storage disease as well as in congenital or acquired abnormalities of hepatic vasculature.

Prevalence and Epidemiology

HCA most frequently occurs in women of reproductive age (male-to-female ratio, 1 : 10). The estimated incidence of HCA in patients undergoing steroid therapy is 4 cases in every 100,000 steroid users.

Occasionally, HCA can be multiple (>10) in patients without commonly associated predisposing factors (liver adenomatosis).[12]

Clinical Presentation

Although HCA can be asymptomatic, it is generally diagnosed as symptoms develop, including an abdominal mass and either acute or chronic abdominal pain after intratumoral hemorrhage. Occasionally, hemorrhage may be severe enough to produce hemorrhagic shock, thus requiring emergency surgery.

Pathophysiology

HCA most commonly originates within the right liver lobe (75% of cases), particularly underneath the hepatic capsule.

Pathology

Typically, HCA manifests as a large, well-demarcated mass.[13] On sectioning, it shows a variegated appearance owing to areas of hemorrhage or necrosis.[13] Multiple lesions are more commonly present in patients with glycogen storage disease type I.

Histologically, HCA consists of normal-appearing hepatocytes arranged in sheets and cords without acinar architecture.[13] Tumor cells typically contain an increased amount of fat and glycogen and are separated by abnormally enlarged sinusoids, which account for the higher risk of intratumoral hemorrhage.[13] Unlike FNH, bile ducts are invariably absent.[13]

Liver Function

Liver function test results are generally unremarkable. Increased α-fetoprotein levels are suggestive of malignant transformation.

Imaging

Contrast-enhanced CT and MRI and, more recently, contrast-enhanced ultrasonography represent the modalities of choice for preoperative assessment of HCA.

Radiography

Plain abdominal radiographs do not usually provide any information in patients with HCA.

CT

CT findings of HCA correspond to its appearance at gross inspection. At precontrast CT, most tumors manifest as large, heterogeneous masses due to hemorrhage, necrosis, and calcification,[14] although smaller lesions may be isoattenuating relative to liver.

Because of the increased arterial supply, HCA is usually hypervascular and appears as a hyperattenuating lesion compared with the surrounding liver at contrast-enhanced CT during the hepatic arterial phase, with the only exception of intratumoral areas of hemorrhage, fat, and necrosis. HCA generally shows variable wash out during the portal venous and delayed phases (Fig. 63-7).[14]

When occurring in the setting of diffuse fatty liver disease, HCA is hyperattenuating relative to the liver either before or after administration of a contrast agent.

MRI

MRI findings of HCA closely resemble those of either primary or secondary malignant liver lesions. Compared with the adjacent liver, HCA typically shows mild hyperintensity and hypoisointensity on T2- and T1-weighted

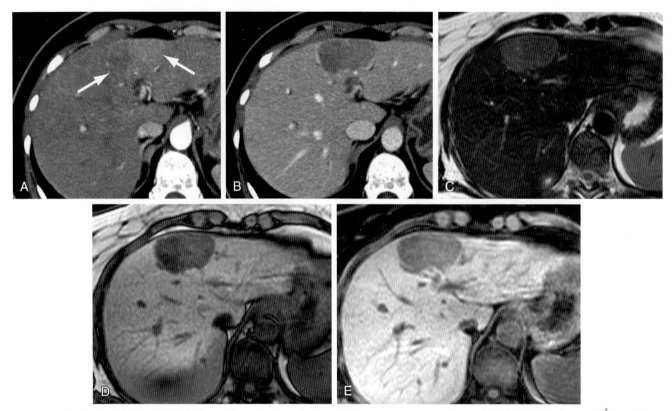

■ **FIGURE 63-7** Typical CT and MRI findings of hepatic adenoma. **A** and **B,** Transverse contrast-enhanced CT during hepatic arterial phase (**A**) shows a 4-cm, heterogeneously and mildly hypervascular lesion (*arrows*) in the left liver lobe. **B,** Note marked wash out during portal venous phase. **C,** Corresponding T2-weighted turbo spin-echo MR image shows mild hyperintensity of the lesion in comparison to the surrounding liver. **D** and **E,** Dual-echo T1-weighted gradient-recalled-echo MR image demonstrates substantial signal loss of the lesion on opposed-phase image (**D**) compared with in-phase image (**E**) due to increased content of cytoplasmic lipids within tumor cells.

images, respectively.[15,16] Because of intracellular deposition of fat, opposed-phase MR images can demonstrate substantial drop of signal of HCA (see Fig. 63-7). Occasionally, a reversal signal intensity pattern may be observed when lesions occur in the setting of diffuse fatty liver disease.

On gadolinium-enhanced MRI, the tumor enhancement pattern is substantially comparable to that at CT (see Fig. 63-7).[15,16]

Unlike FNH, HCA cannot take up hepatobiliary liver-specific contrast agents owing to absence of biliary ductules within the lesion and thus appear as hypointense masses against the highly enhanced background liver on delayed phase images.[17]

Ultrasonography

HCA shows a variable, nonspecific appearance on gray-scale ultrasonography. By providing insights into the vascular enhancement pattern of liver lesions, microbubble contrast agents have been shown to provide reliable differentiation between HCA and FNH. Unlike FNH, HCA is characterized by a mixed filling without the typical stellate vascularity.[18]

Nuclear Medicine

Findings at radionuclide scintigraphy are rarely diagnostic for HCA.

PET/CT

The role of PET/CT in the diagnosis of HCA has not been explored.

Imaging Algorithm

An ideal algorithm is presented in Figure 63-15.

Classic Signs: Hepatocellular Adenoma
■ More common in women
■ Associated with use of oral contraceptives
■ Hypervascular
■ Wash out
■ Signal drop on out-of-phase imaging
■ Heterogeneous
■ Rupture
■ Degeneration
■ Associated with other benign hepatic tumors

Differential Diagnosis

Tumor interval growth with or without increased α-fetoprotein levels is highly suggestive of hepatocellular carcinoma (HCC) or, alternatively, malignant degeneration of HCA. Although larger HCA can be easily differentiated from FNH based on the heterogeneous appearance (see Fig. 63-7), the differential diagnosis can be challenging at imaging and even at histopathology when the lesions are small (see Table 63-4). Liver-specific MR contrast agents with hepatobiliary excretion have been shown to be accurate in differentiating HCA from FNH, because the absence of biliary ductules precludes active contrast uptake on delayed imaging by tumor cells in HCA.[17]

Because HCA cannot be differentiated with confidence from both HCC and hypervascular liver metastases, hepatic biopsy is warranted for diagnosis (see Table 63-4).

Treatment

Medical Treatment

Discontinuation of steroid medication is indicated in the conservative management of smaller lesions (<5.0 cm).

Surgical Treatment

Because of the increased risk of complications (i.e., rupture or malignant transformation), surgical resection is warranted for larger lesions (>5.0 cm). Emergency surgery is required in the event of lesion rupture.

What the Referring Physician Needs to Know: Hepatocellular Adenoma

- Women of reproductive age with a long-term history of use of oral contraceptives are affected.
- Smaller lesions (<5.0 cm) can be treated conservatively with discontinuation of contraceptive medication and follow-up.
- Larger lesions (>5.0 cm) generally require surgery.

Focal Nodular Hyperplasia

Etiology

Rather than a neoplastic process, FNH is considered to be a hyperplastic response of the hepatic parenchyma to a congenital or acquired anomaly of the arterial blood supply leading to focal hyperperfusion.[19] Unlike hepatic adenoma, oral contraceptives do not play a role for the development of FNH but their use may stimulate its growth.

Prevalence and Epidemiology

FNH most frequently occurs in women of childbearing age (male-to-female ratio, 1:8). After hemangioma, FNH is the second most common benign tumor of the liver, with an estimated incidence of 3% to 8% in the general population.

Clinical Presentation

Typically, FNH is an incidental finding in asymptomatic patients. Rarely, larger lesions may manifest as an abdomi-

nal mass and/or abdominal discomfort, which is occasionally associated with pain.

Pathophysiology

FNH can occur on all liver segments. In 25% of cases FNH is multiple.

Pathology

Characteristically, FNH manifests as a single, well-circumscribed, unencapsulated mass, varying in size from few millimeters to several centimeters. On sectioning, lobulated margins are seen. A stellate fibrous scar (either central or eccentric) represents a hallmark for the diagnosis.

Association of FNH with hepatic hemangioma[7,20] and HCA[21] has been described.

At histology, FNH consists of multiple monoacinar nodules (approximately 1 mm in diameter) composed of normal-appearing hepatocytes arranged in cell plates 1 to 2 mm thick.[13,19] Nodules are clustered around a fibrous core with radiating septa that contain enlarged feeding arteries and numerous capillaries.[13,19] At the interface between hepatocytes and fibrous bands, a cholangiolar proliferation surrounded by an inflammatory infiltrate of variable amount is usually present. Occasionally, lesions show some degree of fatty infiltration.

Different histologic variants of FNH have been described (i.e., the telangiectatic type, the mixed hyperplastic and adenomatous form, and the variety with cytologic atypia).[20]

Liver Function

Liver function test results are generally unremarkable.

Imaging

With current advances in modern cross-sectional imaging, an increasing number of lesions of FNH are incidentally detected in asymptomatic patients.

Radiography

A plain abdominal radiograph does not provide any clinical information in the investigation of patients with FNH.

CT

At precontrast CT, most FNH is isoattenuating relative to the adjacent liver and, thus, cannot be reliably detected. When occurring in the setting of diffuse fatty liver disease, FNH is typically hyperattenuating because of uniformly decreased attenuation of the hepatic parenchyma.

With the only exception of the central fibrous scar, FNH shows vivid enhancement at contrast-enhanced CT during the hepatic arterial phase[21] and manifests as homogeneous hyperattenuating lesions compared with the surrounding liver. Whereas lesions gradually fade during the

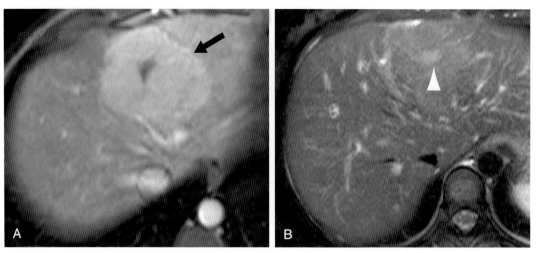

■ **FIGURE 63-8** Typical MRI findings of focal nodular hyperplasia (FNH). **A,** Gadolinium-enhanced T1-weighted gradient-recalled-echo MR image during hepatic arterial phase shows strong and homogeneous hyperintensity of FNH (*arrow*), with the exception of a central hypointense scar. **B,** Corresponding T2-weighted turbo spin-echo MR image shows hyperintensity of the central scar (*arrowhead*). Homogeneous enhancement on hepatic arterial phase and hyperintensity of central scar on T2-weighted imaging are useful features in differentiating FNH from fibrolamellar hepatocellular carcinoma.

portal venous and delayed phases, thus becoming isoattenuating relative to the liver, the central scar typically shows delayed enhancement (5 to 10 minutes from the start of injection of contrast medium).

Although most lesions can be confidently diagnosed based on this characteristic enhancement pattern, in a limited number of cases FNH may show atypical imaging findings, such as wash out (i.e., hypoattenuating to liver parenchyma) during the portal venous and delayed phases, peripheral rim enhancement, absence of a central scar (particularly for lesions <3.0 cm), or lack of delayed enhancement of the central scar.[22] Atypical FNH may simulate either primary or secondary hypervascular malignant liver tumors and, thus, warrant further investigation with liver biopsy.

MRI

Because FNH is almost entirely composed of normal hepatocytes, lesions are nearly isointense compared with the adjacent liver on both T1- and T2-weighted MR images,[23] with the only exception of the central scar, which is typically hypointense on T1-weighted images and hyperintense on T2-weighted images owing to an abundance of myxomatous stroma.

On gadolinium-enhanced MRI, the tumor enhancement pattern is substantially comparable to that at CT (Figs. 63-8 and 63-9).[24] Notably, unlike most malignant liver tumors, FNH shows normal uptake of either hepatobiliary or reticuloendothelial system liver-specific MR contrast agents.[24]

Telangiectatic FNH can be distinguished from typical FNH because of absence of a central fibrous scar, increased signal intensity on T2- and T1-weighted images, and heterogeneous contrast enhancement during the hepatic arterial phase, which persists during the portal venous and delayed phases.[25] Several genetic similarities between telangiectatic FNH and hepatocellular adenoma have, however, been identified recently. Therefore, "telangiec-

tatic hepatocellular adenoma" has been proposed as a more appropriate definition for this lesion.

Ultrasonography

According to recent reports, FNH can be reliably diagnosed at ultrasonography with microbubble contrast agents based on the distinctive enhancement characterized by centrifugal filling of the lesion during the hepatic arterial phase (the so-called spoke-wheel appearance). In addition, FNH shows sustained enhancement in the late parenchymal phase.[18]

Nuclear Medicine

On hepatobiliary scintigraphy with tracers that simulate the behavior of bilirubin, such as ^{99m}Tc diethyl-iminodiacetic acid, FNH manifests as an area of increased and prolonged uptake of the radiopharmaceutical ("hot spot") into the abnormally developed biliary ducts of the tumor.

On ^{99m}Tc-labeled sulfur colloid imaging, two thirds of FNH show normal uptake of the tracer due to a normal number of Kupffer cells.

PET/CT

On FDG-PET, tumor metabolic activity is comparable to that of the normal liver.

Imaging Algorithm

An ideal algorithm is presented in Figure 63-15.

Differential Diagnosis

Clinical findings usually do not contribute to the diagnosis of FNH. Although FNH can be easily differentiated from

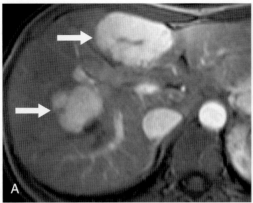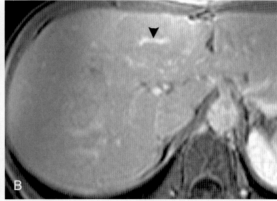

■ **FIGURE 63-9** MRI findings of multiple FNH. **A,** Gadolinium-enhanced T1-weighted gradient-recalled-echo MR image obtained during hepatic arterial phase shows two FNH lesions (*arrows*) with homogeneous bright enhancement in comparison to adjacent liver parenchyma. A central hypointense scar is noted in the larger lesion. **B,** Corresponding image obtained during delayed phase shows lesion isointensity compared with the background hepatic parenchyma and hyperintensity (*arrowhead*) of the central scar. Strong and homogeneous enhancement of the tumor on hepatic arterial phase and scar hyperintensity on delayed phase are key findings for a confident diagnosis.

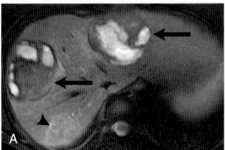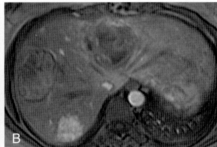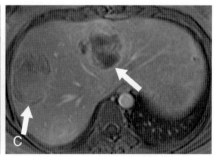

■ **FIGURE 63-10** MRI findings and differential diagnosis between FNH and bleeding hepatic adenomas coexisting in the same liver. Axial T2-weighted (**A**), hepatic arterial phase T1-weighted (**B**), and delayed phase T1-weighted (**C**) MR images. Typical imaging findings of FNH include slight hyperintensity (*arrowhead,* **A**) in comparison with the surrounding liver on T2-weighted image and strong and homogeneous enhancement on T1-weighted gradient-recalled-echo MR image during the hepatic arterial phase, which fades to isointensity on the corresponding delayed phase image, with the exception of the enhancing central scar. On the other side, adenomas (*arrows*) demonstrate heterogeneous signal intensity on a T2-weighted image, which correspond to areas of intralesional bleeding. Lesions show minimal, heterogeneous enhancement on hepatic arterial phase and wash out on delayed phase images, with the exception of a peripherally enhancing capsule.

Classic Signs: Focal Nodular Hyperplasia

- Homogeneous, bright enhancement on hepatic arterial phase
- Same enhancement of background "nonfatty" liver on non-contrast images and portal venous and delayed phases
- Contrast retention of scar on delayed phase images
- Hyperintense scar on T2-weighted images
- Association with other benign liver neoplasms

HCA based on characteristic imaging findings (Fig. 63-10), their appearance may overlap in smaller lesions. Liver-specific MR contrast agents[17] and, more recently, dynamic evaluation of the lesion perfusion at contrast-enhanced ultrasonography[18] may provide additional clues for differential diagnosis at imaging.

Liver-specific MR contrast agents also enable discrimination of FNH from either primary or secondary hypervascular malignant liver tumors (see Table 63-1).

In comparison to large benign regenerative nodules, FNH usually manifests as solitary, larger lesions originating within a normal liver (see Tables 63-3 and 64-4).

Because of rapid and homogeneous enhancement, small hemangiomas can mimic FNH during the hepatic arterial phase (the so-called flash-filling hemangiomas). However, marked hyperintensity on T2-weighted images, as well as isointensity to blood vessels on contrast-enhanced images during different vascular phases, usually allows a confident diagnosis of hemangioma (see Table 63-3). Differential diagnosis between FNH and cavernous hemangioma is usually not a challenge based on the characteristic enhancement pattern and intensity of both lesions (Fig. 63-11) (see Tables 63-3 and 63-4).

Treatment

Medical Treatment

Withdrawal of oral contraceptive medication usually results in lesion size reduction.

Surgical Treatment

Because of the lack of malignant potential and the extremely low complication rate, FNH warrants conservative management.

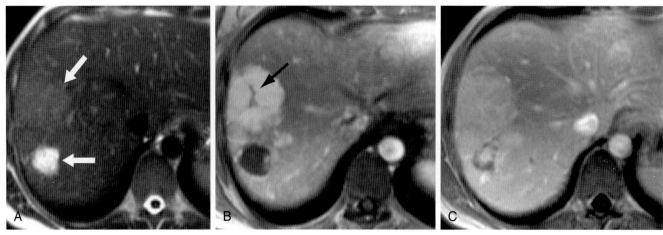

■ **FIGURE 63-11** MRI findings and differential diagnosis between FNH and cavernous hemangioma coexisting in the same liver. **A,** Unlike FNH (*oblique arrow*), which is only mildly hyperintense compared with the liver, hemangioma (*horizontal arrow*) demonstrates marked hyperintensity on this transverse T2-weighted MR image, which is comparable to cerebrospinal fluid intensity ("light-bulb" sign). **B** and **C,** On gadolinium-enhanced T1-weighted gradient-recalled-echo MR images, hemangioma shows nodular peripheral enhancement with progressive, centripetal fill while FNH demonstrates strong, immediate enhancement apart from the central hypointense scar (*arrow*) on hepatic arterial phase (**B**). FNH is nearly isointense to surrounding liver during the delayed phase (**C**).

What the Referring Physician Needs to Know: Focal Nodular Hyperplasia

- Young women are affected.
- Conservative management is warranted owing to lack of malignant potential and extremely low complication rate.
- Discontinuation of contraceptive medication is recommended owing to its stimulating effect on lesion growth.
- Atypical lesions may require further investigation with liver biopsy.

Large Benign Regenerative Nodules

Etiology

Large benign regenerative nodules represent a hyperplastic response of the liver in areas with preserved blood supply secondary to impaired perfusion of the remaining hepatic parenchyma. Although several liver disorders may lead to the development of large benign regenerative nodules, most cases have been reported in patients with Budd-Chiari syndrome.

Prevalence and Epidemiology

Large benign regenerative nodules most frequently occur in young to middle-aged women, perhaps reflecting the gender prevalence of the underlying disorders. They are infrequently reported in childhood. Large benign regenerative nodules almost invariably coexist with diffuse nodular regenerative hyperplasia (NRH) of the liver, which is characterized by diffuse micronodular transformation of the hepatic parenchyma with minimal or no fibrosis.

Clinical Presentation

Although NRH and large benign regenerative nodules may be completely asymptomatic, occasionally patients may develop symptoms, such as portal hypertension and hepatic failure.

Pathophysiology

Large benign regenerative nodules may occur anywhere within the liver.

Pathology

Characteristically, large benign regenerative nodules manifest as multiple, rounded, well-circumscribed, unencapsulated masses, varying in size from 0.5 to 4.0 cm.[13] Histologically, large benign regenerative nodules consist of multiacinar nodules that are composed of normal-appearing hepatocytes arranged in cell plates 1 to 2 mm thick and are supplied by enlarged feeding arteries.[13]

Liver Function

Liver test results are usually normal or mildly abnormal due to mild elevation of alkaline phosphatase and gamma-glutamyl transpeptidase. As a general rule, α-fetoprotein levels are unremarkable.

Imaging

Although large benign regenerative nodules have been considered a rare entity, their reported frequency is rising as a result of higher-resolution contrast-enhanced CT and MRI performed with multiphasic acquisition protocols.

Radiography

A plain abdominal radiograph will not provide any information in patients with large benign regenerative nodules.

CT

Like FNH, large benign regenerative nodules are isoattenuating compared with the adjacent liver at precontrast CT

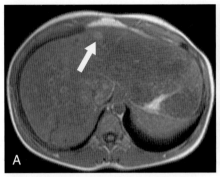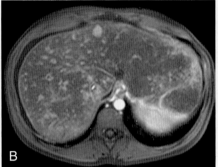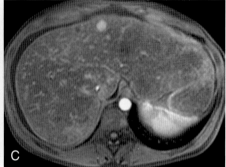

■ **FIGURE 63-12** Typical imaging findings of large benign regenerative nodules in Budd-Chiari syndrome. **A,** Lesion (*arrow*) is hyperintense compared with the adjacent liver on precontrast T1-weighted image. **B,** On gadolinium-enhanced T1-weighted gradient-recalled-echo MR image, lesion shows bright enhancement during hepatic arterial phase. **C,** There is sustained enhancement during portal venous phase. Note the small amount of ascites surrounding the enlarged liver.

and show marked, homogeneous enhancement at contrast-enhanced CT during the hepatic arterial phase.[26,27] During the portal venous and delayed phases, large benign regenerative nodules show sustained enhancement and persistent hyperattenuation relative to the hepatic parenchyma.[26,27]

MRI

Unlike FNH, which is almost invariably isointense relative to the liver on precontrast MRI, large benign regenerative nodules usually show hypointensity and hyperintensity on T2- and T1-weighted images, respectively. This finding has been related to increased content of paramagnetic metal ions (e.g., copper) within lesion hepatocytes.[26,27]

On gadolinium-enhanced MRI, the tumor enhancement pattern is substantially comparable to that at CT (Fig. 63-12).[26,27] Like FNH, large benign regenerative nodules show normal or increased uptake of hepatobiliary MR contrast agents.[27]

Ultrasonography

Large benign regenerative nodules show a variable echoic pattern at ultrasonography with most lesions (53% of cases) being hyperechoic compared with the surrounding liver.

Nuclear Medicine

Findings at radionuclide scintigraphy are rarely diagnostic for large benign regenerative nodules.

PET/CT

The role of PET/CT in large benign regenerative nodules has not been explored.

Imaging Algorithm

An ideal algorithm is presented in Figure 63-15.

Differential Diagnosis

Large benign regenerative nodules should be strongly suspected when multiple, small, hypervascular liver lesions

---

Classic Signs: Large Benign Regenerative Nodules

- Multiple
- Hypointense on T2-weighted images
- Hyperintense on T1-weighted images
- Hypervascular
- Sustained enhancement on portal venous and delayed phases

---

are discovered in association with Budd-Chiari syndrome. Because the same initiating mechanism (i.e., focal hyperperfusion of the liver) seems to precede the development of large benign regenerative nodules and FNH, in a substantial number of cases both lesions may not be differentiated at either imaging evaluation or histopathologic analysis (Fig. 63-13). Unlike FNH, large benign regenerative nodules are usually multiple, are almost invariably associated with vascular disorders of the liver (especially Budd-Chiari syndrome), and rarely show a central scar. In addition, owing to increased content of paramagnetic metal ions, large benign regenerative nodules are characteristically hypointense and hyperintense on T2- and T1-weighted MR images, respectively.

Although HCA can be confidently differentiated from large benign regenerative nodules in the majority of cases based on typical imaging findings (see Table 63-3), preserved lesion uptake of hepatobiliary excreted liver-specific MR contrast agents can be the only imaging clue for differentiating large benign regenerative nodules from liver adenomatosis.

Increased uptake of liver-specific MR contrast agents as well as sustained enhancement during the portal venous and delayed phases usually enable confident discrimination of large benign regenerative nodules from primary and secondary hypervascular malignant liver tumors (see Table 63-3).

Treatment

Medical Treatment

Because of the low malignant potential,[28] Large benign regenerative nodules warrant imaging follow-up. Therapeutic approaches are usually directed toward the

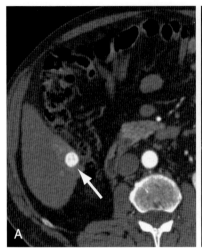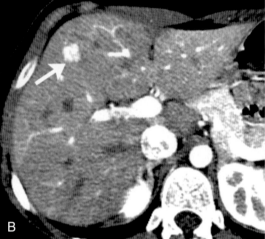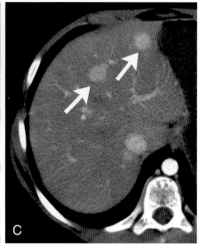

■ **FIGURE 63-13** Imaging findings and differential diagnosis between small (<2 cm) hypervascular liver lesions, including capillary hemangioma, FNH, and large benign regenerative nodules. Although all lesions demonstrate strong, homogeneous enhancement during hepatic arterial phase, some clues can be used for a differential diagnosis. **A,** Capillary hemangioma (*arrow*) demonstrates well-defined margins and characteristic enhancement comparable to aorta. Note the small, wedge-shaped, hyperattenuating area surrounding this lesion, which corresponds to an arteriovenous shunt (*arrow*). **B,** Unlike hemangioma, FNH (*arrow*) shows finely lobulated margins and a very thin central fibrous scar, which represents its diagnostic hallmark. **C,** Large benign regenerative nodules are typically multiple (*arrows*), as in this case, and almost invariably occur in the setting of impaired perfusion abnormalities of the liver (more commonly Budd-Chiari syndrome).

management of portal hypertension and include β-blocker medication and sclerotherapy for esophageal varices.

Surgical Treatment

In patients with refractory portal hypertension, mesenteric-caval shunt and transjugular intrahepatic portosystemic shunt (TIPS) are the treatments of choice. Liver transplantation represents the only potential curative therapy in patients with end-stage liver disease and progressive hepatic failure.

What the Referring Physician Needs to Know: Large Benign Regenerative Nodules

- Large benign regenerative nodules are almost invariably associated with an underlying liver disorder, most commonly Budd-Chiari syndrome.
- Because of the low malignant potential, conservative management and follow-up are warranted.

Hepatic Abscess

Etiology

Hepatic abscesses are caused by bacteria in pyogenic abscesses, *Entamoeba histolytica* in amebic abscesses, and *Candida albicans* in fungal abscesses. Choledocholithiasis, benign or obstructive malignancy, and postsurgical strictures cause extrahepatic biliary obstruction leading to ascending cholangitis and bacterial proliferation and are the most common causes of pyogenic liver abscess formation. Biliary-enteric anastomoses, pylephlebitis from appendicitis and diverticulitis, perforated gastric or duodenal ulcer, infection of infarcted hepatic parenchyma, blunt or penetrating injuries, and septicemia from bacte-

rial endocarditis have also been associated with a high incidence of liver abscesses.

Prevalence and Epidemiology

Liver abscesses are defined as localized collection of pus in liver due to an infectious process, with destruction of hepatic parenchyma and stroma. Roughly 90% are pyogenic, 9% are amebic, and 1% are fungal. Fungal abscesses occur in individuals with prolonged exposure to antibiotics, hematologic malignancies, solid-organ transplants, and immunodeficiencies. Patients are typically middle-aged or elderly.

Clinical Presentation

Patients typically present with fever and right upper quadrant pain.

Pathophysiology

Infections in organs draining into the portal system can cause a localized septic thrombophlebitis, which can lead to the development of liver abscesses. Septic emboli can result in formation of microabscesses that are initially multiple ("cluster" sign) but usually coalesce into a solitary lesion.[29]

Pathology

At gross pathology, sectioning through the pyogenic abscess cavity usually reveals multiple loculated foci, varying in size from a few millimeters to several centimeters. The cavities are usually filled with thick, purulent material and lined by pale fibrous tissue. The fibrous cuff around the abscess is often a centimeter or more thick and gradually merges into the liver parenchyma. Microscopic sections of the abscesses show necrotic fibrinopurulent debris. The edges of the cavities are lined by a chronic inflammatory infiltrate consisting of epithelioid macrophages, lymphocytes, eosinophils, and neutrophils. The fibrous tissue around the abscess cavity can contain a sparser infiltrate as well as small necrotizing and non-necrotizing granulomas.[30]

Liver Function

The white blood cell count is usually above normal, and the sedimentation rate is elevated in virtually all cases. Alkaline phosphatase is greater than the age-appropriate level in 50% of cases.

Imaging

Tender hepatomegaly, hypoalbuminemia, chills, anorexia, malaise, nausea, vomiting, weight loss, cough due to diaphragmatic irritation, atelectasis, and pleural effusion are commonly observed in patients harboring hepatic abscesses. Laboratory data reveal increased leukocytes and serum alkaline phosphatase level (67% to 90%).

Radiography

Plain abdominal radiographs might show hepatomegaly, elevation of the right hemidiaphragm, and right pleural effusion. If gas-forming organisms are present, evidence of intrahepatic air, portal venous gas, air/fluid levels, or air in the biliary tree will also be evident.

CT

On precontrast CT images, abscesses are lower in attenuation than the surrounding liver. On postcontrast images, abscesses typically show capsule and septal enhancement with central hypovascularity (Fig. 63-14). Small abscesses aggregate to coalesce into a single, usually septated, larger cavity. Air bubbles and fluid/debris levels might be seen. Intense enhancement of liver parenchyma adjacent to the abscess, when present, is caused by venous compression and poor venous drainage.[30]

MRI

On T1-weighted MR images, abscesses show low signal intensity relative to the surrounding liver. On T2-weighted images, abscesses show moderately high signal intensity. Intense enhancement of abscesses appears as a uniform ring of high signal intensity on post-gadolinium T1-weighted MRI.[30]

Ultrasonography

On ultrasonography, abscesses appear hypoechoic and heterogeneous in echotexture.

Nuclear Medicine

The role of nuclear medicine has been replaced by cross-sectional imaging. Pyogenic liver abscesses will, however,

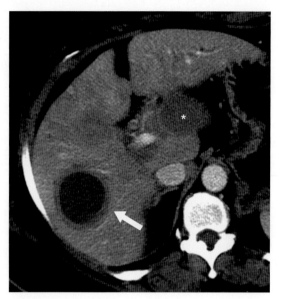

■ **FIGURE 63-14** CT findings of pyogenic abscess. Transverse contrast-enhanced CT image shows a round, well-defined, hypoattenuating lesion (*arrow*) in the right hepatic lobe, with a thick, peripherally enhancing capsule. Note bulky lymph node (*asterisk*) at the hepatic hilum. In this case, the differential diagnosis between either pyogenic or amebic abscess is not possible based on imaging criteria alone.

appear as areas of high radiotracer concentration in gallium-67 citrate studies and as cold defects on indium-111 white blood cell scintigraphy.

PET/CT

At PET/CT, all liver abscesses will show definite uptake, raising problems in differential diagnosis with malignant liver tumors.

Imaging Algorithm

An ideal algorithm is presented in Figure 63-15.

Classic Signs: Hepatic Abscess

- Small abscesses coalesce into big cavity: "cluster" sign
- Thick capsule
- Nonenhancing fluid content
- Presence of central gas or fluid level (see Table 63-2)

Differential Diagnosis

If hepatic abscess is associated with weight loss and anemia, malignancy often is the initial consideration. Metastases, however, are not associated with fever or leukocytosis. Metastases after ablative treatment or infarction in liver transplant can mimic the appearance of a pyogenic abscess at imaging; therefore, knowing the patient's history is important for the differential diagnosis. A history of diarrhea with mucus in the stool of recent immigrants and homosexuals is more suggestive of amebic rather than pyogenic abscess.

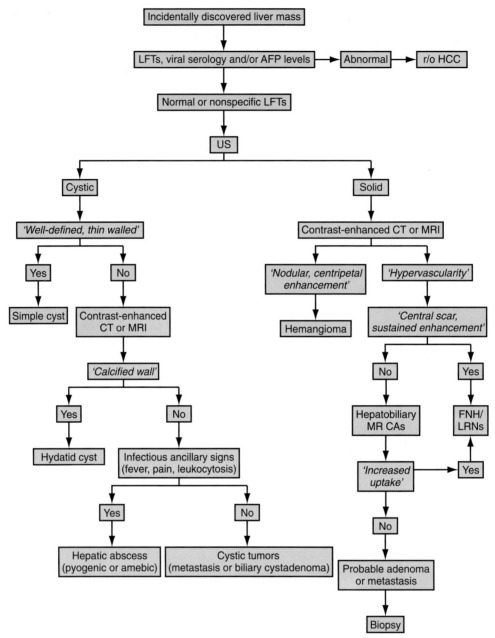

■ **FIGURE 63-15** Flow chart of a practical diagnostic approach to management of benign hepatic lesions. CAs, contrast agents; LFTs, liver function tests; AFP, α-fetoprotein; HCC, hepatocellular carcinoma; FNH, focal nodular hyperplasia; LRNs, large regenerative nodules.

A cluster of small cystic lesions or a single large cavity surrounded by a capsule is the classical presentation of pyogenic abscess. Simple hepatic cysts usually have a thin wall and homogeneous content. Liver malignancies are more commonly solid and more enhancing. However, nonliquefied abscess may simulate solid tumor. Metastases usually do not appear as a cluster or septated cystic mass. Treated necrotic metastases may be indistinguishable from abscess. Amebic abscess is usually sharply defined, of hypoechoic or low attenuation, and most often solitary and shows a thicker wall in comparison to pyogenic abscesses. Hepatic hydatid cyst consists of a large cystic liver mass with peripheral daughter cysts and curvilinear or ring-like pericyst calcification. They can cause dilated intrahepatic bile ducts owing to mass

effect and/or rupture into bile ducts. Biliary cystadenocarcinoma is a rare, multiseptated, water-density cystic mass that can be difficult to differentiate from abscess based on imaging alone. Infarction in liver transplant due to hepatic artery thrombosis with hepatic and biliary necrosis can be indistinguishable from pyogenic abscess (see Table 63-2).

Treatment

Medical Treatment

Intravenous antibiotics and percutaneous drainage are the standard of care. Depending on the etiology, medical treatment consists of antibiotic or antifungal therapy.

TABLE 63-5   Accuracy, Limitations, and Pitfalls of the Modalities Used in Imaging of Benign Focal Hepatic Lesions

Modality	Accuracy	Limitations	Pitfalls
Radiography	Poor	Insensitive Nonspecific	Unable to directly visualize soft tissue masses in the liver
CT	Sensitivity 69%-71% Specificity 86%-91% 76% hemangioma from fibrolamellar HCC and FNH 76% FNH from fibrolamellar HCC and hemangioma 47% sensitivity and 95% specificity in differentiating small hemangiomas from malignant tumors	Radiation Limited use in patients with allergy or renal insufficiency Potential for anaphylactoid reaction	Lesion detection and characterization may be difficult in fatty liver
MRI	80%	Motion artifact in uncooperative patients Claustrophobic patients Patients with cardiac pacemaker Risk of nephrogenic systemic fibrosis in patients with renal insufficiency High costs	Calcifications not well visualized
Ultrasonography	35% B-mode 78% contrast-enhanced ultrasonography	Poor performance in the case of obesity or overlying bowel gas Operator dependent	Calcifications not well visualized
Nuclear medicine	No utility unless hemangioma	Poor spatial resolution	Numerous false-negative and false-positive findings
PET/CT	No utility	Radiation High cost	Mismatches between the fused images, for example due to respiratory movement

Surgical Treatment

Aggressive surgical management with débridement or enucleation of the abscesses is favored if abscesses are not amenable to percutaneous drainage secondary to location, if there is coexistence of other intra-abdominal disease requiring operative management, or if combined treatment with antibiotic therapy and percutaneous drainage has failed. Surgery is, however, contraindicated in the presence of multiple abscesses, of associated malignancy or immunosuppressive disease, or of coexistence of other multiple complicated medical conditions.

What the Referring Physician Needs to Know: Hepatic Abscess

- Hepatic abscess is associated with elevated white blood cell count, fever, and right upper quadrant pain.
- Causes are an ascending infection in the biliary tract (ascending cholangitis), direct invasion from a nearby source, trauma, diverticulitis, or appendicitis.
- Life-threatening sepsis can develop.
- CT is the most useful imaging technique.
- A cluster of small pyogenic abscesses coalesces into a single large cavity.
- Check for history of transplantation, ablation, or chemotherapy for liver tumor.
- Hepatic abscesses must be differentiated from metastases, hepatic amebic abscess, biliary cyst, biliary cystadenocarcinoma, hydatid cyst, and infarction.

SUMMARY

Assessment of focal liver abnormalities typically relies on several cross-sectional imaging modalities, such as ultrasonography, CT, and MRI, which may be used independently or, even more commonly, in combination (Table 63-5). Although guidelines have been developed for the optimal diagnostic strategy in the diagnosis of most common malignant liver tumors, especially HCC, there is still no consensus on how to optimize the radiologic investigation of incidentally discovered benign liver lesions. Commonly, the diagnostic approach relies on the request of referring physicians, availability of equipment, and experience of the radiologists.

Because of low costs and wide availability, ultrasonography should be considered the first line in the evaluation of an incidentally discovered liver lesion. Despite its inherent limitations, ultrasonography can confidently diagnose two among the most common benign hepatic tumors: simple cysts and hemangioma. Although recently introduced microbubble-based ultrasound contrast agents can provide insights into hemodynamics of a liver lesion, most incidentally discovered solid liver lesions are still investigated with contrast-enhanced CT or MRI. Although both techniques provide reproducible image quality with excellent anatomic detail and have been demonstrated to be equally useful for lesion detection and characterization, CT still represents the modality of choice, owing to its broad availability and overall lower costs compared with MRI. Despite the fact that most benign liver lesions can be definitely characterized at contrast-enhanced CT, taking account of their enhancement pattern as well as the patient clinical history, in a limited number of cases imaging findings may overlap between benign and malignant liver tumors (see Tables 63-3 and 63-4). Owing to the introduction of liver-specific contrast agents and the inherent greater accuracy in exploring tissue characteristics, MRI can provide a more comprehensive workup of focal liver lesions. Because of improved diagnostic and decision-making processes, MRI has been recently proposed as a cost-effective, first-line imaging modality in the evaluation of liver disease. In addition, because of the lack of hazards of ionizing radiation, the use of MRI should be preferred in young patients. The role of PET/CT in the evaluation of benign liver lesions is still under investigation. Finally, lesion biopsy should still be performed in a limited number of undetermined cases.

What the Referring Physician Needs to Know: Benign Focal Liver Lesions

The role of imaging in the approach to benign focal liver lesions is to determine (see Table 63-5):

■ Whether background liver is cirrhotic or noncirrhotic to narrow the differential diagnosis
■ Whether lesion is solid or cystic
■ Enhancement pattern
■ Number, size, and location of liver lesions
■ Whether a lesion can be confidently characterized as benign and therefore managed conservatively

---

KEY POINTS

Simple Cysts

■ Well defined
■ Thin walled
■ Anechoic with posterior acoustic enhancement at ultrasonography
■ Water attenuating at precontrast CT
■ Markedly high signal intensity on T2-weighted MR images
■ No enhancement after intravenous injection of a contrast agent

Hemangiomas

■ Usually solitary
■ Peripheral, nodular, centripetal enhancement
■ Isoattenuation to vessels on all phases
■ Capillary hemangioma: homogeneous, rapid ("flash filling") enhancement
■ Association with focal nodular hyperplasia

Hepatocellular Adenoma

■ Heterogeneous
■ Hypervascular
■ Wash out
■ Intratumoral hemorrhage, necrosis, and calcification
■ Signal drop on out-of-phase imaging
■ Lack of active uptake of liver-specific, hepatobiliary MR contrast agents

Focal Nodular Hyperplasia

■ Intense, homogeneous enhancement during hepatic arterial phase (either contrast-enhanced CT, MRI, or ultrasonography)
■ Difficult to recognize from surrounding liver during unenhanced, portal venous, and delayed phases
■ Delayed enhancement of central fibrous scar (at 5 to 10 minutes post contrast administration)
■ Either normal or increased uptake of both hepatobiliary and reticuloendothelial system liver-specific MR contrast agents

Large Regenerative Nodules

■ Usually found in patients with Budd-Chiari syndrome
■ Intense, homogeneous enhancement during hepatic arterial phase
■ Sustained enhancement during portal venous and delayed phases
■ Hypointensity on T2-weighted and hyperintensity on T1-weighted MR images

Hepatic Abscess

■ Single or multiple
■ History of appendicitis, diverticulitis, or biliary obstruction
■ Fever and right upper quadrant pain
■ CT is the most useful imaging technique

SUGGESTED READINGS

Brancatelli G, et al. Benign regenerative nodules in Budd-Chiari syndrome and other vascular disorders of the liver: radiologic-pathologic and clinical correlation. RadioGraphics 2002; 22:847-862.

Brancatelli G, et al. CT and MR imaging evaluation of hepatic adenoma. J Comput Assist Tomogr 2006; 30:745-750.

Chiche L, et al. Liver adenomatosis: reappraisal, diagnosis, and surgical management: eight new cases and review of the literature. Ann Surg 2000; 231:74-81.

Choi BY, et al. The diagnosis and management of benign hepatic tumors. J Clin Gastroenterol 2005; 39:401-412.

Federle MP, et al. Imaging of benign hepatic masses. Semin Liver Dis 2001; 21:237-249.

Grazioli L, et al. Hepatic adenomas: imaging and pathologic findings. RadioGraphics 2001; 21:877-892.

Horton KM, et al. CT and MR imaging of benign hepatic and biliary tumors. RadioGraphics 1999; 19:431-451.

Valls C, et al. Hyperenhancing focal liver lesions: differential diagnosis with helical CT. AJR Am J Roentgenol 1999; 173:605-611.

Vilgrain V, et al. Imaging of atypical hemangiomas of the liver with pathologic correlation. RadioGraphics 2000; 20:379-397.

Vilgrain V. Focal nodular hyperplasia. Eur J Radiol 2006; 58:236-245.

REFERENCES

1. Jones EC, et al. The frequency and significance of small (less than or equal to 15 mm) hepatic lesions detected by CT. AJR Am J Roentgenol 1992; 158:535-539.
2. Dai Y, et al. Focal liver lesions: can SonoVue-enhanced ultrasound be used to differentiate malignant from benign lesions? Invest Radiol 2007; 42:596-603.
3. Ishak KJ, et al. Benign cholangiocellular tumors. In Ishak KJ, Goodman ZD, Stocsker JT (eds). Tumours of the Liver and Intrahepatic Bile Ducts, 3rd ed. Washington, DC, Armed Forces Institute of Pathology, 2001, pp 113-114.
4. Mortelé KJ, et al. Cystic focal liver lesions in the adult: differential CT and MR imaging features. RadioGraphics 2001; 21:895-910.
5. Ishak KJ, et al. Benign mesenchymal tumors and pseudotumors. In Ishak KJ, Goodman ZD, Stocsker JT (eds). Tumours of the Liver and Intrahepatic Bile Ducts, 3rd ed. Washington, DC, Armed Forces Institute of Pathology, 2001, pp 113-114.
6. Brancatelli G, et al. Hemangioma in the cirrhotic liver: diagnosis and natural history. Radiology 2001; 219:69-74.
7. Vilgrain V, et al. Prevalence of hepatic hemangioma in patients with focal nodular hyperplasia: MR imaging analysis. Radiology 2003; 229:75-79.
8. Marsh JI, et al. Hepatic hemangioma in the presence of fatty infiltration: an atypical sonographic appearance. Gastrointest Radiol 1989; 14:262-264.
9. Nelson RC, et al. Diagnostic approach to hepatic hemangiomas. Radiology 1990; 76:11-13.
10. Quinn SF, et al. Hepatic cavernous hemangiomas: simple diagnostic sign with dynamic bolus CT. Radiology 1992; 182:545-548.
11. McFarland EG, et al. Hepatic hemangiomas and malignant tumors: improved differentiation with heavily T2-weighted conventional spin-echo MR imaging. Radiology 1994; 193:43-47.
12. Grazioli L, et al. Liver adenomatosis: clinical, histopathologic, and imaging findings in 15 patients. Radiology 2000; 216:395-402.
13. Ishak KJ, et al. Benign hepatocellular tumors. In Ishak KJ, Goodman ZD, Stocsker JT (eds). Tumours of the Liver and Intrahepatic Bile Ducts, 3rd ed. Washington, DC, Armed Forces Institute of Pathology, 2001, pp 113-114.
14. Ichikawa T, et al. Hepatocellular adenoma: multiphasic CT and pathologic findings in 25 patients. Radiology 2000; 214:861-868.
15. Paulson EK, et al. Hepatic adenoma: MR characteristics and correlation with pathologic findings. AJR Am J Roentgenol 1994; 163:113-116.
16. Arrivé L, et al. Hepatic adenoma: MR findings in 51 pathologically proved lesions. Radiology 1994; 193:507-512.
17. Grazioli L, et al. Accurate differentiation of focal nodular hyperplasia from hepatic adenoma at gadobenate dimeglumine-enhanced MR imaging: prospective study. Radiology 2005; 236:166-177.
18. Kim TK, et al. Focal nodular hyperplasia and hepatic adenoma: differentiation with low-mechanical-index contrast-enhanced sonography. AJR Am J Roentgenol 2008; 190:58-66.
19. Wanless IR, et al. On the pathogenesis of focal nodular hyperplasia of the liver. Hepatology 1985; 5:1194-2000.
20. Nguyen BN, et al. Focal nodular hyperplasia of the liver: a comprehensive pathologic study of 305 lesions and recognition of new histologic forms. Am J Surg Pathol 1999; 23:1441-1454.
21. Brancatelli G, et al. Focal nodular hyperplasia: CT findings with emphasis on multiphasic helical CT in 78 patients. Radiology 2001; 219:61-68.
22. Choi CS, et al. Triphasic helical CT of hepatic focal nodular hyperplasia: incidence of atypical findings. AJR Am J Roentgenol 1998; 170:391-395.
23. Vilgrain V, et al. Focal nodular hyperplasia of the liver: MR imaging and pathologic correlation in 37 patients. Radiology 1992; 184:699-703.
24. Grazioli L, et al. Focal nodular hyperplasia: morphologic and functional information from MR imaging with gadobenate dimeglumine. Radiology 2001; 221:731-739.
25. Attal P, et al. Telangiectatic focal nodular hyperplasia: US, CT, and MR imaging findings with histopathologic correlation in 13 cases. Radiology 2003; 228:465-472.
26. Vilgrain V, et al. Hepatic nodules in Budd-Chiari syndrome: imaging features. Radiology 1999; 210:443-450.
27. Brancatelli G, et al. Large regenerative nodules in Budd-Chiari syndrome and other vascular disorders of the liver: CT and MR imaging findings with clinico-pathologic correlation. AJR Am J Roentgenol 2002; 178:877-883.
28. Moucari R, et al. Hepatocellular carcinoma in Budd-Chiari syndrome: characteristics and risk factors. Gut 2008; 57:828-835.
29. Jeffrey RB Jr, et al. CT of small pyogenic hepatic abscesses: the cluster sign. AJR Am J Roentgenol 1988; 151:487-489.
30. Mortelé KJ, et al. The infected liver: radiologic-pathologic correlation. RadioGraphics 2004; 24:937-955.

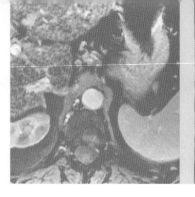
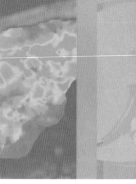

CHAPTER 64

Malignant Focal Lesions

Daniele Marin and Giuseppe Brancatelli

ETIOLOGY

Malignant liver tumors can be classified either by cell of origin as hepatocellular, cholangiocellular, or mesenchymal or by site of origin as primary or secondary. In this chapter we will describe the most frequently encountered malignant hepatic tumors arising in noncirrhotic liver, including hepatocellular carcinoma (HCC), fibrolamellar HCC, epithelioid hemangioendothelioma (EHE), angiosarcoma, and metastatic disease. Also discussed are other rare primary liver tumors, such as lymphoma and hepatoblastoma. HCC arising in cirrhosis and intrahepatic cholangiocarcinoma are discussed elsewhere in this text.

PREVALENCE AND EPIDEMIOLOGY

Metastases are the most common malignant neoplasm of the liver, with an incidence of 40% in cancer patients at the time of death. Although HCC—one of the most common causes of cancer death worldwide—usually occurs in the setting of cirrhosis, in about 10% of cases this tumor can occur without cirrhosis or other known risk factors. Other primary malignant mesenchymal (i.e., angiosarcoma and EHE), hepatocellular (i.e., hepatoblastoma), or lymphoid (i.e., primary or secondary lymphoma) tumors are much rarer, accounting for only 1% to 2% of all primary malignant liver neoplasms.

CLINICAL PRESENTATION

Clinical presentation is usually nonspecific and includes fever of unknown origin, abdominal pain, malaise, weight loss, a palpable abdominal mass, or cachexia. Jaundice is not common.

PATHOPHYSIOLOGY

Malignant liver lesions may occur anywhere in the liver. The ability of CT and MRI to show hepatic tumors is enhanced by the dual blood supply of the liver. Although liver tumors generally receive nearly all their blood supply from the hepatic artery, after bolus intravenous injection of a contrast agent some of them will enhance more than the surrounding liver parenchyma (hypervascular tumors) on hepatic arterial phase, whereas others will be best depicted as low-density or low-intensity lesions (hypovascular) against the background of enhanced liver during the portal venous phase.

PATHOLOGY

Pathologic findings vary greatly according to the specific tumor type and degree of differentiation.

LIVER FUNCTION

Tumor markers such as α-fetoprotein, protein induced from the absence of vitamin K (PIVKA), carcinoembryonic antigen (CEA), and cancer antigen 19-9 (CA19-9) are commonly used for differentiating focal liver lesions, although their role for diagnosis is controversial. Laboratory examination is nonspecific and can reveal increased levels of alkaline phosphatase and transaminases or minor elevation of bilirubin levels.

IMAGING

Radiography

Because of the poor soft tissue resolution, a plain abdominal radiograph does not provide any clinical information in the investigation of patients with malignant hepatic tumors, although larger lesions may be occasionally suspected based on deformation of a visible liver border, mass effect on adjacent structures, or calcifications.

CT

The multiphasic imaging capability of MDCT allows one to set different protocols for both hypovascular and hypervascular lesions. The advantages of MDCT include high speed with less motion artifact (i.e., improved temporal resolution), submillimeter slice thickness with true isotropic imaging, ease of image interpretation, and the ability to cover large volumes and to create multiplanar reformatted images. Sagittal, coronal, or curved multiplanar reformatted images can better delineate those small subcapsular lesions in the dome of the liver that might not be well depicted with transverse imaging alone. In those patients who are candidate for hepatic resection, CT angiography yields an excellent depiction of the relationship of the lesion to intrahepatic vessels.

MRI

Major advantages of MRI over CT are higher contrast resolution; better ability to detect, characterize, and quantify both intrahepatic and intralesional fat and iron; and the use of both extracellular and liver-specific contrast agents. There is some evidence in the recent literature that MRI has higher diagnostic accuracy than CT for liver lesion detection and characterization. The most diagnostically important information is usually obtained from multiphase gadolinium-enhanced fat-suppressed 3D T1-weighted gradient-recalled-echo MRI, including a properly timed hepatic arterial phase, followed by portal venous and delayed phases. Specifically, the hepatic arterial phase enables investigation of lesion perfusion as well as excellent depiction of vascular anatomy with multiplanar capabilities. T2-weighted imaging is not used for lesion detection but rather for lesion characterization. Precontrast T1-weighted in-phase and opposed-phase imaging allows assessment of lipid and iron content within the liver or lesion. With the advent of liver-specific MR contrast media, which include reticuloendothelial system–specific contrast agents and hepatocyte-selective contrast agents, MRI currently represents the modality of choice for the detection of hepatic metastases with reported diagnostic accuracy values exceeding those of either ultrasonography or MDCT.

Ultrasonography

Although ultrasonography is frequently the first-line modality for imaging of the liver due to low costs and widespread availability, its role is currently limited in the evaluation of patients with malignant liver tumors and must be invariably supplemented by either MDCT or MRI. By providing insights on lesion vascularity, ultrasound contrast agents have recently shown the potential to improve both detection and characterization of a lesion.

Nuclear Medicine

The role of nuclear medicine for detection and characterization of malignant liver lesions has been largely replaced by cross-sectional imaging, with the exception of the use of somatostatin receptor scintigraphy for neuroendocrine liver metastasis.

PET/CT

Because most malignant tumors show enhanced glycolysis, PET allows differentiation of metabolically active tumors from benign lesions. Major pitfalls include false-positive results in a minority of abscesses and false-positive results in smaller or well-differentiated HCC. Besides its well-established role in lesion detection, PET can also provide important clues for tumor staging as well as early detection of tumor recurrence after therapy.

What the Referring Physician Needs to Know: Malignant Focal Liver Lesions

The role of imaging in the approach to malignant focal liver lesions is to determine (Table 64-1):

- Number, size, and location of liver lesions
- Enhancement pattern (hypervascular or hypovascular)
- Tissue characterization (fat, blood, necrosis, cystic or solid areas)
- Differentiation of benign versus malignant
- Differentiation of primary versus secondary
- Whether the background liver shows normal or altered morphology (e.g., chronic liver disease)
- Whether the background liver shows fatty infiltration
- Indications for biopsy (especially in smaller lesions)
- Suitability of resection (relationship of the tumor to surrounding vessels)
- Tumor staging (rule out extrahepatic metastatic disease)
- Reliable follow-up after treatment

SPECIFIC LESIONS

Epithelioid Hemangioendothelioma

Etiology

There are no known risk factors for hepatic EHE.

Prevalence and Epidemiology

Hepatic EHE is a low-grade malignant vascular neoplasm with an intermediate clinical course between that of cavernous hemangioma and malignant angiosarcoma. EHE shows a slight female predominance (male-to-female ratio, 2:3), with a peak incidence around 50 years of age.[1]

Clinical Presentation

Clinical manifestations are nonspecific and vary from asymptomatic patients to patients with portal hypertension or hepatic failure. Most common findings are weakness, anorexia, weight loss, right upper quadrant pain, and hepatomegaly. Unusual presentation includes acute abdomen from rupture of the tumor with hemoperitoneum, Budd-Chiari–like syndrome, portal hypertension, and liver failure due to extensive replacement of liver parenchyma by the tumor.[1]

Pathophysiology

Characteristically, EHE demonstrates a peripheral, subcapsular location, although in advanced cases lesions may grow to almost replace the entire liver. Compensatory hypertrophy of unaffected hepatic parenchyma can be seen in patients with extensive liver involvement.[2]

TABLE 64-1 Clinical and Radiologic Features of Malignant Focal Liver Tumors

Tumor	Sex	Age	Capsule	Size	Number	Calcification	Fat	Scar	Bleed	Necrosis	Associated Signs and Predisposing Factors
Epithelioid hemangioendothelioma	F > M	4-5th decade	No	Variable	Multifocal	13%	No	No	No	No	Capsular retraction Subcapsular location
Angiosarcoma	M > F	6-7th decade	No	Variable	Multiple nodules or large mass	Rare	No	No	Yes	Yes	Thorotrast
Fibrolamellar carcinoma	M = F	2-3rd decade	35%	Large	Usually solitary	Central (68%)	No	Yes (80%) Hypo on T2W	No	Yes	Lymphadenopathy
HCC in noncirrhotic liver	M > F	5-6th decade	51%	Large	One or few	Peripheral (28%)	10%	No	Rare	Yes	Hepatitis B and C
Hepatoblastoma	M > F	Infants and children < age 3 yr	No	Large	Single or multinodular	30%	No	No	Yes	Yes	Genetic
Lymphoma	M > F	6-7th decade	No	Variable	Usually solitary	Rare (10%)	No	No	No	No	Multiorgan involvement and lymphadenopathy
Hypervascular metastases	M = F	Variable	No	Variable	Multiple	Rare (neuroendocrine)	No	Rare (neuroendocrine)	No	Yes	Primary malignancy
Hypovascular metastases	M = F	Variable	No	Variable	Multiple	Rare (colon)	No	No	No	Yes	Primary malignancy

Pathology

Typically, EHE manifests as multiple lesions, ranging from 1 to 3 cm in diameter. On sectioning, lesions are white to tan and firm, with a fibrous, relatively hypocellular center surrounded by a rim of hyperemic, actively proliferating viable tissue. An additional peripheral hypovascular halo may be observed at the interface between the tumor and the surrounding hepatic parenchyma and has been related to a narrow avascular zone secondary to tumor occlusion of hepatic sinusoids and small vessels.[2,3] Larger lesions are generally confluent, thus forming aggregate masses that may sometimes contain coarse calcifications. Demonstration of the vascular or endothelial origin of the tumor is critical for diagnosis and requires immunostaining for endothelial markers, including factor VIII–related antigen, CD31, and CD34.[1]

Liver Function

Increased alkaline phosphatase activity may be present in about two thirds of patients. Tumor marker levels, such as α-fetoprotein and CA19-9 levels, are generally unremarkable.[1]

Imaging

Radiography

Calcifications, elevated diaphragm, and mass effect, although uncommon, are the most important findings evident on plain abdominal radiography.[1]

CT

CT findings reflect the gross appearance of the tumor and typically demonstrate multiple, peripheral, and partially confluent liver masses. Capsular retraction can be seen when lesions abut the liver surface. At precontrast CT, EHE is generally hypoattenuating compared with the liver, with the only exception of occasional intralesional calcifications. At contrast-enhanced CT, EHE shows a very characteristic target-type enhancement pattern (the so-called bull's eye appearance) with a central hypoattenuating area, which corresponds to the central fibrous core, surrounded by a peripheral thick enhancing ring and an outer hypoattenuating halo, which corresponds to the peripheral viable tumor and the avascular zone of transition, respectively (Fig. 64-1).[1-4]

MRI

At precontrast MRI, EHE shows nonspecific imaging findings with hypointensity and mild hyperintensity on T1- and T2-weighted MR images, respectively (see Fig. 64-1). On gadolinium-enhanced MRI, the tumor enhancement pattern is substantially comparable to that at CT.[2,3]

Ultrasonography

EHE appears as lobulated confluent hepatic lesions with variable echotexture on gray-scale ultrasonography.[1]

Nuclear Medicine

Among 18 scintigraphic studies found in the literature performed with technetium-99m, gallium-67, and indium-111—labeled leukocytes, 78% of EHE lesions demonstrated low uptake.[1]

PET/CT

Fluorodeoxyglucose (FDG)-PET/CT has shown some utility for detection of EHE recurrence after resection.

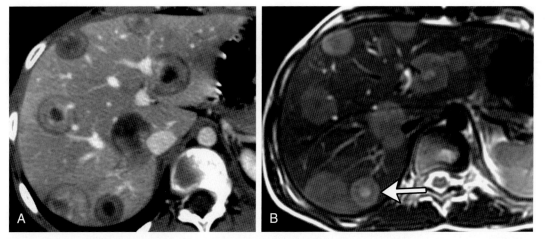

■ **FIGURE 64-1** Typical CT and MRI findings of epithelioid hemangioendothelioma. **A,** Transverse contrast-enhanced CT image during portal venous phase shows multiple round masses with a typical target appearance due to a hypoattenuating center surrounded by a hyperattenuating inner rim and a thin hypoattenuating outer halo. **B,** On this T2-weighted turbo spin-echo MR image the central area appears markedly hyperintense compared with the adjacent liver and is surrounded by a mildly hyperintense rim (*arrow*), which corresponds to viable tumor.

Imaging Algorithm

An imaging algorithm is provided in Figure 64-14 at the end of this discussion.

Classic Signs: Epithelioid Hemangioendothelioma

- Multiple round lesions or large confluent masses
- Target appearance ("bull's eye")
- Compensatory hypertrophy of unaffected hepatic parenchyma
- Subcapsular location
- Capsular retraction

Differential Diagnosis

Absence of a known history of a primary tumor may be helpful in ruling out metastatic disease. Because EHE may occasionally show delayed enhancement, lack of a history of primary sclerosing cholangitis helps in differentiating it from peripheral cholangiocarcinoma. Positive imaging findings, in addition to features such as occurrence in younger adults, relative indolent progression of the disease, and the presence of numerous intrahepatic tumors with a good clinical condition are suggestive of EHE.[1]

EHE can be confidently differentiated from hemangioma based on tumor enhancement as well as demonstration of retraction of the adjacent liver capsule (Table 64-2). In those cases in which retraction of the liver capsule overlying a lesion is noted, absence of morphologic changes of cirrhosis and regenerative nodules are helpful to differentiate these lesions from confluent hepatic fibrosis and absence of biliary dilatation is key to differentiate them from peripheral cholangiocarcinoma (Table 64-3; Fig. 64-2). The definitive diagnosis requires core biopsy and histologic analysis, because the typical target sign observed in EHE can be mimicked by metastatic disease (Fig. 64-3).[1]

Treatment

Medical Treatment

At present, the roles of radiation and chemotherapy are still undetermined.

Surgical Treatment

Surgical resection and liver transplantation are considered the treatments of choice. Liver transplantation is

---

TABLE 64-2 Differential Features among Mesenchymal Liver Tumors (Hemangioma, Epithelioid Hemangioendothelioma (EHE), and Angiosarcoma)

	Hemangioma	EHE	Angiosarcoma
Sex	F > M	F ≥ M	M > F
Age	2-5th decade	4-5th decade	6-7th decade
Location	Variable	Subcapsular	Diffuse liver involvement
Shape	Round/oval	Round	Ill-defined
Number	Single > multiple	Multiple	Multiple
Capsular Retraction	No	Yes	No
Central Scar	Rare (larger lesions)	No	No
Calcifications	Only large lesions	Uncommon	Uncommon
Enhancement	Centripetal	Low degree	Bizarre, centrifugal
Necrosis	No	No	Yes

TABLE 64-3 Differential Features Associated with Retraction of the Liver Capsule (Peripheral Cholangiocarcinoma, Focal Confluent Fibrosis, Epithelioid Hemangioendothelioma, Metastases, and Hemangioma)

	Peripheral Cholangiocarcinoma	Focal Confluent Fibrosis	EHE	Metastases	Hemangioma
Sex	F = M	M > F	F ≥ M	F = M	F > M
Age	6-8th decade	6-7th decade	4-5th decade	Any age	2-5th decade
Predisposing Factors	Primary sclerosing cholangitis	End-stage cirrhosis	None	Primary malignancy	None
Number	Single	Single	Multiple	Multiple	Single > multiple
Delayed Enhancement	++	++	±	±	+++
Central Calcifications	No	No	Uncommon	Uncommon (mucinous primary)	Uncommon (larger lesions)
Capsular Retraction	++	++ (advanced cirrhosis)	++	After chemotherapy	No
Necrosis	++	−	±	++	−
Enhancement on Portal Venous Phase	+ (ring)	Rare (trapped vessels)	−	±	++ (nodular, peripheral, discontinuous)

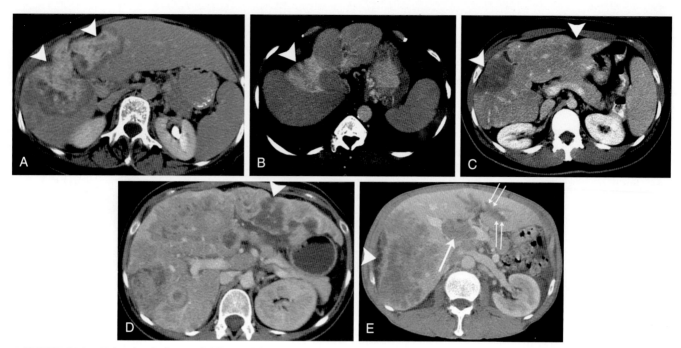

■ **FIGURE 64-2** CT imaging findings and differential diagnosis among liver lesions associated with capsular retraction, including peripheral cholangiocarcinoma, focal confluent fibrosis, epithelioid hemangioendothelioma, and treated metastases from breast and rectal adenocarcinoma. All these conditions show capsular retraction (*arrowheads*) when abutting the liver surface. Peripheral cholangiocarcinoma (**A**) and focal confluent fibrosis (**B**) characteristically demonstrate enhancement during the delayed phase owing to abundance of fibrotic tissue. **C,** Epithelioid hemangioendothelioma can also manifest as an infiltrative mass owing to the confluence of multiple lesions. **D,** Patients with metastatic breast carcinoma characteristically show a pseudocirrhotic appearance after chemotherapy. **E,** Note massive thrombosis into the main portal vein (*arrow*) and moderate left intrahepatic biliary duct dilatation (*double arrows*) due to neoplastic infiltration in this patient with metastatic rectal carcinoma.

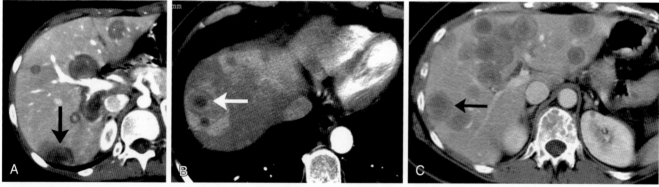

■ **FIGURE 64-3** CT imaging findings of epithelioid hemangioendothelioma (**A**), pancreatic (**B**), and breast (**C**) adenocarcinoma metastases. Lesions are multiple, are partially confluent, and have a "target" appearance (*arrows*) in all cases. The "target sign" is therefore not specific for epithelioid hemangioendothelioma.

What the Referring Physician Needs to Know: Epithelioid Hemangioendothelioma

- EHE is a low-grade malignant primary tumor
- The etiology is unknown.
- There is a nonspecific clinical presentation.
- The course is variable.
- CT and MRI are the best diagnostic tools but cannot provide a definitive diagnosis.
- Biopsy is required for definitive diagnosis.
- Liver resection and transplantation are the treatments of choice.

beneficial in patients with multiple lesions and extensive involvement of liver parenchyma.

Angiosarcoma

Etiology

Although several conditions, such as hemochromatosis, von Recklinghausen's disease, and environmental carcinogens (i.e., vinyl chloride, thorium dioxide, and arsenic), may favor the development of angiosarcoma, currently most cases occur in patients without known associated risk factors.[5,6]

Prevalence and Epidemiology

Angiosarcoma is a high-grade malignant neoplasm of endothelial cells. This tumor represents the most common sarcoma of the liver. The peak age incidence is in the sixth and seventh decades, with a male-to-female ratio of 3 : 1.[5,6]

Clinical Presentation

Angiosarcomas typically present at an advanced stage with hepatomegaly, ascites, abdominal pain, and weight loss. Sudden onset with acute symptoms may result from spontaneous tumor rupture and subsequent hemoperitoneum.[5,6]

Pathophysiology

Angiosarcoma is usually multifocal or diffuse and involves both liver lobes.[5,6]

Pathology

Typically, angiosarcoma manifests as an ill-defined lesion with a variegated appearance due to areas of hemorrhage and necrosis. At histology, tumor cells demonstrate a preferential growth along sinusoids, terminal hepatic venules, and portal vein branches that lead to progressive disruption of liver cell plates with the development of blood-filled cavitary spaces of varied size. Invasion of terminal hepatic venules and portal vein branches also leads to atrophy, infarction, and necrosis of hepatic parenchyma.[5,6]

Liver Function

The most reliable abnormalities include bromosulphthalein retention, increased serum alkaline phosphatase activity, hyperbilirubinemia, and prolonged prothrombin time.

Imaging

Angiosarcomas show an aggressive behavior with metastatic spread to spleen, lung, bone marrow, portohepatic nodes, and peritoneum. A rare complication is tumor rupture, which results in acute hemoperitoneum. Because of the tumor vascularity and associated coagulopathy and thrombocytopenia, liver biopsy is associated with significantly high morbidity and mortality rates.[5,6]

Radiography

Besides generic findings secondary to mass effect by the tumor, focal areas of metallic density with an irregular pattern can be seen in patients with previous exposure to Thorotrast.

CT

At precontrast CT, angiosarcoma is isoattenuating to abdominal vessels and the surrounding liver. Focal hyperattenuating areas can be seen secondary to intralesional hemorrhage. At contrast-enhanced CT, lesions

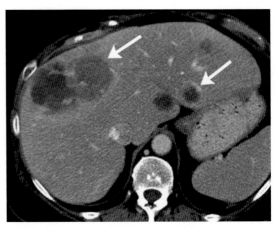

■ **FIGURE 64-4** CT imaging findings of angiosarcoma. Transverse contrast-enhanced CT image during portal venous phase shows multiple, round, solid masses (*arrows*). Because these findings are nonspecific and may also be observed in patients with either metastatic disease or hepatic lymphoma, definitive diagnosis requires biopsy.

can have a variable appearance. In some cases, angiosarcoma can present as an infiltrative pattern (Fig. 64-4), whereas some other times it shows bizarre, heterogeneous enhancement.[5,6]

MRI

Because hemangiosarcomas are predominantly composed of blood-filled tumor cavities, their T1 and T2 values are extremely long, thus explaining the very low signal intensity on T1-weighted images and markedly high signal intensity on T2-weighted images. Intralesional hemorrhagic foci can be seen as focal areas of bright signal intensity on T1-weighted images. On gadolinium-enhanced MRI, the tumor enhancement pattern is substantially comparable to that at CT.[5,6]

Ultrasonography

Because of extensive liver involvement, angiosarcomas generally manifest as ill-defined areas of distorted hepatic echotexture.[5,6]

Nuclear Medicine

Angiosarcoma shows increased uptake at gallium scan. Because of histologic similarities, angiosarcoma can mimic hemangioma on ^{99m}Tc-labeled red blood cell scans ("perfusion-blood pool mismatch").

PET/CT

Lesions show markedly increased accumulation of FDG compared with the surrounding liver parenchyma. This technique is particularly sensitive for the detection of distant metastases.

Imaging Algorithm

An imaging algorithm is provided in Figure 64-14.

Classic Signs: Angiosarcoma

- Multifocal nodules or diffuse liver involvement
- Bizarre, heterogeneous enhancement
- Progressive enhancement over time
- Distant metastases
- Intratumoral hemorrhage

Differential Diagnosis

Association with hemochromatosis, with von Reckling-hausen's disease, or with exposure to Thorotrast and arsenic can raise the suspicion of angiosarcoma.[5,6] Bizarre shape of the enhancing foci, large size of dominant lesions, multifocal distribution, and intratumoral hemorrhage are useful differentiating features from those of cavernous hemangioma (see Table 64-2).[5,6]

Treatment

Medical Treatment

Systemic or hepatic arterial chemotherapy or antiangio-genic therapy may be performed in patients with diffuse liver involvement that is not amenable to surgical treatment.

Surgical Treatment

Combined surgery and radiation therapy can offer the best chance of treatment, although the tumor is invariably associated with a poor outcome (5-year survival rate, 37%).[5,6]

What the Referring Physician Needs to Know: Angiosarcoma

- Angiosarcoma is the most common malignant mesenchymal tumor of the liver.
- It may be difficult to differentiate from other primary or secondary neoplasms.
- Multiphasic contrast-enhanced CT and MRI are the best diagnostic tools.
- Outcome is poor.
- The tumor can recur after surgery.

Hepatocellular Carcinoma in Noncirrhotic Liver

Etiology

Although predisposing factors such as hepatitis, viral infection, or alcohol abuse have been reported in some cases, no specific risk factor can be found in the majority of patients. Nonalcoholic fatty liver disease may represent the underlying causative factor in some instances.[7,8]

Prevalence and Epidemiology

In a substantial number of cases (21%), HCC may arise de novo in an otherwise normal liver. Patients are generally younger and have a better prognosis as well as a longer survival rate than patients with HCC in the cirrhotic liver.[8,9]

Clinical Presentation

Because the disease course is generally indolent and tumor surveillance is not performed, tumor size is typically large at diagnosis. At presentation, most common signs and symptoms include abdominal pain, distention, weight loss, and anorexia. In a limited number of patients without referred symptoms, the tumor may be incidentally discovered at imaging studies for unrelated reasons.[7,9]

Pathophysiology

HCC can occur anywhere in the liver.[7,9]

Pathology

HCC in noncirrhotic liver typically manifests as a large, predominantly solitary or dominant mass with satellite lesions. Lesions may be well defined and partially encapsulated, with areas of hemorrhage, macroscopic fat, and necrosis ("mosaic pattern"). Invasion of the portal vein or the biliary ducts and metastases to abdominal lymph nodes are occasionally observed. Despite the large size of lesions, most HCC arising in noncirrhotic liver is well to moderately differentiated at histologic analysis. This finding correlates well with the favorable prognosis of this tumor compared with "conventional" HCC.[10]

Liver Function

Although serologic levels of α-fetoprotein are abnormally increased in 65% of cases, in a consistent number of patients this tumor marker is within normal values (20 μg/L or less).[7]

Imaging

HCC in noncirrhotic liver comes to clinical attention because of a palpable abdominal mass, abdominal pain, distention, weight loss, anorexia, or cachexia.[7]

Radiography

Although larger lesions may deform one of the visible borders of the liver or cause mass effect on adjacent structures, more commonly a plain abdominal radiograph does not provide any clinical information in patients with HCC.

CT

At precontrast CT, HCC manifests as a large, dominant lesion that is hypoattenuating compared with the surrounding liver with the exception of occasional peripheral calcification. At contrast-enhanced CT, HCC shows heterogeneous, moderate enhancement during the hepatic

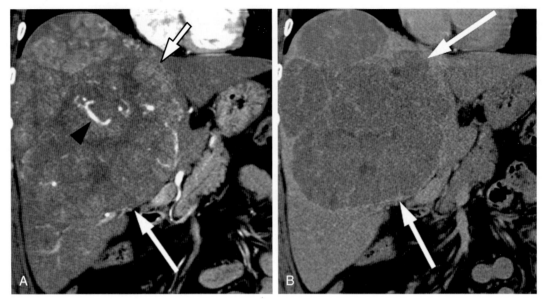

■ **FIGURE 64-5**   Typical CT imaging findings of HCC in a noncirrhotic liver. **A,** Coronal contrast-enhanced CT image during hepatic arterial phase demonstrates a large, heterogeneously enhancing mass (*arrows*) replacing almost the entire right liver lobe. Note prominent vascularity with large feeding arteries (*arrowhead*) entering the lesion. **B,** Corresponding CT image during portal venous phase shows wash out of the tumor, which appears hypoattenuating compared with the adjacent liver. Note enhancement of peripheral fibrous capsule (*arrows*).

arterial phase, followed by rapid wash out (i.e., the lesion is hypoattenuating relative to the liver) during the portal venous and delayed phases. Areas of necrosis or hemorrhage are frequently depicted as nonenhancing intralesional foci (Fig. 64-5). Tumor invasion of the portal vein, hepatic veins, and biliary ducts is common.[8,9]

MRI

At precontrast MRI, HCC shows nonspecific imaging findings with hypointensity and mild hyperintensity on T1- and T2-weighted MR images, respectively. Cystic-like or necrotic areas appear as markedly hypointense and hyperintense on T1- and T2-weighted images, respectively. On gadolinium-enhanced MRI, the tumor enhancement pattern is substantially comparable to that of CT.[10]

Ultrasonography

HCC manifests as large, predominantly hypoechoic masses, with a complex appearance due to areas of necrosis and hemorrhage.

Nuclear Medicine

Nuclear medicine is nonspecific. HCC may present as a "cold" defect on a sulfur colloid study or may demonstrate uptake of radiopharmaceuticals if the mass produces bile. Gallium uptake is seen in 90% of cases.

PET/CT

FDG-PET/CT is useful in the evaluation of HCC metastases, although its role in the diagnosis of primary HCC is more limited.

Imaging Algorithm

An imaging algorithm is provided in Figure 64-14.

Classic Signs: Hepatocellular Carcinoma in Noncirrhotic Liver

- Predominantly affects middle-aged men
- Solitary large lesion or dominant mass with smaller satellite nodules
- Lobulated surface
- Mosaic pattern
- Capsule
- Heterogeneous hypervascularity
- Lymphadenopathy
- Vascular and biliary tract invasion
- Wash out on portal venous and delayed imaging phases

Differential Diagnosis

Lack of history of chronic liver disease and younger age at presentation are helpful to differentiate this lesion from HCC arising in cirrhosis.[7] Absence of a primary tumor such as neuroendocrine, thyroid, or renal carcinoma may contribute to exclude hypervascular metastases.

Larger lesion size as well as a noncirrhotic appearance of the background liver (i.e., regular liver margins and well-preserved liver morphology) represents useful imaging clues to rule out classic HCC. Lack of a "true" central scar with calcification can help in the differential diagnosis with fibrolamellar HCC (Table 64-4). Absence of delayed enhancement and of capsular retraction can

TABLE 64-4 Differential Features between Fibrolamellar HCC and Hepatocellular Carcinoma in Noncirrhotic Liver

	Fibrolamellar HCC	HCC
Sex	M = F	M > F
Average Age	2-3rd decade	5-6th decade
Calcifications	68% (central)	28% (peripheral)
Surface	Lobulated	Lobulated
Capsule	35%	51%
Average Size	13 cm	12.4 cm
Lymphadenopathy	65%	21%
Intralesional Fat	~0%	10%
Scar	Yes	No
Necrosis	Yes	Yes
Enhancement on Hepatic Arterial Phase	Strong	Mild
Homogeneity on Hepatic Arterial Phase	No	No

reduce the likelihood of cholangiocarcinoma and mixed hepatocholangiocarcinoma.

Treatment

Medical Treatment

No medical treatment is effective in HCC occurring in noncirrhotic liver.

Surgical Treatment

Extensive, aggressive surgery is the treatment of choice for HCC in noncirrhotic liver. Because local tumor recurrence within the liver is a frequent occurrence, long-term follow-up is mandatory, because surgery for recurrent disease prolongs survival.[7]

What the Referring Physician Needs to Know: Hepatocellular Carcinoma in Noncirrhotic Liver

- HCC can rarely occur in noncirrhotic liver, usually in middle-aged men.
- HCC in noncirrhotic liver occurs at a younger age in comparison with HCC in cirrhotic liver.
- Hepatic resection can be beneficial.
- CT and MRI are useful for planning hepatic resection, staging, and follow-up.

Fibrolamellar Hepatocellular Carcinoma

Etiology

Etiologic factors for fibrolamellar HCC have not been identified. There are still conflicting theories on whether this malignancy represents either a histologic variant of classic HCC or a different biologic entity.[11]

Prevalence and Epidemiology

Fibrolamellar HCC is a rare primary hepatic malignancy with different epidemiology and clinical course than HCC. Fibrolamellar HCC occurs in younger patients, with most cases diagnosed before the age of 40. Although HCC is more commonly detected in men (74% of cases), fibrolamellar HCC shows no sex predilection. Patients with fibrolamellar HCC show a better resectability rate as well as improved survival rate than those with HCC.[11]

Clinical Presentation

At clinical presentation, most lesions are symptomatic because of their large size. Signs and symptoms include abdominal pain, hepatomegaly, palpable right upper quadrant abdominal mass, and cachexia. Jaundice is an uncommon finding (5% of cases) and results from biliary compression by either the dominant tumor mass or mass effect of metastatic lymphadenopathy. The tumor may also manifest as symptoms related to metastatic dissemination to distant organs.[11]

Pathophysiology

Fibrolamellar HCC occurs predominantly in the left hepatic lobe.[12]

Pathology

Fibrolamellar HCC generally manifests as a large, single, well-defined but nonencapsulated mass. On sectioning, lesions show a lobulated appearance, firm to hard consistency, and a characteristic central fibrous scar with radiating septa. Areas of hemorrhage and necrosis can be seen within the tumor in fewer than half of cases. The background liver is almost invariably normal. At histology, the distinctive features of fibrolamellar HCC are the coexistence of both fibrous stroma and tumor cells, typically arranged in a uniform sheet-like pattern.[12]

Liver Function

Liver function tests may demonstrate mild to moderate elevation of serum aminotransferases, alkaline phosphatase, and bilirubin. Unlike HCC, fibrolamellar HCC is infrequently accompanied by increased circulating levels of α-fetoprotein.[11]

Imaging

Fibrolamellar HCC comes to clinical attention because of either mass effect–related symptoms or nonspecific symptoms of malignancy.[11,12]

Radiography

Although larger lesions may deform one of the visible borders of the liver or cause mass effect on adjacent structures, more commonly a plain abdominal radiograph does not provide any clinical information in patients with fibrolamellar HCC.

CT

At precontrast CT, fibrolamellar HCC manifests as large, solitary, well-demarcated and lobulated masses that are hypoattenuating compared with the surrounding liver. Intratumoral areas of hemorrhage, necrosis, and calcification are present in approximately two thirds of cases. At contrast-enhanced CT, fibrolamellar HCC shows vivid and heterogeneous enhancement with the exception of the central fibrous scar. During the portal venous and delayed phase, lesions show wash out and become hypoattenuating compared with the liver. Notably, unlike other benign liver tumors with a central scar (e.g., focal nodular hyperplasia), there is no delayed enhancement of the central fibrous scar. Multiple, bulky metastatic nodes can frequently be seen at the hepatic hilum and the anterior cardiophrenic angles (Fig. 64-6).[12,13]

MRI

At MRI, fibrolamellar HCC is hypointense and mildly hyperintense on T1- and T2-weighted images, respectively. Because of dense fibrous stroma and calcification, the central fibrous scar is characteristically hypointense on both T1- and T2-weighted images. On gadolinium-enhanced MRI, the tumor enhancement pattern is substantially comparable to that of CT (see Fig. 64-6).[12]

Ultrasonography

Fibrolamellar HCC shows variable appearance on gray-scale ultrasonography, with most lesions being predominantly hypoechoic. A central echogenic area with tiny hyperechoic foci may be frequently seen and corresponds to the central fibrous scar and calcifications at pathologic analysis.

Nuclear Medicine

On sulfur-colloid liver/spleen scans, fibrolamellar HCC typically lacks normal uptake of the radiotracer and appears as a "cold" area within the liver.

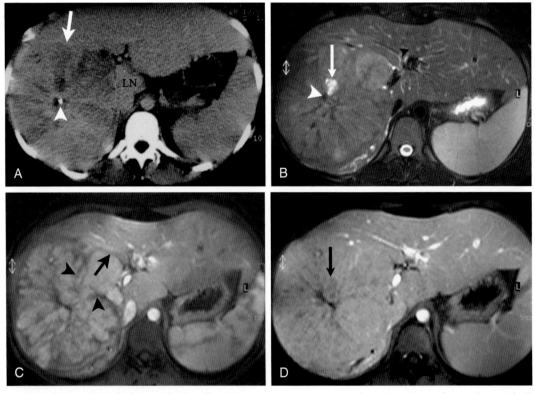

■ **FIGURE 64-6** Typical CT and MRI findings of fibrolamellar HCC. **A,** Transverse contrast-enhanced CT image shows a large right liver lobe mass (*arrow*) with central calcification (*arrowhead*). Bulky lymphadenopathy (LN) is seen at hepatic hilum. **B,** On fat-suppressed T2-weighted turbo spin-echo MR image, the mass demonstrates mild hyperintensity compared with the adjacent liver. The central scar (*arrowhead*) is hypointense. A hyperintense area (*arrow*), which corresponds to tumor necrosis, is also seen. **C,** On fat-suppressed T1-weighted gradient-recalled-echo MR image during hepatic arterial phase, this lesion shows marked, heterogeneous enhancement and is hyperintense relative to the liver, with the only exception of the central fibrous scar, radiating septa (*arrowheads*), and capsule (*arrow*). **D,** On corresponding image during portal venous phase, the tumor becomes isointense compared with the surrounding liver. A central portion of the tumor that was of high signal intensity on T2-weighted imaging is noted as of low-signal intensity (*arrow*) on this sequence. The central fibrous scar remains hypointense. *(From Brancatelli G, Federle MP, et al. Hepatocellular and fibrolamellar carcinoma. In Lencioni R, Cioni D, Bartolozzi C (eds). Focal Liver Lesions: Detection, Characterization, Ablation. Berlin, Springer, 2005, pp 209-217. With kind permission of Springer Science+Business Media.)*

Classic Signs: Fibrolamellar Hepatocellular Carcinoma	**What the Referring Physician Needs to Know: Fibrolamellar Hepatocellular Carcinoma**
■ Large lesion ■ Heterogeneous, strong enhancement ■ Wash out ■ Lobulated margins ■ Central, stellate scar ■ Central calcifications ■ Hypointense scar on T2-weighted imaging ■ Radiating septa ■ Metastatic lymphadenopathy	■ Fibrolamellar HCC typically occurs in patients younger than 40 years of age. ■ It frequently demonstrates aggressive local invasion, with both nodal and distant metastases. ■ The indolent growth rate is relative. ■ Pretherapy imaging is important for staging. ■ Aggressive surgical resection may prolong survival. ■ Imaging after resection is important for surveillance. ■ Prognosis is better than that of HCC when the tumor is resected.

PET/CT

The usefulness of PET/CT in the evaluation of fibrolamellar HCC has not been investigated.

Imaging Algorithm

An imaging algorithm is provided in Figure 64-14.

Differential Diagnosis

Younger age and lack of history of chronic liver disease allow the differential diagnosis with HCC.[11] Because of some similarities in demographic and imaging appearances, the differential diagnosis of fibrolamellar HCC from focal nodular hyperplasia may be challenging (Fig. 64-7; Table 64-5). Besides common signs of malignancy, such as biliary or vascular invasion and metastatic dissemination to lymph nodes or distant organs, additional clues for the diagnosis of fibrolamellar HCC include larger size, heterogeneous enhancement, and low signal intensity on T2-weighted images as well as lack of delayed enhancement of the central fibrous scar.[12] In some cases, giant hemangiomas can also show a central fibrous scar that is usually larger than fibrolamellar HCC. However, hemangiomas can be readily diagnosed based on their typical enhancement pattern (see Table 64-5).

Treatment

Medical Treatment

Several chemotherapeutic regimens have been used, with partial responses.

Surgical Treatment

Partial resection or liver transplantation represents the optimal treatment in patients with fibrolamellar HCC. All series have reported long survival periods after excision, with the longest post-resection survival time of 21 years. The most significant determinant of survival is tumor stage.[14]

Hepatoblastoma

Etiology

Hepatoblastoma has been recently associated with prematurity or low birth weight. The coincidence of hepatoblastoma with familial adenomatous polyposis and Beckwith-Wiedemann syndrome suggests a role in the pathogenesis of hepatoblastoma for chromosomes 5 and 11, respectively.[15]

Prevalence and Epidemiology

Hepatoblastoma is the most frequent liver tumor in children, accounting for half of those that are malignant. Males are twice as commonly affected as females in early childhood, but tumor frequency is nearly equal in older children.[15,16]

Clinical Presentation

Common signs and symptoms include rapidly enlarging abdomen, weight loss or anorexia, nausea, vomiting, abdominal pain, and jaundice. Occasionally, paraneoplastic phenomena, such as precocious puberty with genital enlargement, appearance of pubic hair, and a deepening voice may appear, owing to tumor overproduction of human chorionic gonadotropin.[15,16]

Pathophysiology

Hepatoblastoma occurs more frequently in the right lobe of the liver.[16]

Pathology

At gross inspection, hepatoblastoma generally manifests as a large mass. On sectioning, it is well demarcated, with prominent vascularity and a variegated appearance due to areas of hemorrhage, necrosis, and calcification. Three patterns of hepatoblastoma have been described at histopathologic analysis and include the pure fetal epithelial, the mixed epithelial, and the mesenchymal forms.[16]

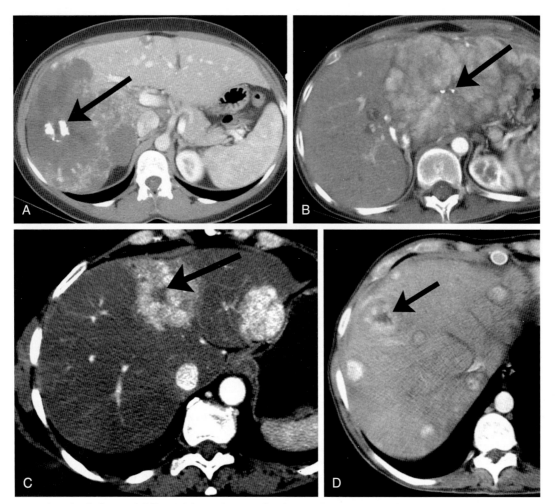

■ **FIGURE 64-7** CT imaging findings and differential diagnosis among liver lesions showing a central fibrous scar, including giant hemangioma, fibrolamellar HCC, focal nodular hyperplasia, and large regenerative nodules. Although all these lesions present a central fibrous scar, the differential diagnosis relies on imaging findings of both the lesion and the scar. **A,** Regardless its size, hemangioma invariably shows peripheral, nodular enhancement that is isoattenuating to vessels and with centripetal progression. Larger lesions may present as a central, calcified scar, as in this case (*arrow*). **B,** Fibrolamellar HCC typically manifests as a large lesion originating in the left liver lobe that demonstrates strong, heterogeneous enhancement during hepatic arterial phase and wash out during portal venous phase. Note coarse calcifications of the central scar (*arrow*) that represent a hallmark for this tumor. **C** and **D,** Unlike fibrolamellar HCC, focal nodular hyperplasia and large regenerative nodules both demonstrate strong enhancement during hepatic arterial phase and no wash out during portal venous phase. Both lesions may show a central fibrous scar (*arrows*) that, as a general rule, does not calcify. Although multiplicity is a characteristic of large regenerative nodules, this finding can also be observed in patients with focal nodular hyperplasia, as in this case. (*B from Brancatelli G, Federle MP, et al. Hepatocellular and fibrolamellar carcinoma. In Lencioni R, Cioni D, Bartolozzi C (eds). Focal Liver Lesions: Detection, Characterization, Ablation. Berlin, Springer, 2005, pp 209-217. With kind permission of Springer Science+Business Media.*)

TABLE 64-5 Differential Features between Lesions with Central Scar (Focal Nodular Hyperplasia, Fibrolamellar Hepatocellular Carcinoma, Giant Hemangioma, Large Regenerative Nodules)

	Focal Nodular Hyperplasia	Fibrolamellar HCC	Giant Hemangioma	Large Regenerative Nodules
Sex	F > M	F = M	F > M	F > M
Age	3-4th decade	2-3rd decade	2-5th decade	3-4th decade
Central Scar	Yes	Yes	Yes	Larger lesions
Enhancement Degree on Hepatic Arterial Phase	Very strong	Strong	Isoattenuatng to aorta	Strong
Homogeneous Enhancement on Hepatic Arterial Phase	Yes	No	No	Yes
Central Calcifications	No	68%	Yes	No
Capsule	No	35%	No	No
Lobulated Shape	Yes	Yes	Yes	No
Lymph Nodes	No	65%	No	No
Delayed Enhancement of Lesion	No	No	Yes	No
Delayed Enhancement of Scar	Yes	No	No	No
Wash Out on Portal Venous and Delayed Phases	No	Yes	No	No
Scar Hyperintensity on T2 Weighting	Yes	No	Yes	Yes
Necrosis	No	Yes	No	No

Liver Function

Laboratory findings almost invariably show elevated α-fetoprotein levels, which is regarded as a reliable predictor of tumor response to chemotherapeutic treatment as well as patient outcome.[15]

Imaging

Hepatoblastoma usually presents as an asymptomatic, firm, irregular mass noted on physical examination in the right abdomen. Because lesions are generally large, they may extend across the midline or down to the pelvic brim. Weight loss, anorexia, emesis, and abdominal pain indicate advanced disease.[15]

Radiography

The most common radiographic finding is hepatomegaly or a soft tissue mass in the right upper quadrant (with or without calcification).[16]

CT

At precontrast CT, hepatoblastoma typically manifests as a large, solitary, predominantly hypoattenuating mass with heterogeneous internal texture due to intralesional hemorrhage, calcifications, and necrosis. At contrast-enhanced CT, the tumor enhancement pattern closely mimics that of conventional HCC, with heterogeneous enhancement during the hepatic arterial phase (Fig. 64-8), followed by substantial wash out during the portal venous and delayed phases. Vascular invasion and peripheral rim of enhancement can also be seen.[16]

MRI

Because hepatoblastoma invariably occurs in children or younger patients, MRI is the modality of choice in the preoperative evaluation of the tumor owing to the lack of hazards of ionizing radiation. At precontrast MRI, hepato-blastoma shows nonspecific imaging findings with hypointensity and mild hyperintensity on T1- and T2-weighted MR images, respectively. Areas of hemorrhage can be seen as intratumoral hyperintense foci on T1-weighted images, whereas calcification is depicted as signal void on T2-weighted images. On gadolinium-enhanced MRI, the tumor enhancement pattern is substantially comparable to that of CT.[16]

Ultrasonography

Hepatoblastomas generally manifest as well-defined, solid, echogenic lesions on gray-scale ultrasonography. Occasionally, tumors may show a spoked-wheel appearance owing to prominent fibrous bands. Calcification and mesenchymal elements can be seen as increased echogenic areas.[16]

Nuclear Medicine

99mTc-sulfur colloid liver/spleen scans show large filling defects in the hepatic parenchyma. Gallium scanning shows avidity for the radiopharmaceutical in the tumor mass.[16]

PET/CT

Preliminary results suggest that PET/CT may enable optimal evaluation of liver parenchyma in patients with either primary or recurrent hepatoblastoma and may also detect metastatic sites not identified by other imaging techniques, thus allowing more precise tumor staging.

Imaging Algorithm

An imaging algorithm is provided in Figure 64-14.

Differential Diagnosis

Patient age is the major clinical discriminator between hepatoblastoma and classic HCC. Elevated α-fetoprotein

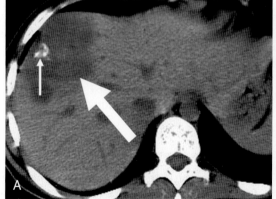
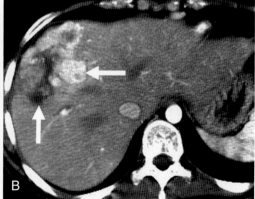

■ **FIGURE 64-8** CT of hepatoblastoma. **A,** Transverse precontrast CT image demonstrates a large, hypoattenuating mass (*arrow*) with a peripheral coarse calcification (*small arrow*) in the right lobe. **B,** On contrast-enhanced CT image during hepatic arterial phase, the mass shows marked, heterogeneous enhancement due to coexistence of both viable tumor (*horizontal arrow*) and necrosis (*vertical arrow*).

Classic Signs: Hepatoblastoma

- Young age (<3 years)
- Right lobe of liver
- Large lesion
- Coarse calcifications
- Internal septa
- Peripheral rim enhancement

What the Referring Physician Needs to Know: Hepatoblastoma

- Hepatoblastoma typically affects infants and children younger than 3 years of age.
- Some imaging features are helpful in differentiating hepatoblastoma from other pediatric tumors.
- Cure of hepatoblastoma can be achieved by surgical resection.
- Orthotopic liver transplantation is a suitable approach in patients with unresectable hepatoblastoma.
- MRI is the preferred modality to define tumor margins, determine tumor resectability, and detect residual or recurrent tumor after surgery.

---

level, but normal serum vanillylmandelic acid levels, may provide a clue for differentiating hepatoblastoma from neuroblastoma.

Although diagnosis of hepatoblastoma can be rarely based on imaging findings, a pattern of coarse and dense calcifications is suggestive of this neoplasm and allows differentiation with the fine granular calcifications of infantile hemangioendothelioma.[16]

Treatment

Medical Treatment

Despite the fact that 40% to 60% of hepatoblastomas are considered to be unresectable at the time of diagnosis, nearly 85% of cases may become resectable after preoperative chemotherapy (i.e., with cisplatin and doxorubicin).[16]

Surgical Treatment

Surgery remains the mainstay in the treatment of hepatoblastoma, with prognosis directly related to tumor stage. Lesions localized to a single lobe can be adequately treated by lobectomy. Liver transplantation has demonstrated promising results and is currently performed in patients with larger lesions, including those requiring preoperative chemotherapy.

Lymphoma

Etiology

Although secondary involvement of the liver by advanced Hodgkin's or non-Hodgkin's lymphoma is relatively common, primary hepatic lymphoma is an exceedingly rare neoplasm. Its frequent association with hepatitis C virus infection suggests that this virus plays some role in the pathogenesis of the neoplasm.[17]

Prevalence and Epidemiology

Unlike secondary involvement of the liver in patients with multiorgan lymphoma, primary hepatic lymphoma is a malignant neoplasm that arises in, and is initially confined to, the liver. In the majority of cases, splenic involvement is also present at the time of detection. This tumor shows a slight predominance in males (male-to-female ratio, 2.5:1) with a peak incidence from the sixth to the seventh decade.[18]

Clinical Presentation

Symptoms are generally nonspecific and include abdominal pain, hepatomegaly, weight loss, and fever. Occasionally, hepatic lymphoma may be incidentally discovered in asymptomatic patients.[18]

Pathophysiology

Patients usually have an enlarged liver containing solitary or multiple masses.

Pathology

Primary and secondary hepatic lymphomas may manifest as either solitary or multifocal disease. Tumor size varies from a few millimeters to several centimeters and is generally larger for solitary lesions. Occasionally, tumors may present as a diffuse, infiltrative growth pattern.

At histology, all hepatic lymphomas are classified as non-Hodgkin's with coexistence of both B- and T-cell lineage. Misdiagnosis—as metastatic carcinoma, chronic hepatitis, or inflammatory pseudotumor—is common.[18]

Liver Function

Serum liver enzymes, lactate dehydrogenase, and β_2-microglobulin levels are usually elevated, whereas α-fetoprotein and CEA levels are within normal range.[18]

Imaging

Presenting complaints consist of abdominal pain, weakness, fatigue, and constitutional symptoms. Hepatomegaly is frequent.

Radiography

Although plain film radiograph gives no diagnostic clue for the diagnosis of hepatic lymphoma, extrahepatic associated findings, such as bulky mediastinal lymphadenopathies or splenomegaly, can be detected in patients with multiorgan disease.

CT

At precontrast CT, hepatic lymphomas are generally isoattenuating to hypoattenuating compared with the surrounding liver. At contrast-enhanced CT, lymphomas manifest as either solitary or multifocal, well-defined hypoattenuating lesions (Fig. 64-9). In cases of diffuse, infiltrative liver involvement, lymphoma manifests as diffuse areas of decreased attenuation with geographic configuration, thus mimicking focal fatty infiltration or hepatic metastases (Fig. 64-10).[18]

MRI

Hepatic lymphomas show a wide spectrum of imaging appearances on MRI. Although lesions are generally mildly to moderately hypointense relative to the liver on T1-weighted images, their appearance can vary from low to moderate hyperintensity on T2-weighted images and may reflect differences in tumor vascularity, size of extracellular space, and presence of necrosis and fibrosis.[19]

Ultrasonography

At gray-scale ultrasonography, primary hepatic lymphomas generally appear as well-defined, either anechoic or hypoechoic lesions that mimic simple hepatic cysts, except for the absence of increased through-transmission.[18]

Nuclear Medicine

Because either necrotic or fibrous tissue usually lacks radiotracer uptake, gallium-67 scintigraphy has proved useful in restaging and determining the need for further therapy in post-treatment evaluation. These findings may be an important indicator of patients who may benefit from a change to a more aggressive treatment.

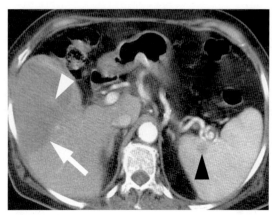

■ **FIGURE 64-9** Typical CT imaging findings of lymphoma. Transverse contrast-enhanced CT image during portal venous phase shows a large, solitary mass (*arrow*) in the right liver lobe that is hypoattenuating compared with the adjacent hepatic parenchyma. A portal venous branch (*white arrowhead*) extending through the lesion is barely visible. A small splenic lesion (*black arrowhead*) is also seen.

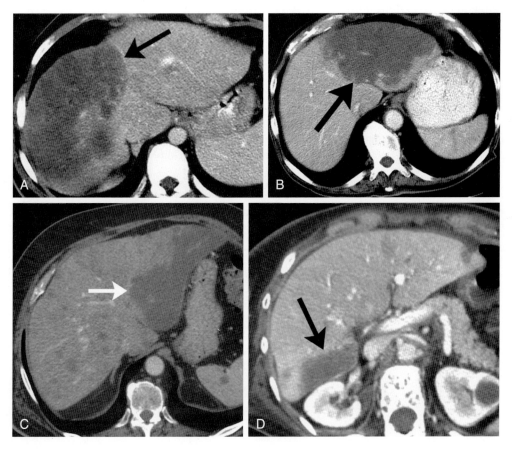

■ **FIGURE 64-10** CT imaging findings of liver lesions showing an infiltrative pattern, including epithelioid hemangioendothelioma (**A**), lymphoma (**B**), fatty infiltration (**C**), and breast metastases (**D**). Although an infiltrative appearance (*arrows*) is generally regarded as a worrisome sign, differential diagnosis among both malignant and benign liver lesions is frequently challenging solely based on imaging findings.

PET/CT

At present, PET/CT is commonly used to stage both Hodgkin's disease and non-Hodgkin's lymphoma. Besides its high sensitivity for detecting nodal disease regardless of the lesion site and size, PET/CT can also accurately demonstrate extranodal involvement, such as liver and splenic lesions. In addition, PET/CT is the modality of choice for evaluating recurrent lymphomas as well as tumor response to therapy.

Imaging Algorithm

An imaging algorithm is provided in Figure 64-14.

Classic Signs: Lymphoma

- Rare
- Unknown etiology
- Solitary
- Large
- Infiltrative pattern
- Decreased attenuation

Differential Diagnosis

Clinical data do not provide any clue for the diagnosis of primary hepatic lymphoma. The absence of increased through-transmission at ultrasonography is helpful for differentiation from simple hepatic cyst.[18] At contrast-enhanced CT and MRI, lymphomas do not show perilesional, continuous rim enhancement followed by centripetal filling that characterize metastases.

Differential diagnosis with other infiltrative liver lesions, such as EHE, infiltrative primary or secondary neoplasms, and focal steatosis, can be challenging (see Fig. 64-10; Table 64-6). Unlike in the setting of fatty liver disease, lymphomas do not show signal drop on opposed-phase MR images.

Treatment

Medical Treatment

Primary lymphoma shows an excellent response rate associated with the use of combination chemotherapy alone.[17]

Surgical Treatment

Surgery alone has been advocated for those patients with small solitary hepatic lesions, although its efficacy is frequently limited by early extrahepatic recurrence.[17]

What the Referring Physician Needs to Know: Lymphoma

- Primary hepatic non-Hodgkin's lymphoma is rare and difficult to diagnose.
- Patients are typically male and middle-aged.
- This is a lymphoproliferative disorder of unknown etiology.
- Typical presenting complaints are right upper quadrant pain, nausea, and emesis with significant weight loss.
- Prognosis in affected patients is dismal, with early disease recurrence at extrahepatic sites and short survival.
- Anthracycline-based chemotherapy is the most appropriate treatment.

Hepatic Metastases

Etiology

The liver provides a prime location for metastases from malignant tumors due to its location, blood supply, anatomy, as well as other poorly understood factors.

Prevalence and Epidemiology

Metastases are by far the most common malignant neoplasm of the liver. In the United States, it has been esti-

---

TABLE 64-6 Differential Features between Lesions with Infiltrative Pattern (Epithelioid Hemangioendothelioma, Lymphoma, Fatty Infiltration, and Metastases)

	Epithelioid Hemangioendothelioma	Lymphoma	Fatty Infiltration	Metastases
Sex	F ≥ M	M > F	F = M	F = M
Age	4-5th decade	6-7th decade	5th decade	Any age
Associated Conditions	None	Multiorgan involvement	Obesity, diabetes	Primary malignancy
Normal Vessels through Lesion	No	Yes	Yes	No
Lymph Nodes	No	Yes	No	Yes
Capsular Retraction	Yes	±	No	Yes if previous chemotherapy
Straight Margins	No	No	Yes	No
Hypertrophy of Unaffected Liver	Yes	No	No	No
Signal Drop on Out-of-Phase MRI	No	No	Yes	No

mated that up to 40% of patients with cancer have metastatic dissemination to the liver at the time of death. After regional lymph nodes, the liver is the predominant site of metastasis. Although liver metastases are fed primarily by arterial blood supply, they have been arbitrarily classified as either hypervascular or hypovascular according to their enhancement pattern compared with that of the surrounding hepatic parenchyma at either multiphasic contrast-enhanced CT or MRI.

The most common primary sites for liver metastases include the gastrointestinal tract, pancreas, gallbladder, breast, lung, eye, and carcinoids.[20-22]

Clinical Presentation

Metastases are often detected during radiologic workup of patients with newly discovered primary tumors. In advanced stages, signs and symptoms are referred to liver involvement and include hepatomegaly, anorexia, weight loss, and right upper quadrant abdominal pain (30% to 40%). Less than 10% of patients may present with a palpable mass.[20-22]

Pathophysiology

Metastases may be found anywhere in the liver but usually occur more in the right lobe than the left. The reason for this distribution is unclear, although possible reasons may be the greater total mass of the right lobe compared with the left lobe as well as underlying differences in laminar portal vein flow patterns, which may guide the distribution of metastatic cells.

Pathology

Liver metastases typically manifest as multiple irregular nodules, with a variable size ranging from a few millimeters to several centimeters. Central areas of avascular necrosis can be frequently seen at the center of the lesions. After chemotherapy, metastases may demonstrate an umbilicated appearance owing to scarring and retraction.

At histology, metastases closely resemble the appearance of primary tumor. By taking advantage of histochemical and immunohistochemical stains, experienced pathologists can often suggest the primary site when unknown.[20-22]

Liver Function

Liver-associated enzymes, such as alkaline phosphatase and gamma-glutamyl transpeptidase, are frequently abnormal in patients with liver metastases. Elevated blood levels of CEA are commonly discovered in patients with liver metastases from colorectal and pancreatic adenocarcinomas.

Imaging

Clinical signs and symptoms referable to the liver are generally associated with far advanced tumor stages as well as extensive liver involvement.

Radiography

Although larger lesions may deform one of the visible borders of the liver or cause mass effect on adjacent structure, more commonly a plain abdominal radiograph does not provide any clinical information in the investigation of patients with liver metastases. Rarely, amorphous calcifications may be seen in metastases from mucinous adenocarcinomas.

CT

Although metastases can be mildly hypoattenuating relative to the liver, lesion conspicuity is relatively poor at precontrast CT. Occasionally, intratumoral calcifications can be seen in mucinous adenocarcinoma metastases (i.e., colon, rectum, or ovary) (Fig. 64-11) or after local or systemic chemotherapy.[23] Hypervascular metastases, such as those from neuroendocrine tumors, thyroid, renal cell carcinoma, pheochromocytoma, and, occasionally, breast,

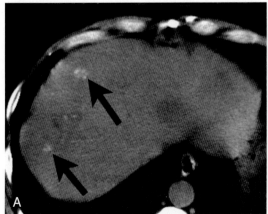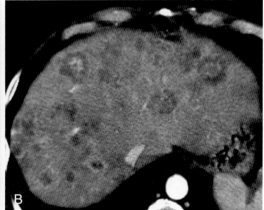

■ **FIGURE 64-11** Typical CT imaging findings of hypovascular liver metastases with calcifications from metastatic mucinous adenocarcinoma of the colon. **A,** Transverse precontrast CT image demonstrates two hepatic lesions with amorphous calcifications (*arrows*). **B,** On contrast-enhanced CT image during portal venous phase, multiple hypoattenuating lesions with peripheral rim enhancement are identified throughout the liver.

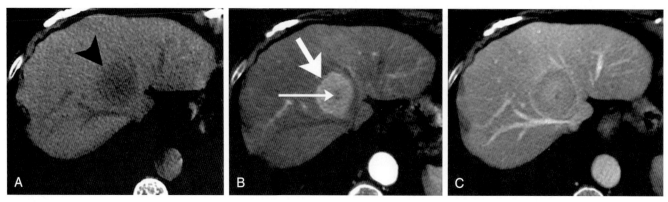

■ **FIGURE 64-12** Typical CT imaging findings of a hypervascular liver metastasis from gastrointestinal stromal tumor. Based on the strong, homogeneous hypervascularity (*arrow*, **B**) on hepatic arterial phase and on the central area of hypoattenuation simulating a central scar (*long thin arrow*, **B**), the lesion enters in differential diagnosis with focal nodular hyperplasia. However, strong hypoattenuation (*arrowhead*) on noncontrast image (**A**), wash out on portal venous phase (**C**), and the history of a known primary neoplasm all favor metastatic disease.

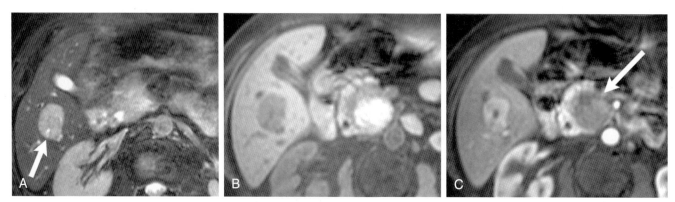

■ **FIGURE 64-13** Typical MR imaging findings of a hypervascular liver metastasis from neuroendocrine tumor of the pancreas. **A**, Transverse fat-suppressed T2-weighted fast spin-echo MR image demonstrates a 3-cm, strongly hyperintense lesion (*arrow*). **B**, The lesion is markedly hypointense on corresponding fat-suppressed T1-weighted gradient-recalled-echo MR image. **C**, On gadolinium-enhanced MRI, the lesion shows marked enhancement during hepatic arterial phase. Note the large primary tumor (*arrow*) in the pancreatic head. Although strong, homogeneous enhancement of the lesion during hepatic arterial phase may resemble focal nodular hyperplasia, other imaging findings, such as marked hypointensity on T1-weighted imaging, strong hyperintensity on T2-weighted imaging, as well as a known history of malignancy, allow a confident diagnosis in this case.

melanoma, and gastrointestinal stromal tumors, are best depicted during the hepatic arterial phase when they manifest as hyperattenuating foci compared with the surrounding liver (Fig. 64-12).[24,25] Hypovascular liver metastases, which encompass the vast majority of cases, such as colorectal tumor metastases, manifest as hypoattenuating lesions during the portal venous phase when the maximum enhancement of hepatic parenchyma occurs (see Fig. 64-11).[26] Early peripheral rim enhancement can also be seen in hypovascular liver metastases and reflects highly vascularized viable tumor at the periphery of the lesion.[27] By providing detailed information of the vascular anatomy, CT arteriography with volumetric 3D rendering is routinely performed in patients with colorectal metastases, which may benefit from local targeted chemotherapy after hepatic artery pump implantation.[28]

MRI

At MRI, metastases show nonspecific imaging findings with hypointensity and mild hyperintensity on T1- and T2-weighted MR images, respectively. In the setting of diffuse fatty liver disease, metastases may appear hyperintense on opposed-phase T1-weighted images owing to substantial signal drop of the surrounding hepatic parenchyma. On gadolinium-enhanced T1-weighted gradient-recalled-echo MRI, the tumor enhancement pattern is substantially comparable to that at CT. Because of increased sensitivity of MRI for gadolinium chelates and the more compact administration of contrast bolus, the conspicuity of hypervascular metastases at MRI (Fig. 64-13) can be higher than at CT. In addition, with the recent introduction of liver-specific MR contrast media, which can further increase both detection and characterization of liver lesions, MRI is currently considered the modality of choice in the investigation of patients with liver metastases.[29]

On diffusion-weighted MRI, the apparent diffusion coefficient values of metastases are slightly higher than those of the liver but significantly lower than those of hemangiomas and simple hepatic cysts.

Ultrasonography

Hepatic metastases show a variable appearance on gray-scale ultrasonography. Although ultrasonography is generally associated with a poor diagnostic performance, recently developed microbubble contrast agents have shown the potential to increase the accuracy of ultrasonography for the detection of liver metastases.

Intraoperative ultrasonography is a crucial adjunct during surgery to accurately define the anatomic relationship between tumors and major vascular and biliary structures and for detection of previously unsuspected liver lesions.

Nuclear Medicine

Somatostatin-receptor scintigraphy is useful for suspected neuroendocrine metastases. Radioimmunoscintigraphy with ^{99m}Tc-labeled anti-CEA monoclonal antibody has been proposed as a useful tool in patients with rising CEA levels by revealing increased tumor uptake. CT has replaced radionuclide imaging as the standard screening tool for liver metastatic disease.

PET/CT

Besides its leading role in the assessment of primary tumor as well as regional lymph node involvement, functional metabolic imaging with PET/CT also plays a key role in the detection of distant metastases. Because of their increased metabolic rate, hepatic metastases typically demonstrate increased FDG uptake compared with the normal liver.[29]

Imaging Algorithm

An imaging algorithm is provided in Figure 64-14.

> ## Classic Signs: Hepatic Metastases
>
> - Multiple lesions
> - Heterogeneous enhancement
> - Rim enhancement
> - Slow, centripetal enhancement
> - Central necrosis
> - Calcifications on unenhanced CT (metastases from primary mucinous adenocarcinoma)
> - Either hypervascular or hypovascular

Differential Diagnosis

A known history of malignancy raises the pre-test probability of a diagnosis of hepatic metastases. Although the peripheral rim enhancement of hypovascular metastases with centripetal progression can be mistaken for cavernous hemangiomas, lesion wash out on delayed images, mild hyperintensity on T2-weighted images, and, more recently, lower apparent diffusion coefficient values on diffusion-weighted images are all indicative findings of liver metastases. Unlike focal nodular hyperplasia, hypervascular metastases are heterogeneous due to areas of necrosis and demonstrate wash out during the portal venous (see Fig. 64-12) and delayed phases. In the setting of diffuse metastatic liver involvement from breast cancer, a macronodular appearance of hepatic margins can be seen after systemic chemotherapy (see Fig. 64-2) and should not be mistaken for cirrhosis (see Tables 64-3 and

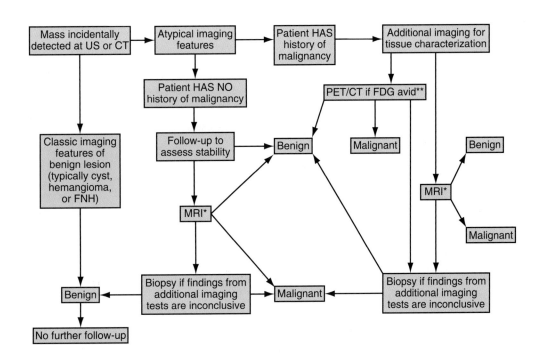

* Presence of focal fat can be ascertained with MRI using in-phase and out-of-phase scanning

** Metastatic disease from melanoma, colon and esophageal cancer, breast cancer, sarcoma

■ **FIGURE 64-14** Flow chart of a practical approach to the diagnosis of malignant hepatic lesions.

64-6).[20] Liver adenomatosis may closely mimic metastatic disease, although adenomas should be suspected when lesions demonstrate a fatty component with substantial signal drop on opposed-phase MR images. Metastases can occasionally present a cystic appearance with extensive necrosis and marked hyperintensity on T2-weighted MR images, lack of metabolic activity on FDG-PET, and high apparent diffusion coefficient values on diffusion-weighted MRI. These findings may not be differentiated from those of simple cyst or hemangioma and require further investigation with liver biopsy.[30]

Treatment

Medical Treatment

Chemotherapy represents the treatment of choice in patients with liver metastases in whom surgical resection cannot be performed. Furthermore, adjuvant chemotherapy is often combined with liver surgery in patients with metastatic disease. Several therapeutic regimens have been developed according to the primary tumor. Targeted delivery of chemotherapy to liver metastases via a surgically placed hepatic artery infusion pump represents an effective treatment in patients with unresectable hepatic colorectal metastases.[28]

Surgical Treatment

Hepatic metastases are surgically resectable if they are confined within a single lobe and if no extrahepatic disease is present. Less invasive alternatives to surgical resection include hepatic artery chemoembolization and percutaneous tumor ablation by using methods such as radiofrequency, cryosurgery, microwaves, ethanol, or interstitial laser thermotherapy.

What the Referring Physician Needs to Know: Hepatic Metastases

- CT is the primary imaging modality for the detection of hepatic metastases.
- Liver dual blood supply contributes to the metastases.
- Metastases are treated with chemotherapy, resection, or ablation techniques.
- CT and MRI are the preferred modalities for diagnosis of liver metastases and assessment of response to treatment.
- FDG-PET is the most sensitive noninvasive imaging method for detection of hepatic metastases from colorectal, gastric, or esophageal cancers.

SUMMARY

The discovery of a focal liver lesion, either incidentally or in a patient at higher risk for a liver tumor, commonly triggers multiple diagnostic tests, including general and liver function tests, circulating tumor markers, virology tests, and several imaging examinations (Table 64-7). Although primary detection may rely on transabdominal ultrasonography, this technique is hampered by poor sensitivity and specificity in the assessment of focal malignant liver tumors, with the only notable exception of intraoperative ultrasound evaluation.

Multiphasic contrast-enhanced CT and MRI currently play a key role in the evaluation of patients with liver tumors. Besides remarkable capabilities for lesion detection, both techniques can also provide excellent depiction of the anatomic relationship of the tumor with major intrahepatic biliary and vascular structures, which

---

TABLE 64-7 Accuracy, Limitations, and Pitfalls of the Modalities Used in Imaging of Malignant Focal Liver Lesions

Modality	Accuracy	Limitations	Pitfalls
Radiography	Poor	Insensitive Nonspecific	Unable to directly visualize soft tissue masses in the liver
CT	Sensitivity 69%-71% Specificity 86%-91% 76% fibrolamellar HCC from hemangioma and FNH	Radiation Limited use in patients with allergy or renal insufficiency Potential for anaphylactoid reaction	Lesion detection and characterization may be difficult in fatty liver
MRI	80%	Motion artifact in uncooperative patients and in patients with ascites Risk of nephrogenic systemic fibrosis in patients with renal insufficiency Claustrophobic patients Patients with cardiac pacemaker High cost	Calcifications not well visualized
Ultrasonography	91% before contrast enhanced ultrasonography)	Poor performances in the case of obesity or overlying bowel gas Operator dependent	Calcifications not well visualized
Nuclear medicine	Not useful except for neuroendocrine liver metastases (somatostatin receptor scintigraphy)	Poor spatial resolution	Numerous false-negative and false-positive findings
PET/CT	85%	Radiation High cost	Mismatches between the fused images, for example due to respiratory movement

is of paramount importance for treatment planning. Although CT is commonly used as the first-line modality owing to its broad availability and relatively limited costs, with the recent introduction of liver-specific MR contrast agents as well as remarkable improvements in image quality, MRI is emerging as the modality of choice, particularly in the evaluation of patients with liver metastases.

Recently, PET/CT is gaining greater popularity because of its capability to couple standard anatomic information with functional assessment of tumor metabolic activity (at the molecular level).

KEY POINTS

Epithelioid Hemangioendothelioma

- Rare
- Vascular origin
- Younger adults
- Good clinical condition
- Slow course of the disease
- Numerous intrahepatic lesions
- Nodules tend to merge into each other
- Peripheral location
- Capsular retraction
- Hypertrophy of the unaffected liver segments

Angiosarcoma

- Heterogeneous enhancement pattern
- Progressive enhancement
- Multifocal
- Hemorrhage and necrosis
- Rapid metastatic dissemination
- Aggressive behavior
- Tend to recur after treatment
- Poor prognosis

Hepatocellular Carcinoma in Noncirrhotic Liver

- Middle-aged men
- Large at diagnosis
- Solitary lesion or dominant mass with smaller satellite lesions
- Heterogeneous
- Lobulated
- Mosaic pattern
- Tumor thrombus
- Biliary invasion

Fibrolamellar Hepatocellular Carcinoma

- Noncirrhotic liver in young adults
- Large
- Often solitary
- Central scar in ~50% (CT: hypointense; MR: hypointense)
- Central calcifications in 68%
- Strong arterial enhancement
- Wash out
- Heterogeneous
- Biliary invasion
- Nodal and distant metastases

Hepatoblastoma

- Most commonly occurs in the first 3 years of life
- Large diameter at diagnosis
- Resection or transplantation can be curative

Lymphoma

- Rare
- Usually solitary
- Infiltrative pattern
- Large at presentation
- Imaging findings are nonspecific

Hepatic Metastases

- More common malignant hepatic lesion
- Usually multiple
- Hypovascular or hypervascular based on enhancement characteristics
- Heterogeneous enhancement

SUGGESTED READINGS

Danet IM, et al. Spectrum of MRI appearances of untreated metastases of the liver. AJR Am J Roentgenol 2003; 181:809-817.

Elsayes KM, et al. Focal hepatic lesions: diagnostic value of enhancement pattern approach with contrast-enhanced 3D gradient-echo MR imaging. RadioGraphics 2005; 25:1299-1320.

Imam K, et al. MR imaging in the evaluation of liver metastases. Magn Reson Imaging Clin North Am 2000; 8:741-767.

Kelekis NL, et al. Focal hepatic lymphoma: magnetic resonance demonstration using current techniques including gadolinium enhancement. Magn Reson Imaging 1997; 15:625-636.

Levy AD. Malignant liver tumors. Clin Liver Dis 2002; 6:147-164.

McLarney JK, et al. Fibrolamellar carcinoma of the liver: radiologic-pathologic correlation. RadioGraphics 1999; 19:453-471.

Pedro MS, et al. MR imaging of hepatic metastases. Magn Reson Imaging Clin North Am 2002; 10:15-29.

Powers C, et al. Primary liver neoplasms: MR imaging with pathologic correlation. RadioGraphics 1994; 14:459-482.

Sica GT, et al. Computed tomography and magnetic resonance imaging of hepatic metastases. Clin Liver Dis 2002; 6:165-179.

Sica GT, et al. CT and MR imaging of hepatic metastases. AJR Am J Roentgenol 2000; 174:691-698.

REFERENCES

1. Mehrabi A, et al. Primary malignant hepatic epithelioid hemangio-endothelioma: a comprehensive review of the literature with emphasis on the surgical therapy. Cancer 2006; 107:2108-2121.

2. Miller WJ, et al. Epithelioid hemangioendothelioma of the liver: imaging findings with pathologic correlation. AJR Am J Roentgenol 1992; 159:53-57.

3. Mermuys K, et al. Epithelioid hemangioendothelioma of the liver: radiologic-pathologic correlation. Abdom Imaging 2004; 29:221-223.

4. Lyburn ID, et al. Hepatic epithelioid hemangioendothelioma: sonographic, CT, and MR imaging appearances. AJR Am J Roentgenol 2003; 180:1359-1364.

5. Peterson MS, et al. Hepatic angiosarcoma: findings on multiphasic contrast-enhanced helical CT do not mimic hepatic hemangioma. AJR Am J Roentgenol 2000; 175:165-170.

6. Koyama T, et al. Primary hepatic angiosarcoma: findings at CT and MR imaging. Radiology 2002; 222:667-673.

7. Bralet MP, et al. Hepatocellular carcinoma occurring in nonfibrotic liver: epidemiologic and histopathologic analysis of 80 French cases. Hepatology 2000; 32:200-204.

8. Iannaccone R, et al. Hepatocellular carcinoma in patients with non-alcoholic fatty liver disease: helical CT and MR imaging findings with clinical-pathologic comparison. Radiology 2007; 243:422-430.

9. Brancatelli G, et al. Hepatocellular carcinoma in noncirrhotic liver: CT, clinical, and pathologic findings in 39 U.S. residents. Radiology 2002; 222:89-94.

10. Winston CB, et al. Hepatocellular carcinoma: MR imaging findings in cirrhotic livers and noncirrhotic livers. Radiology 1999; 210:75-79.

11. El-Serag HB, et al. Is fibrolamellar carcinoma different from hepatocellular carcinoma? A US population-based study. Hepatology 2004; 39:798-803.

12. Ichikawa T, et al. Fibrolamellar hepatocellular carcinoma: imaging and pathologic findings in 31 recent cases. Radiology 1999; 213:352-361.

13. Blachar A, et al. Radiologists' performance in the diagnosis of liver tumors with central scars by using specific CT criteria. Radiology 2002; 223:532-539.

14. Ichikawa T, et al. Fibrolamellar hepatocellular carcinoma: pre- and posttherapy evaluation with CT and MR imaging. Radiology 2000; 217:145-151.

15. Schnater JM, et al. Where do we stand with hepatoblastoma? A review. Cancer 2003; 15;98:668-678.

16. Dachman AH, et al. Hepatoblastoma: radiologic-pathologic correlation in 50 cases. Radiology 1987; 164:15-19.

17. Page RD, et al. Primary hepatic lymphoma: favorable outcome after combination chemotherapy. Cancer 2001; 92:2023-2029.

18. Sanders LM, et al. CT of primary lymphoma of the liver. AJR Am J Roentgenol 1989; 152:973-976.

19. Kelekis NL, et al. Focal hepatic lymphoma: magnetic resonance demonstration using current techniques including gadolinium enhancement. Magn Reson Imaging 1997; 15:625-636.

20. Paulson EK. Evaluation of the liver for metastatic disease. Semin Liver Dis 2001; 21:225-236.

21. Namasivayam S, et al. Imaging of liver metastases: MRI. Cancer Imaging 2007; 7:2-9.

22. Kanematsu M, et al. Imaging liver metastases: review and update. Eur J Radiol 2006; 58:217-228.

23. Valls C, et al. Hepatic metastases from colorectal cancer: preoperative detection and assessment of resectability with helical CT. Radiology 2001; 218:55-60.

24. Paulson EK, et al. Carcinoid metastases to the liver: role of triple-phase helical CT. Radiology 1998; 206:143-150.

25. Braga L, et al. Does hypervascularity of liver metastases as detected on MRI predict disease progression in breast cancer patients? AJR Am J Roentgenol 2004; 182:1207-1213.

26. Soyer P, et al. Detection of hypovascular hepatic metastases at triple-phase helical CT: sensitivity of phases and comparison with surgical and histopathologic findings. Radiology 2004; 231:413-420.

27. Yu JS, et al. Hepatic metastases: perilesional enhancement on dynamic MRI. AJR Am J Roentgenol 2006; 186:1051-1058.

28. Kapoor V, et al. Multidetector CT arteriography with volumetric three-dimensional rendering to evaluate patients with metastatic colorectal disease for placement of a floxuridine infusion pump. AJR Am J Roentgenol 2003; 181:455-463.

29. Bipat S, et al. Colorectal liver metastases: CT, MR imaging, and PET for diagnosis—meta-analysis. Radiology 2005; 237:123-131.

30. Kim T, et al. Discrimination of small hepatic hemangiomas from hypervascular malignant tumors smaller than 3 cm with three-phase helical CT. Radiology 2001; 219:699-706.

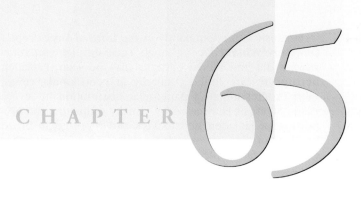
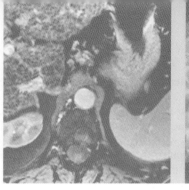
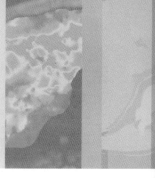

CHAPTER 65

Fatty Liver Disease

Sameer M. Mazhar, Heather M. Patton, Richard T. Scuderi, Takeshi Yokoo, Silvana C. Faria, and Claude B. Sirlin

ETIOLOGY

Fatty liver is a generic term that refers to the accumulation of lipids within hepatocytes. This chapter focuses on *nonalcoholic fatty liver disease* (*NAFLD*), the most common form of fatty liver. Histologically, it resembles alcoholic liver injury but occurs in patients who deny significant alcohol consumption. NAFLD encompasses a spectrum of conditions, ranging from benign hepatocellular *steatosis* to inflammatory *nonalcoholic steatohepatitis* (*NASH*), fibrosis, and cirrhosis.[1] NAFLD is associated with obesity and insulin resistance and is considered the hepatic manifestation of the metabolic syndrome, a combination of medical conditions including type 2 diabetes mellitus, hypertension, hyperlipidemia, and visceral adiposity.[2]

Other conditions associated with fatty liver include alcoholic liver disease, viral hepatitis, effects of certain medications (e.g., corticosteroids, tamoxifen, amiodarone, methotrexate, valproic acid, and select chemotherapy agents), human immunodeficiency virus (HIV) infection with lipodystrophy, total parenteral nutrition, pregnancy, and intestinal bypass surgery for weight loss.[3]

The pathogenesis of NAFLD and its progression to NASH is complex and remains incompletely understood. The most widely accepted paradigm is the so-called two-hit hypothesis.[4] In this model, the initial abnormality ("first hit") is the accumulation of lipids within hepatocytes (steatosis), which is mediated by insulin resistance.[5-8] The majority of hepatocellular lipids are stored as triglycerides, but other lipid metabolites, such as free fatty acids, cholesterol, and phospholipids, may also be present and play a role in disease progression.[9]

The accumulated hepatocellular lipids promote oxidative stress, which is the subsequent insult ("second hit") responsible for the progression from simple steatosis to steatohepatitis (NASH). Inflammatory and hormonal mediators secreted by adipocytes may contribute to the development of hepatic inflammation, apoptosis, and fibrosis.[7]

PREVALENCE AND EPIDEMIOLOGY

NAFLD is the most common form of chronic liver disease among adults and children in the United States and has been reported in many other parts of the world.[1,10] It is thought to be the leading cause of asymptomatic elevations of serum aminotransferase values and likely accounts for the majority of cases of cryptogenic cirrhosis. Determining the prevalence of NAFLD, however, is challenging. This is because it is generally a silent condition, and liver biopsy, which is the "gold standard" for the diagnosis of NAFLD, is not a tenable tool for establishing disease prevalence in the general population. Consequently, serum levels of aminotransferases (alanine aminotransferase [ALT] and aspartate aminotransferase [AST]) and imaging studies (ultrasonography and MR spectroscopy) have been used as surrogate markers to estimate population prevalence in most series.

Depending on the cutoff values used to define the upper limit of normal for aminotransferase levels, the estimated prevalence of NAFLD in the general United States population ranges from 5.4% to 24%, but these values may be underestimations because aminotransferase levels have limited sensitivity for steatosis.[11,12] Histologic estimates of NAFLD prevalence via preoperative or intraoperative liver biopsy, mainly obtained from individuals evaluated as donors for living-donor liver transplantation, are 33% to 88%.[13-15] In children, NAFLD prevalence has been estimated to be 9.6%; of great concern, 2% to 8% of children with NAFLD progress to cirrhosis.[16,17]

Obesity is the most important risk factor for NAFLD; the prevalence of NAFLD is 4.6 times greater in the obese, and up to 74% of obese individuals have fatty livers.[18] Among morbidly obese patients undergoing bariatric surgery for weight loss, 84% to 96% have NAFLD, 25% to 55% have NASH, and 2% to 12% have severe fibrosis or cirrhosis.[19-22] NAFLD is also strongly associated with hepatic and adipose tissue insulin resistance and metabolic syndrome.[23] Although NAFLD is clearly linked to obesity and metabolic syndrome, it may occur in up to 29% of lean patients lacking associative risk factors.[24]

Other factors that influence the development of NAFLD include age, sex, race, and ethnicity.[25-29] The prevalence of NAFLD increases with age in both adults and children.[26] NAFLD is more common among men than women younger than the age of 50; however, higher prevalence rates are seen in women older than the age of 50, perhaps related to hormonal changes occurring after menopause.[12] The highest rates of NAFLD are seen among Mexican-Americans, followed by non-Hispanic whites.[27,28] Non-Hispanic blacks display the lowest rates of NAFLD, despite the high prevalence of obesity and type 2 diabetes in this population.[13]

Metabolic syndrome and its associated conditions are commonly affiliated with NAFLD. The prevalence of NAFLD is estimated to be at least twice as common among individuals who meet criteria for metabolic syndrome.[29] Among individuals with NAFLD, it is estimated that over 90% have some features of metabolic syndrome.[2] Diabetes is reported in 33% to 50% of patients with NAFLD, whereas insulin resistance may occur in as many as 75%.[2,30]

CLINICAL PRESENTATION

The natural history of NAFLD is poorly understood but seems to be related to the severity of histologic disease. In simple steatosis, less than 5% of patients progress to cirrhosis over a 5- to 17-year period; alternatively, 25% of patients with NASH advance to cirrhosis within 10 years.[31] The rate of development of hepatocellular carcinoma is not well characterized but is thought to be lower than in viral liver disease.

Most patients with NAFLD are asymptomatic. When symptomatic, patients may experience malaise and non-specific right upper quadrant discomfort. On physical examination, hepatomegaly may be detected.[3] Patients characteristically have abdominal or visceral obesity. Those who progress to cirrhosis may exhibit stigmata of chronic liver disease and complications of portal hypertension.[3]

Typically, NAFLD is discovered incidentally when routine laboratory studies reveal a mild-to-modest elevation in ALT (less than five times the upper limit of normal), although AST is also often elevated to a milder degree. Serum aminotransferase levels may fluctuate, however, and some patients with NAFLD have normal levels. A careful history should exclude significant alcohol use. Laboratory testing must exclude viral hepatitis and iron overload syndromes. Imaging can be used to noninvasively suggest fatty deposition. Although unnecessary to secure the diagnosis, a liver biopsy may provide staging and prognostic information.

PATHOLOGY

On gross inspection, the fatty liver is enlarged and soft, with a yellowish tinge and greasy consistency. Microscopically, the spectrum of fatty liver disease is assessed on the basis of steatosis, steatohepatitis, cell injury, and fibrosis. These histologic changes are often shared by alcoholic liver disease and NAFLD; at times, only a detailed alcohol history will distinguish the two diagnoses.

Steatosis is predominantly in the form of large-droplet (*macrovesicular*) fat, although small-droplet (*microvesicular*) fat and mixed patterns may be seen. Fat-laden hepatocytes are found primarily in centrilobular areas, with progression to a panlobular distribution in severe cases. Steatosis is assessed by visually estimating the proportion of fat-laden hepatocytes and reported in broad brackets of severity: normal (less than 5% of hepatocytes containing fat droplets), mild (5% to 30% of hepatocytes), moderate (30% to 60% of hepatocytes), and severe (greater than 60% of hepatocytes).

When present, steatohepatitis is usually mild and characterized by a mixed inflammatory infiltrate of neutrophils and mononuclear cells (lymphocytes, macrophages, and Kupffer cells). In adults, the distribution is multifocal and may affect all zones of the liver lobule, which contrasts to the prominent portal inflammation seen in pediatric NASH.[32]

The hallmark feature of cellular injury in fatty liver disease is hepatocellular ballooning, thought by some to be the most important defining criterion in distinguishing NASH from simple steatosis. Ballooning refers to swollen, enlarged hepatocytes with partially cleared cytoplasm, found mainly in centrilobular regions near areas of steatosis.[32] *Mallory's hyaline* (ropy clumps of dense perinuclear cytoplasmic deposits composed of intermediate filaments) and *acidophil bodies* (apoptotic or necrotic hepatocytes with eosinophilic cytoplasmic globules) can be seen in NAFLD, although they are more frequently observed in alcoholic liver disease.

In adults, fibrosis is mainly centrilobular, radiating outward from terminal hepatic veins in a perisinusoidal or pericellular pattern. This "chicken wire" appearance of fibrosis progresses in advanced disease, causing a bridging of fibrous bands and, ultimately, cirrhosis. In advanced disease ("burnt-out NASH"), there is a paucity of fatty deposition because the parenchyma has been replaced by fibrotic tissue. Pediatric fatty liver disease has distinct histologic features, such as predominance of periportal fibrosis, which is rarely seen in adults.[33]

Several scoring systems have been proposed for the histologic grading and staging of fatty liver disease. Recently, the Pathology Committee of the NASH Clinical Research Network proposed a NAFLD activity score (NAS) based on steatosis (0-3), lobular inflammation (0-2), and hepatocellular ballooning (0-2). In this system, NASH is probable if the NAS is greater than 4, unlikely if less than 3, and of intermediate probability if 3 or 4.[34] Staging is based on the extent of fibrosis (0-4).

Differing patterns of steatosis arise in patients with hepatitis C infection or due to medication effects. In hepatitis C, macrovesicular fat droplets have a periportal, rather than centrilobular, distribution. The amount of steatosis increases with disease severity and is most commonly associated with genotype 3 hepatitis C virus. A number of medications lead to steatosis, including cytotoxic/cytostatic drugs, antibiotics, nucleoside analogs, and corticosteroids. The pattern of injury in drug-induced steatosis is nonspecific, typically consisting of macrovesicular fat deposits. Notable exceptions are Reye syndrome, associated with aspirin use in children, and tetracycline, both of which may lead to microvesicular steatosis.

IMAGING

The radiologic features of fatty liver disease stem from the increased fat content of the liver parenchyma. The spatial pattern may be diffuse and homogeneous or heterogeneous, with focal fat deposition in an otherwise normal liver or areas of focal fat sparing in a diffusely fatty liver (Table 65-1). The homogeneous form is the most common; the heterogeneous and focal forms may simulate perfusion abnormalities, diffusely infiltrative disease, nodular lesions, or masses.[35,36] Such findings may be especially problematic in the setting of known malignancy. Therefore, it is not only important to recognize fatty liver on imaging but also to discriminate it from other pathologic processes.

The most important modalities used in the assessment of hepatic steatosis are ultrasonography, CT, and MRI and MR spectroscopy (Table 65-2). These modalities vary in their accuracy to diagnose and grade steatosis, as discussed below. To date, no noninvasive method reliably differentiates NASH from simple steatosis. Several MR techniques (diffusion-weighted and perfusion-weighted MRI, MR elastography, and double-contrast enhanced MRI) show promise for detecting and staging the severity of liver fibrosis, but these techniques have not been validated in large clinical trials and are considered experimental.

Radiography

Plain radiography does not have a significant role in the assessment of fatty liver disease. Hepatomegaly and ascites may be appreciated in patients with early and advanced disease, respectively.

CT

CT has been widely used in the evaluation of fatty liver disease in adults. The use of ionizing radiation precludes its use as a research tool in children, although fatty liver may be observed in children on scans done for clinical purposes.[37]

Fat deposition in the liver is characterized by a reduction in the attenuation of the hepatic parenchyma. On unenhanced CT, normal liver parenchyma has slightly greater attenuation than the spleen or blood. However, with increasing hepatic steatosis, liver attenuation decreases and the liver may become less dense than the intrahepatic vessels, simulating the appearance of that on a contrast-enhanced scan (Fig. 65-1).[38]

A subjective 5-point qualitative grading has been proposed for the degree of hepatic steatosis based on hepatic attenuation and visualization of hepatic vessels (hepatic and portal veins):

TABLE 65-1 Spatial Pattern of Steatosis

Spatial Pattern	Remarks
Diffuse and homogeneous	Most common form
Diffuse and heterogeneous	Ill-defined, geographic, segmental or lobar areas of fatty deposition
Focal deposition or sparing	Typically adjacent to falciform ligament, porta hepatis, gallbladder fossa, and subcapsular regions; speculated to be due to anomalous venous drainage and/or locally variable insulin effects
Multifocal deposition	Multiple round or oval nodular fat depositions in atypical locations
Perivascular	Halos of fat surrounding hepatic veins, portal veins, or both
Subcapsular	Seen in patients receiving peritoneal dialysis with insulin-containing dialysate

TABLE 65-2 Classic Imaging Signs of Fatty Liver Disease

Modality	Diffuse Fat Deposition	Focal Fat Deposition	Focal Fat Sparing
Ultrasonography	Hyperechoic relative to adjacent kidney or spleen; Attenuation of the ultrasound beam; Decreased visualization of hepatic and portal veins; Loss of definition of the diaphragm; Hepatomegaly	Hyperechoic area in an otherwise normal liver; Occurs in specific locations: adjacent to falciform ligament, gallbladder fossa, and porta hepatis; Geographic margins; Absence of mass effect with nondistortion of traversing vessels	Hypoechoic area within a hyperechoic liver
Unenhanced CT	Hypodense liver measuring < 40 HU; Liver-spleen difference ≥ 10 HU; Liver/spleen ratio < 0.9	Hypodense area in an otherwise normal liver	Hyperdense area within a diffusely low attenuated liver
Enhanced CT	Absolute liver attenuation < 40 HU	Hypodense area in an otherwise normally enhancing liver; Enhancement similar to background liver	Isodense/hyperdense area compared with the liver parenchyma
MR spectroscopy	Spectral peak at resonance frequency of fat (e.g., methylene protons $-CH_2-$ at 3.2 ppm).	Not useful for focal fat deposition and/or focal fat sparing unless a multivoxel approach is used	
MRI	Relative signal loss on the fat-saturated image on frequency-selective imaging (fat saturated versus non-fat saturated). Relative signal loss on out-of-phase images compared with in-phase images on phase-interference imaging	Focal area of signal loss on fat-saturated or out-of-phase image	Focal sparing of signal loss on fat-saturated or out-of-phase image

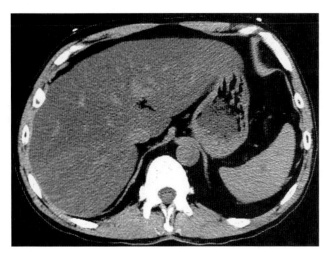

■ **FIGURE 65-1** Diffuse liver steatosis. Axial unenhanced CT scan reveals diffuse low attenuation of the liver compared with the spleen and the intrahepatic vessels. The appearance mimics that of a contrast-enhanced scan.

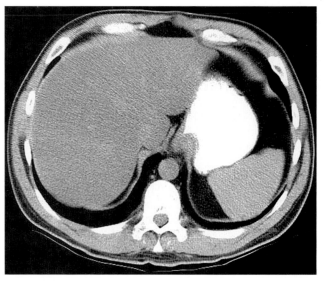

■ **FIGURE 65-2** Diffuse liver steatosis. Axial unenhanced CT scan reveals diffuse low attenuation of the liver. The absolute hepatic attenuation value is 26 HU, considered diagnostic of fatty liver. When comparing liver with spleen (55 HU), the difference between hepatic and splenic attenuations is −29 HU and the liver-to-spleen attenuation ratio is about 0.5. Both parameters indicate steatosis greater than 30% on histology.

Grade 1: hepatic vessels show lower attenuation than the hepatic parenchyma out to the peripheral third of liver

Grade 2: hepatic vessels show lower attenuation than the hepatic parenchyma out to the middle third of liver

Grade 3: hepatic vessels show lower attenuation than hepatic parenchyma in the central third of liver

Grade 4: hepatic vessels show the same attenuation as that of the hepatic parenchyma

Grade 5: hepatic vessels show higher attenuation than the hepatic parenchyma

Several criteria for the diagnosis of hepatic steatosis on unenhanced CT have been proposed. The first such criterion is an absolute liver attenuation of less than 40 HU. However, because the normal hepatic parenchyma attenuation ranges from 60 to 70 HU, the 40-HU cutoff value has high specificity but low sensitivity. Moreover, absolute attenuation values on unenhanced CT are subject to technical variations, such as scanner type. The second and third criteria attempt to overcome this limitation by expressing hepatic steatosis in relation to other organs known to be free of fat, such as the spleen. In these criteria (Hepatic Attenuation Index Criteria), an attenuation difference between liver and spleen of less than −10 HU and liver-to-spleen attenuation ratio of 0.9 indicate steatosis (Fig. 65-2).[39,40] Liver attenuation may be affected by a variety of factors other than liver fat, such as iron, copper, glycogen, fibrosis, edema, or amiodarone use. Assessment of liver fat by CT attenuation may be unreliable, and CT methods are insensitive to mild steatosis. The reported sensitivity and specificity of unenhanced CT for detection of moderate/severe steatosis (>30% on histology) ranges from 73% to 100% and 95% to 100%, respectively.[37]

At enhanced CT, the presence of iodine contrast interferes with attenuation, adding a new confounding factor. Perfusion alterations, timing of acquisitions, and contrast type, dosage, and injection rate all may influence hepatic and splenic attenuation. Nevertheless, criteria have been proposed to detect hepatic steatosis at enhanced CT,

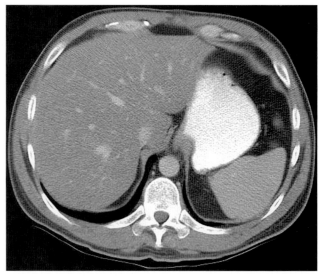

■ **FIGURE 65-3** Diffuse liver steatosis (same patient as in Fig. 65-2). On axial enhanced CT scan during portal venous phase, the difference between hepatic (57 HU) and splenic (101 HU) attenuation is 45 HU, which exceeds the 20-HU threshold proposed by some investigators as diagnostic of fatty liver.

including a liver-spleen attenuation difference of at least 20 HU between 80 to 100 seconds, or at least 18.5 HU between 100 to 120 seconds, after intravenous contrast injection (Fig. 65-3). Sensitivity and specificity of these attenuation differences range from 54% to 93% and 87% to 93%, respectively.[37] Ultimately, however, the quantitative criteria for diagnosing fatty liver at enhanced CT are protocol specific and have significant overlap of liver-spleen attenuation values between normal and fatty liver, thereby limiting its clinical role.

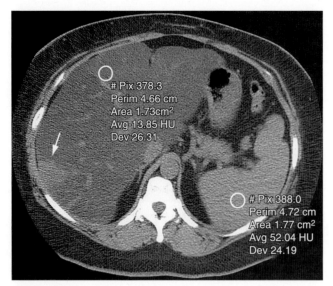

Pix 378.3
Perim 4.66 cm
Area 1.73cm²
Avg-13.85 HU
Dev 26.31

Pix 388.0
Perim 4.72 cm
Area 1.77 cm²
Avg 52.04 HU
Dev 24.19

■ **FIGURE 65-4** Focal fat sparing. Axial unenhanced CT scan reveals a geographically shaped area of high attenuation (*arrow*) in the subcapsular region of the right lobe of a fatty liver consistent with focal fatty sparing.

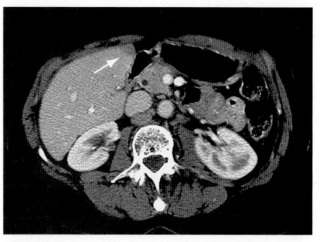

■ **FIGURE 65-5** Focal fat sparing. Axial unenhanced CT scan reveals a focal small high-attenuation area (*arrow*) in a diffuse low-attenuation liver consistent with an area of focal sparing in a fatty liver.

On CT, focal hepatic steatosis appears as a hypodense area in an otherwise normal liver, whereas focal fatty sparing appears as a hyperdense region within a diffusely lowly attenuated liver (Figs. 65-4 and 65-5). Although, areas of focal fat deposition and focal fat sparing are usually geographic in shape and occur at specific locations, in a few cases they be nodular or occur in an atypical region, raising concern for a true hepatic mass.[35] Other characteristic features include geographic margins, absence of mass effect, and nondistortion of the portal and hepatic venous branches traversing through regions of fat deposition or sparing.

Dual-energy CT has also been shown to have a role in the detection of hepatic steatosis. It involves scanning the liver with two different tube potentials (140 kVp and 80 kVp) and has been used for evaluation of focal and diffuse fatty infiltration of liver. The varying attenuation characteristics of different tissues at different energies have been utilized for the differentiation of various body tissue types, such as bone, fat, and soft tissue. Steatotic liver exhibits greater change in attenuation between 80 kVp and 140 kVp than does normal liver. Increase in fatty content leads to decrease in Hounsfield unit number at low energies, and as the kVp increases the fat attenuation increases.

MRI

MRI is generally considered the most definitive radiologic modality for the qualitative and quantitative assessment of fatty liver disease. Visual recognition of fatty liver disease usually is straightforward, because it is most often characterized by diffuse and homogeneous liver involvement. However, atypical fat distribution, like that seen in focal and multifocal fatty disease, may simulate other lesions and presents a diagnostic challenge. Key distinguishing imaging features of fatty liver disease, other than the fat content, include lack of increased gadolinium enhancement (isoenhancing to hypoenhancing compared with normal liver tissue), geographic distribution, ill-defined margins, characteristic locations of focal fat deposition or sparing, and absence of mass effect on surrounding structures.

In fatty liver, both fat and water protons contribute to the observed MR signal. Because of the chemical shift, the fat and water protons resonate and precess at different frequencies. MR spectroscopy, frequency-selective MRI, and phase-interference MRI are three techniques that exploit the fat-water chemical shift to assess fatty liver disease.

Spatially selective proton MR spectroscopy allows the direct measurement of the chemical (proton) composition within a specified volume of the liver.[36] The MR spectrum describes the intensity of MR signal as a function of precession frequency. At field strengths greater than or equal to 1.5 T, the water peak at 4.7 ppm and the dominant fat peak at 1.2 ppm of $-(CH_2)_n-$ can be resolved and identified as distinct spectral peaks. In fatty liver disease, both water and fat spectral peaks are present (Fig. 65-6). In normal (nonfatty) liver, only the water peak is seen.

Frequency-selective imaging applies a saturation (or excitation) radiofrequency pulse to the fat or water frequency range to selectively suppress (or excite) fat or water signals. In particular, fat saturation is a common option for many clinical imaging sequences, including most spin-echo– and gradient-echo–based sequences at 1.5 T and higher. With fat saturation, the images coincide with the water signal alone; without fat saturation, they represent the sum of fat and water signals. Therefore, hepatic fat may be assessed by comparing these two sets of images. In fatty liver disease, the fat-saturated images show relative signal loss compared with unsaturated images (Fig. 65-7). In normal liver, fat saturation has no effect and the two sets of images have similar signal intensities.

Phase-interference imaging takes advantage of the echo time–dependent phase-interference effect between fat and water gradient-echo signals. Because fat and

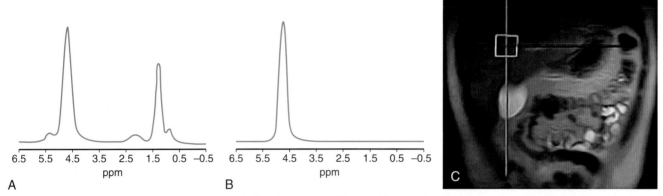

■ **FIGURE 65-6** Liver proton MR spectroscopy. **A,** Findings in a 49-year-old man with severe fatty liver show a large fat signal peak at 1.2 ppm as well as hepatic water at 4.7 ppm; fat fraction = 33%. **B,** Findings in a healthy 14-year-old boy with only hepatic water peak; fat fraction < 1%. **C,** An example of MR spectroscopic voxel placement.

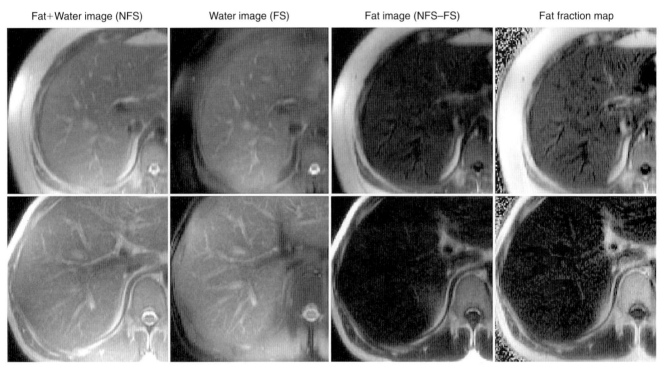

■ **FIGURE 65-7** Frequency-selective MRI. **Top,** Findings in a 48-year-old man with 23% fat fraction by spectroscopy. **Bottom,** Findings in a 34-year-old healthy man with 1% fat fraction. NFS, non–fat saturated; FS, fat saturated. Images were acquired at 1.5 T.

water signals precess at different frequencies, they undergo phase interference at predictable periodicity. Consequently, the fat and water signals cancel at out-of-phase (OP) and add at in-phase (IP) echo times. Hepatic fat may be assessed by comparing sequential OP and IP images. In fatty liver disease, the OP images show relative signal loss due to signal cancellation (Fig. 65-8). In normal liver, the OP and IP images have similar intensities.

The distinct advantage of the various MRI techniques over CT and ultrasonography is the capability to noninvasively quantify steatosis as a "fat fraction." Using a non–T1-weighted (T1W) sequence (long relaxation time and/or low flip angle) and multiple echo-time acquisition, it is possible to estimate individual fat and water proton densities from the spectroscopic or imaging data. The fat fraction can then be calculated as a ratio of fat proton density to total (fat and water) proton density.[36,41] From the proton density of fat and water and prior knowledge of the fatty acids' chemical compositions, the molecular triglyceride concentration can be determined. In spectroscopy, the proton density fat fraction has been validated using biochemical assay of tissue samples.[36,42] Although no direct comparison with biochemical assay has been performed for imaging, a recent study shows close agreement between the proton density fat fraction determined by spectroscopy and by phase-interference imaging.[43]

Ultrasonography

Transabdominal ultrasonography is the most common imaging modality used to initially evaluate and diagnose hepatic steatosis due to its low cost, noninvasiveness, and widespread availability.[38] The echogenicity of the normal liver is similar or minimally exceeds that of the renal cortex or spleen. At ultrasonography, diffuse fatty liver is characterized by hyperechogenicity of the liver parenchyma relative to the adjacent right kidney or spleen (the so-called bright liver) (Fig. 65-9). Focal fat deposition appears as a hyperechoic area in an otherwise normal liver, whereas focal fat sparing is represented by a hypoechoic area within diffusely hyperechoic liver parenchyma.[36] Other frequently described ultrasound features of fatty liver include attenuation of the ultrasound beam, decreased visualization of vascular margins, loss of definition of the diaphragm, and hepatomegaly (Fig. 65-10).[44]

The degree of fat accumulation in the liver can be classified subjectively by ultrasonography as mild, moderate, or severe. The qualitative grading for hepatic steatosis is as follows:

Mild: mild increase in liver echogenicity with visualization of hepatic and portal vein walls

Moderate: increased liver echogenicity obscuring visualization of hepatic and portal vein walls

Severe: increased liver echogenicity with significant posterior attenuation that impairs evaluation of deep liver parenchyma and diaphragm

Ultrasonography has several limitations in the detection of both diffuse and focal hepatic steatosis. It is highly operator dependent, nonreproducible, and limited by abdominal gas and patient body habitus. The last inadequacy is highlighted in this patient population because the majority of cases of fatty liver disease occur in overweight or obese individuals. Similar to CT, however, ultrasonography is not a quantitative method and may be unable to distinguish simple steatosis from advanced fibrosis or early cirrhosis. Ultrasonography has low sensitivity and specificity for detecting small amounts of fat in the liver. For detecting moderate and severe fat accumulation (>30% by histology), ultrasound sensitivity and specificity range from 60% to 95% and 84% to 100%, respectively.[37]

Nuclear Medicine

Scintigraphy with xenon-133 (^{133}Xe) was used to detect hepatic steatosis in the 1980s and 1990s but is now no

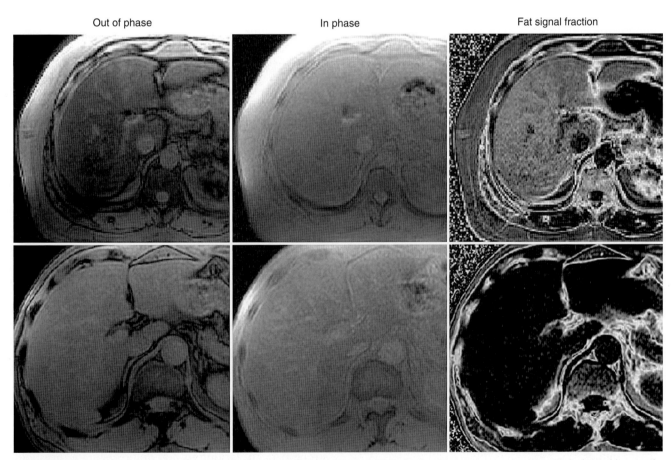

| Out of phase | In phase | Fat signal fraction |

■ **FIGURE 65-8** Phase-interference MRI. **Top,** Findings in a 45-year-old man with 26% fat fraction by spectroscopy show marked signal loss on the out-of-phase image compared with the in-phase image. Fat fraction map demonstrates diffuse fat deposition throughout the liver. **Bottom,** Findings in a 61-year-old healthy man with 1% fat fraction by spectroscopy show no significant signal difference between out-of-phase and in-phase images; fat fraction map demonstrates no fat in the liver. Images were acquired at 1.5 T.

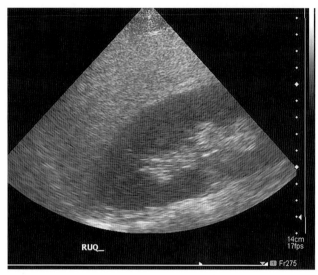

■ FIGURE 65-9 Diffuse liver steatosis. Ultrasound image of the liver shows a hyperechoic liver. The adjacent renal cortex appears hypoechoic by comparison. The intrahepatic vessels are not well depicted, and the diaphragm is poorly delineated.

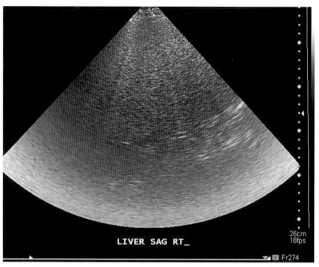

■ FIGURE 65-10 Diffuse liver steatosis. Sagittal ultrasound image of the liver shows a hyperechoic liver, decreased visualization of intrahepatic vessels and vessel walls, posterior darkness, and loss of definition of the diaphragm (posterior beam attenuation).

longer incorporated in diagnostic algorithms. ^{133}Xe is a highly fat-soluble gas that, after being inhaled or injected, remains in the fatty tissue after blood pool clearing. The ^{133}Xe hepatic retention ratio is increased in patients with fatty liver, with reported sensitivity and specificity of 95% and 94%, respectively.[45]

Imaging Algorithm

Ultrasonography is the most inexpensive modality for diagnosis of fatty liver disease but is limited by its low sensitivity and operator, observer, and body habitus dependence (Table 65-3). Although CT is objective, is more reproducible, and may be more sensitive, it involves ionizing radiation and is not suitable for routine examinations, especially in the pediatric population. MRI is the most definitive radiologic modality for hepatic fat assessment but is relatively costly. However, a focused fatty liver protocol can be performed in less than 10 minutes and may be a reasonable option for routine fatty liver screening and follow-up. Such a protocol would include localizing, followed by noncontrast fat detection and quantification sequences. These are detailed as follows:

Hepatic Fat Detection

High T1-weighting (high flip angle or short relaxation time) makes the fat signal more conspicuous for detection and preferentially amplifies the fat signal due to its shorter T1 relative to lean liver. This accentuates the relative signal loss on fat-saturated or OP images and aids visual detection of the fat signal.

Hepatic Fat Quantification

Low T1 weighting is essential to suppress arbitrary T1-dependent fat signal amplification. A long relaxation time ($> 4 \times T1_{liver}$) or low flip angle (5 to 20 degrees)

should be used to minimize T1 weighting. Regardless of the imaging sequence used, multiple echo-time acquisition should be considered to correct for T2(*) signal decay that may confound fat fraction estimation.[46] Such dedicated fat-quantification sequences are becoming commercially available.

DIFFERENTIAL DIAGNOSIS

The clinical differential diagnosis of NAFLD mirrors that of hepatic steatosis. Among patients with elevated serum aminotransferase values, the etiology is usually established through a careful evaluation of their history (medication use, risk factors for viral hepatitis, history of alcohol and drug use, and review of comorbidities), a series of screening blood tests for causes of chronic liver disease (viral serologic studies, iron studies, autoimmune markers, ceruloplasmin, and α_1-antitrypsin), supportive imaging studies (initial evaluation is usually with ultrasonography), and, sometimes, liver biopsy. If other causes of chronic liver disease have been excluded, risk factors for NAFLD have been identified, and the presence of fatty liver is confirmed by imaging studies, the clinician is challenged with establishing the etiology of hepatic steatosis.[47,48]

Alcoholic liver disease encompasses a spectrum of conditions provoked by alcohol ingestion, including fatty liver disease, alcoholic hepatitis, and cirrhosis. It has been estimated that almost all patients with heavy alcohol consumption develop fatty liver, although only 10% to 35% develop alcoholic hepatitis and 8% to 20% progress to alcoholic cirrhosis.[49] In individuals who admit to moderate alcohol intake, the differentiation between NAFLD and alcoholic fatty liver disease is difficult because laboratory, imaging, and histologic findings are similar. Unfortunately, strong data are lacking to determine accurate thresholds for alcohol consumption required to cause fatty liver. Historically, daily alcohol intake of 20 g in women and 30 g in men has been used to distinguish alcoholic fatty liver

TABLE 65-3 Accuracy, Limitations, and Pitfalls of the Modalities Used in Imaging of Fatty Liver Disease

Modality	Accuracy	Limitations	Pitfalls
Unenhanced CT	73%-100% sensitivity for diagnosis of moderate/severe steatosis (histologic steatosis greater than 30%)[38] 95%-100% specificity for diagnosis of moderate/severe steatosis[38]	Radiation exposure No role in pediatric populations for sole purpose of fat assessment	Confounded by multiple variables (see text) Confusion with other hypoattenuating lesions if atypical in distribution (see text)
Enhanced CT	54%-93% sensitivity for diagnosis of moderate/severe steatosis[38] 87%-93% specificity for diagnosis of moderate/severe steatosis[38]	Radiation exposure Because of risks of intravenous contrast agents, no role in any population for sole purpose of fat assessment	
MRI	81% sensitivity and 100% specificity for diagnosis of moderate/severe steatosis[48] 84%-98% sensitivity and 88%-100% specificity for diagnosis of mild steatosis (histologic steatosis of 5%-10%)[49]	Patient cooperation required High costs Not widely available Dedicated pulse-sequence needed for accurate diagnosis and fat grading	Out-of-phase/in-phase imaging has low sensitivity in presence of iron unless T2(*) correction is performed. Frequency-selective imaging unreliable in inhomogeneity (e.g., metal artifact, high susceptibility)
Ultrasonography	60%-95% sensitivity in detection of moderate/severe steatosis[38] 84%-100% specificity in detection of moderate/severe steatosis[38]	Operator dependent Nonreproducible Limited by overlying bowel gas and patient body habitus Subjective	Confusion with other hyperechoic lesions if atypical in distribution (see text) Liver with severe fibrosis or early cirrhosis may mimic the sonographic appearance of mild steatosis, potentially causing gross underestimation of disease severity.
Nuclear medicine (xenon-133)	95% sensitivity and 94% specificity[46]	Poor spatial resolution	

disease from NAFLD, although the validity of these thresholds is unknown.[50] If liver biopsy specimens are obtained, individuals with alcoholic liver disease tend to have more Mallory's hyaline and acidophil bodies and less glycogenated nuclei than those with NAFLD, although these are not reliable findings.

Hepatic steatosis may also occur in chronic hepatitis C virus infection, where it is related to host factors such metabolic syndrome as well as viral factors in those infected with genotype 3 hepatitis C virus. Steatosis in hepatitis C is significant because it contributes to disease progression and decreases response rates to treatment with interferon-based therapy.[51]

Certain drugs may produce de novo steatohepatitis (e.g., amiodarone, perhexiline maleate, diethylaminoethoxyhexestrol) and others may exacerbate NASH (tamoxifen, corticosteroids, diethylstilbestrol, estrogens).[52] Oxiliplatin and irinotecan administered as preoperative chemotherapy before surgical resection of hepatic metastases have been associated with steatohepatitis, with irinotecan-associated steatohepatitis associated with poorer outcomes after hepatic resection.[53,54] Other conditions capable of eliciting fatty liver include intestinal bypass surgery for weight loss (classically seen with jejunoileal bypass surgery), HIV infection with lipodystrophy, and parenteral nutrition.[3] If any of the these secondary causes of fatty liver are excluded (alcohol, viral hepatitis, drug-induced, jejunoileal bypass surgery, HIV infection, and parenteral nutrition support), then a diagnosis of NAFLD can be made.

Because the radiologic findings of hepatic steatosis are common to its diverse causes, the differential diagnosis is largely discriminated on clinical and laboratory grounds.[42]

Special attention needs to be given to the possible imaging overlap between simple steatosis and advanced fibrosis or early cirrhosis; these disparate conditions are often, but not always, easily distinguished clinically.

A major challenge in the differential diagnosis of hepatic steatosis occurs when the radiologic findings of focal fat deposition or focal fat sparing simulate hepatic nodular lesions such as abscess, benign neoplasm, or primary or metastatic malignancy. The diagnosis of focal fat deposition or sparing is supported by their occurrence in typical locations, a wedge shape, the lack of mass effect, and the absence of vascular displacement or distortion inside the lesion. When there is still doubt, MRI may be performed.

TREATMENT

Medical Treatment

The standard of care in managing patients with NAFLD consists of lifestyle modification through diet and exercise, with the goal of gradual weight loss in patients who are overweight or obese. Weight loss and exercise decrease adipose stores and improve insulin sensitivity, thereby targeting the underlying causative factor of insulin resistance. Evidence for the efficacy of this strategy comes from trials that have demonstrated histologic regression of steatosis with weight loss.[55,56] In patients with associated metabolic syndrome, optimal control of diabetes, hyperlipidemia, and hypertension are routinely recommended, although the effects of such treatment on histology are poorly characterized and are unlikely to produce complete resolution of NAFLD in most cases.[3]

To date, no pharmacologic therapy has been approved for the treatment of NAFLD. Based on current understanding of the pathogenesis of NASH, pharmacologic therapy has been attempted with weight-loss promoting medications (orlistat), antioxidants (vitamin E and betaine), cytoprotective agents (ursodeoxycholic acid), and insulin sensitizers (metformin and thiazolidinediones).[57-63] Although some of these agents have promoted decreases in aminotransferase levels and histologic improvement, their trials have often been poorly powered or nonrandomized. Therefore, treatment with these various medications is controversial and not typically pursued in clinical practice. All patients with NAFLD should be treated with lifestyle modification and considered for referral to centers involved in clinical research until definitive pharmacotherapy is approved.

Surgical Treatment

Bariatric surgery is the primary surgical intervention for NAFLD in patients with a body mass index of more than 40 kg/m^2 or of 35 kg/m^2 with comorbidities.[64] Current bariatric surgical techniques include vertical banded gastroplasty, adjustable gastric banding, Roux-en-Y gastric bypass, biliopancreatic bypass, and biliopancreatic diversion with duodenal switch. Based on a recent meta-analysis, bariatric surgery is associated with significant histologic improvements in steatosis, steatohepatitis, and fibrosis, with more than 50% of patients experiencing complete resolution of their fatty liver disease after surgery.[65] Although these results are compelling, these observational studies showed no relationship between histologic improvement and the amount of weight loss.

As with other causes of cirrhosis, liver transplantation is a viable option for patients with end-stage liver disease due to fatty liver disease, although a significant amount of preoperative weight loss in obese patients is necessary to make liver transplantation technically feasible. Post-transplant survival rates are similar to those in patients with transplants performed for other reasons.[66]

What the Referring Physician Needs to Know

- The distinction between simple steatosis and steatohepatitis (NASH) is important in determining prognosis in NAFLD, and, at the present time, this can only be accomplished with liver biopsy.
- Weight loss through diet and exercise is likely to provide some benefit in all patients with NAFLD.
- Obese patients with NASH who are not successful in lifestyle modification and meet criteria for bariatric surgery (body mass index >40 kg/m^2 or >35 kg/m^2 with comorbidities) may benefit from weight loss surgery.
- Among patients with NASH in whom there is risk for progression to cirrhosis, consideration should be given to refer patients for participation in clinical trials.
- Patients with cirrhosis secondary to NASH are at risk for hepatocellular carcinoma and should undergo regular screening examinations, although specific guidelines are lacking.

KEY POINTS

- Patterns of fat accumulation include diffuse and homogeneous (most common), focal fat deposition, focal fat sparing, multinodular, subcapsular, and perivascular.
- In some circumstances, MRI may need to be performed to differentiate focal fat deposition or focal fat sparing from a true liver lesion, particularly in the evaluation of oncology patients.

CT

- A noncontrast study is best for the evaluation of hepatic steatosis.
- With CT there is concern for ionizing radiation, especially in children.
- The diagnosis is potentially confounded by multiple variables.
- Enhanced CT may be unreliable for the diagnosis of steatosis.
- CT has moderate sensitivity and is more reliable than ultrasonography.

Ultrasonography

- Findings depend on equipment, operator, and observer.
- It is not useful for longitudinal assessment of the severity of steatosis.
- Its use is limited in patients with large body habitus.
- Of all the modalities used it is of lowest sensitivity and thus not recommended for screening of early disease.

MRI

- MR spectroscopy is theoretically most accurate but may not be available depending on the center.
- MRI (frequency-selective, phase-interference) is rapid and highly specific for presence of fat.
- Dedicated fat quantification imaging or spectroscopy sequences are necessary for accurate diagnosis and grading of fatty liver disease and are being developed.

SUGGESTED READINGS

Angulo P. Nonalcoholic fatty liver disease. N Engl J Med 2002; 346:1221-1231.

Angulo P, Lindor KD. Non-alcoholic fatty liver disease. J Gastroenterol Hepatol 2002; 17(Suppl):S186-S190.

Clark JM, Brancati FL, Diehl AM. Nonalcoholic fatty liver disease. Gastroenterology 2002; 122:1649-1657.

Hamer OW, Aguirre DA, Casola G, et al. Fatty liver: imaging patterns and pitfalls. RadioGraphics 2006; 26:1637-1653.

Karcaaltinacaba M, Akhan O. Imaging of hepatic steatosis and fatty sparing. Eur J Radiol 2007; 61:33-43.

Lall CG, Aisen AM, Bansal N, Sandrasegaran K. Nonalcoholic fatty liver disease. AJR Am J Roentgenol 2008; 190:993-1002.

Marchesini G, Bugianesi E, Forlani G, et al. Nonalcoholic fatty liver, steatohepatitis, and the metabolic syndrome. Hepatology 2003; 37:917-923.

Rofsky NM, Fleishaker H. CT and MRI of diffuse liver disease. Semin Ultrasound CT MR 1995; 16:16-33.

Valls C, Iannacconne R, Alba E, et al. Fat in the liver: diagnosis and characterization. Eur Radiol 2006; 16:2229-2308.

REFERENCES

1. Kleiner DE, Brunt EM, Van Natta M, et al. Design and validation of a histological scoring system for nonalcoholic fatty liver disease. Hepatology 2005; 41:1313-1321.
2. Marchesini G, Bugianesi E, Forlani G, et al. Nonalcoholic fatty liver, steatohepatitis, and the metabolic syndrome. Hepatology 2003; 37:917-923.
3. Angulo P. Nonalcoholic fatty liver disease. N Engl J Med 2002; 346:1221-1231.
4. Day CP, James OF. Steatohepatitis: a tale of two "hits"? Gastroenterology 1998; 114:842-845.
5. Parekh S, Anania FA. Abnormal lipid and glucose metabolism in obesity: implications for nonalcoholic fatty liver disease. Gastroenterology 2007; 132:2191-2207.
6. Goldberg IJ, Ginsberg HN. Ins and outs modulating hepatic triglyceride and development of nonalcoholic fatty liver disease. Gastroenterology 2006; 130:1343-1346.
7. Edmison J, McCullough AJ. Pathogenesis of non-alcoholic steatohepatitis: human data. Clin Liver Dis 2007; 11:75-104, ix.
8. Rajala MW, Scherer PE. Minireview: the adipocyte—at the crossroads of energy homeostasis, inflammation, and atherosclerosis. Endocrinology 2003; 144:3765-3773.
9. Browning JD, Horton JD. Molecular mediators of hepatic steatosis and liver injury. J Clin Invest 2004; 114:147-152.
10. Patton HM, Sirlin C, Behling C, et al. Pediatric nonalcoholic fatty liver disease: a critical appraisal of current data and implications for future research. J Pediatr Gastroenterol Nutr 2006; 43:413-427.
11. Clark JM. The epidemiology of nonalcoholic fatty liver disease in adults. J Clin Gastroenterol 2006; 40:S5-S10.
12. Clark JM, Brancati FL, Diehl AM. Nonalcoholic fatty liver disease. Gastroenterology 2002; 122:1649-1657.
13. Browning JD, Szczepaniak LS, Dobbins R, et al. Prevalence of hepatic steatosis in an urban population in the United States: impact of ethnicity. Hepatology 2004; 40:1387-1395.
14. Ryan CK, Johnson LA, Germin BI, Marcos A. One hundred consecutive hepatic biopsies in the workup of living donors for right lobe liver transplantation. Liver Transpl 2002; 8:1114-1122.
15. Soejima Y, Shimada M, Suehiro T, et al. Use of steatotic graft in living-donor liver transplantation. Transplantation 2003; 76:344-348.
16. Schwimmer JB, Deutsch R, Kahen T, et al. Prevalence of fatty liver in children and adolescents. Pediatrics 2006; 118:1388-1393.
17. Dunn W, Schwimmer JB. The obesity epidemic and nonalcoholic fatty liver disease in children. Curr Gastroenterol Rep 2008; 10:67-72.
18. Angulo P, Lindor KD. Non-alcoholic fatty liver disease. J Gastroenterol Hepatol 2002; 17(Suppl):S186-S190.
19. Crespo J, Fernandez-Gil P, Hernandez-Guerra M, et al. Are there predictive factors of severe liver fibrosis in morbidly obese patients with non-alcoholic steatohepatitis? Obes Surg 2001; 11:254-257.
20. Dixon JB, Bhathal PS, O'Brien PE. Nonalcoholic fatty liver disease: predictors of nonalcoholic steatohepatitis and liver fibrosis in the severely obese. Gastroenterology 2001; 121:91-100.
21. Beymer C, Kowdley KV, Larson A, et al. Prevalence and predictors of asymptomatic liver disease in patients undergoing gastric bypass surgery. Arch Surg 2003; 138:1240-1244.
22. Gholam PM, Kotler DP, Flancbaum LJ. Liver pathology in morbidly obese patients undergoing Roux-en-Y gastric bypass surgery. Obes Surg 2002; 12:49-51.
23. Bugianesi E, Gastaldelli A, Vanni E, et al. Insulin resistance in non-diabetic patients with non-alcoholic fatty liver disease: sites and mechanisms. Diabetologia 2005; 48:634-642.
24. Angulo P, Keach JC, Batts KP, Lindor KD. Independent predictors of liver fibrosis in patients with non-alcoholic steatohepatitis. Hepatology 1999; 30:1356-1362.
25. Schwimmer JB. Definitive diagnosis and assessment of risk for non-alcoholic fatty liver disease in children and adolescents. Semin Liv Dis 2007; 27:312-318.
26. Fan JG, Zhu J, Li XJ, et al. Prevalence of and risk factors for fatty liver in a general population of Shanghai, China. J Hepatol 2005; 43:508-514.
27. Ruhl CE, Everhart JE. Relation of elevated serum alanine aminotransferase activity with iron and antioxidant levels in the United States. Gastroenterology 2003; 124:1821-1829.
28. Clark JM, Brancati FL, Diehl AM. The prevalence and etiology of elevated aminotransferase levels in the United States. Am J Gastroenterol 2003; 98:960-967.
29. Liangpunsakul S, Chalasani N. Unexplained elevations in alanine aminotransferase in individuals with the metabolic syndrome: results from the third National Health and Nutrition Survey (NHANES III). Am J Med Sci 2005; 329:111-116.
30. Matteoni CA, Younossi ZM, Gramlich T, et al. Nonalcoholic fatty liver disease: a spectrum of clinical and pathological severity. Gastroenterology 1999; 116:1413-1419.
31. Day CP. Natural history of NAFLD: remarkably benign in absence of cirrhosis. Gastroenterology 2005; 129:375-378.
32. Hubscher SG. Histological assessment of non-alcoholic fatty liver disease. Histopathology 2006; 49:450-465.
33. Schwimmer JB, Behling C, Newbury R, et al. Histopathology of pediatric nonalcoholic fatty liver disease. Hepatology 2005; 42:641-649.
34. Kleiner DE, Brunt EM, Van Natta M, et al. Design and validation of a histological scoring system for nonalcoholic fatty liver disease. Hepatology 2005; 41:1313-1321.
35. Karcaaltincaba M, Akhan O. Imaging of hepatic steatosis and fatty sparing. Eur J Radiol 2007; 61:33-43.
36. Hamer OW, Aguirre DA, Casola G, et al. Fatty liver: imaging patterns and pitfalls. RadioGraphics 2006; 26:1637-1653.
37. Rofsky NM, Fleishaker H. CT and MRI of diffuse liver disease. Semin Ultrasound CT MR 1995; 16:16-33.
38. Charatcharoenwitthaya P, Lindor KD. Role of radiologic modalities in the management of non-alcoholic steatohepatitis. Clin Liver Dis 2007; 11:37-45.
39. Valls C, Iannacconne R, Alba E, et al. Fat in the liver: diagnosis and characterization. Eur Radiol 2006; 16:2229-2308.
40. Park SH, Kim PN, Kim KW, et al. Macrovesicular hepatic steatosis in living liver donors: use of CT for quantitative and qualitative assessment. Radiology 2006; 239:105-112.
41. Kodama Y, Ng CS, Wu TT, et al. Comparison of CT methods for determining the fat content of the liver. AJR Am J Roentgenol 2007; 188:1307-1312.
42. Kawamori Y, Matsui O, Takahashi S, et al. Focal hepatic fatty infiltration in the posterior edge of the medial segment associated with aberrant gastric venous drainage: CT, US, and MR findings. J Comput Assist Tomogr 1996; 20:356-359.
43. Matsui O, Kadoya M, Takahashi S, et al. Focal sparing of segment IV in fatty livers shown by sonography and CT: correlation with aber-

rant gastric venous drainage. AJR Am J Roentgenol 1995; 164:1137-1140.

44. Yokoo T, Bydder M, Hamilton G, et al. Hepatic fat quantification by low flip-angle multi-echo gradient-echo MR imaging: a clinical study with validation with MR spectroscopy. Presented before the annual meeting of the International Society for Magnetic Resonance in Medicine. Toronto, Canada, 2008, p 706.

45. Lall CG, Aisen AM, Bansal N, Sandrasegaran K. Nonalcoholic fatty liver disease. AJR Am J Roentgenol 2008; 190:993-1002.

46. Yeh SH, Wu LC, Wang SJ, et al. Xenon-133 hepatic retention ratio: a useful index for fatty liver quantification. J Nucl Med 1989; 30:1708-1712.

47. Itai Y, Saida Y. Pitfalls in liver imaging. Eur Radiol 2002; 12:1162-1174.

48. Rinella ME, McCarthy R, Thakrar K, et al. Dual-echo, chemical shift gradient-echo magnetic resonance imaging to quantify hepatic steatosis: implications for living liver donation. Liver Transpl 2003; 9:851-856.

49. Pilleul F, Chave G, Dumortier J, et al. Fatty infiltration of the liver: detection and grading using dual T1 gradient echo sequences on clinical MR system. Gastroenterol Clin Biol 2005; 29:1143-1147.

50. Lelbach WK. Epidemiology of alcoholic liver disease. In Popper H, Schaffner F (eds). Progress in Liver Disease, vol 5. New York: Grune & Stratton, 1976, pp 494-515.

51. Neuschwander-Tetri BA, Caldwell SH. Nonalcoholic steatohepatitis: summary of an AASLD Single Topic Conference. Hepatology 2003; 37:1202-1219.

52. Patton HM, Patel K, Behling C, et al. The impact of steatosis on disease progression and early and sustained treatment response in chronic hepatitis C patients. J Hepatol 2004; 40:484-490.

53. Hasegawa T, Yoneda M, Nakamura K, et al. Plasma transforming growth factor-beta$_1$ level and efficacy of alpha-tocopherol in patients with non-alcoholic steatohepatitis: a pilot study. Aliment Pharmacol Ther 2001; 15:1667-1672.

54. Fernandez FG, Ritter J, Goodwin JW, et al. Effect of steatohepatitis associated with irinotecan or oxaliplatin pretreatment on resectability of hepatic colorectal metastases. J Am Coll Surg 2005; 200:845-853.

55. Zorzi D, Laurent A, Pawlik TM, et al. Chemotherapy-associated hepatotoxicity and surgery for colorectal liver metastases. Br J Surg 2007; 94:274-286.

56. Huang MA, Greenson JK, Chao C, et al. One-year intense nutritional counseling results in histological improvement in patients with nonalcoholic steatohepatitis: a pilot study. Am J Gastroenterol 2005; 100:1072-1081.

57. Andersen T, Gluud C, Franzmann MB, Christoffersen P. Hepatic effects of dietary weight loss in morbidly obese subjects. J Hepatol 1991; 12:224-229.

58. Harrison SA, Fincke C, Helinski D, et al. A pilot study of orlistat treatment in obese, non-alcoholic steatohepatitis patients. Aliment Pharmacol Ther 2004; 20:623-628.

59. Lavine JE. Vitamin E treatment of nonalcoholic steatohepatitis in children: a pilot study. J Pediatr 2000; 136:734-738.

60. Sanyal AJ, Mofrad PS, Contos MJ, et al. A pilot study of vitamin E versus vitamin E and pioglitazone for the treatment of nonalcoholic steatohepatitis. Clin Gastroenterol Hepatol 2004; 2:1107-1115.

61. Abdelmalek MF, Angulo P, Jorgensen RA, et al. Betaine, a promising new agent for patients with nonalcoholic steatohepatitis: results of a pilot study. Am J Gastroenterol 2001; 96:2711-2717.

62. Lindor KD, Kowdley KV, Heathcote EJ, et al. Ursodeoxycholic acid for treatment of nonalcoholic steatohepatitis: results of a randomized trial. Hepatology 2004; 39:770-778.

63. Bugianesi E, Gentilcore E, Manini R, et al. A randomized controlled trial of metformin versus vitamin E or prescriptive diet in nonalcoholic fatty liver disease. Am J Gastroenterol 2005; 100:1082-1090.

64. Belfort R, Harrison SA, Brown K, et al. A placebo-controlled trial of pioglitazone in subjects with nonalcoholic steatohepatitis. N Engl J Med 2006; 355:2297-2307.

65. NIH conference. Gastrointestinal surgery for severe obesity. Consensus Development Conference Panel. Ann Intern Med 1991; 115:956-961.

66. Mummadi RR, Kasturi KS, Chennareddygari S, Sood G. Effect of bariatric surgery on nonalcoholic fatty liver disease (NAFLD): a meta-analysis. Hepatology 2007; 46:A130.

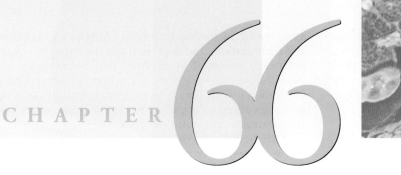
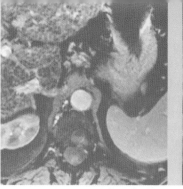
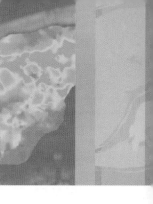

CHAPTER 66

Cirrhosis

Sameer M. Mazhar, Robert Hanna, Michael R. Peterson, and Claude B. Sirlin

Cirrhosis is the pathologic and clinical culmination of chronic liver disease. Characterized by the replacement of normal liver parenchyma with fibrotic scar and regenerative nodules, it leads to progressive loss of liver function, portal hypertension, and, ultimately, liver failure. Once cirrhosis occurs, it is generally thought to be irreversible, with treatment efforts focused on the prevention and management of its myriad complications. Liver transplantation is the only curative therapy.

ETIOLOGY

Virtually any chronic insult to the liver, if sufficiently severe and of long standing, may result in cirrhosis. In the United States the most common causes are hepatitis C and alcohol ingestion, whereas in Asia and sub-Saharan Africa, chronic hepatitis B is the most frequent culprit. Nonalcoholic fatty liver disease is increasing in prevalence and is now the third most common cause of cirrhosis in North America and in parts of Europe and South America. Other common causes in adults include nonviral infections (mainly, parasitic—e.g., schistosomiasis), autoimmune hepatitis, primary biliary cirrhosis, primary sclerosing cholangitis, genetic disorders (hemochromatosis, Wilson's disease, α_1-antitrypsin deficiency, and glycogen storage diseases), medications (e.g., amiodarone and methotrexate), and veno-occlusive disease (especially Budd-Chiari syndrome; sinusoidal obstruction syndrome generally does not cause cirrhosis). Cryptogenic cirrhosis describes cirrhosis of unknown etiology; once a frequent diagnosis, the term has become less common in the past 2 decades with the discovery of the hepatitis C virus and the recognition of nonalcoholic fatty liver disease.[1]

The fundamental pathogenic mechanism of cirrhosis is that of "injury and repair." Hepatocytes may be injured by a variety of etiologic factors, initiating an inflammatory response. Atypical, dysfunctional hepatocytes aggressively multiply to counteract the effects of hepatocyte injury, forming *regenerative nodules.* Isolated insults cause self-limited inflammation, and the liver's wound-healing mechanisms successfully repair the damage. Repetitive or chronic injuries, however, overwhelm these restorative processes, leading to the dysregulated production of cytokines (e.g., transforming growth factor-β) and activation of profibrogenic perisinusoidal stellate cells. The end result is the unchecked deposition of excess macromolecules and collagen in the extracellular matrix (fibrosis).[2]

Fibrosis initially occurs in the space of Disse, where it obliterates normal endothelial fenestrations. Further scar deposition in the perisinusoidal and sinusoidal spaces obstructs sinusoidal blood flow and causes *portal hypertension.* Because of the elevated intrahepatic resistance, portal venous blood is shunted to systemic veins with lower pressures and is returned to the heart without passing through the liver. The microvascular architecture of the liver remodels in response. Abnormal connections develop between the portal vein and terminal hepatic vein, which contribute to the shunting of blood from the hepatic parenchyma. As a result of portal hypertension and microvascular hepatic alterations, varices form, ascites develops, and hypersplenism occurs. Toxins normally metabolized and eliminated by the liver accumulate in the blood and contribute to the development of hepatic encephalopathy.

Loss of hepatocytes impacts hepatic synthetic function, resulting in reduced levels of essential proteins (e.g., blood clotting factors and albumin) and causing coagulation abnormalities as well as reduced intravascular oncotic pressure. Atypical hepatocytes have impaired ability to secrete bile into canaliculi, which not only causes intestinal fat and vitamin malabsorption and steatorrhea but also results in cholestasis (accumulation of bile within hepatocytes), which may perpetuate hepatocellular damage. Because the liver is required for the normal metabolism and supply of glucose and lipids to the rest of the body, hepatocellular dysfunction leads to muscle breakdown, inefficient mobilization of energy stores, and redistribution of adipose tissue. Clearance of estrogens may be reduced, leading to gynecomastia in males.

Systemically, patients with cirrhosis exhibit a *hyperdynamic circulation* due to decreased systemic vascular resistance and peripheral vasodilation, mediated by nitric oxide, among other factors.[3] End consequences include increased cardiac output, splanchnic vasodilation, renal

607

vasoconstriction and hypoperfusion, and salt and water retention. Additionally, the intestinal mucosa becomes hyperpermeable, perhaps related to reduced oncotic pressure; this may account for bacterial translocation from the gut to the peritoneal space, resulting in spontaneous bacterial peritonitis.[4]

PREVALENCE AND EPIDEMIOLOGY

The prevalence of cirrhosis is difficult to ascertain and is probably underestimated because large numbers of patients with compensated cirrhosis go undetected. This is especially the case in patients with cirrhosis due to nonalcoholic fatty liver disease or hepatitis C viral infection, conditions with asymptomatic phases of long duration. In the United States, the prevalence of cirrhosis was estimated to be 0.15%, accounting for roughly 400,000 cases in 1998. This was associated with 25,000 deaths and 375,000 hospital admissions. By comparison, cirrhosis is undoubtedly more frequent in Africa and Asia, where vertically transmitted hepatitis B viral infection is common, although precise estimates are unavailable.

Age, sex, and ethnicity all influence the risk of cirrhosis. Cirrhosis rarely afflicts children (<18 years) or the elderly (>75 years), occurring 80% of the time in patients between the ages of 25 to 64. Sixty-five percent of cases occur in males. Although there is little variation in the prevalence of cirrhosis among different ethnicities, there are differences with regard to cirrhosis-related death. In 2001, chronic liver disease with cirrhosis was the 12th leading cause of death in the United States; however, it was the 6th and 7th most frequent cause of death in Native Americans and Hispanics, respectively.[5,6]

The economic burden of chronic liver disease and cirrhosis has increased substantially in recent years. In 2000, direct health care costs exceeded $1.5 billion, whereas indirect costs contributed an additional $230 million. More than $1 billion was accounted for by inpatient hospitalizations, whereas office visits and cirrhosis-specific medications added $65 million and $17 million, respectively.[7]

CLINICAL PRESENTATION

Cirrhosis is often indolent and unsuspected until its complications arise. Some asymptomatic patients present for the evaluation of unrelated problems and are incidentally found to have cirrhosis based on physical examination, laboratory findings, or imaging. Owing to the large number of abnormalities in liver function caused by cirrhosis and the central role the liver plays in whole-body physiology, symptomatic patients may present with a broad spectrum of clinical manifestations.

Common presenting symptoms of compensated cirrhosis include fatigue, weakness, anorexia, jaundice, itching, and easy bruising. On physical examination, patients may exhibit muscular and temporal wasting, ecchymoses, and jaundice. Dermatologic stigmata of chronic liver disease, such as spider angiomas and palmar erythema, are present in 33% of cases.[8] Gynecomastia occurs in the majority of male patients. Hypogonadism, due to either primary gonadal injury or disruption of the hypothalamic-pituitary

axis, results in testicular atrophy, impotence, infertility, and feminization. The liver itself may be enlarged (characteristically observed in alcoholic and nonalcoholic fatty liver disease, storage diseases, and Budd-Chiari syndrome) or shrunken with firm edges (characteristically observed in viral causes). Portal hypertension frequently causes splenomegaly and caput medusae.[9]

With hepatic decompensation, more advanced signs and symptoms may manifest. Ascites, the most common complication of cirrhosis, occurs as a result of portal hypertension and salt and water retention. Over 60% of patients with cirrhosis develop ascites within 10 years of diagnosis; and once ascites occurs, 2-year survival is only about 50%.[10] Spontaneous bacterial peritonitis is a life-threatening complication of ascites and is one of the reasons for the high ascites-related fatality.

Portosystemic collaterals, or varices, develop as a result of portal hypertension. The most clinically significant varices are located in the distal esophagus and upper stomach. These so-called esophagogastric varices occur in approximately 60% of patients with cirrhosis, with 30% of them experiencing bleeding complications.

Hepatic encephalopathy refers to a spectrum of neuropsychiatric abnormalities caused by the retention of ammonia and other toxic substances normally metabolized and cleared by the liver. Precipitating factors include dehydration, electrolyte and metabolic derangements, gastrointestinal bleeding, infections, and sedating medications. Transjugular intrahepatic portosystemic shunt (TIPS) and surgical shunt procedures hasten the development of hepatic encephalopathy in about 40% of patients.[11]

Hepatorenal syndrome refers to acute renal failure in patients with cirrhosis without underlying renal abnormalities. It is thought to occur because of splanchnic vasodilatation, which results in unremitting, hormone-mediated renovascular vasoconstriction and reduced renal perfusion. Occurring in approximately 40% of patients with cirrhosis and ascites by 5 years, hepatorenal syndrome is a terminal complication of cirrhosis and has a poor prognosis.[12,13]

In the majority of patients, the diagnosis of cirrhosis is based on history, physical examination, basic laboratory studies, and imaging studies. In general, serum aminotransferase levels are mildly elevated (generally, <100 U/L), the total bilirubin level is proportionally elevated, and the albumin value is reduced. Because the liver synthesizes many of the blood clotting factors, the prothrombin time may be prolonged. Hyponatremia, due to impaired free water secretion, and renal insufficiency are seen in advanced cirrhosis and are poor prognostic signs.[14] Serum α-fetoprotein levels are sometimes elevated in those patients presenting with cirrhosis complicated by hepatocellular carcinoma (HCC).

Once diagnosed, the severity of cirrhosis historically has been graded by the Child-Turcotte-Pugh classification (e.g., Child class A, B, or C), with higher point totals coinciding with greater short-term and perioperative fatality. More recently, the Model for End-Stage Liver Disease (MELD) score has gained preference.[15] This score is calculated from a logarithmic formula using the patient's total bilirubin, international normalized ratio (INR), and creatinine concentration.

The natural history of cirrhosis is that of an inexorably progressive condition. Within 10 years, 58% of patients with cirrhosis develop various forms of hepatic decompensation.[10-17] The annual incidence of HCC in patients with cirrhosis is about 5%[18] but ranges from less than 1% to up to 10%, depending on the etiology of cirrhosis and the presence of comorbidities, such as human immunodeficiency virus infection or diabetes, which may increase the hepatocarcinogenesis risk.

PATHOLOGY

Cirrhosis is a diffuse process affecting the architecture of the entire liver; localized scarring does not constitute cirrhosis. In advanced cirrhosis, it is not possible to determine the cause with certainty. However, in early-stage cirrhosis, different hepatic insults may cause varied patterns of cirrhosis.

Gross examination of the cirrhotic liver typically reveals a shrunken and firm organ, although the liver may be enlarged depending on the cause. Cirrhosis is defined histologically by the presence of fibrous septa that divide the liver parenchyma into nodules. The septa range from delicate fibrous bands to large fibrous tracts that obliterate multiple lobules.[19] The fibrous septa may connect portal tracts and centrilobular hepatic terminal veins in portal-portal, portal-central, or central-central patterns. The nodules are variably sized and arbitrarily defined as micronodules (<3 mm) or macronodules (>3 mm).[19]

By far, the most common nodules are regenerative in nature (RNs). These tend to be relatively uniform in size and appearance. Occasionally, nodules may arise that are conspicuous in terms of size, color, texture, or degree of bulging from the cut surface of the liver. These may represent low- or high-grade dysplastic nodules (DNs) or HCC. Low-grade DNs have been alternatively referred to as large RNs and macroregenerative nodules. The hepatocytes in low-grade DNs are essentially indistinguishable from background hepatocytes, although subtle variations in cell size may be seen. High-grade DNs are distinguished microscopically from low-grade DNs via recognition of cytologic alterations (increased nuclear to cytoplasmic ratio) and architectural changes (thickening of hepatocyte cell plates and pseudogland formation). Grossly, high-grade DNs frequently show a "nodule-in-nodule" appearance, reflecting patchy proliferative activity. Low-grade DNs are considered benign, whereas high-grade DNs are thought to be precursors of HCC.[20]

Recently, focal nodular hyperplasia (FNH)–like lesions have been described in cirrhosis.[21] Both macroscopically and microscopically, these lesions appear identical to FNH in the noncirrhotic liver. Unlike true FNH, which is thought to arise in response to congenital arteriovenous malformations, FNH-like lesions are thought to arise from acquired vascular flow perturbations associated with cirrhosis.[21]

IMAGING

Imaging studies, including ultrasonography, CT, and MRI, are used to assess liver size, the biliary tree, patency of hepatic vasculature, and sequelae of portal hypertension (e.g., ascites, varices, and splenomegaly) and to screen for HCC. Although the portosystemic pressure gradient may be directly measured via transjugular cannulation of the hepatic veins, this is invasive and often unnecessary because portal hypertension can be inferred by endoscopic findings of varices and sequelae of portal hypertension seen on imaging.

On cross-sectional imaging, the cirrhotic liver may demonstrate a nodular surface, widened fissures between lobes, and an increase in size of the hypertrophied caudate lobe relative to the atrophied right lobe (>0.6). Depending on the modality and imaging technique, fibrotic reticulations, fatty changes, and the presence of various hepatocellular nodules (RNs, DNs, HCC, FNH-like lesions) may be visible. The critical diagnostic distinction is between malignant nodules (e.g., HCC) and nonmalignant nodules (e.g., RNs, DNs, and FNH-like lesions).[22] Although DNs have higher rates of malignant transformation than RNs, the transformation rate is not sufficiently high to warrant ablation or other intervention, nor to increase imaging surveillance frequency or alter surveillance strategies.[23] The natural history of FNH-like lesions in cirrhosis is unknown, but these lesions are considered benign.[21] Simple hepatic cysts and hemangiomas are observed less frequently in the cirrhotic liver than in the noncirrhotic liver. These lesions are described elsewhere in this text. Peribiliary cysts are serous cysts that are hypothesized to represent obstructed periductal glands in patients who have severe liver disease. Recognition of these cysts on imaging helps radiologists to avoid the incorrect diagnosis of dilated bile ducts, abscesses, or cystic neoplasms.[24]

Classic vascular manifestations of cirrhosis include hepatic artery dilatation, tortuosity of hepatic arteries within the liver ("corkscrew" arteries, which may be observed with high-resolution, state-of-the-art CT and MRI), portal vein dilation in early portal hypertension, portal vein occlusion in late portal hypertension due to sluggish portal flow, and formation of shunts. Intrahepatic shunts (arterioportal and arteriovenous) may manifest on dynamic imaging studies as small (≤2 cm) hypervascular pseudolesions and may be mistaken for nodules.[25] Portosystemic shunts manifest as varices (e.g., esophagogastric and paraumbilical); these are usually located outside the liver, although intrahepatic varices also may occur. In addition to varices, other sequelae of portal hypertension (e.g., ascites, splenomegaly, peribiliary cysts, and Gamna-Gandy bodies) may be noted (Figs. 66-1 to 66-3).[26]

Radiography

On plain radiographs, gynecomastia may be appreciated in males with cirrhosis; and on lateral films a recanalized umbilical vein may be noted as a round shadow in the fatty tissue anterior and inferior to the liver. Other possible findings include dilation of the azygos vein, a shrunken liver, and enlarged spleen. Barium esophagograms may depict large varices as serpentine-like defects at the inferior portion of the esophagus; these characteristically change in size in response to positional maneuvers. Esophagrams have limited sensitivity for small varices. Ultimately, however, radiography is an insufficient modality to assess cirrhosis or its complications.

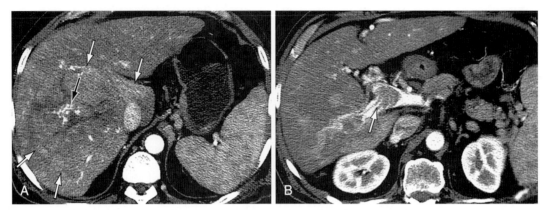

■ **FIGURE 66-1** Hepatocellular carcinoma with invasion into the right portal vein. **A,** Axial CT image during hepatic arterial phase after injection of intravenous contrast agent demonstrates a large, encapsulated mass in the right lobe of the liver (*black arrow*). Note the irregular arteries coursing through the lesion center (*white arrows*), a finding suggestive of hepatocellular carcinoma. **B,** On a more inferior slice, the right portal vein is expanded and contains linear areas of arterial hypervascularity (*arrow*). These represent tumor vessels within a malignant thrombus.

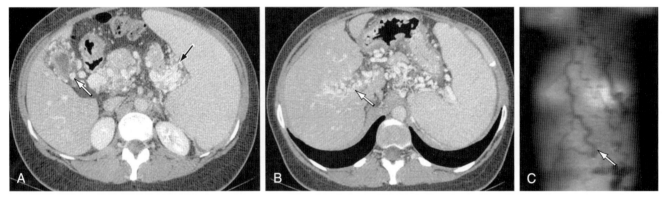

■ **FIGURE 66-2** Extrahepatic manifestations of portal hypertension. **A** and **B,** Axial CT contrast-enhanced images show extensive intra-abdominal varices in a patient with long-standing portal venous thrombosis. Note pericholecystic (**A,** *white arrow*), peripancreatic, perisplenic (**A,** *black arrow*), and left gastric varices as well as cavernous transformation of the right portal vein (**B,** *arrow*). **C,** Coronal single-shot fast spin-echo T2W image in a different patient reveals varices along the anterior abdominal wall (*arrow*).

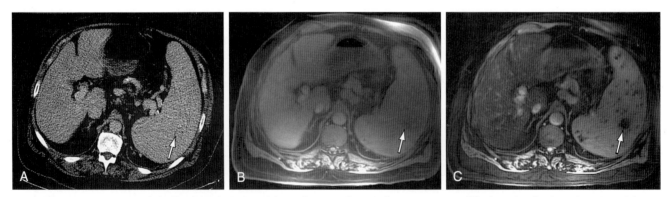

■ **FIGURE 66-3** Gamna-Gandy bodies (GGBs). **A,** On axial portal venous phase CT image, GGBs are difficult to visualize (*arrow*). **B,** On axial unenhanced gradient-recalled-echo MR image with ultrashort echo time (0.08 ms), a 1-cm GGB (*arrow*) and several subcentimeter GGBs are barely perceptible. **C,** On axial unenhanced co-localized gradient-recalled-echo MR image with echo time of 9 ms generated by the same radiofrequency excitation as in **B,** the 1-cm GGB (*arrow*) and several other GGBs are easily visible as focal hypointense lesions with associated blooming artifacts. Signal loss and blooming in GGBs are due to susceptibility from hemosiderin. As illustrated in this case, GGBs are more visible on MR images than on CT images, especially on T2*W gradient-recalled echo acquisitions.

Catheter angiography is used mainly for therapeutic purposes (e.g., transarterial chemoembolization and placement of TIPS). In some centers, it may be used for presurgical planning. It does not play a role in the routine imaging assessment of cirrhotic patients.[27]

CT

Technical Considerations

The primary indications for performing multiphasic CT in patients with cirrhosis are the evaluation of disease progression, surveillance for HCC, and follow-up of known lesions. Contrast enhancement of vessels, liver, and other solid organs may be impaired in patients with cirrhosis owing to third spacing of fluid and leakage of contrast material into the pulmonary interstitium during passage through the right-sided circulation. For this reason, patients with cirrhosis may require higher rates and concentrations of contrast material than patients without cirrhosis. At our institution, iodinated contrast agents with a concentration of 0.5 mol/L are given at 4 to 5 mL/s. The critical phases for image acquisition are the late arterial (typically at 35 to 40 seconds), portal venous (at 60 to 80 seconds), and late venous (at 3 to 5 minutes).[27] Unenhanced images usually are recommended; cirrhotic nodules may be intrinsically hyperdense due to copper or iron deposition or high glycogen content and may appear hyperdense at hepatic arterial phase and be mistakenly characterized as hypervascular if unenhanced images are not acquired first. Some authors also advocate early arterial phase images (typically at 20 to 25 seconds) to detect very early enhancement of malignant lesions and permit more precise characterization of lesion enhancement features, but this strategy has not been proven to be superior for lesion diagnosis in large clinical trials. Owing to its radiation exposure, CT is not an optimal modality for use in children or pregnant women. CT hepatic artery angiography, CT portography, and CT after transarterial administration of iodized oil may be performed in select cases but are not utilized routinely in the assessment of cirrhotic patients and their discussion is beyond the scope of this chapter.

Fibrosis

On unenhanced images, the attenuation of normal liver is typically about 10 HU greater than that of the spleen. However, the density of the cirrhotic liver or of focal lesions may be reduced (e.g., by steatosis, fibrosis, or edema) or increased (e.g., by iron or copper deposition). Fibrosis typically is not visible on nonenhanced CT; if sufficiently severe, fibrosis may manifest as a diffuse lacework of hypoattenuating bands or as mottled areas of decreased density. Regions of confluent fibrosis are characterized as hypoattenuating wedge- or geographically shaped regions, radiating from the portal hilus and causing retraction of the overlying hepatic capsule (Fig. 66-4). Involvement of the medial segment of the left lobe or anterior segment of the right lobe is characteristic, but other segments may be involved as well. Confluent fibrosis is observed more commonly in alcoholic liver disease and primary sclerosing cholangitis than in viral and other liver diseases. On contrast-enhanced CT, fibrosis, especially if confluent, may show progressive enhancement and appear hyperattenuating on delayed images. Confluent fibrosis occasionally may be mass-like and cause diagnostic confusion. Differentiation from HCC is usually possible based on the characteristic capsular retraction, volume loss, and progressive enhancement pattern associated with confluent fibrosis. In difficult cases, follow-up imaging may be necessary: progressive volume loss, if observed, clinches the diagnosis of confluent fibrosis.[28]

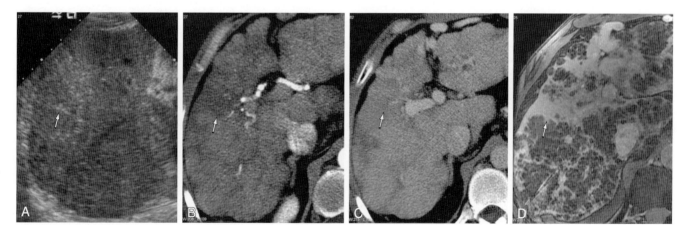

■ **FIGURE 66-4** Confluent fibrosis. Coronal ultrasound (**A**), hepatic arterial phase contrast-enhanced CT (**B**), portal venous phase contrast-enhanced CT (**C**), and double-contrast–enhanced axial 2D spoiled gradient-echo (SGE) (**D**) images obtained at 3.0 T with echo time of 5.8 ms. **A**, On ultrasonography, individual regenerative nodules and reticulations of fibrotic tissue are difficult to delineate but the liver displays patchy areas of increased echogenicity (*white arrow*) suggesting increased fibrotic tissue in the liver. **B** and **C**, Unenhanced and contrast-enhanced CT images show confluent fibrosis as a hypoattenuating geographically shaped region radiating from the portal hilus and causing minimal contraction of the overlying hepatic capsule (*white arrows*). **D**, On the MR image, the fibrotic tissue takes up gadolinium and displays high signal intensity in the same geographically shaped formation that is seen on the CT images, while the surrounding regenerative tissue appears dark due to superparamagnetic iron oxide uptake.

Nodules

FNH-like lesions are small, ranging up to about 1 cm in diameter.[29] Isoattenuating on nonenhanced imaging, these lesions hyperenhance on the arterial phase and then fade to isoattenuation on more delayed images. On both non-enhanced and contrast-enhanced CT, RNs usually are iso-attenuating relative to the surrounding hepatic parenchyma and are difficult to visualize (Figs. 66-5 and 66-6), although siderotic RNs may be hyperdense. On nonenhanced CT, large DNs are hyperattenuating relative to surrounding parenchyma due to the presence of increased iron and glycogen, whereas small DNs remain isoattenuating. Con-versely, DNs enhance simultaneously with normal paren-chyma on contrast-enhanced CT, appearing isoattenuated. With increased dedifferentiation, however, these DNs may appear hyperattenuating owing to increased vascular-ity and consequent increased contrast uptake.[25]

HCCs may have a varied appearance at CT depending on tumor size, vascularity, steatosis, cholestasis, hemor-rhage, and necrosis. On nonenhanced CT, HCCs generally appear as hypoattenuating or heterogeneously attenuating lesions. Intralesional fat or blood products may be difficult to identify on CT; these features are more readily observed on MRI. After administration of contrast agents, HCCs become hyperattenuating or heterogeneously enhancing during the arterial phase, then fade to isoattenuation or wash out to hypoattenuation on venous and delayed phases. If a tumor capsule is present, it often enhances progressively and retains contrast material on delayed images. Vascular invasion, if present, is more easily appre-ciated on contrast-enhanced images.

Perfusional pseudolesions due to arteriovenous or arte-rioportal shunts enhance during the arterial phase and then fade to isoattenuation on images acquired during the portal venous and equilibrium phases. As opposed to true nodules, pseudolesions tend to have ill-defined or straight borders and may have blood vessels running through their center. In diagnostically challenging cases, longitudinal imaging is necessary. At follow-up, pseudolesions regress or are stable but rarely grow.

MRI

Technical Considerations

Whereas MRI provides the best performance characteris-tics for the diagnosis of cirrhosis, it requires longer scan times than CT and is more costly. Therefore, it is generally employed when CT is not definitive or if further charac-terization of a lesion is required. Because of its lack of radiation, it is also used in lieu of CT in children when ultrasound findings raise further concerns.

There is controversy regarding which MR technique is optimal for evaluation of cirrhotic patients.[30] For T1-weighted (T1W) imaging, dual-phase in-phase and out-of-phase gradient-echo images are commonly acquired because these permit assessment of parenchymal and lesional fat content as well as provide characterization based on T1 relaxation. If a tissue contains no fat, it is also possible to infer qualitative $T2^*$ information from the dual-phase echoes: voxels with short $T2^*$ visibly lose signal on the later echo, whereas voxels with long $T2^*$ do not. Multiphase gradient-echo imaging, in which three

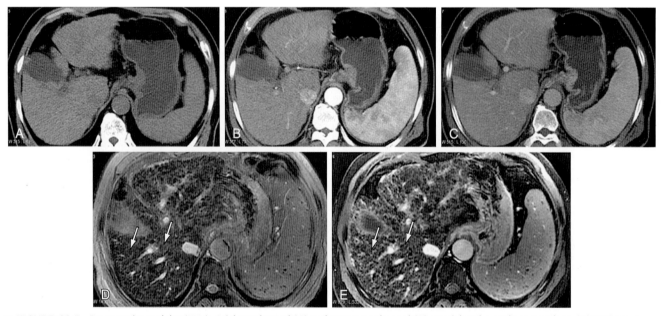

■ **FIGURE 66-5**   Regenerative nodules (RNs). Axial unenhanced (**A**) and contrast-enhanced (**B**) arterial and portal venous phase (**C**) CT images. **A-C,** The liver parenchyma shows minimal heterogeneity, and discrete RNs are not confidently characterized. **D,** At the same level as the CT images, on axial 2D spoiled gradient-echo (SGE) MR image obtained at 3.0 T with echo time of 5.8 ms after SPIO administration, the RNs are visible as sharply demarcated hypointense nodules owing to phagocytic uptake of SPIO, which causes $T2^*$ shortening. **E,** On double-contrast–enhanced MR image after gadolinium administration, fibrotic reticulations display an increase in signal intensity owing to the extracellular accumulation of the low-molecular-weight contrast agent. Enhancement of fibrotic tissue further increases visibility of RNs (*arrows*). Note that this image shows innumerable RNs carpeting the liver. The two representative RNs as labeled for illustrative purposes are examples of SPIO-enhanced and double-contrast–enhanced MRI.

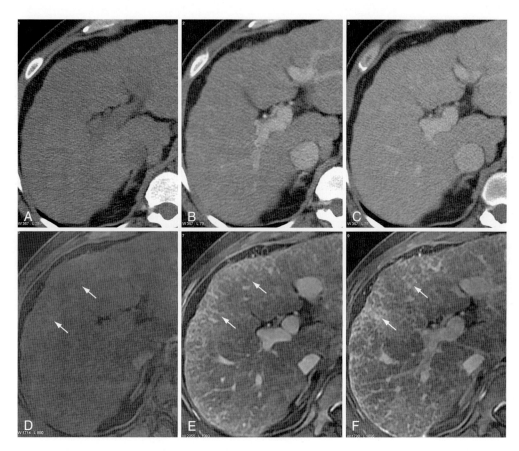

■ **FIGURE 66-6** Dynamic enhancement of fibrotic tissue in the cirrhotic liver. Dynamic contrast-enhanced (**A**), unenhanced portal venous phase (**B**), and delayed phase (**C**) CT images show the nodular liver surface diagnostic of cirrhosis. The liver parenchyma is homogeneous, with neither fibrotic reticulations nor RNs clearly identified. Dynamic gadolinium-enhanced axial gradient-recalled unenhanced (**D**), portal venous (**E**), and delayed (**F**) phase MR images obtained at the same level as the CT images show progressive enhancement of the fibrotic reticulations due to accumulation of the low-molecular-weight gadolinium. Dynamic MR images depict the enhancement of the fibrotic septa (*arrows*) with higher clarity than CT.

or more gradient echoes are acquired after a single radio-frequency excitation, is now available on some scanners and permits more reliable characterization of fat content and T2* relaxation. T2-weighted (T2W) fast spin-echo imaging is useful for evaluating bile ducts, cysts, and fluid collections; single-shot fast spin-echo sequences are particularly useful for this purpose. T2W imaging also helps characterize RNs and DNs but has low sensitivity for detecting HCC. Diffusion-weighted imaging is another available technique and shows promise; HCCs tend to have restricted diffusion and appear bright on diffusion-weighted images.

The most common dynamic technique to evaluate the liver is MRI after a rapid bolus injection of gadolinium-based contrast agents at a rate of about 2 mL/s. The authors typically use the dose indicated in the product insert (0.1 mmol/kg). Because MRI has higher sensitivity to contrast agents than CT, the standard dose usually suffices and higher doses are rarely necessary. Patients with cirrhosis may develop acute renal failure due to hepatorenal syndrome and other mechanisms, which in theory increases their risk for developing nephrogenic systemic fibrosis after exposure to gadolinium-based contrast agents. For this reason, the American College of Radiology recommends assessment of the estimated glomerular filtration rate (eGFR) nearly contemporaneous with gadolinium exposure. If the eGFR exceeds 30 mL/min/1.73 m^2, the risk of nephrogenic systemic fibrosis appears to be miniscule.[31,32]

Volumetric 3D T1W fat-saturated spoiled gradient-echo acquisitions are usually utilized for dynamic imaging. The key phases are the *hepatic arterial phase*, in which the acquisition of the center of K space coincides with peak arterial perfusion of hepatic nodules, *portal venous phase*, acquired 60 to 80 seconds after gadolinium injection (see Fig. 66-6), and *delayed venous phase* image acquisitions (acquired 3 to 5 minutes after injection).[33-35] The delayed venous phase images help to assess venous wash out.

Superparamagnetic iron oxides (SPIOs) may be given to evaluate phagocytic function of hepatic Kupffer cells. The agent is administered as a slow infusion, typically over 30 minutes. Uptake of SPIOs results in T2 and T2*shortening.[36] Lesions with Kupffer cells (most RNs and DNs) lose signal intensity on SPIO-enhanced T2W and T2*W images, whereas lesions deficient in Kupffer cells (most HCCs and cirrhotic scars) do not lose signal intensity and appear relatively hyperintense. There is controversy regarding whether spin-echo or gradient-echo techniques are most well suited for evaluating SPIO uptake.[37] We prefer gradient-echo images, but other institutions may prefer spin-echo images.

In select centers, *double-contrast–enhanced imaging*, in which SPIO followed by gadolinium are administered sequentially in the same examination, is performed. The sequential administration of two agents theoretically improves the characterization of cirrhotic nodules by permitting the assessment of *two* complementary biologic features (phagocytic activity of Kupffer cells *and* vascularity).[30]

Fibrosis

Fibrosis in the cirrhotic liver has low signal intensity on unenhanced T1W images and high signal on T2W images. Similar to its appearance on CT, confluent fibrosis tends to have straight borders and is associated with progressive volume loss over time at follow-up imaging. When gadolinium is administered, fibrotic tissue slowly enhances in the arterial phase and retains contrast on portal venous and delayed images. As a result, fibrosis has relatively high signal on delayed gadolinium-enhanced images (see Figs. 66-4 and 66-5). Fibrosis, which lacks Kupffer cells, also has relatively high signal intensity on T2W and T2*W images after SPIO administration. Double-contrast–enhanced gradient-echo images show the reticulations and bands of liver fibrosis to greatest advantage; the fibrotic tissue appears hyperintense due to gadolinium accumulation while the background liver parenchyma appears hypointense due to SPIO accumulation. Such images also show other features of cirrhosis, including capsular thickening (Fig. 66-7) and nonuniform distribution of fibrosis (Fig. 66-8).

Nodules

FNH-like lesions are typically isointense on both T1W and T2*W imaging. Similar to their appearance on contrast-enhanced CT, these lesions enhance during the hepatic arterial phase after injection of gadolinium-based agents and then fade to isointensity on more delayed phases. RNs have a variable appearance at unenhanced T1W imaging and may be hypointense, isointense, or hyperintense. Some RNs are steatotic and lose signal intensity on out-of-phase compared with in-phase imaging (Fig. 66-9). Most RNs are isointense and not detectable at T2W and T2*W imaging, whereas some RNs, particularly those with high iron concentration, are hypointense at T2W and T2*W imaging.[38,39] High signal intensity on T2W and T2*W images is distinctly unusual for RNs; marked T2 hyperin-

tensity suggests a simple cyst, whereas mild to moderate T2 hyperintensity raises suspicion for HCC. On administration of gadolinium, RNs enhance to a similar degree as surrounding parenchyma and appear isointense. When SPIOs are administered, RNs take up the iron particles and, due to superparamagnetic effects, appear hypointense on T2W and T2*W images (see Fig. 66-5). DNs, like RNs, have variable signal intensity on unenhanced T1W images and appear isointense or hypointense on T2W images. On gadolinium and SPIO-enhanced imaging, low-grade DNs typically are difficult to distinguish from RNs,

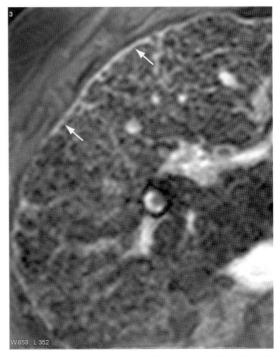

■ **FIGURE 66-7** Hepatic capsular thickening. On this axial double-contrast–enhanced MR image, the hepatic capsule can be seen retaining gadolinium and has high signal intensity similar to the fibrotic reticulations distributed throughout the liver. As illustrated in this case, the fibrotic thickening of the liver capsule (*arrows*) is a frequent manifestation of cirrhosis but it is not always observed on imaging.

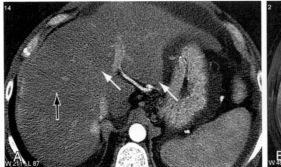
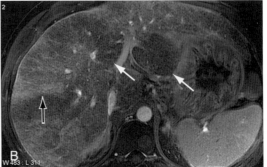

■ **FIGURE 66-8** Nonuniform distribution of fibrosis. **A,** On this axial arterial-phase contrast-enhanced CT image the liver has an unusual contour and there is relative hypertrophy of the posterior portion of the lateral segment of the left lobe (*black arrow*). The liver parenchyma is relatively heterogeneous with areas of hyperattenuation and hypoattenuation (*white arrows*). **B,** The axial double-contrast–enhanced MR image shows to better advantage the nonuniform distribution of fibrosis within this cirrhotic liver. Note that areas of atrophy and volume loss are associated with a higher density of fibrotic tissue (*black arrow*) than areas of hypertrophy (*white arrows*).

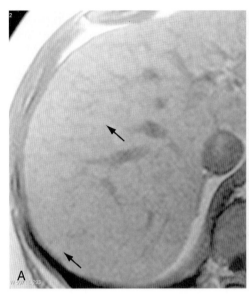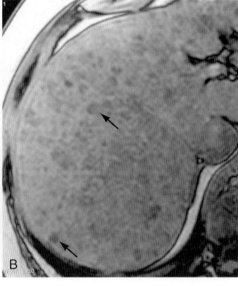

■ FIGURE 66-9 Fatty regenerative nodules (RNs). On axial unenhanced MR in-phase (**A**) and out-of-phase (**B**) images, regenerative nodules can be appreciated (*arrows*). The regenerative nodules lose signal, as evidenced by the decrease in signal intensity on out-of-phase images, indicating the presence of intralesional fat. Innumerable nodules are present in the images.

whereas high-grade dysplastic nodules may resemble well-differentiated HCCs.

HCCs display variable signal intensity on unenhanced T1W imaging. They characteristically appear hyperintense at T2W imaging, but T2W imaging has limited sensitivity for HCCs and may render them invisible or mildly hypointense. After administration of gadolinium, hypervascular HCCs enhance rapidly to high signal intensity on arterial phase images and then become hypointense on portal venous and delayed images. Compared with RNs and DNs, HCCs tend to have a reduced concentration of Kupffer cells and diminished phagocytic capacity. Hence, when SPIOs are administered, HCCs do not take up the particles and have high signal intensity relative to the adjacent non-neoplastic parenchyma. Focal areas of fibrosis also have high signal on such images and may be mistaken for HCCs on low-resolution SPIO-enhanced images. High-resolution SPIO-enhanced imaging usually permits differentiation of fibrosis (reticulated morphology) from HCC (nodular morphology). In challenging cases, gadolinium administration or follow-up imaging is necessary.

Perfusional pseudolesions may be indistinguishable from FNH-like lesions; similar to FNH-like lesions, the pseudolesions hyperenhance during the arterial phase and then fade to isointensity. Differentiation is not clinically important, however, because both FNH-like lesions and perfusional pseudolesions are benign. If these entities are suspected, follow-up imaging rather than intervention is recommended.

Ultrasonography

Technical Considerations

Because of its low cost and lack of radiation, ultrasonography is typically the initial imaging modality performed in patients with cirrhosis. It provides information about liver size and shape and, if high-frequency transducers are used, may detect subtle nodularity along the liver surface to establish the diagnosis of cirrhosis in clinically equivo-cal cases. In patients with established cirrhosis, ultrasonography plays an important role in assessing sequelae of portal hypertension (e.g., splenomegaly and ascites). On gray-scale images, features suggestive of portal hypertension include dilation of the portal vein to greater than 13 mm, splenic vein to greater than 11 mm, and superior mesenteric vein to greater than 12 mm. Color Doppler tracings can be utilized to further characterize portal vein patency and direction of flow. Portal hypertension is associated with increased pulsatility of the portal vein Doppler tracing and loss of the normal triphasic hepatic vein Doppler tracing. When portal flow is hepatofugal, the liver has progressed to end-stage disease and shunt placement or liver transplantation may be required. Color Doppler tracings can also be used to monitor shunt patency as well as patency of vascular anastomoses after transplantation.

In Europe, Asia, and select centers in North America, microbubble-based contrast agents may be administered intravenously to assess lesion vascularity using ultrasonography. Similar to CT and MRI, multiple phases are acquired: *arterial phase* (15 to 30 seconds after injection), *portal phase* (30 to 60 seconds after injection), and *sinusoidal (or blood pool) phase* (60 to 240 seconds after injection).[25]

Nodules

Ultrasonography has limited sensitivity for cirrhosis-associated nodules. Discrete RNs are rarely identified even if they are obvious on other imaging modalities. Coarsening and heterogeneity of the liver echotexture may suggest the presence of RNs, but this finding is neither sensitive nor specific and the liver parenchyma may appear normal even if cirrhosis is advanced (see Figs. 66-4 and 66-10). Another indirect clue to the presence of RNs includes nodularity of the liver surface, most reliably appreciated if high-resolution transducers are used; in this setting, the RNs themselves are usually not visible and their presence is inferred by the bulging of the liver capsule.

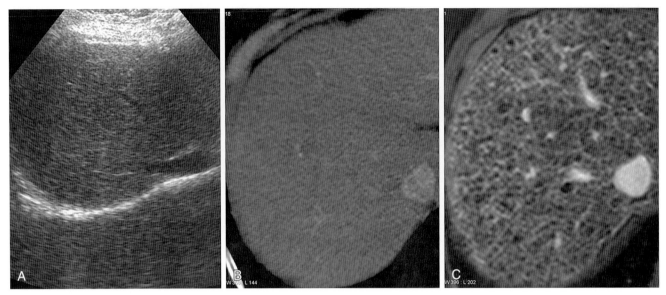

■ **FIGURE 66-10** Ultrasound (**A**), CT (**B**), and MR (**C**) images of the liver of a male patient with cirrhosis. On the ultrasound image the liver has increased echogenicity and heterogeneity, although specific reticulations are difficult to identify. On the axial CT image, reticulations are again difficult to appreciate. However, on the double-contrast–enhanced MR image the fibrotic tissue forms honeycomb-like reticulations of high signal intensity surrounding the low signal regenerative nodules. Of the three modalities, the extent and degree of fibrosis are more easily appreciated with MRI.

Nodules sufficiently large or anomalous to be visible in the cirrhotic liver on ultrasound evaluation are likely to be HCCs. If visible on ultrasonography, HCCs tend to be hypoechoic or have mixed echogenicity. Unenhanced ultrasonography has limited sensitivity for HCC, however, and most HCCs are not visible unless large or associated with vascular invasion. If microbubbles are administered, HCCs typically hyperenhance and become vividly hyperechoic on arterial phase and then wash out to become hypoechoic on the portal and sinusoidal phases.

Fibrosis

Similar to cirrhotic nodules, ultrasonography has low sensitivity for fibrosis. Advanced fibrosis associated with cirrhosis may manifest as diffuse increase in echogenicity, with poor visualization of coursing liver vessels. Findings overlap with those of simple steatosis, and it is common for cirrhosis to be misdiagnosed as fatty liver on the basis of ultrasound findings.

Nuclear Medicine

Nuclear medicine imaging of the cirrhotic liver is limited by poor performance characteristics and is no longer utilized in standard clinical practice. Historically, the primary hepatic radionuclide study was *radiocolloid liver scintigraphy* or, more commonly, the *liver-spleen scan.* Liver-spleen scintigraphy is based on the principle that radiolabeled colloid particles are phagocytosed and localized to the reticuloendothelial system of the liver, spleen, and bone marrow after intravenous injection. The radiopharmaceutical agent most commonly used for liver-spleen scanning is technetium-99m sulfur colloid (^{99m}Tc-SC). The radionuclide has a relatively short half-life of 6 hours, does not release beta radiation, and discharges gamma photons at 140 keV/m.[27] Imaging is performed 15 to 20 minutes after intravenous injection of 3 to 8 mCi of ^{99m}Tc-SC. The normal liver demonstrates greater uptake of radiocolloid than the spleen. In advanced cirrhosis, hepatic uptake may be reduced, leading to relatively greater uptake in the spleen ("colloid shift"). Other scintigraphic findings of advanced cirrhosis include morphologic alterations of the liver (e.g., enlargement of the left lobe and caudate with atrophy of the right lobe) and reduced activity in the distribution of the left portal vein if there is shunting into a recanalized umbilical vein. Splenomegaly may be evident. Ascites may be inferred if there is separation of the liver from the abdominal wall or if a photopenic rim is seen around the liver. Dynamic flow images may be acquired immediately after injection to assess vascularity of hepatic lesions, although this is less accurate than the dynamic images acquired at CT or MRI.

Imaging Algorithm

The most appropriate method for assessing cirrhosis and screening for HCC through imaging is complicated and controversial. The American Association for the Study of Liver Diseases recommends ultrasonographic screening every 6 to 12 months, but ultrasonography has low sensitivity and may fail to detect HCC until advanced stages when it is no longer curable.[40] Therefore, many centers use CT for initial screening, with contrast-enhanced MRI reserved for further characterization of known lesions. Although MRI offers higher sensitivity to contrast agents, higher tissue contrast, and a larger variety of contrast agents with different biologic properties, MR costs and time preclude it from being utilized as a screening modality in most centers. Even so, some academic centers primarily utilize MRI for screening purposes because of its perceived benefits (Table 66-1).

TABLE 66-1 Accuracy, Limitations, and Pitfalls of the Modalities Used in Imaging of Cirrhosis

Modality	Accuracy	Pitfalls	Limitations
CT	Detects morphologic alterations of cirrhosis, which have high specificity but low sensitivity for cirrhosis Low sensitivity for RNs and DNs	Most cirrhosis-associated hepatocellular nodules are not visible. The liver parenchyma may appear normal even if cirrhosis is advanced.	Exposes patient to ionizing radiation. Less intrinsic soft tissue contrast and less sensitivity to contrast agents compared with MRI Vascular and parenchymal enhancement may be suboptimal. Higher contrast agent concentrations and rates may be necessary. Does not assess vascular flow direction
MRI	Like CT, detects morphologic alterations of cirrhosis Sensitivity and specificity for cirrhosis may be improved by using double-contrast techniques. Depending on the imaging technique, hepatocellular nodules (RNs, DNs, and HCC) may be visible with high clarity.	Imaging features of nonmalignant lesions (RNs, DNs, perfusional pseudolesions, confluent fibrosis) may overlap with those of HCC.	More time consuming and expensive than CT Prone to imaging artifacts, especially in uncooperative patients and those with severe ascites Using standard techniques, does not assess vascular flow direction
Ultrasonography	Using high-resolution transducers, can detect subtle nodularity along cirrhotic liver surface Low sensitivity for all cirrhosis-associated hepatocellular nodules (RNs, DNs, HCC) High accuracy for detecting vascular flow direction	Most cirrhosis-associated hepatocellular nodules are not visible. The liver parenchyma may appear normal even if cirrhosis is advanced. If abnormal, the parenchymal findings are nonspecific and ultrasonography does not reliably distinguish fibrosis from steatosis.	Operator dependent Limited evaluation of liver parenchyma

RNs, regenerative nodules; DNs, dysplastic nodules; HCC, hepatocellular carcinoma.

Classic Signs of Cirrhosis

- Classic signs for the diagnosis of cirrhosis include morphologic and textural alterations.
- The most definitive morphologic alteration is surface nodularity, which is due to the presence of regenerative nodules subjacent to the liver capsule. The presence of surface nodularity is highly specific for cirrhosis in the right clinical setting but has low sensitivity for early cirrhosis, in which the liver surface may be smooth.
- Another morphologic alteration is atrophy of certain segments with relative enlargement of others. Characteristically, the right lobe atrophies, often in association with surface notching at the junction of the caudate and segment 6. The left lobe atrophies less and appears large by comparison. Alternatively, there may be atrophy of the central segments (4, 5, and 8), with or without enlargement of other segments.
- As certain portions of the liver atrophy, the hepatic fissures (falciform, venosum), gallbladder fossa, and porta hepatis may widen, and the anterior liver surface may withdraw from the anterior abdominal wall. Focal areas of surface retraction

may develop due to confluent fibrosis. Unless advanced, however, these global contour alterations are nonspecific and there is considerable overlap in the overall shape of the normal and diseased liver.

- Textural alterations consist of meshwork fibrotic reticulations surrounding regenerative nodules. Unlike the morphologic alterations, which may be identified with similar confidence at CT, MRI, and ultrasonography, visualization of textural alterations is technique dependent. These textural alterations tend to be invisible at CT unless disease is markedly advanced, in which case CT may depict nonspecific parenchymal heterogeneity.
- Direct CT visualization of fibrosis or regenerative nodules is relatively uncommon.
- Ultrasonography shows nonspecific coarsening of liver echotexture but, as with CT, rarely permits direct visualization of fibrosis or nodules.
- MRI, by comparison, may show fibrosis and regenerative nodules with exquisite detail, particularly if contrast-enhanced or double-contrast–enhanced techniques are used.

DIFFERENTIAL DIAGNOSIS

Because cirrhosis systemically impacts physiology and has effects on diverse organs, its diagnosis is rarely disputed. Its characteristic physical examination, laboratory findings, and imaging findings infrequently overlap with other conditions; therefore, there is usually no clinical differential diagnosis for cirrhosis. The main diagnostic challenge for the clinician is to determine the etiology of cirrhosis through careful history and laboratory testing. Elucidating the underlying cause is important because it may have implications for management and prognosis. For example, cirrhosis due to hepatitis B or C is more likely to be complicated by HCC than cirrhosis due to nonalcoholic fatty liver disease and, therefore, may warrant more aggressive cancer screening and treatment. Additionally, knowledge of the cause directs preventive measures, including the screening for high-risk behaviors in family members of patients with cirrhosis due to alcohol or hepatitis C and genetic testing in relatives of those diagnosed with an inherited storage disease.[41]

Unlike cirrhosis itself, its complications, namely, ascites, variceal hemorrhage, hepatic encephalopathy, and hepatorenal syndrome, may mimic nonhepatic causes. For example, cardiac and renal ascites, due to heart failure and nephrotic syndrome, respectively, need to be differentiated from hepatic ascites. Other less common confounders include pancreatitis, peritoneal carcinomatosis, peritoneal tuberculosis, portal vein thrombosis, and peritoneal infection. Evaluation of the serum-ascites albumin gradient via paracentesis may differentiate hepatic ascites from other causes.

Aggressive bleeding from esophageal varices may resemble hemorrhage from other sites in the upper gastrointestinal tract, especially peptic ulcers, erosive esophagitis, and Mallory-Weiss tear. Although a history may suggest the cause (e.g., nonsteroidal anti-inflammatory drug use as a cause of peptic ulcer disease), upper endoscopy clearly differentiates the plump, dilated varices at the esophagogastric junction from other causes of bleeding.

The differential diagnosis of hepatic encephalopathy includes metabolic, infectious, psychiatric, and neurologic abnormalities. Considerations should be made for electrolyte imbalances, hypoglycemia, hypercarbia, uremia, toxic encephalopathy due to alcohol ingestion, meningitis or encephalitis, organic brain syndrome, and intracranial masses or hemorrhage. These causes can be distinguished from hepatic encephalopathy on the basis of neuropsychiatric testing, basic laboratory tests, lumbar puncture, and brain imaging.

Hepatorenal syndrome is a challenging diagnosis because there are a number of common causes of renal failure in cirrhosis. These include sepsis, acute tubular necrosis, medication toxicity, contrast nephropathy, prerenal azotemia (due to overdiuresis or poor oral intake), and intrinsic glomerular diseases (e.g., membranoproliferative glomerulonephritis in patients with hepatitis C). These causes can be effectively excluded by examining the clinical scenario and testing the urinary sediment; renal ultrasonography and, occasionally, renal biopsy, may be necessary.

The radiologic differential diagnosis of cirrhosis is limited and includes diseases that mimic the fibrotic and nodular pattern of cirrhosis. Treated metastases may shrink and fibrose, simulating a nodular liver contour. Sarcoid lesions appear as hypoattenuating nodules (usually <2 cm) at CT and are hypointense on T2W MR images, resembling RNs and DNs.

The most common focal lesions in cirrhosis (RNs, DNs, HCCs, FNH-like lesions, perfusional pseudolesions, and confluent fibrosis) are differentiated by CT and MRI.

TREATMENT

Medical Treatment

Because cirrhosis is thought to be irreversible, its management focuses on the prevention and treatment of its complications, with the goal of liver transplantation in select patients. Recent advances, however, suggest that the halting of cirrhosis, or perhaps even its regression, is possible in some cases.[41]

In all patients with cirrhosis, alcohol cessation is stressed to prevent further liver injury. Patients are also vaccinated for hepatitis A and B, as well as for *Streptococcus pneumoniae* and influenza. Adequate nutrition and vitamin supplementation are emphasized. Some patients with well-compensated cirrhosis due to hepatitis B or C virus infection are candidates for antiviral therapy, which may slow the progression of cirrhosis and decrease the risk of development of HCC.[42]

The first-line therapy for ascites is dietary salt restriction, which decreases total-body fluid overload. Resistant cases are managed with diuretics, although aggressive diuresis is hindered by hypotension and renal insufficiency induced by hypovolemia. Periodic large-volume paracentesis is another strategy, with concomitant infusion of albumin to prevent massive fluid shifts. The treatment for spontaneous bacterial peritonitis includes antibiotics and albumin infusion. Once spontaneous bacterial peritonitis occurs, patients require antibiotic prophylaxis to prevent recurrence.

Patients who present with variceal hemorrhage require immediate stabilization with volume resuscitation via intravenous fluids, blood transfusion, reversal of coagulopathy, and intensive care unit monitoring. Administration of somatostatin analogs to lower splanchnic pressure and antibiotics to prevent spontaneous bacterial peritonitis are also mainstays of therapy.[43] Endoscopic management, via band ligation or sclerotherapy, is definitive treatment. Prophylaxis of variceal hemorrhage is attained by periodic surveillance with upper endoscopy and the use of nonselective β blockers, which decrease portal pressure and variceal size.[44]

Management of hepatic encephalopathy centers on the correction of precipitating factors. Adjunctive therapy includes administration of lactulose and nonabsorbable antibiotics to induce osmotic diarrhea, alter gut bacterial flora, and decrease bacteria-mediated conversion of proteins into ammonia.

Pharmacologic therapy of hepatorenal syndrome includes somatostatin or vasopressin analogs to induce splanchnic vasoconstriction and midodrine and albumin to enhance systemic vascular tone and renal perfusion. Dialysis does not improve the already poor prognosis of hepatorenal syndrome and is indicated only in those patients who are candidates for liver transplantation.

Surgical Treatment

Shunt placement is used as a bridge to liver transplantation in patients with adequate hepatic reserve and complications of portal hypertension that are refractory to medical or endoscopic therapy, most notably, varices and ascites. The most common shunts are TIPS, although patients with surgical mesocaval or portocaval shunts are still encountered. TIPS decreases the portosystemic gradient by providing ancillary venous outflow that bypasses the increasing intrahepatic sinusoidal pressure; it is preferred to surgical shunting at most centers because it avoids laparotomy, does not require general anesthesia, has fewer serious complications, and rarely results in procedure-related death. It decompresses the portal circulation in 90% of cases, has a greater than 70% success rate in producing hemostasis in active or recurrent variceal hemorrhage, and resolves ascites 75% of the time.[45,46] Drawbacks include limited long-term TIPS patency and the need for frequent endovascular re-intervention.[46]

Cadaveric or living-donor liver transplantation is the only "cure" for cirrhosis and its complications. In the 1990s, approximately 4500 liver transplants were performed in the United States.[24] Adult recipients are prioritized according to the MELD scoring system and are committed to lifelong immunosuppression.

What the Referring Physician Needs to Know

■ Cirrhosis is the final common clinical and histologic pathway of various chronic conditions affecting the liver, characterized by the replacement of normal hepatic architecture with fibrosis and regenerative nodules and manifested as portal hypertension and liver failure.

■ In the United States, the most common causes of cirrhosis are hepatitis C and alcoholic liver disease, whereas hepatitis B predominates in Asia and sub-Saharan Africa.

■ The main clinical manifestations of cirrhosis are the complications of portal hypertension, including ascites (with or without spontaneous bacterial peritonitis), esophageal varices (with or without hemorrhage), hepatic encephalopathy, and hepatorenal syndrome.

■ In the majority of patients, the diagnosis of cirrhosis is based on history, physical examination, basic laboratory studies, and imaging studies; liver biopsy is generally not required and may in fact be ill advised in these clinically tenuous patients.

■ Cirrhosis is thought to be irreversible; management focuses on treating its various complications, screening for HCC, and evaluating appropriate patients for liver transplantation.

KEY POINTS

■ Classic vascular manifestations of cirrhosis include hepatic artery dilatation, intrahepatic artery tortuosity ("corkscrew" vessels), portal vein dilation in early portal hypertension, portal vein occlusion in late portal hypertension due to sluggish portal flow, and formation of shunts.

■ Because of third spacing of fluid and leakage of contrast material, patients with cirrhosis sometimes require higher rates and concentrations of contrast material than patients without cirrhosis.

■ Confluent fibrosis occasionally may be mass-like and confused for HCC on CT or MRI, but differentiation is usually possible based on its characteristic morphology, associated capsular retraction and volume loss, and progressive enhancement pattern.

■ The administration of superparamagnetic iron oxides in MRI allows for the assessment of a second biologic property of the liver (in addition to the vascularity demonstrated by gadolinium or iodinated contrast with CT), providing complementary information to characterize hepatic masses.

■ Ultrasound imaging of steatosis or fibrosis may result in increased echogenicity and poor visualization of coursing liver vessels; this is a common pitfall for radiologists because it results in frequent misdiagnosis of cirrhosis as simple steatosis.

■ The American Association for the Study of Liver Diseases recommends ultrasonographic screening every 6 to 12 months, but ultrasonography has low sensitivity and may fail to detect HCC until advanced stages when it is no longer curable. Therefore, many centers use CT for initial screening, with contrast-enhanced MRI reserved for further characterization of known lesions.

SUGGESTED READINGS

Bruix J, Sherman M. Management of hepatocellular carcinoma. Hepatology 2005; 42:1208-1236.

Federle M. Liver anatomy and imaging issues. In Federle M, Jeffrey RB, Anne VS (eds). Diagnostic Imaging: Abdomen. Salt Lake City, Amirsys, 2004, pp 2-43.

Gandhi SN, Brown MA, Wong JG, et al. MR contrast agents for liver imaging: what, when, how. RadioGraphics 2006; 26:1621-1636.

Grose RD, Hayes PC. Review article: the pathophysiology and pharmacological treatment of portal hypertension. Aliment Pharmacol Ther 1992; 6:521-540.

Hanna RF, Aguirre DA, Kased N, et al. Cirrhosis-associated hepatocellular nodules: correlation of histopathologic and MR imaging features. RadioGraphics 2008; 28:747-769.

Schuppan D, Afdhal NH. Liver cirrhosis. Lancet 2008; 371:838-851.

Tsai MH. Splanchnic and systemic vasodilatation: the patient. J Clin Gastroenterol 2007; 41(Suppl 3):S266-S271.

REFERENCES

1. Clark JM, Diehl AM. Nonalcoholic fatty liver disease: an underrecognized cause of cryptogenic cirrhosis. JAMA 2003; 289:3000-3004.
2. Morreira RK. Hepatic stellate cells and liver fibrosis. Arch Pathol Lab Med 2007; 131:1728-1734.
3. Blei AT, Mazhar S, Davidson CJ, et al. Hemodynamic evaluation before liver transplantation: insights into the portal hypertensive syndrome. J Clin Gastroenterol 2007; 41(10 Suppl 3):S323-S329.
4. Such J, Runyon BA. Spontaneous bacterial peritonitis. Clin Infect Dis 1998; 27:669-674.
5. US Department of Health and Human Services. National Center for Health Statistics. Series 13. Hyattsville, MD, Centers for Disease Control and Prevention, 2005.
6. Anderson RN, Smith BL. Deaths: leading causes for 2001. Natl Vital Stat Rep 2003; 52:1-85.
7. Sandler RS, Everhart JE, Donowitz M, et al. The burden of digestive diseases in the United States. Gastroenterology 2002; 122:1500-1511.
8. Li CP, Lee FY, Hwang SJ, et al. Spider angiomas in patients with liver cirrhosis: role of alcoholism and impaired liver function. Scand J Gastroenterol 1999; 34:520-523.
9. Reynolds TB, Redeker AG, Geller HM. Wedged hepatic vein pressure: a clinical evaluation. Am J Med 1957; 22:341-350.
10. Gines P, Quintero E, Arroyo V, et al. Compensated cirrhosis: natural history and prognostic factors. Hepatology 1987; 7:122-128.
11. Riggio O, Masini A, Efrate C, et al. Pharmacological prophylaxis of hepatic encephalopathy after transjugular intrahepatic portosystemic shunt: a randomized controlled study. J Hepatol 2005; 42:674-679.
12. Gines A, Escorsell A, Gines P, et al. Incidence, predictive factors, and prognosis of the hepatorenal syndrome in cirrhosis with ascites. Gastroenterology 1993; 105:229-236.
13. Turban S, Thuluvath PJ, Atta MG. Hepatorenal syndrome. World J Gastroenterol 2007; 13:4046-4055.
14. Marti-Llahi M, Guevera M, Gines P. Hyponatremia in cirrhosis: clinical features and management. Gastroenterol Clin Biol 2006; 30:1144-1151.
15. Kamath PS, Wiesner RH, Malinchoc M, et al. A model to predict survival in patients with end-stage liver disease. Hepatology 2001; 33:464-470.
16. Gines P, Quintero E, Arroyo V, et al. Compensated cirrhosis: natural history and prognostic factors. Hepatology 1987; 7:122-128.
17. Sorensen HT, Thulstrup AM, Mellemkjar L, et al. Long-term survival and cause-specific mortality in patients with cirrhosis of the liver: a nationwide cohort study in Denmark. J Clin Epidemiol 2003; 56:88-93.
18. Montalto G, Cervello M, Giannitrapani L, et al. Epidemiology, risk factors, and natural history of hepatocellular carcinoma. Ann NY Acad Sci 2002; 963:13-20.
19. Crawford JM. Basic mechanisms in hepatopathology. In Burt AD, Portmann BC, Ferrell LD (eds). MacSween's Pathology of the Liver, 5th ed. New York: Churchill Livingstone, 2006, p 108.
20. Goodman ZD, Terraciano LM. Tumours and tumour-like lesions in the liver. In Burt AD, Portmann BC, Ferrell LD (eds). MacSween's Pathology of the Liver, 5th ed. New York, Churchill Livingstone, 2006, p 767.
21. Lee YH, Kim SH, Cho MY, et al. Focal nodular hyperplasia-like nodules in alcoholic liver cirrhosis: radiologic-pathologic correlation. AJR Am J Roentgenol 2007; 188:W459-W463.
22. Terminology of nodular hepatocellular lesions. International Working Party. Hepatology 1995; 22:983-993.
23. United Network for Organ Sharing. Policy 3.6 Organ Distribution: Allocation of Livers. Revised December 14, 2006. Available at: http://www.optn.org/policiesAndBylaws/policies.asp. Accessed September 18, 2007.
24. Baron RL, Campbell WL, Dodd GD 3rd. Peribiliary cysts associated with severe liver disease: imaging-pathologic correlation. AJR Am J Roentgenol 1994; 162:631-636.
25. Federle M. Liver anatomy and imaging issues. In Federle M, Jeffrey RB, Anne VS (eds). Diagnostic Imaging: Abdomen. Salt Lake City, Amirsys, 2004, pp 2-43.
26. Seguchi T, Akiyama Y, Itoh H, et al. Multiple hepatic peribiliary cysts with cirrhosis. J Gastroenterol 2004; 39:384-390.
27. Gore RM. Radionuclide imaging of the liver and spleen. In Spies WG (ed). Textbook of Gastrointestinal Radiology, 2nd ed. Philadelphia, WB Saunders, 2000, pp 1442-1464.
28. Ohtomo K, Baron RL, Dodd GD 3rd, et al. Confluent hepatic fibrosis in advanced cirrhosis: appearance at CT. Radiology 1993; 188:31-35.
29. Libbrecht L, Cassiman D, Verslype C, et al. Clinicopathological features of focal nodular hyperplasia-like nodules in 130 cirrhotic explant livers. Am J Gastroenterol 2006; 101:2341-2346.
30. Hanna RF, Kased N, Kwan SW, et al. Double-contrast MRI for accurate staging of hepatocellular carcinoma in patients with cirrhosis. AJR Am J Roentgenol 2008; 190:47-57.
31. Shiehmorteza M, Hanna RF, Middleton MS. Can gadopentetate dimeglumine be safely administered more rapidly than the FDA-approved injection rate for liver imaging? AJR Am J Roentgenol 2007; 189:W231.
32. Mazhar SM, Shiehmorteza M, Kohl CA, et al. Is chronic liver disease an independent risk factor for nephrogenic systemic fibrosis? A comprehensive literature review. Preented before the annual meeting of the International Society of Magnetic Resonance in Medicine, Toronto, Canada, 2008, p 297.
33. Gandhi SN, Brown MA, Wong JG, et al. MR contrast agents for liver imaging: what, when, how. RadioGraphics 2006; 26:1621-1636.
34. Lutz AM, Willmann JK, Goepfert K, et al. Hepatocellular carcinoma in cirrhosis: enhancement patterns at dynamic gadolinium- and superparamagnetic iron oxide–enhanced T1-weighted MR imaging. Radiology 2005; 237:520-528.
35. Vogl TJ, Stupavsky A, Pegios W, et al. Hepatocellular carcinoma: evaluation with dynamic and static gadobenate dimeglumine-enhanced MR imaging and histopathologic correlation. Radiology 1997; 205:721-728.
36. Qayyum A, Thoeni RF, Coakley FV, et al. Detection of hepatocellular carcinoma by ferumoxides-enhanced MR imaging in cirrhosis: incremental value of dynamic gadolinium-enhancement. J Magn Reson Imaging 2006; 23:17-22.
37. Hanna RF, Aguirre DA, Kased N, et al. Cirrhosis-associated hepatocellular nodules: correlation of histopathologic and MR imaging features. RadioGraphics 2008; 28:747-769.
38. Hussain SM, Zondervan PE, Ijzermans JN, et al. Benign versus malignant hepatic nodules: MR imaging findings with pathologic correlation. RadioGraphics 2002; 22:1023-1036; discussion 37-39.
39. Zhang J, Krinsky GA. Iron-containing nodules of cirrhosis. NMR Biomed 2004; 17:459-464.
40. Bruix J, Sherman M. Management of hepatocellular carcinoma. Hepatology 2005; 42:1208-1236.
41. Schuppan D, Afdhal NH. Liver cirrhosis. Lancet 2008; 371: 838-851.
42. Yoshida H, Shiratori Y, Moriyama M, et al. Interferon therapy reduces the risk for hepatocellular carcinoma: national surveillance program of cirrhotic and noncirrhotic patients with chronic hepatitis C in Japan. Ann Intern Med 1999; 131:174-181.
43. Sharara AI, Rockey DC. Gastroesophageal variceal hemorrhage. N Engl J Med 2001; 345:669-681.
44. Garcia-Tsao G. Preventing the development of varices in cirrhosis. J Clin Gastroenterol 2007; 41(10 Suppl 3):S300-S304.
45. Ochs A, Rossle M, Haag K, et al. The transjugular intrahepatic portosystemic stent-shunt procedure for refractory ascites. N Engl J Med 1995; 332:1192-1197.
46. Colombato L. The role of transjugular intrahepatic portosystemic shunt (TIPS) in the management of portal hypertension. J Clin Gastroenterol 2007; 41:S344-S351.

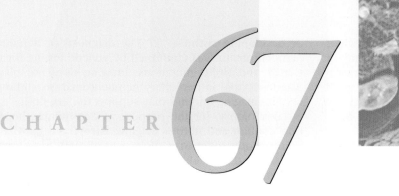
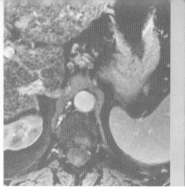
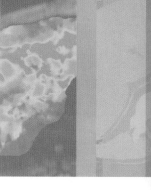

Hepatic Iron Overload

Heather M. Patton, Sameer M. Mazhar, Michael R. Peterson, Robert Hanna,
Karthik Ganesan, and Claude B. Sirlin

ETIOLOGY

Hepatic iron overload is a generic term that refers to the nonphysiologic accumulation of iron within the hepatic parenchyma. The most clinically significant cause of hepatic iron overload is *hereditary hemochromatosis.* Hereditary hemochromatosis is associated with several mutations in genes regulating iron metabolism, the most common of which are in the *HFE* gene. The *HFE* mutations result in dysregulated iron absorption, which may lead to total-body iron overload and accumulation of excess iron in tissue (hemosiderosis), including the liver, heart, and various endocrine organs. The iron accumulation causes tissue damage and, if untreated, may lead to cirrhosis and hepatocellular carcinoma, along with assorted cardiac and endocrine disturbances.

Secondary (acquired) causes of hepatic iron overload include the iron-loading anemias (thalassemia major, sideroblastic anemia, chronic hemolytic anemia, and spur cell anemia), long-term hemodialysis, and dietary iron overload. These usually do not lead to significant liver dysfunction, although they may cause dysfunction in other organs such as the heart. Chronic liver diseases (hepatitis B and C virus infection, alcohol-induced liver disease, nonalcoholic fatty liver disease, and porphyria cutanea tarda) also may be associated with hepatic iron overload, but the clinical picture is dominated by the primary hepatic abnormality and the excess liver iron is of secondary importance.

The average adult stores 1 to 3 g of iron, mainly within the liver and in red blood cells as hemoglobin. In normal persons, about 10% of dietary iron (1 mg/day) is absorbed daily.[1] A similar amount of iron is lost via sloughing of cells from the skin and mucosal surfaces.[2,3] In premenopausal women, menstruation increases the amount of iron loss to about 2 mg/day.[2] Ultimately, however, the body lacks a proficient iron excretion mechanism and pathologic excesses in iron overload are therefore unchecked and progressive. Systemic iron levels are kept within a narrow

homeostatic range due to a complex regulatory mechanism monitoring the absorption of iron via the gastrointestinal tract and its accumulation in the body.[3]

Iron overload in hereditary hemochromatosis occurs when iron absorption via the digestive tract exceeds iron utilization and excretion. The most common cause of hereditary hemochromatosis is a mutation in the *HFE* gene located on chromosome 6 that regulates iron homeostasis.[4-7] It can also result from genetic anomalies corresponding to other genes involved in iron metabolism.[8,9]

Regardless of the underlying genetic abnormality, when iron absorption exceeds the transport capacity of transferrin, excess iron is deposited within parenchymal cells of various tissues, including the liver, heart, and endocrine organs. *Hemosiderosis* refers to this excess parenchymal iron and may cause tissue damage by catalyzing the production of radical oxygen species from hydrogen peroxide. These radical oxygen species attack cell membranes, cellular proteins, and DNA.[10] The pathophysiologic sequelae depend on the organs and tissues involved.

Hepatic dysfunction from secondary hemosiderosis due to these entities is rare, although clinically significant iron deposition in other organs (e.g., the heart) may occur. Chronic liver diseases (hepatitis B and C virus infection, alcohol-induced liver disease, nonalcoholic fatty liver disease, and porphyria cutanea tarda) are sometimes associated with hepatic iron overload; this has been attributed to diminished functional hepatocyte mass and reduced hepcidin production.[11-13] In these diseases, the primary liver condition is the paramount abnormality and the secondary iron overload is of relatively minor clinical relevance.

PREVALENCE AND EPIDEMIOLOGY

Hereditary hemochromatosis is the most common genetic disease in populations of Northern European ancestry. Homozygosity of the C282Y mutation has a prevalence of

1 per 200 persons (0.5%), 10 times higher than that of cystic fibrosis.[6-7,14,15] In the United States, about 1 million people carry the diagnosis of hereditary hemochromatosis; it is estimated that an additional 1.5 million have undiagnosed hereditary hemochromatosis and approximately 5% of individuals with hereditary hemochromatosis have cirrhosis.[16-19]

The development of hereditary hemochromatosis is impacted by ethnicity, race, sex, and age. Hereditary hemochromatosis is typically a disease of Northern European ancestry, with persons of Irish descent at greatest risk. In the United States, C282Y heterozygosity was demonstrated in 9.5% of non-Hispanic whites, 2.3% of blacks, and 2.8% of Hispanics.[15] Because of the countereffects of menstruation on iron accumulation, females are three times less likely to develop hereditary hemochromatosis than males and are two to three times less likely to progress to serious complications (e.g., cirrhosis, diabetes, heart failure). Hereditary hemochromatosis typically manifests in patients older than 40 years of age, and it appears later in women than men.

CLINICAL PRESENTATION

The clinical manifestations of hereditary hemochromatosis range from isolated biochemical abnormalities to multisystem disease involving the liver, heart, endocrine organs (e.g., pancreas and pituitary gland), joints, and skin. Most patients are asymptomatic at the time of diagnosis, which is discovered as a result of screening serum iron studies in individuals with elevated liver function tests or testing of family members of an affected proband.[20] In early disease, symptoms are nonspecific and include weakness, lethargy, and fatigue. Symptoms related to iron deposition within specific organs occur later. Involvement of the liver may be associated with hepatomegaly and right upper quadrant abdominal pain. If the disease progresses to cirrhosis, patients may develop portal hypertension or hepatocellular carcinoma. Other manifestations of hereditary hemochromatosis include arthropathy due to iron deposition in the joints (classically involving the second and third metacarpophalangeal joints and proximal interphalangeal joints); diabetes mellitus due to pancreatic iron deposition; loss of libido, impotence, and amenorrhea due to pituitary involvement; and dilated cardiomyopathy, congestive heart failure, conduction abnormalities, and arrhythmias due to iron deposition in the heart.[4,21] The characteristic darkening of the skin, termed *bronze diabetes,* is caused by increased levels of melanin and is an infrequent manifestation in late disease.[21]

Patients with hepatic involvement demonstrate mild, nonspecific elevations in serum levels of aminotransferases (<200 mg/dL) and bilirubin (<4.0 mg/dL). When hereditary hemochromatosis is suspected, however, serum iron studies hone the diagnosis. In mild disease, the excess iron is mainly in the plasma compartment and is shown by elevated serum iron levels and transferrin saturation and diminished transferrin. In advanced disease, iron is stored within parenchymal cells, shown by an elevated serum ferritin level. If serum ferritin and aspartate aminotransferase (AST) levels both are elevated and platelet counts are low, patients are at high risk for having

or developing cirrhosis.[22,23] The diagnosis of hereditary hemochromatosis is confirmed by genetic testing for the C282Y and H63D mutations. Imaging does not play a diagnostic role in hereditary hemochromatosis, although certain imaging findings may support the diagnosis.

Liver biopsy, for the purpose of determining hepatic iron content and fibrosis staging, is reserved for C282Y homozygotes older than the age of 40 with high ferritin (>1000 mg/L) and elevated serum AST levels. In individuals with results of serum iron studies that are of concern and who are not homozygous for the C282Y mutation, consideration should be given to other causes of liver disease; a liver biopsy in these patients may uncover other causes and determine hepatic iron content, which could guide the decision as to whether to pursue therapeutic phlebotomy.

The natural history of hereditary hemochromatosis varies according to type, and disease progression is accelerated with excess alcohol consumption, overweight and obesity, and viral hepatitis.[24-28] Primary liver cancer is an important complication of advanced hereditary hemochromatosis and is almost exclusively observed in patients with underlying cirrhosis. Importantly, the risk for malignancy persists after therapeutic phlebotomy, so appropriate screening should continue after this intervention. Large population-based studies analyzing the risk of malignancy are lacking, but it is clear that hepatocellular carcinoma is the most common primary liver malignancy in patients with hereditary hemochromatosis, followed by combined hepatocellular carcinoma and cholangiocarcinoma, and cholangiocarcinoma alone.[29]

PATHOLOGY

Iron deposition within the liver varies in distribution according to the cause. Generally, the iron distribution in hereditary hemochromatosis is predominantly within hepatocytes, whereas in most cases of secondary iron overload the iron is situated mainly within the reticuloendothelial system (e.g., Kupffer cells). However, in advanced stages of either of these groups of diseases, stainable iron may be found in both cell types. In microscopic sections, iron is demonstrated via a Perls stain (using acid ferrocyanide), which produces a Prussian blue reaction with ferritin and hemosiderin.

In hereditary hemochromatosis, stainable iron first appears as golden-yellow hemosiderin granules in the cytoplasm of periportal hepatocytes. With disease advancement, the iron deposition progresses in a portal to centrilobular fashion, eventually involving the entire lobule diffusely. When well-developed there is a distinctive pericanalicular "chicken wire" distribution to the stainable iron, a result of accumulation of iron within subapical hepatocyte lysosomes.[30] Although the majority of iron is found within hepatocytes, Kupffer cells and biliary epithelium may contain iron later in the disease course.

Because iron is a direct hepatotoxin, inflammation is characteristically absent; therefore, the identification of significant inflammation should prompt consideration of coexistent causes of chronic liver disease. As iron accumulates, fibrosis slowly develops in a periportal distribution. Eventually, portal-portal bridging fibrosis and cirrhosis ensue, resulting in a diffuse micronodular pattern. With phlebotomy there is steady disappearance of stainable iron in a pattern that is the reverse of its accumulation, from centrilobular areas to portal tracts. Although iron deposition is typically diffuse in cirrhosis secondary to hereditary hemochromatosis, small regions spared by iron deposition have been theorized to represent preneoplastic lesions.[31]

IMAGING

As stated earlier, imaging does not play a role in the diagnosis of hereditary hemochromatosis. Nevertheless, imaging modalities may be used to monitor patients with established hereditary hemochromatosis, and patients with the disorder may undergo imaging studies for unrelated reasons. Patients with advanced disease may progress to cirrhosis (Fig. 67-1), portal hypertension, and hepatocellular carcinoma; findings relevant to these complications are discussed in other chapters. In recent years, interest has grown in developing noninvasive methods to quantify hepatic iron, and a brief description is given of some of the proposed techniques.

Radiography

Radiographs play no role in the routine assessment of the liver in hereditary hemochromatosis but may be used to identify the characteristic arthropathy associated with the disorder. Findings in the hands of patients with hereditary hemochromatosis may include squared-off bone ends and hook-like osteophytes, joint space narrowing, sclerosis, and cyst formation.[32]

CT

Unenhanced CT

The normal liver parenchyma has an attenuation of 45 to 65 HU on unenhanced, standard (single-energy) CT. In hepatic hemosiderosis due to hereditary hemochromatosis or other causes, unenhanced CT reveals elevated hepatic attenuation due to the greater electron density associated with iron atoms compared with normal liver.

The characteristic CT finding is a "white liver" with a diffuse increase in liver density above 70 HU. In general, unenhanced CT accurately detects hepatic iron in advanced disease but is unable to do so for early or mild hepatic iron overload. Unenhanced CT has almost 100% sensitivity in detecting hepatic iron overload more than 5-fold above the upper limit of normal but only 60% sensitivity for detection of hepatic iron concentration 2.5-fold above the upper limit of normal. Increased hepatic attenuation is not specific for iron accumulation and may also be seen in storage disorders, sarcoidosis, Wilson's disease, and drug-induced (amiodarone, methotrexate, and gold) hepatotoxicity.

Contrast-Enhanced CT

Contrast-enhanced CT is not relevant for the detection and monitoring of hepatic iron overload but may be performed for surveillance of hepatocellular carcinoma in patients who have progressed to cirrhosis.

Extrahepatic Findings

Patients with hereditary hemochromatosis may develop iron overload in the pancreas and myocardium. However, these tissues typically have normal attenuation at unenhanced CT and CT has limited sensitivity for detection of extrahepatic manifestations of hereditary hemochromatosis.

CT Quantification of Hepatic Iron Overload

Although iron overload is associated with increased hepatic attenuation, the correlation between CT attenuation and hepatic iron concentration is poor and CT does not permit reliable gradation of hepatic iron overload or accurate quantification of hepatic iron content.[33]

MRI

Unenhanced MRI

Because of susceptibility effects, iron accumulation in tissue leads to T2 and T2* shortening, causing signal loss

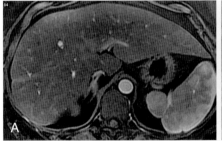 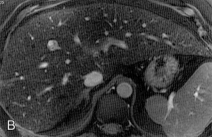 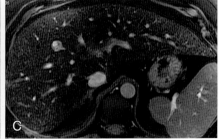

■ **FIGURE 67-1** Cirrhosis secondary to hemochromatosis. **A,** Axial 3D T1W gradient-echo MR image (TE = 1.6 ms) acquired during the late hepatic arterial phase after intravenous gadolinium administration shows heterogeneous parenchyma with scattered regenerative nodules and a focal scar indenting the right lateral surface of the liver. **B** and **C,** Axial 2D intermediate-weighted gradient-echo MR images with echo times of 4 ms (**B**) and 8 ms (**C**) acquired several minutes after gadolinium administration show considerable signal loss with an increase in echo time. The signal loss is due to T2* shortening from endogenous iron accumulation. In standard doses, gadolinium administration does not meaningfully shorten the T2* of the liver. Note that, consistent with mild cirrhosis, there are fibrotic reticulations throughout the liver; these are most pronounced in the left lateral segment.

on T2-weighted (T2W) and T2*-weighted (T2*W) images. Gradient echoes are more sensitive to susceptibility effects than spin echoes, and the signal loss is more pronounced on gradient-echo images. Thus, the affected liver appears relatively hypointense on T2*W images and, to a lesser extent, T2W images (Figs. 67-2 and 67-3). Mild cases of iron overload may be apparent only on gradient-echo imaging. If iron overload is severe, the degree of signal loss may be marked on both types of images. Although iron primarily shortens the T2 and T2* of the liver, it also shortens the T1, and the liver may have increased signal intensity on T1-weighted (T1W) sequences acquired with very short echo times.

In- and out-of-phase gradient-echo imaging typically is used to assess fat accumulation in tissue, but the images can also be used to detect iron (Fig. 67-4): loss of signal

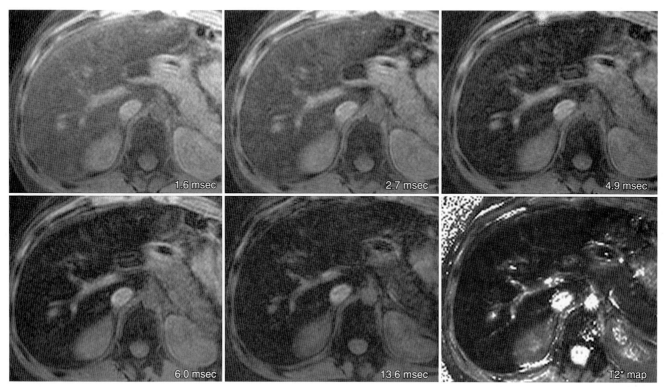

■ **FIGURE 67-2** A T2* map was generated by acquiring 12 co-localized fat-saturated spoiled gradient-recalled-echo MR images. Echo times ranged from 1.6 to 13.6 ms. Five representative images from the series of 12 are demonstrated for illustrative purposes with echo times as shown. The T2* value was calculated assuming monoexponential signal decay from the 12 echoes. The estimated T2* relaxation value, 9 ms, suggests moderate iron overload.

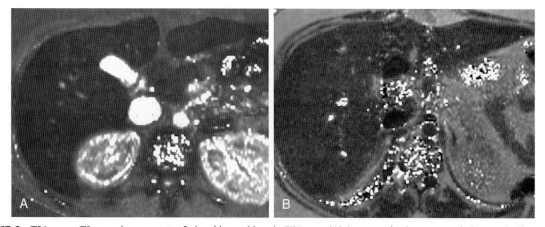

■ **FIGURE 67-3** T2* versus T2 maps in severe transfusional hemosiderosis. T2* map (**A**) (generated using same technique as in Figure 67-2 and T2 map (**B**) (generated in analogous fashion to T2* map but with 9 spin-echo images from 10 to 90 ms) in a patient with severe transfusional hemosiderosis. The estimated T2* value in A is 4.5 ms, markedly less than a normal 25- to 30-ms T2* value typically obtained with this particular imaging sequence and MR scanner. The estimated T2 value, 45 ms, is only slightly lower than the normal 50- to 60-ms T2 measured on this scanner. As shown in this example, a given amount of iron deposition causes greater T2* shortening than T2 shortening.

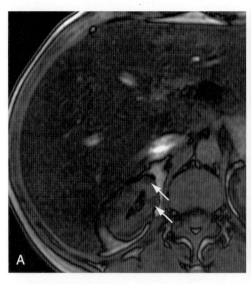 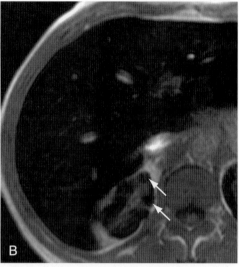

■ FIGURE 67-4 Use of out-of-phase and in-phase imaging for detecting iron overload. Axial spoiled gradient-recalled-echo MR images through the liver at echo times of 2.3 ms (out-of-phase) (**A**) and 4.6 ms (in-phase) (**B**) show marked signal loss of the liver on the later echo, suggesting iron overload. The hepatic findings are consistent with hemochromatosis or secondary hemosiderosis. However, marked signal loss between echoes in the renal cortex (*arrows*) indicates renal parenchymal iron deposition. The involvement of the kidney favors secondary hemosiderosis.

on the second echo (later echo time) compared with the first echo (earlier echo time) indicates short T2* relaxation and suggests the presence of parenchymal iron. Concomitant liver steatosis may confound the interpretation, however, because fat-water phase interference will alter the relative signal intensities of the in-phase and out-of-phase images.[34] To avoid this pitfall, dual-echo images can be acquired at in-phase echo times or after application of chemical fat saturation. Alternatively, multiple gradient echoes can be obtained and the effects of fat-water phase interference and T2* relaxation modeled simultaneously.

Contrast-Enhanced MRI

The administration of gadolinium does not provide additional information regarding hepatic iron accumulation per se but may be necessary to evaluate focal lesions in the liver with iron overload. In general, the infusion of superparamagnetic iron oxides (SPIOs) should be avoided in patients with known hepatic iron overload, mainly because the particles further reduce T2* and may diminish liver signal-to-noise ratio to a subdiagnostic range. In principle, giving SPIOs also may exacerbate the hepatic iron overload.[35]

MR Features of Extrahepatic Iron Overload

T2W and T2*W images may show hypointensity in the pancreas and, if acquired with cardiac gating, the myocardium.

MR Quantification of Hepatic Iron Overload

Two MRI techniques are commonly used for grading the degree of hepatic iron deposition: (1) calculation of T2 or T2* relaxation time constants using multiple echo times and (2) calculation of the signal intensity ratio between the liver and an internal reference tissue known to be unaffected by iron accumulation (e.g., paravertebral muscles).[33] In subjects with high levels of secondary iron overload, relaxation time constants have correlated closely with hepatic iron concentration determined by liver

biopsy (Fig. 67-5). If gradient echoes are used for T2* measurements, it is important to reduce possible phase-interference effects from concomitant fat accumulation by acquiring echoes only at in-phase echo times or obtaining images with frequency selective fat saturation (or water excitation).

A reduced liver to paraspinal signal intensity ratio has been shown to have high sensitivity and specificity for moderate degrees of iron accumulation. The exact ratio used for diagnostic classification depends on the imaging parameters of the sequence.[33]

Ultrasonography

Iron particles are too small to scatter ultrasound waves, and, therefore, ultrasonography does not detect iron overload in tissue (Fig. 67-6). However, although ultrasonography cannot monitor hepatic iron deposition in the liver, it may be the initial imaging modality used in the evaluation for cirrhosis and portal hypertension.

Nuclear Medicine

Liver scintigraphy is of limited clinical use. Uptake of sulfur colloid by the siderotic liver may be reduced due to Kupffer cell damage incurred from iron overload. The colloid scan may be abnormal, but the alteration tends to be mild and may be difficult to appreciate. Iron quantification is not possible.

Imaging Algorithm

Imaging may be used to monitor parenchymal iron in patients with established hereditary hemochromatosis. For this purpose, we rely on T2* relaxometry using MRI, although other centers may prefer T2 relaxometry (Table 67-1). If relaxometry is unavailable, liver-to-muscle signal intensity ratio measurements may suffice. Unenhanced CT is inaccurate for grading iron deposition, exposes the patient to ionizing radiation, and is not recommended. Ultrasonography cannot detect parenchymal iron and plays no routine role.

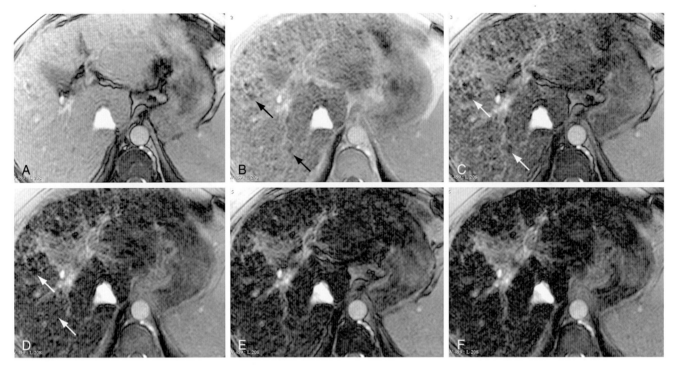

■ **FIGURE 67-5** Acquired hemosiderosis due to cirrhosis in patient with chronic viral hepatitis. Co-localized spoiled gradient-recalled echo MR images acquired at echo times of 2.3 (**A**), 4.6 (**B**), 6.9 (**C**), 9.2 (**D**), 11.5 (**E**), and 13.5 (**F**) ms. The liver parenchyma progressively loses signal as echo time increases, consistent with short T2* relaxation. Note several siderotic nodules on intermediate echoes, at 4.6 to 9.2 ms, which are visibly more hypointense (*arrows*) than the rest of the liver parenchyma. These siderotic nodules have higher concentrations of iron than the rest of the liver. Despite the reduced T2* of the liver, the spleen (*right corner of images*) has normal T2* and does not lose signal, indicating that the spleen is not iron overloaded.

Classic Signs

- The classic imaging features of hepatic iron overload are a diffuse increase in parenchymal attenuation on unenhanced CT images and hypointensity on unenhanced T2W and T2*W MR images.
- T2*W images are more sensitive to mild-to-moderate iron overload than T2W images.

DIFFERENTIAL DIAGNOSIS

The clinical differential diagnosis of hereditary hemochromatosis attempts to distinguish between primary (genetic) and secondary (acquired) causes of iron overload. C282Y/C282Y homozygosity and C282Y/H63D compound heterozygosity, the most common *HFE* mutations, are easily diagnosed via genetic testing. Although genetic testing is not readily available for the non–*HFE*-related mutations, these conditions have characteristic clinical findings. Juvenile hemochromatosis, due to mutations in either *HAMP* or *HFE2,* manifests at a younger age (typically in the teen years) than other non-*HFE* mutations and primarily exhibits cardiac and endocrine abnormalities.[3,7] Abnormalities in ferroportin due to mutations in *SLC40A1* can be diagnosed by pedigree analysis, because this iron overload disorder uniquely is inherited in autosomal dominant fashion.

Secondary causes of hepatic iron overload are ruled out if genetic testing suggests a primary cause. History and review of laboratory tests identify those with transfusional iron overload and iron-loading anemias. In addition, most secondary causes of hepatic iron overload histologically are characterized by iron deposition within Kupffer cells rather than hepatocytes. Histology may also provide evidence for a particular underlying disease (e.g., viral hepatitis and alcoholic and nonalcoholic fatty liver disease).

In patients with hyperattenuation of the liver at CT, the main radiologic differential diagnosis includes hereditary hemochromatosis, secondary hemosiderosis, glycogen storage diseases, and amiodarone therapy. In hereditary hemochromatosis, iron overload is restricted to the liver early in the course of disease with subsequent involvement of the pancreas and myocardium. The reticuloendothelial organs (spleen, marrow, and lymph nodes) are relatively spared. By comparison, secondary hemosiderosis leads to uniform iron deposition in the reticuloendothelial system and also may involve the renal cortex. Patients with hepatic hyperattenuation due to glycogen storage disease may present with massive hepatomegaly as well as multiple hepatic adenomas. In liver disease due to amiodarone therapy, the hyperattenuation of the liver is diffuse and homogeneous on unenhanced CT.

In patients with T2 or T2* shortening of the liver on MRI, the differential diagnosis is limited to hereditary hemochromatosis and secondary hemosiderosis, because neither glycogen storage disease nor amiodarone therapy leads to T2 or T2* shortening. Differentiation of hereditary hemochromatosis from secondary hemosiderosis at MRI is based on the distribution and severity of extrahepatic organ involvement as described for CT.

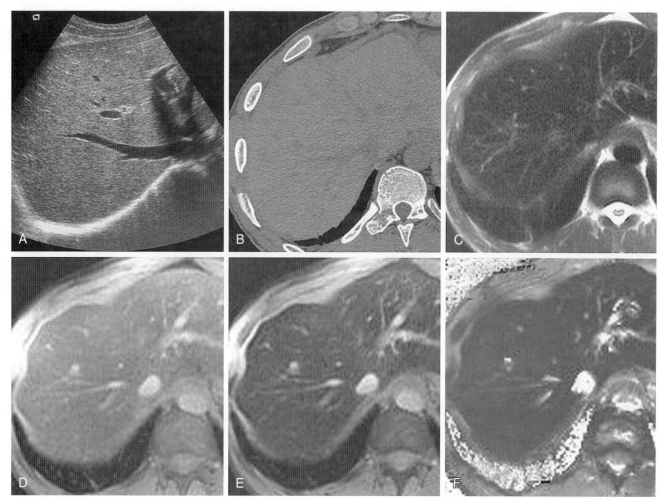

■ **FIGURE 67-6** Varying sensitivity of imaging techniques in patient with moderate to severe transfusional iron overload. **A,** Ultrasound image is normal. **B,** Unenhanced CT is borderline abnormal with CT attenuation of 75 HU. **C,** On axial single-shot fast spin-echo MR image the liver is slightly more hypointense than normal liver parenchyma. On axial gradient-recalled-echo MR images with echo times of (**D**) 1.6 ms and (**E**) 5.9 ms, the liver loses signal with increased echo times in keeping with iron deposition. As calculated in Figure 67-3, the T2* map (**F**) value measures 6 ms. This suggests moderate-to-severe iron overload. As shown in this example, ultrasound cannot detect iron deposition. CT has low sensitivity for moderate overload, and MRI has high sensitivity, particularly with gradient-echo imaging.

TABLE 67-1 Accuracy, Limitations, and Pitfalls of the Modalities Used in Imaging of Hepatic Iron Overload

Modality	Accuracy	Pitfalls	Limitations
CT	Unenhanced CT has high sensitivity for detecting moderate to severe iron overload but low sensitivity for mild iron overload. Using standard CT techniques, it does not accurately grade the degree of overload.	Contrast-enhanced CT increases the liver parenchyma attenuation and makes iron difficult to detect.	Exposes patient to ionizing radiation Insensitive to mild iron overload
MRI	T2*-weighted imaging and in- and out-of-phase imaging is useful for detecting the presence of iron. Multiple-echo T2 and T2* relaxometry and liver-to-muscle signal intensity ratios can also be used to grade the degree of iron overload.	If only in- and out-of-phase imaging is performed, the concomitant presence of fat may be a confounder for the detection of iron.	More costly than CT Accurate calculation of iron load using MRI requires standardized protocols T2 and T2* values obtained using one protocol may not be reproducible using other protocols.

TREATMENT

Medical Treatment

The primary treatment for patients with hereditary hemochromatosis is life-long therapeutic phlebotomy, which aims to remove excess iron and prevent tissue damage related to iron accumulation. Regression of liver fibrosis after therapy has been described.[36] Phlebotomy is initially performed weekly, with longer intervals between sessions once hemoglobin levels decrease or an acceptable serum ferritin and transferrin saturation is achieved.

Iron chelation agents, such as deferoxamine, are used with modest success in patients with secondary hemosiderosis. If successful, reduction in hepatic iron concentrations with chelation therapy significantly reduces the risk of clinical disease caused by iron overload in these patients.

Surgical Treatment

Surgical therapy for iron overload consists of liver transplantation for decompensated cirrhosis or resection of hepatocellular carcinoma. Post-transplantation survival is equivalent in patients who have undergone transplantation for hemochromatosis versus other causes of liver disease.

What the Referring Physician Needs to Know

- Genetic mutations causing hereditary hemochromatosis are prevalent, especially among persons of northern European descent, but phenotypic expression of the disease tends to be low.
- The majority of hereditary hemochromatosis is caused by the C282Y and H63D mutations in the HFE gene, with the large majority of cases seen in C282Y homozygotes.
- Iron overload is caused by excessive iron absorption by duodenal enterocytes.
- Iron overload is initially reflected by an increased transferrin saturation level and later by an increased ferritin level.
- Ferritin levels greater than 1000 mg/L indicate a greater risk for hepatic iron overload.
- Hepatic iron overload may progress to cirrhosis and increases the risk of hepatocellular carcinoma.
- The primary mode of therapy for iron overload is with phlebotomy to deplete iron stores, which may result in regression of hepatic fibrosis.

KEY POINTS

- On unenhanced CT, normal liver attenuation ranges from 45 to 65 HU.
- Iron overload can result in a homogeneously hyperattenuating liver (75 to 135 HU) because of the high electron density associated with iron atoms.
- Iron overload causes T2 and T2* shortening of the liver, which manifests as relative hypointensity on T2W and T2*W images.
- Gradient-echo sequences (T2* relaxation) are more sensitive to mild iron overload than spin-echo sequences (T2 relaxation).
- Steatosis may confound the interpretation of iron overload if only in- and out-of-phase imaging is performed.
- Ultrasound waves are not scattered by iron particles, and ultrasonography cannot detect parenchymal iron.

SUGGESTED READINGS

Adams PC. Review article: the modern diagnosis and management of haemochromatosis. Aliment Pharmacol Ther 2006; 23:1681-1691.

Andrews NC. Disorders of iron metabolism. N Engl J Med 1999; 341:1986-1995.

Bacon BR. Hemochromatosis: diagnosis and management. Gastroenterology 2001; 120:718-725.

Jensen PD. Evaluation of iron overload. Br J Haematol 2004; 124:697-711.

O'Neil J, Powell L. Clinical aspects of hemochromatosis. Semin Liver Dis 2005; 25:381-391.

Pietrangelo A. Hereditary hemochromatosis—a new look at an old disease. N Engl J Med 2004; 350:2383-2397.

Pietrangelo A. Hereditary hemochromatosis. Biochim Biophys Acta 2006; 1763:700-710.

Yen AW, Fancher TL, Bowlus CL. Revisiting hereditary hemochromatosis: current concepts and progress. Am J Med 2006; 119:391-399.

REFERENCES

1. Cook JD, Skikne BS, Lynch SR, Reusser ME. Estimates of iron insufficiency in the US population. Blood 1986; 68:726-731.
2. Bothwell TH, Charlton RW. A general approach to the problems of iron deficiency and iron overload in the population at large. Semin Hematol 1982; 19:54-67.
3. Pietrangelo A. Hereditary hemochromatosis—a new look at an old disease. N Engl J Med 2004; 350:2383-2397.
4. Bacon BR. Hemochromatosis: diagnosis and management. Gastroenterology 2001; 120:718-725.
5. Adams PC. Review article: the modern diagnosis and management of haemochromatosis. Aliment Pharmacol Ther 2006; 23:1681-1691.
6. Rochette J, Pointon JJ, Fisher CA, et al. Multicentric origin of hemochromatosis gene (*HFE*) mutations. Am J Hum Genet 1999; 64:1056-1062.
7. Pietrangelo A. Hereditary hemochromatosis. Biochim Biophys Acta 2006; 1763:700-710.
8. Papanikolaou G, Samuels ME, Ludwig EH, et al. Mutations in *HFE2* cause iron overload in chromosome 1q-linked juvenile hemochromatosis. Nat Genet 2004; 36:77-82.
9. Babitt JL, Huang FW, Wrighting DM, et al. Bone morphogenetic protein signaling by hemojuvelin regulates hepcidin expression. Nat Genet 2006; 38:531-539.
10. Andrews NC. Disorders of iron metabolism. N Engl J Med 1999; 341:1986-1995.
11. Bridle K, Cheung TK, Murphy T, et al. Hepcidin is down-regulated in alcoholic liver injury: implications for the pathogenesis of alcoholic liver disease. Alcohol Clin Exp Res 2006; 30:106-112.
12. Harrison-Findik DD, Schafer D, Klein E, et al. Alcohol metabolism-mediated oxidative stress down-regulates hepcidin transcription and

leads to increased duodenal iron transporter expression. J Biol Chem 2006; 281:22974-22982.

13. Ludwig J, Hashimoto E, Porayko MK, et al. Hemosiderosis in cirrhosis: a study of 447 native livers. Gastroenterology 1997; 112: 882-888.

14. Merryweather-Clarke AT, Pointon JJ, Shearman JD, Robson KJ. Global prevalence of putative haemochromatosis mutations. J Med Genet 1997; 34:275-278.

15. Steinberg KK, Cogswell ME, Chang JC, et al. Prevalence of *C282Y* and *H63D* mutations in the hemochromatosis (*HFE*) gene in the United States. JAMA 2001; 285:2216-2222.

16. Asberg A, Hveem K, Thorstensen K, et al. Screening for hemochromatosis: high prevalence and low morbidity in an unselected population of 65,238 persons. Scand J Gastroenterol 2001; 36:1108-1115.

17. Adams PC, Passmore L, Chakrabarti S, et al. Liver diseases in the hemochromatosis and iron overload screening study. Clin Gastroenterol Hepatol 2006; 4:918-923; quiz 807.

18. Olynyk JK, Cullen DJ, Aquilia S, et al. A population-based study of the clinical expression of the hemochromatosis gene. N Engl J Med 1999; 341:718-724.

19. Powell LW, Dixon JL, Ramm GA, et al. Screening for hemochromatosis in asymptomatic subjects with or without a family history. Arch Intern Med 2006; 166:294-301.

20. Bacon BR, Sadiq SA. Hereditary hemochromatosis: presentation and diagnosis in the 1990s. Am J Gastroenterol 1997; 92:784-789.

21. Yen AW, Fancher TL, Bowlus CL. Revisiting hereditary hemochromatosis: current concepts and progress. Am J Med 2006; 119:391-399.

22. Guyader D, Jacquelinet C, Moirand R, et al. Noninvasive prediction of fibrosis in *C282Y* homozygous hemochromatosis. Gastroenterology 1998; 115:929-936.

23. Beaton M, Guyader D, Deugnier Y, et al. Noninvasive prediction of cirrhosis in *C282Y*-linked hemochromatosis. Hepatology 2002; 36:673-678.

24. Pietrangelo A. Juvenile hemochromatosis. J Hepatol 2006; 45: 892-894.

25. Walsh A, Dixon JL, Ramm GA, et al. The clinical relevance of compound heterozygosity for the *C282Y* and *H63D* substitutions in hemochromatosis. Clin Gastroenterol Hepatol 2006; 4:1403-1410.

26. Gochee PA, Powell LW, Cullen DJ, et al. A population-based study of the biochemical and clinical expression of the *H63D* hemochromatosis mutation. Gastroenterology 2002; 122:646-651.

27. Fletcher LM, Dixon JL, Purdie DM, et al. Excess alcohol greatly increases the prevalence of cirrhosis in hereditary hemochromatosis. Gastroenterology 2002; 122:281-289.

28. Powell EE, Ali A, Clouston AD, et al. Steatosis is a cofactor in liver injury in hemochromatosis. Gastroenterology 2005; 129:1937-1943.

29. Morcos M, Dubois S, Bralet MP, et al. Primary liver carcinoma in genetic hemochromatosis reveals a broad histologic spectrum. Am J Clin Pathol 2001; 116:738-743.

30. Knisely AS, Crawford JM. Inherited and developmental disorders of the liver. In Odze RD, Golblum JR, Crawford JM (eds). Surgical Pathology of the GI Tract, Liver, Biliary Tract, and Pancreas. Philadelphia, WB Saunders, 2004, pp 986-987.

31. Deugnier YM, Guyader D, Crantock L, et al. Primary liver cancer in genetic hemochromatosis: a clinical, pathological, and pathogenetic study of 54 cases. Gastroenterology 1993; 104:228-234.

32. Jordan JM. Arthritis in hemochromatosis or iron storage disease. Curr Opin Rheumatol 2004; 16:62-66.

33. Jensen PD. Evaluation of iron overload. Br J Haematol 2004; 124:697-711.

34. Westphalen AC, Qayyum A, Yeh BM, et al. Liver fat: effect of hepatic iron deposition on evaluation with opposed-phase MR imaging. Radiology 2007; 242:450-455.

35. Hanna RF, Aguirre DA, Kased N, et al. Cirrhosis-associated hepatocellular nodules: correlation of histopathologic and MR imaging features. RadioGraphics 2008; 28:747-769.

36. O'Neil J, Powell L. Clinical aspects of hemochromatosis. Semin Liver Dis 2005; 25:381-391.

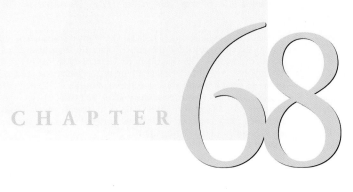
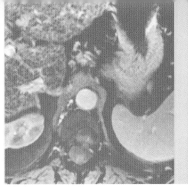
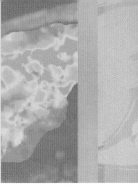

CHAPTER 68

Hepatic Storage Disorders

Sameer M. Mazhar, Lance L. Stein, Silvana C. Faria, Michael R. Peterson, and Claude B. Sirlin

The hepatic storage disorders are genetic conditions characterized by the accumulation of toxic substances within either hepatocytes or the hepatic extracellular matrix. This deposition causes secondary tissue damage, which may eventually progress to cirrhosis, portal hypertension, and hepatocellular carcinoma. As genetic conditions, their manifestations are wide ranging and systemic, with hepatic involvement only one component of the larger illness. The most common of these disorders, hereditary hemochromatosis, is discussed in detail in Chapter 67 on hepatic iron overload. In this chapter the focus is on the other relatively common storage disorders with hepatic manifestations: Wilson's disease, α₁-antitrypsin (A1AT) deficiency, and the glycogen storage diseases (GSDs). Other storage disorders, such as the porphyrias, amyloidosis, and lysosomal storage diseases (Gaucher's and Niemann-Pick diseases), are either very rare or primarily affect extrahepatic tissues. Nonalcoholic fatty liver disease (see Chapter 65) shares some features of the storage disorders but is not inherited in mendelian fashion and so is not included in this disease category.

tocellular carcinoma. It is caused by mutations in the *SERPINA1* (formerly known as *PI*) gene located on chromosome 14, which encodes the A1AT serine protease.[5]

The GSDs are a heterogeneous group of inborn errors of metabolism characterized by excessive glycogen content of the liver and muscles (among other tissues, including the kidneys and spleen) due to enzyme defects in glycogen synthesis or degradation. Enzymatic deficiencies in nearly every step of glycogen processing have been identified, accounting for at least 10 discrete diseases that are grouped into the GSDs (types 0, I, II, III, IV, V, VI, VII, IX, and XI). This chapter focuses on type I GSD (von Gierke's disease), by far the most common GSD associated with hepatic involvement. The other three GSDs associated with liver disease, types 0, III (Cori's or Fanconi's disease), and IV (Andersen's disease), are rare.

Type I GSD is caused by mutations in the *G6PC* gene. Located on chromosome 13, *G6PC* encodes glucose-6-phosphatase, a vital enzyme of glycogenolysis. Individuals heterozygous for the *G6PC* mutation have no phenotypic expression.

ETIOLOGY

Wilson's disease, A1AT deficiency, and the GSDs are familial conditions inherited in autosomal recessive fashion caused by mutations in putative genes.

Wilson's disease, also called hepatolenticular degeneration, is a disorder of copper metabolism. It is characterized by progressive neurologic deterioration and chronic liver disease leading to cirrhosis.[1] The gene responsible for this disease is *ATP7B*, located on chromosome 13. Highly expressed in the liver, kidney, and placenta, it encodes a metal-transporting, copper-dependent P-type adenosine triphosphatase, which functions in the incorporation of copper into ceruloplasmin (plasma protein that binds copper) and excretion of excess copper into bile.[2-4]

A1AT deficiency is associated with the development of pulmonary emphysema, chronic liver disease, and hepa-

PATHOGENESIS

The pathogeneses of Wilson's disease, A1AT deficiency, and the GSDs are explained by the metabolic defects caused by their underlying genetic abnormalities.

Wilson's Disease

The liver is the main organ responsible for copper homeostasis.[3] Normal copper metabolism begins with the absorption of dietary copper (Cu⁺) by duodenal enterocytes and its transportation to hepatocytes via the portal circulation. Hepatocytes then excrete the copper into bile biliary copper excretion, which eventually leads to fecal copper loss.[4]

Genetic defects in the *ATP7B* protein are associated with diminished incorporation of copper into ceruloplasmin and reduced excretion of copper into the bile.

Unincorporated copper accumulates within hepatocytes, where it causes secondary oxidative tissue damage. Some of the excess copper enters the systemic circulation and is deposited in extrahepatic sites such as the brain (especially the basal ganglia and limbic system), cornea, and kidneys. Copper not deposited in tissues is excreted in the urine. Ceruloplasmin not incorporated with copper is released into the bloodstream and rapidly degraded.

α₁-Antitrypsin Deficiency

A1AT is normally synthesized in the liver and released into the blood. An acute-phase reactant, it is elevated during inflammation, infection, and cancer. Its most important physiologic role is to inactivate proteolytic enzymes in the lung (especially, neutrophil elastase), which degrade lung matrix tissue after being released as a byproduct of cellular immune responses to airborne pathogens. A1AT counterbalances this proteolytic activity, preventing the net degradation of the lung matrix and alveoli.

In A1AT deficiency, hepatic production of A1AT is compromised and pulmonary proteolytic activity is unopposed, resulting in chronic obstructive pulmonary disease (COPD) and emphysema. Liver disease is uncommon except in some forms of A1AT deficiency, which leads to a cascade of cellular events, including autophagy, mitochondrial injury, caspase inactivation, and hepatocellular damage. Eventually, fibrosis and cirrhosis may ensue.[6,7]

Glycogen Storage Diseases

Glycogen is a highly-branched glucose polysaccharide. It is found in greatest concentration in the liver, and it functions as the body's primary form of short-term energy storage during fasting periods. In the GSDs, enzyme defects in glycogen metabolism lead to accumulation of glycogen or glycogen metabolites, resulting in hepatocyte swelling, marked hepatomegaly, and hypoglycemia.

In Type I GSD, a deficiency in glucose-6-phosphatase (G6P) results in glycogen accumulation within hepatocytes and causes hepatocellular damage via oxidative reactions. The damaged hepatocytes form neoplasms (hepatic adenomas and hepatocellular carcinomas) with relatively high frequency. Despite the hepatocellular damage and steatosis associated with type I GSD, liver fibrosis and cirrhosis do not occur.

The other GSDs associated with liver disease (types 0, III, and IV) are caused by enzymatic defects at other steps in glycogen metabolism; these disorders are associated with progressive liver disease, leading to cirrhosis and portal hypertension.

PREVALENCE AND EPIDEMIOLOGY

Wilson's disease is present across almost all races and ethnicities, with a roughly even male/female distribution. The prevalence is 1 per 30,000 persons, and the carrier frequency is 1 in 90.[8-10] Clinical presentation is usually in the second or third decade of life, although it has been described in patients younger than 5 years of age[11] and rarely older than age 45.

The incidence of A1AT deficiency is about 1 in 2000 live births.[12-14] Men and women are affected equally. In children, A1AT is the most common genetic cause of liver disease. The mean life span is 65 years in nonsmokers and is reduced to 50 years in smokers.

As a class, the GSDs occur in approximately 1 in 25,000 births; type I GSD has a prevalence of about 1 in 100,000 to 200,000 births.[15] Almost all cases have been identified in individuals from North America, Europe, or the Middle East. There is no predilection for ethnicity, race, or gender. Seventy percent of patients are diagnosed before the age of 2 years, with the development of hepatic adenomas in the second decade of life.

CLINICAL PRESENTATION
Wilson's Disease

Wilson's disease manifests over a wide spectrum and may involve hepatic or neuropsychiatric sequelae, either together or alone. The presentation may be either acute or chronic: acute disease typically manifests as fulminant hepatic failure, whereas chronic disease consists of chronic hepatitis, cirrhosis, and neuropsychiatric illness.[16] Patients who present with neuropsychiatric symptoms typically have asymptomatic hepatic involvement and are generally older than those who present with hepatic disease. Those presenting with hepatic disease typically will develop neuropsychiatric symptoms within 2 to 5 years.[17]

Hepatic involvement occurs as either fulminant hepatic failure or a progressive, indolent chronic hepatitis that may ultimately result in cirrhosis.[18] In the fulminant form, patients undergo rapid hepatic deterioration, with coagulopathy, encephalopathy, and renal failure. The chronic form develops over a period of decades, ultimately leading to the typical findings of cirrhosis and complications of portal hypertension (see Chapter 66). Hepatocellular carcinoma is a rare complication, with fewer than 20 documented cases, but would predictably occur in those with long-standing Wilson's disease. Neuropsychiatric symptoms are the initial presentation in 40% to 50% of patients.[19]

No single test determines the diagnosis of Wilson's disease, although an amalgamation of clinical and biochemical findings, as well as pedigree analysis, is suggestive in the correct clinical scenario. Serum aminotransferase levels are typically mildly elevated (<200 IU/L), with a proportional increase in total bilirubin (<4.0 mg/dL). Interestingly, the serum alkaline phosphatase concentration is reduced in fulminant disease; thus, a ratio of alkaline phosphatase to total bilirubin of less than 2 is highly suggestive of Wilson's disease in patients with fulminant hepatic failure.[21] Copper-specific findings include elevated serum copper and 24-hour urinary copper levels, as well as decreased serum ceruloplasmin levels. In some cases, liver biopsy is indicated with attention placed on the hepatic copper content.

α₁-Antitrypsin Deficiency

Pulmonary disease is usually more severe than hepatic disease and may occur in isolation; hepatic disease in the absence of pulmonary disease is rare. Pulmonary disease is accelerated by noxious stimuli, such as tobacco and air pollutants. Generally manifesting in early adulthood, it eventually progresses to severe panacinar emphysema (predominantly in the lower lobes) and COPD, characterized by bronchial hyperreactivity. Recurrent pulmonary infections are common.

Hepatic manifestations may occur in neonates as isolated disease (e.g., without concurrent pulmonary disease) or in adults with pulmonary disease.[22] The neonatal presentation is that of a hepatitis with cholestasis, resulting in hepatomegaly and jaundice 4 to 8 weeks after birth, which spontaneously resolves after a few weeks. The presence of neonatal disease does not predict hepatic disease in adulthood.[22] In adults, hepatic disease manifests as a hepatitis, eventually progressing to fibrosis and cirrhosis. Cirrhosis develops slowly, typically requiring 20 to 30 years for portal hypertension to occur, and is the most common stage of presentation. Patients may exhibit complications of portal hypertension, including bleeding from varices, hypersplenism, ascites, and hepatic encephalopathy. The incidence of hepatocellular carcinoma is thought to be higher in patients with A1AT deficiency, although its transformation rate has not been well characterized.[23] The diagnosis of A1AT deficiency should be considered in any young patient with obstructive lung disease or in any person with concurrent lung and liver abnormalities; in a patient presenting with hepatomegaly, elevated transaminase or bilirubin levels, or with signs of portal hypertension or cholestasis; or in an individual with chronic hepatitis or cirrhosis of unknown cause.

Glycogen Storage Diseases

Type I GSD clinically manifests in the neonate, usually becoming evident within the first week of life.[24] The chief systemic metabolic abnormality is hypoglycemia, typically in the range of 25 to 50 mg/dL. G6P accumulation in the kidneys causes renomegaly and may result in proteinuria, systemic hypertension, or Fanconi's syndrome. G6P accumulation in the liver causes hepatomegaly. By the second decade of life, hepatic adenomas develop in up to 75% of patients with type I GSD; these adenomas are considered premalignant and may transform into hepatocellular carcinoma in both pediatric and adult patients.[25,26]

PATHOLOGY

Wilson's Disease

The hepatic manifestations of excess copper accumulation are variable and often progressive. In early disease, patients demonstrate nonspecific signs of injury. In fulminant disease, massive hepatic necrosis is seen. In some patients, chronic inflammation may be present with increased numbers of lymphocytes in portal tracts, which can mimic chronic viral hepatitis. In advanced disease, progressive fibrosis leads to portal-portal bridging with eventual macronodular cirrhosis. Histochemical staining with rhodanine may be used to detect cytoplasmic copper; however, staining may be focal and missed on needle biopsy. Electron microscopy reveals characteristic

mitochondrial abnormalities, including swollen cristae and crystalline inclusions.

α₁-Antitrypsin Deficiency

Accumulated hepatocellular A1AT can be detected by histochemical staining with diastase-positive periodic acid–Schiff (PAS-D) or by immunohistochemical staining for A1AT. PAS-D staining reveals characteristic inclusions consisting of round-to-oval, purple-red globules within the cytoplasm of periportal hepatocytes. They may display hepatitis with features of canalicular cholestasis, giant cell transformation, swollen ("ballooning") hepatocytes, and diminished bile ducts. Other histologic findings in the liver are nonspecific and include fatty change and, rarely, Mallory hyaline.

Glycogen Storage Diseases

In type I GSD, accumulation of glycogen metabolites within hepatocytes leads to hepatic enlargement. These metabolites may be seen on light microscopy as intracellular cytoplasmic vacuoles. The hepatocytes take on a pale appearance with prominent cell membranes.

IMAGING

The diagnosis of Wilson's disease is generally based on clinical and laboratory findings; complicated cases are confirmed by increased hepatic copper concentration in biopsy samples of liver tissue. In patients with cirrhosis secondary to Wilson's disease, abdominal imaging may play a role in surveillance for hepatocellular carcinoma and detecting complications of portal hypertension.[3]

A1AT deficiency primarily affects the lungs. Pulmonary manifestations include panlobular emphysema, predominantly involving the lung bases. Liver abnormalities are less frequent and usually less severe. There are no characteristic liver imaging findings.[23] As with Wilson's disease, abdominal imaging is used in advanced disease for the assessment of stigmata of cirrhosis and portal hypertension, as well as surveillance for hepatocellular carcinoma.

Accumulation of glycogen metabolites within the liver, kidneys, and spleen may result in enlarged organs, manifesting as hepatomegaly (Fig. 68-1), bilateral renomegaly (Fig. 68-2), and splenomegaly, respectively.[27,28] The liver is the most frequently involved organ, and hepatomegaly may be massive, fully comprising the abdomen and extending into the pelvis. A variable degree of fat accumulation within the liver parenchyma may also be evident. Because of the high incidence of adenomas and the potential risk of malignant transformation, patients with type I GSD usually undergo periodic imaging studies to assess and monitor hepatic tumors.[29]

CT, MRI, and Ultrasonography

Wilson's Disease

In the early stages of Wilson's disease, the liver usually has a normal imaging appearance, although nonspecific

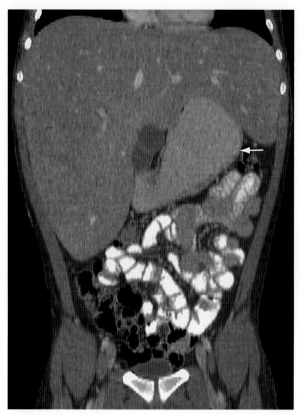

■ FIGURE 68-1 A 19-year-old man presented with a history of type I GSD. Coronal reformatted postcontrast CT image during the portal venous phase reveals massive enlargement of the liver, almost completely filling the abdomen, with the tip of the right lobe of the liver projecting into the pelvis. Note the stomach (*arrow*) displaced inferiorly.

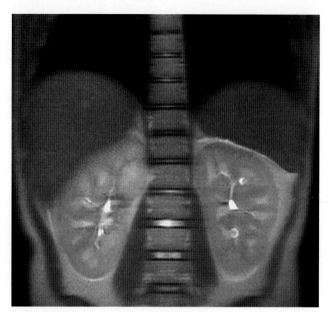

■ FIGURE 68-2 A 19-year-old man presented with a history of type I GSD (see also Fig. 68-1). Coronal single-shot turbo spin-echo image reveals diffuse enlargement of the kidneys bilaterally. The right kidney measures 15.8 cm, and the left kidney measures 15.2 cm.

findings such as hepatomegaly may be observed. On unenhanced CT images, the liver may have increased attenuation due to deposited copper. However, there is no correlation between the degree of CT attenuation and hepatic copper concentration and the CT findings do not permit quantitative assessment of copper deposition. Copper has no ferromagnetic effect on MRI, and the signal intensity of the involved liver is usually normal.[30] Similarly, copper does not scatter the ultrasound beam and the affected liver has normal echogenicity.[30]

In fulminant presentations, necrotic portions of the liver may fail to enhance after intravenous administration of contrast agents.[31] In advanced chronic cases, features of cirrhosis may be evident. These are indistinguishable from those of other causes of end-stage liver disease, with the exceptions of a normal caudate lobe size and high hepatic attenuation on unenhanced CT due to copper deposition (Fig. 68-3).[30]

On brain MRI, high-intensity signal abnormalities on T1-weighted (T1W) and T2-weighted (T2W) images are usually seen in the basal ganglia. The putamen is involved most frequently, with other sites of involvement including the globus pallidus, caudate, and thalami.[32]

α_1-Antitryspin Deficiency

The CT, MRI, and ultrasound findings of patients with A1AT deficiency depend on the severity of liver involve-

ment.[5] In the precirrhotic phase, the liver usually has a normal imaging appearance, although hepatomegaly, heterogeneity of hepatic parenchyma, and heterogeneous enhancement may be apparent.[23] The cirrhotic phase is characterized by findings common to the other causes of end-stage liver disease (Fig. 68-4).

Glycogen Storage Diseases

CT, MRI, and ultrasonography may depict hepatomegaly, splenomegaly, and renomegaly. Hepatic steatosis manifests as hyperechogenicity on ultrasonography, low attenuation on unenhanced CT, and signal loss on out-of-phase MR images (Figs. 68-5 and 68-6). In the absence of significant steatosis, however, the liver parenchyma may be hyperattenuating rather than hypoattenuating on CT owing to the accumulation of excess glycogen.

Adenomas have variable degrees of fat, hemorrhage, and necrosis and may be heterogeneous in imaging appearance on both CT (Fig. 68-7) and MRI (Figs. 68-8 and 68-9).[18] Longitudinal examination is necessary to differentiate between benign hepatic adenomas and those that have transformed to hepatocellular carcinoma. In adenomas examined longitudinally, findings that suggest malignant transformation include rapid interval growth and/or change in imaging features.[17]

Imaging Algorithm

Wilson's Disease and α_1-Antitrypsin Deficiency

Patients with a clinical history suggestive of Wilson's disease or A1AT deficiency may be imaged for signs of cirrhosis and portal hypertension and screened for hepatocellular carcinoma, as described in other chapters. Ultrasonography and CT are usually the imaging studies

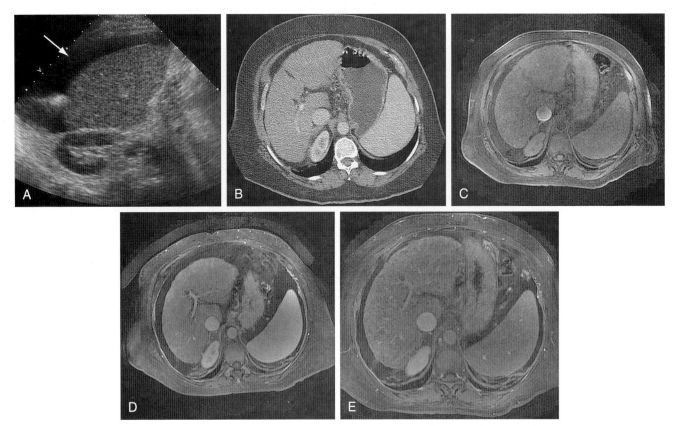

■ **FIGURE 68-3** Wilson's disease in a 56-year-old man. **A,** On the longitudinal sonogram the liver is small and has a heterogeneous echotexture. There is moderate ascites (*arrow*). **B,** Axial contrast-enhanced CT image demonstrates the nodular surface of the liver. The right lobe is relatively diminutive. **C,** Precontrast MR image shows fibrous septa, in addition to the morphologic alterations of cirrhosis (also shown in **A** and **B**). **D,** Appearance of fibrous septa during portal venous phase after intravenous administration of gadolinium administration. **E,** Double-contrast–enhanced MR image shows hyperintense fibrotic reticulations delineating small hypointense regenerative nodules. Note that the discrete regenerative nodules and fibrotic scars are not visible on the ultrasound or CT images.

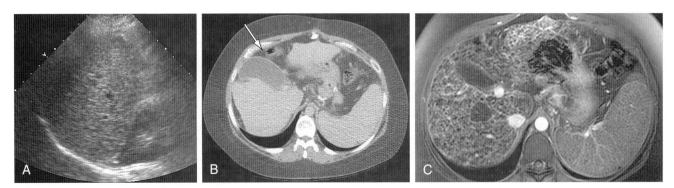

■ **FIGURE 68-4** α₁-Antitrypsin deficiency in a 47-year-old woman with cirrhosis. **A,** Longitudinal ultrasound image shows the diffuse heterogeneous echotexture of the liver parenchyma. **B,** Axial postcontrast CT image during the portal venous phase shows nodularity of the liver surface and an enlarged pericholecystic space (*arrow*) filled with adipose tissue ("expanded gallbladder fossa" sign). **C,** Axial combined contrast-enhanced MR image shows, in addition to the morphologic alterations depicted in **A** and **B**, hyperintense reticulations throughout the liver parenchyma associated with various hypointense regenerative nodules. Also note mild enlargement of the spleen.

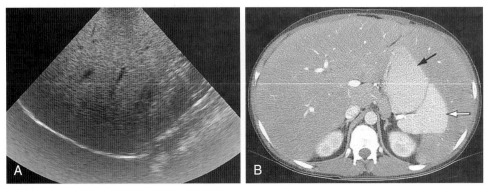

■ **FIGURE 68-5** A 19-year-old man presented with a history of type I GSD (see also Fig. 68-1). **A,** Longitudinal ultrasound image of the liver shows parenchymal hyperechogenicity and posterior beam attenuation. Intrahepatic vessels are poorly visualized. **B,** Axial contrast-enhanced CT image reveals massive hepatomegaly. Note that the left lobe of the liver surrounds and medially displaces the stomach (*black arrow*) and spleen (*white arrow*). The spleen is of normal size.

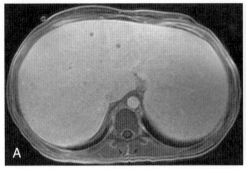
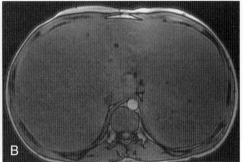

■ **FIGURE 68-6** A 19-year-old man presented with a history of type I GSD (see also Fig. 68-1). In-phase (**A**) and out-of-phase (**B**) T1W gradient-recalled-echo (GRE) axial MR images show loss of signal on the out-of-phase images, indicating fat accumulation within the liver parenchyma.

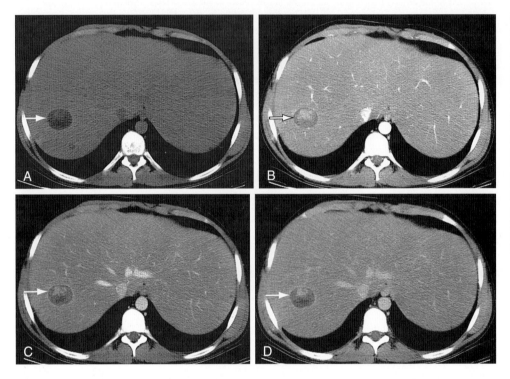

■ **FIGURE 68-7** A 19-year-old man presented with a history of type I GSD (see Fig. 68-1). **A,** Axial unenhanced CT image reveals massive hepatomegaly with diffuse hypoattenuation of the liver parenchyma suggestive of steatosis. Note the hypoattenuating well-defined hepatic lesion (*arrow*) located in segment 7 of the liver, measuring 3.2 cm. The lesion attenuation on the precontrast image is −18 HU, suggesting the presence of intralesional fat. The lesion (*arrows*) enhances heterogeneously during the arterial phase (**B**) and fades during the portal venous (**C**) and delayed phases (**D**). It was resected and proved to be an adenoma.

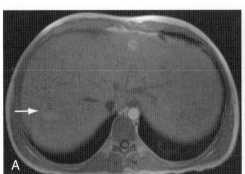
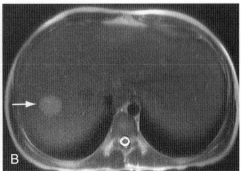

■ **FIGURE 68-8** A 19-year-old man presented with a history of type I GSD (see Fig. 68-1). Axial T1W (**A**) and T2W (**B**) MR images of the liver. The well-defined nodular lesion (*arrows*) located in segment 7 of the liver has high signal intensity.

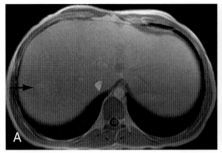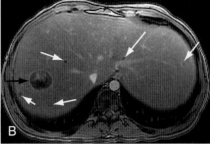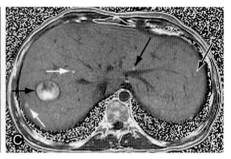

■ **FIGURE 68-9** A 19-year-old man presented with a history of type I GSD (see Fig. 68-1). A 3.2-cm adenoma (*black arrow*) shows loss of signal on the out-of-phase (**B**) compared with the in-phase (**A**) image, indicating the presence of fat within the lesion. The fat signal fraction map (**C**) shows pixel by pixel the percentage of the total MR signal that comes from fat protons. Tissues that contain fat appear hyperintense, and tissues that do not contain fat appear hypointense. The blood vessels and the capsule of the 3.2-cm adenoma are devoid of fat and thus appear hypointense, whereas the liver parenchyma and the adenoma itself (*black arrow*) contain fat and thus appears hyperintense. The adenoma has greater fat content than the liver. Note several other smaller fat-containing adenomas (*white arrows*) that lose signal on the out-of-phase image and appear hyperintense on the fat signal fraction map.

TABLE 68-1 Accuracy, Limitations, and Pitfalls of the Modalities Used in Imaging of Wilson's Disease

Modality	Accuracy	Limitations	Pitfalls
CT	Data on the imaging accuracy for the diagnosis of Wilson's disease are not available.	Ionizing radiation	CT attenuation does not correlate with copper concentration.
MRI	CT may depict increased hepatic attenuation due to copper deposition and probably has higher sensitivity than MR or US.	Copper does not alter liver signal intensity.	
Ultrasonography		Copper does not alter liver echogenicity.	

TABLE 68-2 Accuracy, Limitations, and Pitfalls of the Modalities Used in Imaging for α₁-Antitrypsin Deficiency

Modality	Accuracy	Limitations	Pitfalls
CT	No data on the accuracy of CT, MRI, or US for the diagnosis of α_1-antitrypsin deficiency. In principle, CT may have higher sensitivity and specificity than the other modalities because it can depict the pulmonary manifestations of panlobular emphysema	Ionizing radiation. Risk of IV contrast reactions	Cirrhosis may coexist with emphysema of other causes.
MRI		Cannot assess the pulmonary manifestations (panlobular emphysema) directly	
Ultrasonography		Cannot assess the pulmonary manifestations (panlobular emphysema) directly	

performed initially, with MRI reserved for problem solving or if CT is contraindicated (Tables 68-1 and 68-2). The American Association for the Study of Liver Diseases does not offer specific guidelines for screening for hepatocellular carcinoma in patients with Wilson's disease or A1AT deficiency because the hepatocellular carcinoma transformation rate is poorly understood. Regardless, many institutions advocate semi-annual screening (via ultrasonography or CT); at our institution screening via CT or MRI is recommended every 6 months. In patients with fulminant presentations of Wilson's disease, CT may be performed to assess the extent of necrosis.[3] Imaging does not play a role in assessing the degree of copper deposition.

Imaging techniques to grade the severity of liver fibrosis in precirrhotic stages of chronic liver disease, including Wilson's disease and A1AT deficiency, are under development (see Chapter 69).

An advantage of CT over ultrasonography and MRI for the assessment of patients with A1AT deficiency is that CT can simultaneously evaluate the lung parenchyma and the liver.

Glycogen Storage Diseases

Patients with type I GSD should undergo surveillance imaging to detect and monitor hepatic tumors. MRI is probably the superior modality for this indication, because of its excellent safety profile and high sensitivity for focal lesion detection. Ultrasonography is insensitive for identification of small solid liver tumors, especially in the setting of hepatic steatosis. CT exposes the patient to ionizing radiation and should be avoided if possible in pediatric patients and young adults who may need lifelong monitoring.

Classic Signs

WILSON'S DISEASE

■ The liver parenchyma may be hyperattenuating at unenhanced CT due to deposited copper.

■ In cirrhosis due to Wilson's disease, the caudate lobe is characteristically normal in size.

α₁-ANTITRYPSIN DEFICIENCY

■ The classic signs of liver cirrhosis due to A1AT deficiency are indistinguishable from the imaging findings of cirrhosis from other causes.

■ Cirrhosis in conjunction with panlobular emphysema is suggestive.

GLYCOGEN STORAGE DISEASES

■ There may be marked hepatomegaly with variable renomegaly and infrequent splenomegaly.

■ CT attenuation may be low, normal, or high depending on the balance of fat and glycogen accumulation.

■ Hepatic adenomas are frequent and may contain fat and/or blood.

■ Rapid interval growth or change in imaging features of adenomas suggests malignant transformation. Stigmata of cirrhosis and portal hypertension are absent even in advanced stages of disease.

DIFFERENTIAL DIAGNOSIS

Wilson's Disease

The clinical differential diagnosis for Wilson's disease differs depending on whether the presentation is predominantly hepatic or neuropsychiatric. If the presentation is hepatic, Wilson's disease must be considered in the differential diagnosis of any chronic liver disease of unexplained origin, particularly if the patient is younger than 40 years of age. Wilson's disease is easily differentiated from other causes of chronic liver disease (e.g., viral hepatitis, autoimmune hepatitis, alcoholic or nonalcoholic fatty liver disease) by history and characteristic blood tests (e.g., low ceruloplasmin and high urinary copper levels, lack of serologic findings of viral hepatitis, or autoimmune

markers). Kayser-Fleischer rings and high levels of hepatic copper on liver biopsy are sensitive and specific for Wilson's disease and confirm the diagnosis.

Assessment of the liver usually permits clinical differentiation. Unlike Wilson's disease, which has quiescent hepatic involvement (via elevated aminotransferase levels and hepatic copper deposition on liver biopsy) even in strict neuropsychiatric presentations, these other conditions are not associated with liver disease.

Radiologically, hepatomegaly related to Wilson's disease must be differentiated from hepatomegaly due to other causes, such as acute hepatitis, toxic-metabolic disorders, vascular disorders, and lymphoproliferative diseases. Hepatic hyperattenuation on unenhanced CT, if present, may suggest the correct diagnosis.

The imaging features of patients with cirrhosis secondary to advanced Wilson's disease overlap with the imaging findings of other causes of end-stage liver disease. The presence of cirrhosis associated with hepatic hyperattenuation on CT suggests Wilson's disease, hereditary hemochromatosis, or cirrhosis with secondary hemosiderosis.[33]

α₁-Antitrypsin Deficiency

The clinical differential diagnosis is limited to A1AT deficiency when there is both significant pulmonary and hepatic disease, because this combination of organ involvement is unique. When there is primarily pulmonary involvement, consideration must be given to other causes of chronic airway obstruction, including COPD, smoking-related emphysema and bronchitis, bronchiectasis, and chronic asthma. These diagnoses are differentiated from A1AT deficiency by normal serum A1AT levels and no suggestive factors in a family history.

In adults, the differential diagnosis of predominant hepatic disease due to A1AT deficiency includes all causes of chronic liver disease and/or cirrhosis. If other causes are excluded based on history, serologic findings of viral hepatitis, autoimmune markers, and iron studies, then serum A1AT levels should be checked.

Neonatal A1AT deficiency should be distinguished from other causes of neonatal liver disease, including infection (e.g., Epstein-Barr virus, cytomegalovirus, hepatitis B virus) and biliary atresia.

The imaging findings of end-stage liver disease secondary to A1AT deficiency are nonspecific. However, the presence of cirrhosis in conjunction with panlobular emphysema suggests A1AT deficiency.

Glycogen Storage Diseases

The clinical differential diagnosis of type I GSD is narrow owing to its unique presentation of hypoglycemia, lactic acidosis, hyperuricemia, hyperlipidemia, and hepatomegaly in the neonatal period, along with growth retardation and developmental delay in subsequent years. Depending on the clinical manifestations, consideration may be given to other inborn errors of metabolism (e.g., the remaining

GSDs, particularly types III and IV), fructose-1,6-bisphosphatase deficiency, and various disorders associated with growth retardation (e.g., Crohn's disease and growth hormone deficiency). Hepatoblastoma, a rare malignant hepatic tumor of infancy, causes marked hepatomegaly, which may mimic that of type I GSD.

Massive hepatomegaly, in which the liver comprises the entire abdomen and extends into the pelvis, has a narrower differential diagnosis than mild hepatomegaly. In particular, massive hepatomegaly may be caused by lymphoproliferative diseases such as lymphoma, infectious diseases such as viral hepatitis, and other metabolic disorders such as lysosomal storage diseases. Polycystic liver disease also may cause severe hepatomegaly but is easily distinguished from GSD by the presence of cysts. Hepatomegaly and renomegaly in association with hepatic adenomas suggest the diagnosis of type I GSD because this combination of findings is rarely seen in other conditions.[34]

TREATMENT

Medical Treatment

Wilson's Disease

Treatment of Wilson's disease has been shown to slow the progression of both hepatic and neuropsychiatric disease and limit symptom recurrence. Medical therapy is reserved for those with chronic hepatic and neurologic disease and is of no benefit in patients with a fulminant presentation. The mainstay of treatment is lifelong therapy with a chelating agent, either D-pencillamine or trientine, which absorbs free copper in the bloodstream and enhances its removal in the urine.[35]

α₁-Antitrypsin Deficiency

The treatment of A1AT deficiency focuses on management of pulmonary disease. Smoking cessation is stressed to prevent pulmonary disease progression. Active disease is treated with a variety of inhalers (bronchodilators and corticosteroids), systemic corticosteroids, and antibiotics. Substitution therapy with intravenously administered A1AT has been advocated in patients with pulmonary disease, although rigorous outcome analyses are lacking.[5]

Medical management does not alter the course of hepatic disease. Hepatic disease is supportively managed, with attention to prevention of complications of portal hypertension and screening for hepatocellular carcinoma.

Glycogen Storage Diseases

In type I GSD, the primary treatment goals are to correct systemic metabolic abnormalities, counteract hypoglycemia, and reduce the severity of malnourishment and growth retardation. Nutritional supplementation with nocturnal high-starch feeds through a nasogastric or gastrostomy tube and small, frequent daytime feedings are usually required.[36] Severe cases of acidosis may require infusion of sodium bicarbonate. Allopurinol is used to prevent the joint and renal complications of hyperuricemia.

Surgical Treatment

Wilson's Disease

Liver transplantation is indicated for patients with decompensated liver disease unresponsive to medical therapy and those presenting with fulminant hepatic failure.

α₁-Antitrypsin Deficiency

Surgical therapy for A1AT deficiency may be pursued for end-stage pulmonary or hepatic disease. Lung transplantation is a viable option for those with the most advanced pulmonary disease. Progressive liver dysfunction is an indication for liver transplantation, which has demonstrated survival rates greater than 92% at 5 years after transplantation.[37,38]

Glycogen Storage Diseases

Liver transplantation has been performed in a handful of patients with GSDs, most commonly in patients with cirrhosis due to type IV GSD.[39] Liver transplantation for type I GSD is rarely performed and only in those patients with bulky hepatic adenomas or hepatocellular carcinoma.

What the Referring Physician Needs to Know

WILSON'S DISEASE

■ Also called hepatolenticular degeneration, Wilson's disease is a disorder of copper metabolism characterized by progressive neurologic deterioration and chronic liver disease leading to cirrhosis.

■ Caused by mutations in the *ATP7B* gene, Wilson's disease is a state of copper excess in which copper accumulates in the liver, lentiform nucleus, and other sites.

■ The clinical presentation includes hepatic and neuropsychiatric sequelae, either together or alone.

■ The hepatic presentation may be either as fulminant hepatic failure or progressive, indolent chronic hepatitis, ultimately resulting in cirrhosis.

■ Hepatic copper concentration of sampled liver tissue is a useful diagnostic tool in some circumstances.

■ Hepatocellular carcinoma is a rare complication of long-standing Wilson's disease.

■ Treatment consists of oral chelators, zinc, and, in advanced cases, liver transplantation.

α₁-ANTITRYPSIN DEFICIENCY

■ A1AT deficiency manifests as a combination of pulmonary emphysema and chronic liver disease; neonates may present with solitary hepatitis.

■ Caused by mutations in the *SERPINA1* gene, the A1AT protein accumulates within the liver and is thus unable to counteract the destructive effects of pulmonary proteases on the lung matrix.

What the Referring Physician Needs to Know—Cont'd

- Cirrhosis develops over a period of decades.
- The incidence of hepatocellular carcinoma is thought to be higher than in other causes of end-stage liver disease, although the transformation rate is not well characterized.
- Characteristic histologic inclusions can confirm the diagnosis if gel electrophoresis is unrevealing.
- Whereas there are a few alternatives for the medical therapy of pulmonary disease, no such options exist to prevent the progression of hepatic disease.
- Lung and liver transplantation are viable options in patients with end-stage disease.

GLYCOGEN STORAGE DISEASES

- The GSDs are a heterogeneous group of inborn errors of metabolism characterized by excessive glycogen content of the liver and muscles due to enzyme defects in glycogen synthesis or degradation.
- Type I GSD is the most common GSD associated with hepatic involvement.
- Due to mutations in the *G6PC* gene, glucose-6-phosphatase activity is diminished, resulting in the hepatic accumulation of G6P, its upstream metabolites, and glycogen itself.
- Other features include hepatic steatosis and the formation of hepatic adenomas; the hepatic adenomas may transform into hepatocellular carcinomas.
- Hepatic fibrosis and cirrhosis do not occur.
- Clinical manifestations include massive hepatomegaly, recalcitrant hypoglycemia, lactic acidosis, growth retardation, and developmental delay.

KEY POINTS

Wilson's Disease

- High density of the liver parenchyma at unenhanced CT may be seen due to deposited copper.
- In cirrhosis, the caudate typically is normal in size, but this finding is not specific for Wilson's disease.
- Cirrhosis associated with hepatic hyperattenuation on CT raises the possibility of, but is not specific for, Wilson's disease. The differential diagnosis includes hereditary hemochromatosis and cirrhosis of any cause with secondary hemosiderosis.
- Fulminant hepatic failure may be the first manifestation.
- Copper does not affect liver signal intensity at MRI or echogenicity at ultrasonography.

α_1-Antitrypsin Deficiency

- Liver involvement is less frequent than lung involvement.
- Liver severity is variable and unrelated to lung severity.
- Liver manifestations are nonspecific in the precirrhotic phase.
- In the cirrhotic phase, imaging findings overlap with other causes of end-stage liver disease.
- Cirrhosis in conjunction with panlobular emphysema suggests A1AT deficiency.

Glycogen Storage Diseases

- Liver attenuation on unenhanced CT depends on the balance of glycogen (increases attenuation) and steatosis (reduces attenuation).
- Bilateral renomegaly with increased frequency of calculi is common.
- The spleen is less frequently involved, although splenomegaly may be observed.
- With age, hepatic adenomas tend to increase in both size and number.

SUGGESTED READINGS

Ala A, Schilsky ML. Wilson disease: pathophysiology, diagnosis, treatment, and screening. Clin Liver Dis 2004; 8:787-805.
Ala A, Walker AP, Ashkan K, et al. Wilson's disease. Lancet 2007; 369:397-408.
Fink S, Schilsky ML. Inherited metabolic disease of the liver. Curr Opin Gastroenterol 2007; 23:237-243.
Kohnlein T, Welte T. Alpha-1 antitrypsin deficiency: pathogenesis, clinical presentation, diagnosis, and treatment. Am J Med 2008; 121:3-9.
Medici V, Rossaro L, Sturniolo GC. Wilson disease—a practical approach to diagnosis, treatment and follow-up. Dig Liver Dis 2007; 39:397-408.
Ozen H. Glycogen storage diseases: new perspectives. World J Gastroenterol 2007; 13:2541-2553.
Perlmutter DH. Alpha-1-antitrypsin deficiency: diagnosis and treatment. Clin Liver Dis 2004; 8:839-859.
Roberts EA, Schilsky ML. A practice guideline on Wilson disease. Hepatology 2003; 37:1475-1492.
Talente GM, Coleman RA, Alter C, et al. Glycogen storage disease in adults. Ann Intern Med 1994; 120:218-226.
Teckman JH. Alpha$_1$-antitrypsin deficiency in childhood. Semin Liver Dis 2007; 27:274-281.

REFERENCES

1. Wilson S. Progressive lenticular degeneration: a familial nervous disease associated with cirrhosis of the liver. Brain 1912; 34:295-507.
2. Bull PC, Thomas GR, Rommens JM, et al. The Wilson disease gene is a putative copper transporting P-type ATPase similar to the Menkes gene. Nat Genet 1993; 5:327-337.
3. Ala A, Walker AP, Ashkan K, et al. Wilson's disease. Lancet 2007; 369:397-408.
4. Ala A, Schilsky ML. Wilson disease: pathophysiology, diagnosis, treatment, and screening. Clin Liver Dis 2004; 8:787-805.
5. Kohnlein T, Welte T. Alpha-1 antitrypsin deficiency: pathogenesis, clinical presentation, diagnosis, and treatment. Am J Med 2008; 121:3-9.
6. Teckman JH. Alpha$_1$-antitrypsin deficiency in childhood. Semin Liver Dis 2007; 27:274-281.

7. Ogushi F, Fells GA, Hubbard RC, et al. Z-type alpha 1-antitrypsin is less competent than M1-type alpha 1-antitrypsin as an inhibitor of neutrophil elastase. J Clin Invest 1987; 80:1366-1374.

8. Frydman M. Genetic aspects of Wilson's disease. J Gastroenterol Hepatol 1990; 5:483-490.

9. Lovicu M, Dessi V, Zappu A, et al. Efficient strategy for molecular diagnosis of Wilson disease in the Sardinia population. Clin Chem 2003; 49:496-498.

10. Kusuda Y, Hamaguchi K, Mori T, et al. Novel mutations of the *ATP7B* gene in Japanese patients with Wilson disease. J Hum Genet 2000; 45:86-91.

11. Wilson DC, Phillips MJ, Cox DW, Roberts EA. Severe hepatic Wilson's disease in preschool-aged children. J Pediatr 2000; 137:719-722.

12. Blanco I, de Serres FJ, Fernandez-Bustillo E, et al. Estimated numbers and prevalence of PI*S and PI*Z alleles of alpha 1-antitrypsin deficiency in European countries. Eur Respir J 2006; 27:77-84.

13. Lieberman J, Winter B, Sastre A. Alpha 1-antitrypsin Pi-types in 965 COPD patients. Chest 1986; 89:370-373.

14. de Serres FJ, Blanco I, Fernandez-Bustillo E. Genetic epidemiology of alpha-1 antitrypsin deficiency in North America and Australia/New Zealand: Australia, Canada, New Zealand and the United States of America. Clin Genet 2003; 64:382-397.

15. Talente GM, Coleman RA, Alter C, et al. Glycogen storage disease in adults. Ann Intern Med 1994; 120:218-226.

16. Roberts EA, Schilsky ML. A practice guideline on Wilson disease. Hepatology 2003; 37:1475-1492.

17. Medici V, Mirante VG, Fassati LR, et al. Monotematica AISF 2000 OLT Study Group. Liver transplantation for Wilson's disease: the burden of neurological and psychiatric disorders. Liver Transpl 2005; 11:1056-1063.

18. Ostapowicz G, Fontana RJ, Schiodt FV, et al. U.S. Acute Liver Failure Study Group. Results of a prospective study of acute liver failure at 17 tertiary care centers in the United States. Ann Intern Med 2002; 137:947-954.

19. Walshe JM. Wilson's disease. The presenting symptoms. Arch Dis Child 1962; 37:253-256.

20. Svetel M, Kozic D, Stefanova E, et al. Dystonia in Wilson's disease. Mov Disord 2001; 16:719-723.

21. Sallie R, Katsiyiannakis L, Baldwin D, et al. Failure of simple biochemical indexes to reliably differentiate fulminant Wilson's disease from other causes of fulminant liver failure. Hepatology 1992; 16:1206-1211.

22. Perlmutter DH. Alpha-1-antitrypsin deficiency: diagnosis and treatment. Clin Liver Dis 2004; 8:839-859.

23. Propst T, Propst A, Dietze O, et al. Alpha-1-antitrypsin deficiency and liver disease. Dig Dis 1994; 12:139-149.

24. Sadeghi-Nejad A, Presente E, Binkiewicz A, Senior B. Studies in type I glycogenosis of the liver: the genesis and disposition of lactate. J Pediatr 1974; 85:49-54.

25. Howell RR, Stevenson RE, Ben-Menachem Y, et al. Hepatic adenomata with type 1 glycogen storage disease. JAMA 1976; 236:1481-1484.

26. Limmer J, Fleig WE, Leupold D, et al. Hepatocellular carcinoma in type I glycogen storage disease. Hepatology 1988; 8:531-537.

27. Lin CC, Tsai JD, Lin SP, Lee HC. Renal sonographic findings of type I glycogen storage disease in infancy and early childhood. Pediatr Radiol 2005; 35:786-791.

28. Grossman H, Ram PC, Coleman RA, et al. Hepatic ultrasonography in type I glycogen storage disease (von Gierke disease). Detection of hepatic adenoma and carcinoma. Radiology 1981; 141:753-756.

29. Lee PJ. Glycogen storage disease type I: pathophysiology of liver adenomas. Eur J Pediatr 2002; 161(Suppl 1):S46-S49.

30. Akhan O, Akpinar E, Karcaaltincaba M, et al. Imaging findings of liver involvement of Wilson's disease. Eur J Radiol 2007; Nov 2. [Epub ahead of print.]

31. Williams R. Acute liver failure—practical management. Acta Gastroenterol Belg 2007; 70:210-213.

32. King AD, Walshe JM, Kendall BE, et al. Cranial MR imaging in Wilson's disease. AJR Am J Roentgenol 1996; 167:1579-1584.

33. Abuzetun JY, Hazin R, Suker M, Porter J. A rare case of hemochromatosis and Wilson's disease coexisting in the same patient. J Natl Med Assoc 2008; 100:112-114.

34. Moraru E, Cuvinciuc O, Antonesei L, et al. Glycogen storage disease type I—between chronic ambulatory follow-up and pediatric emergency. J Gastrointest Liver Dis 2007; 16:47-51.

35. Shilsky MN. Treatment of Wilson's disease: what are the relative roles of penicillamine, trientine, and zinc supplementation? Curr Gastroenterol Rep 2001; 3:54-59.

36. Leonard JV, Dunger DB. Hypoglycaemia complicating feeding regimens for glycogen-storage disease. Lancet 1978; 2:1203-1204.

37. Kayler LK, Merion RM, Lee S, et al. Long-term survival after liver transplantation in children with metabolic disorders. Pediatr Transplant 2002; 6:295-300.

38. Bund M, Seitz W, Schafers HJ, et al. Combined lung and liver transplantation. Anesthesiologic management. Anaesthesist 1994; 43:322-329.

39. Starzl TE, Demetris AJ, Trucco M, et al. Chimerism after liver transplantation for type IV glycogen storage disease and type 1 Gaucher's disease. N Engl J Med 1993; 328:745-749.

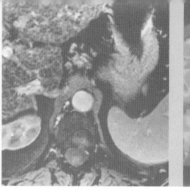
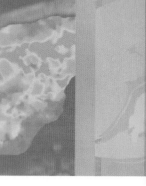

69

Hepatitis

Silvana C. Faria, Sameer M. Mazhar, Michael R. Peterson, Masoud Shiehmorteza, and Claude B. Sirlin

ETIOLOGY

Hepatitis is broadly defined as diffuse inflammation of the liver. More than two thirds of cases of hepatitis are caused by viruses.[1] Hepatotropic viruses, such as hepatitis A (HAV), B (HBV), C (HCV), D (HDV), and E (HEV), are the most commonly implicated, but examples of other possible causes include autoimmune disorders, metabolic conditions (e.g., Wilson's disease), toxic injury, and drug reaction. The focus here is on hepatotropic viral hepatitis, with special attention provided to the most prevalent of these, HBV and HCV.

PREVALENCE AND EPIDEMIOLOGY

HAV is a nonenveloped RNA picornavirus.[1] It is transmitted via a fecal-oral route. HAV is geographically distributed and is most prevalent in Central and South America, Africa, Asia, and the Middle East. The incidence of HAV in the United States in 2005 was 1.5 per 100,000, having dropped substantially since vaccination of at-risk individuals became widespread in 1996.[1]

HBV is the principal member of the DNA family of viruses known as Hepadnaviridae.[2] The prevalence of HBV varies from 0.1% to 2% in the United States and Western Europe to up to 20% in endemic areas such as China, Southeast Asia, and sub-Saharan Africa. The main modes of transmission are via unprotected sexual intercourse and needle sharing during intravenous drug use.

HCV is a small, enveloped, single-stranded RNA virus of the Flaviviridae family.[3] There are approximately 170 million people worldwide infected with HCV.[1] In the United States, HCV is the most common cause of virally transmitted chronic liver disease. About 4.1 million Americans are infected, and about 10,000 Americans die annually of complications related to HCV infection. The two main risk factors for HCV transmission are the sharing of needles during intravenous drug use and receiving a blood transfusion before 1990. Other risk factors include multiple sex partners, tattoos, and needlestick exposure.[3]

HDV comprises an RNA genome and an HDV antigen, both surrounded by a lipoprotein coat provided by HBV surface antigen.[4] As such, concurrent infection with HBV is required for HDV propagation and secretion. HDV is most commonly acquired parenterally via intravenous drug use or tainted blood transfusions, although spread perinatally or through sexual contact is also possible. The geographic distribution of HDV, however, does not follow that of HBV, centering on the Mediterranean, Pacific Islands, and portions of Africa and South America.[4]

HEV is an enterically transmitted, self-limited infection caused by a nonenveloped RNA virus of the Hepeviridae family. Its highest prevalence is in Southeast Asia, the Middle East, North Africa, and Mexico.[5]

CLINICAL PRESENTATION

Clinically, hepatitis can be divided into acute and chronic forms, based on the duration of the disease as assessed via biochemical (e.g., elevations of transaminases) and histologic means.

Severity of acute viral hepatitis ranges from subclinical infection to symptomatic disease and, rarely, fulminant hepatic failure.[6] In acute hepatitis, the viral incubation period may vary from 30 to 60 days, after which symptomatic patients develop a prodrome of malaise, nausea, anorexia, fever, and right upper quadrant abdominal pain that typically lasts 1 week, giving rise to a 2-week-long period of jaundice and pruritus. The most common physical examination findings are jaundice, tender hepatomegaly, and lymphadenopathy. Laboratory tests demonstrate markedly elevated serum aminotransferase enzymes (alanine aminotransferase [ALT] and aspartate aminotransferase [AST]), commonly exceeding 1000 IU/dL, with ALT values usually higher than those of AST, and an increase in bilirubin levels, often greater than 10 mg/dL. The specific virus type can be diagnosed serologically by testing for antiviral antibodies and viral antigens.[1]

Fulminant hepatic failure is a rare manifestation of acute hepatitis. Thought to be secondary to diffuse immune-mediated lysis of infected hepatocytes, it usually occurs 4 to 8 weeks after symptom onset and is marked by encephalopathy, coagulopathy, and multiple organ failure. The case-fatality rate may be as high as 75% without liver transplantation.[6]

In acute viral hepatitis, full clinical and biochemical resolution occurs within 6 months. However, a proportion of patients may proceed to chronic hepatitis, characterized by evidence of hepatocyte damage and inflammation for more than 6 months' duration. The chronic form may manifest decades later as cirrhosis and portal hypertension.[2]

Approximately 5% of immune-competent adults infected with HBV are unable to clear the virus and thus advance to chronic HBV; in contrast, 90% of children who contracted HBV perinatally go on to develop chronic HBV. Approximately 20% of patients with chronic HBV progress to cirrhosis decades after initial infection. Chronic HBV infection is an independent risk factor for the development of hepatocellular carcinoma (HCC), with chronic carriers being 100 times more likely to develop HCC than noncarriers. In contrast to other viral hepatitides, patients with long-standing chronic HBV infection have an elevated risk for HCC development even in the absence of underlying cirrhosis.[2]

As opposed to HBV infection, most patients infected with HCV advance to chronic HCV, with viremia persisting in up to 86% of infected patients and resulting in variable amounts of hepatic inflammation and fibrosis. The natural course of HCV infection is indolent; 20% to 30% of patients with chronic HCV develop cirrhosis in 20 to 30 years. The risk of developing HCC in patients with HCV cirrhosis has been estimated to be approximately 2% per year. In the absence of cirrhosis, the risk for HCC is considered small.[7]

PATHOLOGY

Hepatitis is defined pathologically by hepatocyte necrosis and hepatic inflammation.[8] In nonfulminant acute hepatitis, the liver is typically enlarged and erythematous with a tense capsule. If there is severe cholestasis, the liver has a noticeable yellow-green color. Microscopically, there is hepatocyte swelling (hepatocellular enlargement and cytoplasmic rarefaction), spotty hepatocellular necrosis and apoptosis, lobular disarray (disruption of the normal architecture of the liver), and mononuclear inflammatory infiltrates. The inflammatory infiltrate is composed of lymphocytes, macrophages, occasional eosinophils, and minimal neutrophils and is predominantly lobular, which contrasts to the portal inflammation typically seen in chronic hepatitis. There may be pronounced canalicular cholestasis and formation of so-called cholestatic rosettes, where regenerating hepatocytes form circular

structures around canalicular bile plugs. Kupffer cells in acute hepatitis are more numerous and hypertrophic, sometimes containing phagocytosed cellular debris and/or golden-brown ceroid pigment.

In fulminant acute hepatitis, the liver is shrunken and soft, with a wrinkled capsule and a mottled cut surface. Fulminant acute hepatitis is divided into either submassive or massive variants. Submassive necrosis is characterized by necrosis of portions of the lobule, typically the centrilobular areas; massive or panlobular necrosis refers to cases in which the entire lobule is affected. Microscopically, there is extensive hepatocyte loss, proliferation of bile ductules, and a mixed inflammatory infiltrate.[9]

Chronic hepatitis is characterized microscopically by a combination of portal inflammation, parenchymal or lobular inflammation, interface hepatitis, spotty hepatocyte necrosis, and progressive fibrosis. Lymphoid follicles may be present and are especially prominent in chronic hepatitis due to HCV. Interface hepatitis, also known as piecemeal necrosis, refers to mononuclear inflammation extending from the limiting plate of the portal tract to envelop adjacent hepatocytes. Affected hepatocytes exhibit degenerative changes, including swelling and apoptosis. Ongoing interface hepatitis causes hepatocyte loss and fibrosis. The end stage of this process is cirrhosis, where dense fibrous bands divide the liver into parenchymal nodules. Progressive hepatic fibrosis with the development of cirrhosis is a feature of almost all chronic liver diseases, including chronic hepatitis.[9]

Certain histologic findings may suggest specific causes. Chronic hepatitis due to HCV is most often mild, is associated with patchy macrovesicular steatosis, and often has prominent lymphoid follicles within the portal triads. HBV is classically associated with so-called ground-glass hepatocytes, which are enlarged hepatocytes with faintly granular eosinophilic cytoplasmic inclusions. These inclusions represent endoplasmic reticulum filled with viral particles, as demonstrated via immunohistochemistry.[9]

Currently, liver biopsy is the gold standard for diagnosis, staging, and follow-up of chronic liver disease. However, liver biopsy has limitations, such as high costs, a false-negative rate of up to 24%, a sampling error rate ranging from 25% to 40%, and morbidity and fatality rates of 3% and 0.3%, respectively.[10] These limitations restrict its use as a method for longitudinal monitoring at a population level. Therefore, it is vital that noninvasive methods for the assessment of liver fibrosis be developed and validated.

IMAGING

Acute Hepatitis

Because acute hepatitis is diagnosed by clinical examination and liver function tests, imaging studies play a limited role in evaluating patients with this condition. The imaging findings are nonspecific and may include hepatomegaly and gallbladder wall thickening (Fig. 69-1). If steatohepatitis is present, diffuse fat deposition dominates the imaging findings. Other features may include parenchymal heterogeneity, accentuation of the portal triads, and heterogeneous perfusion (Fig. 69-2).[11]

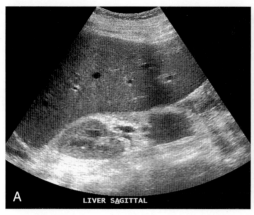
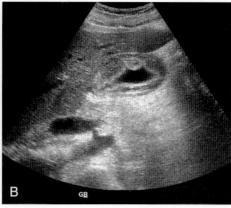

■ **FIGURE 69-1** Acute hepatitis in a 28-year-old woman due to acetaminophen overdose. **A,** Sagittal ultrasound image shows an enlarged liver that measures 21 cm in length. **B,** Oblique ultrasound image through the left lobe of the liver demonstrates a markedly thickened gallbladder.

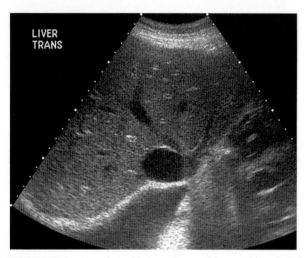

■ **FIGURE 69-2** Acute hepatitis in a 19-year-old man with a clinical history of acute hepatitis. Transverse ultrasound image of the liver shows mild prominence of portal triads.

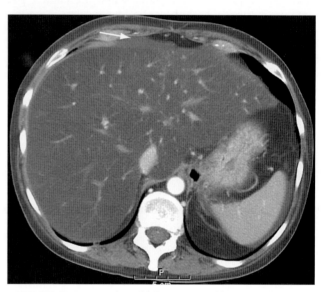

■ **FIGURE 69-3** Acute hepatitis in a 35-year-old woman who presented to the emergency department with acute severe hepatitis. CT shows an enlarged liver with severe fat accumulation. Note that the attenuation of the liver is lower than that of ascites (*arrow*). She died 6 days later of fulminant liver failure.

In patients with an atypical clinical presentation, imaging may be performed to assess for biliary obstruction, cholangitis, or vascular occlusion. In cases with fulminant presentations, imaging may assess the extent of necrosis and exclude complications of acute hepatitis, such as ascites and spontaneous hepatic rupture. Because of its portability, low cost, and widespread availability, transabdominal ultrasonography is the most common imaging modality used initially in these clinical settings, although CT may be performed as well (Fig. 69-3).

CT

The CT findings in acute hepatitis are also nonspecific, including hepatomegaly, gallbladder wall thickening, and periportal edema, which manifests as low attenuation regions along the portal triads. Additionally, after the intravenous injection of contrast material, the liver parenchyma may enhance heterogeneously. Patchy areas of arterial phase hyperenhancement may be visible and superficially resemble the appearance of an infiltrative malignancy. A key distinguishing feature is that perfu-

sional hyperenhancement due to acute inflammation fades to isoattenuation during the venous phases; by comparison, infiltrative malignancies tend to appear heterogeneous and wash out to hypoattenuation during the venous phases.[12]

MRI

MRI is not commonly used in the assessment of patients with acute hepatitis. However, some MRI findings, such as heterogeneous hepatic signal intensity most apparent on T2-weighted (T2W) images, periportal edema presenting as low signal on T1-weighted (T1W) and high signal on T2W images, and irregular patchy areas of abnormal increased heterogeneous enhancement seen on the arterial phase immediately after intravenous contrast agent administration, have been described in patient with acute hepatitis. These MRI findings are analogous to the ones reported with contrast-enhanced CT.[13]

Ultrasonography

There are no specific ultrasonographic findings in acute hepatitis, although hepatomegaly may be appreciated. Other findings may include heterogeneous echotexture, gallbladder wall thickening, and accentuation of the portal triads (see Figs. 69-1 and 69-2). Ultrasonography is operator dependent, however, and these findings have limited reproducibility.[11]

Imaging Algorithm

Patients presenting with a clinical history of malaise, nausea, anorexia, fever, and right upper quadrant abdominal pain associated with jaundice and pruritus should be investigated promptly with liver function tests and an abdominal ultrasound evaluation. When the clinical presentation is atypical or there is a finding of concern evident on ultrasonography, CT is recommended for optimal assessment of the liver and biliary system (Table 69-1). CT is helpful to rule out the presence of biliary obstruction, cholangitis, or vascular occlusion. Meanwhile, in patients with fulminant presentations, CT is also performed to assess the extent of necrosis and to exclude complications such as ascites and spontaneous hepatic rupture. Conversely, MRI is infrequently used in the assessment of patients with acute hepatitis and usually is reserved for patients with contraindications for the use of intravenous iodine contrast and for further imaging characterization.

Classic Signs: Acute Hepatitis

■ There are no reliable signs for acute hepatitis on any modality.

■ The most common findings are nonspecific, such as hepatomegaly and gallbladder wall thickening.

■ Nonspecific findings also include parenchymal heterogeneity, accentuation of the portal triads, periportal edema, and heterogeneous perfusion.

TABLE 69-1 Accuracy and Limitations of the Modalities Used in Imaging of Acute Hepatitis

Modality	Accuracy	Limitations
CT	Performed most frequently in the evaluation of affected patients due to widespread availability and ease of use	Has low sensitivity and specificity for the diagnosis of acute hepatitis
MRI	Infrequently used in the assessment of patients with acute hepatitis	Has low sensitivity and specificity for the diagnosis of acute hepatitis
Ultrasonography	Performed most frequently in the evaluation of affected patients due to widespread availability and ease of use	

Chronic Hepatitis

Until recently, the role of imaging studies in patients with chronic hepatitis was limited to the identification of individuals with cirrhosis or its complications and the early detection of HCC. Using standard ultrasonography, CT, and MRI techniques, the liver usually has a normal imaging appearance in patients with chronic viral hepatitis until cirrhosis has developed. Other possible findings include nonspecific parenchymal heterogeneity, heterogeneous enhancement after intravenous contrast agent administration, and lymphadenopathy. Lymphadenopathy, in particular, is an important consideration because it is present in up to 65% of cases and may be the only indication of chronic active hepatitis in up to 35% of cases.[12] The lymph nodes of the porta hepatis, hepatoduodenal ligament, and retroperitoneum are most commonly involved.

Once cirrhosis becomes evident, the imaging features of end-stage liver disease secondary to chronic hepatitis are similar to those of other causes of cirrhosis (Fig. 69-4). Morphologic changes of cirrhosis are neither sensitive nor specific for precirrhotic liver disease. In some patients, hepatomegaly and heterogeneity of the hepatic parenchyma may be seen during the precirrhotic stages of disease progression, but these findings are nonspecific.

In recent years, the rising prevalence of chronic hepatitis in Western nations has spurred the development of noninvasive, imaging-based techniques to assess parenchymal inflammation, hepatocellular injury (necroinflammation), and liver fibrosis. All such techniques are currently considered experimental, and none has been validated in large clinical trials. This chapter briefly describes experimental techniques that attempt to diagnose and stage liver fibrosis. The reader is referred elsewhere for a discussion of the techniques aimed at assessing inflammation and hepatocellular injury.

CT

CT is frequently used in the assessment and monitoring of patients with chronic liver disease because it accurately demonstrates the intrahepatic and extrahepatic manifestations of cirrhosis and portal hypertension. However, CT is insensitive in assessing precirrhotic liver disease and early stages of fibrosis. Recently, the use of an imaging processing method based on textural analysis for assessing liver fibrosis using unenhanced CT scans ("fibro-CT") was reported.[13] The fibrosis stage estimated by fibro-CT was closely correlated with the histologic fibrosis stage ascertained by biopsy, suggesting a possible role for fibro-CT in the longitudinal monitoring of patients with chronic hepatitis. Validation in independent studies is necessary before this approach can be recommended.

MRI

MRI, due to its intrinsic contrast resolution, is more sensitive than CT in the assessment of patients with chronic liver disease. Conventional MR sequences can easily depict the morphologic changes associated with cirrhosis and the signs suggestive of portal hypertension. During the precirrhotic stages of liver disease, heterogeneity of

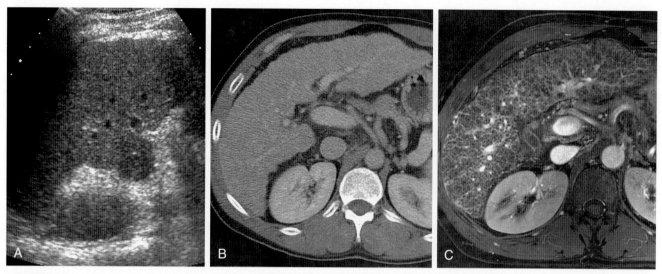

■ **FIGURE 69-4** Ultrasound, CT, and MRI findings in a 59-year-old man with cirrhosis due to chronic hepatitis C. **A,** Transverse ultrasound image shows nodular contours of the liver and a diffusely heterogeneous parenchymal echotexture. **B,** Axial postcontrast CT image during the portal venous phase shows nodularity of the liver surface, atrophy of the right lobe, and widening of the porta hepatis. **C,** Axial combined contrast-enhanced MR image additionally shows hyperintense reticulations throughout the liver parenchyma. Note the innumerable hypointense regenerative nodules carpeting the liver diffusely. Discrete regenerative nodules and fibrotic scars are not visible on ultrasound or CT images.

hepatic parenchyma may be seen after intravenous contrast agent administration; however, this finding is nonspecific and has not been shown to permit noninvasive staging of liver fibrosis.

Recently, diverse experimental MR techniques have been used for assessment of liver fibrosis in chronic hepatitis, including combined double-contrast–enhanced MRI, diffusion-weighted imaging, MR elastography, MR spectroscopy, and MR perfusion.[14]

Double-Contrast–Enhanced MRI

Double-contrast–enhanced MRI refers to MRI after the sequential administration of superparamagnetic iron oxides (SPIOs) and gadolinium chelates. After intravenous administration, SPIOs accumulate in hepatic Kupffer cells, causing hypointensity of the liver parenchyma on appropriately weighted gradient-echo images. Subsequent administration of gadolinium promotes delayed enhancement of hepatic septal fibrosis, which augments the image contrast between the low-signal liver parenchyma and the high-signal fibrotic reticulations (Figs. 69-5 and 69-6). In the relatively rare patient with endogenous iron accumulation in liver due to hemochromatosis or secondary hemosiderosis (see Chapter 67), administration of SPIO is unnecessary and the use of gadolinium alone suffices.

Double-contrast–enhanced MRI has been shown to have high sensitivity, specificity, and accuracy for differentiating patients with advanced fibrosis from those with absent or mild fibrosis.[15] Prospective clinical trials assessing the accuracy of this technique for staging liver fibrosis are being done (Fig. 69-7). An important limitation of this technique is the high cost associated with the use of two contrast agents. In principle, the use of two agents also may increase risk, but preliminary studies suggest the double contrast-enhanced technique is safe. Another limitation is that accurate assessment of liver texture for purposes of staging fibrosis requires the acquisition of

high-quality images with high signal-to-noise ratio and free of breathing and other motion artifacts; the generation of such images is not possible in all patients with current MR technology.

Diffusion-Weighted MRI

Diffusion-weighted imaging assesses the diffusion of protons within tissue and is quantified by the apparent diffusion coefficient (ADC). Diffusion-weighted imaging uses preparatory pulses that cause diffusing protons to lose signal. The amount of signal loss is influenced by the strength of the diffusion weighting (the b-value of the sequence) and the ability of protons to diffuse through tissue (the ADC of the tissue). Brain diffusion-weighted imaging has been performed clinically for nearly 20 years, but liver diffusion-weighted imaging has a much shorter history.[16]

Until recently, high-quality liver diffusion-weighted imaging was not achievable because of the relatively short T2 of liver, unavoidable physiologic motion in the abdomen, susceptibility effects, and other factors. However, the recent implementation of high performance gradients and parallel imaging has improved the quality of diffusion-weighted imaging of the liver.[17] With these advances, diffusion-weighted imaging has emerged as an experimental method for MRI diagnosis of fibrosis. A central hypothesis of this method is that fibrosis restricts water diffusion. Studies using fat-suppressed (or water-excited) diffusion-weighted echoplanar imaging have shown reduced ADC in cirrhosis of various causes (Figs. 69-8 and 69-9).[18]

Mean ADC values have been shown to be significantly lower in cirrhotic patients than in controls (1.11 ± 0.16 vs. $1.54 \pm 0.12 \times 10^{-3}$ mm^2/s, respectively; $P < .0001$) in one study, for example.[19] Additionally, the sensitivity and specificity for a cutoff of 1.31×10^{-3} mm^2/s were 93% and 100%, respectively.[19] Anisotropy has not been observed.

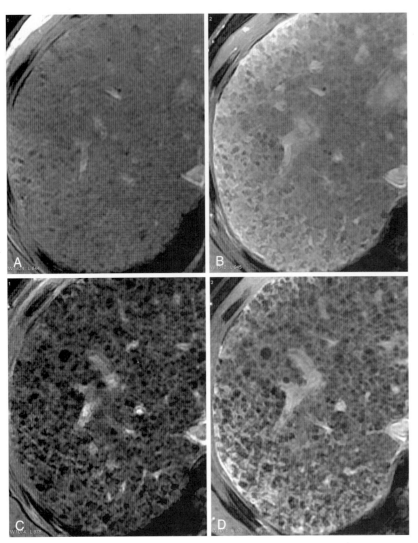

■ **FIGURE 69-5** MRI features of fibrosis and regenerative nodules in a 63-year-old cirrhotic man with hepatitis C. All images were acquired with the same imaging parameters within 1 week of each other. The unenhanced image (**A**) shows mild heterogeneity of the liver, as well as a few scattered regenerative nodules. After gadolinium administration, fibrotic reticulations enhance and appear hyperintense (**B**). Compared with the unenhanced image, regenerative nodules on the image obtained with SPIO enhancement (**C**) have become more hypointense due to T2* shortening from phagocytic uptake by Kupffer cells. Double contrast-enhanced image (**D**) shows hyperintense fibrotic reticulations sharply delineated against hypointense nodules.

Studies assessing the accuracy of diffusion-weighted imaging for staging liver fibrosis over the entire spectrum of disease severity (from normal to cirrhosis) have reported inconsistent results.[20]

A limitation of diffusion-weighted imaging is that it measures a surrogate of fibrosis, ADC, rather than directly visualizing fibrosis in vivo. Clinical diagnosis relies on the quantitative estimation of ADC and may be confounded by motion-related and other artifacts. Reported ADCs are variable, with considerable overlap between normal and abnormal ranges, indicating that technical factors may lead to differences in estimated ADC. This suggests the need to develop site- and technique-specific normal ranges, which may impede widespread implementation of this technique. Perfusion effects also may confound ADC estimations.[19] Other confounders may include hepatic steatosis, hepatic iron, and liver inflammation. The latter may be associated with cellular infiltration or edema, processes that inherently may have opposite effects on ADC.[20]

MR Elastography

MR elastography is an MRI sequence that noninvasively quantifies the mean tissue stiffness.[21] This technique is based on the biologic concept that the rigidity of tissues increases as the severity of disease progresses. In brief, a mechanical driver delivers mechanical oscillatory waves into the patient's abdomen at a predetermined frequency. Images are acquired as the waves propagate through the liver and other abdominal organs, and the shear waves are imaged. The displacement of the shear waves is determined and converted into an MR elastogram, a 2D map of the tissue shear stiffness (in kilopascals) within the abdomen at the level of the slice in which the gradient echoes were obtained. Regions of interest can be placed on the portion of the map corresponding to the liver and the stiffness of the liver recorded (Fig. 69-10).[22]

Studies have shown that liver stiffness measurements correlate with the stage of fibrosis, with mean liver shear stiffness significantly higher in patients with histologic liver fibrosis versus healthy volunteers.[22,23] MR elastography has been advocated by some investigators as an accurate noninvasive method for assessment of liver fibrosis. In one study, MR elastography had a sensitivity of 98% and specificity of 100% at a shear stiffness cutoff value of 2.5 kPa for fibrosis stages greater than or equal to F2 and a sensitivity of 95% and specificity of 100% at a cutoff value of 3.1 kPa for stages greater than or equal to F3.[24]

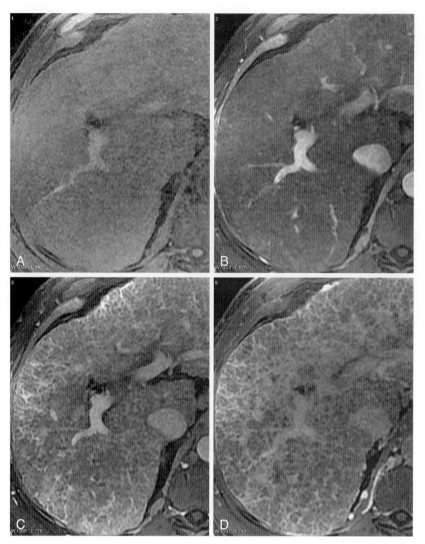

■ **FIGURE 69-6** MRI features of fibrosis. Double contrast-enhanced 3D dynamic gradient-echo images of the liver in a 54-year-old cirrhotic man with chronic hepatitis C. Unenhanced (**A**) and arterial (20 s) (**B**), portal venous (80 s) (**C**), delayed (240 s) (**D**) images were obtained after gadolinium administration. Iron oxides were administered before the dynamic series, and so all images are also enhanced with SPIO. After gadolinium administration, fibrous septa progressively enhance and achieve maximum enhancement at the delayed phase.

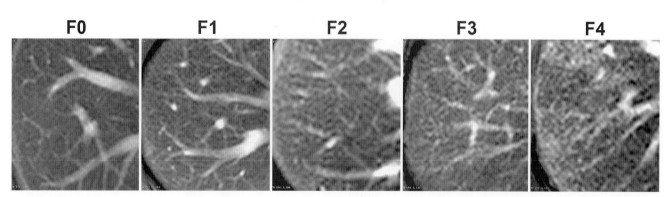

F0 F1 F2 F3 F4

■ **FIGURE 69-7** Noninvasive staging of liver fibrosis. Double-contrast–enhanced gradient-echo MR images show progressive reticulation in liver parenchyma of five different patients with various stages of liver fibrosis ranging from normal (F0) to cirrhosis (F4).

Although promising, MR elastography has some limitations, the main one being that, like diffusion-weighted imaging, it measures a surrogate of liver fibrosis (shear stiffness) rather than the fibrosis itself. Additionally, it requires a purely quantitative approach and is not amenable to qualitative analysis, precluding the radiologist's subjectivity. Another challenge is that the MR elastograms tend to

be heterogeneous, and results may vary depending on the exact location in which the regions of interest are placed.

Moreover, using currently available techniques, MR elastography does not work in patients with moderate or severe iron overload; the imaging technique employs relatively long echo times, and the signal intensity of the iron-overloaded liver is not adequate for imaging the

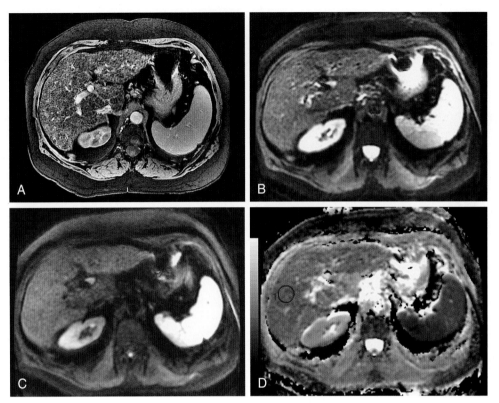

■ **FIGURE 69-8** Diffusion-weighted imaging of liver in a 58-year-old-woman with cirrhosis due to hepatitis C. **A,** Double-contrast–enhanced MR image shows reticulations and regenerative nodules consistent with cirrhosis. Images with b-values of 0 (**B**) and 500 s/mm^2 (**C**) and an apparent diffusion coefficient map (**D**) are seen. The estimated apparent diffusion coefficient in the region of interest was 1.05×10^{-3} mm^2/s. This indicates relatively restricted diffusion.

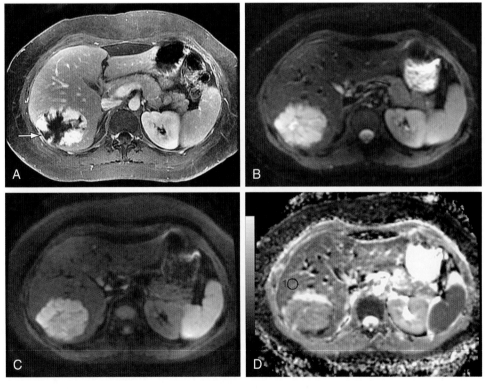

■ **FIGURE 69-9** Diffusion-weighted imaging of a 21-year-old-woman with normal liver except for hemangioma. **A,** Gadolinium-enhanced image during portal venous phase shows large hemangioma with globular peripheral puddles of enhancement (*arrow*). Liver parenchyma is normal. Images have b-values of 0 (**B**) and 500 s/mm^2 (**C**). **D,** Apparent diffusion coefficient map. The estimated coefficient at the region of interest was 1.55×10^{-3} mm^2/s, suggesting normal liver parenchyma.

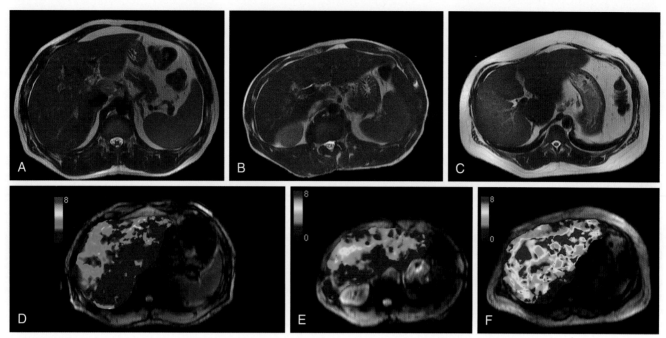

■ **FIGURE 69-10**   MR elastography staging of liver fibrosis. Axial single-shot fast spin-echo (**A-C**) and MR elastographic (**D-F**) images in three different patients with biopsy-proven F0 classification (no fibrosis, **A, D**), F2 (moderate fibrosis, **B, E**), and F4 (cirrhosis, **C, F**). The estimated tissue stiffness was 2, 4, and 6 kPa. As illustrated in this example, liver stiffness appears to correlate with the degree of liver fibrosis.

hepatic shear waves. This limitation may be overcome in the future by using images with shorter echo times. In principle, MR elastographic assessment of liver fibrosis may be confounded by a variety of factors expected to augment liver stiffness, including hepatic inflammation, hepatic congestion, cholestasis, and portal hypertension. Further study will be needed to determine whether these potential confounders affect the accuracy of MR elastography for fibrosis staging.

MR Spectroscopy

MR spectroscopy enables the noninvasive measurement of metabolic processes in vivo.[25] In-vivo MR spectroscopy is most commonly used to assess signals from hydrogen (^{1}H) and phosphorus (^{31}P). ^{1}H MR spectroscopy generates a spectrum of the various resonances of protons that are embedded in different chemical bonds within a variety of tissues.[26]

Some researchers have concluded that ^{1}H MR spectroscopy may be a valid substitute for liver biopsy in the assessment of chronic hepatitis.[25] This is illustrated by findings in which the mean value of the metabolite-to-lipid ratios of glutamate complex, phosphomonoesters, and glucose complex increase significantly with increasing stage of fibrosis seen on liver biopsy. In the end, however, MR spectroscopy is limited because findings such as this have not been reproduced and it is technically difficult to perform and interpret, relegating its use mainly to academic research centers.

MR Perfusion

Another promising MRI method is perfusion imaging. Progressive liver fibrosis gradually obliterates normal intrahe-patic vessels and sinusoids and slows passage of blood through the parenchyma. Additionally, as portal hypertension develops, portal venous flow to the liver decreases, hepatic arterial flow increases, and intrahepatic shunts form. These physiologic alterations can be detected by kinetic models of dynamic image datasets acquired rapidly after bolus intravenous injection of paramagnetic extracellular contrast agents. Several perfusion parameters can be estimated, including absolute portal venous blood flow, absolute arterial blood flow, absolute total liver blood flow, portal venous fraction, arterial fraction, distribution volume, and mean transit time.

A recent study applied a dual-input kinetic model for the noninvasive assessment of liver fibrosis.[27] The dual input approach models two sources of blood flow into the liver, via the hepatic artery and portal vein, and assumes a single tissue compartment. Significant differences were found in several perfusion parameters between patients with and without advanced fibrosis: those with advanced fibrosis had increased absolute arterial blood flow, arterial fraction, distribution volume, and mean transit time. Additionally, the distribution volume parameter demonstrated a sensitivity of 77% and a specificity of 79% for the diagnosis of advanced fibrosis.

Similar to diffusion-weighted imaging and MR elastography, MR perfusion is limited because it measures surrogate markers of liver fibrosis rather than the fibrosis itself. Several factors may confound the correlation between perfusion parameters and fibrosis, including cardiac status, fasting state, hepatic congestion, hepatic inflammation, hepatic lesions, and portal vein disturbances. Other limitations include the need for modeling assumptions, which may be only partially correct, and the requirement of very rapid imaging, which leads to compromises in image quality and/or coverage. Images acquired for perfusion analysis generally are not suitable for assessment of structural abnormalities such as small nodules, and a second contrast injection may be necessary. Additionally, the image analysis is laborious and requires placement of co-localized regions of interest on the input vessels (aorta and portal vein) and tissue of interest (liver) on a large number of different acquisitions. Sophisticated and automatic methods of misregistration correction software will be required before this technique is widely implemented.

Ultrasonography

Ultrasound Perfusion Imaging

Ultrasound perfusion, or contrast-enhanced ultrasonography, is performed after the intravenous administration of a contrast medium containing microbubbles. Contrast-enhanced ultrasonography measures the transit time of the microbubbles from the injection site to the hepatic veins. As opposed to MR perfusion, in which advanced fibrosis was associated with an increase in transit time though the liver,[27] advanced fibrosis via contrast-enhanced ultrasonography as measured by microbubbles is associated with reduced transit time. This apparent paradox is explained by the fact that ultrasound microbubbles are blood pool agents; the reduced transit time probably reflects the presence of intrahepatic shunts, which allow the direct passage of microbubbles from the hepatic artery to the hepatic vein.[28] In comparison, the contrast media used in MR perfusion are extracellular agents; the increased transit time may therefore reflect delayed passage of the agent through the hepatic extracellular space.[27]

Contrast-enhanced ultrasonography is limited in its assessment of liver fibrosis because it is highly specialized and technically difficult to perform and interpret. Additionally, results depend on the size and type of the microbubbles and do not take into consideration potential confounders such as cardiac status, hepatic congestion, hepatic inflammation, and presence of hepatic lesions.

Ultrasound Transient Elastography

Ultrasound transient elastography ("Fibroscan") is a relatively new ultrasound-based technology that involves acquisition of pulse-echo ultrasound signals to measure liver stiffness. The probe transmits a vibration of mild amplitude and low frequency toward the liver, which in turn induces an elastic shear wave that propagates through the liver. Pulse-echo ultrasound acquisitions are performed to follow the propagation of the shear wave and measure its velocity, which is directly related to tissue stiffness. The harder the tissue, the faster the shear wave propagates. As with MR elastography, results are expressed in kilopascals (kPa).[29] However, ultrasound elastography measures the Young modulus of elasticity, whereas MR elastography measures the shear modulus; thus, stiffness measurements made by ultrasound elastography and MR elastography differ.

Several European studies have shown promising performance characteristics of Fibroscan in patients with viral hepatitis. A recent review of Fibroscan in patients with chronic hepatitis C with paired liver biopsies demonstrated that the stiffness cutoff values for diagnosis of significant fibrosis (F ≥ 2), and cirrhosis (F = 4) ranged from 4 to 8.8 kPa and from 11.9 to 16 kPa.[29] Another review reported an accuracy of 84%, 89%, and 94% for the diagnosis of significant fibrosis (F ≥ 2), severe fibrosis (F ≥ 3), and cirrhosis (F = 4), respectively.[30]

Ultrasound elastography is advantageous over other noninvasive techniques described in this chapter because it is rapid, relatively inexpensive, and widely available. However, as with other ultrasound-based techniques, it is operator dependent, is limited by overlying abdominal gas, has reduced penetration in patients with increased subcutaneous fat, and may not be reproducible. Additionally, the technique has a restricted volume of interrogation, has a cylinder about 1 cm in diameter and 2 cm long, and does not permit assessment of the whole liver, allowing for the possibility of sampling errors.[30]

Imaging Algorithm

It is recommended that patients with cirrhosis secondary to chronic hepatitis receive imaging to assess for sequelae of portal hypertension and screen for HCC. Ultrasonography and CT are usually the imaging studies performed initially in patients who have advanced to cirrhosis (Table 69-2). Ultrasonography depicts a liver usually decreased in size with heterogeneous echotexture and is useful for assessing portal venous flow direction and waveforms. CT better demonstrates the hepatic morphologic changes of advanced fibrosis and extrahepatic sequelae of portal hypertension. MRI can subsequently be utilized if the CT is equivocal or to better characterize nodules. Some centers routinely use CT or MRI in their HCC screening and surveillance protocols despite the fact that the American Association for the Study of Liver Diseases (AASLD) advocates the use of ultrasonography.

Imaging-based techniques to noninvasively assess liver fibrosis are in development. Although promising, these techniques have not yet been validated to replace liver biopsy and further investigation in large clinical trials is still necessary.

Classic Signs: Chronic Hepatitis

- Other than the findings associated with cirrhosis, the imaging signs of precirrhotic disease are nonspecific.
- Conventional techniques using ultrasonography, CT, and MRI may show a normal liver, nonspecific parenchymal heterogeneity, lymphadenopathy, and/or heterogeneous enhancement after intravenous contrast agent administration.

DIFFERENTIAL DIAGNOSIS

The clinical differential diagnosis of acute hepatitis includes all hepatic insults resulting in the signs, symptoms, and laboratory abnormalities described in earlier sections. These causes include exposure to various toxins or toxin ingestion (e.g., acetaminophen or alcohol),

TABLE 69-2 Accuracy and Limitations of the Modalities Used in Imaging of Chronic Hepatitis

Modality	Accuracy	Limitations
CT	Conventional CT has low sensitivity for detection of fibrosis and early cirrhosis. CT has high sensitivity for detection of advanced cirrhosis.	Ionizing radiation Risk of intravenous contrast agent reactions
MRI: conventional	Conventional MRI has low sensitivity for detection of fibrosis and early cirrhosis. MRI has high sensitivity for detection of advanced cirrhosis.	Patient-limiting factors (e.g., pacemaker, claustrophobia, cooperation) High cost Not widely available
MRI: double-contrast enhanced	90% sensitivity, specificity, and accuracy for prediction of advanced fibrosis (fibrosis stage ≥ F3)	
MRI diffusion	Sensitivity of 93% and specificity of 100% for differentiating cirrhotic from normal livers (apparent diffusion coefficient cutoff value of 1.31×10^{-3} mm^2/s).	
MR elastography	Sensitivity of 98% and specificity of 100% for detecting fibrosis stages greater than or equal to F2 (shear modulus stiffness cutoff value of 2.5 kPa). Sensitivity of 95% and specificity of 100% in detecting fibrosis stages greater than or equal to F3 (shear modulus stiffness cutoff value of 3.1 kPa).	
MR perfusion	Depending on the perfusion parameter, sensitivity up to 77% and specificity up to 79% for prediction of advanced fibrosis	
Ultrasound elastography	Accuracy ranging from 73% to 84% for detection of fibrosis stages greater than or equal to F2 Accuracy ranging from 87% to 96% for detection of fibrosis stages greater than or equal to F3 Accuracy ranging from 93% to 100% for detection of fibrosis stage F4 Optimal stiffness cutoff values of 8.7 for fibrosis stages greater than or equal to F2 and 14.5 kPa for fibrosis stage F4	Poor performance in the cases of obesity or overlying bowel gas Operator dependent

metabolic disease (Wilson's disease), and autoimmune hepatitis. They are generally easily distinguishable by obtaining a complete history (e.g., ruling out toxin ingestion or exposure, travel history, risk factors for viral hepatitis, presence of other autoimmune diseases) and evaluating copper studies, autoimmune markers, and viral hepatitis serologic studies.

The clinical differential diagnosis of chronic hepatitis is similar to that of the various causes of cirrhosis. As with acute hepatitis, a careful history and evaluation of laboratory studies provides direction. Liver biopsy may also be helpful in distinguishing some processes.

Acute Hepatitis

The imaging findings of acute hepatitis are nonspecific. Hepatomegaly is one of the most frequent findings and has a broad differential diagnosis that can be divided into systemic and local causes. Among the hepatic causes of hepatomegaly, hepatitis is one of the most commonly seen. Additional causes of hepatomegaly may include lymphoproliferative diseases, toxic and drug-related diseases, metabolic disorders, vascular disorders, hematologic disorders, biliary disease, autoimmune liver disease, and other conditions, such as obesity, diabetes mellitus, and connective tissue diseases. The differential diagnosis of gallbladder wall thickening includes primary and secondary causes. The most common secondary causes include liver cirrhosis, hepatitis, congestive heart failure, and pancreatitis. Almost all diseases that affect the liver can cause parenchymal heterogeneity. The ones that interfere with the hepatic vascular supply may also cause heterogeneous perfusion after the intravenous injection of a contrast agent. In cases of hepatic rupture and necrosis, the differential diagnosis includes trauma, fatty liver, acute fulminant liver failure, focal liver lesions such as adenomas and HCCs, acetaminophen overdose, blood dyscrasias, and drug toxicity, among others.

Chronic Hepatitis

Presence of abdominal lymphadenopathy has a wide differential diagnosis. Because abdominal lymphadenopathy is most commonly detected in patients with lymphoproliferative disorders or metastatic disease, knowledge of existence of a primary malignancy is crucial in the differential diagnosis. Additionally, a large number of benign diseases may also present as abdominal lymphadenopathy, such as infectious diseases (abdominal tuberculosis and acquired immunodeficiency syndrome), noninfectious diseases, and other less frequent diseases (e.g., Whipple's and Crohn's diseases). Cirrhosis can be caused by a large number of different causes, including alcohol abuse, chronic viral hepatitis (especially hepatitis B and C), drug toxicity, primary biliary cirrhosis, primary sclerosing cholangitis, nonalcoholic steatohepatitis, autoimmune hepatitis, and hemochromatosis. Other less common causes include congestive changes, both veno-occlusive and secondary to prolonged congestive heart failure; congenital hepatic fibrosis; cryptogenic cirrhosis; and hereditary causes, such as Wilson's disease, α_1-antitrypsin deficiency, tyrosinemia, galactosemia, cystic fibrosis, and glycogen storage diseases. The imaging findings of cirrhosis are better described in Chapter 66. Imaging usually does not permit reliable differential diagnosis of causes of cirrhosis, but some findings may be suggestive of some causes over others, including enlarged liver with cirrhosis in alcoholic and nonalcoholic steatohepatitis, segmental or subsegmental areas of nodular regeneration in primary sclerosing cholangitis, presence of confluent fibrosis in alcoholic steatohepatitis, markedly enlarged caudate in Budd-Chiari syndrome, and portal halos in primary biliary cirrhosis.

TREATMENT

Medical Treatment

The treatment of acute hepatitis is largely supportive, because the symptomatic phases of most cases resolve spontaneously after a few weeks. An exception to this is patients with acute HBV infection, who are often started on antiviral therapy.

Treatment options for chronic hepatitis are reserved for patients with hepatitis B or C (there are no established therapies for HAV or HEV; HDV is managed by treating the underlying hepatitis B co-infection or superinfection). There are a variety of antiviral agents available for the treatment of chronic HBV, including lamivudine, adefovir, entecavir, and others. HCV infection, on the other hand, has a single effective regimen, consisting of interferon and ribavirin.

Surgical Treatment

Liver transplantation is the only accepted surgical treatment for acute hepatitis that has progressed to fulminant hepatic failure or chronic hepatitis that has advanced to cirrhosis and/or HCC. Cirrhosis secondary to HCV is the most common indication of liver transplantation in the United States, accounting for approximately 2000 transplants annually.

What the Referring Physician Needs to Know

ACUTE HEPATITIS

- Acute hepatitis refers to hepatocyte damage and inflammation of less than 6 months' duration.
- The main causes of acute hepatitis are viral, toxin-mediated, metabolic (Wilson's disease), and autoimmune.
- Hepatitis B is the most common viral infection in sub-Saharan Africa and Asia, whereas hepatitis C predominates in the United States.
- Most cases of acute hepatitis resolve spontaneously after a few weeks, although, rarely, some may progress to fulminant disease requiring liver transplantation.

CHRONIC HEPATITIS

- Chronic hepatitis refers to hepatocyte damage and inflammation lasting longer than 6 months; sometimes it may progress to fibrosis and cirrhosis.
- The causes of chronic hepatitis mirror those of cirrhosis in general but, as a rule, are significantly represented by hepatitis B and C infection.
- Regardless of its underlying cause, once cirrhosis develops, patients are at risk for the complications of portal hypertension (e.g., ascites, variceal hemorrhage, hepatic encephalopathy) and HCC.
- Chronic hepatitis B may result in HCC in the absence of underlying cirrhosis.

KEY POINTS

Acute Hepatitis

- Imaging studies have a limited role in the diagnosis of acute hepatitis.
- When performed, imaging findings of acute hepatitis are nonspecific.
- The most common findings, regardless of modality, are hepatomegaly and gallbladder wall thickening, with other nonspecific findings including heterogeneous parenchyma, accentuation of the portal triads, and periportal edema.
- Imaging may be helpful in atypical clinical presentations to assess for biliary obstruction, cholangitis, or vascular occlusion.
- In fulminant presentations, imaging may assess the extent of necrosis and exclude complications such as ascites and spontaneous hepatic rupture.

Chronic Hepatitis

- Imaging studies are performed to monitor development of cirrhosis and permit early diagnosis of HCC.

- Conventional ultrasonography, CT, and MRI techniques do not permit assessment of precirrhotic stages of chronic hepatitis.
- Possible findings of conventional imaging in precirrhotic stages include a normal liver, nonspecific parenchymal heterogeneity, lymphadenopathy in the porta hepatis, hepatoduodenal ligament and/or retroperitoneum, and heterogeneous enhancement after intravenous contrast agent administration.
- MRI is the most accurate noninvasive diagnostic modality for the diagnosis of cirrhosis and, in patients who have advanced to cirrhosis, for depiction of fibrosis and regenerative nodules.
- The imaging findings of cirrhosis due to chronic hepatitis overlap with those of other causes of cirrhosis.
- Experimental techniques to assess liver fibrosis noninvasively are under development and may eventually replace liver biopsy.

SUGGESTED READINGS

Afdhal NH, Nunes D. Evaluation of liver fibrosis: a concise review. Am J Gastroenterol 2004; 99:1160-1174.

Baldwin SL. Diffuse benign liver disease. Radiol Technol 2007; 78:476-490.

Brancatelli G, Federle MP, Ambrosini R, et al. Cirrhosis: CT and MR imaging evaluation. Eur J Radiol 2007; 61:57-69.

Danrad R, Martin DR. MR imaging of diffuse liver diseases. Magn Reson Imaging Clin North Am 2005; 13:277-293, vi.

Fischbach F, Bruhn H. Assessment of in vivo (1)H magnetic resonance spectroscopy in the liver: a review. Liver Int 2008; 28:297-307.

Ito K, Mitchell DG. Imaging diagnosis of cirrhosis and chronic hepatitis. Intervirology 2004; 47:134-143.

Margolis DJ, Hoffman JM, Herfkens RJ, et al. Molecular imaging techniques in body imaging. Radiology 2007; 245:333-356.

Rockey DC. Noninvasive assessment of liver fibrosis and portal hypertension with transient elastography. Gastroenterology 2008; 134:8-14.

Talwalkar JA, Yin M, Fidler JL, et al. Magnetic resonance imaging of hepatic fibrosis: emerging clinical applications. Hepatology 2008; 47:332-342.

Yin M, Talwalkar JA, Glaser KJ, et al. Assessment of hepatic fibrosis with magnetic resonance elastography. Clin Gastroenterol Hepatol 2007; 5:1207-1213.

REFERENCES

1. Wasley A, Miller JR, Finelli L. Surveillance for acute viral hepatitis—United States, 2005. MMWR Surveill Summ 2007; 56:1-24.

2. Ganem D, Prince AM. Hepatitis B viral infection—natural history and clinical consequences. N Engl J Med 2004; 350:1118-1129.

3. Lauer GM, Walker BD. Hepatitis C virus infection. N Engl J Med 2001; 345:41-52.

4. Fattovich G, Giustina G, Christensen E, et al. Influence of hepatitis delta virus infection on morbidity and mortality in compensated cirrhosis type B. The European Concerted Action on Viral Hepatitis (Eurohep). Gut 2000; 46:420-426.

5. Balayan MS. Epidemiology of hepatitis E virus infection. J Viral Hepat 1997; 4:155-165.

6. Taylor RM, Davern T, Munoz S, et al. Fulminant hepatitis A virus infection in the United States: incidence, prognosis, and outcomes. Hepatology 2006; 44:1589-1597.

7. Hu KQ, Tong MJ. The long-term outcomes of patients with compensated hepatitis C virus-related cirrhosis and history of parenteral exposure in the United States. Hepatology 1999; 29:1311-1316.

8. Lamps LW, Washington K. Acute and chronic hepatitis. In Odze RD, Goldblum JR, Crawford JM (eds). Surgical Pathology of the GI Tract, Liver, Biliary Tract, and Pancreas. Philadelphia, Elsevier, 2004, p 783.

9. Theise ND, Bodenheimer HC, Ferrell LD. Acute and chronic viral hepatitis. In Burt AD, Portmann BC, Ferrell LD (eds). MacSween's Pathology of the Liver, 5th ed. Philadelphia, Elsevier, 2007, p 405.

10. Thampanitchawong P, Piratvisuth T. Liver biopsy: complications and risk factors. World J Gastroenterol 1999; 5:301-304.

11. Tchelepi H, Ralls PW, Radin R, Grant E. Sonography of diffuse liver disease. J Ultrasound Med 2002; 21:1023-1032.

12. Gore RM, Vogelzang RL, Nemcek AA Jr. Lymphadenopathy in chronic active hepatitis: CT observations. AJR Am J Roentgenol 1988; 151:75-78.

13. Romero-Gómez M, Gómez-González E, Madrazo A, et al. Optical analysis of computed tomography images of the liver predicts fibrosis stage and distribution in chronic hepatitis C. Hepatology 2008; 47:810-816.

14. Martin DR. Magnetic resonance imaging of diffuse liver diseases. Top Magn Reson Imaging 2002; 13:151-163.

15. Aguirre DA, Behling CA, Alpert E, et al. Liver fibrosis: noninvasive diagnosis with double contrast material-enhanced MR imaging. Radiology 2006; 239:425-437.

16. Chow LC, Bammer R, Moseley ME, Sommer FG. Single breath-hold diffusion-weighted imaging of the abdomen. J Magn Reson Imaging 2003; 18:377-382.

17. Taouli B, Martin AJ, Qayyum A, et al. Parallel imaging and diffusion tensor imaging for diffusion-weighted MRI of the liver: preliminary experience in healthy volunteers. AJR Am J Roentgenol 2004; 183:677-680.

18. Ichikawa T, Haradome H, Hachiya J, et al. Diffusion-weighted MR imaging with single-shot echo-planar imaging in the upper abdomen: preliminary clinical experience in 61 patients. Abdom Imaging 1999; 24:456-461.

19. Girometti R, Furlan A, Bazzocchi M, et al. Diffusion-weighted MRI in evaluating liver fibrosis: a feasibility study in cirrhotic patients. Radiol Med (Torino) 2007; 112:394-408.

20. Taouli B, Tolia AJ, Losada M, et al. Diffusion-weighted MRI for quantification of liver fibrosis: preliminary experience. AJR Am J Roentgenol 2007; 189:799-806.

21. Manduca A, Oliphant TE, Dresner MA, et al. Magnetic resonance elastography: non-invasive mapping of tissue elasticity. Med Image Anal 2001; 5:237-254.

22. Rouvière O, Yin M, Dresner MA, et al. MR elastography of the liver: preliminary results. Radiology 2006; 240:440-448.

23. Yeh WC, Li PC, Jeng YM, et al. Elastic modulus measurements of human liver and correlation with pathology. Ultrasound Med Biol 2002; 28:467-474.

24. Huwart L, Sempoux C, Salameh N, et al. Liver fibrosis: noninvasive assessment with MR elastography versus aspartate aminotransferase-to-platelet ratio index. Radiology 2007; 245:458-466.

25. Cho SG, Kim MY, Kim HJ, et al. Chronic hepatitis: in vivo proton MR spectroscopic evaluation of the liver and correlation with histopathologic findings. Radiology 2001; 221:740-746.

26. Orlacchio A, Bolacchi F, Angelico M, et al. In vivo, high-field, 3-Tesla (1)H MR spectroscopic assessment of liver fibrosis in HCV-correlated chronic liver disease. Radiol Med (Torino) 2008; 113:289-299.

27. Hagiwara M, Rusinek H, Lee VS, et al. Advanced liver fibrosis: diagnosis with 3D whole-liver perfusion MR imaging—initial experience. Radiology 2008; 246:926-934.

28. Searle J, Mendelson R, Zelesco M, et al. Noninvasive prediction of the degree of liver fibrosis in patients with hepatitis C using an ultrasound contrast agent: a pilot study. J Med Imaging Radiat Oncol 2008; 52:130-133.

29. Cobbold JF, Morin S, Taylor-Robinson SD. Transient elastography for the assessment of chronic liver disease: ready for the clinic? World J Gastroenterol 2007; 13:4791-4797.

30. Friedrich-Rust M, Ong MF, Martens S, et al. Performance of transient elastography for the staging of liver fibrosis: a meta-analysis. Gastroenterology 2008; 134:960-974.

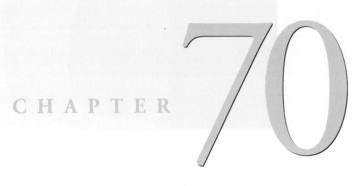
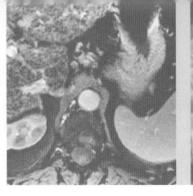
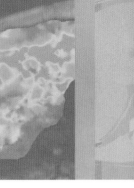

CHAPTER 70

Hepatic Veno-occlusive Diseases

Cynthia S. Santillan, Sameer M. Mazhar, Michael R. Peterson, and Claude B. Sirlin

The hepatic veno-occlusive diseases are a heterogeneous group of circulatory disorders characterized by obstruction of hepatic venous outflow at the sinusoidal or postsinusoidal levels. These disorders uniquely manifest portal hypertension before overt hepatic parenchymal disease and dysfunction, in contrast to other causes of hepatic disease in which hepatic dysfunction precedes portal hypertension.[1] The focus in this chapter is on the most common types of sinusoidal (sinusoidal obstruction syndrome) and postsinusoidal (Budd-Chiari syndrome) veno-occlusive disease.

ETIOLOGY

Sinusoidal Obstruction Syndrome

Sinusoidal obstruction syndrome (SOS) is a toxin-induced, usually iatrogenic, vascular hepatic disorder. Previously thought to require the involvement of the hepatic venules, it is now recognized that SOS primarily afflicts the sinusoids and may spare the hepatic venules.[2]

SOS was first linked to the ingestion of pyrrolizidine alkaloids in teas from *Senecio*, *Heliotropium*, and *Crotalaria*, sometimes resulting in epidemics of SOS in developing areas.[3] In the West, SOS occurs almost exclusively in cancer patients as a complication of chemotherapy and abdominal irradiation. Several chemotherapeutic and immunosuppressive agents have been implicated,[4] but the most serious cases of SOS develop after hematopoietic stem cell transplantation with myeloablative conditioning.[5] In stem cell transplant patients, the risk of developing SOS includes a history of prior stem cell transplantation, hepatitis C with elevated levels of aminotransaminases, underlying hepatic fibrosis or cirrhosis, advanced age, and infection at the time of transplant.[3] Although controversial, there is no convincing evidence to support causation by thrombosis due to clotting and hypercoagulable states.[6]

Budd-Chiari Syndrome

Budd-Chiari syndrome (BCS) refers to postsinusoidal obstruction at any level, from the small hepatic veins to the junction of the inferior vena cava (IVC) with the right atrium.[5] Mechanical obstruction can either be primary or secondary. In primary BCS, the obstruction arises from the venous wall (fibrosis or phlebitis) or lumen (thrombosis). In secondary BCS, the obstruction originates from outside the vein and may be caused by extrinsic compression (abscess, cyst, or solid tumor) or tumor invasion.[7]

Intravascular thrombosis is the most common mechanism of hepatic venous obstruction in primary BCS: at least one acquired or inherited procoagulative disorder is identified in up to 75% of patients.[8] Acquired myeloproliferative disorders, such as polycythemia vera and, less commonly, essential thrombocythemia and myelofibrosis, account for 50% of cases of BCS.[9] In the majority of cases, BCS is the initial manifestation of the underlying myeloproliferative disorder. Other acquired procoagulative states include paroxysmal nocturnal hemoglobinuria, malignancy, anti–phospholipid antibody syndrome, Behçet's disease, pregnancy, and oral contraceptive use. The most common inherited procoagulative disorder is factor V Leiden deficiency, occurring in up to 30% of cases of BCS.[10] Other inherited states result in elevations of prothrombin, factors VII and VIII, and homocysteine and in deficiencies of antithrombin, protein C, and protein S.

Secondary BCS is sometimes seen when a malignant tumor grows within the lumen of its associated venous outflow tract (hepatocellular carcinoma, renal cell carcinoma, Wilms' tumor, and hepatic angiosarcoma). It can also result from extrinsic compression by malignant and benign solid tumors of the liver or adjacent organs, intrahepatic hematomas, hepatic abscesses, hydatid cysts, and hepatic cysts in polycystic kidney disease. No precipitating cause is identified in 10% of cases of BCS.[8]

PATHOGENESIS

Sinusoidal Obstruction Syndrome

The inciting event in SOS is toxin-mediated sinusoidal endothelial injury. The injured endothelial cells undergo a morphologic transformation from their normal spindle shape to a rounder configuration, which narrows the sinusoidal lumen and introduces gaps between the cells. Blood flows through the gaps into the space of Disse, detaching endothelial as well as other perisinusoidal cells. The detached cells embolize downstream, causing further sinusoidal and possibly venular obstruction. Eventually, sinusoidal and centrilobular fibrosis ensues, causing hepatic congestion and manifesting clinically as portal hypertension. Later, the resulting low-flow state causes redistribution of the hepatic microcirculation and focal hepatic ischemia, culminating in centrilobular hepatocyte necrosis.[11]

Budd-Chiari Syndrome

Postsinusoidal obstruction causes sinusoidal (and portal) pressure to increase. Increased sinusoidal pressure promotes centrilobular sinusoidal dilatation and congestion. The congested liver enlarges. Sinusoidal perfusion diminishes, and centrilobular ischemia and necrosis may occur. Stagnant blood flow and an underlying procoagulant state may precipitate concomitant thrombosis of the extrahepatic (10%) and intrahepatic (50%) portal veins. Areas in which there is simultaneous obstruction of the hepatic and portal veins undergo infarction.[12] Perivenular fibrosis develops within weeks of the obstruction.

PREVALENCE AND EPIDEMIOLOGY

SOS occurs after hematopoietic stem cell transplantation. Large-scale epidemiologic studies to assess prevalence, incidence, and demographic factors have not been conducted. The annual incidence of BCS is 1 in 100,000. Women in their third or fourth decades of life are afflicted most commonly.[13]

Veno-occlusive disease refers to a class of hepatic vascular disorders in which obstruction of sinusoidal or postsinusoidal hepatic venous outflow results in portal hypertension. Historically, this term was used to describe SOS only. More recently, the term has been broadened to include BCS as well as SOS.

BCS may be acute (presentation within 4 weeks of obstruction) or chronic (obstruction present for at least 6 months).

CLINICAL PRESENTATION

Sinusoidal Obstruction Syndrome

SOS usually manifests 1 to 2 weeks after stem cell transplantation. The first symptom is abdominal pain, followed by ascites, tender hepatomegaly, jaundice, and weight gain (due to fluid retention). Laboratory abnormalities include direct hyperbilirubinemia initially with subsequent elevations in alkaline phosphatase and aminotransferases. Renal dysfunction (with up to 50% of patients

requiring dialysis), diuretic-resistant fluid retention, recalcitrant thrombocytopenia due to splenic sequestration, and encephalopathy occur later. SOS is an acute or subacute illness that either fully resolves, usually in 2 to 3 weeks, or ends in death. All-cause fatality from SOS varies according to disease severity, with fatality rates in one series reported as 9%, 23%, and 98%, in mild, moderate, and severe disease, respectively.[14] Patients who recover do not develop cirrhosis.

SOS is a clinical diagnosis that utilizes noninvasive criteria devised by groups from Seattle and Baltimore. Both sets of criteria use variable combinations of hyperbilirubinemia, weight gain, ascites, and hepatomegaly within 3 weeks of stem cell transplantation.[15] The diagnosis can be confirmed by liver biopsy. If percutaneous biopsy is contraindicated due to thrombocytopenia, a transjugular approach may be employed, at which time the hepatic venous pressure gradient may also be measured. When elevated above 10 mm Hg, this gradient has a specificity of 90% in the appropriate clinical scenario.[16]

Budd-Chiari Syndrome

The clinical manifestations and severity of BCS depend on the location and acuity of the venous obstruction. Asymptomatic disease occurs in patients with obstruction of only one hepatic vein or more than one hepatic vein with the development of collateral vessels. Slow obstruction of two hepatic veins results in chronic disease, whereas sudden obstruction of all three hepatic veins or the extrahepatic IVC may produce fulminant hepatic failure.

Patients classically present with ascites, hepatosplenomegaly, and right upper quadrant abdominal pain. Lower extremity edema and venous collaterals on the abdominal wall may be evident. The presentation is acute in 20% of patients. Serum values of aminotransferases, alkaline phosphatase, and bilirubin are moderately elevated, whereas those of plasma coagulation factors are diminished. Twenty-five percent of patients with acute BCS progress to fulminant hepatic failure. The presentation is chronic in 80% of patients; 20% of these patients progress to cirrhosis.[17] Laboratory abnormalities are milder than in the acute form. The prognosis of chronic BCS has improved owing to advances in supportive care, with a current 1-year transplant-free survival of 80% and a 10-year transplant-free survival of 60%.[18]

BCS is an imaging diagnosis. Liver biopsy may suggest the diagnosis but is not specific.

PATHOLOGY

SOS and BCS have similar pathologic features. In both conditions, acute venous obstruction is characterized by dilated centrilobular sinusoids filled with erythrocytes. Associated findings include parenchymal compression as well as atrophy and loss of hepatocytes. Erythrocytes may extravasate into the space of Disse and replace the disappearing hepatocytes. In severe cases, blood-filled lakes may form in the centrilobular zone, with little recognizable hepatic parenchyma. Cholestatic changes may develop at the periphery of the injured areas. Hemosiderin-laden macrophages may be present, but inflammation is absent to minimal.

In chronic BCS, fibrosis of the centrilobular zones may develop and may progress to bridging fibrosis between central veins. This form of fibrosis spares the portal tracts, resulting in a pattern termed *reserve lobulation* or *veno-centric cirrhosis,* although end-stage cases may be indistinguishable from cirrhosis from other causes.[19]

A key pathologic difference between SOS and BCS is that thrombus within central veins is characteristic of BCS but not of SOS. The central veins in SOS may contain fibrin deposits, as demonstrated via electron microscopy and immunohistochemistry, but thrombus is rare. Grossly, involvement of the liver tends to be uniform in SOS. Involvement may be uneven in BCS, depending on the sites of venous obstructions; areas of the liver drained by unoccluded hepatic veins may undergo compensatory hypertrophy. BCS may progress to cirrhosis, but SOS does not.

IMAGING

Whereas SOS has a characteristic clinical manifestation and is a unique complication of chemoradiation or hematopoietic stem cell transplantation, hepatic venous obstruction due to BCS can be due to any number of causes, including hepatocellular carcinoma, venous invasion from an extrahepatic malignancy, or occlusion of the intrahepatic or suprahepatic IVC. As such, the imaging evaluation should not only seek to secure the diagnosis of hepatic venous obstruction but also attempt to identify the cause of the obstruction.

Radiography

Plain radiography has no routine role in the assessment of SOS or BCS because hepatomegaly is the only reliable finding.[20,21]

The venographic findings in SOS are not well characterized. In BCS, venography is considered the diagnostic gold standard. In acute BCS, liver edema may cause smooth extrinsic narrowing of the IVC and hepatic veins. In chronic BCS, collaterals may form between the hepatic and systemic veins.[22] These small collateral vessels have a characteristic "spider web" appearance during venography (Fig. 70-1).

CT and MRI

Sinusoidal Obstruction Syndrome

Compared with the unaffected liver parenchyma, the affected portion of the liver may be hypoattenuating at CT and have heterogeneous signal intensity at MRI on unenhanced images. Low attenuation and heterogeneous signal intensity persist after the administration of contrast material.[23] Periportal edema is present and manifests as periportal low attenuation at CT[24] and high signal at T2-weighted (T2W) MRI.[25] Intrahepatic collateral vessels, which can appear as round foci of enhancement on the portal venous and delayed phases of contrast administration, may be observed.[26] Hepatic veins are narrow but patent. In the setting of liver irradiation, the affected region may have a geographic or polygonal morphology that does not conform to an anatomic segment. Other findings include hepatomegaly, gallbladder wall thickening, and ascites.

Budd-Chiari Syndrome

In the acute phase of BCS, the liver is enlarged. The periphery of the liver is hypoattenuating on unenhanced CT and of high signal intensity on T2W MRI (Fig. 70-2).[27] The liver enhances heterogeneously. Relative hypoenhancement of the periphery of the liver is characteristic.[21] Areas of the liver with independent venous drainage, such as the caudate lobe, hyperenhance on the arterial phase. The resulting "fan-shaped" enhancement pattern[28] (Figs. 70-3 and 70-4) may reverse on delayed-phase imaging, with the caudate lobe and central portion of the liver demonstrating lower attenuation or signal intensity than the periphery. If only one or two hepatic veins are

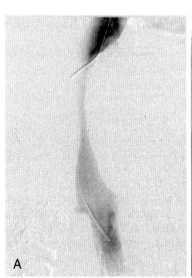
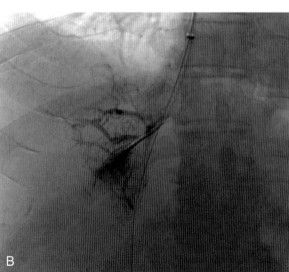

■ **FIGURE 70-1** **A,** Venography of the inferior vena cava in a 61-year-old man with Budd-Chiari syndrome shows smooth extrinsic narrowing of the intrahepatic inferior vena cava. **B,** Injection of the right hepatic vein demonstrates occlusion of the vessel with numerous small collateral vessels in a characteristic "spider web" appearance.

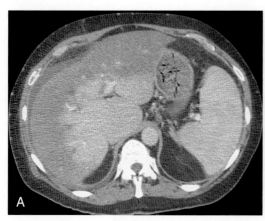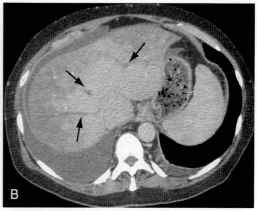

■ **FIGURE 70-2** **A,** CT image of the abdomen in the same patient as in Figure 70-1 during the portal venous phase of administration of iodinated contrast agent demonstrates the hyperenhancement of the central portions of the liver with hypoenhancement of the periphery. **B,** Equilibrium-phase image at the level of the hepatic veins continues to show this pattern of enhancement and demonstrates lack of enhancement of the vessels, consistent with occlusion (*arrows*). Also note the presence of ascites.

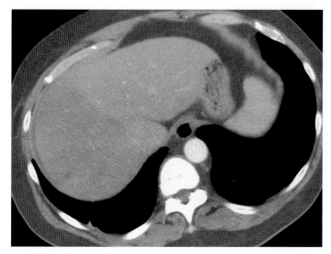

■ **FIGURE 70-3** CT image of the abdomen in the same patient as in Figure 70-2 performed during the portal venous phase of enhancement 2 months before the previous images demonstrates relative hypoattenuation of the right hepatic lobe due to occlusion of the right and middle hepatic veins. Note that the remainder of the liver demonstrates a normal enhancement pattern, because venous drainage of the left hepatic lobe is not obstructed.

occluded, the characteristic enhancement pattern may be confined to the affected portions of the liver (Fig. 70-5). The occluded hepatic veins may be nonvisualized or may show lack of intraluminal enhancement. Coronal imaging may be helpful to assess the IVC for compression or thrombus.[27]

In the chronic phase of BCS, liver fibrosis may be visible as reticulations of low attenuation at unenhanced CT or high signal at T2W MRI. The liver atrophies, particularly in the periphery. If the IVC is not obstructed, there may be compensatory hypertrophy of the caudate lobe due to direct venous drainage into the IVC. Ultimately, the hypertrophied caudate lobe may compress the intrahepatic IVC, exacerbating the outflow obstruction. Large intrahepatic and extrahepatic collateral vessels, as well as ascites and splenomegaly may be present (Fig. 70-6).[29,30] The chroni-

cally thrombosed hepatic veins may be difficult to identify. The enhancement differences between the caudate lobe and the periphery of the liver become less noticeable and may no longer be appreciated.

Regenerative nodules, particularly in portal regions, may develop with long-standing hepatic venous obstruction. These nodules range from 0.5 to 4.0 cm and are sometimes hyperattenuating at unenhanced CT and hyperintense on T1-weighted (T1W) and hypointense on T2W MR images, possibly owing to intralesional copper deposition (Fig. 70-7).[29] The nodules may enhance avidly on the arterial phase and fade to isoattenuation or isointensity on the portal venous and equilibrium phases (Fig. 70-8).[29] Distinguishing these regenerative nodules from hepatocellular carcinoma can be difficult, but hepatocellular carcinomas tend to wash out to hypoattenuation or hypointensity on portal venous and delayed phases. In addition, multiplicity (>10) and smaller size (<4 cm) favor a diagnosis of regenerative nodules.[30]

Ultrasonography

Sinusoidal Obstruction Syndrome

Ultrasonography is frequently performed in suspected SOS, mainly to exclude other causes of hepatic dysfunction.[20] It is usually nonspecific, but some findings suggest the correct diagnosis in the appropriate clinical setting.[31,32] Elevation of the hepatic artery resistive index above 0.75 is characteristic of SOS and helps to differentiate it from graft-versus-host disease (GVHD).[33,34] Abnormalities in the portal vein, including pulsatile, bidirectional, and reversed flow, have also been reported.[35] Gallbladder wall thickening, ascites, hepatomegaly, and narrowing of the hepatic veins are also evident.

Budd-Chiari Syndrome

Doppler ultrasound imaging is highly sensitive and specific for the diagnosis of BCS. Abnormalities of flow within the hepatic veins are present in nearly all cases, often

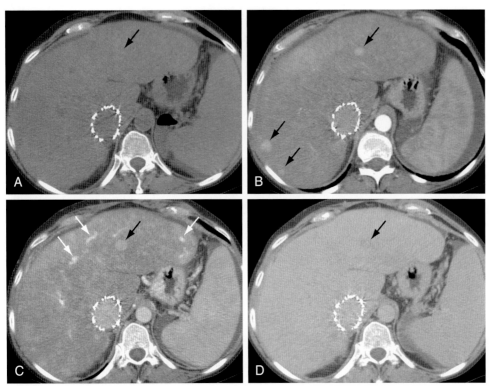

■ **FIGURE 70-4**   **A,** Nonenhanced CT image of the abdomen performed in a 56-year-old woman with chronic hepatic venous obstruction demonstrates a lobular liver with multiple regenerative nodules (*black arrow*). The nodules are slightly hyperattenuating. After the administration of an iodinated contrast agent, the nodules enhance avidly on the arterial (**B**) and portal venous (**C**) phases of the study, becoming slightly hypoattenuating on the equilibrium phase image (**D**). Note the intrahepatic collateral vessels (*white arrows,* **C**), ascites, and stent within the intrahepatic inferior vena cava.

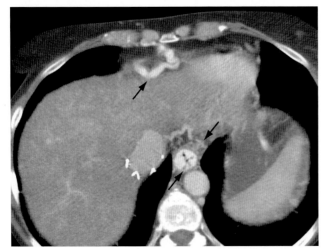

■ **FIGURE 70-5**   Portal venous phase CT image from the same patient as in Figure 70-4 demonstrates extrahepatic collateral vessels (*arrows*), as well as paraesophageal and submucosal esophageal varices.

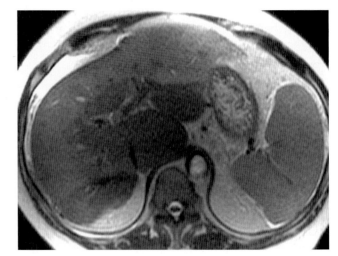

■ **FIGURE 70-6**   T2W MR image in a 61-year-old man with Budd-Chiari syndrome (see also Figs. 70-2 and 70-3) demonstrates increased T2 signal in the periphery of the liver.

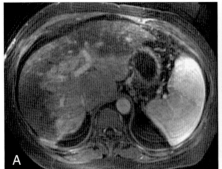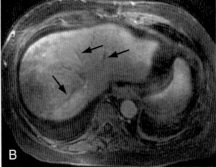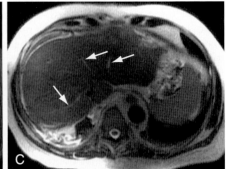

■ **FIGURE 70-7**   **A,** T1W MR image during the arterial phase of administration of a gadolinium chelate in the same patient as in Figures 70-2, 70-3, and 70-6 demonstrates hyperenhancement of the central portion of the liver. **B,** In addition, occlusion of the hepatic veins (*arrows,* **B, C**) is demonstrated both by lack of enhancement during the delayed phase of imaging as well as by the absence of flow voids on the T2W pregadolinium image (**C**).

manifesting as an absent, flattened, or reversed waveform (Fig. 70-9).[36,37] Acutely, thrombus may be detectable in the hepatic veins. Flow in the portal vein may be antegrade (hepatopetal), bidirectional, or retrograde (hepatofugal). In addition, the distribution of the abnormality may vary with the extent of hepatic venous occlusion, with abnormal portal flow present only in the affected segments. Ultrasonography may detect abnormalities of the IVC accounting for venous obstruction, such as thrombus or membranes. Heterogeneity of the liver parenchyma, hepatomegaly, ascites, collateral vessels, and splenomegaly can also be detected.

Nuclear Medicine

Sinusoidal Obstruction Syndrome

Nuclear medicine is not routinely used in the evaluation of SOS, although heterogeneous liver uptake and increased lung uptake of technetium-99m sulfur colloid have been reported.[38,39]

Budd-Chiari Syndrome

Nuclear medicine has a limited role in the diagnosis of hepatic venous occlusion. Hepatobiliary iminodiacetic acid (HIDA) or technetium-99m sulfur colloid scans may demonstrate an appearance very similar to that seen on contrast-enhanced MRI or CT, with poor uptake in the periphery of the liver and normal to increased uptake within the central liver and caudate lobe (Fig. 70-10).[40]

Imaging Algorithms

Suspicion of SOS

Imaging findings are not diagnostic of SOS but may be used to support clinical and laboratory data. A Doppler ultrasound or CT evaluation may initially be obtained to exclude other causes of post–stem cell transplant cholestasis. MRI may be performed if CT is contraindicated but adds little additional information.

Suspicion of BCS

In acute BCS, Doppler ultrasonography is initially performed to detect abnormal flows suggestive of venous obstruction and, in some instances, the thrombus itself. If the ultrasound evaluation is abnormal, further evaluation

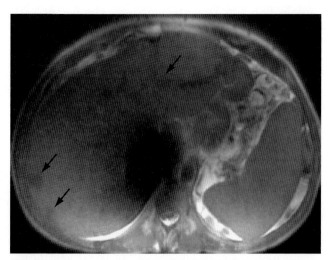

■ **FIGURE 70-8** Proton-density imaging in the 56-year-old woman shown in Figure 70-4 demonstrates numerous regenerative nodules (*arrows*).

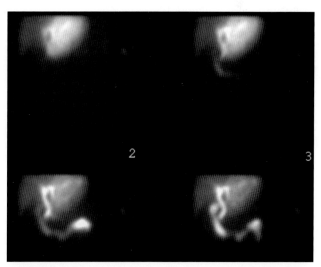

■ **FIGURE 70-10** HIDA scan performed at the time of occlusion of the right and middle hepatic veins in a 61-year-old-man (see also Figs. 70-2, 70-3, 70-6, 70-7, and 70-9) demonstrates decreased uptake of radiotracer within the right hepatic lobe in a pattern similar to that seen on the CT image shown in Figure 70-3.

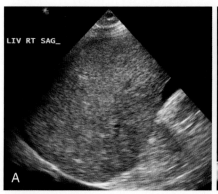
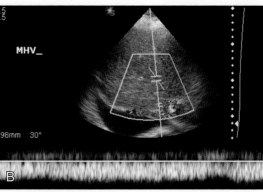

■ **FIGURE 70-9** A, Ultrasound image of the 61-year-old man with Budd-Chiari syndrome (see also Figs. 70-2, 70-3, 70-6, and 70-7) demonstrates a heterogeneous liver. B, Duplex Doppler ultrasound image in the region of the middle hepatic vein shows a flattened waveform with absence of the normal respiratory or cardiac variation.

with CT or MRI is warranted to verify the obstruction and distinguish between intrahepatic and extrahepatic causes. If treatment is desired, venography may provide useful information to guide shunting or stenting.

In chronic BCS, CT or MRI is employed to detect parenchymal abnormalities suggestive of cirrhosis and sequelae of portal hypertension. If cirrhosis is present, patients are at increased risk for developing hepatocellular carcinoma (HCC) and, in our opinion, should be considered for surveillance for this tumor. The incidence of HCC in patients with cirrhosis due to BCS is unknown, however, and the American Association for the Study of Liver Diseases (AASLD) does not provide specific guidelines for HCC surveillance in these patients.

Classic Signs

SINUSOIDAL OBSTRUCTION SYNDROME

- Patent but narrowed hepatic veins
- Elevated hepatic arterial resistive index
- Periportal edema and ascites
- Diffuse involvement of the liver or involvement of the region of the liver that has been irradiated (may not be in an anatomic distribution)

ACUTE BUDD-CHIARI SYNDROME

- Hepatic venous collateral vessels in a "spider web" pattern
- Hyperenhancement of the central liver and caudate lobe on arterial phase imaging, which may reverse on delayed-phase imaging
- Intrahepatic collateral vessels
- Occluded hepatic veins
- Abnormal or absent hepatic venous waveform on Doppler ultrasonography

CHRONIC BUDD-CHIARI SYNDROME

- Hypertrophy of the central liver and caudate with atrophy of the periphery
- Regenerative nodules, which may show arterial phase hypervascularity

---

DIFFERENTIAL DIAGNOSIS

Sinusoidal Obstruction Syndrome

Conditions in the clinical differential diagnosis of SOS are those that may result in post–stem cell transplant cholestasis. The most challenging distinction is from acute hepatic GVHD. Whereas the physical examination and laboratory findings are similar, hepatic GVHD typically occurs as a part of a syndrome that includes a rash and diarrhea. Other causes of post-transplant cholestasis are easily differentiated from SOS on clinical and laboratory findings and include sepsis, viral and fungal hepatic infections, medication toxicity, hemolysis, and total parenteral nutrition.

Imaging findings may help differentiate SOS from GVHD in post–stem cell transplant patients. Periportal edema, narrowing of the hepatic veins, and elevation of the hepatic arterial resistive index suggest SOS, whereas small bowel wall thickening is more often seen in GVHD.

As opposed to BCS, the central portions of the liver and caudate lobe do not demonstrate a different enhancement pattern from the rest of the liver.[24]

Budd-Chiari Syndrome

Acute BCS shares clinical features with other causes of fulminant hepatic failure, such as acetaminophen toxicity, viral hepatitis, or ischemic hepatitis. Typically, however, the other causes of fulminant disease do not demonstrate prominent ascites and have serum aminotransferase values that are two to six times more elevated than what is seen in BCS.

Chronic BCS may resemble the cirrhosis and portal hypertension of any etiology of chronic liver disease, and a comprehensive workup is required to systematically rule out other possibilities. Patients with right-sided heart failure may develop congestive hepatopathy similar to that observed in BCS but have distinguishing features of right-sided heart failure, such as jugular venous distention, and may also have signs of left-sided heart failure, such as pulmonary edema and diminished cardiac ejection fraction.

Acute BCS is associated with outflow obstruction and typically is easily differentiated with imaging from other causes of fulminant hepatic failure.

Distinguishing cirrhosis secondary to parenchymal disease such as hepatitis infection and changes due to chronic BCS can be challenging. In chronic BCS, the hepatic veins may be undetectable on CT or MRI. The regenerative nodules seen in most causes of cirrhosis do not typically demonstrate arterial enhancement and are often smaller than those seen in chronic BCS.

TREATMENT

Sinusoidal Obstruction Syndrome

Because effective therapies are lacking, focus has shifted to preventive strategies. Ultimately, the most successful prevention involves judicious selection of pretransplant conditioning regimens in those patients at highest risk for developing SOS.

Targeted therapy is implemented in those with severe SOS, because most patients with mild or moderate SOS survive with supportive care alone. In severe SOS, dialysis and ventilatory support is often necessary; experimental anticoagulants show promise for salvage therapy.[41]

Transjugular intrahepatic portosystemic shunting (TIPS) may be necessary to control portal hypertension in patients with severe SOS.[42] Liver transplantation may be performed as an option of last resort in patients who received stem cell transplantation for benign conditions.

Budd-Chiari Syndrome

Medical therapy for mild BCS utilizes diuretics to control ascites, anticoagulants to prevent thrombus extension, and thrombolytics to dissolve the clot.

The object of surgical therapy of BCS is to decompress the liver by restoring hepatic outflow, thereby reducing sinusoidal pressure. Minimally invasive techniques, such as angioplasty and stenting, are used in conjunction with either systemic or in-situ thrombolytic therapy. Angioplasty maintains 2-year patency in 50% of patients. The addition of stents improves long-term patency to 90%, but stents generally are not removable and may potentially complicate liver transplantation if placed above the IVC.

Failure of angioplasty and stenting may require the placement of a TIPS or surgical shunt, particularly in the setting of acute hepatic decompensation or as a bridge to transplantation. TIPS alleviates sinusoidal pressure by providing ancillary venous outflow that bypasses the obstruction; it is preferred to surgical shunting at most centers because it avoids laparotomy and has fewer serious complications. Long-term TIPS patency approximates 50%. Portocaval and mesocaval shunts are the two most common surgical shunts. These shunts decompress the liver by inducing hepatofugal blood flow through the portal vein and are most effective when the IVC is patent. Shunt dysfunction occurs in 30% of patients due to thrombosis, stenosis, or compression of the IVC by the growing caudate lobe.[43]

Liver transplantation is an option in patients in whom TIPS or surgical shunting has failed or who present with fulminant hepatic failure or decompensated cirrhosis. Ten-year survival approaches 85% in some series.[44] When anticoagulation is administered, the risk of recurrent BCS post transplant is approximately 10%.[45]

What the Referring Physician Needs to Know

■ As a class, the hepatic veno-occlusive diseases are circulatory disorders that cause portal hypertension by obstructing venous outflow at the sinusoidal or postsinusoidal level.

■ SOS is a toxin-mediated disorder of hepatic sinusoids that occurs as a complication of chemoradiation or myeloablative hematopoietic stem cell transplantation.

■ SOS manifests with varying severity and needs to be differentiated from other causes of post-transplant cholestasis.

■ Treatment strategies for SOS are lacking and thus attention is placed on prevention.

■ BCS represents a postsinusoidal obstruction that may occur from the small hepatic veins to the suprahepatic IVC.

■ Common causes of BCS include intravascular thrombosis, tumor invasion, or extrinsic compression.

■ Treatment of BCS includes medical therapy with anticoagulation and thrombolytics, procedural interventions such as TIPS and surgical shunts, and, in the most severe cases, liver transplantation.

■ Whereas imaging plays an accessory role to clinical presentation in the diagnosis of SOS, it is the primary diagnostic tool in BCS.

KEY POINTS

■ Although the diagnosis of SOS in high-risk patients is primarily based on clinical and laboratory findings, imaging findings supporting the diagnosis include periportal edema, narrowing of the hepatic veins, abnormal attenuation or signal intensity on unenhanced CT or MRI, respectively, and elevation of the hepatic arterial resistive index on Doppler ultrasonography.

■ Although venography remains the gold standard for the diagnosis of BCS, its current role is predominantly for procedural planning, such as before TIPS placement.

■ Hyperenhancement of the central liver and caudate lobe during the arterial and portal venous phases of contrast-enhanced CT or MRI is characteristic of acute occlusion of the hepatic veins.

■ Chronic occlusion of the hepatic veins results in atrophy of the liver, with relative sparing or hypertrophy of the caudate lobe and formation of regenerative nodules and intrahepatic collateral vessels.

■ Abnormalities of flow within the hepatic veins on Doppler ultrasonography are present in nearly all cases of hepatic venous occlusion, manifesting as flattening of the waveform or reversal or absence of blood flow.

SUGGESTED READINGS

Aydinli M, Bayraktar Y. Budd-Chiari syndrome: etiology, pathogenesis and diagnosis. World J Gastroenterol 2007; 13:2693-2696.

Bayraktar UD, Seren S, Bayraktar Y. Hepatic venous outflow obstruction: three similar syndromes. World J Gastroenterol 2007; 13:1912-1927.

Brancatelli G, Vilgrain V, Federle MP, et al. Budd-Chiari syndrome: spectrum of imaging findings. AJR Am J Roentgenol 2007; 188:W168-W176.

Buckley O, O'Brien J, Snow A, et al. Imaging of Budd-Chiari syndrome. Eur Radiol 2007; 17:2071-2078.

DeLeve LD. Vascular liver diseases. Curr Gastroenterol Rep 2003; 5:63-70.

Helmy A. Review article: updates in the pathogenesis and therapy of hepatic sinusoidal obstruction syndrome. Aliment Pharmacol Ther 2006; 23:11-25.

Kumar S, DeLeve L, Kamath PS, Tefferi A. Hepatic veno-occlusive disease (sinusoidal obstruction syndrome) after hematopoietic stem cell transplantation. Mayo Clin Proc 2003; 78:589-598.

McDonald GB, Sharma P, Matthews DE, et al. Veno-occlusive disease of the liver after bone marrow transplantation: diagnosis, incidence, and predisposing factors. Hepatology 1984; 4:116-122.

Senzolo M, Germani G, Cholongitas E, et al. Veno-occlusive disease: update on clinical management. World J Gastroenterol 2007; 13:3918-3924.

REFERENCES

1. DeLeve LD. Vascular liver diseases. Curr Gastroenterol Rep 2003; 5:63-70.
2. Shulman HM, Fisher LB, Schoch HG, et al. Veno-occlusive disease of the liver after marrow transplantation: histological correlates of clinical signs and symptoms. Hepatology 1994; 19:1171-1180.
3. Kumar S, DeLeve L, Kamath PS, Tefferi A. Hepatic veno-occlusive disease (sinusoidal obstruction syndrome) after hematopoietic stem cell transplantation. Mayo Clin Proc 2003; 78:589-598.
4. Dawson LA, Ten Haken RK, Lawrence TS. Partial irradiation of the liver. Semin Radiat Oncol 2001; 11:240-246.
5. McDonald GB, Sharma P, Matthews DE, et al. Veno-occlusive disease of the liver after bone marrow transplantation: diagnosis, incidence, and predisposing factors. Hepatology 1984; 4:116-122.
6. Helmy A. Review article: updates in the pathogenesis and therapy of hepatic sinusoidal obstruction syndrome. Aliment Pharmacol Ther 2006; 23:11-25.
7. Aydinli M, Bayraktar Y. Budd-Chiari syndrome: etiology, pathogenesis and diagnosis. World J Gastroenterol 2007; 13:2693-2696.
8. Denninger MH, Chait Y, Casadevall N, et al. Cause of portal or hepatic venous thrombosis in adults: the role of multiple concurrent factors. Hepatology 2000; 31:587-591.
9. Hirshberg B, Shouval D, Fibach E, et al. Flow cytometric analysis of autonomous growth of erythroid precursors in liquid culture detects occult polycythemia vera in the Budd-Chiari syndrome. J Hepatol 2000; 32:574-578.
10. Deltenre P, Denninger MH, Hillaire S, et al. Factor V Leiden related Budd-Chiari syndrome. Gut 2001; 48:264-268.
11. DeLeve LD, McCuskey RS, Wang X, et al. Characterization of a reproducible rat model of hepatic veno-occlusive disease. Hepatology 1999; 29:1779-1791.
12. Tanaka M, Wanless IR. Pathology of the liver in Budd-Chiari syndrome: portal vein thrombosis and the histogenesis of veno-centric cirrhosis, veno-portal cirrhosis, and large regenerative nodules. Hepatology 1998; 27:488-496.
13. Mahmoud AF, Mendoza A, Meshikhes AN, et al. Clinical spectrum, investigations and treatment of Budd-Chiari syndrome. Q J Med 1996; 89:37-43.
14. McDonald GB, Hinds MS, Fisher LD, et al. Veno-occlusive disease of the liver and multiorgan failure after bone marrow transplantation: a cohort study of 355 patients. Ann Intern Med 1993; 118:255-267.
15. Carreras E, Granena A, Navasa M, et al. On the reliability of clinical criteria for the diagnosis of hepatic veno-occlusive disease. Ann Hematol 1993; 66:77-80.
16. Shulman HM, Gooley T, Dudley MD, et al. Utility of transvenous liver biopsies and wedged hepatic venous pressure measurements in sixty marrow transplant recipients. Transplantation 1995; 59:1015-1022.
17. De BK, Sen S, Biswas PK, et al. Occurrence of hepatopulmonary syndrome in Budd-Chiari syndrome and the role of venous decompression. Gastroenterology 2002; 122:897-903.
18. Murad SD, Valla DC, de Groen PC, et al. Determinants of survival and the effect of portosystemic shunting in patients with Budd-Chiari syndrome. Hepatology 2004; 39:500-508.
19. Wanless IR. Vascular disorders. In Burt AD, Portmann BC, Ferrell LD (eds). MacSween's Pathology of the Liver, 5th ed. New York, Churchill Livingstone, 2006, p 621.
20. Senzolo M, Germani G, Cholongitas E, et al. Veno-occlusive disease: update on clinical management. World J Gastroenterol 2007; 13:3918-3924.
21. Buckley O, O'Brien J, Snow A, et al. Imaging of Budd-Chiari syndrome. Eur Radiol 2007; 17:2071-2078.
22. Cho OK, Koo JH, Kim YS, et al. Collateral pathways in Budd-Chiari syndrome: CT and venographic correlation. AJR Am J Roentgenol 1996; 167:1163-1167.
23. Chiou SY, Lee RC, Chi KH, et al. The triple-phase CT image appearance of post-irradiated livers. Acta Radiol 2001; 42:526-531.
24. Erturk SM, Mortele KJ, Binkert CA, et al. CT features of hepatic veno-occlusive disease and hepatic graft-versus-host disease in

25. van den Bosch MA, van Hoe L. MR imaging findings in two patients with hepatic veno-occlusive disease following bone marrow transplantation. Eur Radiol 2000; 10:1290-1293.
26. Mortele KJ, Van Vlierberghe H, Wiesner W, Ros PR. Hepatic veno-occlusive disease: MRI findings. Abdom Imaging 2002; 27:523-526.
27. Noone TC, Semelka RC, Siegelman ES, et al. Budd-Chiari syndrome: spectrum of appearances of acute, subacute, and chronic disease with magnetic resonance imaging. J Magn Reson Imaging 2000; 11:44-50.
28. Camera L, Mainenti PP, Di Giacomo A, et al. Triphasic helical CT in Budd-Chiari syndrome: patterns of enhancement in acute, subacute and chronic disease. Clin Radiol 2006; 61:331-337.
29. Brancatelli G, Federle MP, Grazioli L, et al. Benign regenerative nodules in Budd-Chiari syndrome and other vascular disorders of the liver: radiologic-pathologic and clinical correlation. RadioGraphics 2002; 22:847-862.
30. Brancatelli G, Vilgrain V, Federle MP, et al. Budd-Chiari syndrome: spectrum of imaging findings. AJR Am J Roentgenol 2007; 188: W168-W176.
31. Teefey SA, Brink JA, Borson RA, Middleton WD. Diagnosis of veno-occlusive disease of the liver after bone marrow transplantation: value of duplex sonography. AJR Am J Roentgenol 1995; 164: 1397-1401.
32. Hommeyer SC, Teefey SA, Jacobson AF, et al. Veno-occlusive disease of the liver: prospective study of US evaluation. Radiology 1992; 184:683-686.
33. Lassau N, Leclere J, Auperin A, et al. Hepatic veno-occlusive disease after myeloablative treatment and bone marrow transplantation: value of gray-scale and Doppler US in 100 patients. Radiology 1997; 204:545-552.
34. Herbetko J, Grigg AP, Buckley AR, Phillips GL. Veno-occlusive liver disease after bone marrow transplantation: findings at duplex sonography. AJR Am J Roentgenol 1992; 158:1001-1005.
35. Brown BP, Abu-Yousef M, Farner R, et al. Doppler sonography: a noninvasive method for evaluation of hepatic venocclusive disease. AJR Am J Roentgenol 1990; 154:721-724.
36. Makuuchi M, Hasegawa H, Yamazaki S, et al. Primary Budd-Chiari syndrome: ultrasonic demonstration. Radiology 1984; 152:775-779.
37. Millener P, Grant EG, Rose S, et al. Color Doppler imaging findings in patients with Budd-Chiari syndrome: correlation with venographic findings. AJR Am J Roentgenol 1993; 161:307-312.
38. Jacobson AF, Marks MA, Kaplan WD. Increased lung uptake on technetium-99m-sulfur colloid liver-spleen scans in patients with hepatic veno-occlusive disease following bone marrow transplantation. J Nucl Med 1990; 31:372-374.
39. Joshi MJ, Ford PV, Vogel JM, Lutrin CL. Grossly abnormal liver-spleen scan in a patient with veno-occlusive disease of the liver that normalized completely on follow-up. Clin Nucl Med 1993; 18:590-593.
40. Meindok H, Langer B. Liver scan in Budd-Chiari syndrome. J Nucl Med 1976; 17:365-368.
41. Richardson PG, Murakami C, Jin Z, et al. Multi-institutional use of defibrotide in 88 patients after stem cell transplantation with severe veno-occlusive disease and multisystem organ failure: response without significant toxicity in a high-risk population and factors predictive of outcome. Blood 2002; 100:4337-4343.
42. Zenz T, Rossle M, Bertz H, et al. Severe veno-occlusive disease after allogeneic bone marrow or peripheral stem cell transplantation—role of transjugular intrahepatic portosystemic shunt (TIPS). Liver 2001; 21:31-36.
43. Panis Y, Belghiti J, Valla D, et al. Portosystemic shunt in Budd-Chiari syndrome: long-term survival and factors affecting shunt patency in 25 patients in Western countries. Surgery 1994; 115:276-281.
44. Ulrich F, Pratschke J, Neumann U, et al. Eighteen years of liver transplantation experience in patients with advanced Budd-Chiari syndrome. Liver Transpl 2008; 14:133-135.
45. Srinivasan P, Rela M, Prachalias A, et al. Liver transplantation for Budd-Chiari syndrome. Transplantation 2002; 7:973-977.

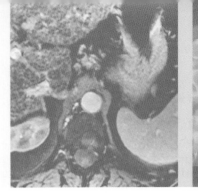
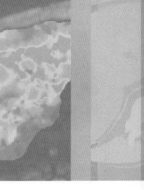

71

Cholestatic Hepatic Disorders

Sameer M. Mazhar, Silvana C. Faria, Michael R. Peterson, and Claude B. Sirlin

Primary biliary cirrhosis (PBC) and primary sclerosing cholangitis (PSC) are the two most common and well-characterized primary cholestatic disorders. In contrast to hepatocellular conditions, such as viral hepatitis and autoimmune hepatitis, the initial insult in cholestatic diseases centers on the bile duct epithelium. Nevertheless, as with other diffuse liver diseases, these disorders may progress to cirrhosis, portal hypertension, liver failure, and/or malignancy.

ETIOLOGY AND PATHOGENESIS

Primary Biliary Cirrhosis

PBC is a chronic, cholestatic disease of presumed autoimmune origin affecting the small-to-medium intrahepatic bile ducts. Pathogenically, this is manifested as immune-mediated destruction and loss of bile ducts ("ductopenia"), as well as portal inflammation. As a result, biliary secretion is impaired, toxins accumulate within the liver, and inflammation is exacerbated. Ultimately, the process progresses to fibrosis and cirrhosis.[1]

The etiology of PBC is multifactorial. Geographic variations in disease prevalence suggest that environmental factors play a role in the pathogenesis. It is thought that an environmental trigger, such as an infection or toxin, either directly causes bile duct injury or initiates the process of autoimmunity.[2] Infectious organisms, including *Helicobacter pylori*, *Escherichia coli*, *Chlamydia pneumoniae*, and retroviruses, as well as toxins containing halogenated hydrocarbons (found in pesticides and cosmetics), have been implicated.

Pathogenically, both cellular and humoral immune mechanisms are involved. CD4[+] and CD8[+] T lymphocytes aggregate in regions of periportal inflammation and trigger cytokine-mediated cytotoxic reactions. The antimitochondrial antibody (AMA) is an autoantibody targeted to the E2

subunit of the pyruvate dehydrogenase complex (PDC-E2), which initiates an immunologic cascade resulting in bile duct cell apoptosis.

Primary Sclerosing Cholangitis

PSC is a chronic, cholestatic disorder associated with inflammatory bowel disease (IBD) and involves the medium-to-large intrahepatic and extrahepatic bile ducts. Pathogenically, the disease manifests as progressive biliary necroinflammation, fibrosis, multifocal stricturing, and obstruction. Prolonged retention of bile and associated toxins, along with inflammation due to recurrent or chronic cholangitis, may ultimately lead to hepatic fibrosis and cirrhosis.

The etiology of PSC is unknown, although it is likely multifactorial. Proposed mechanisms include humoral and cell-mediated immunologic insults to the bile duct epithelium, ischemic ductal injury, and ductal damage induced by chronic cholangitis and recurrent portal phlebitis in IBD patients with increased bacterial permeability across the inflamed colonic wall.[3] As evidenced by familial pedigree studies, genetic factors may make certain patients particularly susceptible to PSC pathogenesis.[4]

The immunologic underpinnings of PSC are supported by the presence of various autoantibodies and immunoglobulins. Autoantibodies, such as antinuclear antibody (ANA), anti-smooth muscle antibody (ASMA), peripheral antineutrophil cytoplasmic antibody (P-ANCA), and autoantibodies to human biliary epithelial cells (BEC), suggest a loss of self-tolerance to autoantigens, whereas hypergammaglobulinemia and increased levels of serum IgM imply a heightened immunologic response. Later stages of the immunologic response are mediated by CD4[+] and CD8[+] T lymphocytes, which are heavily represented in the periportal inflammatory infiltration of PSC.

PREVALENCE AND EPIDEMIOLOGY

Primary Biliary Cirrhosis

The prevalence of PBC varies geographically but is generally thought to be greatest in northern Europeans.[1] Prevalences ranging from 19 to 402 cases per million in Australia and Minnesota, respectively, have been reported.[5,6] All races are affected. There is a strong female predominance, with women accounting for 90% of cases. Disease onset is in adulthood, with a median age at diagnosis of 50 years. In familial pedigree studies, 6% of affected individuals have at least one family member with PBC. The concordance frequency of PBC in monozygotic twins is 63%.[7,8]

Risk factors for PBC pathogenesis include smoking, prior abdominal surgeries or tonsillectomies, urinary tract infections, and the presence of other autoimmune diseases (all with odds ratios of at least 2.0).[9]

Primary Sclerosing Cholangitis

Worldwide, the prevalence of PSC ranges between 10 to 60 cases per million. However, as with PBC, geographic variations exist. For example, the prevalence in Spain is 2 cases per million, compared with 136 cases per million in parts of the United States.[10,11] These geographic differences probably reflect the varying frequency of IBD in the underlying population, as well as discrepancy in access to diagnostic procedures. Approximately 75% of patients with PSC are male, and the average age at diagnosis is 40 years. Family history appears to play an important role: the risk of PSC in first-degree relatives of afflicted patients is roughly 100-fold greater than in the general population.[12]

The most important risk factor for PSC is IBD. About 75% of PSC patients have IBD, with ulcerative colitis (UC) accounting for 90% of the IBD cases. Conversely, in patients with UC, the risk of developing PSC approaches 4%, with the highest risk in male patients with pancolitis.[13] In general, however, there is no correlation between the duration and severity of IBD and the course of PSC.

CLINICAL PRESENTATION

Primary Biliary Cirrhosis

PBC is a progressive disease. About 40% of patients are symptomatic at diagnosis, and an additional 25% develop symptoms within a few years with rapid progression to cirrhosis over a decade.[14]

The most common symptoms are fatigue and pruritus, occurring in 60% and 50% of patients, respectively.[1] PBC is associated with several comorbid conditions, including hypothyroidism, hyperlipidemia, sarcoidosis, renal tubular acidosis, and celiac disease, as well as autoimmune disorders such as Sjögren's syndrome and scleroderma. Malabsorption due to bile salt deficiency may occur in advanced disease and manifest as steatorrhea and fat-soluble vitamin deficiencies. Bone pain and spontaneous fractures due to osteopenia/osteoporosis related to vitamin D deficiency are common. The clinical manifestations of cirrhosis and portal hypertension in PBC are similar to other causes of chronic liver disease, except that variceal hemorrhage may occur earlier in the disease course, before the development of true cirrhosis.[15] In patients who have progressed to cirrhosis, hepatocellular carcinoma occurs with an average yearly incidence of approximately 7%, which is slightly higher than the published incidence for most other causes of cirrhosis.[16]

The serologic hallmark of PBC is AMA positivity. These antibodies have a sensitivity and specificity for PBC of 90% and 95%, respectively.[17] ANAs are found in up to 70% of patients but are nonspecific and do not generally aid in the diagnosis. Characteristically, these patients have striking elevations in the serum alkaline phosphatase level (three to four times the upper limit of normal), as well as elevations in γ-glutamyltransferase (GGT) and abnormalities in immunoglobulins, particularly IgM. Imaging is obtained to exclude biliary obstruction. A liver biopsy is almost always performed for staging and prognostication and as a baseline for evaluating the response to treatment. A definitive diagnosis of PBC requires the presence of AMAs, elevated alkaline phosphatase for 6 months, and characteristic histologic findings; a probable diagnosis requires two of these three criteria.[1]

Primary Sclerosing Cholangitis

As with PBC, PSC, too, is a progressive disease. The most important prognostic factor for predicting the rate of progression is the presence or absence of symptoms at the time of diagnosis. Most patients with PSC are asymptomatic at the time of diagnosis; transplant-free survival in these patients is on average 10 to 12 years, whereas survival is halved in those symptomatic at diagnosis.

Characteristic symptoms of PSC are fatigue and pruritus, which typically do not occur until the disease progresses to more advanced stages. Frequent but nonspecific symptoms include right upper quadrant abdominal pain, nausea, anorexia, weight loss, and jaundice. Malabsorption due to bile salt deficiency, in the form of steatorrhea and fat-soluble vitamin deficiencies, and osteoporosis-related bone disease manifest in the latest stages of disease.

In 10% to 15% of patients, transient episodes of fever, chills, right upper quadrant abdominal pain, and jaundice may occur, which are typically mirrored by fleeting elevations in serum alkaline phosphatase and bilirubin levels. Although blood cultures rarely become positive and antibiotics are not typically prescribed, these occurrences mimic acute bacterial cholangitis and may represent transient occlusions of strictured bile ducts by biliary sludge or small stones.[18] Twenty percent of patients develop a dominant stricture, presenting as mechanical obstruction and acute cholangitis.

The main concern with a dominant stricture is whether it represents a cholangiocarcinoma. Arising in either the intrahepatic or extrahepatic ducts, cholangiocarcinoma is accelerated in PSC patients, generally occurring when patients reach their 40s, roughly 20 years before onset in patients without PSC. The prognosis is grim, with median survival of 6 months after diagnosis. In patients in whom cirrhosis develops, hepatocellular carcinoma occurs at similar rates as in other causes of chronic liver disease.

As stated earlier, another strong association is that between PSC and UC. Although the symptoms of UC may predate or follow the diagnosis of PSC, the majority of patients (>75%) have established UC at the time of their PSC diagnosis. Proctocolectomy for UC has no impact on the course of PSC, and PSC may be detected years after proctocolectomy.[19]

Curiously, compared with patients with UC but without PSC, patients with UC and PSC have less active colitis, remain asymptomatic for longer periods, and require less anti-inflammatory and immunosuppressive medication to achieve disease remission. The rectum is often spared in PSC, which differs from the cardinal finding of rectal inflammation in non-PSC patients. Nevertheless, PSC patients with UC have a five times greater risk for developing colorectal cancer than patients with UC without PSC.[20]

Serologic immunologic markers are abundant in PSC patients: 30% have hypergammaglobulinemia, 50% demonstrate elevated serum IgM titers, and approximately 65% exhibit P-ANCAs, with fewer proportions of patients developing ANAs and ASMAs.[21] In contrast to PBC, PSC patients lack AMAs. In addition to these immunologic measures, PSC is particularly suspected in patients with IBD with markedly elevated serum alkaline phosphatase levels (more than four times the upper limit of normal) and GGT in association with hepatomegaly. The serum aminotransferases are typically elevated to a lesser degree, not exceeding 300 IU/L. The serum bilirubin value is normal early in the disease course but rises in advanced cases. Serum albumin, on the other hand, may be low at the time of diagnosis, especially in instances of severe coexisting IBD.

As discussed further later, radiology plays a vital role in the diagnosis of PSC by elucidating ductal abnormalities, cholangiocarcinoma, and hepatocellular carcinoma. Liver biopsy is obtained for prognostication and staging but may not help with diagnosis because the usual findings of ductopenia and portal inflammation and fibrosis are nonspecific and, owing to their patchy distribution as well as sampling errors unavoidable with biopsy, may be missed.

PATHOLOGY

Primary Biliary Cirrhosis

In the early stages of PBC, the liver is slightly enlarged and is variably bile stained. In later stages, the liver is cirrhotic and has a green hue, reflecting the extensive cholestasis. The microscopic hallmark of PBC is destructive, nonsuppurative cholangitis affecting the interlobular and septal bile ducts, resulting in duct loss and subsequent biliary cirrhosis.[22]

With disease progression, there is patchy necrosis of the periportal hepatocytes and delicate periportal fibrosis, often with ductular proliferation. Florid duct lesions become less common as the disease advances into the later stages. Fibrous septa appear and extend in a portal-portal distribution, later evolving into biliary cirrhosis. This type of cirrhosis results in regenerative nodules with serpentine or garland-like borders, as opposed to the roughly spherical regenerative nodules seen in the usual forms of cirrhosis. The regenerative nodules in biliary cirrhosis have some resemblance to the pieces of a jigsaw puzzle.

Primary Sclerosing Cholangitis

Similar to the gross findings of PBC, the liver in early PSC is slightly enlarged and variably bile stained, progressing to biliary cirrhosis in the later stages. One characteristic gross finding in PSC is the presence in the hilum of cholangiectases, which are cystic collections of bilious, dark green material measuring up to several centimeters in size and representing cystically dilated intrahepatic ducts.[23]

The pathognomonic microscopic finding of PSC is the concentric fibrous replacement of bile ducts in an "onion-skin" pattern. This fibrous cholangitis is characterized by a mixed inflammatory infiltrate that, over time, results in loss of the bile duct in a process called fibrous obliterative cholangitis. As the disease progresses, fibrous septa form between portal tracts and ductopenia becomes more common; inflammation in this stage typically subsides.[24] End-stage PSC is indistinguishable from other causes of biliary cirrhosis, with large irregularly shaped, bile-stained regenerative nodules characteristically arranged in a jigsaw puzzle pattern.

IMAGING

Radiologic imaging is obtained in the initial evaluation of patients with PBC to assist in distinguishing the differential diagnosis of cholestasis. Namely, various radiologic studies are useful in evaluating for biliary obstruction, which is the main condition that needs to be ruled out in the workup of these patients. Radiology also plays an important role in the surveillance of this chronic condition, particularly with regard to the evolution of portal hypertension and detection of hepatocellular carcinoma.

Rather than playing an ancillary role as it does in PBC, imaging has a central diagnostic responsibility in PSC and fundamentally impacts treatment options. Similar to PBC, however, imaging is useful in excluding secondary causes of biliary obstruction and surveillance of complications of portal hypertension, cholangiocarcinoma, and hepatocellular carcinoma. The two principal techniques utilized to highlight the structure of the intrahepatic and extrahepatic ducts are cholangiography and magnetic resonance cholangiopancreatography (MRCP). Cholangiography, in particular, is most commonly accomplished via endoscopic retrograde cholangiopancreatography (ERCP); transhepatic cholangiography is generally pursued only if ERCP is unsuccessful. In all techniques, the characteristic finding of PSC is a beading pattern of short, multifocal strictures with areas of normal or dilated intervening intrahepatic and extrahepatic ducts (Table 71-1).

CT, MRI, Ultrasonography, and Cholangiography

Primary Biliary Cirrhosis

Patients with PBC have a spectrum of disease severity ranging from asymptomatic to cirrhosis. In the initial presentation, the liver may be normal or slightly enlarged.

TABLE 71-1   Accuracy, Limitations, and Pitfalls of the Modalities Used in Imaging of Cholestatic Hepatic Disorders

	Modality	Accuracy	Limitations	Pitfalls
Primary Biliary Cirrhosis	CT	No data on the accuracy of CT in the diagnosis of PBC		
	MRI	In one retrospective study, the "periportal halo" sign had 43% sensitivity and 100% specificity for the diagnosis of PBC in patients with known cirrhosis.	Low sensitivity	
	MRCP	No data on the accuracy of MRCP in the diagnosis of PBC		
	Ultrasonography	No data on the accuracy of US in the diagnosis of PBC		
Primary Sclerosing Cholangitis	CT	No data on the accuracy of CT in the diagnosis of PSC		
	MRCP	Sensitivity of 85% to 88% Specificity of 92% to 97% Positive predictive value of 85% to 94% Negative predicted value of 93% to 94% Overall diagnostic accuracy is 90%.	May be negative in the early stages of PSC Lower spatial resolution than ERCP Does not permit tissue sampling or treatment of stenoses	Secondary causes of chronic cholangitis may be indistinguishable from PSC. Biliary neoplasia and PSC may be difficult to differentiate. Performed in the physiologic nondistended state, lending more difficulty to visualizing small ducts
	ERCP	Considered the gold standard for the diagnosis Overall diagnostic accuracy is 97%	Invasive; may cause complications such as sepsis, hemorrhage, pancreatitis, bowel perforation, and cholangitis	Limited visualization of the peripheral ducts due to central obstruction from stones, strictures, and thick bile
	Ultrasonography	No data on the accuracy of US in the diagnosis of PSC		

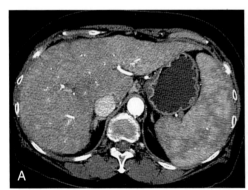

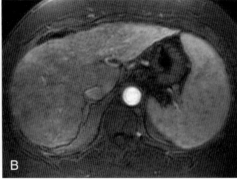

■ **FIGURE 71-1**   A 58-year-old woman presented with cirrhosis due to PBC. Axial contrast-enhanced CT image (**A**) and 3D dynamic gradient-echo MR axial image (**B**) obtained during the arterial phase after intravenous administration of iodine and a gadolinium-based contrast agent, respectively, demonstrate diffuse heterogeneous enhancement of the liver parenchyma.

Splenomegaly, sometimes severe, is a common finding in early stages. Early disease is also associated with periportal hyperintensity on T2-weighted (T2W) MR images, a finding that is less common in late PBC.[25]

With disease progression, the liver demonstrates heterogeneous enhancement that may be associated with small, punctuated arterial-portal shunts in the early phase of dynamic contrast injection (Fig. 71-1). Hepatic fibrosis presenting as either reticular, confluent, or both reticular and confluent patterns may also be observed. In some cases, regenerative nodules of various sizes can be seen intercalated by coarse fibrous reticulations (Fig. 71-2). Additionally, lymphadenopathy, manifesting as enlarged lymph nodes in the porta hepatis, gastrohepatic ligament, portacaval region, and upper retroperito-

neal regions, is a frequent finding, seen in 60% to 80% of patients.[26]

The imaging features of advanced PBC usually resemble those seen in other causes of cirrhosis and portal hypertension. However, one imaging finding that may potentially differentiate cirrhosis secondary to PBC versus other causes is the "periportal halo" sign. This finding was described in 43% of patients with advanced PBC compared with none in cirrhotic patients without PBC, suggesting that this is a specific imaging finding for the diagnosis of PBC.[27] On MRI, the "periportal halo" sign is seen as a low signal intensity abnormality without mass effect on T1-weighted (T1W) and T2W images, measuring 5 to 10 mm (Fig. 71-3). This abnormality is centered on portal venous branches and is more conspicuous on the

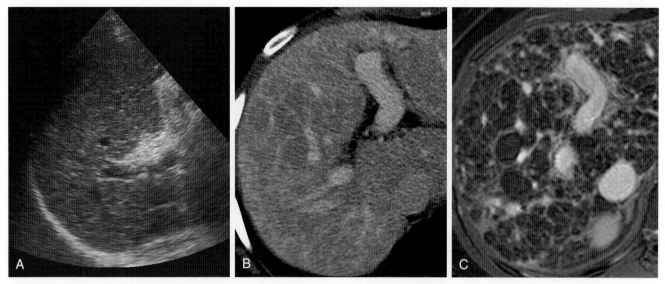

■ **FIGURE 71-2** A 62-year-old woman presented with cirrhosis due to PBC. **A,** Transverse ultrasound image of the liver shows mild nonspecific diffuse heterogeneity of the hepatic parenchyma. **B,** Axial postcontrast CT image acquired during the portal venous phase shows heterogeneity of the liver parenchyma. Note the diffuse reticular pattern, mainly in the periphery of the liver. **C,** Axial double-contrast–enhanced 3D gradient-echo MR image of the liver obtained after intravenous administration of iron oxides and a gadolinium-based contrast agent shows regenerative nodules of various sizes intercalated by coarse fibrous reticulations.

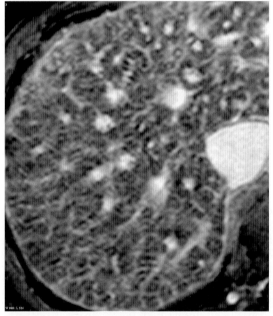

■ **FIGURE 71-3** A 57-year-old woman presented with cirrhosis due to PBC. Axial double-contrast–enhanced 3D gradient-echo MR image of the liver obtained after intravenous administration of iron oxides and a gadolinium-based contrast agent shows innumerable small regenerative nodules intercalated by coarse fibrous reticulations. Note the areas of low signal intensity centered around portal triads in the middle of some of the nodules, characterizing the "periportal halo" sign.

portal venous and equilibrium phases.[27] Additionally, in contrast to other chronic liver diseases, portal hypertension may occur even before cirrhosis has developed; therefore, some patients with severe portal hypertension due to PBC may have an enlarged liver, an unusual finding among other causes of chronic liver disease.[28]

In PBC, cholangiography studies such as ERCP and/or MRCP are usually normal but in some cases demonstrate diffuse attenuation of the bile ducts.[28]

Primary Sclerosing Cholangitis

In the early stages of PSC, CT, MRI, and ultrasonography demonstrate hepatic parenchymal heterogeneity associated with a normal-appearing biliary tree. Nonetheless, in some cases, fine ulcerations of the common bile duct may be seen at ERCP.[3]

As PSC progresses, intrahepatic bile duct dilatation becomes more evident and is a characteristic finding observed in approximately 80% of patients. Additional findings of PSC include intrahepatic and extrahepatic bile duct stenosis in 64% and 50% of cases, respectively, and extrahepatic bile duct wall enhancement and thickening in 67% and 50%, respectively.[29] CT shows scattered dilated intrahepatic ducts, some of which may have no apparent connection to more central bile ducts. Biliary calculi may develop in obstructed ducts as a consequence of biliary stasis and secondary infection.[29] In a small subgroup of patients, the cystic duct or gallbladder may be involved. Ultrasonography depicts intrahepatic and/or extrahepatic bile duct dilatation.

On MRI, heterogeneity of the liver parenchyma, with peripheral wedge-shaped areas and fine reticulations of increased signal intensity on T2W images associated with bile duct dilatation, is suggestive of PSC.[30] Additional MRI findings include increased enhancement of the liver parenchyma on dynamic arterial-phase images, more evident in peripheral areas, in 56% of cases.[29]

A more precise diagnosis of PSC can be obtained with cholangiography, either by ERCP or MRCP. ERCP can demonstrate multifocal areas of strictures and irregularities involving the intrahepatic and/or extrahepatic bile

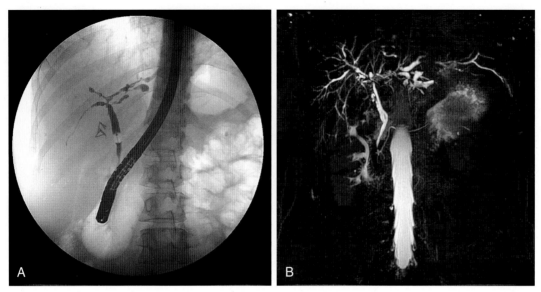

■ FIGURE 71-4   A 48-year-old-man presented with PSC. **A,** ERCP image demonstrates irregularity and narrowing of the intrahepatic and extrahepatic bile ducts intercalated with segments of normal or dilated ducts, producing a "beaded" appearance. Note the nonopacification of the peripheral ducts due to obstructions in the more central ducts, causing a "pruned tree" appearance of the biliary tree. **B,** Oblique coronal collapsed image from a respiratory-triggered 3D MRCP sequence reveals diffuse beading of the intrahepatic ducts. Note that the peripheral ducts, which were nonopacified at ERCP, are visible at MRCP. *(Case courtesy of Scott Reeder, MD, PhD, University of Wisconsin.)*

ducts intercalated with segments of normal or dilated ducts, producing the characteristic beaded appearance of PSC. The strictures can vary in size, ranging from 1 to 2 mm to several centimeters. In some cases, the lack of visualization of the peripheral ducts due to obliteration of the more central ducts causes a "pruned tree" appearance of the biliary tree (Fig. 71-4). Although ERCP is currently the gold standard for diagnosing PSC, it is an invasive procedure that may cause complications such as sepsis, hemorrhage, pancreatitis, bowel perforation, and cholangitis. Transhepatic cholangiography may be performed if ERCP is unsuccessful.[31]

As with ERCP, the key MRCP feature of PSC is the characteristic beaded appearance of the biliary ducts. MRCP is also useful in demonstrating the extent of the strictured segment and displaying the dilated peripheral bile ducts that are not connected to central stenosed ducts (a finding that only can be demonstrated via MRCP) (see Fig. 71-4). Less frequent findings include webs, stones, and diverticula. MRCP has a reported sensitivity of 85% to 88%, a specificity of 92% to 97%, a positive predictive value of 85% to 94%, and a negative predictive value of 93% to 94% in detecting PSC. Unfortunately, these performance characteristics are valid only in advanced disease, because MRCP may be normal in the early stages of PSC. The overall diagnostic accuracy of MRCP in patients with PSC is 90%, compared with 97% for ERCP.[31] MRCP has the advantage of being a noninvasive method with less risk for complications when compared with ERCP. Furthermore, MRCP can depict more strictures, especially of the peripheral intrahepatic ducts, and is better at visualizing bile ducts proximal to obstructed areas and unconnected to the central ducts; direct cholangiography cannot depict these regions because of nonfilling.[32]

In patients with cirrhosis secondary to PSC there is marked lobulation of the hepatic contours. Parenchymal atrophy occurs proximal to the obstructed bile ducts and is more frequently seen in the right lobe of the liver, whereas marked hypertrophy occurs in spared segments. Hypertrophy of the caudate lobe is seen in up to 98% of cases. The hypertrophied caudate lobe, surrounded by the atrophic right hepatic lobe, produces a mass-like or "pseudo tumor" appearance, which is a prominent feature of cirrhosis caused by PSC (Fig. 71-5).[33] Although published reports emphasize hypertrophy of the caudate lobe, hypertrophic "pseudotumors" also may occur in other portions of the liver. Long broad scars of fibrosis may surround the hypertrophied segments that, in some cases, may show paucity of bile ducts (Fig. 71-6).

Many PSC cases are complicated by cholangitis. Heterogeneous enhancement of the liver associated with biliary ductal dilatation and mural contrast enhancement of the bile duct are seen in patients with acute cholangitis and may predispose to hepatic abscess formation.[29]

Cholangiocarcinoma may occur in up to 20% of PSC patients. The tumor is usually multifocal. Cholangiographic findings that suggest the presence of a superimposed cholangiocarcinoma include rapid progression of strictures, asymmetrically thickened bile duct walls, irregular luminal narrowing causing marked dilatation of ducts proximal to strictures, and development of intraluminal masses or polyps evident after delayed contrast enhancement.[34]

Imaging Algorithms

Primary Biliary Cirrhosis

Ultrasonography is the initial modality used to evaluate patients with cholestatic serologic markers. If biliary

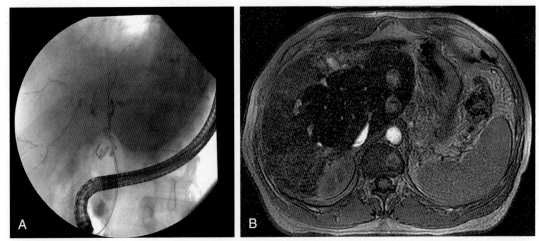

■ **FIGURE 71-5** A 50-year-old man presented with cirrhosis due to PSC. **A,** ERCP image demonstrates multifocal strictures of the intrahepatic and extrahepatic bile ducts intercalated with segments of normal-caliber ducts, producing the characteristic beaded appearance of PSC. **B,** Axial iron oxides–enhanced 2D T2*W gradient-echo MR image of the liver shows a "pseudotumor" appearance of the markedly hypertrophic caudate lobe. Note the incidental ghost artifacts from the aorta over the left lobe of the liver.

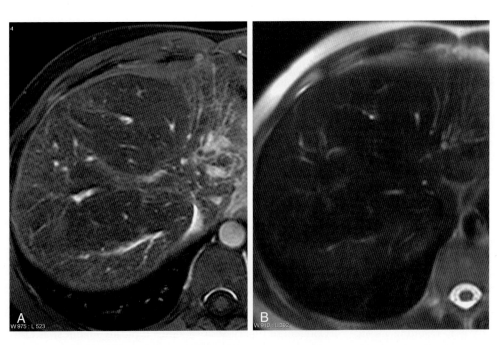

■ **FIGURE 71-6** A 56-year-old-man presented with cirrhosis due to PSC. **A,** Axial double-contrast-enhanced 3D gradient-echo MR image of the liver obtained after intravenous administration of iron oxides and a gadolinium-based contrast agent shows hypertrophy of the central portions of segments 8 and 4a. The peripheral portion of segment 8 is atrophic, as are segments 7 and 2. The atrophic parenchyma has coarse reticulations consistent with fibrosis. **B,** Axial T2W single-shot turbo spin-echo MR image reveals a paucity of bile ducts within the hypertrophic segments.

obstruction is suggested, further characterization is achieved by CT or MRI. Because patients with cirrhosis related to PBC are at risk for the development of hepatocellular carcinoma, the American Association for the Study of Liver Diseases (AASLD) recommends regular screening; although the AASLD suggests biannual ultrasound examinations, some institutions, including ours, perform CT or MRI screening every 6 months.

Primary Sclerosing Cholangitis

As with PBC, ultrasonography is the initial modality used to evaluate cholestasis. Confirmation and further charac-

terization of biliary obstruction is achieved by CT or MRI. The gold standard for PSC diagnosis is ERCP. If ERCP is contraindicated (particularly in elderly patients with comorbid conditions), MRCP is a valid alternative. However, it should be noted that MRCP is not therapeutic: if a dominant stricture is present, ERCP should be performed because of its capabilities in sampling the stricture for malignancy and dilating the narrowed region.

Patients with PSC are at risk for the development of cholangiocarcinoma. However, regular screening with imaging is not advocated because no studies have demonstrated a benefit in patient outcomes using this strategy. As with other causes of chronic liver disease, patients with PSC are at risk for hepatocellular carcinoma. Because the rate of transformation to hepatocellular carcinoma is poorly characterized, the AASLD does not provide strict screening guidelines. However, some institutions, including ours, pursue CT or MRI screening every 6 months.

Classic Signs

PRIMARY BILIARY CIRRHOSIS

■ In its initial presentation, the liver of a patient with PBC may appear normal or slightly enlarged, with concomitant splenomegaly.

■ On MRI, there is periportal hyperintensity on T2W images. As the disease progresses, heterogeneous enhancement of the liver and lymphadenopathy may be seen. The biliary system is usually normal. Portal hypertension may develop early in the disease course, before the onset of cirrhosis.

■ Findings in end-stage liver disease due to PBC are nonspecific; the "periportal halo" sign, if observed, may suggest a diagnosis of PBC.

PRIMARY SCLEROSING CHOLANGITIS

■ Many imaging findings in cirrhosis secondary to advanced PSC are similar to those seen in other causes of end-stage liver disease.

■ Findings more specific for PSC include biliary duct dilatation in the setting of the characteristic beaded appearance of the biliary tree and marked hypertrophy and "pseudotumor" appearance of spared segments of the liver, characteristically including the caudate lobe.

DIFFERENTIAL DIAGNOSIS

Primary Biliary Cirrhosis

The diagnosis of PBC is strongly suggested in a middle-aged woman presenting with fatigue and/or pruritus in the setting of cholestatic laboratory findings. The primary alternate diagnosis to be excluded is that of extrahepatic biliary obstruction in the form of a neoplasm, stricture, or choledocholithiasis. Neoplasms may involve either the common bile duct or ampulla of Vater, resulting in secondary biliary obstruction. Choledocholithiasis is common in certain groups, especially obese females older than the age of 40. These mechanical biliary obstructions generally are easily identifiable with noninvasive imaging (CT, MRI, MRCP). If liver biopsy is performed, mechanical obstructions are characterized histologically by the presence of ductal proliferation (rather than duct dropout) and neutrophilic (rather than lymphocytic) infiltration.

PBC also needs to be distinguished from PSC. The presence of AMA confirms the diagnosis of PBC, whereas the presence of IBD favors PSC. Histologic differences between these two conditions are slight and do not usually permit reliable differentiation.

Although granulomas are a histologic hallmark of PBC, other hepatic conditions, such as hepatic sarcoidosis and some cases of hepatitis C (HCV) infection, also may be associated with granuloma formation and cholestatic liver function tests. The presence of AMA excludes these conditions.

Another diagnostic consideration is drug hepatotoxicity. Various ingestions or exposures (e.g., phenytoin, anabolic steroids, estrogens), may result in both hepatocellular and cholestatic biochemical profiles. Affected patients have a suggestive ingestion/exposure history and absent AMA and other autoimmune markers.

At the time of diagnosis, patients with PBC usually have a normal or enlarged liver with splenomegaly. When presenting with hepatomegaly, PBC needs to be differentiated from other causes of hepatomegaly, including hepatitis, lymphoproliferative diseases, toxic and drug-related diseases, metastatic diseases, metabolic disorders, and vascular disorders. In cirrhotic patients secondary to PBC, the imaging findings overlap with other causes of end-stage liver disease. However, portal hypertension may occur even before cirrhosis, and some patients with portal hypertension may have an enlarged liver, a useful finding in the differential diagnosis of PBC. Additionally, the "periportal halo" sign, if present, suggests the diagnosis of PBC.

Primary Sclerosing Cholangitis

PSC is highly suggested in a patient with UC, cholestatic serologic tests, and characteristic cholangiographic findings. However, UC may be associated with hepatic abnormalities other than PSC. Such abnormalities may occur in the setting of normal bile ducts and include hepatic steatosis, as well as varying degrees of portal inflammation and fibrosis. These latter findings are differentiated on liver biopsy.

Distinguishing PSC from secondary biliary cirrhosis is sometimes arduous. Causes of secondary biliary cirrhosis that may be confused with PSC include choledocholithiasis, ischemic bile duct injury, prior biliary surgery, and congenital biliary abnormalities. Choledocholithiasis is frequent in certain groups, especially obese females older than the age of 40. Ischemic bile duct injury is most common after liver transplantation, although it has also been identified after transcatheter arterial chemoembolization therapy for hepatocellular carcinoma.[34] Biliary surgery may be complicated by mechanical stricturing. Congenital biliary abnormalities typically manifest as cholestasis in early life. Differentiating between these various concerns requires careful history-taking and radiologic investigation.

PSC may be difficult to differentiate from cholangiocarcinoma, particularly if there is a single or dominant stricture. Cytology or biopsy via ERCP is diagnostic for cholangiocarcinoma in some instances, although underlying PSC may be present. PSC is suggested if concomitant IBD is present, along with a history of cholestatic serologic liver tests.

Other confounding conditions include AIDS cholangiopathy, PBC, autoimmune hepatitis, and drug reactions. AIDS cholangiopathy occurs in human immunodeficiency virus (HIV)-infected patients with CD4 counts below 100/mm³ and within the context of concomitant infection; the most common infection is by intestinal *Cryptosporidium*, which yields nonbloody diarrhea (an infrequent symptom of PSC). PBC is associated with AMA positivity but not IBD. Autoimmune hepatitis may overlap with PSC and can be diagnosed via typical histologic findings of periportal plasma cell and eosinophilic infiltration. Drug hepatotoxicity may produce cholestatic liver tests and requires a careful exposure/ingestion history.

Most imaging findings in cirrhosis secondary to advanced PSC are similar to those in other causes of end-stage liver disease. However, PSC is suggested by a "beaded" biliary tree and marked hypertrophy of spared segments.

Conditions that may mimic the cholangiographic findings of PSC include ascending cholangitis, AIDS cholangiopathy, recurrent pyogenic cholangitis, and biliary ischemia due to intra-arterial chemotherapy or liver transplantation surgery. Ascending cholangitis, due to bacterial contamination of an obstructed duct, is a clinical diagnosis in which patients generally present with abdominal pain, fever, and jaundice, in the setting of a leukocytosis and positive blood cultures. AIDS cholangiopathy is best discriminated from PSC by its unique combination of intrahepatic ductal strictures and papillary stenosis. In chemotherapy-induced cholangitis, the most common cholangiographic findings are strictures of the bifurcation of the common hepatic duct with sparing of the distal common bile duct; this contrasts to PSC, which demonstrates diffuse involvement of the intrahepatic and extrahepatic bile ducts.[31]

TREATMENT

Medical Treatment

Primary Biliary Cirrhosis

Promoting the delivery of bile acids into the bile canaliculi, ursodeoxycholic acid (ursodiol; UDCA) is the only treatment approved by the U.S. Food and Drug Administration (FDA) for PBC. It slows the progression of disease, delaying advancement to cirrhosis and the need for liver transplantation. In approximately 25% of patients treated with UDCA, serum biochemical markers of cholestasis normalize and histology stabilizes or improves.[35] Patients successfully treated with UDCA have similar 20-year survival compared with matched controls.[36] If laboratory tests or histologic findings do not improve on UDCA monotherapy, some clinicians advocate adding anti-inflammatory or immunosuppressant agents such as corticosteroids, colchicine, methotrexate, or cyclosporine. Specific therapy should also be directed at the various symptoms associated with PBC, such as pruritus.

Liver transplantation is a viable option in patients with PBC-induced liver failure. Five-year survival of transplanted patients is 85%, although PBC recurs in 30% of patients at 10 years.[37] Re-transplantation is required in 10% of cases. Indications for liver transplantation include hepatic decompensation, development of appropriate-stage hepatocellular carcinoma, and debilitating fatigue or pruritus.

Primary Sclerosing Cholangitis

No therapy has been shown to increase transplant-free survival or reverse the severity of histologic disease. Management focuses on treating the complications related to chronic cholestasis (e.g., pruritus, malabsorption), controlling associated conditions (e.g., IBD), and, once cirrhosis develops, monitoring complications of portal hypertension and hepatocellular carcinoma. Various bile acids and anti-inflammatory and immunosuppressive agents have been investigated, including corticosteroids, methotrexate, cyclosporine, etanercept, and tacrolimus.

Surgical management of PSC covers four areas: treatment of biliary strictures, proctocolectomy for concomitant UC, management of cholangiocarcinoma, and liver transplantation.

Twenty percent of patients develop a dominant stricture in the common bile duct, common hepatic duct, or left/right hepatic ducts, presenting with mechanical obstruction, progressive jaundice, and acute cholangitis. Endoscopic treatment via ERCP is the treatment of choice in these patients with symptomatic dominant strictures. Endoscopic management with balloon dilatation and stenting is most successful in the case of common bile duct strictures; these strategies are less effective if the stricture is in an intrahepatic duct. Stent placement is associated with recurrent stent occlusion and cholangitis. Stents may need to be exchanged at regular intervals. Endoscopic therapy may yield prolonged biochemical and symptomatic improvement for several years and is a reasonable "bridge" to liver transplantation. Cytologic brushings and/or endoscopic biopsies can be performed if there is a concern for cholangiocarcinoma. When endoscopic therapy for a dominant stricture is unavailable or unsuccessful, surgical intervention is an option. Biliary tract reconstructive procedures, such as the bilioenteric bypass, are sometimes performed. Because of infectious complications, external biliary drains are not viable long-term options although they may be used in acute cholangitis when rapid biliary decompression is required.

Patients with concomitant UC are at high risk for colorectal cancer, and proctocolectomy is frequently performed prophylactically. As discussed earlier, proctocolectomy has no impact on the course of PSC.

The surgical management of cholangiocarcinoma does not typically involve liver transplantation owing to the high risk of tumor recurrence. However, in select patients, transplantation remains a possibility. The Mayo Clinic protocol permits liver transplantation after a course of neoadjuvant chemotherapy and irradiation for perihilar cholangiocarcinoma without lymph node involvement; a 5-year survival rate of 82% has been reported.[38]

Liver transplantation has replaced biliary-enteric reconstruction as the surgical treatment of choice in patients with PSC. Five-year survival of transplanted patients is approximately 85%.[39] Recurrence of PSC post transplant occurs in about 20% of patients, usually manifesting within the first year.[40] The impact of liver transplantation on the course of concurrent IBD is variable; some patients experience regression of colitis and long-term remission, whereas others progress rapidly to colectomy.

What the Referring Physician Needs to Know

PRIMARY BILIARY CIRRHOSIS

- Autoimmune-mediated destruction occurs of small and medium-sized intrahepatic bile ducts.
- This chronic, cholestatic condition is marked by fatigue, pruritus, jaundice, bone disease, and progressive liver disease.
- Pathogenesis is multifactorial, with genetic, environmental, and infectious underpinnings.
- AMA is the serologic hallmark.
- The diagnosis is strongly suggested in a middle-aged woman presenting with fatigue or jaundice who has cholestatic laboratory findings and AMA positivity.
- Annual incidence of hepatocellular carcinoma in patients with cirrhosis related to PBC is approximately 7%.
- UDCA is the only FDA-approved medical treatment, with liver transplantation reserved for those patients with progressive, decompensated liver failure, hepatocellular carcinoma, and/or intractable symptoms.

PRIMARY SCLEROSING CHOLANGITIS

- This chronic, cholestatic disorder associated with IBD involves the medium and large intrahepatic and extrahepatic bile ducts.

- It is characterized by pruritus, jaundice, recurrent episodes of cholangitis, cholangiocarcinoma, and progressive liver disease.
- There is a strong association with IBD: 75% of PSC patients have IBD, 90% of whom have UC.
- There is no serologic hallmark, although a variety of autoantibody and immunoglobulin levels may be elevated.
- The diagnosis is strongly suggested in a patient with UC, cholestatic serologic tests, and characteristic cholangiographic findings.
- Patients with cirrhosis due to PSC are at increased risk for hepatocellular carcinoma.
- Cholangiocarcinoma develops in up to 20% of patients.
- No medical treatment has proven to be reliably effective; endoscopic and surgical approaches, including liver transplantation, are commonly used in the setting of a dominant biliary stricture, decompensated liver failure, hepatocellular carcinoma, and/or cholangiocarcinoma.

KEY POINTS

Primary Biliary Cirrhosis

- Periportal hyperintensity is seen on T2W MR images at earlier stages.
- "Periportal halo" sign is seen in 43% of advanced cases.
- Lymphadenopathy occurs in 60% to 80% of cases.
- Cholangiographic studies are usually normal, although diffuse attenuation of the bile ducts may be observed.
- Portal hypertension may precede cirrhosis.
- In cirrhosis secondary to PBC, the liver may be enlarged.

Primary Sclerosing Cholangitis

- Characteristic finding is multiple areas of biliary duct strictures intercalated with segments of normal or dilated ducts, producing the characteristic beaded appearance.
- "Pruned tree" appearance of the biliary tree at ERCP is due to nonopacification of the peripheral ducts.
- There is a hypertrophic "pseudotumor" appearance of the caudate lobe.

SUGGESTED READINGS

Bambha K, Kim WR, Talwalkar J, et al. Incidence, clinical spectrum, and outcomes of primary sclerosing cholangitis in a United States community. Gastroenterology 2003; 125:1354-1369.

Ernst O, Asselah T, Sergent G, et al. MR cholangiography in primary sclerosing cholangitis. AJR Am J Roentgenol 1998; 171:1027-1030.

Ito K, Mitchell DG, Outwater EK, Blasbalg R. Primary sclerosing cholangitis: MR imaging features. AJR Am J Roentgenol 1999; 172:1527-1533.

Kaplan MM, Gershwin ME. Primary biliary cirrhosis. N Engl J Med 2005; 353:1261-1273.

Lee YM, Kaplan MM. Primary sclerosing cholangitis. N Engl J Med 1995; 332:924-933.

Prince MI, Chetwynd A, Craig WL, et al. Asymptomatic primary biliary cirrhosis: clinical features, prognosis, and symptom progression in a large population-based cohort. Gut 2004; 53:865-870.

Wenzel JS, Donohoe A, Ford KL 3rd, et al. Primary biliary cirrhosis: MR imaging findings and description of MR imaging periportal halo sign. AJR Am J Roentgenol 2001; 176:885-889.

REFERENCES

1. Kaplan MM, Gershwin ME. Primary biliary cirrhosis. N Engl J Med 2005; 353:1261-1273.
2. Bogdanos DP, Baum H, Grasso A, et al. Microbial mimics are major targets of crossreactivity with human pyruvate dehydrogenase in primary biliary cirrhosis. J Hepatol 2004; 40:31-39.
3. Lee YM, Kaplan MM. Primary sclerosing cholangitis. N Engl J Med 1995; 332:924-933.
4. Bergquist A, Lindberg G, Saarinen S, Broome U. Increased prevalence of primary sclerosing cholangitis among first-degree relatives. J Hepatol 2005; 42:252-256.

5. Kim WR, Lindor KD, Locke GR III, et al. Epidemiology and natural history of primary biliary cirrhosis in a US community. Gastroenterology 2000; 119;1631-1636.

6. Prince MI, James OF. The epidemiology of primary biliary cirrhosis. Clin Liver Dis 2003; 7:795-819.

7. Bittencourt PL, Farias AQ, Abrantes-Lemos CP, et al. Prevalence of immune disturbances and chronic liver disease in family members of patients with primary biliary cirrhosis. J Gastroenterol Hepatol 2004; 19:873-878.

8. Selmi C, Mayo MJ, Bach N, et al. Primary biliary cirrhosis in monozygotic and dizygotic twins: genetics, epigenetics, and environment. Gastroenterology 2004; 127:485-492.

9. Parikh-Patel A, Gold EB, Worman H, et al. Risk factors for primary biliary cirrhosis in a cohort of patients from the United States. Hepatology 2001; 33:16-21.

10. Bambha K, Kim WR, Talwalkar J, et al. Incidence, clinical spectrum, and outcomes of primary sclerosing cholangitis in a United States community. Gastroenterology 2003; 125:1354-1369.

11. Escorsell A, Pares A, Rodes J, et al. Epidemiology of primary sclerosing cholangitis in Spain. Spanish Association for the Study of the Liver. J Hepatol 1994; 21:787-791.

12. Bergquist A, Lindberg G, Saarinen S, Broome U. Increased prevalence of primary sclerosing cholangitis among first-degree relatives. J Hepatol 2005; 42:252-256.

13. Olsson R, Danielsson A, Jarnerot G, et al. Prevalence of primary sclerosing cholangitis in patients with ulcerative colitis. Gastroenterology 1991; 100:1319-1323.

14. Prince MI, Chetwynd A, Craig WL, et al. Asymptomatic primary biliary cirrhosis: clinical features, prognosis, and symptom progression in a large population-based cohort. Gut 2004; 53:865-870.

15. Thornton JR, Triger DR, Losowsky MS. Variceal bleeding is associated with reduced risk of severe cholestasis in primary biliary cirrhosis. Q J Med 1989; 71:467-471.

16. Nijhawan PK, Therneau TM, Dickson ER, et al. Incidence of cancer in primary biliary cirrhosis: the Mayo experience. Hepatology 1999; 29:1396-1398.

17. Van de Water J, Cooper A, Surh CD, et al. Detection of autoantibodies to recombinant mitochondrial proteins in patients with primary biliary cirrhosis. N Engl J Med 1989; 320:1377-1380.

18. Kaplan MM. Medical approaches to primary sclerosing cholangitis. Semin Liver Dis 1991; 11:56-63.

19. Cangemi JR, Wiesner RH, Beaver SJ, et al. Effect of proctocolectomy for chronic ulcerative colitis on the natural history of primary sclerosing cholangitis. Gastroenterology 1989; 96:790-794.

20. Soetikno RM, Lin OS, Heidenreich PA, et al. Increased risk of colorectal neoplasia in patients with primary sclerosing cholangitis and ulcerative colitis: a meta-analysis. Gastrointest Endosc 2002; 56:48-54.

21. Duerr RH, Targan SR, Landers CJ, et al. Neutrophil cytoplasmic antibodies: a link between primary sclerosing cholangitis and ulcerative colitis. Gastroenterology 1991; 100:1385-1391.

22. Portmann BC, Nakanuma Y. Diseases of the bile ducts. In Burt AD, Portmann BC, Ferrell LD (eds). MacSween's Pathology of the Liver, 5th ed. New York, Churchill Livingstone, 2006, p 539.

23. Batts KP. Autoimmune and cholestatic disorders of the liver. In Odze RD, Goldblum JR, Crawford JM (eds). Surgical Pathology of the GI Tract, Liver, Biliary Tract, and Pancreas. Philadelphia, WB Saunders, 2006, p 826.

24. Portmann BC, Nakanuma Y. Diseases of the bile ducts. In Burt AD, Portmann BC, Ferrell LD (eds). MacSween's Pathology of the Liver, 5th ed. New York, Churchill Livingstone, 2006, p 554.

25. Kobayashi S, Matsui O, Gabata T, et al. MRI findings of primary biliary cirrhosis: correlation with Scheuer histologic staging. Abdom Imaging 2005; 30:71-76.

26. Blachar A, Federle MP, Brancatelli G. Primary biliary cirrhosis: clinical, pathologic, and helical CT findings in 53 patients. Radiology 2001; 220:329-336.

27. Wenzel JS, Donohoe A, Ford KL 3rd, et al. Primary biliary cirrhosis: MR imaging findings and description of MR imaging periportal halo sign. AJR Am J Roentgenol 2001; 176:885-889.

28. Kumagi T, Heathcote EJ. Primary biliary cirrhosis. Orphanet J Rare Dis 2008; 3:1.

29. Ito K, Mitchell DG, Outwater EK, Blasbalg R. Primary sclerosing cholangitis: MR imaging features. AJR Am J Roentgenol 1999; 172:1527-1533.

30. Revelon G, Rashid A, Kawamoto S, Bluemke DA. Primary sclerosing cholangitis: MR imaging findings with pathologic correlation. AJR Am J Roentgenol 1999; 173:1037-1042.

31. Vitellas KM, El-Dieb A, Vaswani KK, et al. MR cholangiopancreatography in patients with primary sclerosing cholangitis: interobserver variability and comparison with endoscopic retrograde cholangiopancreatography. AJR Am J Roentgenol 2002; 179:399-407.

32. Ernst O, Asselah T, Sergent G, et al. MR cholangiography in primary sclerosing cholangitis. AJR Am J Roentgenol 1998; 171:1027-1030.

33. Dodd GD 3rd, Baron RL, Oliver JH 3rd, Federle MP. End-stage primary sclerosing cholangitis: CT findings of hepatic morphology in 36 patients. Radiology 1999; 211:357-362.

34. Yu JS, Kim KW, Jeong MG, et al. Predisposing factors of bile duct injury after transcatheter arterial chemoembolization for hepatic malignancy. Cardiovasc Intervent Radiol 2002; 25:270-274.

35. Leuschner M, Dietrich CF, You T, et al. Characterisation of patients with primary biliary cirrhosis responding to long term ursodeoxycholic acid treatment. Gut 2000; 46:121-126.

36. Corpechot C, Carrat F, Bahr A, et al. The effect of ursodeoxycholic acid therapy on the natural course of primary biliary cirrhosis. Gastroenterology 2005; 128:297-303.

37. Neuberger J. Liver transplantation for primary biliary cirrhosis: indications and risk of recurrence. J Hepatol 2003; 39:142-148.

38. De Vreede I, Steers JL, Burch PA, et al. Prolonged disease-free survival after orthotopic liver transplantation plus adjuvant chemoirradiation for cholangiocarcinoma. Liver Transpl 2000; 6:309-316.

39. Graziadei IW, Wiesner RH, Marotta PJ, et al. Long-term results of patients undergoing liver transplantation for primary sclerosing cholangitis. Hepatology 1999; 30:1121-1127.

40. Graziadei IW, Wiesner RH, Batts KP, et al. Recurrence of primary sclerosing cholangitis following liver transplantation. Hepatology 1999; 29:1050-1056.

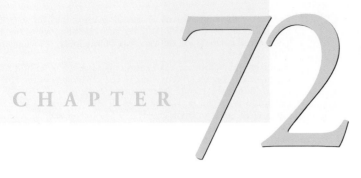
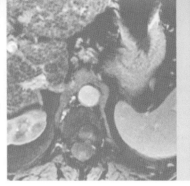
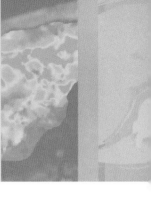

CHAPTER 72

Hepatic Variants

Onofrio Catalano and Dushyant V. Sahani

TECHNICAL ASPECTS

Diagnostic imaging of the hepatobiliary system, with multidetector CT (MDCT) and MRI, plays a major role in hepatobiliary surgery, helping to choose the best therapeutic approach, to reduce complications, and to identify the anatomy requiring special attention at surgery.

Anatomic variants of the biliary and hepatic vascular anatomy are common; they dictate the surgical technique and may also predict the risk of postsurgical complications, both in the case of complex surgeries, such as liver transplantation, and of more common procedures, such as laparoscopic cholecystectomy.

MDCT and MRI, especially when contrast agents excreted into the biliary system are used (e.g., mangafodipir trisodium, Gd-EOB-DTPA, Gd-BOPTA), clearly visualize both biliary and arterial anatomic variants, with a high degree of correlation with intraoperative cholangiography and digital subtraction angiography.[1-5]

PROS AND CONS

Contrast-enhanced MDCT and MRI are noninvasive techniques that permit angiographic and parenchymal evaluation of the liver.

MDCT and MR angiography have shown excellent correlation with catheter angiography but are devoid of its invasiveness and of many of its complications. Moreover, the radiation burden is reduced in MDCT, when compared with catheter angiography, and absent in the case of MRI.

Because of the availability of biliary excreted contrast agents, cholangiography can now be performed in a noninvasive way by both MDCT and MRI. Currently, MDCT cholangiography, owing to the higher spatial resolution, allows better visualization of second-order bile ducts than MR cholangiography.

MDCT and MR angiography and cholangiopancreatography (MRCP) protocols, used at our institution, are summarized in Tables 72-1 to 72-3. Raw data, obtained from MDCT and MRI are postprocessed to maximize the information they can provide; and multiplanar reformatted, 3D reconstruction, maximum intensity projection (MIP), and volume rendering (VR) images are obtained.[1-7]

CONTROVERSIES

Which is the best modality to assess hepatic variants, between MDCT and MRI, is still unclear. Both methodologies are subject to rapid improvements, and each one shows advantages and disadvantages over the other. Currently the choice of a specific modality over the other is mainly dictated by institutional preferences.

NORMAL ANATOMY

Anatomic variants of the biliary, hepatic arterial, hepatic venous, and portal venous anatomy are common. Classic biliary and hepatic arterial anatomy is found in only 58% and 55% of the population, respectively. To understand anatomic variants, a brief description of normal anatomy is provided.[2,4-6]

Liver

The liver (Fig. 72-1) is a large, wedge-shaped parenchymal organ that occupies most of the right hypochondrium and epigastrium and extends to the left epigastrium with its narrow end. Peritoneal reflections, constituting the falciform ligament, the coronary ligament, and the right and left triangular ligaments, provide attachment to the anterior abdominal wall and diaphragm. The hepatic inferior surface is attached to the stomach and duodenum through the gastrohepatic and hepatoduodenal ligaments, within whose free margin the hepatic artery, portal vein, hepatic duct, and lymphatic vessels run toward the porta hepatis. The falciform ligament, the ligamentum teres, and the ligamentum venosum divide the liver into a large right lobe and a smaller left lobe. A groove in the posterior surface of the liver circumscribes the inferior vena cava (IVC), in which the hepatic veins empty.

A sharp fissure, named the umbilical fissure, is present on the inferior surface of the liver, its anterior part nests

TABLE 72-1	MDCT Angiography Scanning Protocol	
	Hepatic Arterial Phase	**Venous Phase**
Range	Entire liver	Entire liver
Scan Delay	20-25 s after start of bolus injection	60-65 s
Empirical Bolus Tracking	Automatically triggered at 125 HU in aorta at the celiac artery level	
Pitch	1-1.5	1-1.5
Slice Thickness	1-2 mm	2-5 mm
Kilovoltage Peak	120-140	120-140
Milliamperes	200-280	200-280
Image Reconstruction Thickness	1-2 mm and 50% overlap	2-5 mm and 50% overlap

TABLE 72-2	MR Angiography Protocol		
	Hepatic Arterial Phase	**Venous Phase**	**Delayed Venous Phase**
Scan Delay	15-18 s	60 s	180 s
TR/TE	Minimum/ 15 ms	Minimum/ 15 ms	Minimum/ 15 ms
Flip Angle	100 degrees	100 degrees	100 degrees
Field of View	400 mm	400 mm	400 mm
Effective Section	2-4 mm	2-4 mm	2-4 mm
Matrix	160 × 256	160 × 256	160 × 256

TABLE 72-3	MRCP Protocol	
	T2-Weighted MRCP	**3D SPGR**
Scan Delay	None	Gd-BOPTA: 60 min Mangafodipir: 15-30 min
TR/TE	2800-3300/900-1100 ms	6.5/2.1 ms
Flip Angle	0 degrees	15 degrees
Field of View	400 mm	400 mm
Effective Section	60 mm	2.4 mm
Orientation	Coronal oblique	Axial and coronal
Matrix	160 × 256	160 × 256

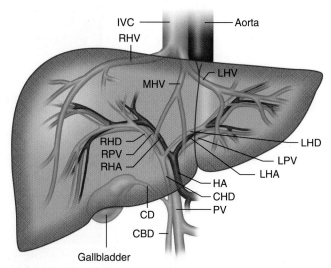

■ **FIGURE 72-1** Drawing of normal anatomy of the liver. RHV, right hepatic vein; MHV, middle hepatic vein; LHV, left hepatic vein; IVC, inferior vena cava; HA, hepatic artery; RHA, right hepatic artery; LHA, left hepatic artery; PV, portal vein; RPV, right portal vein; LPV, left portal vein; CD, cystic duct; CBD, common bile duct; CHD, common hepatic duct; LHD, left hepatic duct; RHD, right hepatic duct.

the ligamentum teres, and its posterior part harbors the ligamentum venosum. Two prominences can be seen on the inferior surface of the organ to the right of the umbilical fissure: the quadrate lobe, anteriorly, and the caudate lobe, posteriorly, separated by the transverse fissure for the porta hepatis. To the right of the quadrate lobe there is a shallow depression, the gallbladder fossa, in which that viscus is allocated. The classic macroscopic anatomy just described does not correlate with functional hepatic anatomy, and therefore it is inadequate for interventional radiology and surgery. Functional anatomy of the liver is based on the vascular and biliary territories (Fig. 72-2). Cantlie's line, running on a coronal oblique plane oriented 75 degrees toward the left, from the middle of the gallbladder to the left side of the IVC, divides the liver into right

and left. The right liver and the left liver, which do not correspond to the classic macroscopic right and left lobes, are two separate functional units, with independent vascular inflows and outflows and with autonomous biliary drainages. The middle hepatic vein (MHV) lies along the cranial continuation of Cantlie's line. The right hepatic vein (RHV), MHV, and left hepatic vein (LHV) divide the liver into four sectors, each one supplied by an independent portal pedicle. They are the posterolateral and anteromedial sectors in the right liver and the posterior and anterior sectors in the left liver. The posterior sector is undivided and constitutes segment II. The anterior sector is divided by the umbilical fissure into a medial segment (IV) and a lateral segment (III). A transverse plane at the level of the main portal bifurcation divides the posterolateral sector into a posterior (VII) and an anterior segment (VI), the anteromedial sector into an anterior (V), and a posterior segment (VIII) and subdivides segment IV into a posterior (IVa) and an anterior segment (IVb). The caudate lobe constitutes segment I or the Spigel lobe, which, owing to its autonomous vascularization, is considered separate from the others.

An ultrasound image of normal liver presents a homogeneous pattern of low-level echoes. Vessels and biliary ducts are anechoic (Fig. 72-3).

On nonenhanced MDCT, the liver exhibits homogeneous intermediate attenuation (50 to 75 HU), similar to the spleen (Fig. 72-4). Vessels and biliary ducts are hypodense. During contrast-enhanced imaging, liver attenuation values progressively increase, with peak enhancement occurring during the portal (PV) and hepatic venous (HV) phases of enhancement. Maximal arterial enhancement occurs during hepatic arterial (HA) phase, usually around 30 seconds after the start of contrast agent injection; the portal and hepatic veins maximally enhance at approximately 70 seconds after contrast agent

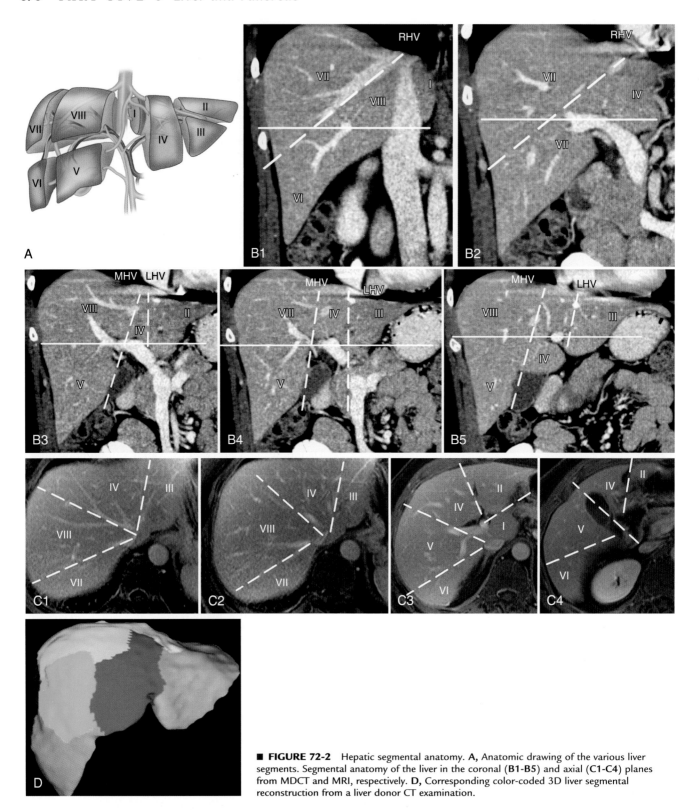

■ **FIGURE 72-2** Hepatic segmental anatomy. **A,** Anatomic drawing of the various liver segments. Segmental anatomy of the liver in the coronal (**B1-B5**) and axial (**C1-C4**) planes from MDCT and MRI, respectively. **D,** Corresponding color-coded 3D liver segmental reconstruction from a liver donor CT examination.

injection. Biliary ducts are nonopacified, unless contrast media with biliary excretion are administered.

At MRI, the signal intensity of the normal liver varies with the sequence used. It presents hyperintense to the spleen on T1-weighted (T1W) images, hypointense on T2-weighted (T2W) images, and always homogeneous (Fig. 72-5).

Normal liver enhances homogeneously and transiently after administration of nonspecific gadolinium (Gd)-based contrast media.

If hepatic-specific contrast agents (Mn-DPDP, Gd-BOPTA, Gd-EOB-DTPA) are used, they are selectively taken up by hepatocytes, with resultant progressive increased signal intensity on delayed T1W images and

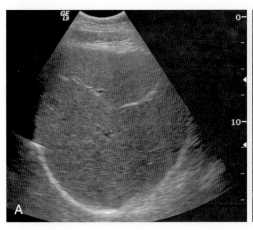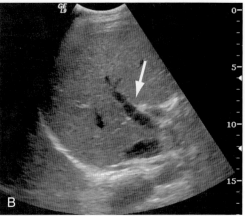

■ **FIGURE 72-3** Ultrasound images of normal liver. **A** and **B,** Normal hepatic parenchyma presents as a homogeneous pattern of low-level echoes. Vessels and bile ducts appear anechoic. Right portal vein is indicated by *arrow.*

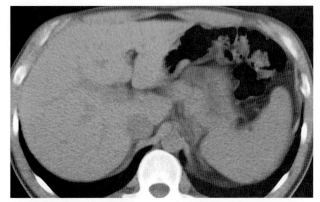

■ **FIGURE 72-4** CT image of normal liver. On nonenhanced MDCT, the liver exhibits homogeneous intermediate attenuation and appears similar to the spleen.

subsequent excretion into and enhancement of the biliary system.

Reticuloendothelial system (RES)–specific contrast agents, composed of iron microparticles, are taken up by Kupffer cells, with resultant reduction of the signal intensity of the liver on T2*W images.

Hepatic Arterial Anatomy

The classic hepatic arterial anatomy, characterized by the proper hepatic artery dividing into right and left hepatic arteries, is observed in about 55% of the population (Fig. 72-6). The Michel classification of hepatic arterial variant anatomy is illustrated in Table 72-4.

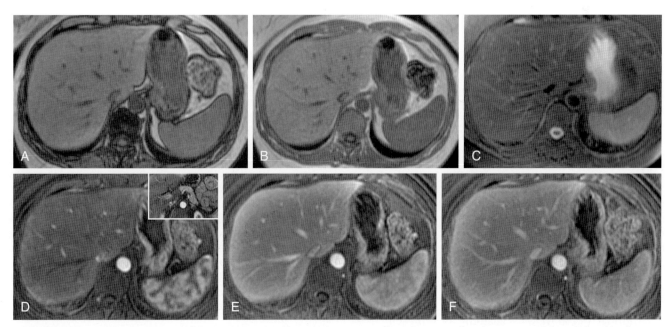

■ **FIGURE 72-5** MR images of normal liver. On MRI, normal hepatic tissue presents hyperintense to the spleen on out-of-phase (**A**) and in-phase (**B**) T1W images, is hypointense on T2W images (**C**), and enhances homogeneously after administration of nonspecific gadolinium-based contrast media. In the arterial dominant phase of contrast enhancement, hepatic veins are nonopacified (**D**), whereas contrast medium is detectable in the liver parenchyma and portal vein (*inset*). During the portal (**E**) and late (**F**) phases of contrast enhancement, both hepatic veins and parenchyma are enhanced.

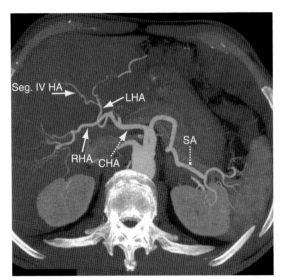

■ **FIGURE 72-6** Normal hepatic arterial anatomy. Axial MIP image shows the normal anatomy of the hepatic artery. CHA, common hepatic artery; RHA, right hepatic artery; LHA, left hepatic artery; Seg. IV HA, segment IV hepatic artery; SA, splenic artery.

TABLE 72-4 Hepatic Arterial Variants According to Michel's Classification

Type	Frequency (%)	Description
I	55	RHA, MHA, LHA arise from CHA
II	10	RHA, MHA, and LHA from CHA; replaced LHA from LGA
III	11	RHA and MHA from CHA, replaced RHA from SMA
IV	1	Replaced RHA and LHA
V	8	RHA, MHA, LHA arise from CHA; accessory LHA from LGA
VI	7	RHA, MHA, LHA arise from CHA; accessory RHA
VII	1	Accessory RHA and LHA
VIII	4	Replaced RHA and accessory LHA or replaced LHA and accessory RHA
IX	4.5	Entire hepatic trunk from SMA
X	0.5	Entire hepatic trunk from LGA

RHA, right hepatic artery; MHA, middle hepatic artery; LHA, left hepatic artery; CHA, common hepatic artery; SMA, superior mesenteric artery; LGA, left gastric artery.

Hepatic Venous Anatomy

Classic hepatic venous anatomy is characterized by three main hepatic veins—LHV, MHV, and RHV—draining into the IVC. The LHV drains segments II and III; the MHV drains segments IV, V, and VIII; and the RHV drains segments V to VII. The MHV and LHV join to form a common trunk in about 60% of the population (Fig. 72-7).

Portal Venous Anatomy

The normal portal venous anatomy is represented by the main portal vein branching, at the porta hepatis, into the right (RPV) and left (LPV) portal veins. The RPV subsequently divides into anterior and posterior branches (Fig. 72-8).

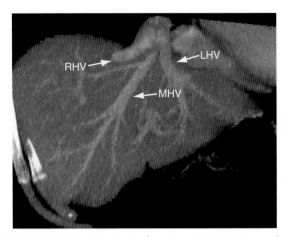

■ **FIGURE 72-7** Hepatic vein confluence on MDCT MIP coronal image. RHV, right hepatic vein; MHV, middle hepatic vein; LHV, left hepatic vein.

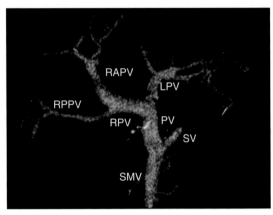

■ **FIGURE 72-8** Normal portal venous branching from 3D CT portography. SMV, superior mesenteric vein; SV, splenic vein; PV, portal vein; LPV, left portal vein; RPV, right portal vein; RAPV, right anterior portal vein; RPPV, right posterior portal vein.

Hepatic Biliary Anatomy

The classic biliary anatomy, found in about 58% of the population, consists of the right hepatic duct (RHD) and the left hepatic duct (LHD) draining the right and left liver, respectively (Fig. 72-9). The RHD divides into the right posterior hepatic duct (RPHD) and the right anterior hepatic duct (RAHD). The RPHD, draining the posterior segments VI and VII, has a horizontal course and runs posterior to the RAHD, draining the anterior segments V and VIII, which is more vertically oriented. The RPHD fuses with the RAHD from a medial approach to form a short RHD. Segmental tributaries draining left lobe segments II to IV form the LHD. The RHD and LHD fuse to constitute the common hepatic duct (CHD). The caudate lobe biliary radicles drain into the origin of the LHD or of the RHD. The cystic duct usually fuses with the CHD from its lateral aspect, below its origin.[2,5,8-15]

PATHOPHYSIOLOGY

Hepatic variants can be divided into parenchymal variants and hepatic vascular and biliary variants.

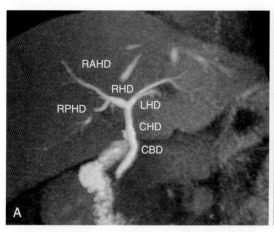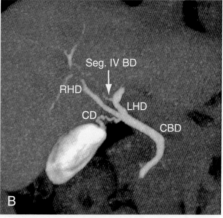

■ **FIGURE 72-9** Normal biliary anatomy from contrast-enhanced 3D T1W MR cholangiography (**A**) and MDCT cholangiography (**B**) in two different cases. CBD, common bile duct; CHD, common hepatic duct; CD, cystic duct; LHD, left hepatic duct; RHD, right hepatic duct; RAHD, right anterior hepatic duct; RPHD, right posterior hepatic duct; Seg. IV BD, segment IV draining biliary duct.

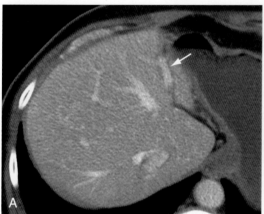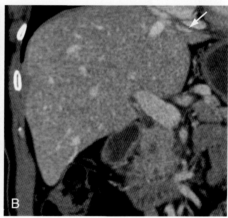

■ **FIGURE 72-10** Left lobe hypoplasia. Axial (**A**) and coronal (**B**) MDCT. Left lobe hypoplasia is characterized by a reduced volume of the left lobe of the liver. Corresponding biliary ducts and hepatic arterial, venous, and portal vessels are present but reduced in caliber. *Arrow* indicates left hepatic vein.

Parenchymal Variants

Hepatic parenchymal variants are devoid of clinical implications unless they are confused with a mass lesion or hepatic volume is reduced, rendering the subject unsuitable to donate part of his or her liver for living-donor liver transplantation.

Liver can undergo defective development, with resultant absence (agenesis) or small size (hypoplasia) of segments or even of an entire lobe (Fig. 72-10), or excessive development, with resultant formation of accessory lobes, parenchymal bridges, or hyperplastic papillary lobes. Agenesis of the right or left hepatic lobe is characterized by absence of the involved lobe and of the corresponding branches of the hepatic artery, portal vein, and biliary system; hypertrophy of the residual hepatic lobe and of the caudate; and possible malposition of the gallbladder, colon, and spleen. Accessory lobes may be connected to the main liver or may be ectopic, in which case they are thought to arise from the extrahepatic biliary tract. Parenchymal bridges may circumscribe the gallbladder or envelop the IVC.

Papillary hyperplasia mainly occurs from the caudate lobe and from the anteroinferior margin of the liver. In the latter case the tongue-like parenchymal projection is named Riedel's lobe.

Diaphragmatic indentations are pseudolesions commonly confused with focal liver lesions. They appear as peripheral wedge-shaped hypodense areas, indenting the liver surface, devoid of contrast enhancement, and closely following the ribs. Coronal images may be useful in uncertain cases (Fig. 72-11).

Vascular and Biliary Variants

Hepatic vascular and biliary variants per se are usually not responsible for any clinical symptomatology but, in the case of hepatobiliary surgery, may strongly influence patient management and prognosis. Their surgical relevance varies greatly depending on the surgical procedure that needs to be performed (e.g., liver transplantation or laparoscopic cholecystectomy). Therefore, hepatic vascular and biliary variants are subsequently described according to their implications on specific surgeries. They comprise anomalies in the number, origin, and travel of the involved vasculature.

Living-Donor Liver Transplantation

For living-donor liver transplantation adequate metabolic vitality to both the hepatic lobe left in the donor and the one transplanted into the recipients must be ensured. The

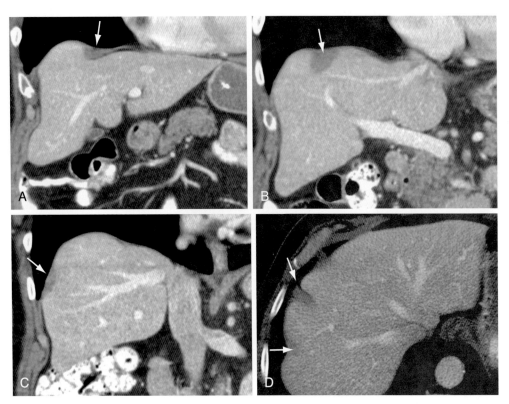

■ **FIGURE 72-11** Diaphragmatic indentations. Coronal (**A-C**) and axial (**D**) MDCT. Diaphragmatic indentations (*arrows*) are caused by close apposition of the diaphragm to the liver. They present as wedge-shaped hypodense areas around the periphery of the liver, devoid of contrast enhancement. In uncertain cases their nature is more easily appreciated on coronal images.

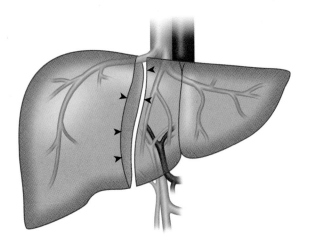

■ **FIGURE 72-12** Anatomic drawing to demonstrate hemihepatectomy plane (*arrowheads*), which runs 1 cm to the right of the middle hepatic vein and connects the gallbladder fossa and the inferior vena cava.

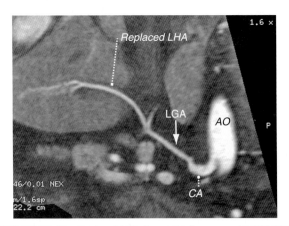

■ **FIGURE 72-13** Replaced LHA from LGA from curved MIP MDCT. Replaced LHA arises from left gastric artery (LGA). AO, aorta; CA, celiac artery.

hemihepatectomy is performed along a relatively avascular plane, close to Cantlie's line, that separates the left and right liver. It runs 1 cm to the right of the MHV and connects the gallbladder fossa and the IVC (Fig. 72-12). The left liver is left in the donor; the right is harvested into the recipient.

The balance between the blood supply and venous drainage of the graft as well as adequate biliary drainage are prerequisites for successful liver transplantation. Inadvertent arterial or venous transection or ligation, with resultant hepatic arterial infarction or venous congestion, can seriously damage the graft, causing its failure; there-

fore, vessels running along the dissection plane need to be preoperatively identified to ascertain if the surgery is feasible and in that case to guide the choice of the best technique to adopt.

The level of importance of anatomic variants depends on whether they are found in the donor or in the recipient. For example, a replaced or accessory left hepatic artery from the left gastric artery is relevant in a recipient, owing to the extra steps required to ligate it at the origin during native liver removal, but it is not important in a donor (Figs. 72-13 and 72-14). On the other hand, a variant origin of the artery to segment IV is extremely relevant in

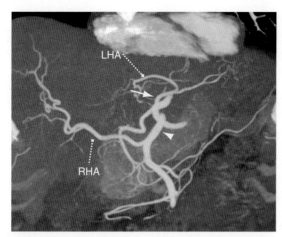

■ **FIGURE 72-14** Replaced RHA and LHA from coronal MDCT MIP. Coronal MIP shows replaced LHA from gastric artery (*arrow*) and replaced RHA from SMA (*arrowhead*).

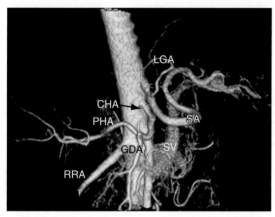

■ **FIGURE 72-15** Variant hepatic artery anatomy from 3D-VR MDCT. Common hepatic artery (CHA), splenic artery (SA), and left gastric artery (LGA) arise separately from the aorta. PHA, proper hepatic artery; GDA, gastroduodenal artery; SV, splenic vein; RRA, right interlobar renal artery.

TABLE 72-5 Hepatic Arterial Variants and Liver Transplantation

Variant	Implications for Surgery
Arterial Variants Relevant in Donors	
MHA from RHA	Hepatic plane would cut this artery, compromising arterial supply to left lobe of the liver
CHA trifurcation into RHA, LHA and GDA	Clamping or ligation of CHA can cause gastric or duodenal hypoperfusion.
RHA or LHA from CHA before the origin of GDA	Clamping or ligation of CHA can cause gastric or duodenal hypoperfusion.
Arterial Variants Relevant in Recipients	
Short RHA	Increases surgical complexity and can lead to difficult anastomosis
Celiac artery stenosis	Increases risks of graft failure and biliary complications
Replaced or accessory LHA (Michel II, V), replaced hepatic trunk arising from SMA (Michel IX)	Increases complexity of the surgery

MHA, middle hepatic artery; RHA, right hepatic artery; CHA, common hepatic artery; GDA, gastroduodenal artery; LHA, left hepatic artery; SMA, superior mesenteric artery.

the donor because the hepatectomy plane would cut its arterial supply, but it is not important in the recipient. Other variants may require extra surgical steps in both the donor and the recipient (Fig. 72-15). Arterial variants relevant in donors and in recipients are summarized in Table 72-5.

Among hepatic venous anomalies, variations in MHV and presence of accessory hepatic veins have profound impact on transplantation surgery. The branching pattern of the MHV influences the location of the hepatectomy plane. Hepatic venous branches draining segments VIII and V may empty into the MHV. Drainage of the right superior anterior segment (segment VIII) into the MHV requires extra surgical steps to avoid venous congestion of the same segment (medial sector venous congestion), necrosis, and atrophy (Fig. 72-16).

An accessory inferior RHV draining directly into the IVC is found in 47% of cases and is relevant in donors. When its distance along the IVC from the main hepatic venous drainage is more than 40 mm, it may be difficult

to implant both veins into the recipient. Hepatic venous variants relevant in donors and in recipients are summarized in Table 72-6.

Of the many portal variants, trifurcation (Fig. 72-17), found in 10% to 16% of patients, although not a surgical contraindication, requires extra surgical steps. Moreover, the distance between the bifurcation of the LPV and that of the RPV must be evaluated preoperatively because of its implications on the surgical technique. Portal venous variants relevant in liver transplantation are summarized in Table 72-7.

Biliary complications, which include bile leakage and bile duct stricture, occurring in 7% to 10% of donors, represent the most common cause of morbidity in living-donor liver transplantation. Preoperative imaging of biliary anatomic variants is useful to prevent this type of complication (Fig. 72-18). For this purpose, T2W MRCP is less adequate than Mn-DPDP 3D MRCP, which accurately identifies variants of the intrahepatic bile ducts.

RPHD drainage into the LHD, one of the most common bile duct variants (15.6% of cases), can lead to inadvertent biliary tract injury in the donor. Other surgically relevant anatomic variants of the biliary tract include a posteroinferior branch of the RHD draining into the LHD and biliary trifurcation (Fig. 72-19). Presurgical imaging evaluation of biliary anatomy variants (Fig. 72-20), using MDCT cholangiography or MRCP helped to prevent biliary tract injuries (1.9%) in one series. Biliary variants relevant in donors and in recipients are summarized in Table 72-8.

Hepatic Tumor Resection

Hepatic tumor resection is mainly performed to treat hepatic metastasis. It strongly benefits from preoperative vascular and biliary anatomy evaluation.

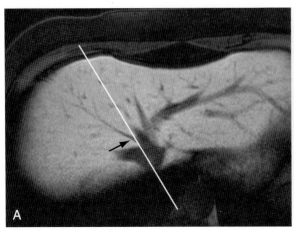
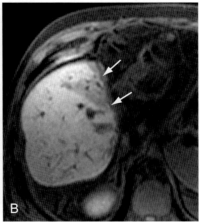

■ **FIGURE 72-16** Segment VIII venous tributary into MHV. **A,** Axial T1W MR image in the donor shows segment VIII tributary vein (*arrow*) emptying into the MHV. The hemihepatectomy plane (*white line*) intersects the accessory segment VIII hepatic vein before its confluence into the IVC. **B,** Postoperative axial T1W MR image in the recipient shows atrophy of the corresponding liver segment (*arrows*).

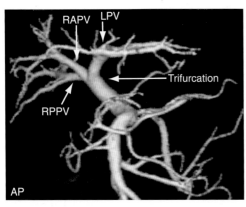

■ **FIGURE 72-17** Portal vein trifurcation from 3D-VR MDCT. CT angiography demonstrates trifurcation of the portal vein (*arrow*) into LPV, right anterior (RAPV), and right posterior (RPPV) portal veins.

TABLE 72-7 Portal Venous Variants and Liver Transplantation

Variant	Implications for Surgery
Portal Venous Variants Relevant in Donors	
Trifurcation of the portal vein	Surgical planning must be modified because of the lack of a portal segment to clamp during surgery and to prevent bleeding in the donor and a difficult anastomosis in the recipient.
Portal venules to segment V	Surgical planning must be modified to avoid bleeding and ischemia.
Portal Venous Variants Relevant in Recipients	
Dorsal branch of segment VII supplying posterosuperior area of right lobe	Surgical planning must be modified to prevent ischemia in the recipient.
Trifurcation of the portal vein	Surgical planning must be modified because of the lack of a portal segment to clamp during surgery and to prevent bleeding in the donor and a difficult anastomosis in the recipient.
Acute angle of portal vein branching	The liver during regeneration may engulf the veins and reduce blood supply, causing ischemia in the graft.
Short length of portal vein	May cause allograft failure

TABLE 72-6 Hepatic Venous Variants and Liver Transplantation

Variant	Implications for Surgery
Hepatic Venous Variants Relevant in Donors	
Accessory inferior RHV larger than 3 mm	Increases surgical complexity and surgical technique must be modified
Hepatic Venous Variants Relevant in Recipients	
Accessory inferior RHV draining into IVC more than 3 cm from the main hepatic venous confluence with the IVC	Increases surgical complexity and surgical technique must be modified
Early branching of segment VIII vein	Increases surgical complexity and surgical technique must be modified
Anomalous drainage of segments V and VII into the MHV	Risk of medial sector congestion and atrophy
Early confluence of hepatic veins	Increases surgical complexity and surgical technique must be modified

RHV, right hepatic vein; IVC, inferior vena cava; MHV, middle hepatic vein.

About 50% of patients suffering from colorectal cancer develop hepatic metastases. They are responsible for death in at least two thirds of them. Liver resection represents the best treatment, with a 5-year survival rate of 37% to 58% in selected patients.

Accurate preoperative patient selection and surgical planning are invaluable for hepatic tumor resection in an otherwise healthy liver, and it is more important in the case of small residual liver volume or in patients with compromised hepatic function, where even minor complications such as bile leakage or partial hepatic necrosis may be fatal. Diagnostic imaging is therefore required to assess the metastases, to define their number, size, location, and surgical margins (see Fig. 72-8) and the hepato-

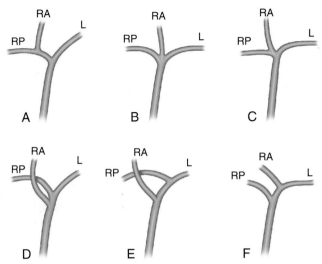

■ **FIGURE 72-18** Drawing representing biliary variants. **A,** Normal bile duct anatomy. **B,** Trifurcation pattern. **C,** Short RHD. **D,** RAHD continuation into the CHD. **E,** RPHD drainage into LHD. **F,** RAHD drainage into LHD.

biliary anatomy, and to identify patients who can undergo a procedure aimed to resect the lesions while preserving functionality of the remaining liver. For this purpose, anticipated remaining liver needs to be evaluated to assess the chance to preserve sufficient remnant liver (>20% in a healthy liver), adequate vascular inflow and outflow as well as biliary drainage, and two contiguous hepatic segments.

Areas at risk for devascularization or venous congestion need to be preoperatively identified so that surgical feasibility can be ascertained and appropriate techniques can be adopted. The spatial relationship of the arterial and/or venous variant to the tumor dictates the level of importance and influence on surgical technique. A summary of the most important vascular variants relevant to hepatic tumor surgery is provided in Tables 72-9 to 72-11.

Biliary complications constitute an important cause of major morbidity in hepatic tumor resection (3.6% to 8.1%) and are important risk factors for liver failure (35.7%) and operative mortality (39.3%). One of the most serious complications is bile leakage. The complexity of bile duct

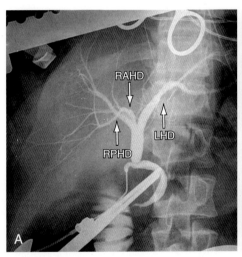

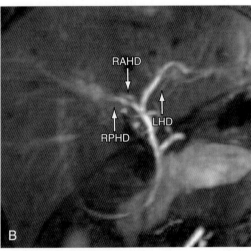

■ **FIGURE 72-19** Biliary trifurcation from conventional and Mn-DPDP–enhanced MR cholangiography. Intraoperative cholangiogram (**A**) and mangafodipir-enhanced MR cholangiography MIP image (**B**) shows biliary trifurcation. LHD, left hepatic duct; RAHD, right anterior hepatic duct; RPHD, right posterior hepatic duct.

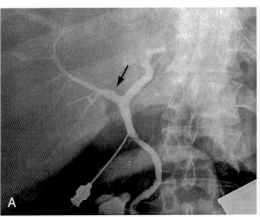

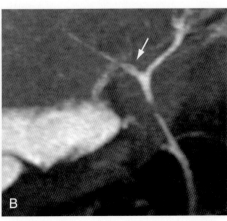

■ **FIGURE 72-20** Early branching RHD from conventional and Mn-DPDP–enhanced MR cholangiography. Intraoperative cholangiogram (**A**) and mangafodipir-enhanced MR cholangiography MIP image (**B**) demonstrate early branching RHD (*arrows*).

TABLE 72-8 Biliary Duct Variants and Liver Transplantation

Biliary Duct Variants Relevant in Donors	
RPHD draining directly into LHD	13-19%
Trifurcation: simultaneous emptying of RAHD, RPHD, LHD into CHD	11%
RPHD draining directly into CHD	5%
Accessory hepatic ducts	2%
Biliary Duct Variants Relevant in Recipients	
LHD draining into RAHD	4%
Trifurcation: simultaneous emptying of RAHD, RPHD, LHD into CHD	11%
Cystic duct draining into RHD	Very unusual
Accessory hepatic ducts	2%

RPHD, right posterior hepatic duct; LHD, left hepatic duct; RAHD, right anterior hepatic duct; CHD, common hepatic duct.

TABLE 72-9 Arterial Variants and Influence on Tumor Resection

	Right Lobe Tumor Resection	Left Lobe Tumor Resection
Replaced LHA from LGA (Michel II)	−	+
Replaced RHA from SMA (Michel III)	+	−
Replaced RHA and LHA (Michel IV)	−	+
Accessory LHA from LGA (Michel V)	−	+
Accessory RHA (Michel VI)	+	−
Accessory RHA and LHA (Michel VII)	+	+
Replaced RHA and accessory LHA or replaced LHA and accessory RHA (Michel VIII)	+	+
Entire hepatic trunk from SMA (Michel IX)	+	+
Entire hepatic trunk from LGA (Michel X)	+	+

LHA, left hepatic artery; SMA, superior mesenteric artery; RHA, right hepatic artery; LGA, left gastric artery.

TABLE 72-10 Hepatic Venous Variants and Tumor Resection Surgery

	Right Lobe Tumor Resection	Left Lobe Tumor Resection
Segment VIII drainage into MHV	−	+
Segment V and VI accessory inferior hepatic veins draining directly into IVC	+	−
Accessory MHV draining directly into IVC	−	+

MHV, middle hepatic vein; IVC, inferior vena cava.

TABLE 72-11 Portal Venous Variants and Tumor Resection Surgery

	Right Lobe Tumor Resection	Left Lobe Tumor Resection
Trifurcation of portal vein	−	+
Right and left portal branches supplying segment VIII	+	−

TABLE 72-12 Biliary Variants and Tumor Resection Surgery

	Right Lobe Tumor Resection	Left Lobe Tumor Resection
RPHD draining directly into LHD	−	+
LHD draining directly into RHD	+	−
Trifurcation: simultaneous emptying of RAHD, RPHD, LHD into CHD	+	+

RPHD, right portal hepatic duct; LHD, left hepatic duct; RAHD, right anterior hepatic duct; CHD, common hepatic duct.

Cholecystectomy

Although bile duct injuries can occur during either open or laparoscopic cholecystectomy, they are more common with the latter technique. An aberrant RHD (3.2% to 18.0% of population), draining part of the right lobe of the liver into the extrahepatic biliary tree, is associated with such injuries. Being close to the cystohepatic angle it may be inadvertently transected or ligated during cholecystectomy, with resultant biliary fistula, biloma, sepsis, pain, cholangitis, and even biliary atrophy with jaundice.

In about 10% of the population the cystic duct runs for a long distance with the CHD in a common fibrous sheath. In this situation the CHD may be misinterpreted as the cystic duct, with resultant inadvertent transection or ligation of the CHD. The extrahepatic bile duct may also undergo stricture in case the long parallel cystic duct is ligated too close to the CHD.

Another potential complication is related to an excessively long cystic duct remnant left after surgery, which can predispose to calculus formation and postcholecystectomy syndrome.

Intra-arterial Chemotherapy

In the case of colorectal metastases, after hepatic tumor resection a combination of hepatic intra-arterial chemotherapy and systemic chemotherapy is useful to treat micrometastases in the remaining liver and to prevent extrahepatic spread.

Hepatic metastases derive most of their blood supply from the hepatic artery, whereas normal liver is mainly nourished by the portal vein. Therefore, hepatic arterial

confluence and the variability of the left intrahepatic bile ducts account for the higher incidence of biliary complications after left-sided hepatectomy. A summary of relevant bile duct variants in partial hepatic resection for tumor treatment is shown in Table 72-12.

infusion pumps, delivering the maximal amount of che- motherapeutics to hepatic malignancies and reduced dosages to the normal liver and other organs, can mini- mize chemotherapeutic toxicity while exerting stronger effects against liver metastases.

Accurate patient selection and surgical expertise in the placement of hepatic arterial infusion pumps are prereq- uisites for successful chemotherapy. The catheter must ensure adequate and homogeneous delivery of chemo- therapeutic agents to the liver without perfusion of extra- hepatic tissues; moreover, to preserve its patency and to reduce the risk of arterial thrombosis, the tip must not create turbulence in the hepatic artery.

In patients with normal arterial anatomy, the hepatic arterial infusion pump is inserted in the proper hepatic artery after the origin of the gastroduodenal artery. In patients with variant arterial anatomy, the pump should be placed within the dominant hepatic artery, as proximal as possible but distal to the origin of the gastroduodenal artery. In patients with arterial variants, such as the replaced RHA and LHA (Michel types II, III, and IV), modi- fication of the technique may be required. Complications of hepatic arterial infusion pumps such as chemotoxicity of normal liver, extrahepatic misperfusion, chemical chol- angitis, bleeding, and duodenitis, can be reduced by pre- operative vascular evaluation.[1-11,14-30]

IMAGING

Radiography

Conventional radiology is unable to assess parenchymal and vascular variants of the liver. Catheter angiography represents the gold standard for vascular evaluation but, owing to its invasiveness, radiation burden, and the improved accuracy of MDCT and MR angiography, its use is mainly restricted to interventional procedures.

CT

MDCT allows accurate evaluation of parenchymal variants in the liver, demonstrating anatomic continuity and baseline and contrast-enhanced features of the accessory lobe paralleling those of the remaining liver. If the accessory lobe is ectopic, the cause can be difficult to ascertain.

MDCT angiography and MDCT cholangiography, pro- viding detailed images of the vascular anatomy of the liver, permit noninvasive detection of vascular and biliary variants.[1-7,14,15]

MRI

MRI has the same potentialities as MDCT in evaluation of parenchymal, vascular, and biliary variants. Moreover, owing to the availability of hepatic-specific contrast agents, such as Gd-BOPTA and Gd-EOB-DTPA, which are selectively taken up by the hepatocytes, it potentially can be used in the evaluation of suspected ectopic accessory hepatic lobes.[1,2,5,7,11,22,25]

Ultrasonography

In many clinical scenarios, ultrasonography is the first diagnostic imaging tool used to evaluate the liver. It can correctly identify parenchymal variants of the liver, dis- closing their continuity with the remaining organ and same echostructure. On the other hand, it is limited in evaluation and characterization of vascular anatomy.

PET/CT

PET/CT does not play a role in assessment of vascular hepatic variants. In the rare case of diagnostic imaging uncertainty regarding the nature of a parenchymal variant, PET/CT may be useful to disclose its benign nature.

Imaging Algorithm

MDCT and MR angiography and cholangiography are accurate imaging tools in hepatic anatomy assessment (Table 72-13). Careful evaluation of raw data and postpro- cessed images allows recognition of normal anatomy and identification of variant anatomy.

TABLE 72-13 Accuracy, Limitations, and Pitfalls of the Modalities Used in Imaging of Hepatic Variants

Modality	Accuracy	Limitations	Pitfalls
Radiography	Conventional angiography 95.8%	Radiation exposure Invasiveness Possible procedural complications	
CT	93.2%	Radiation exposure	Analysis of raw data and of postprocessed images to avoid diagnostic errors
MRI	93%	Patient cooperation High cost	Analysis of raw data and of postprocessed images to avoid diagnostic errors
Ultrasonography	N/A	Poor performance in the case of obesity or overlying bowel gas Operator dependent Comprehensive imaging difficult	Incomplete evaluation of vascular anatomy
Nuclear medicine	N/A	Radiation exposure Currently no role	Unable to evaluate vascular anatomy
PET/CT	N/A	Radiation exposure High cost	Unable to evaluate vascular anatomy

What the Referring Physician Needs to Know
■ Hepatic vascular and biliary anatomic variants are common.
■ They are not responsible for clinical symptoms.
■ They may strongly impact on a patient's management in the case of surgery.

KEY POINTS
■ The role of hepatic vascular and biliary anatomic variants is dictated by the surgical procedure that needs to be performed.
■ Preoperative imaging evaluation is mandatory for patient selection, surgical planning, and avoidance of complications.
■ MDCT and MR angiography and cholangiography are as accurate as catheter angiography and intraoperative cholangiography.
■ Postprocessed imaging is mandatory.

SUGGESTED READINGS

Bismuth H. Surgical anatomy and anatomical surgery of the liver. World J Surg 1982; 6:3-9.

Catalano OA, Singh AH, Uppot RN, et al. Vascular and biliary variants in the liver: implications for liver surgery. RadioGraphics 2008; 28:359-378.

Limanond P, Raman S, Ghobrial M, et al. Preoperative imaging in adult-to-adult living related liver transplant donors: what surgeons want to know. J Comput Assist Tomogr 2004; 28:149-157.

Mortelé KJ, Ros PR. Anatomic variants of the biliary tree: MR cholangiographic findings and clinical applications. AJR Am J Roentgenol 2001; 177:389-394.

Sahani D, D'souza R, Kadavigere R, et al. Evaluation of living liver transplant donors: method for precise anatomic definition by using a dedicated contrast-enhanced MR imaging protocol. RadioGraphics 2004; 24:957-967.

Sahani D, Mehta A, Blake B, et al. Preoperative hepatic vascular evaluation with CT and MR angiography: implications for surgery. RadioGraphics 2004; 24:1367-1380.

Turner MA, Fulcher AS. The cystic duct: normal anatomy and disease processes. RadioGraphics 2001; 21:3-22; questionnaire 288-294.

REFERENCES

1. Sahani D, D'souza R, Kadavigere R, et al. Evaluation of living liver transplant donors: method for precise anatomic definition by using a dedicated contrast-enhanced MR imaging protocol. RadioGraphics 2004; 24:957-967.
2. Sahani D, Mehta A, Blake B, et al. Preoperative hepatic vascular evaluation with CT and MR angiography: implications for surgery. RadioGraphics 2004; 24:1367-1380.
3. Sahani D, Saini S, Pena C, et al. Using multidetector CT for preoperative vascular evaluation of liver neoplasms: technique and results. AJR Am J Roentgenol 2002; 179:53-59.
4. Limanond P, Raman S, Ghobrial M, et al. Preoperative imaging in adult-to-adult living related liver transplant donors: what surgeons want to know. J Comput Assist Tomogr 2004; 28:149-157.
5. Catalano OA, Singh AH, Uppot RN, et al. Vascular and biliary variants in the liver: implications for liver surgery. RadioGraphics 2008; 28:359-378.
6. Pannu HK, Maley WR, Fishman EK. Liver transplantation: preoperative CT evaluation. RadioGraphics 2001; 21:S133-S146.
7. Yeh BM, Breiman RS, Taouli B, et al. Biliary tract depiction in living potential liver donors: comparison of conventional MR, mangafodipir trisodium-enhanced excretory MR, and multi-detector row CT cholangiography—initial experience. Radiology 2004; 230:645-651.
8. Cheng YF, Huang TL, Chen CL, et al. Variation of the intrahepatic portal vein; angiographic demonstration and application in living-related hepatic transplantation. Transplant Proc 1996; 28:1667-1668.
9. Lerut JP, Laterre PF, Goffette P, et al. Adult liver transplantation and abnormalities of splanchnic veins: experience in 53 patients. Transpl Int 1997; 10:125-132.
10. Sugarbaker PH, Nelson RC, Muray DR, et al. A segmental approach to computerized tomographic portography for hepatic resection. Surg Gynecol Obstet 1990; 171:189-195.
11. Mortelé KJ, Ros PR. Anatomic variants of the biliary tree: MR cholangiographic findings and clinical applications. AJR Am J Roentgenol 2001; 177:389-394.
12. Gray H. Gray's Anatomy: The Anatomical Basis of Medicine and Surgery, 38th ed. Edinburgh, Churchill Livingstone, 1995, pp 1795-1802.
13. Bismuth H. Surgical anatomy and anatomical surgery of the liver. World J Surg 1982; 6:3-9.
14. Coskun M, Kayahan E, Ozbek O, et al. Imaging of hepatic arterial anatomy for depicting vascular variations in living related liver transplant donor candidates with multidetector computed tomography: comparison with conventional angiography. Transplant Proc 2005; 37:1070-1073.
15. Bassignani MJ, Fulcher AS, Szucs RA, et al. Use of imaging for living donor liver transplantation. RadioGraphics 2001; 21:39-52.
16. Adams RB, Haller DG, Roh MS. Improving resectability of hepatic colorectal metastases: expert consensus statement by Abdalla et al. Ann Surg Oncol 2006; 13:1281-1283.
17. Allen PJ, Nissan A, Picon AI, et al. Technical complications and durability of hepatic artery infusion pumps for unresectable colorectal liver metastases: an institutional experience of 544 consecutive cases. J Am Coll Surg 2005; 201:57-65.
18. Allen PJ, Stojadinovic A, Ben-Porat L, et al. The management of variant arterial anatomy during hepatic arterial infusion pump placement. Ann Surg Oncol 2002; 9:875-880.
19. Bipat S, van Leeuwen MS, Comans EF, et al. Colorectal liver metastases: CT, MR imaging, and PET for diagnosis—meta-analysis. Radiology 2005; 237:123-131.
20. Capussotti L, Ferrero A, Vigano L, et al. Bile leakage and liver resection: where is the risk? Arch Surg 2006; 141:690-694; discussion 695.
21. Charnsangavej C, Clary B, Fong Y, et al. Selection of patients for resection of hepatic colorectal metastases: expert consensus statement. Ann Surg Oncol 2006; 13:1261-1268.

22. Goldman J, Florman S, Varotti G, et al. Noninvasive preoperative evaluation of biliary anatomy in right-lobe living donors with mangafodipir trisodium-enhanced MR cholangiography. Transplant Proc 2003; 35:1421-1422.

23. Itamoto T, Emoto K, Mitsuta H, et al. Safety of donor right hepatectomy for adult-to-adult living donor liver transplantation. Transpl Int 2006; 19:177-183.

24. Kamel IR, Lawler LP, Fishman EK. Variations in anatomy of the middle hepatic vein and their impact on formal right hepatectomy. Abdom Imaging 2003; 28:668-674.

25. Kapoor V, Peterson MS, Baron RL, et al. Intrahepatic biliary anatomy of living adult liver donors: correlation of mangafodipir trisodium-enhanced MR cholangiography and intraoperative cholangiography. AJR Am J Roentgenol 2002; 179:1281-1286.

26. Kemeny N, Huang Y, Cohen AM, et al. Hepatic arterial infusion of chemotherapy after resection of hepatic metastases from colorectal cancer. N Engl J Med 1999; 341:2039-2048.

27. Lo CM, Fan ST, Liu CL, et al. Biliary complications after hepatic resection: risk factors, management, and outcome. Arch Surg 1998; 133:156-161.

28. Soyer P, Heath D, Bluemke DA, et al. Three-dimensional helical CT of intrahepatic venous structures: comparison of three rendering techniques. J Comput Assist Tomogr 1996; 20:122-127.

29. Taguchi K, Anno H. High temporal resolution for multislice helical computed tomography. Med Phys 2000; 27:861-872.

30. Turner MA, Fulcher AS. The cystic duct: normal anatomy and disease processes. RadioGraphics 2001; 2:3-22; questionnaire 288-294.

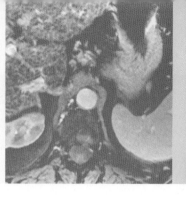
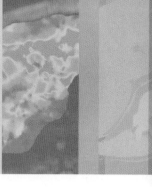

CHAPTER 73

Imaging of the Pancreas

Riccardo Manfredi, Massimiliano Motton, Mirko D'Onofrio,
Rossella Graziani, Giovanni Carbognin, and Marco Testoni

MULTIDETECTOR COMPUTED TOMOGRAPHY

MDCT has become established as a fundamental means of imaging the pancreas. Today, higher image quality can be obtained in abdominal imaging, and this is even more significant in pancreatic imaging, where the reduction of acquisition time, the possibility of multiple phases of enhancement imaging, and higher-resolution images in all three spatial planes with the possibility of excellent multiplanar image reconstructions permit MDCT to provide excellent images of the anatomic layout of the pancreas and its vasculature. Thus this technique is now used to diagnose a variety of congenital, neoplastic, inflammatory, and traumatic lesions of the pancreas.

Pre-examination Considerations

MDCT imaging of the pancreas is largely based on the study of the enhancement pattern of the lesions and the anatomic alterations of the normal pancreas.

The first step of a MDCT study of the pancreas should be the administration of negative oral contrast medium to the patient, to distend the stomach and duodenum. This makes it easier to study the pancreatic area. Negative oral contrast medium should be preferred because it permits an easier evaluation of gastric and duodenal wall lesions and does not mask possible radiopaque stones in the common bile duct or any pancreatic calcifications.[1]

Contrast-enhanced imaging of the pancreas is based on different contrast medium parameters, such as iodine concentration, volume administration, and injection rate.

The use of intravenous iodinated contrast media is routine with MDCT, and the dose and rate of contrast injection must be adapted to the higher scanning speeds of MDCT.

The maximum amount of iodine should not exceed 35 to 45 g, independently from the concentration of the contrast medium used.[2]

Achieving high concentrations of contrast enhancement to study the pancreas is possible either with increasing the increment of the injection rate or the increment in the iodine concentration of the contrast medium used (total iodine dose being kept constant); the latter is more important because it is not dependent on the intravenous access and vessel diameter as the first is.

The contrast enhancement of the extracellular/extravascular space depends on the concentration gradient between intravascular and extracellular/extravascular spaces, the volume of the extracellular/extravascular space, the permeability of organ microvasculature and cellular interfaces, and surface area and time.[3] A high concentration gradient between intravascular and extracellular/extravascular spaces allows a high influx of contrast material into the extracellular/extravascular space and contributes to high organ enhancement.

Keeping the rate of contrast injection and the total dose of iodine constant, the use of contrast medium with higher concentration improves significantly the arterial and portal venous phase enhancement compared with contrast medium with lower concentration.[4]

As a result, the use of high concentrations of contrast medium improve conspicuity of hypovascular and hypervascular lesions in the pancreas.[5]

Scanning Technique

A plain CT of the upper abdomen is performed using 10-mm slice collimation to cover the pancreas (Fig. 73-1). Depending on the scanner type, a pancreatic phase is performed using 1- to 2-mm slice collimation. Acquisition of the pancreatic phase is usually at a delay of 35 to 40 seconds after a bolus of 125 to 150 mL of iodinated contrast medium injected at a rate of 4 to 5 mL/s. The scanned area extends from the diaphragm to below the transverse duodenum in a single breath-hold.[6] A weight-based approach to intravenous contrast medium administration is now considered more appropriate to optimize the iodine dose for a study. An iodine dose of 550 mg/kg

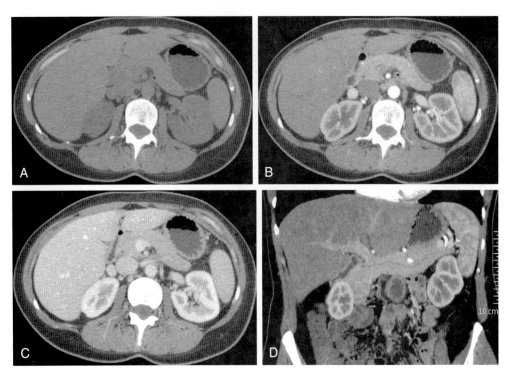

■ FIGURE 73-1 CT anatomy of the pancreas. Precontrast axial CT image of the pancreas (**A**) shows normal glandular thickness. On the pancreatic phase of the dynamic study (**B**), pancreatic parenchyma shows intense, homogeneous enhancement similar to the renal cortex, with wash out during the portal venous phase (**C**). On coronal curved reformatted image (**D**), the whole main pancreatic duct can be depicted.

can be used for both pancreatic and vascular enhancement, which translates into 1.8 to 2.0 mL/kg.

For the next phase, the patient is instructed to breathe deeply after the pancreatic phase acquisition, and a second spiral acquisition is performed at a 70- to 80-second scan delay (see Fig. 73-1). This is the portal venous phase, which covers the entire upper abdomen using 2.5- to 5-mm slice collimation, depending on the patient's body habitus. This phase is critical for the detection of small hypodense liver metastases and in the diagnosis of venous encasement by a tumor. Early arterial phase scans can be performed if a CT angiogram is desired.

Dynamic Imaging

Contrast-enhanced imaging of the pancreas is usually performed in three distinct phases.[7] The first phase is the early arterial phase, which is obtained approximately 20 seconds after contrast administration (see Fig. 73-1). In this phase, contrast medium is preferentially concentrated within the arterial tree with almost no enhancement of the pancreatic parenchyma. The delayed arterial phase, also called the pancreatic phase, is acquired nearly 35 to 40 seconds after contrast agent administration. In this phase we obtain the optimal enhancement of the pancreatic parenchyma and excellent delineation of the arterial vascular system.[7] On the third phase, the portal venous phase, usually acquired at 65 to 70 seconds after contrast agent administration, we have the highest contrast uptake by the portal venous vessels, as well as a good enhancement of the liver parenchyma (see Fig. 73-1).

The bolus tracking techniques, performed by placing a region of interest (ROI) in the aorta just above the level of the pancreas and starting to acquire images when arterial enhancement peaks reach a predetermined Hounsfield unit (HU) trigger value (usually 120 to 130 HU), helps to determine the exact timing of scan delay for a precise individual study for each patient.

Scanning for the pancreatic phase starts 15 seconds after threshold is reached.

Image Postprocessing

To determine resectability of a lesion, the radiologist can also count on various types of image postprocessing. The possibility to obtain high-quality 2D and 3D reconstructions is based on the ability of MDCT to acquire a volumetric dataset with near-isotropic voxels. A large variety of image processing options are available, such as curved reformatted images, minimum intensity projections, volume-rendered images, standard coronal and sagittal plane reformatted images, and coronal oblique reformatted images (see Fig. 73-1). Among these, curved reformatted images give important information about vascular involvement and ductal abnormalities[8]; minimum intensity projections can be used to visualize low-attenuation structures, such as pancreatic and common bile ducts,[9] whereas maximum intensity projections can evaluate high-attenuation structures, such as peripancreatic vasculature. Volume-rendered images are of great aid in visualization of the peripancreatic vessels and tumor encasement.

Such additional 2D and 3D reformatted images provide fundamental information about tumor extent, peripancreatic vascular involvement, or ductal abnormalities, which may be difficult to evaluate on axial images and are also useful to display the lesion characteristics to surgeons and gastroenterologists.[8]

MRI

Recent technologic innovations to both hardware and software have made MRI a reliable technique for studying the pancreas. MRI is potentially the only diagnostic tool that makes it possible to simultaneously image the pancreatic parenchyma and focal (neoplasms, autoimmune pancreatitis) or diffuse (acute/chronic pancreatitis) pathologic processes and to reveal dilatation of pancreatic and bile ducts and to identify gallstones, peripancreatic or hemorrhagic fluid accumulations, lymphadenopathies, hepatic metastases, and vascular anomalies.

In many centers, MRI is currently considered the third method for studying the pancreas, after ultrasonography and CT, not so much because of the technical problems but because of the high costs and, above all, the limited "machine time" useable by departments dealing with pancreatic disease.

Technical Aspects

To achieve the best possible abdominal evaluation with MRI, it is important to use a high-intensity magnetic field (>1.0 T) that guarantees high signal-to-noise ratio (SNR), phased-array surface coils, automatic injectors, powerful gradients, and rapid sequences that can provide images without artifacts due to movement/breathing.[10]

The phased-array surface coils integrate the signal arriving from several coils, reconstructing the final image with a high SNR that ensures greater spatial resolution for the images acquired.[11] The recent development of high-power gradients has made it possible to obtain rapid sequences that ensure better images of the abdomen during breath-holding, thus eliminating the artifacts due to breathing that decrease image quality.[12]

The fat saturation obtained with high field units improves the latitude for nonadipose tissues and reduces the artifacts along the phase-ecoding direction due to movement of subcutaneous adipose tissues during scanning.[13]

The improvement in gradient performance and the development of new pulse sequences (e.g., the T1-weighted volumetric sequences with fat suppression or the half-Fourier rapid acquisition with relaxation enhancement [RARE] sequences) augment the possibility of obtaining better anatomic coverage with more homogeneous saturation of the signal emitted by the adipose tissue.[14]

The development of rapid sequences, associated with fat saturation, enables dynamic imaging of the upper abdomen during the administration of gadolinium chelates in order to study pancreatic parenchyma vascularization, to identify and characterize focal lesions, to evaluate any infiltration or involvement of the peripancreatic vessels, and to identify and characterize focal lesions in the liver.[14]

Protocol

The present protocol calls for use of the following techniques: T1-weighted, gradient-recalled-echo (GRE) sequence axial imaging with "in-phase" and "out-of-phase" echo time (TE); T2-weighted RARE axial imaging; T2-weighted half-Fourier RARE axial and coronal thin slice (5-6 mm) imaging; axial and coronal MR cholangiopancreatography (MRCP); and T1-weighted GRE precontrast axial imaging with fat suppression on the axial plane, possibly with the 3D technique, before and during intravenous administration of gadolinium chelates.[15]

MRCP, an MRI technique that permits noninvasive study of the bile and pancreatic ducts without the use of a contrast medium, has replaced direct cholangiography in most diagnostic indications.[16] The underlying principle behind MRCP is the use of T2-weighted sequences with very long TE (>800 ms) so that, when the echo is detected, only the present stationary fluids (bile and pancreatic juices) are able to provide a signal; the parenchymatous organs, on the other hand, are completely relaxed and, as such, do not emit any signal.[17] This results in good contrast resolution between the bile and pancreatic ducts and the parenchymatous organs. During intravenous administration of secretin, dynamic MRI improves visualization of the principal pancreatic and secondary ducts, thus permitting functional imaging of the pancreas.

Imaging Appearance

T1-Weighted Images

The pancreas is intrinsically endowed with high signal intensity in T1-weighted images, with values higher than other hypochondriac organs (Fig. 73-2). The reason for such signal hyperintensity in T1-weighted images is not fully known. The hypotheses advanced are the high quantity of the proteins in the pancreatic juice located in the pancreas glands; the presence of large quantities of endoplasmic reticula in the acinar cells; or the presence of paramagnetic ions such as manganese.[13] In the elderly, the high signal intensity of the pancreas can be lower than that of the liver, most likely because of the fibrosis incurred by aging.

The T1-weighted GRE images can be used with a fat suppression pulse (Fig. 73-3). Eliminating the signal emitted by the adipose tissues, which has a short T1 relaxation time, redistributes the gray scale over a narrower range, thus making the sequence more sensitive to minor variations in signal intensity.

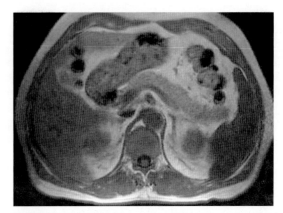

■ **FIGURE 73-2** Normal MRI anatomy of the pancreas: T1-weighted image. Axial T1-weighted gradient-echo image (TR/TE: 145/4.2 ms) shows pancreatic parenchyma of normal thickness. The intensity of pancreatic parenchyma is higher compared with the liver and the spleen.

The T1-weighted GRE images are used for dynamic imaging of the pancreas during the intravenous administration of gadolinium chelates (Fig. 73-4). The dynamic imaging is performed by acquiring 25- to 30-second images (arterial-capillary phase), 45-second images (pancreatic phase), and 80- to 90-second images (portal vein phase) (see Fig. 73-4). The study is completed with T1-weighted coronal images with fat suppression, taken 5 to 10 minutes after administration of gadolinium.[15]

Because of its glandular nature, the pancreas is a highly vascularized organ. For this reason it produces 76% to 115% higher signal intensity during the first minute after gadolinium administration.[13] In the delayed images, the pancreas shows signal intensity similar to that of the liver.

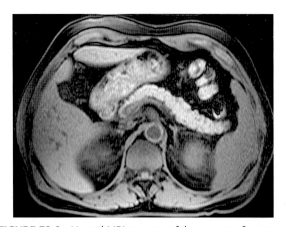

■ FIGURE 73-3   Normal MRI anatomy of the pancreas: fat-saturated T1-weighted image. The application of a fat-saturating pulse eliminates the high signal intensity fat on T1-weighted images, improving in this manner the dynamic range of the image.

The T1-weighted GRE images with fat saturation and the arterial phase after c.m. administration are the most sensitive sequences for identifying focal pancreatic lesions. The portal vein phase is the most useful in evaluating portal vein pathologic processes and identifying lymphadenopathies. The delayed images, obtained 10 minutes after administration of the contrast medium, are instead more useful in identifying cholangiocarcinoma, ascending cholangitis, peritoneal abscesses, and metastases.

The T1-weighted images in GRE sequences, obtained with "in-phase" and "out-of-phase" echo times, are useful in identifying hepatic steatosis, lymphadenopathy, infiltration of the peripancreatic adipose tissue in acute pancreatitis, accumulation of fluids with high methemoglobin or protein concentrations, and adrenal adenoma.

T2-Weighted Images

In T2-weighted images, the parenchymal signal is generally hypointense versus the hepatic parenchyma (Fig. 73-5). Under physiologic conditions, the T2-weighted images provide excellent visualization of the bile and pancreatic duct anatomy and pathology as well as of any peripancreatic fluid accumulations, neuroendocrine tumors, and hepatic metastases.

Other uses of T2-weighted images include the identification of signal hypointensity of fibrosis and iron deposited during hemochromatosis, responsible for the marked hypointensity of the pancreatic gland signal.

MRCP Images

MRCP is an imaging technique that is able to noninvasively assess bile and pancreatic ducts, in a multiplanar fashion,

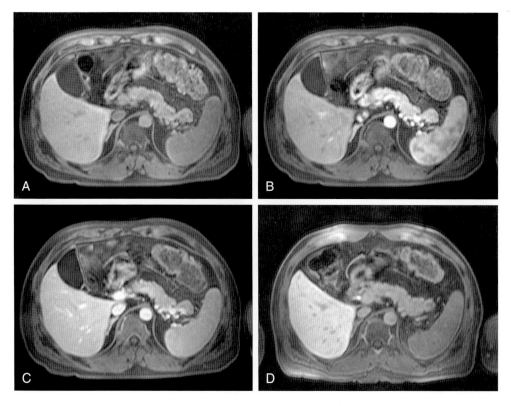

■ FIGURE 73-4   Normal MRI anatomy of the pancreas: dynamic imaging during intravenous administration of gadolinium chelates. **A,** Axial T1-weighted gradient-echo image before the administration of gadolinium chelates. **B,** Axial T1-weighted gradient-echo images during the arterial (**B**), portal venous (**C**), and delayed phase (**D**) of the dynamic study. Of note is the marked signal intensity enhancement of the pancreatic parenchyma during the arterial/pancreatic phase, reflecting its glandular architecture.

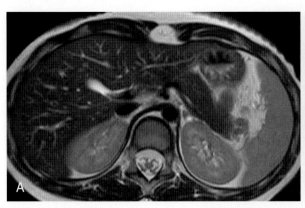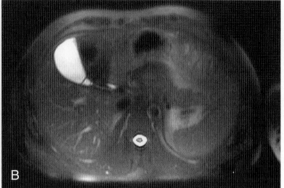

■ **FIGURE 73-5** Normal MRI of the pancreas: T2-weighted imaging. **A,** Axial T2-weighted rapid acquisition with relaxation enhancement (RARE) image (TR/TE: 3500/80 ms) of the pancreas shows the signal intensity of the pancreatic gland is lower compared with the liver and the spleen. **B,** The signal intensity changes are better appreciated on the fat-saturated half-Fourier single-shot turbo spin-echo (HASTE) T2-weighted image (TR/TE: ∞/90 ms).

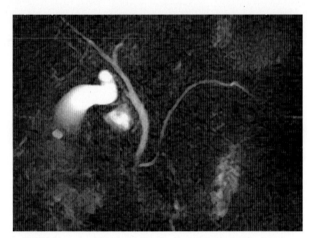

■ **FIGURE 73-6** Normal MRI anatomy of the pancreas: MR cholangiopancreatography (MRCP). Coronal T2-weighted HASTE MRCP image (TR/TE: ∞/1100 ms) shows a normal-sized common bile duct and main pancreatic duct that reaches the duodenum at the major papilla, indicating a Wirsung duct.

without injection of contrast material (Fig. 73-6). MRCP takes advantage of the inherent contrast properties of stationary fluid in the biliary and pancreatic ducts.

The interest in MRCP in the past 5 years is due to its accuracy, its safety, and its availability with nearly all modern scanners, so that MRCP has replaced diagnostic endoscopic retrograde cholangiopancreatography in most of the indications.

The basic principle underlying MRCP is that body fluids, such as bile and pancreatic secretions, have high signal intensity on T2-weighted MR images whereas background signal generates no or little signal. The images of the pancreaticobiliary tree produced by MRCP are similar in appearance to those obtained by direct cholangiographies (i.e., endoscopic retrograde cholangiopancreatography [ERCP] or percutaneous transhepatic cholangiography [PTC]).

MRCP has been initially applied in investigating the biliary ducts; the first reports have focused on the accu-

racy of MRCP in detection of biliary duct dilatation and choledocholithiasis. The application of MRCP to the assessment of the pancreatic duct is less common because pancreatic disease is less frequent compared with biliary disease and the size of the main pancreatic duct is smaller compared with the common bile duct, resulting in signal-to-noise ratios that are less advantageous. Therefore, the visualization of the pancreatic ducts is more challenging compared with that of the biliary ducts.

As a matter of fact, with the use of a surface coil, MRCP clearly showed the main pancreatic duct in the head, body, and tail of the gland, respectively, in 79%, 64%, and 53% of the cases. Furthermore, in patients with chronic pancreatitis, MRCP showed a moderate to high agreement with ERCP in assessing ductal abnormalities. In this group of patients, a high number of false-negative results have been reported because of the small size of the main pancreatic duct, especially in the tail of the pancreas and of the side branches.

MRCP images are able to demonstrate bile and pancreatic duct lithiasis, stenosis, pancreatic cysts, and accumulations of peripancreatic fluids. As opposed to direct cholangiography, the T2-weighted MRCP images can also study the ducts above a tight stenosis.

The exogenous administration of secretin also improves the visualization of pancreatic ducts on MRCP (S-MRCP).[18,19] To obtain better results, MRCP images should employ a slice thickness that encompasses the entire pancreatic ducts, their emergence in the duodenum, and the common bile ducts. A negative contrast agent consisting of 200 mL of superparamagnetic iron oxide particles should be employed routinely to eliminate overlapping fluid-containing organs (Fig. 73-7).

Therefore, secretin can be employed as a contrast agent because it improves the visualization of the pancreatic ducts (Fig. 73-8).[20] But, at the same time, because it physiologically stimulates the exocrine pancreas, when its use is combined with high temporal resolution imaging, functional studies can be performed assessing the dynamics of pancreatic secretion and the pancreatic exocrine reserve.[21,22] Thus, S-MRCP enables morphologic and functional evaluation of the pancreas.

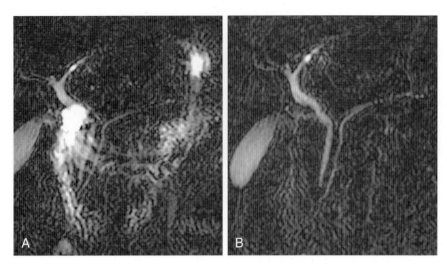

■ FIGURE 73-7 Coronal MRCP before (**A**) and after (**B**) oral administration of superparamagnetic contrast media. **A,** On coronal MRCP single-shot RARE image (TR/TE: ∞/800 ms), the visualization of the main pancreatic duct is impaired by the presence of fluid inside the stomach and duodenum. **B,** The oral administration of superparamagnetic contrast medium improves main pancreatic duct visualization and enables the assessment of duodenal filling.

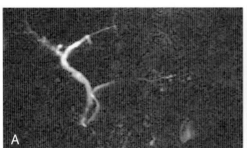 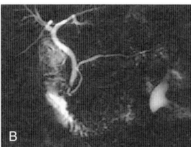 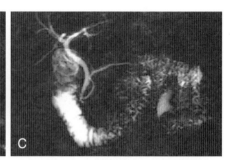

■ FIGURE 73-8 Normal MRI anatomy of the pancreas: dynamic MRCP before and 3 and 10 minutes after secretin administration. **A,** On pre-secretin coronal T2-weighted HASTE MRCP image (TR/TE: ∞/1100 ms) the main pancreatic duct is not completely visualized. **B,** At 3 minutes after secretin administration the main pancreatic duct can be visualized in its whole length. **C,** At 10 minutes after secretin administration the main pancreatic duct caliber decreases and there is duodenal filling.

Evaluation of the Response to Secretin

Morphologic Evaluation

Secretin improves the visualization of the full length of the main pancreatic duct (see Fig. 73-8). This is more evident in patients with normal or minimally dilated pancreatic ducts. In this group of patients there was a significant improvement in main pancreatic duct visualization: 65% (164/252) of the segments before secretin and 97% (245/252) after secretin. An improvement in main pancreatic duct visualization was observed also in the group of patients with severe chronic pancreatitis, from 91% (85/93 segments) to 100% (93/93 segments); this improvement, however, was not significant. This is probably related to the enlargement of the main pancreatic duct, which represents the most frequent sign of severe chronic pancreatitis.[22]

The hallmark of ERCP diagnosis of early chronic pancreatitis is represented by the dilatation of side branches. Because of the small size of these branches, MRCP is not able to routinely recognize dilated side branches, therefore leading to a high false-negative rate. Secretin administration improves the visualization of the side branches (from 4% to 63% of the patients), thus aiding in diagnosing chronic pancreatitis in its early stage (Fig. 73-9). This improved visualization of dilated side branches makes S-MRCP a promising alternative to diagnostic ERCP, with the endoscopic approach indicated only for therapeutic purposes.

Secretin administration also improves visualization of endoluminal filling defects. This improvement, however, is not significant in patients with severe chronic pancreatitis, because the main pancreatic duct is enlarged, containing a larger amount of fluid that encompasses the low-intensity protein plugs along most or all of their circumference. This improvement is therefore particularly important in mild or moderate chronic pancreatitis with a minimally dilated main pancreatic duct where there might be insufficient pancreatic secretion to delineate the whole circumference of the protein plugs. The detection of endoluminal filling defects, namely, their dimension and position, is important in planning adequate treatment, such as interventional ERCP and/or lithotripsy.

Pancreas divisum, a congenital abnormality that results from the failure of fusion of the dorsal and ventral ducts during organogenesis, has a prevalence of 12% at MRCP. In addition to pancreas divisum there are other anatomic variants that share the feature of egression of the major fraction of pancreatic secretions via the dorsal duct orifice. These variants, characterized by a dominant dorsal duct, are found in nearly 10% of the population, double the prevalence of pancreas divisum. Dynamic MRCP after secretin stimulation improved detection of pancreas divisum in 23% of the patients.[20,21]

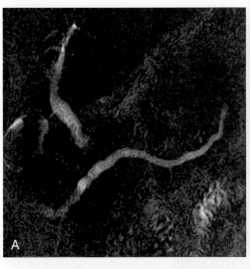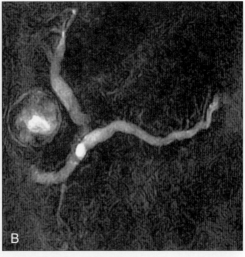

■ **FIGURE 73-9** Dilated side branches. **A,** On coronal MRCP single-shot RARE image (TR/TE: ∞/800 ms) before the administration of secretin, a slight dilation of the main pancreatic duct is observed. **B,** After secretin, dilated side branches in the body and tail of the pancreas are visualized.

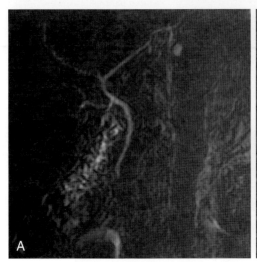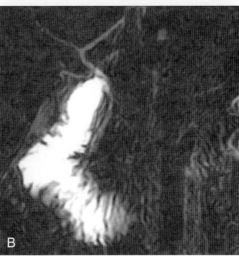

■ **FIGURE 73-10** Duodenal filling after dynamic MRCP, after secretin stimulation: preserved pancreatic exocrine reserve. Coronal T2-weighted HASTE MRCP images (TR/TE: ∞/1100 ms) before (**A**) and 10 minutes after (**B**) secretin administration show duodenal filling beyond the genu inferius.

Besides a better visualization of the morphology of pancreatic abnormalities, secretin also improves the accuracy of MRCP in assessing ductal abnormalities. When comparing MRCP and S-MRCP findings with those from ERCP in patients with recurrent episodes of acute pancreatitis, MRCP showed an overall sensitivity, specificity, and diagnostic accuracy of 53%, 100%, and 93%, respectively, whereas S-MRCP showed an overall sensitivity, specificity, and diagnostic accuracy of 94%, 97%, and 97%, respectively. The slight reduction in specificity of S-MRCP compared with MRCP is due to three false-positive findings.

Functional Evaluation

The dynamic assessment obtainable with rapid imaging after secretin administration gives information on the main pancreatic duct flow dynamics and on the hydrodynamic changes induced by the increased fluid secretion and subsequent elimination into the duodenum (Figs. 73-10 to 73-12).

Papillary stricture can be detected by means of S-MRCP. Papillary stenosis is responsible for persistent dilation of the main pancreatic duct on delayed MRCP images after secretin administration. Ten minutes after secretin admin-

istration, the mean maximal diameter of the main pancreatic duct in patients with papillary stenosis was significantly larger that that in the control subjects in patients without papillary stenosis; furthermore, there was no overlap between observed individual values for the patients with papillary stenosis and for the control subjects (Fig. 73-13).

Another treatable cause of impeded pancreatic secretion outflow is santorinicele, which occurs in patients with pancreas divisum. Santorinicele is a cystic dilatation of the distal dorsal duct, just proximal to the minor papilla. It is termed *santorinicele* in analogy with ureteroceles and choledochoceles, and it is believed to result from a combination of relative obstruction and weakness of the distal duct wall, either acquired or congenital. Santorinicele has been suggested as a possible cause of relative stenosis of the accessory papilla,[23] which in association with unfused dorsal and ventral ducts results in high intraductal pressure. The increased intraductal pressure may be responsible for individual attacks of recurrent acute pancreatitis, which may be caused by temporary obstruction of the minor papilla during passage of protein aggregates. The hypothesis of reduced pancreatic outflow is further sustained by the remarkable reduction in size of the main pancreatic duct and of the santorinicele in patients who

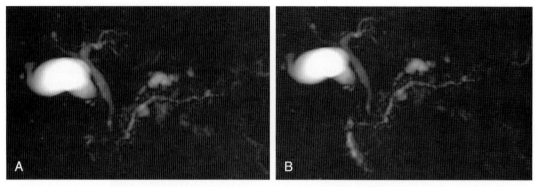

■ **FIGURE 73-11** Duodenal filling after dynamic MRCP, after secretin stimulation: impaired pancreatic exocrine reserve. Coronal T2-weighted HASTE MRCP images (TR/TE: ∞/1100 ms) before (**A**) and 10 minutes after (**B**) secretin administration show duodenal filling up to the genu inferius.

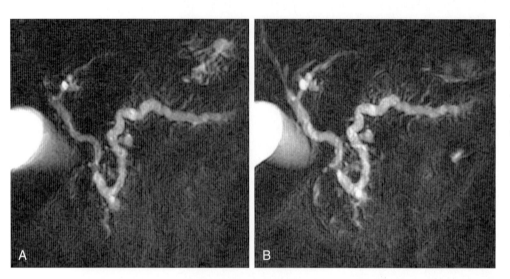

■ **FIGURE 73-12** Duodenal filling after dynamic MRCP, after secretin stimulation: markedly reduced pancreatic exocrine reserve. Coronal T2-weighted HASTE MRCP images (TR/TE: ∞/1100 ms) before (**A**) and 10 minutes after (**B**) secretin administration show absent duodenal filling.

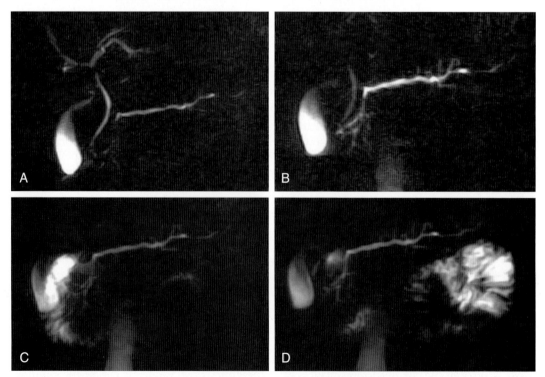

■ **FIGURE 73-13** Dynamic MRCP after secretin stimulation in papillary stenosis. **A,** Coronal MRCP single-shot RARE image (TR/TE: ∞/800 ms) before the administration of secretin shows a normal main pancreatic duct. **B,** At 3 minutes after the administration of secretin the main pancreatic duct enlarges and side branches are visualized. There is very limited duodenal filling. **C,** At 5 minutes after the administration of secretin the duodenal filling starts. **D,** At 10 minutes after the administration of secretin there is persistent dilation of the main pancreatic duct.

underwent sphincterotomy of the minor papilla on follow-up S-MRCP. Furthermore, patients who underwent endoscopic sphincterotomy also had clinical improvement with remission of symptoms.

Papillary stenosis, either idiopathic or due to santorinicele, is responsible for a delay in duodenal filling after the administration of secretin. This duodenal filling after secretin stimulation can be used to semiquantitatively evaluate the pancreatic secretion, which represents an indirect index of the pancreatic exocrine reserve (see Fig. 73-10). The evaluation of the pancreatic exocrine reserve may be important because it can be used to help establish the clinical diagnosis and to monitor the disease and its treatment. Currently, the most valuable pancreatic function tests are the duodenal and intraductal secretin tests with sampling of the duodenal juice or pure pancreatic juice. With invasive techniques, such as those just mentioned, the evaluation of the pancreatic exocrine function is given by measuring bicarbonate output and concentration in the pure pancreatic juice collected after secretin stimulation.

Duodenal filling assessed by dynamic MRCP after secretin administration is a noninvasive means to assess pancreatic exocrine reserve. Patients with severe chronic pancreatitis showed a duodenal filling that was significantly inferior to that of patients with suspected chronic pancreatitis ($P < .001$), probably reflecting a reduced pancreatic exocrine reserve in the advanced phase of the disease.

Dynamic MRCP with secretin administration, however, is not able to perform a qualitative assessment of the pancreatic juice, and this represents a limitation of S-MRCP compared with invasive modalities. Cappeliez and colleagues detected that only maximal bicarbonate concentration is associated with all grades of duodenal filling.[19]

Therefore, the combination of MRCP and secretin administration is able to improve pancreatic duct visualization, reducing in this manner the high false-negative ratio of MRCP. The improved side-branch visualization in S-MRCP, in patients with suspected pancreatic disease, will probably allow an earlier diagnosis of early chronic pancreatitis, making S-MRCP a valid, noninvasive alternative to diagnostic ERCP in this group of patients.

Furthermore, the dynamic assessment of the pancreatic duct enables detection of causes of impeded pancreatic secretion outflow, such as papillary stenosis or santorinicele. Finally, by grading duodenal filling on dynamic MRCP images during secretin administration, a noninvasive assessment of the pancreatic exocrine reserve can be obtained.

ULTRASONOGRAPHY

Conventional ultrasonography is a noninvasive imaging modality that can be considered the technique of choice in the initial evaluation of the pancreas (Fig. 73-14). The pancreas can be visualized by ultrasonography in a high percentage of patients.[23] Nevertheless, it is sometimes difficult to visualize the pancreatic area owing to poor contrast between fat and pancreas and bowel meteorism.

Study of the pancreas is a new and promising application of contrast-enhanced ultrasonography. The dynamic observation of the enhancement allows the evaluation of

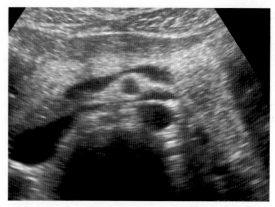

■ **FIGURE 73-14** Anatomy of the pancreas: ultrasonography. The pancreas is identified in front of the splenic vein and the splenomesenteric junction. The pancreatic parenchyma shows moderate hyperechoic structure.

the perfusion of abdominal organs. The parenchymography of the pancreas on contrast-enhanced ultrasonography is well correlated to the semeiology of the gland. Contrast-enhanced ultrasonography can be used to better identify pancreatic lesions with respect to conventional ultrasonography as well as to characterize pancreatic lesions already visible on ultrasonography.[24]

Technical Aspects

The use of multifrequency transducers allows the study of the pancreas with the correct frequencies for any depth. Furthermore, new technologies have improved pancreatic ultrasonographic imaging. Conventional imaging based not only on the amplitude information but also on the phase information of the return echo for the formation of images results in images with more information and greater resolution of detail.

The image quality can also be improved by using compound technology, which reduces speckle in the B-mode image, thus improving contrast resolution and border detection. Speckle is acoustic noise caused by the nature of ultrasound imaging and can be reduced by generating several images or frames of data with independent information and then averaging these several frames of independent or partially independent information.

B-mode technology also optimizes the image by differentiating vascular anatomy from acoustic artifacts and surrounding tissue.

The introduction of 3D and 4D technology opens new clinical possibilities for more complete evaluation of the pancreas in the future.

Harmonic microbubble-specific imaging with a low acoustic ultrasound pressure is required for a dynamic contrast-enhanced ultrasound examination using a second-generation contrast medium. While the background tissue signals are filtered by a specific algorithm of ultrasound image reconstruction, vascular enhancement signals in the regions of interest are related to the presence and the harmonic responses of the microbubbles. The enhancement at low-mechanical index harmonic imaging is immediately visible using second-generation ultrasonographic contrast media. Dynamic observation of the contrast-enhanced phases (early arterial, arterial, pancreatic, portal venous, and late sinusoidal phases) begins immediately after the injection of a second-generation contrast medium. Real-time evaluation of the enhancement is possible maintaining the same scanning frame rate as in the previous conventional B-mode examination.[24] Moreover, contrast-enhanced ultrasonography is the only imaging method that allows monitoring of the enhancement during the dynamic phases.

In general, the correct application of these new technologies in the ultrasonographic study of the pancreas results in very high spatial and contrast resolution.

Examination Protocols

In the study of the pancreas, ultrasound scan planes include transverse, longitudinal, and angled oblique scans. Bowel gas can be displaced by moving the transducer and applying compression when necessary. To obtain complete visualization of all the portions of the pancreatic gland it is possible, and sometimes convenient, to employ different scanning techniques, such as filling the stomach with water, examining the patient with suspended inspiration or expiration, and changing the patient position to erect, supine, and left and right decubitus.[23]

Ultrasound examination of the pancreas is performed after a minimum fast of 6 hours. The purposes of the fast are to improve visualization of the pancreas, limit bowel gas, and ensure an empty stomach. Successful visualization of the pancreas is directly linked to the skill and persistence of the examiner. It is necessary to identify all portions of the pancreas—head, with the uncinate process, neck, body, and tail—in both the longitudinal and the transverse planes. The pancreatic examination begins with the patient in the supine position. If the pancreas is poorly visualized, the water technique can be added.[25] The patient is asked to drink 100 to 300 mL of water through a straw while in the erect or the left lateral decubitus position.

The texture, size, and contour of the pancreas should always be evaluated. The echo pattern of the normal pancreas is isoechoic or hyperechoic compared with that of the normal liver.

During ultrasound examination of the pancreatic gland it is very important to identify the main pancreatic duct but also the common bile duct, especially the intrapancreatic terminal tract. The splenic, superior mesenteric, and portal veins together with the celiac and superior mesenteric arteries must also be identified.

Considering that the blood supply of the pancreas is entirely arterial, the enhancement of the gland begins almost together with the aortic enhancement. On contrast-enhanced ultrasonography the enhancement reaches its peak between 15 and 20 seconds after contrast medium injection. Contrast-enhanced ultrasonography of the pancreas shows a marked parenchymal enhancement in the early contrast-enhanced phases[26]; afterward, there is a progressive wash out of contrast medium with loss of gland echogenicity. The technique of contrast-enhanced ultrasonography of the pancreas should vary according to the clinical indications. To detect or study a small pancreatic lesion, to cover all the glandular sectors in the earliest contrast-enhanced phases, two boluses, each of 2.4 mL of contrast medium, and the "enhancement cancellation"

technique by means of high-acoustic pressure flash can be employed.[26] To study and stage a pancreatic lesion, a complete evaluation of the liver during the late "sinusoidal" phase must be performed to exclude the presence of liver metastases.[27,28,29]

Endoscopic ultrasonography is a novel technique in which the ultrasound probe is placed in close proximity to the pancreas by attaching it to the end of a standard gastrointestinal endoscope and passing the scope in the mouth, down to the duodenum.

Advantages of this technique are in identification and morphologic characterization of lesions as small as 1 cm and in the ability to perform ultrasound-guided fine-needle aspiration cytology for focal lesions.

PROS AND CONS

Pros and cons of the individual modalities used to image the pancreas are listed in Table 73-1.

CLINICAL APPLICATIONS

Inflammatory Pathologic Processes

MDCT

Role of CT in Acute Pancreatitis

● Establishes the diagnosis of acute pancreatitis
● Helps in determining the underlying cause of acute pancreatitis (identifies choledocholithiasis and biliary ductal dilatation associated with biliary pancreatitis)

TABLE 73-1 Pros and Cons of Modalities Used in Imaging the Pancreas

Modality	Pros	Cons
MDCT	High accuracy for diagnosis, characterization, and identification of complications Local and general staging High accuracy in detection of calcifications Parenchymal and vascular visualization Imaging postprocessing	Radiation dose
MRI and MRCP	Higher contrast resolution Parenchymal, vascular, and ductal visualization (MRCP) Functional study (secretin) Higher sensibility for early inflammatory modifications	Less sensitive for calcification characterization Needs high patient cooperation Absolute contraindications
Ultrasonography and contrast-enhanced ultrasonography	Low cost Dynamic microcirculation study (contrast-enhanced)	Operator dependent

● Grades the severity of the disease and detects complications such as pancreatic necrosis, abscess, or pseudocysts

● Serves as an imaging modality for performing percutaneous interventions

MRI

MRI can also be more sensitive than CT in identifying acute pancreatitis, particularly when mild, thanks to its greater contrast resolution.[27,28] Currently, however, the role of MRI in the evaluation of severe acute pancreatitis is not clear because the greatest drawback in this group of patients is the fact that they are generally too ill to cooperate.

Role of MRI in Acute Pancreatitis

● Identifies the underlying causes of the pancreatitis such as choledocholithiasis, pancreas divisum, or pancreatic carcinoma

● Detects early peripancreatic inflammatory infiltration and the accumulation of peripancreatic fluids

● Identifies early stages of pancreatic necrosis, which gives an inhomogeneous appearance to the pancreas on contrast studies

● Detects acute hemorrhagic pancreatitis

● Helps identify complications of acute pancreatitis such as rupture of the main pancreatic duct, formation of pseudocysts or abscesses, fistulas, portal and splenic vein thromboses, and pseudoaneurysms of the splenic artery

Role of MRI in Chronic Pancreatitis

Chronic pancreatitis is a chronic inflammation of the pancreas that results in exocrine and endocrine gland dysfunction.

● MRI is, nevertheless, more sensitive in identifying the initial phase of pancreatitis and/or those cases that do not present calcifications (50%)[30,31]; under basic conditions and during the administration of secretin, MRCP sequences can be used to identify the initial alterations in the secondary ducts.[20,22]

● MRI is able to detect the following duct alterations associated with chronic pancreatitis: dilatation, stenosis, parietal irregularities, twisting, secondary pancreatic duct ectasia, pseudocysts, and intraductal calculi. In addition, association with the section images makes it possible to detect the related morphologic modifications, such as parenchymal atrophy or focal enlargement of the pancreatic parenchyma.

● Intraductal pancreatic calculi are better identified with T2-weighted images where they appear as endoluminal filling defects, surrounded by the high intensity signal of the pancreatic juice. The normal diameter of the main pancreatic duct is approximately 2 mm, whereas the normal secondary pancreatic ducts cannot be viewed by MRCP. The secondary pancreatic ducts are only visible after administration of secretin.[20,22] When visualized, they make it possible to diagnose mild chronic pancreatitis. In severe chronic pancreatitis, the

marked dilatation of the main pancreatic duct and the secondary ducts makes the ductal system look like "rosary beads."

Ultrasonography

Abdominal CT is the technique of choice in the evaluation of patients who present with clinical features suggestive of pancreatitis. However, ultrasonography is widely used. Biliary stones, peripancreatic collections, and pseudocysts can be detected.[32-35] Normal ultrasound findings can be seen in patients with mild acute pancreatitis. Although the pancreas can appear normal in acute pancreatitis, the most frequent findings are enlargement of the gland and a diffuse decrease in normal echogenicity.[26] Acute pancreatitis can be focal or diffuse, depending on the distribution. Focal pancreatitis generally occurs in the pancreatic head and presents as a hypoechoic mass that is sometimes difficult to differentiate from a tumor, especially when focal acute pancreatitis occurs over chronic pancreatitis and the clinical findings are not clear or evident.[26,32,36,37]

The inflamed pancreatic segment shows increased contrast enhancement on contrast-enhanced ultrasonography.[26,32,36,37]

In severe acute pancreatitis, contrast-enhanced ultrasonography may improve the identification and delimitation of areas of parenchymal necrosis, which appear as nonvascular areas.[26,33]

Contrast-enhanced ultrasonography improves the ultrasonographic diagnosis of pseudocyst: the differential diagnosis between pseudocysts and cystic tumors of the pancreas is more reliable thanks to the evaluation of intralesional inclusion vascularization.[37-39]

Abscesses consist of encapsulated collections of purulent material within or near the pancreas. By ultrasonography they are seen as an anechoic or heterogeneous mass containing bright echoes from pus, debris, or gas bubbles. A pancreatic abscess should be suspected on the clinical evidence and when changes in the echogenicity of the content of pseudocysts are documented at ultrasound examination. Vascular complications including pseudoaneurysms and venous thrombosis may be seen in both acute and chronic pancreatitis. Hemorrhage may occur as a consequence of vascular injury.[33]

Chronic pancreatitis is an inflammatory disease characterized by the replacement of the glandular elements of the pancreas by fibrous tissue. The most significant ultrasound findings of chronic pancreatitis are pancreatic duct dilatation, intraductal calcifications, and pseudocysts.

Solid Lesions

MDCT

● Detects and characterizes the lesion based on the enhancement pattern on dynamic imaging. For example, adenocarcinomas appear hypodense in the pancreatic phase and the neuroendocrine tumors are characterized by their intense enhancement pattern in the arterial phase.[40-42]

● Helps in staging of the lesion and determining its resectability criteria such as vascular invasion, hepatic and omental metastasis, and regional lymph node involvement.

MRI

- Is a problem-solving modality to confirm suspicious lesions on CT or ultrasonography[40]
- Characterizes lesions based on their morphology
- Detects masses in the setting of inflammation in and around the pancreas
- Characterizes pancreatic duct stricture and differentiates benign from malignant ones
- Detects liver lesions and characterizes them in patients with pancreatic neoplasm

Ultrasonography

Ultrasonography is often the first technique performed when pancreatic adenocarcinoma is suspected. Pancreatic adenocarcinoma is most common in the pancreatic head (65%) and usually presents as a hypoechoic solid mass. General enlargement from associated pancreatitis is uncommon (15%). Ductal adenocarcinoma shows poor enhancement[36] on all phases of contrast-enhanced ultrasonography. On the contrast-enhanced study this lesion appears as a hypoechoic mass compared with the adjacent normally enhancing pancreatic parenchyma; the margins and size of the lesion are better visualized as is its relationship with peripancreatic arterial and venous vessels for local staging. Contrast-enhanced ultrasonography demonstrates the vascularization of the neoplastic tissue with enhancement seen in the earliest phases of the dynamic study.

On color and power Doppler ultrasonography a "spot pattern" can be demonstrated inside endocrine tumors. However, Doppler "silence" can be present in hypervascular endocrine tumors because of the small size of the lesion or of the tumoral vascular network. On contrast-enhanced ultrasonography different enhancement patterns can be observed in relation to the dimension of the tumor and tumoral vessels. Endocrine tumors show a rapid intense enhancement in the early contrast-enhanced phases, with exclusion of the necrotic intralesional areas and contrast entrapment in the late phase.[26]

Contrast-enhanced ultrasound examination may improve the identification and characterization of endocrine tumors and also improves locoregional and hepatic staging of endocrine tumors.[26,43]

Cystic Lesions

MDCT

- MDCT with its superior resolution helps in detection of the cystic lesions and their morphologic characterization such as size, presence of calcification, septa, central scar, solid mass wall thickness, and enhancement pattern[44]
- Determination of the status of the pancreatic duct dilatation, stricture, or any communication with cyst
- Categorization of patients into surgical and nonsurgical groups

- For follow-up in patients in whom surgery is not indicated initially
- For postoperative management and follow-up

MRI

- Enables better cyst characterization than CT because of superior soft tissue resolution[44]
- For pancreatic duct evaluation, to detect any mural nodules or septations
- For follow-up in patients having higher radiation risk (e.g., those <age 50 years)
- In patients with contraindications for iodinated contrast agents (e.g., patients in renal failure)
- Identifies hemorrhagic complications within the cyst in different stages
- Defines the communication with the pancreatic duct on MRCP images, thus establishing the diagnosis of side-branch intraductal papillary mucinous tumor of the pancreas in the majority of cases[45,46]

Ultrasonography

The contents of serous cystadenomas is a glycogen-rich serous fluid, which makes this tumor visible on ultrasonography. Microcystic lesions may have a solid appearance. Further characterization of the cyst is possible by detection of the presence of an echogenic scar or calcification. Contrast-enhanced ultrasonography improves the ultrasound characterization of serous cystadenoma, showing the enhancement of intralesional septa, with better identification of the microcystic features of the lesion.[47]

However, demonstration of the absence of communication is impossible by ultrasonography and is a specific issue for MRI and ERCP.[48]

KEY POINTS

- Different diagnostic imaging modalities have been evaluated in assessing pancreatic diseases.
- Ultrasonography, although inexpensive and readily available, is limited by patient body habitus and bowel gas for a complete evaluation of the pancreas.
- MDCT is the modality of choice for the initial evaluation of pancreatic diseases, staging, and presurgical planning.
- MRI shows high contrast resolution in evaluating the pancreatic parenchyma for detection of small lesions and is useful in problem-solving situations.
- Liver lesions can be detected and evaluated in patients with pancreatic neoplasms. All imaging modalities are suitable for this purpose.
- MRCP is the diagnostic modality of choice for detailed, noninvasive evaluation of the pancreatic ducts and cystic lesions.
- Secretin-enhanced MRCP is able both to better assess pancreatic ducts and to evaluate pancreatic function.

SUGGESTED READINGS

Rha SE, Jung SE, Lee KH, et al. CT and MR imaging findings of endocrine tumor of the pancreas according to WHO classification. Eur J Radiol 2007; 62:371-377.

Schima W, Ba-Ssalamah A, Goetzinger P, et al. State-of-the-art magnetic resonance imaging of pancreatic cancer. Top Magn Reson Imaging 2007; 18:421-429.

Sidden CR, Mortele KJ. Cystic tumors of the pancreas: ultrasound, computed tomography, and magnetic resonance imaging features. Semin Ultrasound CT MR 2007; 28:339-356.

Siddiqi AJ, Miller F. Chronic pancreatitis: ultrasound, computed tomography, and magnetic resonance imaging features. Semin Ultrasound CT MR 2007; 28:384-394.

Vanbeckevoort D. Solid pancreatic masses: benign or malignant. JBR-BTR 2007; 90:487-489.

REFERENCES

1. Tunaci M. Multidetector row CT of the pancreas. Eur J Radiol 2004; 52:18-30.
2. Fenchel S, Boll DT, Fleiter TR. Multislice helical CT of the pancreas and spleen. Eur J Radiol 2003; 45:S59-S72.
3. Bae KT, Heiken JP, Brink JA. Aortic and hepatic contrast medium enhancement at CT. I. Prediction with a computer model. Radiology 1998; 207:647-655.
4. Fenchel S, Fleiter TR, Aschoff AL, et al. Effect of iodine concentration of contrast media on contrast enhancement in multislice CT of the pancreas. Br J Radiol 2004; 77:821-830.
5. Sahani D, Shah ZK. Soft-organ MDCT imaging: pancreas and spleen. In Saini S, Rubin GD, Kalra MK (eds). MDCT: A Practical Approach. Berlin, Springer, 2006.
6. Fishman EK, Jeffrey RB Jr. Multidetector CT: Principles, Techniques and Clinical Applications. Philadelphia, Lippincott Williams & Wilkins, 2004.
7. McNulty NJ, Francis IR, Platt JF, et al. Multidetector row helical CT of tbc pancreas: effect of contrast enhanced multiphasic imaging on enhancement of the pancreas, peripancreatic vasculature, and pancreatic adenocarcinoma. Radiology 2001; 220:97-102.
8. Nono-Murcia M, Jeffrey RB Jr, Beaulieu CF, et al. Multidetector CT of the pancreas and bile duct system: value of curved planar reformations. AJR Am J Roentgenol 2001; 176:689-693.
9. Raptopoulos V, Prassopoulos P, Chuttani R, et al. Multiplanar CT pancreatography and distal cholangiography with minimum intensity projections. Radiology 1998; 207:317-324.
10. Thoeni RF, Blankenberg F. Pancreatic imaging: computed tomography and magnetic resonance imaging. Radiol Clin North Am 1993; 31:1085-1113.
11. Ferrucci JT. Advances in abdominal MR imaging. RadioGraphics 1998; 18:1569-1586.
12. Semelka RC, Ascher SM. MRI of the pancreas—state of the art. Radiology 1993; 188:593-602.
13. Siegelman ES, Outwater EK. MR imaging techniques of the liver. Radiol Clin North Am 1998; 36:263-286.
14. Rofsky NM, Lee VS, Laub G, et al. Abdominal MR imaging with a volume interpolated breath-hold examination. Radiology 1999; 212:876-884.
15. Hamed MM, Hamm B, Ibrahim ME, et al. Dynamic MR imaging of the abdomen with gadopentetate dimeglumine: normal enhancement patterns of the liver, spleen, stomach, and pancreas. AJR Am J Roentgenol 1992; 158:303-307.
16. Fulcher AS, Turner MA. MR pancreatography: a useful tool for evaluating pancreatic disorders. RadioGraphics 1999; 19:5-24.
17. Cova M, Stacul F, Cester G, et al. MR cholangiopancreatography: comparison of 2D single-shot fast spin-echo and 3D fast spin-echo sequences. Radiol Med 2003; 106:178-179.
18. Matos C, Metens T, Devière J, et al. Pancreatic duct: morphologic and functional evaluation with dynamic MR pancreatography after secretin stimulation. Radiology 1997; 203:435-441.
19. Cappeliez O, Delhaye M, Devière J, et al. Chronic pancreatitis: evaluation of pancreatic exocrine function with MR pancreatography after secretin stimulation. Radiology 2000; 215:358-364.
20. Manfredi R, Costamagna G, Vecchioli A, et al. Dynamic pancreatography with magnetic resonance after functional stimulus with secretin in chronic pancreatitis. Radiol Med 1998; 96:226-231.
21. Nicaise N, Pellet O, Metens T, et al. Magnetic resonance cholangiopancreatography: interest of IV secretin administration in the evaluation of pancreatic ducts. Eur Radiol 1998; 8:16-22.
22. Manfredi R, Costamagna G, Brizi MG, et al. Dynamic magnetic resonance pancreatography after secretin stimulation: severe chronic pancreatitis vs suspected pancreatic disease. Radiology 2000; 214:849-855.
23. Mittelstaedt CA. Abdominal Ultrasound. New York, Mosby, 1987, pp 163-176.
24. Weissleder R, Rieumont MJ, Wittenberg J. Primer of Diagnostic Imaging, 2nd ed. New York, Mosby–Year Book, 1997, pp 220-228.
25. Lev-Toaff AS, Bree RL, Lund PJ, et al. Use of simethicone-coated cellulose suspension to improve pancreatic ultrasound: experience in 55 patients with pancreatic pathology. Radiology 1998; 209(Suppl):310.
26. D'Onofrio M, Zamboni G, Malagò R, et al. Pancreatic pathology. In Quaia E (ed). Contrast media in ultrasonography. Berlin, Springer-Verlag, 2005, pp 335-347.
27. Sahani D, Kalva SP, Farrell J, et al. Autoimmune pancreatitis: imaging features. Radiology 2004; 233:345-352.
28. Robinson PJA, Sheridan MB. Pancreatitis: computed tomography and magnetic resonance imaging. Eur Radiol 2000; 10:401-408.
29. Balthazar EJ, Robinson DL, Megibow AJ, et al. Acute pancreatitis: value of CT in determining prognosis. Radiology 1990; 174:331-336.
30. Luetmer PH, Stephens DH, Ward EM. Chronic pancreatitis reassessment with current CT. Radiology 1989; 171:353-357.
31. Pavone P, Laghi A, Catalano C, et al. The assessment of chronic pancreatitis by magnetic resonance and MR cholangiopancreatography. II. The semeiotics and results. Radiol Med 1999; 98:373-378.
32. Loren I, Lasson A, Fork T, et al. New sonographic imaging observations in focal pancreatitis. Eur Radiol 1999; 9:862-867.
33. Baron HT, Morgan ED. The diagnosis and management of fluid collections associated with pancreatitis. Am J Med 1997; 102:555-563.
34. Bolondi L, Priori P, Gullo L, et al. Relationship between morphological changes detected by ultrasonography and pancreatic esocrine function in chronic pancreatitis. Pancreas 1987; 2:222-229.
35. Furukawa N, Muranaka T, Yasumori K, et al. Autoimmune pancreatitis: radiologic findings in three histologically proven cases. J Comput Assist Tomogr 1998; 22:880-883.
36. Numata K, Ozawa Y, Kobayashi N, et al. Contrast enhanced sonography of autoimmune pancreatitis: comparison with pathologic findings. J Ultrasound Med 2004; 23:199-206.
37. Freeny P, Lawson T. Radiology of the Pancreas. New York, Springer-Verlag, 1982, p 449.
38. Boland GW, O'Malley ME, Saez M, et al. Pancreatic-phase versus portal vein–phase helical CT of the pancreas: optimal temporal window for evaluation of pancreatic adenocarcinoma. AJR Am J Roentgenol 1999; 172:605-608.
39. Lu DS, Reber HA, Krasny RM, et al. Local staging of pancreatic cancer: criteria for unresectability of major vessels as revealed by pancreatic phase, thin-section helical CT. AJR Am J Roentgenol 1997; 168:1439-1443.

40. Ichikawa T, Haradome H, Hachiya J, et al. Pancreatic ductal adeno-carcinoma: preoperative assessment with helical CT versus dynamic MR imaging. Radiology 1997; 193:655-662.

41. Procacci C, Carbognin G, Accordini S, et al. Nonfunctioning endocrine tumors of the pancreas: possibilities of spiral CT characterization. Eur Radiol 2001; 11:1175-1183.

42. Semelka RC, Cumming MJ, Shoenut JP, et al. Islet cell tumors: comparison of dynamic contrast-enhanced CT and MR imaging with dynamic gadolinium enhancement and fat suppression. Radiology 1993; 186:799-802.

43. Galiber AK, Reading CC, Charboneau JW. Localization of pancreatic insulinoma: comparison of pre- and intraoperative ultrasound with computer tomography and angiography. Radiology 1988; 166:405-408.

44. Ros PR, Mortele KJ. Imaging features of pancreatic neoplasms. JBR-BTR 2001; 84:239-249.

45. Manfredi R, Mehrabi S, Motton M, et al. Magnetic resonance (MR) imaging and MR cholangiopancreatography (MRCP) of multifocal intraductal papillary mucinous tumors (IPMT) of the side branches: MR pattern and its evolution. Radiol Med 2008; 113:414-428.

46. Irie H, Honda H, Aibe H, et al. MR cholangiopancreatography differentiation of benign and malignant intraductal mucin-producing tumors of the pancreas. AJR Am J Roentgenol 2000; 174:1403-1408.

47. Bennett GL, Hann LE. Pancreatic ultrasonography. Surg Clin North Am 2001; 81:259-281.

48. Procacci C, Schenal G, Dalla Chiara E, et al. Intraductal papillary mucinous tumors: imaging. In Procacci C, Megibow AJ (eds). Imaging of the Pancreas: Cystic and Rare Tumors. Berlin, Springer-Verlag, 2003, pp 97-137.

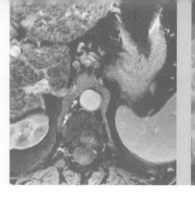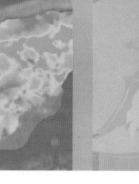

CHAPTER 74

Pancreas—Normal Variants

Onofrio Catalano and Dushyant V. Sahani

TECHNICAL ASPECTS

Many different diagnostic imaging techniques are useful in the evaluation of congenital variants of the pancreas. Ultrasonography is usually the first method used to image the pancreas and the upper abdomen, but it rarely allows a specific diagnosis of pancreatic lesion to be achieved. Multidetector CT (MDCT) and MRI, with the added value of postprocessed images and MR cholangiopancreatography (MRCP), are able to provide a very detailed evaluation of the pancreas, which is useful not only to detect but also to characterize most of the lesions. PET/CT is not indicated in the study of suspected congenital variants of the pancreas unless differentiation with malignancy has not been achieved with other imaging methods. Endoscopic retrograde cholangiopancreatography (ERCP) is usually reserved for selected cases; it allows direct visualization of the pancreatic duct and of its side branches.

PROS AND CONS

Pros and cons of each imaging method are outlined in Tables 74-1 and 74-2.

CONTROVERSIES

An ideal imaging technique to study the pancreas should be devoid of side effects for the patient, able to discriminate benign from malignant lesions, provide accurate images with high temporal and spatial resolution, not be affected by artifact, be reproducible, and not be expensive. At the moment no imaging technology satisfies all these requirements. In our opinion, MDCT and MRI are the technologies better able to study the pancreas, although MDCT is limited by radiation exposure and MRI by dependence on patient cooperation.

ANATOMY

The pancreas (Fig. 74-1) is a mixed exocrine-endocrine retroperitoneal gland located in the anterior pararenal space. It has a grossly oblong shape and a coronal oblique orientation, extending from the splenic hilum, where it is thinner, to the midline of the body, where it enlarges. It is divided into the uncinate process, head, neck, body, and tail. The uncinate process is the triangular inferiormost portion of the head of the pancreas and lies

TABLE 74-1 Pros and Cons of Commonly Utilized Imaging Modalities for Pancreatic Anomalies

Modality	Pros	Cons
Ultrasonography	Inexpensive, noninvasive, easily available	Highly operator dependent Body habitus and bowel gas may reduce its usefulness.
MDCT	High spatial and temporal resolution MPR and 3D postprocessing possible Non–operator dependent	Ionizing radiation exposure
MRCP	High spatial and temporal resolution High signal-to-noise ratio 3D postprocessing possible	Expensive Not widely available Artifacts in the case of poor patient cooperation
ERCP	Detailed evaluation of pancreatic ductal system Intervention possible	Invasive Risk of complications such as bleeding, perforation, sepsis, pancreatitis Operator dependent Ionizing radiation exposure
PET/CT	Functional and imaging evaluation Useful in the case of suspected malignancy	Expensive Radiation exposure Not widely available

TABLE 74-2 Accuracy, Limitations, and Pitfalls of the Modalities Used in Imaging of Normal Variants of the Pancreas

Modality	Accuracy	Limitations	Pitfalls
Radiography	Conventional radiography: poor ERCP: considered the gold standard for many congenital variants	Conventional radiography: insensitive, nonspecific ERCP: invasive, risk of complications	Unable to directly visualize soft tissue masses in the pancreas
CT	Data not available to specify accuracy	Radiation exposure	Characterization of small lesions may be difficult.
MRI	73% in the case of pancreas divisum Data not available to specify accuracy in the case of other variants	Patient cooperation High cost	Calcifications not well visualized
Ultrasonography	Data not available to specify accuracy	Poor performance in the case of obesity or overlying bowel gas Operator dependent Comprehensive imaging difficult	Detection and characterization of small lesions may be difficult.
Nuclear medicine	No role	Poor spatial resolution	
PET/CT	Data not available to specify accuracy Used to differentiate benign from malignant lesions	Radiation exposure High cost	

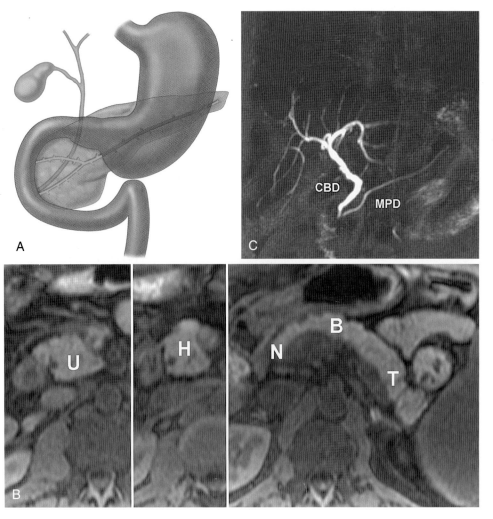

■ **FIGURE 74-1** Normal pancreatic duct system. **A,** Drawing. **B,** T1W fat-saturated axial composite MR image. **C,** MRCP. The pancreas is divided into the uncinate process (U), head (H), neck (N), body (B), and tail (T). The normal duct system is characterized by the main pancreatic duct (MPD) draining the dorsal pancreas and joining the common bile duct (CBD) to empty into the major papilla.

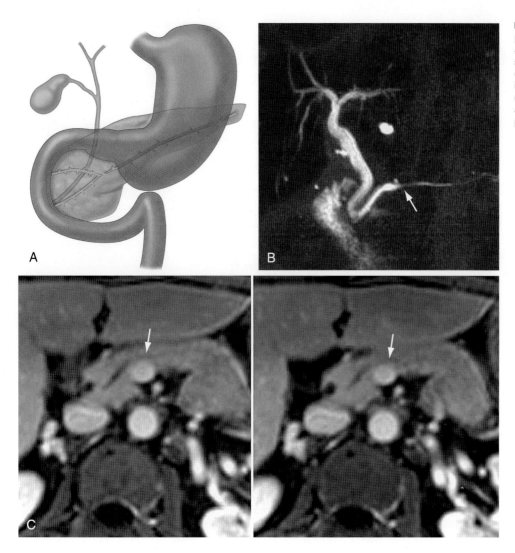

posterior to the superior mesenteric vessels. The head is the thickest portion of the pancreas, located in the "C" loop of the duodenum and to the right of the portal vein. The neck is the short transition between the head and the body; it is located just anterior to the portal vein and superior mesenteric artery. The body and tail extend to the left toward the splenic hilum, with the body representing the medial half and the tail the remaining latter half.

The pancreas is about 15 cm in length and its antero-posterior diameter decreases from the head to the tail. The ratio of the head to the body remains almost constant through life, despite the reduction in size of the organ with advancing age. Variable amounts of adipose and fibrous tissue are present along the margins of the gland and within the parenchyma, giving it a lobular architecture.

The main pancreatic duct (Wirsung's) and the accessory pancreatic duct (Santorini's) drain pancreatic secretions into the duodenum. The former runs into and drains the body, tail, lower head, and uncinate process. It joins the common bile duct at the ampulla of Vater and empties through the major papilla. The latter, which can also

undergo atrophy, runs into and drains the upper portion of the head of the pancreas into the minor papilla. At the fusion point of the ducts of Santorini and Wirsung in the pancreatic neck the duct may be reduced in caliber or demonstrate a loop configuration (Fig. 74-2).

The imaging appearance of the pancreas, using different technologies, is detailed in Chapter 73.[1]

Pancreatic variants and developmental anomalies can be divided into ductal, ductal and parenchymal, parenchymal, and miscellaneous (Fig. 74-3). The most common include pancreas divisum, annular pancreas, congenital short pancreas (pancreatic hypoplasia—agenesis of the dorsal pancreas), pancreatic head lobulation, uneven pancreatic lipomatosis, and ectopic pancreas.[1,2]

PATHOPHYSIOLOGY

Congenital anomalies of the pancreas derive from altered embryogenic development. At the 4th week of gestation, dorsal and ventral endodermal anlagen arise from the foregut, near the junction with the yolk sac. The ventral anlage gives rise to the liver, gallbladder, bile ducts, and the ventral pancreas; meanwhile, the dorsal anlage gives

Pancreatic Variants

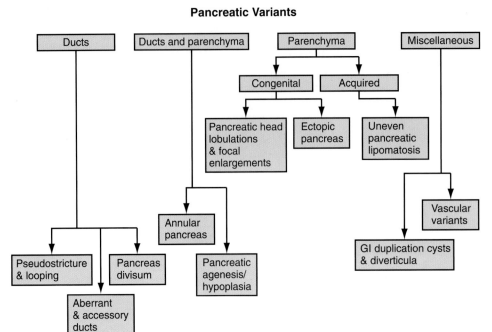

■ **FIGURE 74-3** Classification of pancreatic variants and developmental anomalies.

origin to the dorsal pancreas (Fig. 74-4). The caudal portion of the ventral anlage divides into two ventral buds: the right bud enlarges and develops along with the primitive bile duct; the left bud undergoes atrophy and in some studies its persistence is implicated in annular pancreas development. During the 5th week of gestation, the ventral pancreatic bud rotates clockwise to the right, along with the common bile duct, and the dorsal anlage rotates to the left. At the beginning of the 6th week of gestation, after the rotation process is completed, the right ventral pancreatic bud lies medially to the descending portion of the duodenum and below the dorsal pancreatic anlage (Fig. 74-5).

Most of the pancreas (upper part of the head, the neck, body, tail, dorsal pancreatic duct, and the accessory pancreatic duct of Santorini which drains into the minor papilla) arises from the dorsal pancreatic anlage. The remainder of the organ (the uncinate process, the caudal portion of the head, the corresponding ventral pancreatic duct that drains into the major papilla) arises from the ventral pancreas.

By the end of the 6th week of gestation the ventral and dorsal pancreatic buds, along with their corresponding ducts, fuse. After fusion process has been completed, the dorsal duct system upstream to the point of fusion is named the main pancreatic duct; the remaining portion,

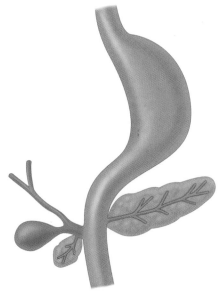

■ **FIGURE 74-4** Drawing displaying separate origin of ventral and dorsal pancreatic anlagen from the foregut at the 4th week of gestation. Note how the ventral anlage shares origin with the biliary system and liver.

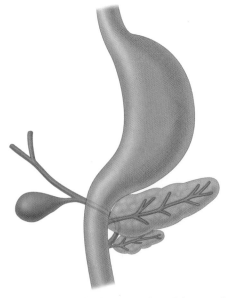

■ **FIGURE 74-5** Drawing displaying rotation of the ventral pancreatic bud and subsequent fusion with the dorsal pancreatic bud, at the 6th week of gestation, to form the adult pancreas.

draining into the minor papilla, is called the accessory duct of Santorini. The latter usually undergoes atrophy. The ventral duct, from the drainage into the major papilla to the fusion point with the dorsal duct, is named the duct of Wirsung. Usually most of the pancreatic juice drains into the major papilla through the fused dorsal and ventral pancreatic ducts. If the contrary happens, the condition is termed *pancreas divisum.*[1-3]

IMAGING

Pancreas Divisum

Pancreas divisum, the most common congenital variant of the pancreas (5% to 14% of the population), is characterized by a failure of fusion of the dorsal and ventral ducts, with predominant drainage occurring through the dorsal duct system into the duct of Santorini.

Pancreas divisum is classified into three types: type 1 or the classic form, with complete lack of fusion between the dorsal and ventral duct systems (Fig. 74-6); type 2, in which the duct of Wirsung is absent (Fig. 74-7); and type 3, or the partial form, in which a small branch connects the dorsal and ventral duct system, with most of the organ being drained through the dorsal system (Fig. 74-8).

The relationship of pancreas divisum to pancreatic diseases is unclear; pancreas divisum may be devoid of any symptoms or be associated with minor abdominal pain or acute, acute recurrent, or chronic pancreatitis.

In some studies, 25% of patients undergoing pancreatography for idiopathic pancreatitis presented with pancreas divisum. Usually these patients were young, female, and nonalcoholic. Moreover, pathology changes circumscribed to the dorsal part of the pancreas have been found at autopsy and pancreatography.

A disproportion between the caliber of the minor papilla and the amount of pancreatic juice drained into it, through the dorsal duct system, could be responsible for a relative outflow obstruction. The reduced size of the minor papilla could be a constant finding, due to anatomic stenosis, or a transient event related to intermittent protein secretion plugging.[2-14]

Radiography

The gold standard for evaluation of pancreas divisum is ERCP. In type 1, ERCP demonstrates a shorter than normal (1 to 4 cm) ventral duct, which does not cross the midline, is normally tree-like branched, and empties into the major papilla, and a dorsal duct system that drains the neck, body, and tail of the pancreas into the minor papilla. In type 2, only the dorsal system is demonstrated and no duct of Wirsung can be found. In type 3, the small filamentous connection between the dominant dorsal duct system and the duct of Wirsung is disclosed.[3-6,8-13]

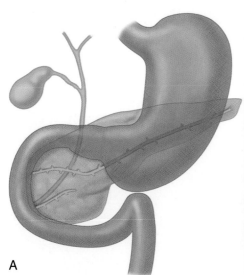
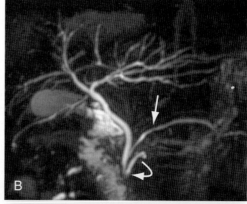
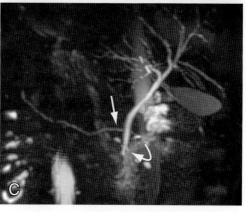

■ **FIGURE 74-6** **A,** Drawing of pancreas divisum type 1. 3D MRCP images (**B** and **C**) show complete separation of the dorsal and ventral duct system with the dorsal system (*straight arrow*) draining into the minor papilla and the ventral system (*curved arrow*) draining in conjunction with the common bile duct into the major papilla. The separate entry of the dorsal duct system, above the major papilla, is better appreciated on the oblique coronal image (**C**).

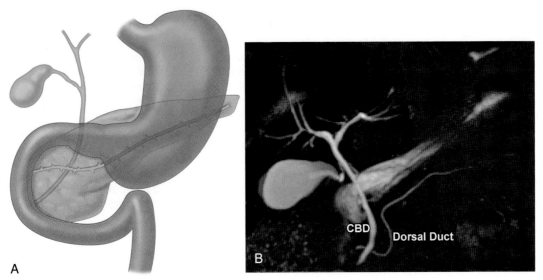

■ **FIGURE 74-7** **A,** Drawing of pancreas divisum type 2. **B,** 3D MRCP demonstrates absent duct of Wirsung and a dominant dorsal duct system, draining into the minor papilla, above the common bile duct (CBD) opening into the major papilla.

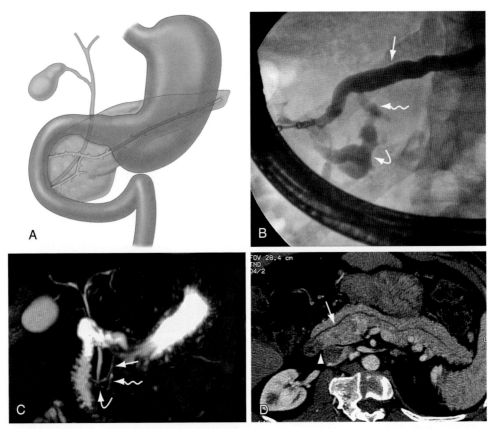

■ **FIGURE 74-8** **A,** Drawing of pancreas divisum type 3. ERCP (**B**), 3D MRCP (**C**), and MDCT pancreatogram (**D**) in different patients show a small filamentous communication (*wavy arrow*) between the dorsal duct system (*straight arrow*), draining into the minor papilla, and the ventral duct system (*curved arrow*), draining along with the common bile duct (*arrowhead*) into the major papilla.

CT

MDCT, with the aid of the high-quality multiplanar reconstructions, including MDCT pancreatograms, may be helpful to diagnose pancreas divisum. The ventral duct is smaller or not visualized; the dorsal pancreatic duct is visualized in its course, through the anterior portion of the organ, draining directly into the minor papilla (see Fig. 74-8).[4-6,8-13]

MRI

MRCP is 73% accurate in the case of complete pancreas divisum, demonstrating a dominant dorsal duct system that crosses the distal bile duct and empties through the accessory duct of Santorini into the minor papilla (see Figs. 74-6 to 74-8). No communication with the ventral duct system can be found. The latter is located below the dorsal duct system, joining with the common bile duct to enter the major papilla.

In the case of incomplete pancreas divisum, MRCP usually allows for suspected dorsal duct system dominance but does not clearly demonstrate the short ventral pancreatic duct as well as the small connecting branch.

Secretin MRCP increases MRCP diagnostic accuracy in pancreas divisum but, because prolonged pancreatic ductal dilatation occurs both in pancreas divisum and in the non–pancreas divisum population, it does not clearly distinguish between patients who can benefit from surgery from those who cannot.[4,5,7,8,10-12]

Imaging Algorithm

Pancreas divisum may enter in the differential diagnosis with pancreatic cancer causing obstruction of the duct of Wirsung and upstream dilatation of the main pancreatic duct. In the case of pancreas divisum, direct continuation of the dorsal duct system with the duct of Santorini, which drains through the minor papilla above to the opening of the bile duct, is pathognomonic. If the ventral duct system is present, it should demonstrate a normal branching pattern. Pancreatic parenchyma is homogeneous; there is no vessel encasement and no infiltrations are observed.[3-8,10-13]

Classic Signs: Pancreas Divisum

- Dorsal pancreatic duct system that drains separately and above the common bile duct
- Ventral duct system that is absent or not connected to the dorsal duct system or connected through a small filamentous communication.[3-8,10-13]

Annular Pancreas

Annular pancreas, a rare congenital anomaly (1/20,000 births), is characterized by the presence of a portion of pancreatic tissue that partially or completely encircles the duodenum (Fig. 74-9). The annular parenchyma usually circumscribes the descending portion of the duodenum (74% of the cases) and can be associated with duodenal anomalies such as atresia, atrophy, or stenosis. Pancreas divisum has been reported in up to 36% of patients with annular pancreas. Persistence of the left ventral pancreatic bud or failure of rotation of the right ventral pancreatic bud have been proposed to explain the occurrence of annular pancreas.

Annular pancreas is usually diagnosed in childhood because of upper gastrointestinal obstruction and less often in adulthood due to symptoms of gastrointestinal obstruction, of peptic ulcer disease, or of pancreatitis. In some cases annular pancreas can be misinterpreted as a tumor.[2,4-6,15-17]

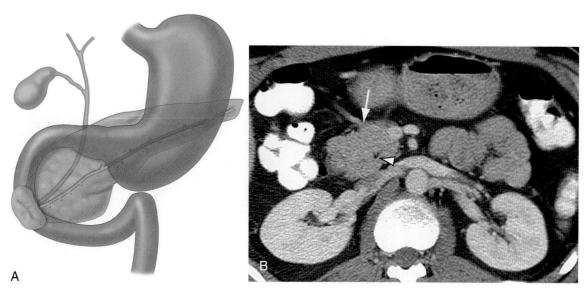

A

B

■ **FIGURE 74-9** **A,** Drawing of annular pancreas. **B,** Axial MDCT image shows an extension of the pancreatic head (*arrow*) partially or completely encircling the duodenum (*arrowhead*), usually the second portion. The annular pancreas is homogeneous, with preserved lobulation, and parallels attenuation of the remaining pancreas.

Radiography

Radiographic signs of annular pancreas are those of duodenal obstruction or stenosis. They are more evident and specific in the youngest children.

Plain films of the abdomen may show a "double bubble" sign from dilation of the duodenum and stomach or a duodenal cutoff sign. Upper gastrointestinal contrast studies confirm duodenal obstruction. Dilation and reverse peristalsis of the proximal duodenum may also be encountered.

ERCP reveals an aberrant pancreatic duct encircling the duodenum. Its site of drainage is variable, but drainage usually occurs in the main pancreatic duct or in the common bile duct near the ampulla of Vater.[4-6,15-18]

CT

MDCT shows homogeneous pancreatic head tissue encircling the duodenum (see Fig. 74-9). MDCT-3D pancreatography, performed after ERCP, can display the aberrant duct and its anatomic relationships.[2,4-6,15-17,19]

MRI

MRI demonstrates soft tissue encircling the duodenum (Fig. 74-10). It is connected to the head of the pancreas, with which it shares the same density and signal intensity, both at the baseline examination and after administration of a contrast agent, unless pancreatitis or other diseases have occurred.

MRCP can demonstrate the aberrant duct encircling the duodenum and the extrinsic stenosis of the second portion of the duodenum.[4-6,15-17,19]

Ultrasonography

Ultrasonography can demonstrate a soft tissue mass, isoechoic to the pancreas, circumscribing the duodenum. Usually this anatomic variant is misinterpreted as an upper abdominal neoplasm. Cross-sectional imaging is the next step to better characterize the lesion.[4-6,15-17,19]

PET/CT

PET/CT may be useful in the case of annular pancreas misinterpreted as a neoplasm. PET/CT, combining the functional and imaging capabilities of both PET and MDCT technologies, reveals absence of uptake of fluorodeoxyglucose (FDG), similar density and contrast enhancement as remaining pancreas, and continuity with the pancreas. Therefore, diagnosis of annular pancreas is easily undertaken.

Imaging Algorithm

In adulthood, annular pancreas must be differentiated from pancreatic or duodenal cancer. The diagnosis may be difficult in the case of associated inflammation. In this case, visualization of an aberrant annular duct encircling the duodenum, at MDCT-3D pancreatography or MRCP or ERCP, is fundamental.

Otherwise, demonstration of annular tissue in continuity with the head of pancreas, with which it shares the same tissue characteristics, both on baseline images and after contrast agent administration, allows the diagnosis to be determined (see Table 74-2).[2,4-6,15-17,19]

Classic Signs: Annular Pancreas

- Soft tissue encircling the duodenum
- Continuity with head of pancreas
- Homogeneity
- Same echogenicity, density, signal intensity, and enhancement features as pancreatic parenchyma
- No vessel encasement
- No infiltration into surrounding structures

Agenesis of the Dorsal Pancreas

Agenesis of the pancreas can be complete, and not compatible with life, or restricted to the ventral or dorsal pancreas, with the latter relatively more common. Both

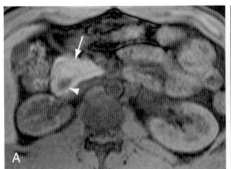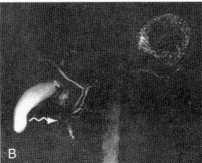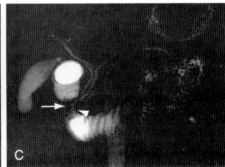

■ FIGURE 74-10 Axial T1W fat-saturated MR image (**A**), 2D MRCP (**B**), and 3D MRCP (**C**) demonstrate an annular pancreas (*arrow*) completely encircling the second portion of the duodenum (*arrowhead*) in **A** and **C**. An aberrant duct draining the annular pancreas (*wavy arrow*) and encircling the duodenum, which is stenosed, can be seen on the MRCP in **B**. (*Courtesy of Professor R. Manfredi, University of Verona, Italy.*)

the ventral and dorsal pancreatic agenesis can be complete or partial.

In the complete form of agenesis of the dorsal pancreas, the body, tail, and dorsal duct system, including the minor papilla and the accessory duct, are completely absent. In the partial form, which is relatively more common, the distal part of the pancreatic body or a remnant of the accessory duct and the minor papilla are present (Fig. 74-11).

Dorsal pancreatic agenesis is usually associated with other congenital anomalies, the most common being polysplenia, lobulation of the liver, and intestinal malrotation.

Dorsal pancreatic agenesis can be completely asymptomatic or associated with recurrent pancreatitis, diabetes, and exocrine pancreatic insufficiency.[2,4-6,20-25]

Radiography

Although conventional radiography does not play any role in imaging this entity, other congenital anomalies, such as malrotation, can be detected. ERCP may disclose a pancreatic duct shorter than normal, with preserved side branching.[4-6,20-25]

CT

MDCT displays a pancreas shorter than normal, with homogeneous density and without vessel encasement and infiltration into surrounding structures (Figs. 74-11 and 74-12). No peripancreatic halo nor any loss of lobulations is found.[4-6,20-25]

MRI

In complete dorsal pancreatic agenesis only the head of the pancreas is visible; and although it may appear rounded and enlarged, it retains the normal pancreatic lobulation pattern. Parenchymal signal intensity is homogeneous at baseline and after contrast agent administration. On MRCP the pancreatic duct is short and present in the head of the organ only. The dorsal pancreatic duct and the accessory

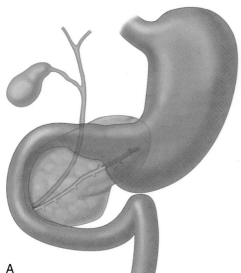

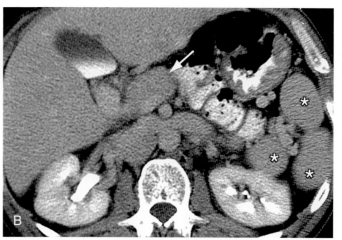

■ **FIGURE 74-11** **A,** Drawing of agenesis of the dorsal pancreas. **B,** Axial MDCT image demonstrates the short and rounded pancreas (*arrow*), with preserved lobulation. Polysplenia (*asterisks*) is one of the developmental anomalies associated with this condition.

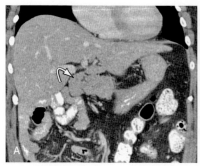

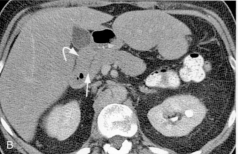

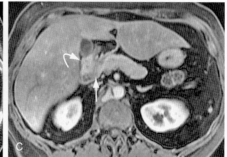

■ **FIGURE 74-12** Partial dorsal pancreatic agenesis. Coronal (**A**) and axial MDCT (**B**) images and postcontrast T1W MR image (**C**) demonstrate a shortened and truncated pancreas. The short pancreas circumscribes the first portion of the duodenum (*straight arrow*), like in the case of an annular pancreas. Note the same lobulation and signal intensity of the annulus (*curved arrow*) as the remaining pancreas.

duct are absent. In the case of a partial dorsal agenesis, at least part of the accessory duct and the neck of the organ are visualized (see Fig. 74-12).[4-6,20-25]

Ultrasonography

Ultrasonography can disclose a shorter than normal pancreas, devoid of any alteration in its echogenicity. Associated polysplenia can be demonstrated.[4-6,20-25]

PET/CT

PET/CT is usually not indicated in the evaluation of this anomaly. In case it is performed, normal FDG uptake is observed.

Imaging Algorithm

Many causes of reduction in size of the pancreas enter in the differential diagnosis with agenesis of the dorsal pancreas. These include autoimmune pancreatitis, chronic dorsal pancreatitis in a pancreas divisum, pancreatitis of the pancreatic body, pancreatic cancer with upstream atrophy of the organ, and normal age-related decrease in the size of the pancreas. Demonstration of a normal pancreatic duct at MRCP rules out agenesis of the dorsal pancreas. In this setting each of the other possible diagnoses need to be evaluated.

Agenesis of the dorsal pancreas is often associated with other congenital anomalies; polysplenia is one of the most common (see Figs. 74-11 and 74-12).[4-6,20-25]

Classic Signs: Agenesis of the Dorsal Pancreas

- Shorter than normal pancreas, usually rounded
- Preserved lobulations
- Homogeneous structure, with preserved echogenicity, density, signal intensity and contrast enhancement features
- No peripancreatic halo
- Associated congenital anomalies, most commonly polysplenia

Pancreatic Head Lobulations and Focal Enlargements of the Pancreas

Discrete lobulations of the head of the pancreas, greater than 1 cm, have been reported in 35% of the general population. They are composed of normal pancreatic tissue, which causes a contour deformity of the organ.

According to their relationships to the gastroduodenal or pancreatic duodenal artery, pancreatic head lobulations are usually classified into three types: in type 1 the lobulation is directed anteriorly to the artery; in type 2 it is oriented posteriorly; and in type 3 it is directed horizontally and laterally (Fig. 74-13). Other forms of focal pancreatic enlargements, composed of normal pancreatic tissue, are frequently reported in the body or tail. They may deform the contour of the organ and focally enlarge the gland (Fig. 74-14).

These lobulations are not responsible for any clinical symptoms but can be misinterpreted as a pancreatic neoplasm.[4-6,26]

Radiography

There is no role for conventional radiography and even for ERCP in these variants.

CT

Both at the baseline study and after contrast agent administration, pancreatic head lobulations and focal pancreatic enlargements in the body and tail of the organ share the same density as the remaining normal pancreas.

There is no infiltration into the surrounding structures, no bile duct dilatation, and no vascular encasement. Margins are well defined (see Figs. 74-13 and 74-14).[4-6,26]

MRI

On MRI, pancreatic head lobulations and focal pancreatic enlargements in the body and tail present the same signal intensity as remaining normal pancreas (see Fig. 74-14). Vessel encasement, infiltration, and inhomogeneity are lacking.[4-6,26]

Ultrasonography

Pancreatic head lobulations and focal pancreatic enlargements in the body and tail may not be detected on ultrasound imaging or may present as contour abnormalities, which usually require cross-sectional imaging to be characterized.

PET/CT

PET/CT can be useful in selected cases, when the differential diagnosis of pancreatic head lobulation or focal pancreatic enlargements in the body and tail versus neoplasm of the pancreatic head has not been achieved with other imaging modalities. Lack of FDG uptake is a reassuring criterion favoring the benign nature of focal pancreatic enlargements.

Imaging Algorithm

Pancreatic head lobulations and focal pancreatic enlargements in the body and tail can be distinguished from pancreatic neoplasms if the previously described diagnostic criteria are satisfied.[4-6,26]

Classic Signs: Pancreatic Head Lobulations and Focal Enlargements of the Pancreas

- Focal lobulation of the head of pancreas
- Focal pancreatic enlargements in the body and tail
- Same echogenicity, density, signal intensity, and contrast enhancement features as remaining normal pancreas
- No vessel encasement and no infiltration into surrounding structures

---

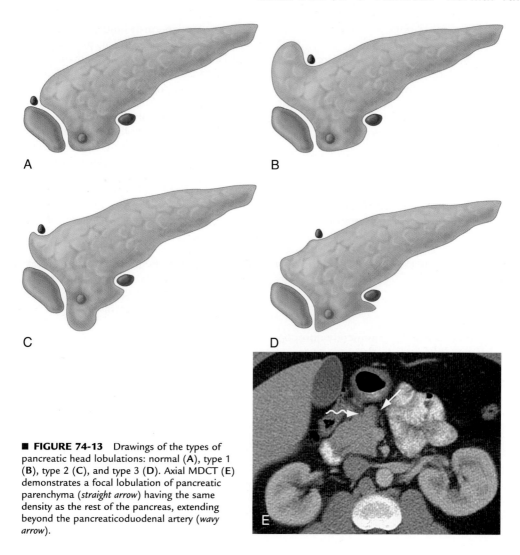

■ **FIGURE 74-13** Drawings of the types of pancreatic head lobulations: normal (**A**), type 1 (**B**), type 2 (**C**), and type 3 (**D**). Axial MDCT (**E**) demonstrates a focal lobulation of pancreatic parenchyma (*straight arrow*) having the same density as the rest of the pancreas, extending beyond the pancreaticoduodenal artery (*wavy arrow*).

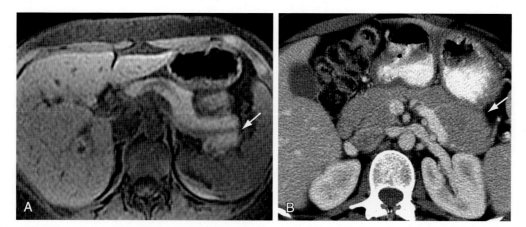

■ **FIGURE 74-14** T1W fat-saturated MR image (**A**) and MDCT image (**B**) of two different patients show focal enlargement of the pancreas causing contour abnormality (*arrows*). Preserved lobulation, structural homogeneity, attenuation and signal intensity values similar to the remaining pancreas, and absence of infiltration and vessel encasement are important clues to correctly identify these morphologic abnormalities as variants.

Ectopic Pancreas

Ectopic pancreatic tissue may be found in different sites along the gastrointestinal tract, most commonly in the proximal tract and in Meckel's diverticulum. Secretion of pancreatic enzymes may cause local inflammation and, therefore, clinical symptoms.[22]

Radiography

Ectopic pancreas has been described from upper gastro-intestinal series as a small, sharply marginated, round or oval, broad-based submucosal mass lesion that is difficult to differentiate from other submucosal lesions on imaging. Although central umbilication of ectopic pancreas has sometimes been described as a useful diagnostic feature on barium studies, radiography does not play any role in imaging of this entity.[22]

CT

On MDCT, ectopic pancreas may be completely unrecognized if small and if not inflamed. In the case of larger lesions and/or of associated inflammatory changes, ectopic pancreas may present as a solid mass lesion or as an area of inflammation. Usually, MDCT is unable to reach a specific diagnosis.[22]

MRI

This entity is difficult to characterize even on MRI. Large or inflamed lesions may be appreciated, but an etiologic diagnosis is usually difficult to achieve. Spontaneous hyperintensity of T1-weighted (T1W) fat-saturated images may be a suggestive, although not pathognomonic, clue.

PET/CT

Although PET/CT may not be able to help reach an etiologic diagnosis of ectopic pancreas, it may be useful in the imaging evaluation of this process. Lack of FDG uptake in the lesion is a useful supportive finding of benignity.

Imaging Algorithm

Diagnostic imaging is usually unable to detect small or noninflamed lesions and is unable to characterize larger lesions.

Although spontaneous hyperintensity on T1W fat-saturated images may be a clue to the proper diagnosis, many different pathologic processes, other than ectopic pancreatic tissue, may present as the same features. Therefore, surgical exploration is usually indicated to rule out malignancy and treat the patient's symptoms.

Uneven Pancreatic Lipomatosis

Uneven pancreatic lipomatosis does not constitute a congenital anomaly of the pancreas but is a histologic variant, which sometimes can be misinterpreted as a neoplasm. It represents the most common histologic change of the pancreas. Usually it is age related, involves the whole organ homogeneously, and gives rise to a reduction in the size of the pancreas and to an increased evidence of its lobulations. Cystic fibrosis or diabetes may be associated with increased fatty replacement. When the fatty replacement is focal, or unevenly distributed throughout the organ, it is named uneven pancreatic lipomatosis. Usually the peribiliary region is spared.

Uneven pancreatic lipomatosis is divided into four different subtypes, according to the affected area: in type 1 the uncinate process is spared; in type 2 the uncinate process is involved. In the subtype a, the head only is involved; in the subtype b, the body and tail are also affected (Fig. 74-15).[4,27]

Radiography

Conventional radiography does not play any role in this entity. ERCP may be useful in selected cases, disclosing a normally branched main pancreatic duct, without amputation, and of preserved length.[4,27]

CT

MDCT appearance of uneven pancreatic lipomatosis varies according to the extent of fatty infiltration. Fatty areas present hypodense relative to uninvolved pancreas both at baseline and contrast enhanced studies, with negative Hounsfield unit values. Pancreatic contour is preserved, although it may be difficult to see in the case of marked lipomatosis in which lipomatous pancreas exhibits the same attenuation values as surrounding retroperitoneal fat (see Fig. 74-15). In the case of extreme lipomatosis, the pancreas may not even be appreciable at MDCT.[4,27]

MRI

The pancreas appears of inhomogeneous signal intensity and preserved shape on MRI. In the case of extensive fatty infiltration it may even be difficult to detect because of the similarity in signal intensity with retroperitoneal fat tissue.

The fatty nature of the pancreatic inhomogeneity is readily diagnosed owing to the higher signal on T1W in-phase imaging and lower signal on T1W out-of-phase imaging and T1W/T2-weighted (T2W) fat-saturated images. The main pancreatic duct is normal in caliber and length.[4,27]

Ultrasonography

On ultrasonography, in the case of uneven pancreatic lipomatosis normal pancreatic areas appear hypoechoic when compared with fatty hyperechoic areas, therefore simulating a neoplastic process.

PET/CT

Although PET/CT is usually not required to make the diagnosis of uneven pancreatic lipomatosis, in selected cases, owing to absent FDG uptake, it can further corroborate the diagnosis of benignity.

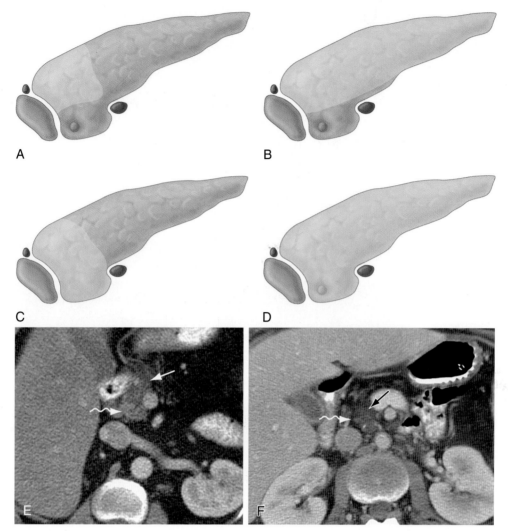

■ **FIGURE 74-15** Drawings illustrate different types of uneven pancreatic lipomatosis: types 1a (**A**), 1b (**B**), 2a (**C**), 2b (**D**). Axial MDCT images (**E** and **F**) show uneven fatty infiltration of the pancreas (*straight arrow*) with sparing of the peribiliary region (*wavy arrow*).

Imaging Algorithm

The differential diagnosis is with dorsal pancreatic agenesis in the case of type 1b and with complete pancreatic agenesis in the case of type 2b. Sometimes a pancreatic mass enters in the differential diagnosis. Important clues, which allow the correct diagnosis of uneven pancreatic lipomatosis to be undertaken, are sparing of the peribiliary region and a normally developed pancreatic duct at MRCP.

Differential diagnosis with complete pancreatic agenesis is not required in humans because it is not compatible with life and represents an autopsy finding in fetuses.[4,27]

Classic Signs: Uneven Pancreatic Lipomatosis

- Focal areas of fatty replacement similar to retroperitoneal fat
- Preserved main pancreatic duct caliber and length
- No infiltration or vascular encasement

Miscellaneous Variants

Many peripancreatic anatomic variants may be misinterpreted as pancreatic lesions, sometimes prompting unnecessary laparotomies. They mainly include duodenal diverticula, gastrointestinal duplication cysts, and accessory spleens. These entities are described more accurately in the pertinent chapters, to which the reader is referred.

Radiography

Conventional radiography may play a role in the case of duodenal diverticula, displaying an air-fluid level in the peripancreatic region. Upper gastrointestinal series may be particularly useful by showing barium filling the diverticulum, a pathognomonic finding (Fig. 74-16).[28-30]

CT

MDCT with multiplanar reconstructions displays the epicenter of the lesion to be outside the pancreas both for duodenal diverticula and gastrointestinal duplication

■ **FIGURE 74-16** A, Drawing of a duodenal diverticula. Upper gastrointestinal series (**B**), coronal T2W MR image (**C**), and contrast-enhanced axial T1W fat-saturated MR image (**D**) show a focal outpouching from the medial aspect of the second part of the duodenum. Duodenal diverticula (*arrow*) may be misinterpreted as pancreatic lesions. Epicenter outside the pancreas, continuity with the duodenum, and air-fluid level are important findings to reach the correct diagnosis.

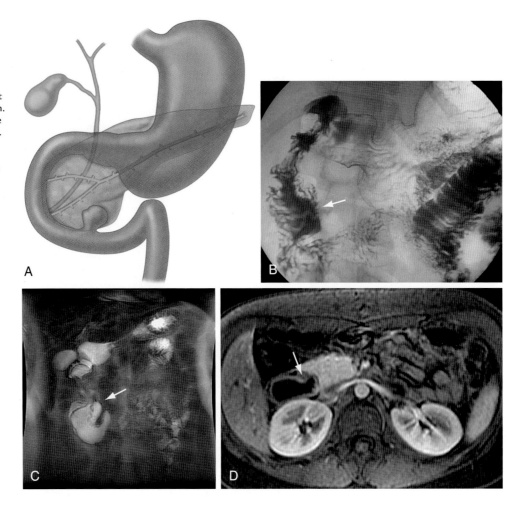

cysts. In the case of duodenal diverticula, air-fluid levels, an enhancement pattern paralleling that of the duodenal wall, and direct continuity with the duodenal wall are important findings. In the case of gastrointestinal duplication cysts, lack of enhancement and closeness to the gastrointestinal tract of origin are supportive imaging criteria. In the case of accessory spleens, the mass is round or ovoid and well circumscribed and the enhancement pattern parallels that of the spleen. All these pseudolesions do not infiltrate or cause vascular encasement.[28-30]

MRI

MRI features of duodenal diverticula, duplication cysts, and accessory spleens are similar to those found on MDCT, with the added value of the better tissue characterization, provided by a combination of different MRI sequences and of the superior contrast resolution of MRI (see Fig. 74-16). For example, duplication cysts may present low in signal intensity on both T1W and T2W sequences and clearly lack contrast enhancement (Fig. 74-17).

Ultrasonography

On ultrasonography, an air-fluid level within the peripancreatic lesion may suggest the diagnosis of duodenal diver-

ticulum. Although the cystic nature of gastrointestinal duplication cysts can be achieved by ultrasonography, this is not an easy task. Accessory spleens can be correctly diagnosed because of their closeness to the splenic hilum, round or ovoid shape, well-defined margins, and stability over time.

Nuclear Medicine

Nuclear medicine is not useful in the case of duodenal diverticulum or duplication cysts. Rarely it may play a role in the case of accessory spleens.

PET/CT

Although PET/CT is usually not required to make the correct diagnosis of these entities, in selected cases, owing to absent FDG uptake, it can further confirm their benign nature.

Imaging Algorithm

The differential diagnosis is mainly with cystic and solid pancreatic neoplasms. To achieve the correct diagnosis one should note if the epicenter of the lesion is located outside the pancreas, the continuity with the duodenum

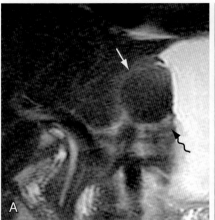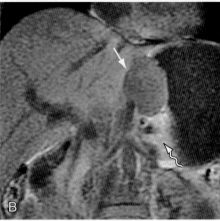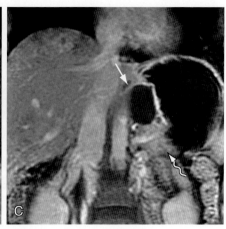

■ **FIGURE 74-17** Esophageal duplication cyst. Coronal T2W (**A**), T1W fat-saturated (**B**), and contrast-enhanced T1W fat-saturated (**C**) MR images. Duplication cysts may be confused with pancreatic cystic lesions. Epicenter of the lesion outside the pancreas (*wavy arrow*), low signal intensity on both T1W and T2W images, and absence of contrast enhancement are important features to exclude their pancreatic origin and suspect the proper diagnosis, as in this case of esophageal duplication cyst (*straight arrow*).

Classic Signs: Miscellaneous Variants

- Continuity or closeness with the organ of origin
- Contrast enhancement paralleling the organ of origin, in the case of duodenal diverticula and accessory spleens
- Filling with oral contrast material, in the case of duodenal diverticula
- No infiltration or vascular encasement

(in the case of diverticula), and the closeness to the gastrointestinal tract and spleen (in the case of duplication cysts and accessory spleens, respectively). Additionally, do the contrast imaging features parallel those of the organ of origin (in the case of duodenal diverticula and accessory spleens) and is there the presence of air-fluid levels or of filling with oral contrast material (in the case of duodenal diverticula)?

What the Referring Physician Needs to Know

- Congenital anomalies of the pancreas, although usually detected in childhood, may also present in adulthood.
- Pancreas divisum and annular pancreas may be symptomatic; others are usually asymptomatic.
- Differential diagnosis includes hepatic neoplasms and autoimmune pancreatitis (dorsal pancreatic agenesis).

KEY POINTS

- Although congenital anomalies may simulate mass lesions, their baseline and contrast enhancement features are similar to those of normal pancreas.
- There is no inhomogeneity.
- There is no vascular encasement or infiltration.
- No stenosis or dilatation of the main pancreatic duct is seen.
- Other developmental abnormalities may be associated.

SUGGESTED READINGS

Kamisawa T, Tu Y, Egawa N, et al. MRCP of congenital pancreaticobiliary malformation. Abdom Imaging 2006; Sep 12 [Epub ahead of print].

Mortele KJ, Rocha TC, Streeter JL, Taylor AJ. Multimodality imaging of pancreatic and biliary congenital anomalies. RadioGraphics 2006; 26:715-731.

Yu J, Turner MA, Fulcher AS, Halvorsen RA. Congenital anomalies and normal variants of the pancreaticobiliary tract and the pancreas in adults: II. Pancreatic duct and pancreas. AJR Am J Roentgenol 2006; 187:1544-1553.

REFERENCES

1. Clemente D. The pancreas. In Clemente D (ed). Gray's Anatomy, 30th ed. Philadelphia, Williams & Wilkins, 1985, pp 1502-1507.
2. Larsen WJ. Development of the gastrointestinal tract. In Larsen WJ (ed). Human Embryology, 2nd ed. Philadelphia, Churchill Livingstone, 1997, pp 235-238.
3. Klein SD, Affronti JP. Pancreas divisum, an evidence-based review: I. Pathophysiology. Gastrointest Endosc 2004; 60:419-425.
4. Mortele KJ, Rocha TC, Streeter JL, Taylor AJ. Multimodality imaging of pancreatic and biliary congenital anomalies. RadioGraphics 2006; 26:715-731.
5. Rizzo RJ, Szucs RA, Turner MA. Congenital abnormalities of the pancreas and biliary tree in adults. RadioGraphics 1995; 15:49, 68; quiz 147-148.
6. Skandalakis JE, Skandalakis LJ, Colborn GL. Congenital anomalies and variations of the pancreas and the pancreatic extrahepatic bile ducts. In Beger HG, Warshaw AL, Buchler MW, et al (eds). The Pancreas. Oxford, UK, Blackwell Science, 1998, pp 27-55.
7. Kamisawa T, Tu Y, Egawa N, et al. MRCP of congenital pancreaticobiliary malformation. Abdom Imaging 2006; Sep 12 [Epub ahead of print].
8. Morgan DE, Logan K, Baron TH, et al. Pancreas divisum: implications for diagnostic and therapeutic pancreatography. AJR Am J Roentgenol 1999; 173:193-198.
9. Quest L, Lombard M. Pancreas divisum: opinio divisa. Gut 2000; 47:317-319.
10. Yu J, Turner MA, Fulcher AS, Halvorsen RA. Congenital anomalies and normal variants of the pancreaticobiliary tract and the pancreas in adults: II. Pancreatic duct and pancreas. AJR Am J Roentgenol 2006; 187:1544-1553.
11. Lowes JR, Lees WR, Cotton PB. Pancreatic duct dilatation after secretin stimulation in patients with pancreas divisum. Pancreas 1989; 4:371-374.
12. Matos C, Metens T, Deviere J, et al. Pancreas divisum: evaluation with secretin-enhanced magnetic resonance cholangiopancreatography. Gastrointest Endosc 2001; 53:728-733.
13. Soto JA, Lucey BC, Stuhlfaut JW. Pancreas divisum: depiction with multi-detector row CT. Radiology 2005; 235:503-508.
14. Davenport M, Howard ER. Acute pancreatitis associated with congenital anomalies. In Beger HG, Warshaw AL, Buchler MW, et al (eds). The Pancreas. Oxford, UK, Blackwell Science, 1998, pp 343-353.
15. Choi JY, Kim MJ, Kim JH, et al. Annular pancreas: emphasis on magnetic resonance cholangiopancreatography findings. J Comput Assist Tomogr 2004; 28:528-532.
16. Cunha JE, de Lima MS, Jukemura J, et al. Unusual clinical presentation of annular pancreas in the adult. Pancreatology 2005; 5:81-85.
17. Paraskevas G, Papaziogas B, Lazaridis C, et al. Annular pancreas in adults: embryological development, morphology and clinical significance. Surg Radiol Anat 2001; 23:437-442.
18. Lieber A, Schaefer JW, Belin RP. Hypotonic duodenography: diagnosis of annular pancreas in an adult. JAMA 1968; 203:425.
19. Ueki T, Yao T, Beppu T, et al. Three-dimensional computed tomography pancreatography of an annular pancreas with special reference to embryogenesis. Pancreas 2006; 32:426-429.
20. Lingareddy S, Duvvuru NR, Guduru VR, et al. Dorsal agenesis of pancreas: CT and ERCP. Gastrointest Endosc 2007; 65:157-158; discussion 158.
21. Schnedl WJ, Reisinger EC, Schreiber F, et al. Complete and partial agenesis of the dorsal pancreas within one family. Gastrointest Endosc 1995; 42:485-487.
22. Haaga JR, Lanzieri CF, Gilkeson RC. The pancreas. In Haaga JR (ed). Computed Tomography and Magnetic Resonance Imaging of the Whole Body, 4th ed. Philadelphia, Elsevier, 2003, pp 1395-1485.
23. Sempere L, Aparicio JR, Martinez J, et al. Role of endoscopic ultrasound in the diagnosis of agenesis of the dorsal pancreas. JOP 2006; 7:411-416.
24. Fukuoka K, Ajiki T, Yamamoto M, et al. Complete agenesis of the dorsal pancreas. J Hepatobiliary Pancreat Surg 1999; 6:94-97.
25. Du J, Xu GQ, Xu P, et al. Congenital short pancreas. Chin Med J (Engl) 2007; 120:259-262.
26. Ross BA, Jeffrey RB Jr, Mindelzun RE. Normal variations in the lateral contour of the head and neck of the pancreas mimicking neoplasm: evaluation with dual-phase helical CT. AJR Am J Roentgenol 1996; 166:799-801.
27. Matsumoto S, Mori H, Miyake H, et al. Uneven fatty replacement of the pancreas: evaluation with CT. Radiology 1995; 194:453-458.
28. Eisenberg RL, Levine MS. Miscellaneous abnormalities of the stomach and duodenum. In Gore RM, Levine SL (eds). Textbook of Gastrointestinal Radiology, 3rd ed. Philadelphia, WB Saunders, 2008, pp 679-706.
29. Macari M, Lazarus D, Israel G, Megibow A. Duodenal diverticula mimicking cystic neoplasms of the pancreas: CT and MR imaging findings in seven patients. AJR Am J Roentgenol 2003; 180: 195-199.
30. Mortelé KJ, Mortelé B, Silverman SG. CT features of the accessory spleen. AJR Am J Roentgenol 2004; 183:1653-1657. Erratum in AJR Am J Roentgenol 2005; 184:348.

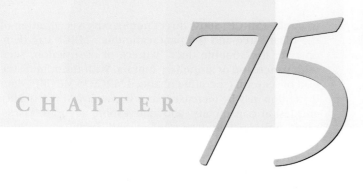
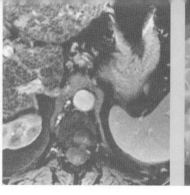
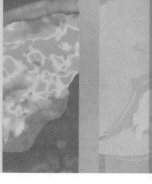

Solid Pancreatic Masses

Onofrio Catalano and Dushyant V. Sahani

ETIOLOGY

The term *solid pancreatic masses,* in its wide meaning, encompasses neoplastic lesions and non-neoplastic masses, ranging from anatomic variants, such as pancreatic head lobulations, to focal inflammatory processes and neoplasms. In this chapter we will mainly discuss solid pancreatic neoplasms and we will provide differential diagnoses with other solid lesions, such as variants and focal inflammatory lesions, which are described in detail in other chapters.

The etiology of pancreatic neoplasms varies accordingly to their specific histotype and will be discussed in each subsection. Most pancreatic neoplasms occur sporadically, but some are genetically transmitted, and different genes are involved. Usually both environmental factors, such as cigarette smoking and dye exposure, and genetic factors are implicated in a multistep process of progressive genetic deregulation and increased biologic aggressiveness, which can lead to the onset of malignant lesions.[1-3]

PREVALENCE AND EPIDEMIOLOGY

Statistical data regarding the prevalence and incidence of all benign and malignant neoplasms of the pancreas are not available in the literature. Statistical data for invasive pancreatic cancer, derived from the Surveillance Epidemiology and End Results of the National Cancer Institute (http://seer.cancer.gov) show an estimated prevalence percent of 0.008% for all ages, an estimated prevalence percent of 0.041% in the age range 70 to 79 years, and an overall incidence of 11.4 per 100,000 persons. The most commonly encountered solid tumors of the pancreas are represented by adenocarcinomas, endocrine tumors, metastases, and lymphomas. Other tumors, which occur less often, include acinar cell tumors, pancreatoblastomas, and lipomas.[1-3]

CLINICAL PRESENTATION

Clinical presentation of pancreatic solid lesions is extremely variable and mainly depends on histotype, location, and size of the lesion.

Unless the neoplasm is responsible for hormone overproduction, resulting in specific clinical symptoms at an early stage, the first symptoms of pancreatic neoplasms are often too vague to be considered. Therefore, the majority of patients seek medical attention late in the course of the disease when abdominal pain, jaundice, and weight loss result.[1-4]

PATHOPHYSIOLOGY

Pancreatic neoplasms tend to affect every region of the pancreas but, owing to the higher amount of pancreatic tissue in the head of the organ, this is where tumors tend to occur more often. The site of occurrence may also be influenced by the specific histotype.[1-3]

PATHOLOGY

The pathology is extremely variable from one neoplasm to another, and on its basis the different lesions are differentiated and classified.[1-3]

IMAGING

The imaging techniques for evaluation of solid masses in the pancreas include ultrasonography, contrast-enhanced multidetector CT (MDCT), MRI, combined PET/CT, endoscopic cholangiopancreatography (ERCP), and endoscopic ultrasonography (EUS). Diagnostic imaging of pancreatic solid lesions is aimed at (1) confirming or excluding the presence of a pancreatic mass; (2) differentiating a benign from a malignant lesion and narrowing the differential diagnosis; (3) staging the neoplastic process, in case it is malignant, and providing a road map for surgery, in case the tumor is considered resectable; and (4) assisting in follow-up of patients after medical and/or surgical treatment.[1,3,4]

Radiography

Because of the poor soft tissue resolution, poor sensitivity, and low specificity of conventional and digital radiography, solid lesions of the pancreas are usually not detected by radiographic studies, unless late in their course, when they are responsible for widening of the duodenal loop; compression, displacement, and infiltration of surrounding structures; or gastrointestinal obstruction. Cross-sectional imaging is far more sensitive and specific than conventional radiographic studies. Therefore, nowadays, conventional radiography does not play any role in diagnosing solid lesions of the pancreas.

CT

MDCT allows the pancreas to be imaged at a high spatial and temporal resolution, within a single breath-hold, with thin-slice collimation and multiphasic imaging. Contrast enhancement time is crucial in tumor detection, and when possible it should be planned in accordance with the suspected type of lesion. Usually, pancreatic tumor detection is suboptimal during the arterial phase of enhancement owing to low tumor-to-pancreas contrast difference, but in the case of a suspected endocrine neoplasm or renal/breast cancer metastases to the pancreas the arterial phase may be the only one in which one is able to detect and characterize the lesion. In the case of adenocarcinoma, a dual-phase pancreatic protocol MDCT is considered sensitive for detection and staging of the primary cancer and for evaluation of metastases to the liver and peritoneum (see Chapter 73).[4,5]

MRI

MRI is usually used as a second-line imaging modality in patients with a high clinical suspicion for a pancreatic tumor or in those with a suspected pancreatic mass and indeterminant finding on high-quality MDCT. MRI, owing to its inherent high soft tissue contrast and resolution, can improve detection of subtle pancreatic lesions even when they are small and do not deform the organ. MRI, through T2-weighted (T2W) and gadolinium-enhanced T1-weighted (T1W) sequences, performs better than MDCT in the detection and characterization of liver metastases and peritoneal implants, especially in the setting of the smallest lesions. Regional vascular anatomy can be mapped by 3D contrast-enhanced dynamic MR angiography and reconstructions to assess for vascular involvement. If mangafodipir trisodium is administered, it is taken up by the normal pancreatic parenchyma, which is enhanced on T1W images, in comparison with the relative lack of enhancement of pancreatic masses whose conspicuity is therefore increased. The sensitivity of mangafodipir trisodium–enhanced MRI for detection of pancreatic cancer may reach 100%. Both 2D and 3D MR cholangiopancrea-tography (MRCP) allow direct noninvasive visualization of the biliary tree and the pancreatic duct. MRCP can demonstrate the "double duct" pattern of obstruction, seen with pancreatic or ampullary tumors. With the administration of secretin (secretin-enhanced MRCP [S-MRCP]), duct distention may be increased, thus improving MRCP quality and lesion conspicuity, allowing a more accurate assessment of pancreatic duct stenosis, and potentially helping to differentiate benign from malignant strictures (see Chapter 73).[4-9]

Ultrasonography

Transabdominal ultrasonography is a relatively inexpensive, noninvasive, and widely available modality often used as a first-line diagnostic imaging tool for disorders of the abdomen, but it is highly operator dependent, nonreproducible, and limited by abdominal gas and patient body habitus.

EUS, on the other hand, is an expensive technique, not available in every center, and requires highly specialized personnel. It provides high-resolution images of the pancreas and allows lesion biopsy.[4-9]

Nuclear Medicine

Nuclear medicine plays a role only (1) in the case of functional endocrine tumors when, using a specific radiopharmaceutical, it can allow the diagnosis to be undertaken and (2) in the study of suspected bony metastases. Otherwise it has no current application in the diagnosis of solid pancreatic neoplasms.

PET/CT

Although MDCT is characterized by high spatial resolution, differentiating benign from malignant processes is often challenging, mainly in the case of small lesions. On the other hand, fluorodeoxyglucose (FDG)-labeled PET has a high accuracy in discriminating benign from malignant lesions but its spatial resolution is limited, compromising precise anatomic localization. PET/CT integrates morphologic and functional data in a single test, overcoming some of these limitations.

Normal pancreatic tissue does not show avid FDG uptake on PET, and therefore a region of increased uptake in the pancreas is considered abnormal.

PET/CT may be useful in the case of small lesions (<1 cm), which are frequently missed with nonfunctional imaging, and of early tumor recurrence. Because FDG accumulation does not depend on tumor size, cancer can be detected even in normal-sized lymph nodes. However, false-negative PET findings can be observed, mostly in patients with insulin-dependent diabetes mellitus; meanwhile, false-positive PET findings can occur in inflammatory benign lesions. New tumor-specific radioisotopes, such as σ-receptor ligands and ^{18}F-FLT (fluorothymidine), are being used to improve specificity and sensitivity for the detection of primary and metastatic tumors, mainly adenocarcinomas. ^{11}C-labeled L-dopa and ^{11}C-labeled 5-hydroxytryptophan are more sensitive and specific radioligands in the setting of functional endocrine pancreatic tumors, but they are less sensitive in detection of nonfunctional neoplasms.[4-9]

Imaging Algorithm

The most used diagnostic imaging techniques for solid neoplasms of the pancreas are MDCT and MRCP, which provide high spatial and contrast resolution images and allow dynamic acquisition and postprocessing image reconstruction. Lesion morphology, epicenter location, relationships with the pancreatic duct, and ancillary findings can be evaluated, providing clues for diagnosis, management planning, and preoperative strategy.

MDCT and MRI have been demonstrated to be nearly equally accurate in establishing the diagnosis of malignancy, in characterizing pancreatic lesions, and in their staging.

Through MRCP and MDCT images and reconstructions, the entire course of the main pancreatic duct (MPD) can be displayed and its relationships with the lesion can be evaluated. In case the patient is considered a surgical candidate, multiplanar image reconstructions, displaying the extent of the lesions and their anatomic relationships to surrounding structures, can be useful.

The role of PET/CT is still under investigation.

An ideal algorithm is summarized in Figure 75-1.[4-9] The different types of solid lesions of the pancreas will be described in the corresponding sections; the most important features are summarized in Table 75-1.

DIFFERENTIAL DIAGNOSIS

Differential diagnosis of solid pancreatic masses is aimed to differentiate benign masses, including anatomic variants, from malignant lesions and to try to characterize the histotype. It relies on a combination of clinical, laboratory, and imaging findings and, in most cases, on information derived from tissue biopsy.

Important clinical factors include age, sex, weight loss, recent onset of diabetes, abdominal pain, jaundice, bloating, gastrointestinal obstruction, thrombophlebitis migrans, diarrhea, depression, history of smoking and of exposure to carcinogenic agents, and family and/or personal history of breast, pancreatic, and endocrine neoplasms and of Peutz-Jaegers syndrome and nonpolyposis familial colon cancer syndrome.

Many laboratory findings and tumor serum markers are available. They include specific hormones, which are overproduced in the case of functional endocrine tumors, or oncologic markers, such as CA 19-9, which is one of the most useful for the diagnosis of adenocarcinoma of the pancreas.[1-4]

Many anatomic variants and pseudolesions may be confused with pancreatic neoplasms. Their differential diagnosis is described in the corresponding sections. Alteration in pancreatic contour, lobulations, and changes in the course and size of the MPD, as well as epicenter, margin, and contrast enhancement characteristics of the lesions are some of the most important imaging features to take into account in the approach to management of pancreatic masses.[4]

TREATMENT

Medical Treatment

Medical treatment differs according to the type of cancer and its stage. Its goals are to treat the neoplasm, to palliate the patient in the case of untreatable tumors, and to improve the quality of life.

Patients who are not fit for surgery usually undergo radiation therapy and/or chemotherapy. Patients with distant metastases are considered ineligible for radiation treatment and undergo chemotherapy alone.[2]

Surgical Treatment

Although complete surgical resection remains the best curative treatment for many tumors, including pancreatic adenocarcinoma, currently only a small percentage of patients are recommended for surgical resection, and the small tumors that can undergo curative surgery are the most difficult to detect. The treatment approach is based on tumor histotype, location in the pancreas (e.g., head versus tail), and whether the tumor is resectable or nonresectable at presentation.

Usually, tumors of the pancreatic head are treated with the Whipple procedure, which includes cephalopancreatectomy and duodenectomy, whereas body and tail tumors are treated with distal pancreatectomy and splenectomy.[2]

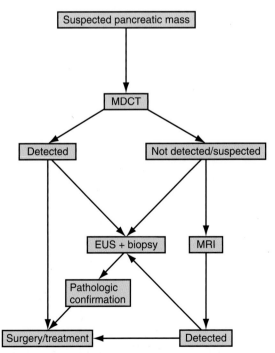

■ **FIGURE 75-1** Diagnostic imaging algorithm for solid pancreatic masses. MDCT, multidetector CT; EUS, endoscopic ultrasonography.

TABLE 75-1 Clinical and Radiologic Features of Solid Neoplasms in the Pancreas

	Sex	Age	Location	Size	Shape/Borders	Ca²⁺	Enhancement	MPD	Peculiar Features	Clinical History
Adenocarcinoma	M > F	7th-8th decades	Head (75%)	Usually <5 cm, mean size 3 cm head location, 5 cm body-tail	Infiltrating	Rare	Poor	Stenosed or obstructed, upstream dilatation	Usually advanced even when small in size	Abdominal pain radiating to the back Jaundice Weight loss
Pancreatic endocrine neoplasm	M = F	5th-6th decades	Tail (60%)	>5 cm, unless functional	Well defined/infiltrating	22%	Intense, early	Usually normal	Strongly enhancing lesions	Endocrinology syndromes may be found. Serum chromogranin A elevated in 70%
Metastases	M = F	6th decade	Head	Usually <5 cm, mean size 4.6 cm	Well defined	Rare	Variable, same as that of the primary tumor	Usually normal	In the setting of widespread malignancy	Positive oncologic history
Lymphoma	M > F	4th-8th decades	Head (80%)	>5 cm, mean size 8 cm	Well defined	Rare	Mild, homogeneous	Usually normal	Lymph node enlargement below renal veins Large homogeneous mass without MPD abnormalities Diffuse enlargement of the gland with loss of its lobular structure	Nonspecific
Acinar cell carcinoma	F > M	7th decade	Head/uncinate (60%)	>5 cm, mean size 7 cm	Well defined	Common 50%	Mild, heterogeneous (cystic areas often coexist)	Usually normal	Mn-DPDP uptake	Serum lipase usually high Hyperlipasemia syndrome in 15%
Alcohol mass-forming pancreatitis	M > F	5th-6th decades	Head (70%)	N/A	Ill defined	Common	Homogeneous	Stenosed, obstructed, normal, dilated	Parenchymal and ductal calcifications	Acute pancreatitis-like pain, history of alcohol abuse
Autoimmune mass-forming pancreatitis	M > F	7th-8th decades	Head (55%)	<5 cm, mean size 3.8 cm	Well defined	Rare	Homogeneous, late enhancement	Usually stenosed	Homogeneous late enhancement Upstream MPD not dilated	IgG4, other autoimmune diseases, response to steroids

MPD, main pancreatic duct; N/A, not applicable.

What the Referring Physician Needs to Know: Pancreatic Masses

■ Solid lesions may be difficult to differentiate on morphology alone.

■ The most important questions in the approach to solid lesions in the pancreas involve differentiation of:
  ● Pseudolesions from true lesions
  ● Benign versus malignant lesions
  ● Adenocarcinomas from nonadenocarcinomas
  ● Resectable versus nonresectable neoplasms

KEY POINT

■ Diagnosis of pancreatic masses usually requires correlation of clinical, laboratory, imaging, and pathology data.

SPECIFIC LESIONS

Adenocarcinoma

Etiology

Both environmental and genetic factors are involved in a multistep process of progressive genetic deregulation and increased biologic aggressiveness, which can lead to the onset of malignant lesions.

Cigarette smoking, diets high in meat, and solvent exposure are among the most well-known environmental factors.

Different DNA alterations have been implicated in the onset of pancreatic adenocarcinomas. They cause inactivation of multiple anti-oncogenes (*CDKN2A, TP53, SMADH4*), activation of oncogenes (*KRAS, HERB2, BRAF*), and interference with DNA mismatch repair (*BRCA2*). Multiple mutations coexist in a single adenocarcinoma.[1,2]

Prevalence and Epidemiology

Pancreatic adenocarcinoma is an invasive malignant epithelial neoplasm with ductal differentiation and without predominance of other types of carcinomas. Its age-adjusted incidence rate is 11/100,000, and it constitutes more than 90% of the malignant tumors of the pancreas. Pancreatic adenocarcinoma is one of the most ominous malignancies: it represents the fifth leading cause of cancer death in Western countries, with a poor overall 5-year survival rate of only 4%, which is nearly equal to the incidence rate. Its peak incidence is in the 7th and 8th decades, and it is slightly more common in men (56%).[1-3]

Clinical Presentation

Clinical presentation varies according to the site of origin of the cancer and its stage, but many patients recall a history of long-standing abdominal pain, asthenia, reduced appetite, and weight loss. New-onset diabetes mellitus is present in 10% of cases. Painless jaundice is found in 75% at presentation, mostly resulting from cancers arising from the head of the organ. Tumors in the pancreatic body and tail tend to manifest as back pain related to tumor infiltration into the surrounding retroperitoneal structures and nerves. Because of its silent course, late clinical symptoms, and rapid growth, it has been named the "silent killer."[1-3]

Pathophysiology

About two thirds of pancreatic adenocarcinomas occur in the head of the pancreas; the remainder are found in the body (5% to 15%) or tail (10% to 15%) or diffusely infiltrate the organ (5% to 15%).[1,2]

Pathology

It is believed that pancreatic intraepithelial neoplasms (PanINs) may represent its precursors. Normal ductal cells progress to flat hyperplasia (PanIN type 1A), to ductal hyperplasia with pseudostratification (PanIN type 1B), to hyperplasia with atypia (PanIN type 2), and to carcinoma in situ (PanIN type 3). PanIN type 3 is associated with a high risk to evolve into invasive carcinoma.

Resected adenocarcinomas arising in the head of the pancreas, because of the earlier occurrence of clinical symptoms, tend to be smaller at resection (3 cm) than those in the body and tail (5 cm).

Pancreatic adenocarcinomas present as poorly defined, firm masses that may focally enlarge the organ and tend to blend with the remaining pancreatic parenchyma. Cystic changes rarely occur due to central necrosis or ductal obstruction with retention cyst formation. The disease is associated with an intense desmoplastic reaction, and, because of its ductal origin, it tends to obstruct the pancreatic duct, with subsequent upstream duct dilatation and associated chronic pancreatitis/parenchymal atrophy. If it arises in the pancreatic head, the common bile duct (CBD) can be stenosed with subsequent biliary tree dilatation.

Pancreatic adenocarcinomas tend to infiltrate early into the retroperitoneum, even when smaller than 2 cm, and invade into the surrounding anatomic structures, including nerves and vessels, which are stenosed and/or thrombosed, and to disseminate to the lymph nodes (mainly the superior head, pancreaticoduodenal, hepatoduodenal, perimesenteric, and para-aortic chains), liver, and peritoneum. Therefore, less than 10% to 20% of cancers are deemed surgically resectable, and many of them present in an advanced stage at pathology.[1,2]

Imaging

The diagnostic imaging approach to pancreatic adenocarcinoma depends on the clinical scenarios: (1) diagnostic imaging proof of the presence or absence of disease for patients with a suspicion of pancreatic cancer, (2) staging for patients with a known pancreatic adenocarcinoma, (3) follow-up of patients with treated adenocarcinoma of the pancreas, and (4) screening of patients at high risk for this tumor. The TNM classification for pancreatic cancer staging is presented in Table 75-2.[4]

CT

A dual-phase pancreatic protocol MDCT is a sensitive technique for both detection and staging of pancreatic adenocarcinoma. The pancreatic phase allows optimal tumor detection and mapping of the vascular structures; in this phase, the pancreatic adenocarcinoma appears as a low-density lesion compared with the normally enhancing pancreatic parenchyma (Figs. 75-2 and 75-3). In the portovenous phase, owing to contrast diffusion into the interstitial spaces of the tumor, its conspicuity may be reduced but the detection of metastases to the liver and peritoneum, as well as the visualization of portal venous structures, is improved. In about 10% of cases, pancreatic adenocarcinoma is not directly visualized, being isoattenuating during dynamic contrast imaging. In these cases, the diagnosis relies on indirect signs, such as focal or diffuse loss of pancreatic parenchyma lobulation, contour deformity, stenosis of the pancreatic duct with upstream ductal dilatation, parenchymal atrophy, stenosis of the distal CBD, and the "double duct" sign (stenosis of both the CBD and the pancreatic duct with subsequent upstream dilatation), which are also useful to support the diagnosis in the case of directly visualized adenocarcinomas (Figs. 75-4 to 75-6).

CT sensitivity in tumor detection inversely correlates with tumor size and is influenced by technology; it can be as low as 63% with single detector scanners and ranges from 88% to 99% with MDCT technology. The assessment of overall tumor resectability with MDCT is accurate, with a negative predictive value of 87%. MDCT is the modality with the highest accuracy in the assessment of vascular invasion. The likelihood of vascular infiltration by pancreatic adenocarcinoma increases as the tumor to vessel circumference contact increases, being less than 3% when the tumor to vessel circumference contact is less than 90 degrees, between 29% and 57% for a contact between 90 and 180 degrees, and more than 80% for a contact of more than 180 degrees. Other imaging criteria for vascular

TABLE 75-2   TNM Classification for Pancreatic Cancer Staging

Classification	Description
T (Tumor)	
Tx	Primary tumor not assessed
Tis	Carcinoma in situ
T1	Tumor is ≤2 cm in maximum diameter and confined to the pancreas
T2	Tumor is >2 cm and confined to the pancreas
T3	Tumor extends beyond the pancreas but does not involve celiac axis or superior mesenteric artery
T4	Tumor involves either celiac axis or superior mesenteric artery
N (Nodal Involvement)	
Nx	Regional lymph nodes not assessed
N0	No involvement of regional lymph nodes
N1	Involvement of regional lymph nodes
M (Metastases)	
Mx	Distant metastases not assessed
M0	No distant metastases
M1	Distant metastases

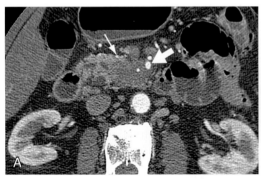
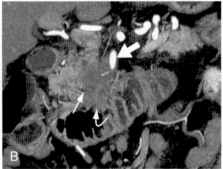

■ **FIGURE 75-2**   Locally invasive pancreatic adenocarcinoma arising from the uncinate process on axial (**A**) and coronal (**B**) MDCT images, presenting as a hypodense mass (*thin arrow*), which circumscribes the superior mesenteric artery (*thick arrow*) for more than 180 degrees and invades the duodenum (*curved arrow*, **B**), rendering the tumor inoperable.

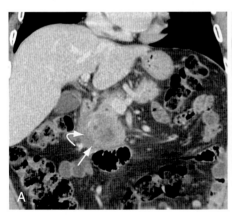
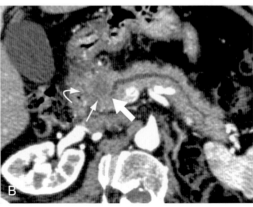

■ **FIGURE 75-3**   Adenocarcinoma of the pancreas shown on coronal (**A**) and curved reconstructed (**B**) MDCT images. Note a poorly enhancing mass (*thin arrow*) that obstructs the main pancreatic duct (*thick arrow*) and infiltrates the duodenum (*curved arrow*).

invasion are violation of the fat plane around the vessels, the "tear drop" sign, which refers to a tear drop shape of the portal vein or the superior mesenteric vein, and dilatation of the pancreaticoduodenal veins (see Figs. 75-1, 75-2, and 75-7).[4-12]

MRI

MRI, because of its high soft tissue and contrast resolution, can facilitate detection of subtle pancreatic lesions and

small, non–organ-deforming masses; therefore, sensitivity and specificity for adenocarcinoma detection with MRI alone are high, 83% and 98%, respectively. On MRI, pancreatic adenocarcinoma appears hypointense on unenhanced T1W images, particularly if 2D fat-saturated sequences are employed. The lobular architecture is

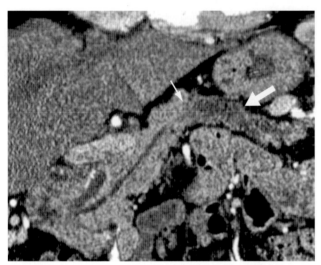

■ **FIGURE 75-4** MDCT-pancreatogram image showing abrupt obstruction of the main pancreatic duct with upstream dilatation (*thick arrow*) due to a small tumor (*thin arrow*).

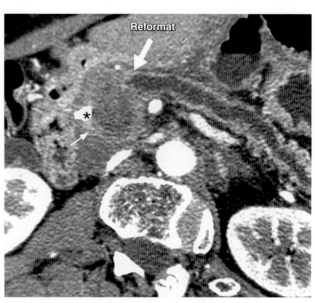

■ **FIGURE 75-6** Adenocarcinoma of the pancreas. MDCT pancreatogram displays obstruction of the main pancreatic duct with upstream dilatation (*thick arrow*) induced by a poorly defined pancreatic adenocarcinoma (*thin arrow*) along with atrophic parenchyma. *Asterisk* indicates a biliary stent.

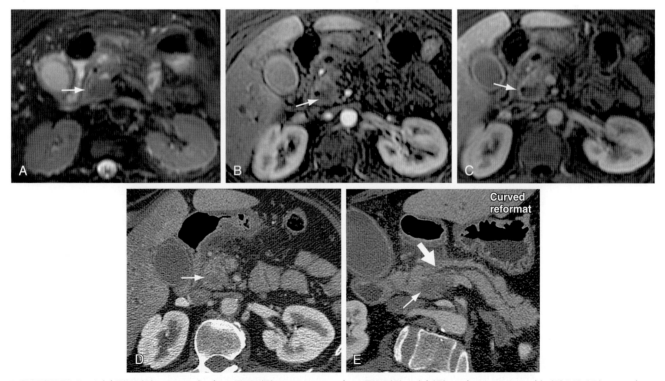

■ **FIGURE 75-5** Axial T2W (**A**), pancreatic phase T1W (**B**), portovenous phase T1W (**C**), axial (**D**), and pancreatographic (**E**) MDCT images show a poorly enhancing pancreatic adenocarcinoma (*thin arrow*) with abrupt obstruction of MPD (*thick arrow,* **E**). The tumor may present as hypointense on T2W images, as in this case, which can render it difficult to be detected, unless contrast medium is injected.

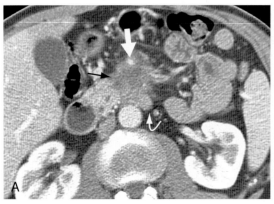
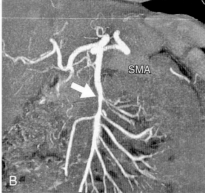

■ **FIGURE 75-7** Axial (**A**) and coronal maximum intensity projection (**B**) MDCT images show an advanced adenocarcinoma (*thin arrow*) infiltrating the superior mesenteric artery (SMA) (*thick arrow*) that appears as the "tear drop" sign. Lymph node metastases are present (*curved arrow*).

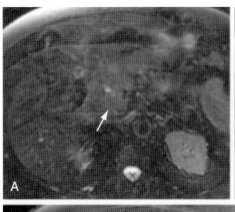
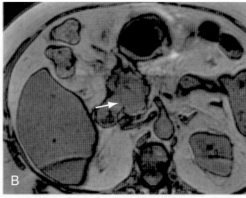
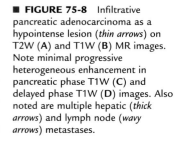
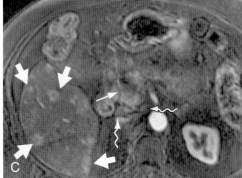
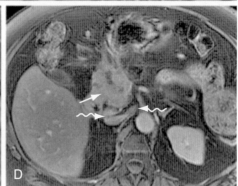

■ **FIGURE 75-8** Infiltrative pancreatic adenocarcinoma as a hypointense lesion (*thin arrows*) on T2W (**A**) and T1W (**B**) MR images. Note minimal progressive heterogeneous enhancement in pancreatic phase T1W (**C**) and delayed phase T1W (**D**) images. Also noted are multiple hepatic (*thick arrows*) and lymph node (*wavy arrows*) metastases.

effaced. Because of the different degrees of associated desmoplastic response, adenocarcinomas of the pancreas demonstrate variable signal intensity on T2W images and enhance relatively less than the background pancreatic parenchyma in the early phases of dynamic contrast imaging but show progressive enhancement in the subsequent phases (Figs. 75-8 and 75-9). If mangafodipir trisodium is administered, the relative lack of enhancement of the adenocarcinoma, which will appear hypointense in comparison to normal enhanced parenchyma, leads to increased tumor detection, with a sensitivity that may be close to 100%.

On 2D and 3D MRCP the pancreatic and biliary ducts can be accurately studied and the typical "double duct" sign, often seen with pancreatic or ampullary tumors can be demonstrated (Fig. 75-10). Moreover, S-MRCP, increas-

ing duct distention, improves the quality of the MRCP and the lesion conspicuity; therefore, pancreatic duct stenosis can be better evaluated and duct irregularities demonstrated.

MRI, with a combination of T2W and T1W fat-saturated gadolinium-enhanced images, performs better than MDCT in the detection and characterization of liver lesions and peritoneal implants, especially for the smallest ones, which tend to parallel the signal intensity of the primary cancer.[4,6-10,13-16]

Ultrasonography

Although transabdominal ultrasonography is usually the first diagnostic imaging tool in the evaluation of the abdomen, it is highly operator dependent and limited by

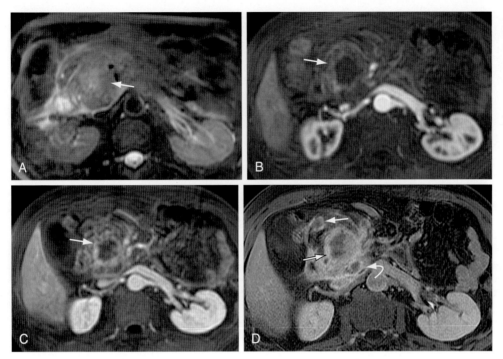

■ **FIGURE 75-9** Advanced pancreatic adenocarcinoma seen on T2W (**A**) and pancreatic phase (**B**), portovenous phase (**C**), and late phase (**D**) contrast-enhanced T1W MR images as a heterogeneously hyperintense infiltrating lesion (*thin arrow*) on T2W imaging and showing poor, heterogeneous, progressive contrast enhancement over time. Peritoneal metastases coexist (*long thin arrow,* **D**), and necrotic lymph node metastases (*curved arrow,* **D**) are also noted.

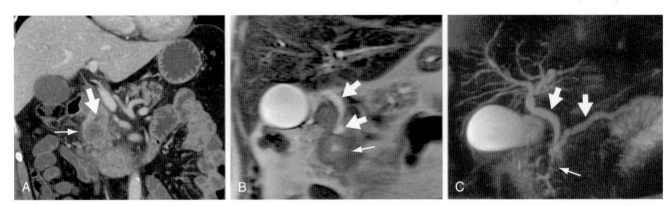

■ **FIGURE 75-10** Infiltrating pancreatic adenocarcinoma (*thin arrow*) causing obstruction and upstream dilatation of both the main pancreatic duct and the common bile duct (*thick arrows*) and showing the "double duct" sign on coronal MDCT (**A**), coronal steady-state fast spin-echo T2W (**B**) MR image, and 3D-MRCP (**C**).

abdominal gas and patient body habitus. Therefore, despite very few single institution studies that demonstrated ultrasonography to be more accurate than CT in tumor diagnosis and as accurate as CT in staging, a negative ultrasound examination does not reliably rule out a solid pancreatic mass. Adenocarcinoma of the pancreas can appear on ultrasound images as a focal, solid, contour-deforming, hypoechoic mass within the pancreas. The MPD may be dilated and surrounding parenchyma atrophic. Peripancreatic lymph nodes may appear enlarged, and their echogenicity reflects that of the primary cancer.

EUS, on the other hand, provides high-resolution images of the pancreas and allows lesion biopsy. EUS is the most accurate imaging technique for lymph node staging and for detection of duodenal infiltration by the cancer (EUS, 76%; CT, 74%; MRI, 67%).[7]

Nuclear Medicine

Nuclear medicine does not play a major role in adenocarcinoma evaluation unless differential diagnosis with functional endocrine tumors or evaluation of bone metastases is required.

PET/CT

PET/CT integrates both functional and morphologic imaging data in a single test. Because the normal pancreas is not visualized on PET, any region of intense FDG uptake is considered abnormal. Initial studies identified pancreatic adenocarcinomas in 95% of patients as discrete foci of increased uptake (Fig. 75-11). Lymph node metastases, especially if small (<1 cm in diameter), are frequently

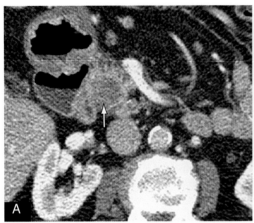
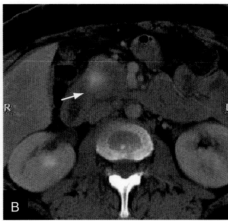

■ **FIGURE 75-11** Axial MDCT **(A)** and fused PET/MDCT **(B)** images show a pancreatic adenocarcinoma (*arrow*) that avidly takes up FDG, highlighting it against normal pancreatic parenchyma.

TABLE 75-3 Accuracy, Limitations, and Pitfalls of Modalities Used in Imaging of Adenocarcinoma

Modality	Accuracy	Limitations	Pitfalls
Radiography	Poor	Insensitive Nonspecific	Unable to directly visualize soft tissue masses in the pancreas
CT	89%-99% tumor diagnosis 86%-91% overall locoregional extension 77%-99% vascular invasion 58%-73% lymph node involvement	Radiation exposure	Difficult detection in the setting of background chronic pancreatitis Characterization of small lesions may be difficult.
MRI	82%-91% tumor diagnosis 63%-89% overall locoregional extension 85%-94% vascular invasion 75%-88% lymph node involvement	Patient cooperation High cost	Calcifications not well visualized
Ultrasonography	<70% US 65%-74% (EUS) locoregional extension	Poor performance in the case of obesity or overlying bowel gas Operator dependent Comprehensive imaging difficult	Detection and characterization of small lesions may be difficult.
Nuclear medicine	Data are not available to specify accuracy. No role at the moment unless in the differential diagnosis with suspected functional endocrine neoplasms or for bone metastases	Poor spatial resolution	
PET/CT	88%-95% tumor diagnosis	Radiation exposure High cost	Diabetes and inflammation may give rise to false results.

missed with CT or ultrasonography and may be responsible for early tumor recurrence after surgery. Because FDG uptake is related to tumor metabolism and not strictly to lesion size, cancer can be detected even in normal-sized lymph nodes. Currently, many new radiopharmaceutical agents are under investigation.[4,17,18]

Imaging Algorithm

An imaging algorithm is provided in Figure 75-1; see also Table 75-3.

Differential Diagnosis

Clinical data are useful to suspect pancreatic adenocarcinoma and contribute to rule out other conditions. Abdominal pain radiating to the back and partially reduced leaning forward, weight loss, jaundice, a palpable gallbladder, thrombophlebitis migrans, recent onset of diabetes, depression, history of smoking and of exposure to carcinogenic agents, and a family and/or personal history of

---

Classic Signs: Pancreatic Masses

- Focal solid pancreatic mass, usually less than 5 cm in diameter
- MPD stenosis/obstruction with upstream dilatation
- CBD dilatation if the tumor is in the pancreatic head
- "Double duct" sign (CBD and MPD dilatation) if the tumor is in the pancreatic head
- Poor enhancement of the mass in the arterial and pancreatic phases of dynamic imaging
- Infiltration into the retroperitoneum
- Lymph node, liver, and peritoneal metastases

---

breast, colon, and pancreatic neoplasms and of hereditary oncologic syndromes may suggest the occurrence of adenocarcinoma of the pancreas.

Laboratory data, mainly increased serum levels of CA 19-9, may provide some support to the diagnosis, but imaging provides the key to the diagnosis.[1,2]

Many anatomic variants may be confused with pancreatic adenocarcinoma. Their differential diagnosis is described in the corresponding sections. Collapsed duodenum or small bowel and duodenal diverticula can be misinterpreted as pancreatic adenocarcinoma, but filling with positive oral contrast agent, air-fluid levels, and enhancement characteristic like that of the intestinal wall suggest the correct diagnosis.

Chronic pancreatitis, usually of alcoholic or autoimmune etiology, may present as a focal mass clinically and radiologically similar to adenocarcinoma. The differential diagnosis with mass-forming chronic pancreatitis is difficult, and different clinical and imaging findings must be carefully satisfied.

Mass-forming chronic pancreatitis (MFP) tends to blend imperceptibly with surrounding parenchyma in the case of alcoholic MFP and to be better defined in the case of autoimmune MFP, but it has infiltrating margins in the case of adenocarcinoma. MFP tends to enhance more homogeneously and to a higher degree than adenocarcinomas. The MPD is obstructed less often in the case of alcoholic MFP and autoimmune MFP; in the case of MPD stenosis, the length of the affected segment is less than 30 mm in 75% of adenocarcinomas and more than 30 mm in nearly all the cases of autoimmune MFP.

The most reliable differentiating finding is the "duct penetrating" sign, characterized by visualization of the MPD traversing the pancreatic mass, without stenosis and ductal wall irregularities. If this criterion is satisfied, it is highly specific (96%) for MFP. On the other hand, MPD with an irregular wall, while traversing a mass, is not considered predictive of a benign etiology. S-MRCP, due to the distention of the pancreatic duct, may potentially help to achieve a correct diagnosis.

FDG-PET/CT may be useful to differentiate pancreatic adenocarcinoma, which shows an avid FGD uptake, from MFP, which demonstrates relatively low levels of FDG uptake. New radioisotopes, such as σ-receptor ligands and ^{18}F-labeled fluorothymidine (^{18}F-FLT), are more tumor specific and potentially of better use in the differential diagnosis. Table 75-4 summarizes the most useful differential features (see also Figs. 75-12 to 75-14).

TABLE 75-4 Differential Diagnosis of Alcoholic Mass-Forming Pancreatitis, Autoimmune Mass-Forming Pancreatitis, and Adenocarcinoma of the Pancreas

Factor	Alcoholic Mass-Forming Pancreatitis	Autoimmune Mass-Forming Pancreatitis	Adenocarcinoma
Age	6th-7th decades	7th-8th decades	7th-8th decades
Lesion margins	Blending with surrounding parenchyma	Defined (67%)	Infiltrative (82%)
Homogeneity, early contrast enhancement	Common (71%)	Uncommon (25%)	Rare (5%)
Homogeneity, late contrast enhancement	Common (82%)	Usual (100%)	Rare (8%)
MPD obstruction	Uncommon (18%)	Uncommon (11%)	Common (60%)
MPD stenosis > 30 mm	Common 50%	Usually 100%	22% may be found
Penetrating duct sign	Common (86%)	Common (50%)	Rare
Upstream MPD < 4 mm	Uncommon (33%)	Common (67%)	Rare (4%)
Downstream MPD irregularity	Usual (100%)	Uncommon (25%)	Uncommon (25%)
Side branches	Usually dilated (100%)	Commonly dilated (50%)	Uncommonly dilated (37%)
CBD	Normal	Stenosed (>20 mm length)	Stenosed (<20 mm length)
Artery encasement	Absent	Common (57%)	Common (81%)
Pseudocysts	Common	Absent	Rare (retention cysts)
Acute pancreatitis–like pain	Common	Uncommon	Rare
CA 19-9	Normal	May be elevated (33%)	Frequently elevated (77%)
IgG4	Normal	Increased	Normal
Corticosteroid response	Absent	Present	Absent

MPD, main pancreatic duct; CBD, common bile duct.

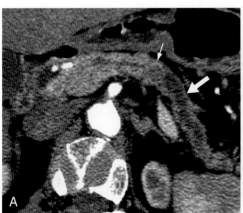
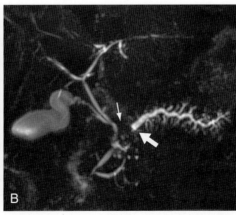

■ **FIGURE 75-12** Pancreatic adenocarcinoma in two different patients on MDCT pancreatogram (**A**) and 3D MRCP (**B**) as a small and barely visible lesion (*thin arrow*) causing abrupt narrowing of the main pancreatic duct and upstream dilatation (*thick arrow*). The main pancreatic duct dilatation is better evaluated on MRCP images.

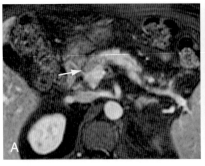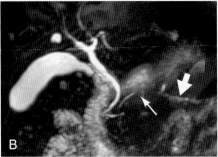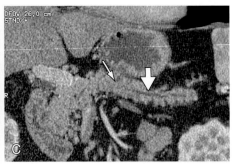

■ **FIGURE 75-13** Autoimmune MFP presents as smooth reduction in the main pancreatic duct over a long segment without any features of obstruction within the lesion (*thin arrow*) and absent upstream dilatation (*thick arrow*) in axial pancreatic phase, contrast-enhanced T1W (**A**) image, 3D-MRCP (**B**), and MDCT pancreatogram (**C**).

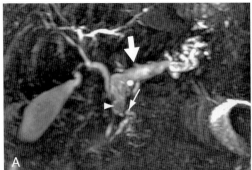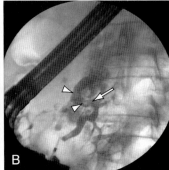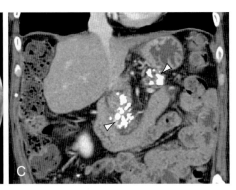

■ **FIGURE 75-14** Benign stricture (*thin arrow*) due to alcoholic chronic pancreatitis appears as smooth narrowing over a short segment along with upstream dilatation of the main pancreatic duct (*thick arrow*) and intraparenchymal and intraductal stones (*arrowheads*) in 3D-MRCP (**A**), ERCP (**B**) and coronal MDCT (**C**) images.

TABLE 75-5 Differential Diagnosis: Adenocarcinoma versus Nonadenocarcinoma of the Pancreas

	Adenocarcinoma	Nonadenocarcinoma
Size	Medium-small (3-5 cm)	Large (>5 cm, unless functional pancreatic endocrine neoplasm)
Necrosis	Rare	Common
Calcifications	Rare	Common
Enhancement	Poor	Mild-intense
Signal Intensity (T2W)	Low-moderate	Moderate-high
Main Pancreatic Duct	Stenosed or obstructed, upstream dilatation	Normal or displaced
Vascular Encasement	Common	Rare

Other neoplasms, such as lymphoma, endocrine tumors, and acinar tumors, enter in the differential diagnosis with pancreatic adenocarcinomas (see later). They all tend to spare the MPD, which is not dilated or stenosed; moreover, their size tends to be larger than that of an adenocarcinoma. A lymphoma is usually sharply circumscribed, if focal, and associated with prominent extrapancreatic nodal disease. Endocrine tumors show intense contrast enhancement, and acinar cell tumors are large at presentation and enhance more than adenocarcinomas. Table 75-5 provides a summary of the most useful features

to differentiate adenocarcinoma versus nonadenocarcinoma of the pancreas (Figs. 75-15 to 75-17).[4,17-20]

Treatment

Medical Treatment

For locally advanced pancreatic cancer, chemotherapy and radiation therapy, alone or in conjunction, are considered alternatives to surgery. Patients with distant metastases are considered ineligible for radiation therapy and

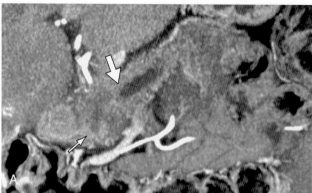
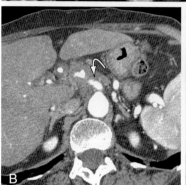
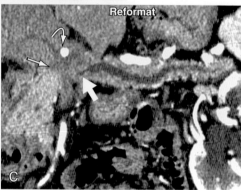
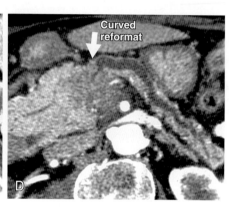

■ **FIGURE 75-15** Staging MDCT for pancreatic adenocarcinoma in two different patients shows a hypodense heterogeneous mass (*thin arrow*), causing abrupt obstruction of the main pancreatic duct (*thick arrow*) with upstream dilatation on coronal (**A**), axial (**B**), and MDCT pancreatograms (**C, D**) images. Also noted in **B** and **C** is atrophy of the corresponding parenchyma and encasement of the superior mesenteric artery (*curved arrow*). Note normal, strong parenchymal enhancement in the pancreatic head, proximal to the tumor.

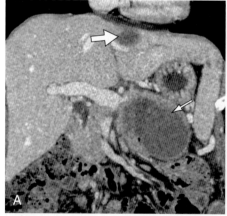
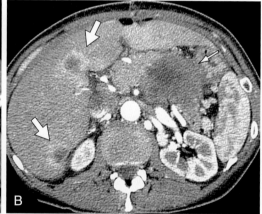

■ **FIGURE 75-16** Colonic metastases to the pancreas are seen on coronal (**A**) and axial (**B**) MDCT as a well-defined mass (*thin arrow*) lacking infiltrative changes, associated main pancreatic duct dilatation, and regional lymphadenopathy. Hepatic metastases are indicated by *thick arrows*.

undergo chemotherapy alone, although the traditional chemotherapy regimen for pancreatic adenocarcinoma offers only a small survival advantage and a slight improvement in the quality of life.[1,2]

Surgical Treatment

Complete surgical resection remains the best curative treatment for adenocarcinoma of the pancreas, with a 5-year survival rate approaching 20% if performed with curative intent; however, owing to late clinical presentation at an advanced stage, and to the biologic aggressiveness, less than 20% of the cases include surgical intervention and of these most reveal node or liver metastases or local infiltration during surgery. Pancreatic adenocarcinoma is considered unresectable in the case of invasion of major arterial vessels (tumor-to-vessel contiguity > 50%) such as the celiac artery, hepatic artery, or superior mesenteric

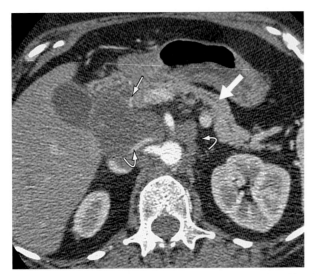

■ **FIGURE 75-17** Primary pancreatic lymphoma in the region of head on axial MDCT presents as a large, minimally enhancing homogeneous mass (*thin arrow*) with regional lymphadenopathy (*curved arrow*). However, the main pancreatic duct (*thick arrow*) is of normal caliber despite the size of the lesion.

artery; in the case of massive venous invasion into the portal vein or superior mesenteric vein; and in the presence of distant metastasis to the liver, regional lymph nodes, or peritoneum (see Figs. 75-1, 75-7, 75-8, 75-15, and 75-18). A tumor with limited invasion into the superior mesenteric vein is still considered resectable.[1,2,4]

What the Referring Physician Needs to Know: Adenocarcinoma

- Adenocarcinomas of the pancreas are malignant lesions with an incidence that usually peaks in the seventh and eighth decades; the 5-year survival rate is only 4%.
- Because of the nonspecific symptoms when at an early stage, the disease is usually advanced when the tumors are detected.
- Even lesions smaller than 2 cm tend to infiltrate locally and disseminate distally.
- MRI and MDCT plus reformatted imaging are the most accurate noninvasive diagnostic modalities.
- Vascular infiltration can be accurately evaluated noninvasively.

KEY POINTS: ADENOCARCINOMA

- Malignant
- Solid
- Usually less than 5 cm
- Poorly defined
- MPD stenosis within the mass and upstream MPD dilatation
- Poor enhancement
- Retroperitoneal infiltration
- Lymph node, liver, and peritoneal metastases

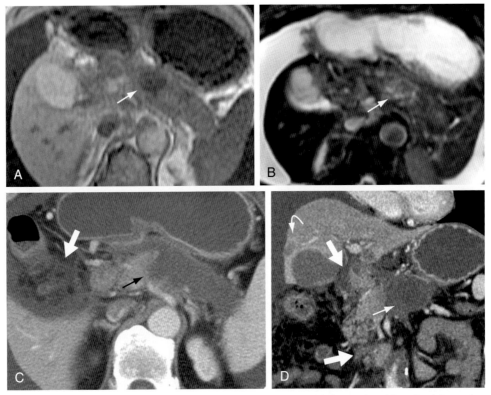

■ **FIGURE 75-18** An advanced case of adenocarcinoma of the pancreas with peritoneal (*thick arrows*) and liver (*curved arrows*) metastases on axial T1W (**A**), T2W (**B**), axial (**C**), and coronal (**D**) MDCT images appears as a mass (*thin arrow*) in the body of the pancreas. MRI is superior to MDCT in detecting the mass when it coexists with postobstructive inflammatory changes.

Endocrine Tumors

Etiology

Many different chromosomal losses have been reported in pancreatic endocrine neoplasms (PENs); some of them are associated with more aggressive biologic behavior. Usually, larger PENs harbor more genetic alterations than smaller lesions. PENs usually occur sporadically but may also arise in patients with von Hippel-Lindau syndrome and multiple endocrine neoplasia (MEN).[1,2]

Prevalence and Epidemiology

PENs are epithelial neoplasms with an organoid growth of cells that resemble pancreatic islet cells or other hormone-producing cells. PENs, which are usually well differentiated, are divided into functional and nonfunctional categories on the bases of associated clinical endocrine paraneoplastic syndrome and are named by the predominantly produced hormone as insulinomas, gastrinomas, VIPomas, glucagonomas, and somatostatinomas. Therefore, in the case of a hormone-secreting PEN, if it is not responsible for any endocrine paraneoplastic syndrome, it falls into the nonfunctional category.

PENs constitute 1% to 2% of pancreatic neoplasms, with the functional category representing between 50% and 85%.

Although PENs may occur at any age, they are found more often between 40 and 60 years of age (mean, 58 years) and at a similar rate between men and women.[1,2]

Clinical Presentation

Clinical presentation varies according to presence or absence of an associated endocrine paraneoplastic syndrome.

Functional PENs are usually small at diagnosis. Nonfunctional PENs tend to be discovered late, when large or locally infiltrating and/or metastatic, with nonspecific features such as abdominal pain, nausea, vomiting, and sometimes jaundice or, in about 15% of the cases, on imaging studies performed for other reasons, in which case they tend to be small.

Elevated serum levels of chromogranin A are associated with PENs in 70% of the cases. Serum hormones do not strictly correlate with hormone type production in the neoplasm as assessed by immunohistochemistry.[1,2]

Pathophysiology

Sixty percent of PENs present in the tail of the pancreas. Functional PENs occur more often in the head and tail, whereas nonfunctional PENs prefer the tail.[1,2]

Pathology

PENs are vascularized neoplasms that present as well circumscribed when small and multinodular with some features of local invasiveness when large. They may contain areas of hemorrhage and fibrosis. Usually PENs are well differentiated, and most of them are malignant; only lesions less than 5 mm are deemed to be completely benign.

PENs are characterized by uniform nuclei, clear cytoplasm, and secretory granules; they stain positive for neuron-specific enolase (NSE) and chromogranin A.

A summary of the classification of functional PENs is provided in Table 75-6.[1,2]

Imaging

PENs may be clinically suspected due to the specific signs and symptoms of the related endocrine paraneoplastic syndrome, may be discovered during workup imaging for nonspecific abdominal complaints or for a suspected malignancy, or may be discovered incidentally during unrelated imaging studies.[1,2]

TABLE 75-6 Functional Pancreatic Endocrine Neoplasms

	Insulinoma	Glucagonoma	Somatostatinoma	Gastrinoma*	VIPoma
Syndrome	Insulinoma syndrome (hypoglycemia)	Glucagonoma syndrome (diabetes, rash, stomatitis, weight loss)	Somatostatinoma syndrome (Hypochlorhydria, diabetes, cholelithiasis)	Zollinger-Ellison syndrome (diarrhea, peptic ulcer disease)	Verner-Morrison syndrome (achlorhydria, watery diarrhea, hypokalemia)
Location	Tail (40%), head (30%), body (30%)	Tail (52%), head (26%), body (22%)	Head (63%), tail (27%), body (10%)	Head (55%), tail (27%), body (18%)	Tail (47%), head (23%), body (19%)
Size	<2 cm	7-8 cm	5-6 cm	2-4 cm	4-5 cm
Malignant Risk	Low	High	High	High	High
Structure†	Homogeneous, solid	Heterogeneous, cystic areas in large lesions	Heterogeneous, cystic areas in large lesions	Homogeneous, solid	Heterogeneous, cystic areas in large lesions
Ca²⁺	Rare	Common	Common		Common
Enhancement	Homogeneous> heterogeneous	Heterogeneous	Heterogeneous	Ring > homogeneous	Heterogeneous
Other Features	Hypoglycemia Increased serum insulin and proinsulin	Elevated fasting serum glucagon	Somatostatin	Serum gastrin > 1000 pg/mL Secretin stimulation test	Serum VIP > 60 pg/mL Elevated serum peptide histidine, methionine

*Gastrinomas often occur in extrapancreatic location in the "gastrinoma triangle" delimited by hepatic hilum cranially, junction of II and III portion of duodenum inferiorly, and junction of neck-body of the pancreas medially. Gastric wall thickening is frequently multiple.
†Structural heterogeneity and cystic areas increase with increasing size of the lesions.

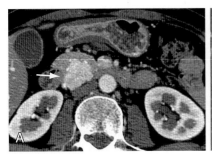
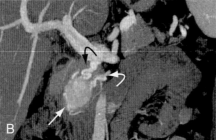
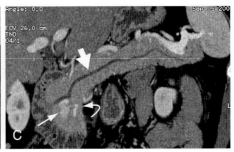

■ **FIGURE 75-19** Functional pancreatic endocrine neoplasm (VIPoma) in the head of the pancreas seen on axial (**A**) and reconstructed (**B** and **C**) MDCT images as a lobulated, well-defined strongly enhancing mass (*thin arrow*) with normal main pancreatic duct (*thick arrow*). Note hypertrophic feeding vessels (*curved arrow*).

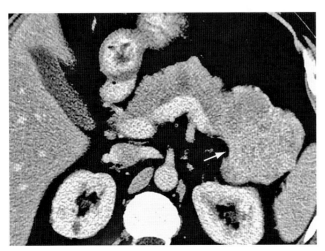

■ **FIGURE 75-20** Nonfunctional pancreatic endocrine neoplasm seen on an axial MDCT as a large, strongly enhancing heterogeneous mass (*arrow*) in the tail of the pancreas.

Radiography

As stated in the introduction, radiography does not play a role in evaluation of PENs.

CT

The imaging appearance of PENs is strongly influenced by their size at presentation. Because of specific clinical symptoms, functional PENs are investigated early in their course and therefore are small and homogeneous at presentation; meanwhile, nonfunctional neoplasms, owing to the lower index of suspicion, are diagnosed late and present larger and nonhomogeneously.

Classically, small PENs present as non–contour-deforming masses, isoattenuating to normal pancreas before contrast agent administration, and strongly enhancing during dynamic imaging (Fig. 75-19). Sometimes, especially if malignant, they may present cystic features, enhance poorly, and contain calcifications. Insulinomas can also appear hyperattenuating before use of a contrast agent.

Large PENs tend to present as large heterogeneous masses at baseline and enhance in a nonhomogeneous fashion during dynamic imaging. The degree of heterogeneity parallels their size (Fig. 75-20).

In the case of malignant behavior, areas of central necrosis, calcifications, and retroperitoneal invasion can

be detected. The imaging features of metastases to regional lymph nodes and to the liver tend to parallel those of the primary tumor and usually enhance early after contrast agent administration.[21-23]

MRI

MRI, owing to its high soft tissue and contrast resolution, can facilitate detection of small, non–organ-deforming masses, especially if strongly enhancing, as in the case of small PENs.

Although PENs, independently of their size, present hypointense on T1W sequences and hyperintense on T2W sequences, in larger lesions there is a higher incidence of hemorrhage, necrosis, and cystic degeneration, which influences their signal intensity. Moreover, lesions smaller than 2 cm display a homogeneous enhancement; meanwhile, larger tumors tend to present as a ring-like peripheral enhancement.

On 2D and 3D MRCP, the MPD is not stenosed or obstructed, although large lesions may cause its displacement.[21-23]

Ultrasonography

On ultrasonography PENs tend to present as focal, solid, sharply demarcated, hypoechoic masses within the pancreas that tend to markedly enhance after contrast agent administration. The MPD is not dilated.[22]

Nuclear Medicine

Nuclear medicine plays a significant role in detection of PENs detection. Scintigraphy with ^{111}In-octreotide, a somatostatin analog, is highly sensitive (67% to 100% of all PENs) and has been proven useful for diagnosis, staging, and follow-up of PENs. Moreover, it helps to identify associated unsuspected lesions.[22,23]

PET/CT

PET/CT and scintigraphy with ^{111}In-octreotide have complementary roles in the case of PENs. PET/CT may be unable to visualize well-differentiated, slowly growing PENs whose metabolic rate is low, providing false-negative results. These same tumors are those easily detected by scintigraphy with ^{111}In-octreotide. On the other hand,

TABLE 75-7 Accuracy, Limitations, and Pitfalls of the Modalities Used in Imaging of Pancreatic Endocrine Tumors

Modality	Accuracy	Limitations	Pitfalls
Radiography	Poor	Insensitive Nonspecific	Unable to directly visualize soft tissue masses in the pancreas
CT	92%	Radiation exposure	Proper contrast-enhancement technique is mandatory to visualize small lesions.
MRI	Specific data regarding MRI accuracy are not available; reported sensitivity ranges from 84% to 94%.	Patient cooperation High cost	Calcifications not well visualized
Ultrasonography	Specific data regarding accuracy are not available; reported sensitivity ranges from 20% to 86%.	Poor performance in the case of obesity or overlying bowel gas Operator dependent Comprehensive imaging difficult	Detection and characterization of small lesions may be difficult.
Nuclear medicine	83%	Poor spatial resolution	^{111}In-octreotide uptake is reduced in the case of poorly differentiated pancreatic endocrine neoplasms.
PET/CT	Specific data regarding PET/CT accuracy are not available; reported sensitivity ranges from 53% to 57%.	Radiation exposure High cost	FDG uptake is poor in well-differentiated pancreatic endocrine neoplasms.

PET/CT is useful in the case of poorly differentiated PENs that scarcely express somatostatin receptors, for which scintigraphy with ^{111}In-octreotide is falsely negative (10% to 20%). PET/CT proves particularly useful in the assessment of malignant PENs, poorly differentiated PENs, and metastatic disease.[23]

Imaging Algorithm

An imaging algorithm is provided in Figure 75-1; see also Table 75-7.

Classic Signs: Pancreatic Endocrine Tumors

- Homogeneous solid pancreatic mass less than 5 cm in diameter
- Heterogeneous pancreatic mass more than 5 cm in diameter
- Calcifications
- Strong enhancement in the arterial and pancreatic phases of dynamic imaging
- No MPD stenosis or obstruction

Differential Diagnosis

In the case of functional PENs, clinical and laboratory data are useful to strongly suspect the neoplasms; therefore, diagnostic imaging is requested to confirm the clinical suspicion (Fig. 75-21).

In the case of nonfunctional PENs the nonspecificity of the clinical picture does not help to reach an early diagnosis and to differentiate against other neoplasms.[1,2]

Differential diagnosis with anatomic variants and pseudolesions is described in the corresponding sections. The differential diagnosis with other neoplasms of the pancreas mainly includes adenocarcinoma of the pancreas and metastases from renal cancer.

Calcifications (found in 22% of the cases), central necrosis or cystic degeneration, higher signal intensity on T2W images, and lack of MPD obstruction and vascular encasement are features suggestive of PENs. Moreover, in the case of glucagonomas and somatostatinomas, metastases to the spleen are characteristic. A negative oncologic history for a renal primary tumor is a useful criterion to rule out intrapancreatic metastases from kidney cancer.[1,2,21-23]

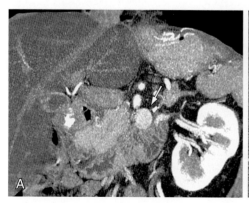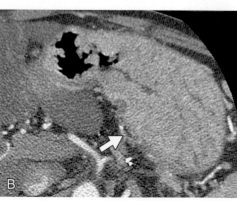

■ **FIGURE 75-21** Extrapancreatic gastrinoma seen on coronal (**A**) and axial (**B**) MDCT images as a well-defined, intensely enhancing lesion (*arrow,* **A**) in the pancreatoduodenal groove during the arterial phase. Also noted in the same patient is marked thickening of the gastric folds (*thick arrows*).

Treatment

Medical Treatment

The role of chemotherapy for metastatic and locally advanced PENs is still debated; it is usually restricted to symptomatic patients, with only some partial responses reported. Octreotide is frequently used to palliate symptoms.[1,2]

Surgical Treatment

Surgical resection represents the best curative treatment for solitary PENs; in the case of a single functional PEN, limited pancreatectomy is the treatment of choice. In the setting of PENs associated with MEN type 1, the treatment is particularly complicated, owing to the occurrence of multiple neoplasms in the pancreas and in other organs (Fig. 75-22).[1,2]

What the Referring Physician Needs to Know: Pancreatic Endocrine Neoplasms

- PENs are deemed benign if less than 5 mm in diameter and harbor malignant potential if larger.
- Peak incidence is usually in the fifth and sixth decades.
- If functional, PENs are suspected at an early stage; otherwise, they are usually diagnosed when advanced.
- In the case of malignancy they can infiltrate locally and disseminate distally, by the lymphatic and hematologic routes.
- MRI and MDCT with reformatted imaging are accurate noninvasive diagnostic modalities.
- ^{111}In-octreotide scintigraphy is highly sensitive in detection of PENs (67%-100%) and has been proven useful for diagnosis, staging, and follow-up.

Intrapancreatic Metastases

Etiology

Intrapancreatic metastases usually occur in the setting of widespread malignancies. The pancreas may be second-arily involved through direct invasion or hematogeneous and lymphatic dissemination or be part of systemic hematologic malignancies, such as leukemias and lymphomas.[1,2]

Prevalence and Epidemiology

Intrapancreatic metastases are rare, accounting for 2% of pancreatic tumors. The mean age at presentation is 60 years. At autopsy the malignancies most commonly implicated are lung (25%), breast (13%), melanoma (11%), gastric (10%), colorectal (6%), renal (4%), and ovarian (4%).[1]

Clinical Presentation

Intrapancreatic metastases usually occur in the setting of disseminated malignancies. They lack a specific symptomatology, are detected during routine oncologic follow-up, and do not constitute a relevant clinical and management problem.

In less than 8.5% of the cases they are clinically suspected, and in less than 4% they undergo biopsy or resection.[1,2,24,25]

Pathophysiology

Intrapancreatic metastases may be single (25%) or multiple (75%). In the case of focal involvement, the pancreatic head is the most common location.

KEY POINTS: PANCREATIC ENDOCRINE NEOPLASMS

- Potentially malignant or malignant
- Solid
- Usually well defined
- Usually less than 5 cm if functional and more than 5 cm if nonfunctional
- Enhancing
- No MPD stenosis
- Lymph node and liver metastases

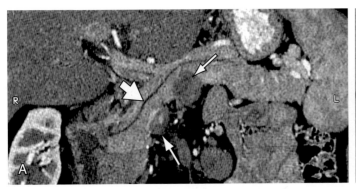
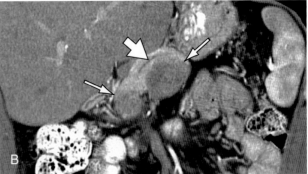

■ **FIGURE 75-22** Multiple pancreatic endocrine neoplasms seen on MDCT pancreatogram (**A**) and coronal (**B**) MDCT images as two well-defined, mildly enhancing solid masses (*thin arrows*) in the body deforming the contour of the organ without causing any obstruction and dilatation of the main pancreatic duct (*thick arrows*).

Pathology

Pathology of intrapancreatic metastases is extremely variable and reflects that of the primary tumor. Mean size at diagnosis is 4.6 cm.

Renal cancer metastases, most often of the clear cell type, tend to present as solitary, well-circumscribed solid masses with prominent vascularization. They can undergo necrosis, hemorrhage, and cystic degeneration. Lymphomatous involvement of the pancreas, reported in a third of the cases of systemic disease, occurs more often in the form of a focal mass than of a diffuse infiltration.[1]

Imaging

Intrapancreatic metastases do not usually pose specific imaging problems because they are discovered during imaging follow-up for a known primary tumor. In the very few cases in which oncologic history is apparently negative, diagnostic imaging is usually inadequate to reach the diagnosis and biopsy or even resection is required.[1,2,24,25]

CT

There is no imaging feature that is specific for intrapancreatic metastases. Besides the fact that small lesions appear homogeneous whereas large masses display internal heterogeneity, and may contain necrotic areas, these lesions tend to reflect the appearance of their tumor of origin.

Metastases from a hypervascular primary tumor such as breast or clear cell renal cancer strongly enhance during the arterial phase of dynamic imaging (Fig. 75-23). Metastases from colorectal cancers tend to enhance poorly and may mimic pancreatic adenocarcinomas (see Fig. 75-16).[24,25]

MRI

In the case of intrapancreatic metastases, the information obtained from MDCT can also be provided by MRI, with the added benefits of superior contrast resolution, which could allow the detection of smaller hypervascularized metastases and the possibility of identifying chemical shift phenomenon and melanin hyperintensity in the case of intrapancreatic metastases from clear cell renal cancer and melanoma, respectively.[24,25]

Ultrasonography

Transabdominal ultrasonography is not the most sensitive and specific imaging tool to evaluate intrapancreatic metastases, which tend to present as focal, well-circumscribed hypoechoic masses.

PET/CT

Although there are no specific studies to address PET/CT of intrapancreatic metastases, in our personal experience, and from case reports, they tend to exhibit increased uptake of FDG, highlighting the lesion against the normal background pancreas.

Imaging Algorithm

An imaging algorithm is provided in Figure 75-1; see also Table 75-8.

Classic Signs: Intrapancreatic Metastases

- No specific imaging sign
- History of primary tumor nearly always present
- Usually in the setting of widespread malignancy
- Single or multiple solid pancreatic masses, with 4.5-cm mean diameter
- Baseline and enhancement features paralleling those of the tumor of origin
- Homogeneous if small lesions
- Heterogeneous if large lesions
- Normal MPD
- Normal CBD; dilatation possible if lesion located in pancreatic head

---

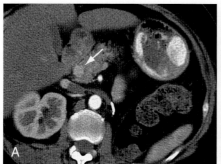 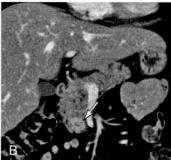 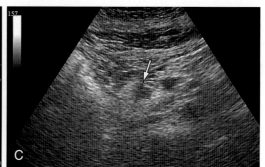

■ FIGURE 75-23 Intrapancreatic metastases seen on axial (**A**) and coronal (**B**) MDCT images as a well-defined enhancing mass (*arrow*) in the uncinate process on CT and as a hypoechoic lesion on ultrasonography (**C**). Note the empty left renal fossa and surgical vascular clip due to previous nephrectomy for clear cell renal cancer.

TABLE 75-8 Accuracy, Limitations, and Pitfalls of the Modalities Used in Imaging of Intrapancreatic Metastases

Modality	Accuracy	Limitations	Pitfalls
Radiography	Poor	Insensitive Nonspecific	Unable to directly visualize soft tissue masses in the pancreas
CT	No studies are available to specifically address CT accuracy in intrapancreatic metastases.	Radiation exposure	Detection and characterization of small lesions may be difficult.
MRI	No studies are available to specifically address MRI accuracy in intrapancreatic metastases.	Patient cooperation High cost	Calcifications not well visualized
Ultrasonography	No studies are available to specifically address accuracy in intrapancreatic metastases.	Poor performance in the case of obesity or overlying bowel gas Operator dependent Comprehensive imaging difficult	Detection and characterization of small lesions may be difficult.
Nuclear medicine	Although no studies are available to specifically address the accuracy of nuclear medicine in intrapancreatic metastases, its role is supposed to be poor.	Poor spatial resolution	
PET/CT	No studies are available to specifically address PET/CT accuracy in intrapancreatic metastases.	Radiation exposure High cost	

Differential Diagnosis

Clinical data are necessary to suspect the metastatic nature of the intrapancreatic lesions and to rule out a pancreatic primary tumor. Clinical history of a primary tumor is found in virtually all patients, with the possible exception of melanoma, which can be unknown to the patient. Pancreatic symptoms are usually absent at presentation or at least overwhelmed by the manifestations of the associated disseminated oncologic disease.[1,2,24,25]

No imaging feature is specific for intrapancreatic metastases. Their imaging appearance varies strongly, according to the primary tumor of origin.

The differential diagnosis from adenocarcinoma of the pancreas is usually prompted by the normal appearance of the MPD and in the case of renal or breast primary tumors by the strong enhancement of the lesions. The most difficult differential diagnosis is with PENs. In these cases, history of a renal/breast primary tumor, absence of endocrinologic abnormalities, and a negative finding on ^{111}In-octreotide scintigraphy are important differential criteria.[24,25]

Treatment

Medical Treatment

Intrapancreatic metastases are treated with the same chemotherapy regimen used to treat the remaining localizations of the disseminated malignancy.[1,24,25]

What the Referring Physician Needs to Know: Intrapancreatic Metastases

- Intrapancreatic metastases usually occur in the setting of widely spread malignancies.
- They are usually detected incidentally.
- Imaging features reflect those of the primary tumor.
- Small lesions tend to be homogeneous, large ones tend to appear nonhomogeneous.

KEY POINTS: INTRAPANCREATIC METASTASES

- Multiple or single
- Solid if small
- Cystic areas may coexist in the case of large lesions
- Mean diameter: 4.6 cm
- Baseline and enhancing features parallel those of the primary tumor
- No MPD/CBD stenosis

Surgical Treatment

Surgical resection is not considered in the case of intrapancreatic metastases, unless it is the case of solitary lesions not associated with other metastases.[1,24,25]

Pancreatic Lymphoma

Etiology

Pancreatic lymphoma is usually of the non-Hodgkin's type of both B- and T-cell lineage.[1]

Prevalence and Epidemiology

Primary pancreatic lymphomas are rare, comprising 0.5% of all pancreatic neoplasms, tend to occur in the fourth to eighth decades (mean age, 55 years), and are more common in men (male-to-female ratio, 7:1).[1,2,26-28]

Clinical Presentation

Clinical presentation is not specific, with abdominal pain present in all the patients. Other symptoms are weight loss and jaundice (<50%); the CA 19-9 value may be elevated.[1]

Pathophysiology

The most common location is the head of the pancreas (80%).[1,26-28]

Pathology

Lymphomas may present as a mass-forming focal lesion (mean diameter, 8 cm) or as a diffuse replacement of the organ, which appears globally enlarged. In both cases, pancreatic lymphomas tend to diffusely infiltrate the retroperitoneal structures and the gastrointestinal tract, not respecting anatomic boundaries.[1,26-28]

Imaging

Primary pancreatic lymphoma is rarely clinically suspected, owing to the nonspecificity of the associated symptoms. It is usually discovered during imaging for nonspecific abdominal complaints or for a suspected abdominal malignancy or may be discovered incidentally during unrelated imaging studies.[1]

CT

On MDCT, primary pancreatic lymphoma presents as a large (usually >7 cm) homogeneous mass or as diffuse enlargement of the gland with effacement of its lobular structure. On baseline CT, lymphomas tend to be hypodense to the pancreas and enhance poorly during dynamic imaging. The MPD is usually not affected. Peripancreatic and infrarenal lymph node enlargement often coexist (see Fig. 75-17).[26-28]

MRI

Pancreatic lymphomas, despite their size, which can be large at presentation, tend to appear homogeneous. They are hypointense on T1W imaging, are hypointense to isointense on T2W sequences, and tend to enhance poorly and homogeneously during dynamic imaging (Figs. 75-24 and 75-25).[26-28]

Ultrasonography

On transabdominal ultrasonography, primary pancreatic lymphomas may present as a large well-defined hypoechoic lesion or as diffuse enlargement of the organ, with reduced echogenicity.[26-28]

PET/CT

Although there are no specific studies dedicated to PET/CT of primary pancreatic lymphomas, from case reports and our personal experience these neoplasms tend to present as large focal masses of increased uptake or as a diffusely increased uptake involving the entire pancreas. Usually, FDG-avid lymph nodes are discovered in the peripancreatic region.

Imaging Algorithm

An imaging algorithm is provided in Figure 75-1; see also Table 75-9.

Classic Signs: Pancreatic Lymphoma

- Solitary mass or diffuse infiltration of the pancreas
- Large diameter, usually >7 cm
- Homogeneity of the lesion despite its large size
- Normal MPD

Differential Diagnosis

In the case of primary pancreatic lymphoma, although clinical data are usually not specific enough to suspect the etiology of the intrapancreatic lesion, they are suggestive for nonadenocarcinoma. Imaging and biopsy are the cornerstones of the diagnosis.[1,2,26-28]

Primary pancreatic lymphomas must be differentiated from pancreatic adenocarcinoma, PENs, and lymphoma with secondary involvement of the organ. A relatively small pancreatic mass with an obstructed MPD favors

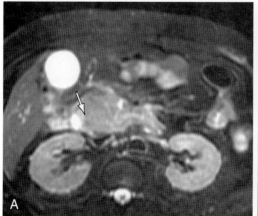
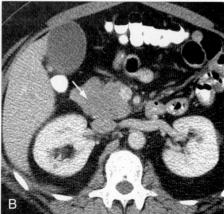

■ **FIGURE 75-24** Primary pancreatic lymphoma on axial T2W (**A**) and MDCT (**B**) images seen as a poorly enhancing mass in the head of pancreas with internal homogeneity and moderately increased signal on the T2W image.

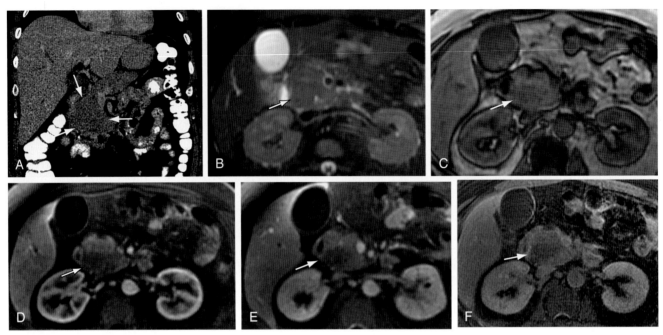

■ **FIGURE 75-25** MDCT and MR images of non-Hodgkin's lymphoma of the pancreas. Coronal MDCT (**A**) image shows a mass in the head of pancreas with lack of main pancreatic duct and intrahepatic bile duct dilatation. The mass is isointense to pancreas on T2W (**B**) and T1W (**C**) images and shows minimal enhancement on gadolinium-enhanced images in the pancreatic phase (**D**), portovenous phase (**E**), and delayed phase (**F**) images.

TABLE 75-9   Accuracy, Limitations, and Pitfalls of the Modalities Used in Imaging of Pancreatic Lymphoma

Modality	Accuracy	Limitations	Pitfalls
Radiography	Poor	Insensitive Nonspecific	Unable to directly visualize soft tissue masses in the pancreas
CT	No studies are available to specifically address CT accuracy in primary pancreatic lymphoma.	Radiation exposure	Detection and characterization of small lesions may be difficult.
MRI	No studies are available to specifically address MRI accuracy in primary pancreatic lymphoma.	Patient cooperation High cost	
Ultrasonography	No studies are available to specifically address accuracy in primary pancreatic lymphoma.	Poor performance in the case of obesity or overlying bowel gas Operator dependent Comprehensive imaging difficult	Detection and characterization of small lesions may be difficult.
Nuclear medicine	Although no studies are available to specifically address the accuracy of nuclear medicine in primary pancreatic lymphoma, its role is supposed to be very limited.	Poor spatial resolution	
PET/CT	No studies are available to specifically address PET/CT accuracy in primary pancreatic lymphoma.	Radiation exposure High cost	

adenocarcinoma of the pancreas; in the case of lymphoma the lesion tends to be large at presentation. The MPD is nonobstructed; and if lymph nodes are enlarged, this occurs below the renal veins.

On the other hand, PENs are suspected in the case of more pronounced hyperintensity on T2W sequences, intense arterial contrast enhancement, calcifications, and necrosis. Diffuse lymph node enlargement not limited to the peripancreatic region, but involving other sites, such as the mediastinum and superficial chains, and splenomegaly, hepatomegaly, and changes in the leukocyte count favor secondary involvement. A fine-needle aspiration biopsy is usually required for a definite histologic diagnosis if the just-mentioned signs are not evident.[1,2,26-28]

Treatment

Medical Treatment

Primary pancreatic lymphomas tend to respond well to chemotherapy and/or radiation therapy.[1,26,27]

Surgical Treatment

Surgery is not routinely performed in the case of primary lymphoma of the pancreas; it is usually done if a preoperative diagnosis has not been undertaken.[1,26,27]

What the Referring Physician Needs to Know: Pancreatic Lymphoma

- The clinical presentation is nonspecific.
- The tumor is usually detected incidentally.
- A large homogeneous mass without MPD dilatation is evident.
- Diffuse enlargement of the pancreas with effacement of its lobular architecture occurs.

KEY POINTS: PANCREATIC LYMPHOMA

- Solitary lesion or diffuse infiltration
- Large size (>7 cm)
- Homogeneity
- Well demarcated if mass-like
- Low to intermediate signal intensity on T2W imaging
- Mild enhancement
- No MPD stenosis/upstream dilatation

Acinar Cell Carcinoma

Etiology

Mutations in the adenomatous polyposis coli (*APC*)/β-catenin gene and losses on chromosome 11 have been implicated as etiologic factors in acinar cell carcinoma (ACC).[1]

Prevalence and Epidemiology

ACC is a rare pancreatic tumor characterized by pancreatic enzyme production by the tumor cells. It accounts for about 1% of all adult exocrine pancreatic neoplasms and about 15% of all pediatric pancreatic tumors. It occurs more often in women, with its incidence peak in the seventh decade.[1]

Clinical Presentation

The clinical presentation is variable. Symptoms can be induced by mass effect and/or local infiltration (jaundice, abdominal pain, vomiting, and weight loss) or by hyperlipase production in 10% to 15% of the cases (polyarthritis and/or subcutaneous fat necrosis). The serum lipase value is elevated in nearly all the patients, even in the absence of associated symptoms. The serum marker CA 19-9 is increased in 30% of patients.[1,29]

Pathophysiology

ACC tends to arise more often in the uncinate process and head of the pancreas (60% of the cases) as a solitary mass. In about 80% of the cases this tumor grows exophytically.[1]

Pathology

ACC presents as a well-defined solid mass, surrounded by a fibrous pseudocapsule, which can harbor focal areas of discontinuity and infiltration. The mean tumor size at presentation is 7 cm. Large ACCs may exhibit a variable amount of necrosis with cystic degeneration that can encompass even more than 75% of the mass.

Neoplastic cells present in an acinar arrangement and acinar differentiation, as demonstrated by zymogen granules and confirmed by immunohistochemistry. Endocrine and ductal components, although commonly present, constitute less than 25% of the mass.[1,29]

Imaging

ACC tends to infiltrate locally and metastasize to regional lymph node and hepatic parenchyma (about 50% of the cases at presentation). Recurrence is common (79% after curative resection); and although the 5-year survival rate is 5.9%, the median survival is higher than that for adenocarcinoma (19 months).[1,29]

CT

ACC presents as a well-circumscribed, mildly enhancing, predominantly solid mass (Figs. 75-26 and 75-27); an enhancing capsule may be demonstrated. Areas of capsular discontinuity and infiltration can be detected. Central necrosis is common (80% of the cases) and may be responsible for a cystic or mixed cystic-solid appearance (Fig. 75-28). Calcifications in the form of central punctuate or stellate calcifications or peripheral calcified punctuations or plaques are found in 50% of the cases.[29,30]

MRI

MRI confirms the same imaging findings detected by MDCT, although calcifications are more difficult to appreciate. It is useful to rule out macroscopic intratumoral hemorrhage, a rare finding in ACC.[29,30]

Ultrasonography

Transabdominal ultrasonography is usually unable to provide an etiologic diagnosis. Usually, ACC presents as a large, well-defined hypoechoic solid or mixed solid-cystic mass.

PET/CT

ACC is rare, and currently there are no specific PET/CT studies to address this entity.

■ **FIGURE 75-26** MDCT images of acinar cell cancer. Axial (**A**) and coronal (**B**) MDCT images show a well-defined, lobulated, predominantly exophytic mass (*arrow*) in the head of the pancreas invading the superior mesenteric vein (*arrowhead*).

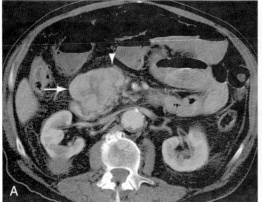
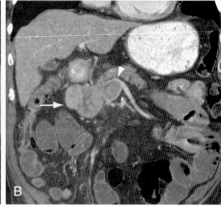

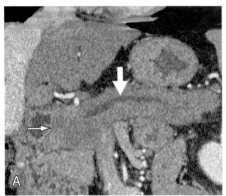
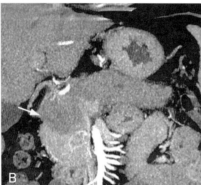
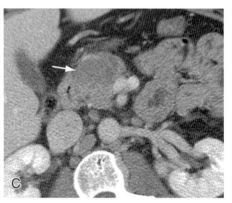

■ **FIGURE 75-27** Acinar cell cancer. Coronal (**A, B**) and axial (**C**) MDCT images demonstrate a well-defined hypoattenuating mass (*thin arrow*) in the head of the pancreas with mild pancreatic ductal dilatation (*thick arrow*). The presence of mild duct dilatation and lack of parenchymal atrophy despite the critical location and size and of the mass differentiate it from pancreatic adenocarcinoma.

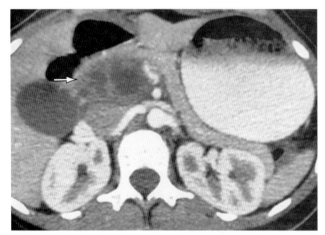

■ **FIGURE 75-28** Axial MDCT image shows a solid and cystic acinar cell tumor (*arrow*) in the head of the pancreas with absence of main pancreatic duct dilatation and parenchymal atrophy.

Classic Signs: Acinar Cell Carcinoma

- Single, large, predominantly solid pancreatic mass with 7-cm mean diameter
- Tendency to esophytic growth
- Areas of necrosis
- Central and/or peripheral calcifications
- Normal MPD and CBD

Differential Diagnosis

Hyperlipasemia syndrome, which occurs in less than 15% of the cases and is characterized by coexistence of subcutaneous fat necrosis, polyarthralgias, and serum hyperlipasemia, prompts the search for an ACC.

If hyperlipasemia syndrome is absent, the tumor may be unsuspected or may cause nonspecific symptoms due to compression, infiltration, and dissemination. Even in this situation the serum lipase level is commonly elevated and may be useful to support the diagnosis.[1,2,29-30]

ACC needs to be differentiated from adenocarcinoma of the pancreas, PENs, and pseudopapillary epithelial neoplasms (SPENs).

Large size at presentation, exophytic growth, calcifications, central necrosis, well-circumscribed appearance,

Imaging Algorithm

An imaging algorithm is provided in Figure 75-1; see also Table 75-10.

TABLE 75-10 Accuracy, Limitations, and Pitfalls of the Modalities Used in Imaging of Acinar Cell Carcinoma

Modality	Accuracy	Limitations	Pitfalls
Radiography	Poor	Insensitive Nonspecific	Unable to directly visualize soft tissue masses in the pancreas
CT	Specific data regarding CT accuracy are not available.	Radiation exposure	Detection and characterization of small lesions may be difficult.
MRI	Specific data regarding MR accuracy are not available.	Patient cooperation High cost	Calcifications not well visualized
Ultrasound	Specific data regarding accuracy are not available.	Poor performance in the case of obesity or overlying bowel gas Operator dependent Comprehensive imaging difficult	Detection and characterization of small lesions may be difficult.
Nuclear medicine	Although specific data regarding the accuracy of nuclear medicine are not available, it currently does not play any role in diagnosis of acinar cell carcinoma.	Poor spatial resolution	
PET/CT	Specific data regarding PET/CT accuracy are not available.	Radiation exposure High cost	

lesion enhancement, and normal size of the MPD are typical for ACCs and rare in adenocarcinomas. Both ACCs and PENs may be large at presentation, display calcifications and central necrosis, and be well circumscribed; but ACCs enhance less than PENs, and take up mangafodipir trisodium. On the other hand, ^{111}In-octreotide uptake is specific for PENs. Differential diagnosis with SPEN is extremely difficult. SPENs may present as central necrosis, be circumscribed by capsule, display calcifications, and enhance as ACCs. SPENs almost invariably present as macroscopic hemorrhage, which is less common, although not rare, in ACCs. The most important differentiating features are the occurrence of SPENs in young females and the increased serum level of lipase in ACCs.[1,2,29,30]

Treatment

Medical Treatment

Chemotherapy alone or combined with irradiation is reserved for patients not deemed surgical candidates because of widespread disease at presentation or poor medical conditions.[1]

Surgical Treatment

Surgical resection is considered the treatment of choice in the case of resectable neoplasms. Large size at presentation, due to the expansive grow pattern, is not a contraindication to surgery.[1]

What the Referring Physician Needs to Know:
Acinar Cell Carcinoma

■ A solitary, large mass is evident.
■ The tumor may infiltrate and metastasize.
■ Detection is incidental or symptomatic.
■ Mass effect is present.
■ Hyperlipasemia syndrome is associated.
■ The prognosis is better than with adenocarcinoma.

KEY POINTS: ACINAR CELL CARCINOMA

■ Single
■ Predominantly solid or cystic
■ Mean diameter: 7 cm
■ Well circumscribed
■ Exophytic growth
■ Necrotic areas in the case of large lesions
■ Calcifications
■ Mildly enhancing
■ No stenosis of MPD or CBD

SUGGESTED READINGS

Biankin AV, Kench JG, Dijkman FP, et al. Molecular pathogenesis of precursor lesions of pancreatic ductal adenocarcinoma. Pathology 2003; 35:14-24.

Cardenes HR, Chiorean EG, Dewitt J, et al. Locally advanced pancreatic cancer: current therapeutic approach. Oncologist 2006; 11:612-623.

Hines OJ, Reber HA. Pancreatic surgery. Curr Opin Gastroenterol 2006; 22:520-526.

Katz MH, Savides TJ, Moossa AR, Bouvet M. An evidence-based approach to the diagnosis and staging of pancreatic cancer. Pancreatology 2005; 5:576-590.

Kostakoglu L, Agress H Jr, Goldsmith SJ. Clinical role of FDG-PET in evaluation of cancer patients. RadioGraphics 2003; 23:315-340.

Mittendorf EA, Shifrin AL, Inabnet WB, et al. Islet cell tumors. Curr Probl Surg 2006; 43:685-765.

Sahani DV, Shah ZK, Catalano OA, et al. Radiology of pancreatic adenocarcinoma: current status of imaging. J Gastroenterol Hepatol 2008; 23:23-33.

Saif MW. Primary pancreatic lymphomas. JOP 2006; 7:262-273.

Semelka RC, Custodio CM, Cem Balci N, Woosley JT. Neuroendocrine tumors of the pancreas: spectrum of appearances on MRI. J Magn Reson Imaging 2000; 11:141-148.

REFERENCES

1. Hruban RH, Pitman Bishop M, Klimstra DS. Tumors of the pancreas. In Armed Forces Institute of Pathology: Atlas of Tumor Pathology, 4th series. Washington, DC, AFIP, 2007.
2. Yamada T, Alpers DH, Kountz WB, et al. Textbook of Gastroenterology. Philadelphia, Lippincott William and Wilkins. Online edition.
3. Surveillance Epidemiology and End Results of the National Cancer Institute (SEER) Cancer Statistics Review, 2000-2004. Bethesda, MD, National Cancer Institute, 2008.
4. Sahani DV, Shah ZK, Catalano OA, et al. Radiology of pancreatic adenocarcinoma: current status of imaging. J Gastroenterol Hepatol 2008; 23:23-33.
5. Fletcher JG, Wiersema MJ, Farrell MA, et al. Pancreatic malignancy: value of arterial, pancreatic, and hepatic phase imaging with multidetector row CT. Radiology 2003; 229:81-90.
6. Schima W, Ba-Ssalamah A, Kolblinger C, et al. Pancreatic adenocarcinoma. Eur Radiol 2007; 17:638-649.
7. Soriano A, Castells A, Ayuso C, et al. Preoperative staging and tumor resectability assessment of pancreatic cancer: prospective study comparing endoscopic ultrasonography, helical computed tomography, magnetic resonance imaging, and angiography. Am J Gastroenterol 2004; 99:492-501.
8. Irie H, Honda H, Kaneko K, et al. Comparison of helical CT and MR imaging in detecting and staging small pancreatic adenocarcinoma. Abdom Imaging 1997; 22:429-433.
9. Mehmet Erturk S, Ichikawa T, Sou H, et al. Pancreatic adenocarcinoma: MDCT versus MRI in the detection and assessment of locoregional extension. J Comput Assist Tomogr 2006; 30: 583-590.
10. Vargas R, Nino-Murcia M, Trueblood W, Jeffrey RB Jr. MDCT in pancreatic adenocarcinoma: prediction of vascular invasion and resectability using a multiphasic technique with curved planar reformations. AJR Am J Roentgenol 2004; 182:419-425.
11. Li H, Zeng MS, Zhou KR, et al. Pancreatic adenocarcinoma: the different CT criteria for peripancreatic major arterial and venous invasion. J Comput Assist Tomogr 2005; 29:170-175.
12. Mertz HR, Sechopoulos P, Delbeke D, Leach SD. EUS, PET, and CT scanning for evaluation of pancreatic adenocarcinoma. Gastrointest Endosc 2000; 52:367-371.
13. Birchard KR, Semelka RC, Hyslop WB, et al. Suspected pancreatic cancer: evaluation by dynamic gadolinium-enhanced 3D gradient-echo MRI. AJR Am J Roentgenol 2005; 185:700-703.
14. Schima W, Fugger R, Schober E, et al. Diagnosis and staging of pancreatic cancer: comparison of mangafodipir trisodium-enhanced MR imaging and contrast-enhanced helical hydro-CT. AJR Am J Roentgenol 2002; 179:717-724.
15. Fulcher AS, Turner MA, Capps GW, et al. Half-Fourier RARE MR cholangiopancreatography: experience in 300 subjects. Radiology 1998; 207:21-32.
16. Fukukura Y, Fujiyoshi F, Sasaki M, Nakajo M. Pancreatic duct: morphologic evaluation with MR cholangiopancreatography after secretin stimulation. Radiology 2002; 222:674-680.
17. Kostakoglu L, Agress H Jr, Goldsmith SJ. Clinical role of FDG-PET in evaluation of cancer patients. RadioGraphics 2003;23:315-340.
18. Bares R, Klever P, Hauptmann S, et al. F-18 fluorodeoxyglucose PET in vivo evaluation of pancreatic glucose metabolism for detection of pancreatic cancer. Radiology 1994; 192:79-86.
19. Ichikawa T, Sou H, Araki T, et al. Duct-penetrating sign at MRCP: usefulness for differentiating inflammatory pancreatic mass from pancreatic carcinomas. Radiology 2001; 221:107-116.
20. Wakabayashi T, Kawaura Y, Satomura Y, et al. Clinical and imaging features of autoimmune pancreatitis with focal pancreatic swelling or mass formation: comparison with so-called tumor-forming pancreatitis and pancreatic carcinoma. Am J Gastroenterol 2003; 98: 2679-2687.
21. Noone TC, Hosey J, Firat Z, Semelka RC. Imaging and localization of islet-cell tumours of the pancreas on CT and MRI. Best Pract Res Clin Endocrinol Metab 2005; 19:195-211.
22. Rockall AG, Reznek RH. Imaging of neuroendocrine tumours (CT/MR/US). Best Pract Res Clin Endocrinol Metab 2007; 21:43-68.
23. Kaltsas G, Rockall A, Papadogias D, et al. Recent advances in radiological and radionuclide imaging and therapy of neuroendocrine tumours. Eur J Endocrinol 2004; 151:15-27.
24. Law CH, Wei AC, Hanna SS, et al. Pancreatic resection for metastatic renal cell carcinoma: presentation, treatment, and outcome. Ann Surg Oncol 2003; 10:922-926.
25. Ghavamian R, Klein KA, Stephens DH, et al. Renal cell carcinoma metastatic to the pancreas: clinical and radiological features. Mayo Clin Proc 2000; 75:581-585.
26. Nayer H, Weir EG, Sheth S, Ali SZ. Primary pancreatic lymphomas: a cytopathologic analysis of a rare malignancy. Cancer 2004; 102:315-321.
27. Saif MW. Primary pancreatic lymphomas. JOP 2006; 7:262-273.
28. Psatha EA, Hyslop WB, Woosley JT, et al. Immunoblastic large B-cell lymphoma of the peripancreatic head region: MR findings. Magn Reson Imaging 2004; 22:1053-1057.
29. Chiou YY, Chiang JH, Hwang JI, et al. Acinar cell carcinoma of the pancreas: clinical and computed tomography manifestations. J Comput Assist Tomogr 2004; 28:180-186.
30. Tatli S, Mortele KJ, Levy AD, et al. CT and MRI features of pure acinar cell carcinoma of the pancreas in adults. AJR Am J Roentgenol 2005; 184:511-519.

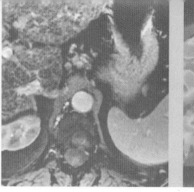
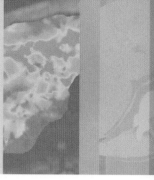

CHAPTER *76*

Cystic Lesions of the Pancreas

Onofrio Catalano and Dushyant V. Sahani

ETIOLOGY

Cystic lesions of the pancreas encompass a wide spectrum of different pathologic entities, ranging from developmental, to inflammatory, to neoplastic cysts. Neoplastic cystic lesions, which are the most important, owing to their profound impact on patient prognosis and the frequent necessity of surgical treatment, are described in detail in this chapter.

Although every pancreatic tumor may undergo central necrosis and presents predominantly cystic, the term *cystic neoplasm* properly refers to a cyst lined by a neoplastic epithelium, which identifies the tumor as a serous cystic neoplasm (SCN), mucinous cystic neoplasm (MCN), and intraductal papillary mucinous neoplasm (IPMN). These lesions account for more than 90% of the whole spectrum of cystic neoplasms. The remaining 10% are represented by neoplasms undergoing cystic degeneration, such as solid and pseudopapillary epithelial neoplasms (SPENs), cystic pancreatic endocrine neoplasms (CPENs), acinar cell cystoadenocarcinomas, cystic metastases, and few other even rarer tumors.[1,2]

PREVALENCE AND EPIDEMIOLOGY

Owing to the increased awareness, improved diagnostic imaging technology, and intensive use of diagnostic imaging, neoplastic cystic lesions of the pancreas have been increasingly diagnosed recently, often at smaller size than in the past and in asymptomatic patients. Therefore, their actual prevalence and size at presentation are not accurately reflected in the literature.

CLINICAL PRESENTATION

Most neoplastic pancreatic cysts are infrequently associated with any symptomatology, and several are inciden-

tally discovered during imaging for an unrelated medical problem. However, few patients can present with symptoms related to mass effect, such as abdominal pain, early satiety, vomiting, and jaundice or with symptoms due to obstruction or communication with the pancreatic duct, such as recurrent pancreatitis. Moreover, advanced cystic malignancies may present as pain, weight loss, and jaundice and be clinically indistinguishable from pancreatic adenocarcinoma.[1-4]

PATHOPHYSIOLOGY

Although lesions can occur in every portion of the pancreas, some histotypes tend to have a predilection for specific regions of the organ.

PATHOLOGY

Pathologic findings vary greatly, according to the specific type of cystic lesion.

IMAGING

The most commonly encountered neoplastic cystic lesions of the pancreas are represented by serous cystic neoplasms, mucinous cystic neoplasms, intraductal papillary neoplasms, solid and papillary epithelial neoplasms, and cystic pancreatic endocrine neoplasms.[1-4]

Radiography

Because of the poor soft tissue resolution, poor sensitivity, and low specificity of the modality, cystic lesions of the pancreas are usually not detected by conventional radiographic studies, unless late in their course when they are large enough to cause compression and displacement of surrounding structures or gastrointestinal obstruction.

Even in the uncommon event of cystic calcification, cross-sectional imaging is far more sensitive and specific than conventional radiographic studies. Therefore, nowadays, conventional radiography does not play any role in the diagnosis of cystic lesions of the pancreas.[1-5]

CT

Because of the widespread availability of multidetector CT (MDCT), its capability to image the whole abdomen and pelvis in a single breath-hold, the superb spatial and temporal resolutions, the nearly isotropic voxels obtainable with the current technology, and the robustness to breathing artifact, it is considered the mainstay of diagnostic imaging to assess patients with suspected pancreatic lesions. Moreover, aesthetically pleasing and clinically useful multiplanar reformatted images, including 3D and angiographic reconstructions of the MDCT data and MDCT-pancreatographic images, facilitate accurate preoperative staging.[1-5]

MRI

Although the role of MRI in assessing pancreatic malignancy is evolving, and new sequences allow faster imaging acquisition, some factors continue to limit its use as a first-line diagnostic tool for imaging of the pancreas. These factors are mainly related to the need of patients' cooperation to reduce motion and breathing artifacts, which can severely degrade and compromise the quality of the examination, the reduced availability of the technique on the territory, its inherent costs, and the more consolidated and widespread knowledge and experience with CT than with MRI.

Currently, MRI is used as a "problem solving" tool in patients with an inconclusive CT diagnosis. MRI can also be considered an alternative preoperative staging examination in patients who are allergic to iodinated contrast agents and in patients with renal insufficiency.

Because of an inherent high soft tissue contrast and resolution achieved with MRI, detection of subtle pancreatic lesions and evaluation of their internal details can be enhanced. Similar to CT, a 3D contrast-enhanced dynamic MR angiography can also be performed to map the regional vascular anatomy to enable assessment of vascular involvement from the tumor. In addition, MR cholangiopancreatography (MRCP) can allow excellent noninvasive visualization of the entire extrahepatic biliary tract and the pancreatic duct. When MRCP is used in combination with a dynamic MR examination of the pancreas, comprehensive preoperative imaging can be accomplished to facilitate detection and preoperative staging of the pancreatic malignancy.[1-6]

Ultrasonography

Transabdominal ultrasonography, which is a relatively inexpensive, noninvasive, and widely available modality, is highly operator dependent, nonreproducible, and limited by abdominal gas and patient body habitus. Endoscopic ultrasonography (EUS), on the other hand, provides high-resolution images of the pancreas and detailed assessment of cyst morphology. Moreover, EUS allows both aspiration of cystic fluid and sampling of cyst wall or mural nodules. Cystic fluid analysis can provide relevant insights into the nature of the cyst. Extracellular mucin or high viscosity usually favor mucinous neoplasms, whereas high amylase concentration, indicating a communication with the pancreatic duct, can be observed both in pseudocysts and in intraductal papillary mucinous neoplasms, with very high levels usually found in the case of pseudocysts. Moreover, tumor markers in the cystic fluid can render the diagnosis of malignancy feasible in selected cases.[1-5]

Nuclear Medicine

Nuclear medicine plays a role only in the case of functional endocrine tumors, whereby the use of a specific radiopharmaceutical can allow the diagnosis to be undertaken.

PET/CT

The role of PET/CT in the evaluation of cystic lesions of the pancreas is still under investigation. Usually, PET/CT is used as an additional imaging functional test to help differentiate benign from malignant neoplasms. In some studies it demonstrated a diagnostic accuracy as high as 83%, but larger studies are needed.[7]

Imaging Algorithm

The most used diagnostic imaging technique for cystic neoplasms of the pancreas are MDCT and MRI/MRCP, which provide high spatial and contrast resolution images and allow dynamic acquisition and postprocessing image reconstruction. Cyst morphology, relationships with the pancreatic duct, and ancillary findings can be evaluated, providing clues for diagnosis, management planning, and preoperative strategy.

MDCT and MRI have been demonstrated to be equally accurate in establishing the diagnosis of malignancy and in characterizing pancreatic cystic lesions.

Through MRCP and MDCT images and reconstructions, the entire course of the main pancreatic duct can be displayed and its relationships with the cystic lesion can be evaluated. If the patient is considered a surgical candidate, multiplanar image reconstructions displaying the extent of cystic lesions and their anatomic relationships to surrounding structures can be useful.

For selected cases, when MRCP and MDCT pancreatograms have been unable to provide the required information regarding cystic lesion relationships with the main pancreatic duct, invasive endoscopic retrograde cholangiopancreatography (ERCP) and/or EUS can be performed. The role of PET/CT is still under investigation.[1-6]

An ideal algorithm is shown in Figure 76-1; see also Table 76-1.

The different types of cystic lesions of the pancreas are described in the corresponding sections; the most important features are shown in Table 76-2.

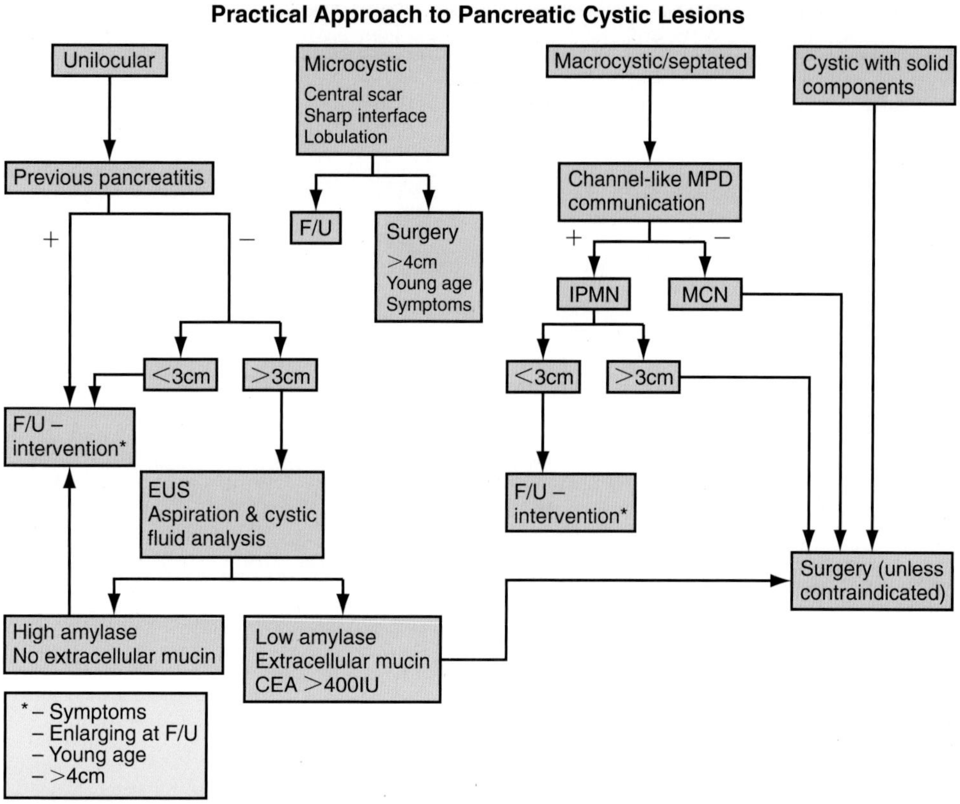

Practical Approach to Pancreatic Cystic Lesions

■ **FIGURE 76-1** Practical approach to diagnosis of cystic lesions in the pancreas. F/U, follow-up; EUS, endoscopic ultrasonography; CEA, carcinoembryonic antigen; MPD, main pancreatic duct; MCN, mucinous cystic neoplasm; IPMN, intraductal papillary mucinous neoplasm.

TABLE 76-1 Accuracy, Limitations, and Pitfalls of the Modalities Used in Imaging of Pancreatic Cysts

Modality	Accuracy	Limitations	Pitfalls
Radiography	Poor	Insensitive Nonspecific	Unable to directly visualize soft tissue masses in the pancreas
CT	80% malignant from benign lesions 100% SCN from MCN 90% SCN from IPMN 69.8%-81.1% IPMN from other lesions 56%-94.5% malignant MCN from benign lesions 43% in diagnosing histotype	Radiation exposure	20% of SCNs, usually when <3 cm, may appear solid on CT. Characterization of small cysts may be difficult. Small mural nodules not easy to be appreciated Difficulty in discriminating between carcinoma in situ and borderline or benign lesions.
MRI	Similar to CT, but in the case of IPMN higher accuracy than CT in differentiating IPMN from other lesions (86.8%-94.3%) More accurate than CT in evaluation of septa, small mural nodules, and duct communications	Patient cooperation High cost	Calcifications not well visualized Tumor can masquerade as nodule
Ultrasonography	Not assessed	Poor performance in the case of obesity or overlying bowel gas Operator dependent Comprehensive imaging difficult	SCN may present as solid lesions in the case of "honeycomb pattern." In IPMN, communication with main pancreatic duct difficult to appreciate
Nuclear medicine PET/CT	No utility unless functional PEN 83% in diagnosing malignancy Morphologic plus functional information Data limited; larger studies needed	Poor spatial resolution Radiation exposure High cost	Difficult differentiation of benign from borderline neoplasms

TABLE 76-2 Clinical and Radiologic Features of Cystic Neoplasms in the Pancreas

Factor	SCN	MCN	IPMN	SPEN	PEN	Pseudocysts	Cystic Adenocarcinoma
Sex	F > M	F	M > F	F	F = M	M > F	M > F
Age*	6th-7th decades	4th-5th decades	6th-7th decades	2nd-3rd decades	5th-6th decades	4th-6th decades	5th-7th decades
Location	Head/body/tail	Tail/body	Head/uncinate	Body/tail	No predilection	Head/tail/body	Head > body/tail
Shape and borders	Lobulated	Oval	Grape-like (branch) Focal or diffuse main pancreatic duct dilatation (main type) Both (combined)	Oval	Oval	Oval	Oval/irregular
Cystic appearance	Microcystic dense stroma	Macrocystic	Macrocystic or cystic with solid component	Cystic with solid component	Cystic with solid component	Unilocular	Cystic with solid component Septa uncommon
Size*	5-11 cm	6-10 cm	1-4 cm (branch type) >5 mm (main type)	5-9 cm	2-10 cm	4-8 cm	4-9 cm
Main pancreatic duct	Normal or rarely compressed	Normal or rarely compressed	Dilated	Normal	Normal	Normal (acute pancreatitis) Dilated (chronic pancreatitis)	Obstructed Upstream dilatation
Calcification	Central stellate in 30%	Peripheral/Septal	Intraductal (or in the case of mucin plug calcification)	Peripheral, nonlaminated	Sometimes	Parenchymal (chronic pancreatitis)	No
Signal intensity	T1 low T2 high	T1 high/low T2 high	T1 low/high T2 high	T1 high T2 high	T1 high/low T2 high	T1 low T2 high	T1 low T2 high
Wall	Occasionally thick	Uniformly thick, variable enhancement	Dilated	Thick, variable enhancement	Thick, strongly enhancing	Thin, occasionally thick	Thick, variable enhancement
Solid components	No Small (<3 cm) may appear solid	If malignant	If malignant	Yes	Yes	No	Yes
Clinical history	Noncontributory	Noncontributory	Noncontributory	Noncontributory	± Endocrine syndromes	Pancreatitis	Weight loss Back and abdominal pain Jaundice (head)

*Due to increased diagnostic imaging use and improved technology, lesions are currently discovered at a younger age and at a smaller size than reported in the literature.

What the Referring Physician Needs to Know: Pancreatic Cystic Lesions

■ Cysts may be difficult to differentiate on morphology alone.
■ Most important answers to be asked in the approach to cystic lesions in the pancreas are differentiation of:
   ● True cyst from pseudocyst
   ● Mucinous versus nonmucinous
   ● Benign versus malignant lesions

SPECIFIC LESIONS

Serous Cystic Neoplasms

Etiology

Biallelic inactivation of the von Hippel-Lindau (VHL) gene has been reported both for the sporadic and the VHL-associated form of SCNs.[1]

Prevalence and Epidemiology

SCNs, which account for 30% to 39% of all pancreatic cystic neoplasms, are slowly growing, benign lesions with a very low malignant potential. They occur predominant in women (75%), and the mean age at presentation is 62 years.[1-5]

Clinical Presentation

They are usually incidentally discovered, unless large enough to be responsible for compression of the surrounding organs.[1-5]

Pathophysiology

SCNs are usually discovered in the head (42%) or body/tail (48%), less often in the proximal body (7%) or diffusely through the pancreas (3%).[1-5]

Pathology

At gross pathology, SCNs present as large (average diameter, 2 to 11 cm), well-circumscribed, lobulated cystic masses that lack a capsule or a definite wall. SCNs do not communicate with the pancreatic duct and are devoid of peripheral wall calcifications. Cystic fluid is watery, without mucin.

SCNs are usually microcystic and, less commonly (10%), macrocystic/oligocystic. The classic microcystic SCNs have a "sponge-like" or "honeycomb"-like morphology, characterized by innumerable small cysts of a few millimeters in size. Larger cysts, if present, are less than 2 cm in diameter and peripheral. Microcystic SCNs tend to exhibit a central stellate fibrous scar, a feature considered specific for SCNs; they can present as stellate calcifications in about 30% of the cases. Macrocystic SCNs are composed of a countable number of larger cysts, between 2 and 7 cm, or even by a single large cyst and usually affect a younger population.

At histopathology, SCNs are lined by a monomorphic epithelium, made up of cuboidal or flat cells, rich in glycogen, that stain with periodic acid–Schiff.[1-5,8,9]

Imaging

SCNs are usually asymptomatic and incidentally discovered. Less often, in the case of large lesions, they may come to clinical attention because of mass-effect symptoms.[1-5,8,9]

Radiography

Because of the high spatial and contrast resolution and the added information provided by contrast administration to cross-sectional imaging, conventional radiography does not play a role in SCN evaluation.

CT

On both MDCT and MRI, the appearance of SCNs is similar to that of gross pathology. Fine, external lobulations and a central fibrous scar (Fig. 76-2), with a stellate pattern of calcification (Fig. 76-3), are suggestive. Enhancement of septa, cyst wall, and the central fibrous scar is best appreciated in the portal and delayed phases of contrast enhancement, respectively. The main pancreatic duct is normal unless compressed by a large SCN.

On MDCT, 20% of SCNs, due to a honeycombed microcystic composition, appear as well-defined, "spongy," soft tissue or mixed density lesions, sharply demarcated from

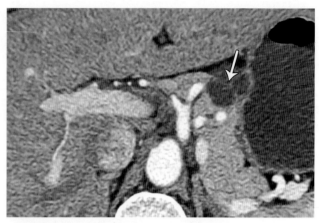

■ **FIGURE 76-2** Typical presentation of SCN in an axial contrast-enhanced MDCT image as a lobulated, microcystic lesion, with a central scar (*arrow*) and radiating septa.

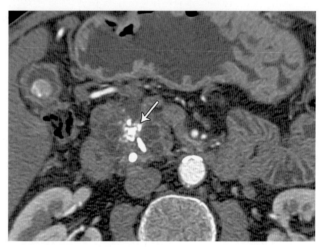

■ **FIGURE 76-3** Axial MDCT image shows the typical SCN with central stellate calcifications (*arrow*).

the adjacent structures and difficult to differentiate from a solid pancreatic mass on MDCT.[1-5,8,9]

MRI

The features of SCNs on MRI are very similar to those on MDCT. The main differences are in better detection of calcification on MDCT than on MRI and in improved visualization of cyst internal architecture and contrast enhancement by MRI. In the case of SCNs appearing solid on MDCT, MRI may provide useful insights into the microcystic nature of the lesions, revealing numerous discrete hyperintense cysts with bright signal on T2-weighted (T2W) sequences and allowing the correct diagnosis to be undertaken (Fig. 76-4).[1-5,8,9]

Ultrasonography

On transabdominal ultrasonography, owing to the innumerable acoustic interfaces of microcystic SCNs, they can present as hyperechoic, lobulated, sharply demarcated masses, lacking posterior acoustic enhancement. In the case of macrocystic/oligocystic SCNs, internal septa are visualized.

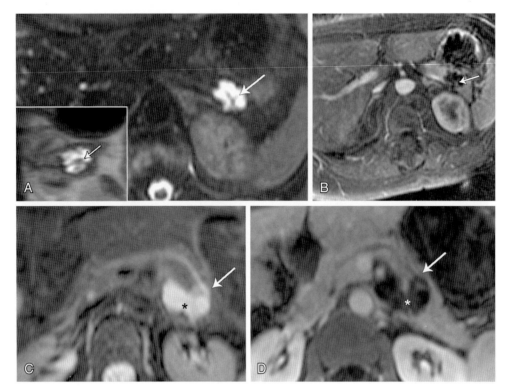

■ **FIGURE 76-4** **A**, Axial fat-suppressed T2W MR image demonstrates a typical SCN with external lobulations and a hypointense central scar (*arrow*). **B**, Note enhancement on postcontrast image. **C** and **D**, External lobulations of SCN may mimic BD-IPMN (*asterisk*), which can be differentiated by communication with the main pancreatic duct (*arrow*) and lack of a central scar.

TABLE 76-3 Accuracy, Limitations, and Pitfalls of the Modalities Used in Imaging of Serous Cystic Neoplasms

Modality	Accuracy	Limitations	Pitfalls
Radiography	Poor	Insensitive Nonspecific	Unable to directly visualize soft tissue masses in the pancreas
CT	100% SCN from MCN 90% SCN from IPMN	Radiation exposure	20% of SCNs, usually when <3 cm, may appear solid on CT. Characterization of small cysts may be difficult. Thin septa not easy to be appreciated
MRI	Although data are not available to specify accuracy, no relevant differences are expected between MRI and MDCT.	Patient cooperation High cost	Calcifications not well visualized
Ultrasonography	Data are not available to specify accuracy.	Poor performance in the case of obesity or overlying bowel gas Operator dependent Comprehensive imaging difficult	SCN may present as solid lesions in the case of "honeycomb pattern."
Nuclear medicine	Data not available to specify accuracy; no current role in diagnosis	Poor spatial resolution	
PET/CT	Data not available to specify accuracy	Radiation exposure High cost	

EUS, which can resolve the fine details of the internal structure of SCNs, is particularly useful in uncertain cases.[1-5,8,9]

PET/CT

Although there is no currently established role for PET/CT in the characterization of SCNs, based on our experience these lesions do not take up fluorodeoxyglucose (FDG). This could be a useful diagnostic finding in selected cases.

Imaging Algorithm

An imaging algorithm is provided in Figure 76-1; see also Table 76-3.

Classic Signs: Serous Cystic Neoplasms

- External lobulations
- More than six loculations, each less than 2 cm
- Central scar, with/without stellate calcifications
- Absence of communication with the main pancreatic duct

Differential Diagnosis

Clinical data usually are not helpful in discriminating SCNs from other cystic neoplasms of the pancreas. Lobulations, microcysts, and a central scar are present in the classic form of SCN and suggest the diagnosis.

Macrocystic SCNs are usually difficult to differentiate from mucinous cystic tumors, with which they share many morphologic features. However, external lobulations or a central scar support the diagnosis of SCN (Table 76-4 and Fig. 76-5).

More than six loculations, a loculation diameter less than 2 cm, a central scar, and absence of channel-like communication with the main pancreatic duct are useful to differentiate SCNs from branch duct IPMNs (Table 76-5).[1-5,8,9]

Treatment

Medical Treatment

Medical treatment is neither advocated nor available for SCNs.

Surgical Treatment

SCNs are usually regarded as benign, slowly growing lesions, with an estimated growth of 4 to 12 mm per year. The decision to operate is often based on size at presentation, patient age, clinical presentation, and location. In younger patients, owing to the increase in size over time, lesions larger than 4 cm are usually resected. In other cases the cysts should be observed with imaging at 6-month intervals for the first year, then annually for a

What the Referring Physician Needs to Know: Serous Cystic Neoplasms

- SCNs are regarded as benign lesions, usually occurring in asymptomatic middle-aged women.
- They may grow over time; therefore, if detected in young patients with a size at presentation greater than or equal to 4 cm, surgery is advocated; in other cases they should be observed by periodic imaging.
- MRI is the most accurate noninvasive diagnostic modality for SCNs.
- Macrocysts are difficult to characterize with imaging; therefore, if lobulations or a central scar is not detected, these patients should undergo EUS and/or biopsy.

TABLE 76-4 Differential Features between Macrocystic SCN and MCN

Feature	Macrocystic SCN	MCN
Sex	Female/Male (75%/25%)	Female almost exclusively
Age	6th-7th decades	4th-5th decades
Location	Head/body/tail	Body/tail 85%
Shape	Lobulated	Oval
Wall	Absent	Present, usually thick
Number of loculations	>6	<6
Coexisting microcysts (<2 cm)	Present	Absent
Central scar	May be found	Absent
Calcifications	Central if present	Peripheral

TABLE 76-5 Differential Features between SCN and BD-IPMN

Feature	SCN	BD-IPMN
Sex	Female/male (75%/25%)	Male > female (60%/40%)
Age	6th-7th decades	6th-7th decades
Morphology	Lobulated	Uncommonly lobulated
Scar	Central	Absent
Loculations	Smaller	Larger
Main pancreatic duct communication	No	Present

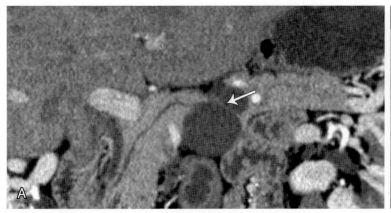
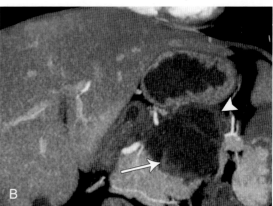

■ **FIGURE 76-5** Curved reformatted MDCT image (**A**) shows an oligocystic/macrocystic SCN with characteristic features of external lobulations and central scar (*arrow*) that needs to be differentiated from MCN (**B**), which lacks external lobulation and shows thick septa (*arrow*) and wall (*arrowhead*).

period of 3 years. If the cyst remains stable and the patient is symptom free, no further workup may be needed.[1-5,8,9]

KEY POINTS: SEROUS CYSTIC LESIONS

■ Benign
■ Microcysts
■ Lobulations
■ Central scar with or without calcification
■ Absence of solid components
■ No communication with main pancreatic duct

Mucinous Cystic Neoplasms

Etiology

Closeness of the left primordial gonad to the dorsal pancreatic anlage during the early stages of development, with the possibility that ovarian stroma can be incorporated into the developing pancreatic bud, has been suggested to play a role in the etiology of MCNs in the pancreas. This observation could explain the female occurrence and the predilection for the tail and body of the pancreas.[1]

Prevalence and Epidemiology

MCNs account for 10% to 45% of the cystic neoplasms of the pancreas and encompass a spectrum ranging from adenomas to invasive adenocarcinomas. They occur almost exclusively in middle-aged women (mean age, 47 years), with only extremely rare cases reported in men.[1,10]

Clinical Presentation

MCNs can be diagnosed incidentally in the case of small lesions, or, in the case of larger lesions, they may be responsible for mass-effect symptoms. In the setting of malignant MCNs, jaundice, weight loss, and abdominal pain may be present.[1,10]

Pathophysiology

MCNs are usually diagnosed in the tail (72%) or body of the pancreas (13%), and less frequently they replace the organ (9%) or are located in the pancreatic head (6%).[1,2,11-13]

Pathology

At gross pathology MCNs present as large (average diameter, 6 to 10 cm), round or oval cystic masses surrounded by a fibrous pseudocapsule, which may contain calcifications. Typically, they are multilocular and macrocystic and occasionally unilocular. Cystic fluid is thick and rich in mucin; hemorrhage may be present. They do not communicate with the pancreatic duct.

Benign MCNs have a smooth internal surface; on the other hand, malignant MCNs contain mural nodules, solid components, and/or papillary projections. Invasive adenocarcinomas are found in 33% of the cases.

At histology, the wall of MCNs contains an ovarian-like stroma that is considered specific for the diagnosis. The epithelial lining exhibits mucin-producing features and may display different degrees of dysplasia, according to which lesions are classified as adenomas, borderline tumors, or carcinomas.[1,2,13]

Imaging

MCNs are usually asymptomatic and incidentally discovered. Less often, in the case of large lesions or of malignant invasive neoplasms, they may come to clinical attention because of mass-effect symptoms or of signs and symptoms of pancreatic malignancy.[1,2,12,13]

Radiography

Because of the high spatial and contrast resolution and the added information provided by contrast administration to cross-sectional imaging, conventional radiography does not play a role in MCN evaluation.

CT

The complex architecture of the cysts is well depicted on both MDCT and MRI. MCNs present as multilocular (less than six loculations) macrocystic lesions, with individual compartments larger than 2 cm (Fig. 76-6). Hemorrhage and/or debris is uncommonly present. Infrequently, MCNs may present unilocular (Fig. 76-7). MCNs do not communicate with the pancreatic duct. Cystic fluid appears hypodense.

Peripheral eggshell or septal calcifications are an infrequent but specific finding for MCNs and are predictive of malignancy.

Differentiation of benign from malignant lesions is not always feasible on imaging, but some findings, such as wall thickening (see Fig. 76-7) or irregularity, mural nodules, papillary projections, and peripheral calcification, suggest malignant behavior.[2,10,11,13-16]

MRI

MRI, by virtue of superior soft tissue and contrast resolution, may better display the internal characteristics of MCN, including thin septa and mural nodules, if present, and their enhancement after administration of gadolinium.

The cystic fluid, owing to the high mucin content, appears hyperintense on T2W sequences and hypointense to minimally hyperintense on T1-weighted (T1W) sequences. Because of different mucin concentration, it is not unusual to observe differences in signal intensity among the different loculations (Fig. 76-8).

MRCP is particularly important to rule out communications with the main pancreatic duct (Table 76-6). Careful scrutiny of 3D MRCP raw data and of thin-section 2D MRCP is required.[2,10,11,13-16]

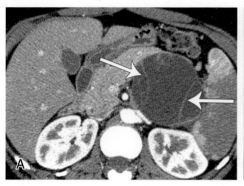 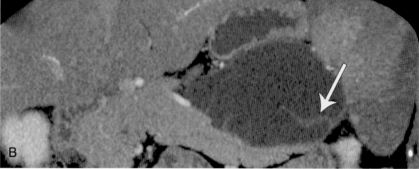

■ **FIGURE 76-6** Axial (**A**) and curved reconstructed (**B**) MDCT images show a typical MCN as a nonlobulated, oval cystic lesion (>2 cm) with enhancing internal septa (*arrows*). Note the lack of central scar.

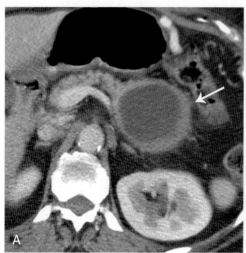 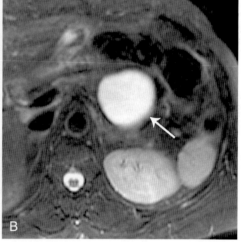

■ **FIGURE 76-7** Axial MDCT (**A**) and corresponding T2W MR image (**B**) show a thick fibrous wall (*arrow*) that is typical of unilocular MCN.

TABLE 76-6 Differential Features: MCN, BD-IPMN, and Pseudocysts

Feature	MCN	BD-IPMN	Pseudocysts
Sex	Female almost exclusively	Male > Female (60%/40%)	Male > female (68-78%/32-22%)
Location	Body/tail only	Head > body/tail	No preferences
Epicenter	Intra/extraparenchymal	Intraparenchymal	Extraparenchymal
Serum amylase	Normal	Normal	Elevated/normal
Loculations	Multilocular, less often oligolocular or unilocular	Multilocular, less often oligolocular or unilocular	Unilocular
Wall	Thick	Nondetectable	Detectable, can be thick in long-lasting cases
Main pancreatic duct communication	Absent	Present Channel-like configuration	Present but rarely seen on imaging Direct opening on pancreatic duct
Cystic fluid content	Mucin	Mucin	Hemorrhagic debris
Parenchyma	Normal	Normal	Often inflammatory changes, calcifications
History of pancreatitis	Negative/uncommon	Negative/uncommon	Positive

Ultrasonography

At transabdominal ultrasonography, MCNs tend to present as round or oval, well-defined multilocular cystic masses, circumscribed by a wall. The cystic components exhibit a variable degree of hypoechogenicity and of through-transmission. Dependent echoes, related to mucin and/or hemorrhage, may also be detected.

EUS is particularly useful to assess the internal architecture of the lesion, to rule out communications with the pancreatic duct, and to obtain fluid and tissue samplings for subsequent analysis. High extracellular levels of mucin and low amylase levels support the diagnosis of MCNs; a high carcinoembryonic antigen value and a high CA 19-9 are suggestive of malignant behavior.[1,2,15]

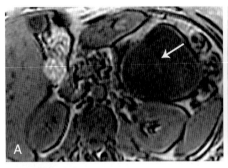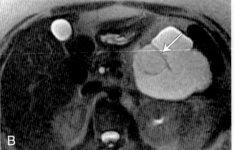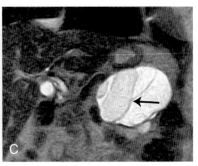

■ **FIGURE 76-8** Axial T1W (**A**) and axial (**B**) and coronal (**C**) T2W MR images show the typical MCN with internal septations (*arrow*) that are better appreciated on the T2W images.

TABLE 76-7 Accuracy, Limitations, and Pitfalls of the Modalities Used in Imaging of Mucinous Cystic Neoplasms of the Pancreas

Modality	Accuracy	Limitations	Pitfalls
Radiography	Poor	Insensitive Nonspecific	Unable to directly visualize soft tissue masses in the pancreas
CT	100% SCN from MCN 56%-94.5% malignant MCN from benign lesions	Radiation exposure	Characterization of small cysts may be difficult. Thin septa not easy to be appreciated
MRI	Although data are not available to specify accuracy, no relevant differences are expected between MRI and MDCT.	Patient cooperation High cost	Calcifications not well visualized Tumor can masquerade as nodule.
Ultrasonography	Data not available to specify accuracy	Poor performance in the case of obesity or overlying bowel gas Operator dependent Comprehensive imaging difficult	Difficult to rule out communication with main pancreatic duct
Nuclear medicine	Data not available to specify accuracy; no current role in diagnosis	Poor spatial resolution	
PET/CT	Data limited; larger studies needed to specify accuracy Morphologic plus functional information	Radiation exposure High cost	Difficult differentiation of benign from borderline neoplasms

PET/CT

Despite the limited data currently available on the role of PET/CT in MCNs, it appears that whereas FDG uptake strongly favors malignancy in cystic lesions, absence of uptake might suggest a benign tumor.

Imaging Algorithm

An imaging algorithm is provided in Figure 76-1; see also Table 76-7.

Classic Signs: Mucinous Cystic Neoplasms

- Oval lesions
- Identifiable wall
- Less than six loculations
- Loculations more than 2 cm in diameter
- No communication with the main pancreatic duct

Differential Diagnosis

The strong association with female sex and middle age at presentation help to differentiate MCNs from SCNs and IPMNs. The presence of a capsule and peripheral calcifications and the absence of communication with the pancreatic duct are useful differential signs from IPMNs (see Table 76-5 and Fig. 76-9).

Useful differentiating features include oval shape, capsule, and peripheral calcifications; absence of external lobulations; lack of a central scar; and less than six loculations, whose diameter is more than 2 cm (see Table 76-4). Absence of arterially enhancing rim/solid components is useful to exclude a CPEN. Absence of fluid-fluid levels and of blood degradation products helps to rule out SPEN.[2,10,11,13,15,16]

Treatment

Medical Treatment

Currently no medical treatment is indicated for MCNs, unless they are malignant, metastatic, or not able to be resected.

Surgical Treatment

Because of the malignant potential, relatively young age at presentation, and postoperative 5-year survival rate of 38%, even in the case of invasiveness, surgery is advocated in all the cases of MCNs, unless it is contraindicated for

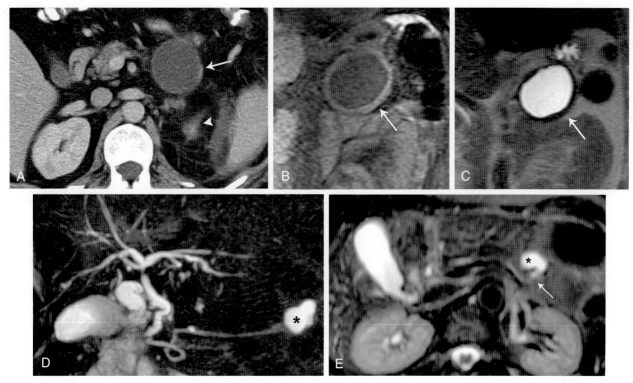

■ **FIGURE 76-9** **A,** Axial MDCT image demonstrating a pseudocyst in the tail of the pancreas that is predominantly extrapancreatic with adjacent inflammatory changes, indicated by *arrowhead*. These cystic lesions need to be differentiated from MCN, which is an intrapancreatic lesion (arrow, **B, C**) with thick walls and internal septations. Another differential diagnosis for this would be a BD-IPMN, which is seen as a cystic lesion (*asterisk*, **D, E**) communicating with the main pancreatic duct.

other reasons. Patients with MCNs without invasive features have excellent survival, and recurrence is rare.[1,2,12-16]

What the Referring Physician Needs to Know: Mucinous Cystic Neoplasms

- MCNs occur almost exclusively in young middle-aged women (30-50 years).
- All MCNs have malignant potential.
- Solid components, thick septa, and cyst size more than 5 cm are predictive of malignancy.
- Surgery is indicated, due to the relatively good survival, even in the case of invasiveness.

KEY POINTS: MUCINOUS CYSTIC NEOPLASMS

- Capsulated
- Oval
- Multilocular
- Macrocystic
- No communication with main pancreatic duct
- Malignant behavior suggested by peripheral calcifications, mural nodularity, solid areas, papillary projections, and FDG uptake

---

Intraductal Papillary Mucinous Neoplasms

Etiology

A large number of different genetic mutations have been reported in IPMNs, including inactivation of tumor suppressor genes, such as *TP53*, and activation of oncogenes, such as *KRAS*. Probably a multiple-step process is involved in the progression from hyperplasia to the invasive carcinoma.[1]

Prevalence and Epidemiology

IPMNs account for 21% to 33% of all pancreatic cystic neoplasms. They more often affect men (60%) and have a mean age at presentation of 65.5 years.

IPMNs are characterized by intraductal papillary growths of mucin-producing neoplastic cells. According to the site of involvement they are classified as main duct (MD) IPMNs, branch duct (BD) IPMNs, and combined IPMNs.[1,2,15-17]

Clinical Presentation

MD-IPMNs are usually symptomatic owing to low-grade pancreatitis, caused by thick mucin occluding the pancreatic duct. Jaundice can be found in the case of malignancy. BD-IPMNs are usually asymptomatic and incidentally detected.[1,2,15-17]

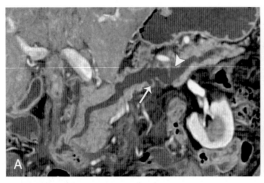
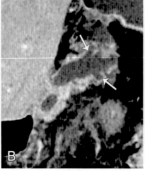
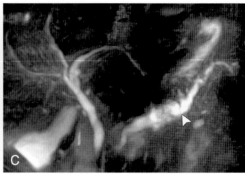

■ **FIGURE 76-10**   MDCT pancreatogram (**A**), MDCT miniP (**B**), and corresponding 2D-MRCP image (**C**) demonstrate MD-IPMN seen as segmental involvement of main pancreatic duct in the body and tail of pancreas (*arrowheads,* **A, C**) with associated dilated side branches (*arrows,* **A, B**) and proportional parenchymal atrophy.

Pathophysiology

MD-IPMNs usually occur in the head (58%) or body (23%) of the pancreas. In 12% of the cases the pancreas is diffusely involved, and in 7% of the cases the tail is affected. The pancreatic head and the uncinate process are the most common locations (about 60%) for BD-IPMN.[1,2,14-17]

Pathology

IPMNs tend to progress through an adenoma-carcinoma sequence and can exhibit a wide spectrum of biologic behaviors, ranging from hyperplasia to adenoma to carcinoma in situ to invasive carcinoma, which can coexist in the same patient.

MD-IPMNs usually produce thick mucin with resultant dilatation of the pancreatic duct, either focally or diffusely. In the case of long-standing processes, a low-grade obstruction with associated features of chronic pancreatitis can also result.

BD-IPMNs usually present as a single cyst or as grape-like communicating cysts, connected, through a channel-like conduit, to the pancreatic duct, which may be dilated. Cysts are in the range of 11 to 40 mm (median diameter, 20 mm); they are septated and contain fluid, mucin, and neoplastic cells.

Side-branch and main pancreatic duct lesions often coexist as independent or combined lesions.[1,2,15-22]

Imaging

MD-IPMNs are usually symptomatic, owing to low-grade pancreatitis. BD-IPMNs are usually asymptomatic and incidentally detected.[1,2,15-22]

Radiography

Because of the high spatial and contrast resolution and the added information provided by contrast agent administration to cross-sectional imaging, conventional radiography does not play a role in IPMN evaluation.

CT

On MDCT, MD-IPMNs exhibit diffuse or segmental dilatation of the main pancreatic duct, usually up to the papilla;

absence of a transition point; and proportional atrophy of the parenchyma (Fig. 76-10). The duodenal papilla may bulge. BD-IPMNs present as one or more lobulated and septated cystic lesions.

Channel-like communication with the pancreatic duct is a requisite for diagnosis, and it can be demonstrated through MDCT-pancreatographic reconstructions (Fig. 76-11).

Some imaging features are strong predictors of malignancy, including main pancreatic duct diameter exceeding 10 mm, nodules, and invasiveness. Moderate predictors of malignancy are side branch IPMNs greater than 4 cm, thick septa, and irregular walls (Fig. 76-12).[1,2,15-23]

MRI

MRI/MRCP in addition to providing the information obtainable through MDCT is characterized by a higher soft tissue and contrast resolution. Therefore, it is particularly

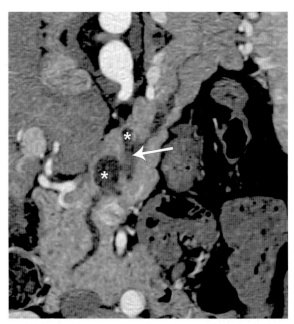

■ **FIGURE 76-11**   MDCT pancreatogram clearly shows multiple BD-IPMNs as cystic lesions (*asterisks*) in the pancreas, connected to the main pancreatic duct through channel-like conduits (*arrow*).

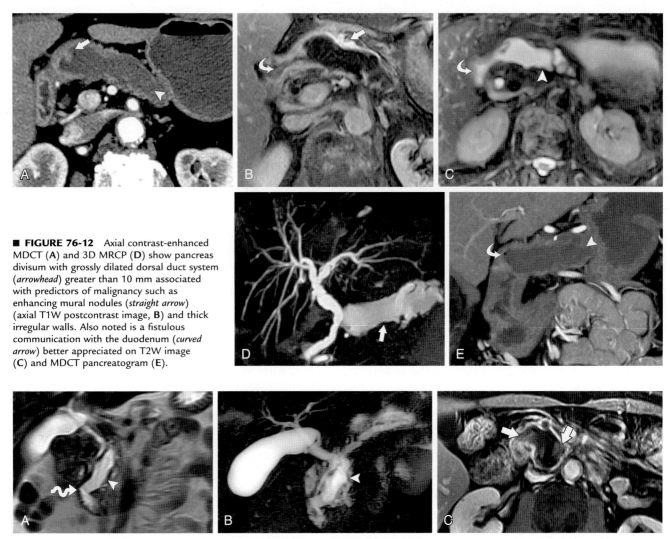

■ **FIGURE 76-12** Axial contrast-enhanced MDCT (**A**) and 3D MRCP (**D**) show pancreas divisum with grossly dilated dorsal duct system (*arrowhead*) greater than 10 mm associated with predictors of malignancy such as enhancing mural nodules (*straight arrow*) (axial T1W postcontrast image, **B**) and thick irregular walls. Also noted is a fistulous communication with the duodenum (*curved arrow*) better appreciated on T2W image (**C**) and MDCT pancreatogram (**E**).

■ **FIGURE 76-13** Coronal T2W (**A**), 2D MRCP (**B**), and axial T1W contrast-enhanced (**C**) images demonstrating MD diameter greater than 10 mm (*arrowhead*) and solid enhancing components (*arrows*) where the major papilla bulges into duodenum (*wavy arrow,* **A**). Features are representative of malignant MD-IPMN.

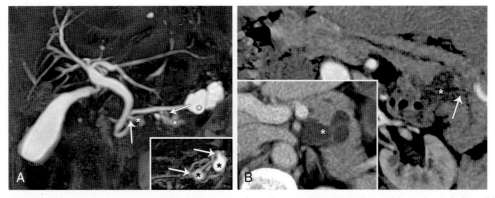

■ **FIGURE 76-14** 3D-MRCP (**A**) and reconstructed MDCT (**B**) images show the typical BD-IPMN (*asterisks*) as a cystic lesion with a channel-like communication with the main pancreatic duct (*arrows*). The communications are better appreciated on the reconstructed images seen in the *inset*.

useful to demonstrate septa, to assess neoplastic mural nodules, and to differentiate them from thick mucin or calcification. In fact, although they all present as areas of low signal intensity on T2W MR images, only neoplastic mural nodules enhance after gadolinium administration (Figs. 76-12 and 76-13).

Both MRCP and ERCP can show fine internal details. ERCP, due to mucus plugging, may be unable to demonstrate a channel-like communication between a BD-IPMN and the pancreatic duct (Fig. 76-14). Therefore, MRCP is the preferred initial modality to evaluate IPMNs.[1,2,6,14-24]

Ultrasonography

Evaluation of BD-IPMNs and MD-IPMNs is usually inadequate on ultrasonography. Imaging differentiation of MD-IPMN from other causes of pancreatic duct dilatation, or BD-IPMN from other pancreatic cystic lesions, is usually difficult. Likewise, papillary projections and mural nodules are difficult to be appreciated.

In the case of large volumes of thick mucin, the pancreatic duct may appear echogenic and indistinguishable from surrounding parenchyma. Therefore, the dilatation of the pancreatic duct may go unrecognized.

In BD-IPMNs, owing to the marked hypoechogenicity of the lesions, their cystic nature is usually demonstrated. On the other hand, communication with main pancreatic duct is difficult to be ascertained.[15]

PET/CT

The usefulness of PET/CT in the case of IPMNs has not been fully investigated at the present time. According to our experience, malignant IPMNs are more likely to exhibit FDG uptake than their benign counterpart, and this could play a role in management of the lesions in selected cases.

Imaging Algorithm

An imaging algorithm is provided in Figure 76-1; see also Table 76-8.

Classic Signs: Intraductal Papillary Mucinous Neoplasms

MD-IPMNs

■ Segmental or diffuse dilatation of the pancreatic duct, without areas of stenosis
■ Intraductal mural nodules
■ Proportional parenchymal atrophy
■ Side branch dilatation
■ Bulging of duodenal papilla with diffuse IPMN or head/uncinate process IPMN

BD-IPMNs

■ Grape-like cystic structure
■ Channel-like communication with the pancreatic duct
■ Intraparenchymal location, more often the head/uncinate process

---

Differential Diagnosis

In the case of BD-IPMNs, male sex is a useful differential feature from MCNs. In the case of BD-IPMNs, absence of clinically significant previous episodes of pancreatitis is useful to rule out postinflammatory pseudocysts. In MD-IPMNs, absence of alcohol consumption and of malabsorption may be contributing factors to rule out chronic pancreatitis.[1,2,10-16,19-22,24]

Absence of a transition point is a useful imaging criterion to rule out adenocarcinoma of the pancreas and to

---

TABLE 76-8 Accuracy, Limitations, and Pitfalls of the Modalities Used in Imaging of Intraductal Papillary Mucinous Neoplasms

Modality	Accuracy	Limitations	Pitfalls
Radiography	Poor	Insensitive Nonspecific	Unable to directly visualize soft tissue masses in the pancreas
CT	90% SCN from IPMN 69.8%-81.1% IPMN from other lesions	Radiation exposure	Characterization of small cysts may be difficult. Thin septa and small mural nodules not easy to be appreciated Difficulty in discriminating between carcinoma in situ and borderline and benign lesions
MRI	Similar to CT, but in the case of IPMN higher accuracy than CT in differentiating IPMN from other lesions (86.8%-94.3%) More accurate than CT in evaluation of septa, small mural nodules, and duct communications	Patient cooperation High cost	Calcifications not well visualized Tumor can masquerade as nodule.
Ultrasonography	Data not available to specify accuracy	Poor performance in the case of obesity or overlying bowel gas Operator dependent Comprehensive imaging difficult	In IPMN, communication with main pancreatic duct difficult to appreciate
Nuclear medicine	Data not available to specify accuracy; no current role in diagnosis	Poor spatial resolution	
PET/CT	Morphologic plus functional information Data limited; larger studies needed to specify accuracy	Radiation exposure High cost	Difficult differentiation of benign from borderline neoplasms

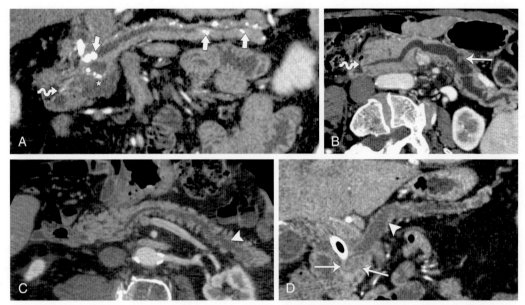

■ **FIGURE 76-15** Multiple reformatted MDCT images depicting the differential diagnosis for pancreatic duct (PD) dilatation. **A,** In chronic pancreatitis PD dilatation is associated with parenchymal atrophy out of proportion to ductal dilatation, ductal calculi (*arrows*), and lack of papillary bulge (*wavy arrow*). In IPMN either diffuse (**B**) or segmental IPMN (**C**) PD dilatation presents as proportional parenchymal atrophy without abrupt PD narrowing. Also in diffuse form, bulging papilla (*wavy arrow,* **B**) is seen. **D,** In adenocarcinoma PD dilatation presents as abrupt change in ductal diameter with a focal stenosis (*arrowhead*) and obstructing mass (*arrows*).

favor the diagnosis of an MD-IPMN. Absence of parenchymal calcifications and proportional atrophy of the parenchyma are suggestive findings of MD-IPMNs and are useful for the differential diagnosis with chronic pancreatitis (see Table 76-2).

Demonstration of a communication with the pancreatic duct is the most important imaging feature used to differentiate BD-IPMNs from other cystic lesions of the pancreas, including MCNs and SCNs (Tables 76-5, 76-6, and 76-9; Fig. 76-15).[1,2,10-24]

Treatment

Medical Treatment

Currently there is no medical treatment for IPMNs, unless they are malignant, metastatic, or nonresectable.

Surgical Treatment

The management of MD-IPMNs and BD-IPMNs is very different owing to their diverse risk of malignant degeneration and to the absence of symptoms in BD-IPMNs.

MD-IPMNs bear a high risk of malignancy (57% to 92%), and in 50% of the cases they show invasive features. Despite this, their 5-year survival rate is excellent (80%); and therefore surgery is usually advocated.

BD-IPMNs have lower risks of malignancy: 6% to 46% in lesions less than 3 cm. Moreover, about 85% of BD-IPMNs, if devoid of mural nodules, remain stable over time. Therefore, in the absence of clinical symptoms and of clinical/radiologic signs of malignancy, BD-IPMNs should undergo close observation.

Combined-IPMNs are regarded and treated as MD-IPMNs (Fig. 76-16).[1-3,16,17]

TABLE 76-9 Differential Features: Chronic Pancreatitis, MD-IPMN, Adenocarcinoma of the Pancreas

Feature	Chronic Pancreatitis	MD-IMPN	Adenocarcinoma
Sex	Male > Female (83%/17%)	Male > Female (60%/40%)	Male > Female (57%/43%)
Age	4th-7th decades	6th-7th decades	5th-7th decades
Location	Diffuse	Body/tail > head	Head > body/tail
Duct dilatation	Diffuse	Segmental: smooth return to normal caliber Diffuse: entire pancreatic duct until papilla	Dilatation upstream to the transition point
Obstructing mass/focal stenosis	Absent	Absent If mass present: small and nonobstructing	Present at site of transition
Intraductal lesions	Absent	Present	Absent
Papilla	Nonbulging	Bulging	Nonbulging
Calcifications	Parenchymal Ductal	Absent (unless coexistent chronic pancreatitis)	Absent
Parenchymal atrophy	Pronounced	Proportional	Mild, unless long lasting

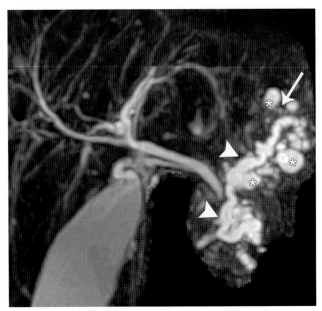

■ **FIGURE 76-16** 3D MRCP displays a typical combined IPMN lesion as diffuse dilatation of MD (*arrowheads*) and multiple cystic lesions (*asterisks*) due to BD-IPMN. Note channel-like communications (*arrow*) between BD-IPMN and main pancreatic duct.

What the Referring Physician Needs to Know: Intraductal Papillary Mucinous Neoplasms

- Because of the high risk of malignancy of MD-IPMNs, surgery is the treatment of choice.
- In the absence of signs of malignancy and of symptoms, BD-IPMNs can be closely observed.
- Combined IPMNs are treated as MD-IPMNs.

KEY POINTS: INTRADUCTAL PAPILLARY MUCINOUS NEOPLASMS

MD-IPMNs

- High risk of malignancy
- Diffusely dilated pancreatic duct without an obstruction point

BD-IPMNs

- More benign behavior
- Cystic lesions communicating with the main pancreatic duct through a channel-like conduit

Combined IPMNs

- Treated as MD-IPMNs

Predictors of Malignancy

- Main pancreatic duct diameter exceeding 9 mm, nodules, and invasiveness

---

Solid and Pseudopapillary Epithelial Neoplasms

Etiology

Mutations in exon 3 of the β-catenin gene have been found in almost all solid and pseudopapillary neoplasms of the pancreas (SPENs), probably interfering with the ubiquitin-mediated degradation of β-catenin proteins.[1]

Prevalence and Epidemiology

SPENs account for 9% of the cystic neoplasms of the pancreas. They usually have low malignant potential but can be locally aggressive. Metastases, although uncommon, have been reported to the liver and regional lymph nodes. They affect more often nonwhite, young (mean age, 27 years) women (78%).[1-3,25-26]

Clinical Presentation

Abdominal pain/discomfort and other symptoms related to mass effect are often present.[1-3,25-26]

Pathophysiology

SPENs usually present in the body/tail of the pancreas.[1-3,25-26]

Pathology

At gross pathology, SPENs present as a large (mean diameter, 5 to 9 cm), well-circumscribed mass. At cut section, an admixture of solid, cystic and papillary components, along with hemorrhagic and necrotic areas, is found. On histology, pseudopapillary architecture is observed.[1-2,25,26]

Imaging

SPENs are usually symptomatic owing to the large size they reach and the subsequent mass-effect symptoms.[1-3,25-26]

Radiography

Because of the high spatial and contrast resolution and the added information provided by contrast agent administration to cross-sectional imaging, conventional radiography does not play a role in SPEN evaluation.

CT

Because of the different proportion of solid and cystic areas in different tumors, the appearance of a SPEN greatly varies on MDCT from a solid mass to an almost cystic structure. The proportion of solid and cystic components dictates imaging features of SPENs on MDCT.

Peripheral calcifications, although present in a third of lesions on pathology, are uncommonly seen on imaging (Fig. 76-17).

Lesions are ill-defined if aggressive, and eventual liver metastases have similar morphology as the primary lesion.[25-27]

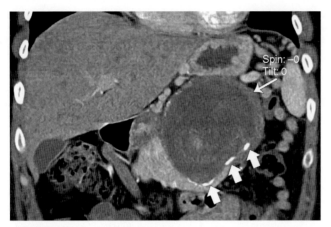

■ **FIGURE 76-17** Reformatted MDCT image showing a typical SPEN (*thin arrow*) as large, ovoid, predominantly cystic lesions in the body and tail of the pancreas. They appear heterogeneous due to the presence of solid, cystic, and hemorrhagic components. The wall can be calcified (*thick arrows*) in up to a third of the cases.

MRI

The MRI presentation of SPEN mirrors that observed on MDCT, although enhancement of solid components and internal hemorrhage are better seen. Hemorrhage, when present, can appear hyperintense on both T1W and T2W sequences, and internal fluid-debris levels can be suggestive, although nonspecific, findings.[25-27]

Ultrasonography

Evaluation of SPENs is usually inadequate on ultrasonography, and differentiation from other pancreatic cystic or solid lesions is usually difficult; therefore, cross-sectional imaging is usually the required next step in the diagnostic imaging protocol.

PET/CT

Because of the rarity of the disease and of relatively recent introduction of PET/CT in the clinical setting, the role of PET/CT in the case of SPENs has not been fully elucidated. According to a few published case reports and our experience, SPENs may show significant uptake of FDG, independently of their biologic behavior.

Imaging Algorithm

An imaging algorithm is provided in Figure 76-1; see also Table 76-10.

Classic Signs: Solid and Papillary Epithelial Neoplasms

- Young women (<30 years)
- Body/tail of pancreas
- Large lesions
- Solid and cystic components

Differential Diagnosis

Young age and female sex are suggestive of SPENs. Fluid-fluid levels and blood degradation products, although not invariably present, are typical of SPENs. Cystic pancreatic endocrine neoplasms, metastases, and adenocarcinomas of the pancreas enter in the differential diagnosis with SPENs (Fig. 76-18 and Table 76-11).

Treatment

Medical Treatment

Medical treatment is reserved for cases of advanced, metastatic SPENs.

Surgical Treatment

Because of their tendency to infiltrate locally and metastasize distally, the young age at presentation, and a 5-year survival rate of 95%, surgical treatment is advocated in all cases of SPENs, even in the cases of metastatic disease.[25,26]

TABLE 76-10 Accuracy, Limitations, and Pitfalls of the Modalities Used in Imaging of Solid and Pseudopapillary Epithelial Neoplasms

Modality	Accuracy	Limitations	Pitfalls
Radiography	Poor	Insensitive Nonspecific	Unable to directly visualize soft tissue masses in the pancreas
CT	Data not available to specify accuracy	Radiation exposure	Characterization of small cysts may be difficult. Thin septa and small mural nodules not easy to be appreciated
MRI	Data not available to specify accuracy	Patient cooperation High cost	Calcifications not well visualized Tumor can masquerade as nodule.
Ultrasonography	Data not available to specify accuracy	Poor performance in the case of obesity or overlying bowel gas Operator dependent Comprehensive imaging difficult	Small lesions may be undetected.
Nuclear medicine	Data not available to specify accuracy	Poor spatial resolution	
PET/CT	Morphologic plus functional information Data limited; larger studies needed to specify accuracy.	Radiation exposure High cost	Difficult differentiation of benign from borderline neoplasms

TABLE 76-11 Differential Features between SPEN, PEN, Metastases, and Adenocarcinoma of the Pancreas

Feature	SPEN	PEN	Metastases (Kidney, Breast)	Adenocarcinoma
Sex	Female > male (78%/22%)	Male = female	Male/female (33%-85%/ 67%-15%)	Male > Female (57%/43%)
Age	2nd-3rd decades	5th-6th decades	5th-7th decades	5th-7th decades
Morphology	Solid and cystic-necrotic areas	Rarely necrotic Septa can be present Thick rind	Rarely necrotic Thick rind	Solid, central necrosis may be present If colloid, predominantly cystic
Main pancreatic duct changes	Typically absent	Usually absent	Absent/mild prominence	Dilated until obstruction point
Fluid content	Hemorrhagic debris (Fluid-fluid level, high T1W)	Necrotic	Necrotic	Necrotic
Contrast enhancement	Moderate	Usually intense	Intense/moderate	Poor
Endocrine abnormalities	Absent	Nonfunctional 70% Functional neoplasms 30%	Absent	Absent
History of previous malignancies	Negative	Negative/positive (MEN)	Positive	Negative

---

What the Referring Physician Needs to Know: Solid and Pseudopapillary Epithelial Neoplasms

- Young women (usually <30 years) are affected.
- Even in the case of metastatic or locally advanced disease, surgery is advocated.

KEY POINTS: SOLID AND PSEUDOPAPILLARY EPITHELIAL NEOPLASMS

- Young women (usually < age 30 years)
- Heterogeneous appearance
- Variable imaging appearance based on different proportion of solid and cystic areas
- Fluid-fluid levels when hemorrhagic
- Hemorrhagic products

Cystic Pancreatic Endocrine Neoplasm

Etiology

Many different chromosomal losses have been reported in pancreatic endocrine neoplasms (PENs); some of them are associated with more aggressive biologic behavior. Usually larger PENs harbor more genetic alterations than smaller lesions.[1]

Prevalence and Epidemiology

PENs, in the case of insufficient blood supply, may undergo necrosis, hemorrhage, and cystic degeneration, resulting in cystic PENs (CPENs), which account for 2% of all pancreatic cystic lesions.

CPENs occur at about the same rate in men and women, at a mean age of 55 years. They may be single or multiple, and solid PENs may coexist. They may be part of multiple endocrine neoplasia (MEN) syndromes.[1,2,28]

Clinical Presentation

They can be functional, if associated with hormonal overproduction, or more often nonfunctional. Actually about 30% of the nonfunctional endocrine neoplasms present cystic.[1,2,28]

Pathophysiology

These lesions tend to be located in the body/tail of the pancreas.[1,2,28]

Pathology

CPENs present as solid neoplasms with cystic degenerations or as a thick-walled cyst, between 2 and 10 cm (median, 3.7 cm). No correlation has been proven between the proportion of cystic and solid components and the biologic behavior. At histology they match the appearance of the corresponding noncystic PEN.[1,2,28]

Imaging

CPENs may be functional and come to clinical attention because of hormonal associated symptoms when still at early stages and small at presentation, or they may be nonfunctional and asymptomatic. In the latter case, they can be discovered incidentally or, more often, when large enough to cause mass-effect symptoms.[1,2,28,29]

Radiography

Because of the high spatial and contrast resolution and the added information provided by contrast agent administration to cross-sectional imaging, conventional radiography does not play a role in SCN evaluation.

CT

On MDCT, CPENs present as mixed solid-cystic masses (Figs. 76-18, 76-19, and 76-20) or as well-defined, unilocular cysts with thick walls. Internal septations, if present,

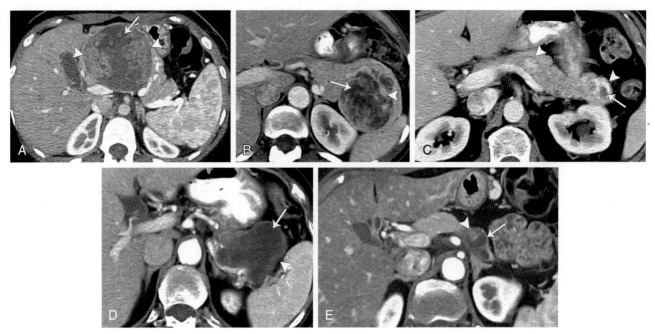

■ **FIGURE 76-18** Differential diagnosis, axial contrast-enhanced MDCT images: SPEN (**A**), CPEN (**B**), cystic metastases (**C**), oncocytic adenocarcinoma (**D**), and cystic adenocarcinoma (**E**). These neoplasms can appear strikingly similar on diagnostic imaging, showing a mixture of cystic (*arrows*) and solid elements (*arrowheads*). Age, sex, clinical features, morphology, and pancreatic duct changes can be helpful to narrow the differential diagnosis. Usually, biopsy is necessary.

■ **FIGURE 76-19** CPEN, classic features. CPEN may present as large cystic lesions with solid components (*arrows*), demonstrating arterial enhancement, as shown on this MDCT image.

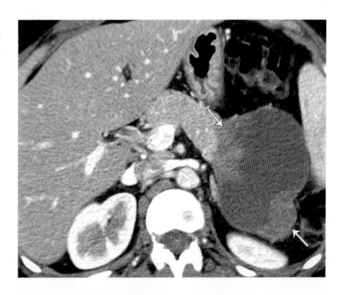

■ **FIGURE 76-20** CPEN, classic features. Typically, CPENs (*arrow*) present as cystic lesions with thick walls and/or solid components, demonstrating intense arterial enhancement, as shown on the MDCT (**A**) and the corresponding MR (**B**) images.

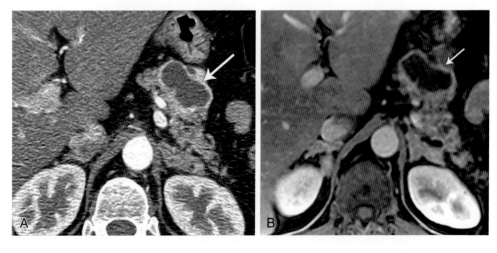

tend to be thick. The intense contrast enhancement of the solid portions of the cystic lesions (wall, solid nodules, septations) is the most important differential imaging feature. However, this finding is not invariably present.[2,3,28,29]

MRI

MRI features closely parallel those found on MDCT, with the added benefit of superior soft tissue and contrast resolution.[2,3,28,29]

Ultrasonography

When the quality of transabdominal ultrasonography is adequate, CPENs tend to present as thick-walled cystic lesions or as solid lesions with cystic areas. In the case of contrast-enhanced ultrasonography, the solid components exhibit strong enhancement.

Nuclear Medicine

Nuclear medicine, using specific radiopharmaceuticals, has a role in the evaluation of functional cystic neoplasms of the pancreas.

PET/CT

Although FDG uptake is poor in well-differentiated neuroendocrine tumors, it is increased in less-differentiated tumors, in lesions with high proliferative activity, and in metastasizing neoplasms. The use of new radiopharmaceuticals, such as ^{11}C-labeled 5-hydroxytryptophan (5-HTP) and L-dihydroxyphenylalanine (L-DOPA), seems promising in the detection of primary and metastatic PEN.[30]

Imaging Algorithm

An imaging algorithm is provided in Figure 76-1; see also Table 76-12.

Classic Signs: Cystic Pancreatic Endocrine Neoplasm

- Solid and cystic components, thick rind
- Strongly enhancing solid components

Differential Diagnosis

In the case of hyperfunctional tumors, clinical and laboratory data may aid in the final diagnosis.[1-3,28-30] Arterially hyperenhancing rim/solid components, although not invariably present, are suggestive of CPEN (see Table 76-11).[28-29]

Treatment

Medical Treatment

Advanced cancers, not amenable to surgical treatment, can be treated with chemotherapy.

Surgical Treatment

Despite the fact that about 80% of CPENs are nonmalignant and nonfunctional, they can be locally invasive and can also metastasize to the liver and regional lymph nodes. Therefore, surgery represents the treatment of choice. The 5-year survival rate is 96%.[28,29]

What the Referring Physician Needs to Know: Cystic Pancreatic Endocrine Neoplasm

- Surgery represents the treatment of choice.
- Solid and cystic components are seen.

TABLE 76-12   Accuracy, Limitations, and Pitfalls of the Modalities Used in Imaging of Cystic Pancreatic Endocrine Neoplasm

Modality	Accuracy	Limitations	Pitfalls
Radiography	Poor	Insensitive Nonspecific	Unable to directly visualize soft tissue masses in the pancreas
CT	Specific data regarding CPEN not available to specify accuracy	Radiation exposure	Characterization of small cysts may be difficult. Thin septa and small mural nodules not easy to be appreciated Difficult discriminating between carcinoma in situ and borderline and benign lesions
MRI	Specific data regarding CPEN not available to specify accuracy	Patient cooperation High cost	Calcifications not well visualized Tumor can masquerade as nodule
Ultrasonography	Specific data regarding CPEN not available to specify accuracy	Poor performance in the case of obesity or overlying bowel gas Operator dependent Comprehensive imaging difficult	Small lesions may be undetected.
Nuclear medicine	Specific data regarding CPEN not available to specify accuracy; can be useful in the case of functional CPEN	Poor spatial resolution	
PET/CT	Specific data regarding CPEN not available to specify accuracy	Radiation exposure High cost	Difficult differentiation of benign from borderline neoplasms

> ## KEY POINTS: CYSTIC PANCREATIC ENDOCRINE NEOPLASM
>
> - Occurs in mid life (usually < age 50 years)
> - 70% of nonfunctional tumors
> - Solid and cystic areas
>
> - Arterially enhancing solid components and/or peripheral rind

SUGGESTED READINGS

Brugge WR, et al. Cystic neoplasms of the pancreas. N Engl J Med 2004; 351:1218-1226.

Demos TC, Posniak HV, Harmath C, et al. Cystic lesions of the pancreas. AJR Am J Roentgenol 2002; 179:1375-1388.

Lim JH, Lee G, Oh YL. Radiologic spectrum of intraductal papillary mucinous tumor of the pancreas. RadioGraphics 2001; 21:323-337; discussion 337-340.

Mittendorf EA, Shifrin AL, Inabnet WB, et al. Islet cell tumors. Curr Probl Surg 2006; 43:685-765.

Noone TC, Hosey J, Firat Z, Semelka RC. Imaging and localization of islet-cell tumours of the pancreas on CT and MRI. Best Pract Res Clin Endocrinol Metab 2005; 19:195-211.

Sahani D, Prasad S, Saini S, Mueller P. Cystic pancreatic neoplasms evaluation by CT and magnetic resonance cholangiopancreatography. Gastrointest Endosc Clin North Am 2002; 12:657-672.

Sahani DV, et al. Cystic pancreatic lesions: a simple imaging-based classification system for guiding management. RadioGraphics 2005; 25:1471-1484.

Sarr MG, et al. Primary cystic neoplasms of the pancreas: neoplastic disorders of emerging importance—current state-of-the-art and unanswered questions. J Gastrointest Surg 2003; 7:417-428.

Sheehan MK, Beck K, Pickleman J, Aranha GV. Spectrum of cystic neoplasms of the pancreas and their surgical management. Arch Surg 2003; 138:657-660; discussion 660-662.

Tanaka M. Intraductal papillary mucinous neoplasm of the pancreas: diagnosis and treatment. Pancreas 2004; 28:282-288.

REFERENCES

1. Hruban RH, Pitman Bishop M, Klimstra DS. Tumors of the pancreas. In Armed Forces Institute of Pathology. Atlas of Tumor Pathology, 4th series. Washington, DC, AFIP, 2007, pp 33-376.
2. Brugge WR, et al. Cystic neoplasms of the pancreas. N Engl J Med 2004; 351:1218-1226.
3. Sahani DV, et al. Cystic pancreatic lesions: a simple imaging-based classification system for guiding management. RadioGraphics 2005; 25:1471-1484.
4. Sheehan MK, Beck K, Pickleman J, Aranha GV. Spectrum of cystic neoplasms of the pancreas and their surgical management. Arch Surg 2003; 138:657-660; discussion 660-662.
5. Galanis C, et al. Resected serous cystic neoplasms of the pancreas: a review of 158 patients with recommendations for treatment. J Gastrointest Surg 2007; 11:820-826.
6. Irie H, et al. MR cholangiopancreatographic differentiation of benign and malignant intraductal mucin-producing tumors of the pancreas. AJR Am J Roentgenol 2000; 174:1403-1408.
7. Sperti C, et al. F-18-fluorodeoxyglucose positron emission tomography in differentiating malignant from benign pancreatic cysts: a prospective study. J Gastrointest Surg 2005; 9:22-28; discussion 28-29.
8. Goh BK, et al. Pancreatic serous oligocystic adenomas: clinicopathologic features and a comparison with serous microcystic adenomas and mucinous cystic neoplasms. World J Surg 2006; 30:1553-1559.
9. Carbognin GT, Petrella M, Fuini E, Procacci A. Serous cystic tumors. In Procacci AJ, Megibow AJ (eds). Imaging of the Pancreas: Cystic and Rare Tumors. Berlin, Springer, 2003, pp 31-55.
10. Sarr MG, et al. Primary cystic neoplasms of the pancreas: neoplastic disorders of emerging importance—current state-of-the-art and unanswered questions. J Gastrointest Surg 2003; 7:417-428.
11. Scott J, et al. Mucinous cystic neoplasms of the pancreas: imaging features and diagnostic difficulties. Clin Radiol 2000; 55:187-192.
12. Goh BK, et al. A review of mucinous cystic neoplasms of the pancreas defined by ovarian-type stroma: clinicopathological features of 344 patients. World J Surg 2006; 30:2236-2245.
13. Zamboni G, et al. Mucinous cystic tumors of the pancreas: clinicopathological features, prognosis, and relationship to other mucinous cystic tumors. Am J Surg Pathol 1999; 23:410-422.
14. Suzuki Y, et al. Cystic neoplasm of the pancreas: a Japanese multi-institutional study of intraductal papillary mucinous tumor and mucinous cystic tumor. Pancreas 2004; 28:241-246.
15. Biasiutti CF, Venturini F, Pagnotta N, et al. Mucinous cystic tumors. In Procacci AJ, Megibow AJ (eds). Imaging of the Pancreas: Cystic and Rare Tumors. Berlin, Springer, 2003, pp 57-74.
16. Tanaka M, et al. Clinicopathologic study of intraductal papillary-mucinous tumors and mucinous cystic tumors of the pancreas. Hepatogastroenterology 2006; 53:783-787.
17. Tanno S, Nakano Y, Nishikawa T, et al. Natural history of branch duct intraductal papillary-mucinous neoplasms of the pancreas without mural nodules: long-term follow-up results. Gut 2008; 57:339-343.
18. Lim JH, Lee G, Oh YL. Radiologic spectrum of intraductal papillary mucinous tumor of the pancreas. RadioGraphics 2001; 21:323-337; discussion 337-340.
19. Loftus EV Jr, et al. Intraductal papillary-mucinous tumors of the pancreas: clinicopathologic features, outcome, and nomenclature. Members of the Pancreas Clinic, and Pancreatic Surgeons of Mayo Clinic. Gastroenterology 1996; 110:1909-1918.
20. Pais SA, et al. Role of endoscopic ultrasound in the diagnosis of intraductal papillary mucinous neoplasms: correlation with surgical histopathology. Clin Gastroenterol Hepatol 2007; 5:489-495.
21. Tanaka M. Intraductal papillary mucinous neoplasm of the pancreas: diagnosis and treatment. Pancreas 2004; 28:282-288.
22. Tanaka M, et al. Clinical aspects of intraductal papillary mucinous neoplasm of the pancreas. J Gastroenterol 2005; 40:669-675.
23. Taouli B, et al. Intraductal papillary mucinous tumors of the pancreas: helical CT with histopathologic correlation. Radiology 2000; 217:757-764.
24. Procacci CS, Schenal G, Chiara ED, Fuini A, Guarise A. Intraductal papillary mucinous tumors: imaging. In Procacci C, Megibow AJ (eds). Imaging of the Pancreas: Cystic and Rare Tumors. Berlin, Springer, 2003, pp 97-137.
25. Geers C, et al. Solid and pseudopapillary tumor of the pancreas—review and new insights into pathogenesis. Am J Surg Pathol 2006; 30:1243-1249.
26. Hernandez JM, Centeno BA, Kelley ST. Solid pseudopapillary tumors of the pancreas: case presentation and review of the literature. Am Surg 2007; 73:290-293.
27. Casadei R, et al. Pancreatic solid-cystic papillary tumor: clinical features, imaging findings and operative management. JOP 2006; 7:137-144.
28. Goh BK, et al. Clinico-pathological features of cystic pancreatic endocrine neoplasms and a comparison with their solid counterparts. Eur J Surg Oncol 2006; 32:553-556.
29. Ligneau B, et al. Cystic endocrine tumors of the pancreas: clinical, radiologic, and histopathologic features in 13 cases. Am J Surg Pathol 2001; 25:752-760.
30. Bombardieri E, Maccauro M, De Deckere E, et al. Nuclear medicine imaging of neuroendocrine tumours. Ann Oncol 2001; 12(Suppl 2):51-61.

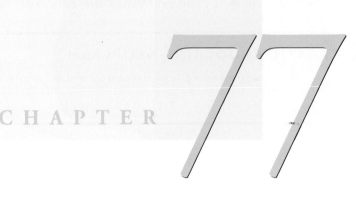
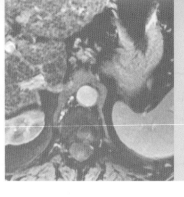
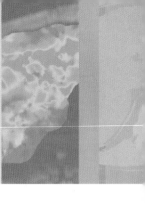

CHAPTER 77

Imaging of Acute Pancreatitis

Anuradha S. Rebello and Dushyant V. Sahani

ETIOLOGY

Acute pancreatitis is an acute inflammatory disorder of the pancreas that has numerous causes (Table 77-1). The most common risk factors are chronic alcohol consumption and choledocholithiasis.[1] In 20% of cases no cause can be found.[1]

PREVALENCE AND EPIDEMIOLOGY

In the United States, up to 210,000 patients per year are admitted to a hospital for acute pancreatitis.[2] The spectrum of acute pancreatitis ranges from mild to severe and fatal.

In 1992, the International Symposium on Acute Pancreatitis in Atlanta, Georgia, established a clinical-based classification and defined certain terminologies commonly associated with acute pancreatitis.[3] Acute pancreatitis is classified as *mild* and *severe* based on the presence of local complications and organ failure.[3,4] This classification helped identify patients with severe disease who required close monitoring and intensive unit care. Mild acute pancreatitis has a mortality rate of less than 1%, whereas the death rate for severe pancreatitis is much higher: 10% with sterile and 30% with infected pancreatic necrosis.[1]

CLINICAL PRESENTATION

The hallmark symptom of acute pancreatitis is the acute onset of persistent upper abdominal pain, usually with nausea and vomiting. The pain may radiate to the back, chest, flanks, and lower abdomen. Physical examination findings include fever, hypotension, severe abdominal tenderness, guarding, respiratory distress, and abdominal distention.[2]

PATHOPHYSIOLOGY

The inflammatory process in acute pancreatitis is triggered by the premature activation of pancreatic enzymes with resultant autodigestion of the pancreatic paren-

chyma. The inflammatory process may remain localized to the pancreas, spread to regional tissues, or even involve remote organ systems, resulting in multiple organ failure and occasionally death.

Mild acute pancreatitis (also known as interstitial or edematous pancreatitis) is more common and a self-limiting disease with minimal organ dysfunction and an uneventful recovery. Pathologically, the mild form of acute pancreatitis is characterized by interstitial edema and infrequently by microscopic areas of parenchymal necrosis.[3]

Severe acute pancreatitis (also known as necrotizing pancreatitis) occurs in 20% to 30% of all patients and is associated with organ failure and/or local complications, such as necrosis, abscess, or pseudocyst.

PATHOLOGY

Pathologic findings include macroscopic areas of focal or diffuse pancreatic necrosis, fat necrosis, and hemorrhage in the pancreas and peripancreatic tissues.[3]

IMAGING

CT and abdominal ultrasonography are routinely used in the setting of an acute abdomen to identify the source of pain.[5] Both these imaging modalities help in confirming the diagnosis of acute pancreatitis and exclude other causes of acute abdomen such as gastrointestinal perforation, acute cholecystitis, acute aortic dissection, and mesenteric artery occlusion, which can clinically mimic acute pancreatitis. In established cases of acute pancreatitis, contrast-enhanced CT is considered the gold standard for evaluating morphologic changes of acute pancreatitis, particularly in the assessment of pancreatic necrosis.[3,6] MRI with MR cholangiopancreatography (MRCP), endoscopic retrograde cholangiopancreatography (ERCP), endoscopic ultrasonography, and angiography have specific indications in a patient with known acute pancreatitis.

TABLE 77-1 Causes of Acute Pancreatitis
Gallstones (45%)
Alcohol (35%)
Others (10%)
Medications
Hypercalcemia
Hypertriglyceridemia
Duct obstruction (e.g., tumor)
Post ERCP
Hereditary
Trauma
Viral
Post cardiac bypass
Idiopathic (10%-20%)

TABLE 77-2 CT Parameters

	Vascular Phase (40-45 s)	Portal Venous Phase (65-70 s)
Intravenous Contrast Range	4-5 cm³/s Celiac through entire pancreas	3 cm³/s Dome of diaphragm to symphysis pubis
Automated Bolus Tracking	+ (150-HU threshold in the aorta at the level of celiac artery and 8- to 10-s diagnostic delay)	+ (55-HU threshold in the right lobe of liver at the level of the right portal vein)
Slice Thickness	1-3 mm	5 mm
Spacing	1-3 mm	5 mm
Kilovoltage peak	120-140	120-140
Milliamperage	240-280	240-280
Time	0.5-0.8 s	0.5-0.8 s
Field of View	28	Based on size of patient

Radiography

Plain abdominal radiographs can be completely normal in patients with acute pancreatitis. Air in the duodenal C-loop, a "sentinel loop" (focally dilated jejunal loop in the left upper quadrant) or the "colon cutoff" sign (distention of the colon to the transverse colon with a paucity of gas distal to the splenic flexure) may be seen on plain radiographs in patients with pancreatitis. However, these findings are never specific enough to confirm the diagnosis.

Barium or water-soluble contrast studies of the gastrointestinal tract have no role except in the rare case of suspected colonic fistula, which can develop late in the course of the disease.

CT

Role of CT in Acute Pancreatitis

CT can establish the diagnosis of acute pancreatitis. It helps in determining the underlying cause of acute pancreatitis (identifies choledocholithiasis and biliary ductal dilatation associated with biliary pancreatitis). It grades the severity of the disease and detects complications such as pancreatic necrosis, abscess, or pseudocysts. CT also serves as an imaging modality when percutaneous interventions are performed.

When Is the Optimal Time to Perform CT?

CT is not necessary in a patient with a clinical diagnosis of mild acute pancreatitis, especially if the clinical course improves. In established cases of severe acute pancreatitis, contrast-enhanced CT helps in grading the severity of the disease and in determining the extent of necrosis. Because necrotic areas of pancreatic parenchyma become better defined 2 to 3 days after the onset of symptoms, contrast-enhanced CT performed 48 to 72 hours after the onset of an acute attack gives more reliable information. CT findings can be equivocal if the scan is obtained during the initial 12 hours.[6]

Scanning Technique

Multidetector CT scanners allow high-resolution, multiphase imaging of the pancreas performed using short scanning times. Table 77-2 depicts the CT scanning parameters used in our institution.[7]

A single-phase contrast-enhanced CT in the portal venous phase (approximately 70 seconds after the injection of intravenous contrast) is usually adequate to make the diagnosis and assess the complications of acute pancreatitis. Normal pancreatic tissue should demonstrate homogeneous increase in attenuation to 100 to 150 HU after contrast agent administration. Lack of contrast enhancement or minimal contrast enhancement of less than 30 HU of a portion of the pancreas or the entire pancreas indicates decreased blood perfusion and necrosis.[6] Precontrast attenuation of the pancreas is 40 to 50 HU. Because unenhanced CT is routinely not performed, qualitative assessment performed by "eyeballing" the enhancement of the pancreas and spleen is generally adequate. In the absence of pancreatic necrosis, the pancreas and spleen should be similar in attenuation on the portal venous phase.[6]

When vascular complications are suspected, an additional vascular phase can be added to the imaging protocol, which is performed approximately 45 seconds after the injection of the contrast agent. Automated bolus tracking can be used to determine optimal timing of image acquisition. Unenhanced CT could be added to the imaging protocol if there is a strong clinical suspicion of hemorrhage.

Imaging Findings

As mentioned earlier, CT is not required in mild, self-limiting cases of acute pancreatitis. In these cases, CT of the pancreas could be normal or the pancreas may be enlarged or low in attenuation, indicating interstitial edema (Fig. 77-1A). The role of CT is primarily in patients with severe acute pancreatitis, in assessing the degree of pancreatic necrosis, and in detecting local retroperitoneal complications such as pseudocyst and abscess formation.

The definitions, pathogenesis, and imaging appearance of the different types of "fluid collections" seen in acute pancreatitis are discussed in this section. These terminologies have been standardized by the 1992 International

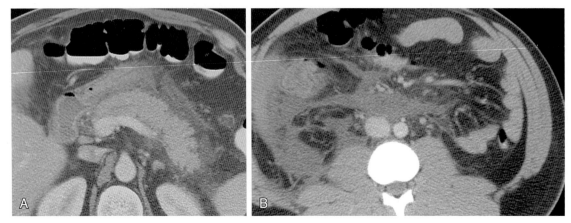

■ FIGURE 77-1 Acute edematous pancreatitis. **A,** Axial contrast-enhanced CT image showing a diffusely enlarged pancreas and peripancreatic inflammatory fat stranding. **B,** Axial CT image of another patient with mild pancreatitis showing an acute fluid collection inferior to the pancreas. Note that, unlike a pseudocyst, acute fluid collections do not have a well-defined wall.

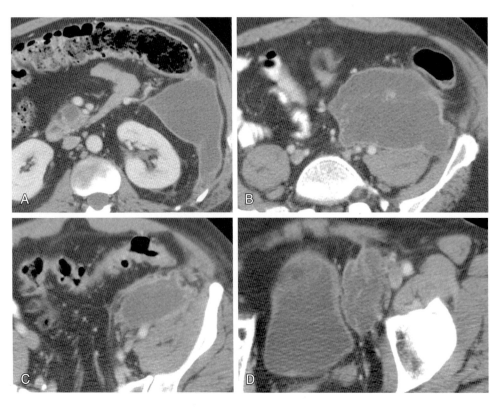

■ FIGURE 77-2 Pancreatic pseudocyst. **A** to **D,** Axial contrast-enhanced CT images show a large pseudocyst extending inferiorly from the left pararenal space into the pelvis and left groin.

Symposium on Acute Pancreatitis[3] and should be included in the radiology reports.

Acute Fluid Collections

Acute fluid collections occur early in the course of acute pancreatitis (within 48 hours). These consist of enzyme-rich pancreatic juices and lack a wall of fibrous or granulation tissue. These usually occur in or near the pancreas and may dissect in the lesser sac, anterior pararenal spaces (commonly on the left), transverse mesocolon, and the mesenteric root (see Fig. 77-1B). Acute fluid collections are seen in 30% to 50% of cases and resolve spontaneously

in approximately 50% of patients. In the remainder, they can get walled off and progress to become pseudocysts or abscesses.[8,9]

Acute Pseudocyst

A *pseudocyst* is defined as a collection of pancreatic juices enclosed by a wall of fibrous or granulation tissue. Pseudocysts are formed approximately 4 weeks after the onset of acute pancreatitis.[8] On CT, a pseudocyst appears as a well-circumscribed, low-attenuation collection commonly occurring in the vicinity of the pancreas (Fig. 77-2). On rare occasions they can be seen in unusual locations such

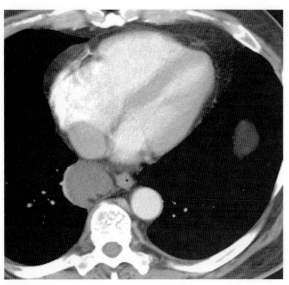

■ **FIGURE 77-3** Mediastinal pseudocyst. Axial contrast-enhanced CT image showing an unusual location of a pancreatic pseudocyst in the posterior mediastinum.

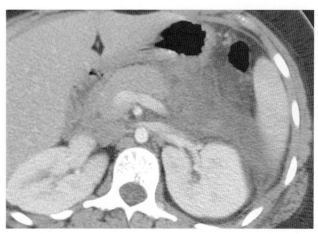

■ **FIGURE 77-5** Acute necrotizing pancreatitis. Axial contrast-enhanced CT image demonstrating nonenhancement of the distal body and tail of pancreas, suggesting necrosis. Note that the head and proximal body of the pancreas demonstrate normal enhancement.

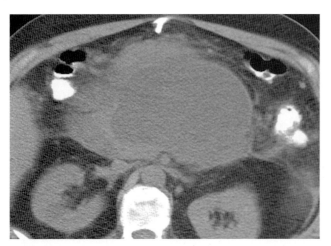

■ **FIGURE 77-4** Pancreatic abscess. Axial CT image of a large thick-walled peripancreatic collection in a patient with severe acute pancreatitis and high fever. Percutaneous needle aspiration of this collection yielded pus.

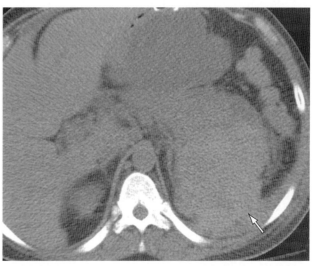

■ **FIGURE 77-6** Severe necrotizing pancreatitis. Axial unenhanced CT image of a patient with necrotizing pancreatitis shows areas of increased attenuation (50-60 HU) (*arrow*) suggesting the presence of hemorrhage.

as the mediastinum and groin (Fig. 77-3).[10,11] A typical pseudocyst is sterile. If there is pus in the pseudocyst, the lesion is termed a *pancreatic abscess.*

Pancreatic Abscess

A pancreatic abscess consists of a circumscribed intra-abdominal collection of pus, usually in proximity to the pancreas, and contains little or no pancreatic necrosis. Like pseudocysts, pancreatic abscesses occur later in the course of severe acute pancreatitis, often 4 weeks or more after the onset.[3] On contrast-enhanced CT, the presence of a thick, irregular wall helps in differentiating a pancreatic abscess from a pseudocyst, which generally has a thin, well-delineated wall (Fig. 77-4).

Pancreatic Necrosis

Pancreatic necrosis is defined as focal or diffuse areas of nonviable pancreatic parenchyma and is typically associated with peripancreatic fat necrosis.[3] On contrast-enhanced CT, pancreatic necrosis appears as one or more focal areas of nonenhancing pancreatic parenchyma (Fig. 77-5). Pancreatic necrosis is often hemorrhagic because of leakage from small veins and is seen on CT as areas of increased attenuation within the pancreas (Fig. 77-6). Retroperitoneal fat necrosis is invariably seen in patients with pancreatic necrosis, but the converse is not true. CT cannot reliably diagnose retroperitoneal fat necrosis, and thus all heterogeneous peripancreatic collections should be considered as areas of fat necrosis until proven otherwise (Fig. 77-7).[6]

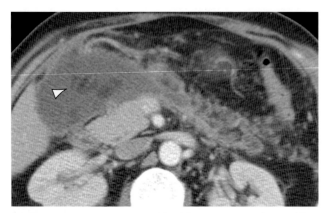

■ **FIGURE 77-7** Acute pancreatitis with peripancreatic fat necrosis. Collection in the peripancreatic tissue with islands of fat (*arrowhead*) suggests fat necrosis.

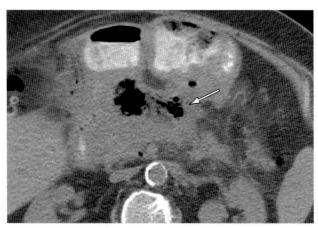

■ **FIGURE 77-8** Axial unenhanced CT image of a patient with known necrotizing pancreatitis. During the course of hospitalization, the patient's condition worsened clinically and the patient appeared septic. CT was performed and demonstrated air in the pancreatic bed (*arrow*) diagnostic of infected necrotic tissue.

TABLE 77-3 Balthazar Grading System and CT Severity Index

Grade	Description
A	Normal-appearing pancreas
B	Focal or diffuse enlargement of the pancreas
C	Pancreatic gland abnormalities accompanied by mild peripancreatic inflammatory changes
D	Fluid collection in a single location
E	Two or more fluid collections near the pancreas or gas in or adjacent to the pancreas

CT Grade	Score	Necrosis (%)	Score
A	0	0	0
B	1	<30	2
C	2	30-50	4
D	3	>50	6
E	4		

CT severity index (maximum score 10) = CT grade (0-4) + necrosis (0-6).

There are a few pitfalls that can lead to a false-positive diagnosis of pancreatic necrosis. In individuals with fatty infiltration of the pancreas and in those with edematous or interstitial pancreatitis, the decreased enhancement of the pancreas should not be mistaken for pancreatic necrosis.[6] Also, small, focal intrapancreatic fluid collections that are sometimes seen in acute pancreatitis should not be mistaken for focal necrosis. This distinction can be difficult in the absence of prior or follow-up imaging.[6]

Can Imaging Differentiate Sterile versus Infected Necrosis?

The differentiation of sterile from infected pancreatic necrosis is important from the management perspective because the latter necessitates necrosectomy.[12-14] The mortality rates increase from 10% in those with sterile necrosis to 30% in the presence of infected necrosis.[1] Distinguishing sterile from infected necrosis based solely on imaging is virtually impossible, the only exception being the presence of gas bubbles within the collection suggesting the presence of infection (Fig. 77-8).[6] Percutaneous needle aspiration under CT or ultrasound guidance is helpful in detecting the presence of infection.

CT Severity Index

Balthazar and colleagues graded the severity of acute pancreatitis based on CT findings and described the term *CT severity index (CTSI)*.[15,16] CT grading of acute pancreatitis is depicted in Table 77-3. These investigators reported 0% and 48% mortality and morbidity rates, respectively in patients who had less than 30% necrosis on CT. Larger areas of necrosis (30% to 50% and >50%) were associated with a morbidity rate of 75% to 100% and a mortality rate of 11% to 25%.[16] Additionally, patients with a CTSI of 0 to 3 showed a 3% mortality rate and an 8% morbidity rate, whereas in patients with a CTSI of 7 to 10, the mortality and morbidity rates were 17% and 92%, respectively.[15]

Extrapancreatic Findings in Acute Pancreatitis

Because of the close proximity of the spleen to the tail of the pancreas, the inflammatory process can spread into the spleen with formation of an intrasplenic pseudocyst or abscess (Fig. 77-9).[17] Splenic infarction can occur as a result of compression of the splenic vessels. Erosion of small intrasplenic vessels can cause parenchymal hemorrhage, and the blood may dissect beneath the splenic capsule, resulting in a subcapsular hematoma. If the hemorrhage is large, splenic laceration and catastrophic rupture of the spleen can occur.

Spread of the inflammatory process near the liver and gallbladder can produce transient areas of enhancement in the liver, typically seen near the gallbladder fossa and the left lobe of the liver.[18] Likewise, the inflammatory process can extend into the perinephric space, resulting in subcapsular and perirenal fluid collections and pseudocysts (Fig. 77-10). Extensive inflammation around the renal vessels can cause renal vein compression and thrombosis. The inflammatory exudates can compress the renal artery, causing asymmetric enhancement of the renal parenchyma.[19]

The colon can rarely be affected, owing to the close relationship of the pancreas with the transverse and the

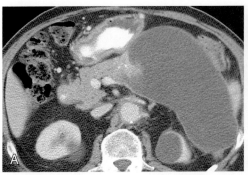
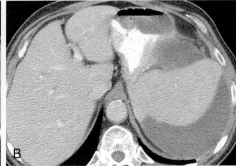

■ **FIGURE 77-9**   **A** and **B,** Axial CT images of a patient with necrotizing pancreatitis involving the body and tail of the pancreas. Owing to the close proximity of the tail of the pancreas and spleen, the inflammatory process has extended laterally and superiorly to the perisplenic tissues.

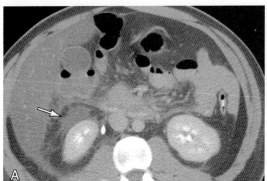
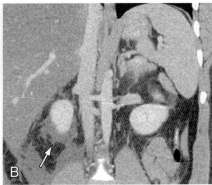

■ **FIGURE 77-10**   Axial (**A**) and coronal (**B**) contrast-enhanced CT images in a patient with acute pancreatitis depicting the spread of the inflammatory process to the right perirenal space (*arrows*).

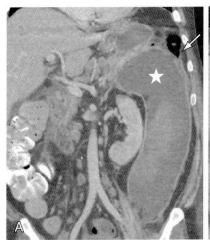
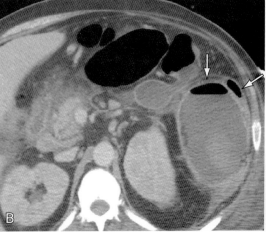
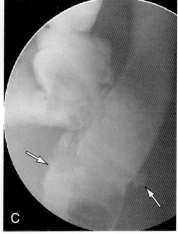

■ **FIGURE 77-11**   **A,** Coronal CT image of a patient with severe pancreatitis shows a large pseudocyst in the left pararenal space (*star*) closely related to the colon (*arrow*). **B,** Axial CT image of the same patient performed 10 days later shows new air within the pseudocyst, suggesting either infection or bowel fistulization. **C,** Water-soluble contrast enema performed the next day shows leakage of contrast agent from the descending colon into the pseudocyst (*arrows*), indicating that the pseudocyst has eroded the large bowel.

splenic flexure of the colon. Direct extension of the inflammatory process or a pseudocyst may compress, inflame, or erode the large bowel, resulting in fistula formation and progressive narrowing of the colonic lumen (Fig. 77-11).[20] Large bowel involvement may present weeks or months after an attack of acute pancreatitis.

Vascular Complications

Arterial complications of acute pancreatitis result from the proteolytic effects of the pancreatic enzymes that cause erosion of blood vessels, which often results in pseudoaneurysm formation or free hemorrhage from the erosion site.[21,22] The splenic artery, followed by the pancreaticoduodenal and gastroduodenal arteries, are affected most commonly.[21,22] The left gastric, hepatic, and small intrapancreatic arteries are involved less often. Arterial bleeding is one of the most life-threatening complications. On imaging, a pseudoaneurysm can be seen as a completely or partially vascular cystic mass (Fig. 77-12). In patients who have a history of acute pancreatitis, one should suspect a pseudoaneurysm when a cystic pancreatic mass

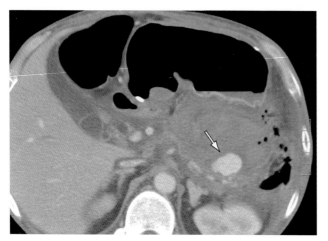

■ **FIGURE 77-12** Splenic artery pseudoaneurysm after an episode of severe acute pancreatitis. Axial contrast-enhanced CT image shows an enhancing structure (*arrow*) in the pancreatic bed with attenuation matching that of the aorta, suggesting a pseudoaneurysm.

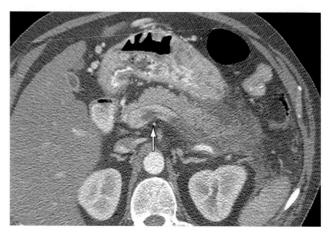

■ **FIGURE 77-13** Axial contrast-enhanced CT image shows inflammation of the body and tail of pancreas and peripancreatic tissues with splenic vein thrombosis (*arrow*).

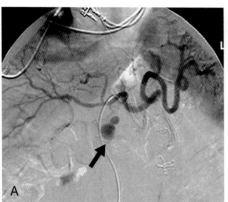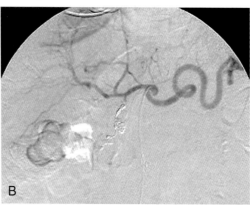

■ **FIGURE 77-14** **A,** Celiac artery angiogram performed in a patient with severe acute pancreatitis and upper gastrointestinal hemorrhage demonstrates a pseudoaneurysm (*arrow*) arising from the gastroduodenal artery. **B,** After coiling there is complete occlusion of the pseudoaneurysm.

demonstrates transient vascular enhancement. CT or MR angiography and 3D reconstructions can demonstrate precisely the specific vessel involved.

In addition to arterial complications, venous thrombosis in the portal-mesenteric circulation can occur. In order of frequency, the splenic vein is involved most often, followed by the portal and the superior mesenteric veins (Fig. 77-13).

Angiography

If acute hemorrhage or pseudoaneurysm is suspected or diagnosed by contrast-enhanced CT or ultrasonography, a celiac/superior mesenteric arteriogram should be performed to definitively assess the extent of vascular involvement (Fig. 77-14). Once the site of pseudoaneurysm or source of active bleeding is identified, it can be treated by Gelfoam embolization, various coil occlusion devices, or tissue adhesives (e.g., bucrylate). Venous thrombosis may be diagnosed via selective angiography.

The primary contraindication for angiography is a hemodynamically unstable patient. Complications of celiac/superior mesenteric arteriography and embolization include arterial injury such as thrombosis, dissection,

or rupture; distal embolization; ischemia of visceral organs such as the spleen and bowel; coil malpositioning; and rebleeding.

MRI

MRI is comparable to CT in the demonstration of morphologic changes associated with acute pancreatitis, including the extent of pancreatic necrosis and peripancreatic fluid collections (Fig. 77-15).[23,24] MRI of the pancreas is best performed with a 1.5-T MR scanner and phased-array coils. The MRI parameters used in our institution are shown in Tables 77-4 and 77-5.[7]

T2-weighted (T2W) sequences accurately depict fluid collections, pseudocysts, and hemorrhage. T2W images are more sensitive than CT in the demonstration of the contents of fluid collections and therefore in the assessment of the drainability of the collection.[25] T1-weighted (T1W) images are useful to depict pancreatic and peripancreatic edema. Dynamic gadolinium-enhanced MRI is useful for depicting viable from nonviable pancreatic parenchyma. The dynamic contrast-enhanced sequence is also useful in demonstrating vascular complications.

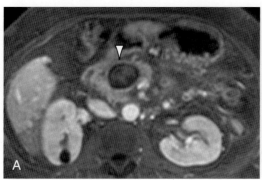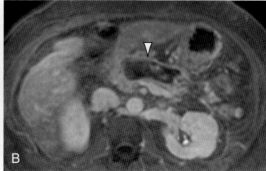

■ **FIGURE 77-15** A and B, Gadolinium-enhanced T1W gradient-echo images show lack of enhancement of the head and body of the pancreas (*arrowheads*) suggesting the presence of necrosis. Contrast-enhanced MRI is equivalent to CT for the demonstration of pancreatic necrosis.

TABLE 77-4 MRI Parameters

	Fast Spin-Echo with Fat Saturation	Fast Spin-Echo without Fat Saturation	T1-Weighted Gradient-Echo (Spoiled Gradient Recalled)	3D Dynamic Precontrast and Postcontrast
Imaging Plane	Axial	Axial	Axial	Axial
TR	4000-4500 ms	2100 ms	200 ms	150 ms
TE	68 ms	60 ms	Minimum	2.4 ms
Flip Angle	90 degrees	90 degrees	80 degrees	15 degrees
Field of View	36	36	36	36
Matrix	128 × 256	128 × 256	256 × 512	160 × 256
Thickness	3 mm	3 mm	4 mm	4 mm
Gap (mm)	0	0	0	Not applicable
Respiration	Triggered	Breath-hold	Breath-hold	Breath-hold (three acquisitions)

TABLE 77-5 MRCP Parameters

	2D SSFSE		3D FRFSE
	Thin Section	Thick Section	
Acquisition Plane	Coronal	Coronal	Coronal
TR	Minimum	4849 ms	1717 ms
TE	180 ms	874 ms	500-600 ms
Bandwidth	62.5	31.25	19
Field of View	48	35	36
Matrix	160 × 384	256 × 256	256 × 256
Thickness	5 mm	40 mm	3 mm
Gadolinium	±	±	±

FRFSE, fast-recovery fast spin-echo; SSFSE, single-shot fast spin-echo.

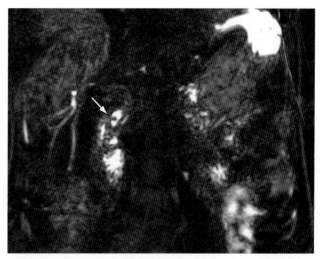

■ **FIGURE 77-16** MRCP performed in a patient with acute pancreatitis demonstrates a stone causing a filling defect (*arrow*) in the common bile duct.

MRCP is highly sensitive and specific for diagnosing choledocholithiasis and hence in establishing the underlying cause of acute pancreatitis (Fig. 77-16).[26,27] Also, pancreatic ductal abnormalities such as dilatation, disruption, or leakage as well as duct communication with a pancreatic pseudocyst can be well demonstrated by MRCP.[27] Structural abnormalities of the pancreas such as pancreas divisum and anomalous pancreaticobiliary junction with an abnormally long common channel that can cause recurrent attacks of pancreatitis can be depicted by MRCP.[27] Secretin-enhanced MRCP has proved to be beneficial in improving the visualization of the pancreatic ductal system.[27] Exogenous administration of secretin stimulates secretion of pancreatic juice, notably the fluid and bicarbonate, which consequently results in transient distention of the pancreatic duct. Secretin-enhanced MRCP enhances the ability of MRI to identify structural anomalies such as pancreas divisum and to make an early diagnosis of ductal disruption.[28,29]

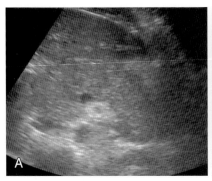
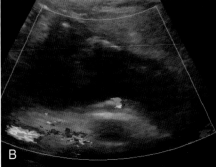
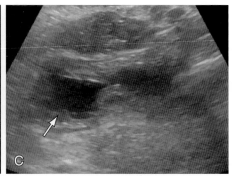

■ **FIGURE 77-17** **A,** Transverse ultrasound image shows an enlarged hypoechoic pancreas seen in acute edema pancreatitis. **B,** Transverse ultrasound image of a patient with elevated amylase and lipase levels shows a complex fluid collection in the epigastrium conforming to the shape of the pancreas. This patient had extensive pancreatic necrosis on a contrast-enhanced CT scan performed a few days later. Ultrasonography is not very reliable in distinguishing pancreatic necrosis from other fluid collections seen in patients with acute pancreatitis. **C,** Transverse ultrasound image of a patient with known acute pancreatitis showing a pancreatic/peripancreatic pseudocyst (*arrow*).

Ultrasonography

In a patient with suspected biliary pancreatitis, ultrasound is helpful for the assessment of biliary dilatation and gallbladder and common bile duct stones.

The assessment of the pancreas by ultrasound is limited, secondary to bowel gas and associated paralytic ileus. The ultrasonographic findings in acute pancreatitis can range from a normal-appearing gland, a diffusely enlarged hypoechoic pancreas, or the presence of intrapancreatic or peripancreatic fluid collections, particularly in the lesser sac and anterior pararenal space (Fig. 77-17). Ultrasonography cannot reliably differentiate these fluid collections from pancreatic necrosis, thus limiting its role in the assessment of the severity of pancreatitis.

The role of endoscopic ultrasonography in the management of acute pancreatitis is limited in everyday practice. There have been reports suggesting that it is accurate in identifying common bile duct stones and in detecting pancreatic necrosis.[14] Diagnostic endoscopic ultrasonography is helpful before performing therapeutic endoscopic interventions such as cystogastrostomy for the management of pseudocysts.

ERCP

ERCP is not used to make the diagnosis of acute pancreatitis. It is used with endoscopic sphincterotomy to extract impacted gallstones in patients with severe gallstone pancreatitis.[30] The morbidity and mortality is reduced with the use of early selective ERCP. ERCP is indicated in patients at risk of or with evidence of biliary sepsis, cholangitis, biliary obstruction, elevated bilirubin, and worsening and persistent jaundice. Endoscopic interventions such as cystogastrostomy and cystoduodenostomy are used for the treatment of pseudocysts.

Imaging Algorithm

See Figure 77-18 for an imaging algorithm and also Table 77-6.

Classic Signs

- Lack of contrast enhancement or minimal contrast enhancement of less than 30 HU indicates pancreatic necrosis.
- If a cystic pancreatic mass demonstrates transient vascular enhancement, one should suspect a pseudoaneurysm.

DIFFERENTIAL DIAGNOSIS

The clinical diagnosis of acute pancreatitis is based on abdominal pain, which often radiates to the back and is accompanied by nausea and vomiting. The diagnosis is confirmed by laboratory studies, namely, elevation of serum amylase and lipase (more than three times the upper limits of normal).[1] Serum amylase and, less commonly, serum lipase levels can be elevated in many other nonpancreatic disorders (Table 77-7). Therefore, in equivocal cases, imaging is helpful in establishing the diagnosis of acute pancreatitis.

CT and ultrasonography are useful in confirming the diagnosis of acute pancreatitis and ruling out other intraabdominal conditions as the cause of pain (Table 77-8).

TREATMENT
Medical Treatment

The severity of pancreatitis is clinically assessed by different scoring systems that assess inflammation and organ failure.[3,6,30] The commonly used Ranson scoring system comprises five clinical criteria measured at admission and six measured after 48 hours.[6,30] The APACHE II monitoring system is considered more reliable, with an accuracy of about 75% for the assessment of the severity of pancreatitis at admission.[6,30] Unlike the Ranson scoring system, the APACHE II system is complex and more cumbersome.

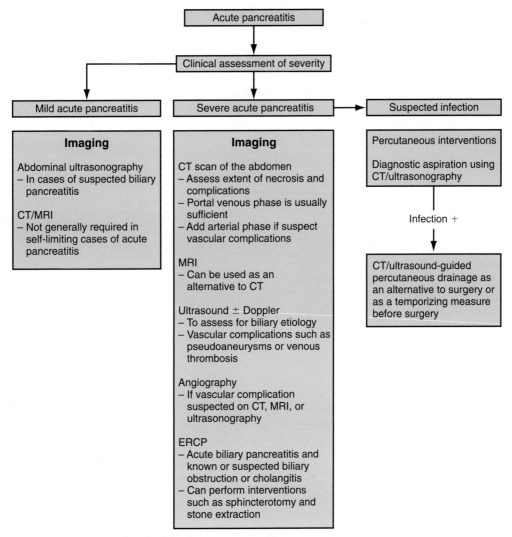

■ **FIGURE 77-18** Imaging algorithm for acute pancreatitis.

TABLE 77-6 Accuracy and Limitations of the Modalities Used in Imaging of Acute Pancreatitis

Modality	Accuracy	Limitations
Radiography	Not very useful	
CT	Establishing diagnosis Establishing etiology Assessing severity and complications Guiding percutaneous interventions	Cannot reliably differentiate sterile from infected necrosis
MRI	Comparable to CT in assessing pancreatic necrosis and complications Superior to CT in assessing the contents of fluid collections and hence is a better predictor of drainability of collections by percutaneous techniques MRCP useful in assessing choledocholithiasis and pancreatic ducal abnormalities	Long scanning times limit its use in severely ill patients.
Ultrasonography	Useful in determining the etiology of acute pancreatitis, mainly choledocholithiasis and biliary dilatation Portable nature of the modality is occasionally helpful in performing simple diagnostic aspirations in critically ill patients.	Limited use in assessing severity of pancreatitis

TABLE 77-7 Common Nonpancreatic Causes of Elevated Amylase and Lipase Levels

Etiology	Amylase	Lipase
Biliary disease	↑	↑
Common bile duct obstruction		
Acute cholecystitis		
Intestinal ischemia, obstruction, perforation	↑	↑
Acute appendicitis	↑	↑
Gynecologic conditions	↑	Normal
Ectopic pregnancy		
Acute salpingitis		
Ovarian cysts and malignancies		
Renal insufficiency	↑	↑
Salivary gland disease including mumps	↑	Normal

TABLE 77-8 Clinical Mimickers of Acute Pancreatitis

Gastritis and peptic ulcer disease
Esophageal spasm
Perforated viscus*
Intestinal obstruction*
Acute cholecystitis*
Leaking abdominal aortic aneurysm or acute aortic dissection*
Mesenteric ischemia*

*Imaging, particularly CT, is useful in establishing the diagnosis.

Mild pancreatitis can be managed conservatively with hydration and analgesics.[30] Right upper quadrant ultrasonography to look for gallstones and biliary dilatation make up the standard of care.[30] Severe acute pancreatitis requires a more aggressive approach, including admission to an intensive care unit and possible surgical, endoscopic, and percutaneous interventions.

Surgical Treatment

Surgical management of acute pancreatitis is indicated in two clinical settings: infected necrosis and gallstone pancreatitis. Surgery, consisting of débridement of all devitalized pancreatic and surrounding tissue, is clearly indicated in infected necrosis; its benefit in sterile necrosis is controversial.[14,30] Recent studies suggest that a delayed approach to surgical necrectomy improves outcomes.[14]

Endoscopic Interventions

In the acute phase of gallstone-induced pancreatitis, if biliary duct obstruction, biliary sepsis, or cholangitis is suggested, then endoscopic sphincterotomy, biliary calculus removal, and common bile duct drainage are done.[30] Eventually, cholecystectomy is recommended in all cases of biliary pancreatitis to prevent recurrence.[30]

Percutaneous Image-Guided Interventions

Both diagnostic and therapeutic percutaneous interventions are often performed in patients with acute pancreatitis. Diagnostic aspiration for Gram stain and culture is performed on fluid collections, pseudocysts, or pancreatic necrosis when there is a clinical suspicion of infection (Fig. 77-19). Although most pseudocysts regress spontaneously, large (>5 cm), unresolving (>6 weeks), or symptomatic pseudocysts (pain, gastric outlet obstruction, or biliary obstruction) require drainage, which can be done either by percutaneous or endoscopic techniques.[30] Pancreatic abscesses and infected necrosis often require multicatheter drainage either as definitive treatment or as a temporizing measure before surgery (Fig. 77-20).[14,30]

CT is commonly used to guide percutaneous interventions. It demonstrates the size, location, and relationship of the collection to the adjacent vasculature and critical

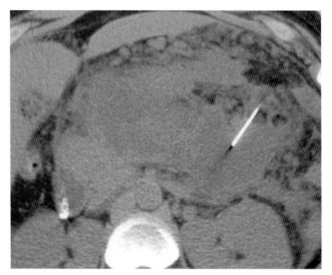

■ **FIGURE 77-19** Axial CT image of a patient with known necrotizing pancreatitis who developed a high-grade fever. Percutaneous diagnostic aspiration of the necrotic material performed under CT guidance with a 20-gauge Chiba needle yielded pus. CT cannot reliably distinguish sterile from infected pancreatic necrosis, and percutaneous aspiration is often performed when there is a strong clinical suspicion of infection.

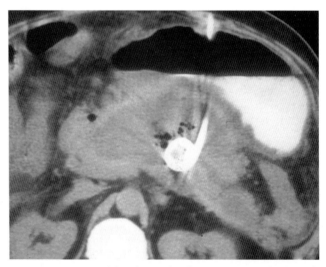

■ **FIGURE 77-20** Axial CT image showing a 14-gauge catheter used to drain extensive pancreatic necrosis. Catheter drainage could be performed as a temporizing measure before definitive surgery for pancreatic necrosis. Large-bore catheters are required if drainage of pancreatic necrosis is attempted.

organs. Ultrasonography can be used as a guidance modality when there are large collections and is particularly useful in the critically ill patient.

Once a drainage procedure has been performed, follow-up CT is critical in assessing the success of the procedure. Once the drain output diminishes, CT helps in assessing residual or new collections. Persistent collections lasting for months may suggest pancreatic ductal communication.

What the Referring Physician Needs to Know

- CT of the abdomen helps to establish the diagnosis of acute pancreatitis if the diagnosis is equivocal based on clinical presentation or laboratory values. Other causes that mimic acute pancreatitis can be excluded.
- CT is not required in mild, self-limiting cases of acute pancreatitis.
- Contrast-enhanced CT is the gold standard for assessing pancreatic necrosis and other complications of acute pancreatitis. CT performed in the portal venous phase is generally sufficient, and an additional vascular phase may be required if one suspects vascular complications.
- Imaging cannot reliably distinguish infected from sterile necrosis. Percutaneous image-guided interventions are helpful if there is suspicion of infection.
- Ultrasonography is helpful in assessing for gallstones and biliary dilatation.
- Gadolinium-enhanced MRI can be used as an alternative to CT for assessing pancreatic necrosis and complications of acute pancreatitis.
- MRCP can be used as a noninvasive alternative to ERCP for evaluation of choledocholithiasis and pancreatic ductal abnormalities.

KEY POINTS

- Chronic alcohol consumption and gallstones are the leading causes of acute pancreatitis. In 20% of cases the etiology may remain unclear.
- The clinical diagnosis of acute pancreatitis is supported by an elevation of the serum amylase and lipase levels in excess of three times the upper limit of normal.
- Appropriate terminology should be used in radiology reports when describing different "fluid collections" that occur in the setting of pancreatitis.
- Contrast-enhanced CT is not required in mild, self-limiting cases of acute pancreatitis.
- Contrast-enhanced CT is considered the gold standard in the assessment of pancreatic necrosis and complications of acute severe pancreatitis.
- The utility of ultrasonography in acute pancreatitis is limited to the evaluation of gallstones and biliary dilatation. Ultrasonography is not very helpful in evaluating pancreatic necrosis.
- MRI can be used as an alternative to CT for the assessment of pancreatic necrosis, especially if the risk of radiation exposure is an issue in younger patients.
- MRI is superior to CT in evaluating the nature of fluid collections and hence in the assessment of its drainability by percutaneous techniques.
- Imaging cannot reliably distinguish infected from sterile necrosis. Diagnostic aspiration under CT or ultrasound guidance is helpful to confirm or rule out infection.
- Infected necrosis is an indication for surgery. Percutaneous drainage can be used as a temporizing measure in cases of infected pancreatic necrosis or pancreatic abscess.
- MRCP is a useful noninvasive method to assess for biliary stones and pancreatic ductal abnormalities.
- Urgent ERCP with sphincterotomy and stone extraction is recommended in cases of gallstone pancreatitis presenting as cholangitis or biliary ductal obstruction.

SUGGESTED READINGS

Balthazar EJ. Acute pancreatitis: assessment of severity with clinical and CT evaluation. Radiology 2002; 223:603-613.

Banks PA. Practice guidelines in acute pancreatitis. Am J Gastroenterol 1997; 92:377-386.

Fulcher AS, Turner MA. MR pancreatography: a useful tool for evaluating pancreatic disorders. RadioGraphics 1999; 19:5-24.

Saokar A, Rabinowitz CB, Sahani DV. Cross-sectional imaging in acute pancreatitis. Radiol Clin North Am 2007; 45:447-460.

Whitcomb DC. Clinical practice: acute pancreatitis. N Engl J Med 2006; 354:2142-2150.

REFERENCES

1. Whitcomb DC. Clinical practice: acute pancreatitis. N Engl J Med 2006; 354:2142-2150.
2. Swaroop VS, Chari ST, Clain JE. Severe acute pancreatitis. JAMA 2004; 291:2865-2868.
3. Bradley EL 3rd. A clinically based classification system for acute pancreatitis. Summary of the International Symposium on Acute Pancreatitis, Atlanta, GA, September 11 through 13, 1992. Arch Surg 1993; 128:586-590.
4. Banks PA. A new classification system for acute pancreatitis. Am J Gastroenterol 1994; 89:151-152.
5. Rosen MP, Sands DZ, Longmaid HE 3rd, et al. Impact of abdominal CT on the management of patients presenting to the emergency department with acute abdominal pain. AJR Am J Roentgenol 2000; 174:1391-1396.
6. Balthazar EJ. Acute pancreatitis: assessment of severity with clinical and CT evaluation. Radiology 2002; 223:603-613.
7. Saokar A, Rabinowitz CB, Sahani DV. Cross-sectional imaging in acute pancreatitis. Radiol Clin North Am 2007; 45:447-460.
8. Bradley EL III, Gonzalez AC, Clements JL Jr. Acute pancreatic pseudocysts: incidence and implications. Ann Surg 1976; 184:734-737.
9. Siegelman SS, Copeland BE, Saba GP, et al. CT of fluid collections associated with pancreatitis. AJR Am J Roentgenol 1980; 134:1121-1132.

10. Yamamura M, Iki K. Mediastinal extension of a pancreatic pseudocyst. Pancreatology 2004; 4:90.

11. Salvo AF, Nematolahi H. Distant dissection of a pancreatic pseudocyst into the right groin. Am J Surg 1973; 126:430-432.

12. Buchler MW, Gloor B, Muller CA, et al. Acute necrotizing pancreatitis: treatment strategy according to the status of infection. Ann Surg 2000; 232:619-626.

13. Buchler P, Reber HA. Surgical approach in patients with acute pancreatitis. Is infected or sterile necrosis an indication—in whom should this be done, when, and why? Gastroenterol Clin North Am 1999; 28:661-671.

14. Shankar S, van Sonnenberg E, Silverman SG, et al: Imaging and percutaneous management of acute complicated pancreatitis. Cardiovasc Intervent Radiol 2004; 27:567-580.

15. Balthazar EJ, Robinson DL, Megibow AJ, et al. Acute pancreatitis: value of CT in establishing prognosis. Radiology 1990; 174:331-336.

16. Balthazar EJ, Ranson JH, Naidich DP, et al. Acute pancreatitis: prognostic value of CT. Radiology 1985; 156:767-772.

17. Fishman EK, Soyer P, Bliss DF, et al. Splenic involvement in pancreatitis: spectrum of CT findings. AJR Am J Roentgenol 1995; 164:631-635.

18. Arita T, Matsunaga N, Takano K, et al. Hepatic perfusion abnormalities in acute pancreatitis: CT appearance and clinical importance. Abdom Imaging 1999; 24:157-162.

19. Mortele KJ, Mergo PJ, Taylor HM, et al. Renal and perirenal space involvement in acute pancreatitis: spiral CT findings. Abdom Imaging 2000; 25:272-278.

20. Gardner A, Gardner G, Feller E. Severe colonic complications of pancreatic disease. J Clin Gastroenterol 2003; 37:258-262.

21. Vujic I. Vascular complications of pancreatitis. Radiol Clin North Am 1989; 27:81-91.

22. Burke JW, Erickson SJ, Kellum CD, et al. Pseudoaneurysms complicating pancreatitis: detection by CT. Radiology 1986; 161:447-450.

23. Ward J, Chalmers AG, Guthrie AJ, et al. T2-weighted and dynamic enhanced MRI in acute pancreatitis: comparison with contrast enhanced CT. Clin Radiol 1997; 52:109-114.

24. Saifuddin A, Ward J, Ridgway J, et al. Comparison of MR and CT scanning in severe acute pancreatitis: initial experiences. Clin Radiol 1993; 48:111-116.

25. Morgan DE, Baron TH, Smith JK, et al. Pancreatic fluid collections prior to intervention: evaluation with MR imaging compared with CT and US. Radiology 1997; 203:773-778.

26. Fulcher AS, Turner MA. MR pancreatography: a useful tool for evaluating pancreatic disorders. RadioGraphics 1999; 19:5-24.

27. Matos C, Cappeliez O, Winant C, et al. MR imaging of the pancreas: a pictorial tour. RadioGraphics 2002; 22:e2.

28. Fukukura Y, Fujiyoshi F, Sasaki M, et al. Pancreatic duct: morphologic evaluation with MR cholangiopancreatography after secretin stimulation. Radiology 2002; 222:674-680.

29. Arvanitakis M, Delhaye M, De Maertelaere V, et al. Computed tomography and magnetic resonance imaging in the assessment of acute pancreatitis. Gastroenterology 2004; 126:715-723.

30. Banks PA. Practice guidelines in acute pancreatitis. Am J Gastroenterol 1997; 92:377-386.

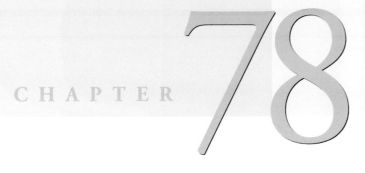
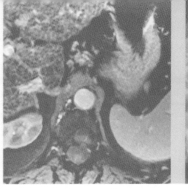
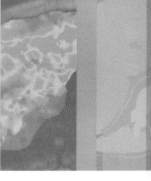

CHAPTER 78

Imaging of Chronic Pancreatitis

Hemali Desai and Naveen M. Kulkarni

ETIOLOGY

Chronic pancreatitis is defined as an ongoing prolonged inflammatory disease characterized by progressive irreversible structural changes resulting in permanent loss of endocrine and exocrine function. The Cambridge classification of 1983 acknowledged that chronic pancreatitis is typically associated with abdominal pain but can occasionally be painless and could recur.[1] According to the revised pancreatic classification of pancreatitis from the Marseille symposium of 1984, acute and chronic pancreatitis are very different diseases and rarely does acute pancreatitis lead to chronic pancreatitis.[2]

Prolonged alcohol abuse is the most common cause (70%) of chronic pancreatitis in the United States. Other causes are familial occurrence with hyperlipidemia, hyperparathyroidism, cystic fibrosis, trauma, cholelithiasis, and pancreas divisum.[3] There is a familial form of pancreatitis termed *hereditary pancreatitis* that is thought to be inherited in an autosomal dominant fashion with variable penetrance.

Thirty to 40 percent of patients with chronic pancreatitis have no apparent underlying cause and are considered to have idiopathic chronic pancreatitis.[4]

Patients with idiopathic chronic pancreatitis have been noted to cluster in a younger group (peak incidence, 15 to 30 years of age) and an older group (peak incidence, 50 to 70 years of age). Autoimmune chronic pancreatitis is an increasingly recognized condition frequently coexisting with other autoimmune diseases such as Sjögren's syndrome and primary sclerosing cholangitis.[5] An independent effect of tobacco smoking on the development of chronic pancreatitis has been suggested by several epidemiologic studies.[6] In certain parts of developing regions such as Africa, India, and South America a particular type of chronic pancreatitis occurs in children and adolescents. It is thought to be caused by dietary toxins and micronutrient deficiencies and results in tropical pancreatitis endemic in these regions (Table 78-1).[7]

PREVALENCE AND EPIDEMIOLOGY

Due to varied clinical presentation, recent increase in alcohol consumption, and improved sensitivity of diagnostic tests, the true prevalence of chronic pancreatitis is unknown, although estimates range from 0.04 to 5%.[4] Earlier reports from Copenhagen, the United States, and Mexico City are nearly the same, with the incidence of chronic pancreatitis reported as 4 cases per year per 100,000 inhabitants. Several retrospective studies have reported an annual incidence of 3 to 9 cases per year per 100,000 population.[8]

CLINICAL PRESENTATION

Chronic abdominal pain is the most frequent presentation in most patients with alcohol-induced disease.[9] Chronic pain is mainly epigastric but may be present in the left or right upper quadrant and often radiates to the back. The pain is described as severe, deep, and penetrating and is characteristically relieved by assuming a stooped or jack-knife posture. In some patients there is spontaneous remission of pain as organ failure sets in (burnout).[10]

Exacerbation of pain may be associated with nausea and vomiting. Two patterns of pain have been described in chronic pancreatitis[11]:

- Type A: short relapsing episodes lasting days to weeks, separated by a pain-free interval
- Type B: prolonged, severe, unrelenting pain

As the disease advances, around one fifth of the patients present without pain but with pancreatic exocrine (fat and vitamin malabsorption) or endocrine failure, manifesting as steatorrhea, diabetes mellitus, or weight loss.[12,13] Severe weight loss should raise concerns for pancreatic carcinoma.

Structural complications of chronic pancreatitis such as pseudocysts and stricture of the common bile duct in the pancreatic head are frequently seen. Thrombosis of the

TABLE 78-1 Classification System for Chronic Pancreatitis

Classification	Risk Factors	Comments
Toxic-metabolic (70%)	Alcoholic	
	Tobacco smoking	
	Hypercalcemia	Associated hyperparathyroidism
	Hyperlipidemia	
	Chronic renal failure	
	Medications	e.g., Phenacetin abuse
	Toxins	e.g., Organotin compounds
Idiopathic (20%)	Early onset	
	Late onset	
	Tropical	Tropical calcific and fibrocalculous pancreatic diabetes
	Other	
Others (10%)		
Genetic	Autosomal dominant	Cationic trypsinogen gene
	Autosomal recessive/modifier genes	*CFTR* mutations, *SPINK1* mutations, cationic trypsinogen, α_1-antitrypsin deficiency (possible)
Autoimmune	Isolated autoimmune chronic pancreatitis	
	Syndromic	Sjögren's syndrome, inflammatory bowel disease, primary biliary cirrhosis, sclerosing cholangitis
Recurrent and severe acute pancreatitis	Postnecrotic	Severe acute pancreatitis
	Recurrent acute pancreatitis	
	Vascular disease/ischemic	
	Radiation injury	
Obstructive	Pancreas divisum	
	Sphincter of Oddi disorders	Not universally accepted
	Duct obstruction	e.g., Tumor
	Periampullary	
	Duodenal wall cysts	
	Post-traumatic	
	Pancreatic duct scars	

splenic or the portal vein with gastric or esophageal varices, arterial pseudoaneurysm formation, pancreatic abscess, ascites, and duodenal obstruction are seen less frequently.

PATHOPHYSIOLOGY AND PATHOLOGY

The pathophysiology of chronic pancreatitis includes chronic inflammation, irregular and patchy loss of acinar and ductal tissue, glandular atrophy, duct changes, and fibrosis. The pathogenesis of chronic pancreatitis is not well elucidated. Several theories have been developed for alcoholic pancreatitis.

1. Stone and duct obstruction: disturbance of acinar and ductular function with formation of intraductal protein plugs, stones, and duct obstruction with subsequent inflammation and fibrosis.
2. Toxic metabolic theory: results in early- and late-phase inflammatory responses and production of profibrotic cells, including stellate cells, with progressive lipid deposition, periacinar fibrosis, and inflammatory and fibrotic changes.
3. Oxidative stress theory: excess free radicals ultimately result in peroxidation of lipid components of the membrane within the pancreatic acinar cell leading to mast cell degranulation, platelet activation, and an inflammatory response.[14]
4. Necrosis-fibrosis sequence: chronic contact of the stones with duct epithelial cells produces ulceration and scarring. Eventually, atrophy and fibrosis result from chronic obstruction of the acini. The necrosis-

fibrosis theory emphasizes that acute and chronic pancreatitis represent a spectrum of disease. New research and discoveries about hereditary pancreatitis have supported the necrosis-fibrosis sequence.[15] The genetic defect of hereditary pancreatitis produces recurrent acute pancreatitis beginning in early childhood, almost invariably leading to chronic pancreatitis in early adulthood.

IMAGING

Radiography

On abdominal radiographs calcification can be found in 30% to 70% of patients at presentation, which suggests the diagnosis with 95% confidence. Pancreatic calcification is nearly 10% specific but poorly sensitive (30% to 70%) for the diagnosis of chronic pancreatitis. In alcoholic pancreatitis, calcification occurs earlier in the course of disease than in idiopathic pancreatitis. It is important to differentiate parenchymal or ductal calcification from calcified pancreatic cysts or occasionally from heavily calcified peripancreatic vasculature (Fig. 78-1).

Ultrasonography

Transabdominal ultrasonography is a noninvasive, easily accessible imaging modality for evaluation of the pancreas. However, it is limited in its evaluation of the pancreas owing to overlying bowel gas and patient body habitus and is operator dependent. Most ultrasound findings of chronic pancreatitis are not sensitive or specific

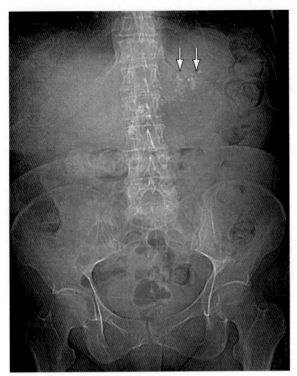

■ **FIGURE 78-1** Diffuse coarse irregular calcification (*arrows*) in the upper abdomen in the expected location of the pancreas suggestive of chronic pancreatitis.

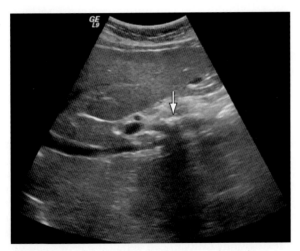

■ **FIGURE 78-2** Ultrasound image of abdomen shows dense calcification within pancreatic body (*arrow*) with posterior acoustic shadowing consistent with chronic calcific pancreatitis.

for the diagnosis. Early diagnosis of chronic pancreatitis is difficult. The size of the gland may be normal, enlarged, or reduced, depending on the amount of active inflammation and fibrosis. Other ultrasound features include altered echotexture of the gland, parenchymal and ductal calcifications, pancreatic duct dilatation and irregularity, biliary dilatation, and, occasionally, pseudocysts.

Pancreatic calcifications are a classic ultrasound finding and appear as multiple punctate, hyperechoic foci, which may be focal or distributed throughout the gland, seen in 40% of patients (Fig. 78-2).[16] These may or may not demonstrate posterior acoustic shadowing, depending on

the size. Intraductal calcification can cause obstruction and lead to persistent recurrent pancreatitis. Pancreatic calcification is believed to be the most specific ultrasound finding for chronic pancreatitis.[17] As the disease progresses, the pancreatic parenchyma demonstrates a heterogeneous echotexture with areas of increased and decreased echogenicity. Areas of increased echogenicity result from fibrosis and calcification, whereas areas of decreased echogenicity result from inflammation. The pancreas may be normal in size, enlarged, or atrophic depending on the amount of fibrosis and active inflammation. Most commonly, the gland atrophies in advanced disease. When the inflammatory process is focal, chronic pancreatitis also presents as a focal mass in up to 40% of patients. The mass may demonstrate increased or decreased echogenicity, irregular dilatation, and tortuosity of the pancreatic duct, mimicking a neoplasm. The presence of calcification within the mass favors an inflammatory process over malignancy. Areas of narrowing and dilatation of the main pancreatic duct are caused by short strictures and post-stenotic dilatation, giving the pancreatic duct a beaded appearance, also referred to as the "chain of lakes" sign. Ultrasonography can be useful in detecting complications of chronic pancreatitis. It has been described as 97% sensitive for pseudocysts larger than 3 cm. Pancreatic pseudocysts are reported in 25% to 40% of patients.[16] Doppler ultrasonography is useful for vascular complications such as portal and splenic vein thrombosis, varices, and splenic artery pseudoaneurysm.

Endoscopic Ultrasonography

Endoscopic ultrasonography (EUS) was introduced in the early 1980s and with advances in its technology it has emerged as a front-line diagnostic tool for detection of early chronic pancreatitis. The proximity of the pancreas to the stomach and duodenum allows acquisition of high-resolution imaging, thus overcoming the limitations of transabdominal ultrasonography, namely, bowel gas and body habitus. The normal pancreas has homogeneous echogenicity with fine granularity and reticulation. The pancreas shows increased echogenicity relative to the liver. The margins are smooth without side-branch ectasia. The average pancreatic duct diameter in the body is 1.9 mm, and normal side branches are visible in 32% of patients.

The parenchymal abnormalities demonstrated with endoscopic ultrasonography are heterogeneous echogenicity with hyperechoic foci, prominent interlobular septa appearing as echogenic strands (due to fibrosis), hypoechoic foci (1 to 3 mm) due to small cystic changes in the parenchyma, lobular outer gland margins, and large echo-poor cavities (>5 mm). The ductal abnormalities include main pancreatic duct (MPD) dilatation more than 3 mm, irregularity, intraductal echogenic foci, hyperechoic margins of the pancreatic duct, side-branch ectasia, and intraductal calculi (Table 78-2).[18]

CT

Contrast-enhanced CT of the abdomen is the imaging modality of choice and a front-line tool in the diagnosis of

TABLE 78-2 Endoscopic Ultrasound Features of
Chronic Pancreatitis

Parenchymal Features	Ductal Features
Gland atrophy	Narrowing
Hyperechoic foci	Dilation
Hyperechoic stranding	Irregularity
Cysts	Calculi
Lobularity	Side branch dilation
	Hyperechoic walls

From Stevens T, Conwell DL. Chronic pancreatitis. In Ginsberg GG, Ahmad
NA (eds). The Clinician's Guide to Pancreaticobiliary Disorders.
Thorofare, NJ, Slack Inc., 2006, p 195.

chronic pancreatitis. The CT features pathognomonic of chronic pancreatitis are scattered coarse parenchymal calcifications, intraductal calcification, ductal dilatation, and parenchymal atrophy.[18] In a retrospective study by Luetmer and colleagues, pancreatic ductal dilatation was reported in 68%, parenchymal atrophy in 54%, and pancreatic calcification in 50%.[19]

Dilatation of the main pancreatic duct and the side branches is the most common feature of chronic pancreatitis. Ductal dilatation can be smooth, beaded, or irregular; no single pattern is predominant, and more than one pattern can be seen in the same gland. Ductal dilatation is nonspecific as an isolated finding because it is also seen with distal common bile duct cholangiocarcinoma and pancreatic and ampullary carcinoma.

Altered glandular size is another key finding in chronic pancreatitis. Parenchymal atrophy was seen in 54% in a retrospective study conducted by Luetmer and colleagues.[19] Parenchymal atrophy is frequently seen in association with ductal dilatation. Most patients with exocrine insufficiency have parenchymal atrophy or ductal dilatation.[17] Atrophy is a common feature in advanced or late chronic pancreatitis. Atrophy, however, is a less sensitive finding in the elderly, in whom it may represent a normal aging process. Occasionally, either focal or diffuse enlargement of the pancreas is present. A more reliable and the most specific sign of chronic pancreatitis is pancreatic calculi.[19] Intraductal calcifications result in obstruction, ductal ectasia, and periductal fibrosis. Intraductal calculi range in size from microscopic to greater than 1 cm in diameter. Calcifications result from inspissation of pancreatic secretions within the duct and subsequent deposition of calcium carbonate on the intraductal protein plugs. Parenchymal calcifications vary in size and can be fine and stippled to large and coarse. The distribution may be focal, involving only one portion of the gland or diffuse throughout the gland. The head of the pancreas is more prominently involved than the tail.[20] Pancreatic calcifications when present are pathognomonic and virtually diagnostic of chronic pancreatitis and occur late in the course of the disease and in advanced disease. However, in hereditary pancreatitis, calculi are seen early in the course of disease. They are large and rounded, and in the dilated main pancreatic duct they tend to be arranged in a linear pattern.[21]

CT also has the advantage of detecting complications of chronic pancreatitis. Fluid collections are seen in 30% and may be within the pancreas or adjacent to the pancreas. They may be seen in the retroperitoneum and rarely in distant sites. Extrapancreatic fluid collections are mostly seen in the lesser sac or anterior pararenal spaces. Most fluid collections in chronic pancreatitis are well-encapsulated mature pseudocysts that are present in 25% of cases. These occur in both acute and chronic pancreatitis. Ductal dilatation and intraductal calculi favor chronic pancreatitis as the underlying cause. Unencapsulated fluid collections are seen only with associated superimposed acute pancreatitis. Most pseudocysts resolve spontaneously but can be complicated by hemorrhage, superinfection, and spontaneous rupture. Pseudocysts may rupture into the peritoneal cavity, the extraperitoneal spaces, the pleural cavity, or the gastrointestinal tract.

Dilatation of the main pancreatic duct is strongly associated. The dilated common bile duct demonstrates smooth gradual tapering as opposed to the abrupt cutoff shown in malignancy. It is often associated with an inflammatory mass in the pancreatic head.

Arterial pseudoaneurysms (pancreatic duodenal and splenic arteries) and splenic vein thrombosis are the most frequently encountered vascular complications. Pseudoaneurysms are seen near the pancreatic head and splenic hilum. They are caused by destruction of the vascular wall by pancreatic inflammation and appear as rounded areas isoattenuating to vascular structures. They can also be diagnosed with MRI and pulsed Doppler ultrasonography without intravenous administration of a contrast agent.[3] The attenuation is similar to hematoma on noncontrast CT.[17] Chronic pancreatitis is also associated with splenic, portal, and superior mesenteric vein thrombosis and accounts for 65% of cases of splenic vein thrombosis. Thrombus is seen as a filling defect in the vein. Venous thrombosis can result in prehepatic portal hypertension with venous collaterals and gastric varices.

Pancreaticopleural fistulas are commonly associated with chronic alcoholic pancreatitis. Patients present with chest symptoms more often than abdominal symptoms. Pancreatic secretions from a ruptured pancreatic duct dissect through the aortic and esophageal hiatus or through the diaphragm and gain access to the pleural cavity and mediastinum.[18] CT and MRI with MR cholangiopancreatography (MRCP) can depict the fistula and ductal anatomy in these patients. Endoscopic retrograde cholangiopancreatography (ERCP) combined with CT can delineate the cause of recurrent pleural effusion and rare complications such as pancreaticobronchial fistula (Figs. 78-3 to 78-8).

Endoscopic Retrograde Cholangiopancreatography

ERCP is performed by cannulation of the ampulla of Vater and ingestion of iodinated contrast. ERCP allows visualization of the pancreatic ductal system, including the side branches, and is often considered the gold standard for defining the disease in its early stages.[22]

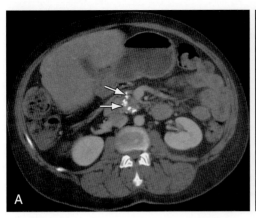
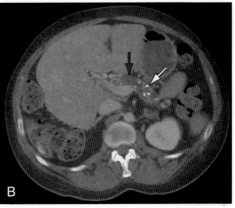

■ **FIGURE 78-3** Chronic pancreatitis. **A** and **B,** CT shows scattered coarse calcifications (*white arrows*) throughout the pancreas with dilatation of the main pancreatic duct (*red arrow*).

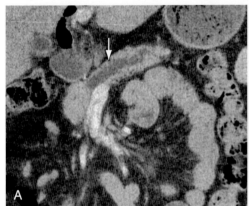
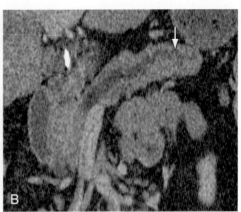

■ **FIGURE 78-4** Known cystic fibrosis. **A** and **B,** CT shows chronic pancreatitis changes with duct dilatation (**A,** *arrow*) and stricture (**B,** *arrow*).

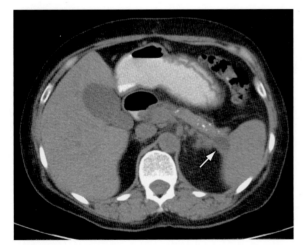

■ **FIGURE 78-5** CT shows chronic pancreatitis changes with a stable pseudocyst in the pancreatic tail (*arrow*).

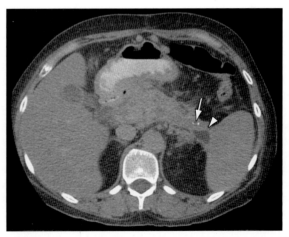

■ **FIGURE 78-6** CT shows features of acute-on-chronic pancreatitis with calcification (*arrow*) and small pseudocyst (*arrowhead*) in the pancreatic tail.

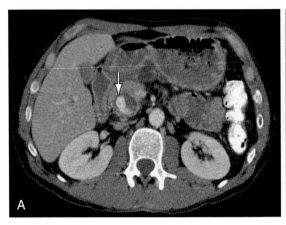
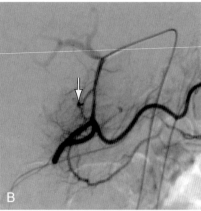

■ FIGURE 78-7 Gastroduodenal artery pseudoaneurysm in a middle-aged man with chronic pancreatitis and upper gastrointestinal tract hemorrhage. **A,** Contrast-enhanced CT arteriogram demonstrates pseudoaneurysm (*arrow*) probably originating from gastroduodenal artery. **B,** Arteriogram of the gastroduodenal artery demonstrates a pseudoaneurysm (*arrow*) originating from the gastroduodenal artery.

TABLE 78-3	Classification of Disease Severity on ERP	
Findings	**MPD**	**Side Branches**
Equivocal	Normal	Fewer than 3 side branches abnormal
Mild	Normal	≥3 side branches abnormal
Moderate	Abnormal	>3 side branches abnormal
Marked	Abnormal	Moderate disease and one of the following: a large cavity, ductal obstruction, filling defects, severe dilatation, or irregularity

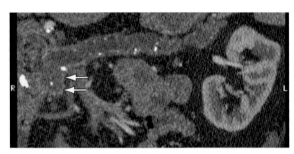

■ FIGURE 78-8 Curved planar reconstruction of pancreas showing chronic pancreatitis changes with a mass in the head of the pancreas (*arrows*).

The normal main pancreatic duct dimension varies between 95 to 25 mm in length. It has the greatest diameter in the pancreatic head with progressive narrowing toward the tail. The average normal diameter is 3 to 4 mm in the head, 2 to 3 mm in the body, and 1 to 2 mm in the tail. There is progressive increase in the overall diameter with aging due to parenchymal atrophy. Normal physiologic narrowing is seen at the junction of the major and minor ducts in the pancreatic head and in the mid gland as the pancreas crosses the mesenteric vessels and the spine. The side branches average 20 to 30 in number and join the main pancreatic duct at right angles alternating above and below. There are fewer branches in the body than in the head and tail. The branches taper toward the periphery from the point of junction.[17] ERCP first demonstrates changes in the side branches and subsequently in the main pancreatic duct. The ERCP features of chronic pancreatitis include dilatation, irregularity, clubbing, and stenosis of the side branches as well as opacification of small cavities.[23] The main pancreatic duct demonstrates diffuse duct dilatation, mural irregularity, loss of normal tapering, and multiple segmental areas of stenosis and dilatation. ERCP may also demonstrate pseudocysts communicating with the main duct. The distal common bile duct may show elongated smooth compression.[23] Solitary stricture of the main pancreatic duct caused by pseudocyst is shorter, is smooth, and shows gradual tapering (Table 78-3; Fig. 78-9).[24]

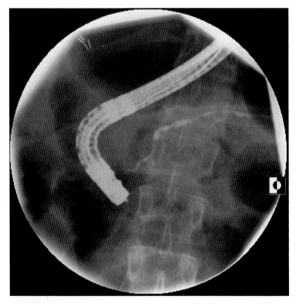

■ FIGURE 78-9 ERCP shows diffuse irregular dilatation of the main pancreatic duct secondary to chronic pancreatitis.

MRI

Recent advances in MR technology have significantly contributed to high-resolution noninvasive evaluation of the pancreatic parenchyma before and after intravenous administration of gadolinium, evaluation of the ducts using MRCP with or without secretin administration, and evaluation of pancreatic exocrine function by measuring duodenal fluid volume after secretin administration.

MRI can depict the diagnosis of chronic pancreatitis based on signal intensity and enhancement as well as morphologic abnormalities in the pancreatic parenchyma, pancreatic duct, and biliary tract. The normal pancreas appears isointense to slightly hyperintense to the liver on T1-weighted (T1W) non–fat-suppressed images. On T1W fat-suppressed images, the pancreas is hyperintense to all solid organs of the abdomen. On T2-weighted (T2W) images, the pancreas has signal intensity similar to the liver and appears hyperintense relative to the spleen and kidneys.

The normal pancreas shows maximum enhancement during the arterial phase after intravenous gadolinium. There is rapid washout during the portal venous and delayed phase when it appears isointense to the liver.[25]

Because of its excellent soft tissue contrast MRI is sensitive in detecting signal intensity and enhancement abnormalities in early chronic pancreatitis before morphologic changes occur.[26]

Early MRI findings of chronic pancreatitis include a low signal intensity of the pancreas on T1W fat-suppressed images owing to decreased proteinaceous fluid content from chronic inflammation and fibrosis.[26] Also noted is diminished heterogeneous enhancement of the pancreas in the arterial phase and progressive enhancement in the delayed phases.[26] There is also dilatation of the side branches. However, CT may demonstrate a normal appearance and enhancement of the pancreas even in advanced disease.

Later in the disease there is evidence of parenchymal atrophy; pseudocysts; dilatation, irregularity, and beading of the main pancreatic duct; and intraductal and parenchymal calcifications. Intraductal calcifications can cause pancreatic duct obstruction and are better defined on MRI.

MRCP

MRCP is an excellent noninvasive imaging technique that utilizes a heavily T2W pulse sequence to selectively display static or slow-moving fluid-filled structures as areas of high intensity.

Technique

3D MRCP sequences are obtained using fast recovery sequences or steady-state free precession in suspended respiration or with respiratory gated techniques. The near-isotropic volume data from 3D MRCP are processed using maximum intensity projection (MIP) or volume-rendered technique to display the pancreatic duct and biliary tree (Table 78-4; Fig. 78-10).

MRCP demonstrates side-branch abnormalities, dilatation and irregularity of the main pancreatic duct, strictures, and pseudocysts. Intraductal calcifications are seen as filling defects surrounded by intraductal fluid. It clearly shows the site of obstruction and the upstream dilatation of the main pancreatic duct, and it is also highly accurate in the diagnosis of pancreas divisum.[27] In

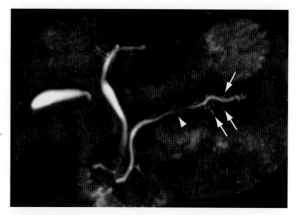

■ **FIGURE 78-10** MRCP image from a middle-aged patient with recurrent pancreatitis shows mild prominence of the side ductal branches (*arrows*) and decreased caliber of long ductal segment (*arrowhead*) suggestive of changes of chronic pancreatitis.

TABLE 78-4 Routinely Used Parameters for 2D and 3D MRCP

Technique	TE (ms)	TR	Thickness (mm)
2D MRCP			
Oblique radial SSFSE T2 weighted (14 slices)	500	Minimum	40
Oblique right anterior SSFSE T2 weighted	160	Minimum	5
Oblique left anterior SSFSE T2 weighted	160	Minimum	5
3D MRCP			
3D MRCP fat saturated	500-600	4000	1.4

advanced disease, the beaded main pancreatic duct with marked dilated side branches may result in a "chain of lakes" appearance.[28]

MRCP also demonstrates other abnormalities of the duct, including clubbing, sacculation, and ectasia of the side radicles; strictures; ductal obstruction; pseudocysts; and fistula formation. It also has the advantage of demonstrating biliary dilatation secondary to inflammatory stricture or compression of the bile duct.[29]

MRCP has a sensitivity of 60% to 80% and a high specificity of 95.5% to 100% in the diagnosis of filling defects.[30] The images can be viewed on a modern workstation as rotational MIP images, and it is possible to differentiate intraductal lesions within a dilated pancreatic duct from partial volume effects.

Functional/Secretin MRCP

A new pharmaceutical agent (Secreflo, Repligen Corporation, Waltham, MA) is now available that allows secretin functional MRCP and exocrine evaluation of the pancreas.

Technique

Intravenous administration of 1 mL of secretin per 10 kg of body weight is followed by thick-slab MRCP in the

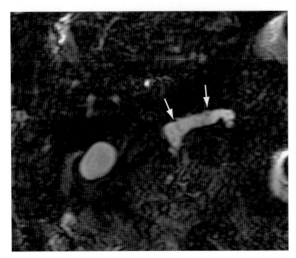

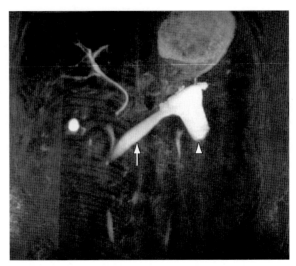

■ **FIGURE 78-11** MRCP shows diffuse pancreatic duct dilatation related to changes of chronic pancreatitis with multiple filling defects (*arrows*) within the duct representing intraductal calculi.

■ **FIGURE 78-12** MRCP image from a patient with chronic pancreatitis shows dilated pancreatic duct (*arrow*) and pseudocyst (*arrowhead*) communicating through pancreatic duct fistula.

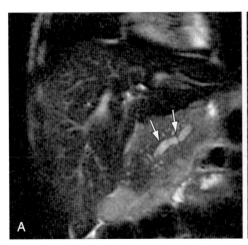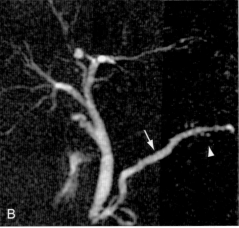

■ **FIGURE 78-13** Secretin MRCP. **A,** Dilated irregular duct with alternating areas of dilatations and narrowing (*arrows*) is seen. **B,** Early side branch dilatation (*arrow* and *arrowhead*) is seen in another case suggestive of changes secondary to chronic pancreatitis.

coronal plane repeated every 15 to 30 seconds for 10 to 15 minutes. The effect of secretin stimulation starts almost immediately after intravenous administration. Measurable dilatation of the main pancreatic duct is observed mostly within 2 to 6 minutes of secretin injection.[31] Around 10 minutes after injection, the caliber of the main pancreatic duct returns to baseline value as the pancreatic juice flows out through the papilla and progressively fills the duodenum. MRCP after secretin administration shows an increase in caliber of the pancreatic duct in patients with chronic pancreatitis. The normal progressive tapering of the duct toward the tail is lost in patients with severe chronic pancreatitis, and secretin improves the detection of this alteration in duct morphology. The time taken to reach peak pancreatic duct diameter after secretin administration is longer in patients with chronic pancreatitis than in normal patients. *Acinar filling* is a term used to describe progressive increase in signal intensity of the pancreatic parenchyma and may be a sign of early chronic pancreatitis.[32]

There have been reports suggesting better visualization of the pancreatic duct after intravenous administration of secretin. In addition, secretin MRCP is also useful for functional evaluation of exocrine pancreas based on quantification of duodenal filling, which with chronic pancreatitis is decreased.[31,33] Investigators are optimistic that secretin MRCP might demonstrate early ductal changes in patients with clinical suspicion of chronic pancreatitis in whom other imaging studies have been normal. However, presently the role of MRCP is limited to the diagnosis and follow-up of advanced cases (Figs. 78-11 to 78-14).

PET/CT

[18]Fluorodeoxyglucose (FDG)-labeled PET combined with CT is increasingly being used to differentiate benign from malignant masses. Maldonado and associates described a sensitivity of 100%, specificity of 91%, negative predictive value of 100%, positive predictive value of 96%, and

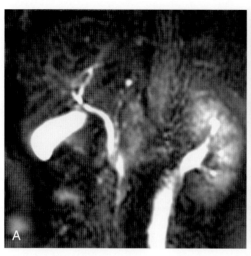
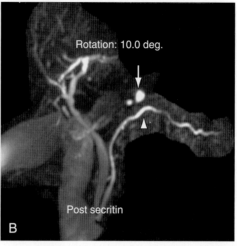

■ **FIGURE 78-14** Secretin MRCP. **A,** On pre-secretin view the relation of the cystic structure to main pancreatic duct is not well demonstrated. **B,** On post-secretin MRCP the relationship between pancreatic duct (*arrowhead*) and pseudocyst (*arrow*) is well seen and there is no communication of pseudocyst to main duct.

TABLE 78-5 Sensitivity and Specificity of Various Imaging Modalities

Modality	Sensitivity	Specificity
Plain radiographs	30-70%	100%
Ultrasonography	60-70%	80-90%
Endoscopic ultrasonography	97%	60%
Contrast-enhanced CT	75-90%	84-100%
MRI/MRCP	85%	100%
ERCP	71%-93%	89-100%

accuracy of 97% in detection of pancreatic lesions.[34] FDG-PET/CT also can be used to distinguish pancreatic carcinoma from a focal inflammatory pancreatic mass (Table 78-5).

Imaging Algorithm

See Figure 78-15 and Table 78-6.

Classic Signs

- Coarse, focal, or diffuse calcifications
- Ductal dilatation
- Pancreatic atrophy
- Pseudocysts

DIFFERENTIAL DIAGNOSIS

Common upper abdominal pathologic processes include acute pancreatitis, acute cholecystitis, choledocholithiasis, pancreatic tumor, and peptic ulcer disease. A finding on plain radiography and CT of pancreatic calcifications is highly suggestive of chronic pancreatitis. The cardinal CT findings of chronic pancreatitis include main pancreatic duct dilatation, calcifications, and pancreatic atrophy.

Pseudocysts, venous thrombosis, and pseudoaneurysms can also be detected with CT.

Evaluation of pancreatic duct and parenchyma with contrast-enhanced MRI and MRCP also offers differentiation of inflammatory and neoplastic masses. Endoscopic ultrasonography has emerged as a first-line modality for evaluation of early chronic pancreatitis and cystic and mass lesions.

TREATMENT

Medical Treatment

The medical management of chronic pancreatitis consists of management of abdominal pain and complications and includes:

1. Analgesics
2. Abstinence from alcohol and tobacco
3. Nerve blockade
4. Pancreatic enzymes with proton-pump inhibitors or histamine-2 blockers
5. Insulin
6. Corticosteroids in autoimmune pancreatitis
7. Vitamin supplements (A, D, E, K, and B_{12})
8. Antidepressants and psychiatric counseling for nonvisceral pain

Surgical Treatment

Endoscopy

Endoscopic duct decompression techniques include pancreatic sphincterotomy, removal of intraductal calculi, and placement of stents. Transampullary or transgastric drainage of pseudocysts can be done.

Decompression Procedures

Large or symptomatic pseudocysts can be drained through cystenterostomy. Lateral pancreaticojejunostomy may be necessary in large-duct disease. Sphincterotomy or sphincteroplasty may be needed.

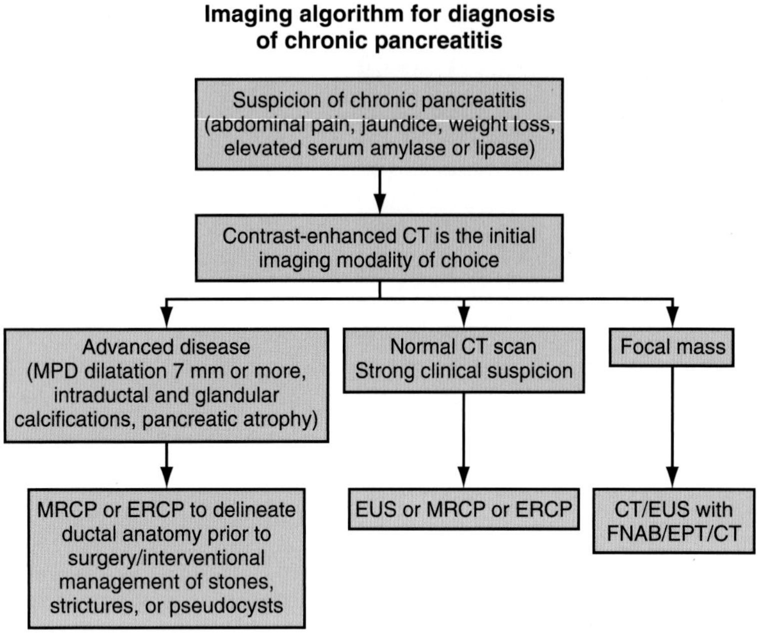

Imaging algorithm for diagnosis of chronic pancreatitis

```
┌─────────────────────────────────────────┐
│ Suspicion of chronic pancreatitis        │
│ (abdominal pain, jaundice, weight loss,  │
│ elevated serum amylase or lipase)        │
└─────────────────────────────────────────┘
                    │
                    ▼
┌─────────────────────────────────────────┐
│ Contrast-enhanced CT is the initial      │
│ imaging modality of choice               │
└─────────────────────────────────────────┘
       │                │              │
       ▼                ▼              ▼
┌──────────────┐ ┌─────────────┐ ┌──────────┐
│ Advanced     │ │ Normal CT   │ │ Focal    │
│ disease      │ │ scan Strong │ │ mass     │
│ (MPD         │ │ clinical    │ └──────────┘
│ dilatation   │ │ suspicion   │
│ 7 mm or      │ └─────────────┘
│ more,        │
│ intraductal  │
│ and          │
│ glandular    │
│ calcifica-   │
│ tions,       │
│ pancreatic   │
│ atrophy)     │
└──────────────┘
       │                │              │
       ▼                ▼              ▼
┌──────────────┐ ┌─────────────┐ ┌──────────┐
│ MRCP or ERCP │ │ EUS or MRCP │ │ CT/EUS   │
│ to delineate │ │ or ERCP     │ │ with     │
│ ductal       │ └─────────────┘ │ FNAB/    │
│ anatomy      │                 │ EPT/CT   │
│ prior to     │                 └──────────┘
│ surgery/     │
│ interven-    │
│ tional       │
│ management   │
│ of stones,   │
│ strictures,  │
│ or           │
│ pseudocysts  │
└──────────────┘
```

■ FIGURE 78-15 Imaging algorithm for diagnosis of chronic pancreatitis. EPT, endoscopic papillotomy; FNAB, fine-needle aspiration biopsy.

TABLE 78-6 Accuracy, Limitations, and Pitfalls of the Modalities Used in Imaging of Chronic Pancreatitis

Modality	Accuracy	Limitations	Pitfalls
Radiography	Poor	Not sensitive	
CT		Radiation	
MRI		Claustrophobia and patient motion	Calcifications difficult to visualize
		High cost	
Ultrasonography		Limited by bowel gas and obesity	Difficulty in differentiating small foci of calcification from small cysts
		Operator dependent	
Nuclear medicine	NA	NA	
PET/CT	NA	Radiation	
		High cost	

Resection

Distal pancreatectomy is done if the disease is confined to the tail of the gland. Otherwise, total pancreatectomy is performed. Whipple's procedure is also an option.

KEY POINTS

- Prolonged alcohol abuse is evident with calcifications, ductal dilatation, atrophy, and a focal mass; carcinoma may be present.
- Imaging modalities of benefit include contrast-enhanced CT, endoscopic ultrasonography, MRI, and secretin MRCP.

What the Referring Physician Needs to Know

- Contrast-enhanced CT is the initial imaging modality of choice.
- Endoscopic ultrasonography is a first-line tool in early chronic pancreatitis and evaluation of cystic and solid masses.
- Contrast-enhanced MRI and MRCP are excellent for non-invasive evaluation of parenchyma, ductal system, and complications of chronic pancreatitis.
- Chronic pancreatitis can present as a focal inflammatory mass mimicking pancreatic carcinoma.

REFERENCES

1. Banks PA. Classification and diagnosis of chronic pancreatitis. J Gastroenterol 2007; 42(Suppl 17):148-151.
2. Singer MV, Gyr K, Sarles H. Revised classification of pancreatitis. Report of the Second International Symposium on the Classification of Pancreatitis in Marseille, France, March 28-30, 1984. Gastroenterology 1985; 89:683-685.
3. Lee JK, Sagel SS, Stanley RJ, Heiken JP (eds). Computed Body Tomography with MRI Correlation, 4th ed. Philadelphia, Lippincott Williams & Wilkins, 2003.
4. Steer ML, Waxman I, Freedman S. Chronic pancreatitis. N Engl J Med 1995; 333:1482-1492.
5. Kim KP, Kim MH, Song MH, et al. Autoimmune chronic pancreatitis. AJR Am J Roentgenol 2004; 99:1605-1616.
6. Lin Y, Tamakoshi A, Hayakawa T, et al. Cigarette smoking as a risk factor for chronic pancreatitis: a case-control study in Japan. Research Committee on Intractable Pancreatic Diseases. Pancreas 2000; 21:109-114.
7. Layer P, Singer MV. Non-alcoholic–related etiologies in chronic pancreatitis. In Beger HG, Buchler M, Ditschuneit H, Malfertheiner P (eds). Chronic Pancreatitis. Berlin, Springer Verlag, 1990, pp 35-40.
8. Otsuki M. Chronic pancreatitis in Japan: epidemiology, prognosis, diagnostic criteria, and future problems. J Gastroenterol 2003; 38:315-326.
9. Layer P, Yamamoto H, Kalthoff L, et al. The different courses of early- and late-onset idiopathic and alcoholic chronic pancreatitis. Gastroenterology 1994; 107:1481-1487.
10. Warshaw AL, Banks PA, Fernandez-Del Castillo C. AGA technical review: treatment of pain in chronic pancreatitis. Gastroenterology 1998; 115:765-776.
11. Ammann RW, Muellhaupt B. The natural history of pain in alcoholic chronic pancreatitis. Gastroenterology 1999; 116:1132-1140.
12. Haaber AB, Rosenfalck AM, Hansen B, et al. Bone mineral metabolism, bone mineral density, and body composition in patients with chronic pancreatitis and pancreatic exocrine insufficiency. Int J Pancreatol 2000; 27:21-27.
13. Malka D, Hammel P, Sauvanet A, et al. Risk factors for diabetes mellitus in chronic pancreatitis. Gastroenterology 2000; 119:1324-1332.
14. Braganza JM. The pathogenesis of chronic pancreatitis. Q J Med 1996; 89:243-250.
15. Schneider A, Whitcomb DC. Hereditary pancreatitis: a model for inflammatory diseases of the pancreas. Best Pract Res Clin Gastroenterol 2002; 16:347-363.
16. Alpern MB, Sandler MA, Kellman GM, Madrazo BL. Chronic pancreatitis: ultrasonic features. Radiology 1985; 155:215-219.
17. Remer EM, Baker ME. Imaging of chronic pancreatitis. Radiol Clin North Am 2002; 40:1229-1242.
18. Siddiqi AJ, Miller F. Chronic pancreatitis: ultrasound, computed tomography, and magnetic resonance imaging features. Semin Ultrasound CT MR 2007; 28:384-394.
19. Luetmer PH, Stephens DH, Ward EM. Chronic pancreatitis: reassessment with current CT. Radiology 1989; 171:353-357.
20. Lesniak RJ, Hohenwalter MD, Taylor AJ. Spectrum of causes of pancreatic calcifications. AJR Am J Roentgenol 2002; 178:79-86.
21. Kattwinkel J, Lapey A, Di Sant'Agnese PA, Edwards WA. Hereditary pancreatitis: three new kindreds and a critical review of the literature. Pediatrics 1973; 51:55-69.
22. Clain JE, Pearson RK. Diagnosis of chronic pancreatitis. Is a gold standard necessary? Surg Clin North Am 1999; 79:829-845.
23. Miller F, Keppke AL, Balthazar E. Pancreatitis. In Laufer I (ed): Textbook of Gastrointestinal Radiology, vol 2, 3rd ed. Philadelphia, WB Saunders, 2007, pp 1767-1795.
24. Axon ATR, Classen M, Cotton PB, et al. Pancreatography in chronic pancreatitis: internal definitions. Gut 1984; 25:1107-1112.
25. Ito K, Koike S, Matsunaga N. MR imaging of pancreatic diseases. Eur J Radiol 2001; 38:78-93.
26. Semelka RC, Shoenut JP, Kroeker MA, Micflikier AB. Chronic pancreatitis: MR imaging features before and after administration of gadopentetate dimeglumine. J Magn Reson Imaging 1993; 3:79-82.
27. Ward J, Chalmers AG, Guthrie AJ, et al. T2-weighted and dynamic enhanced MRI in acute pancreatitis: comparison with contrast enhanced CT. Clin Radiol 1997; 52:109-114.
28. Miller FH, Keppke AL, Wadhwa A, et al. MRI of pancreatitis and its complications: part 2, chronic pancreatitis. AJR Am J Roentgenol 2004; 183:1645-1652.
29. Leyendecker JR, Elsayes KM, Gratz BI, Brown JJ. MR cholangiopancreatography: spectrum of pancreatic duct abnormalities. AJR Am J Roentgenol 2002; 179:1465-1471.
30. Varghese JC, Masterson A, Lee MJ. Value of MR pancreatography in the evaluation of patients with chronic pancreatitis. Clin Radiol 2002; 57:393-401.
31. Cappeliez O, Delhaye M, Deviere J, et al. Chronic pancreatitis: evaluation of pancreatic exocrine function with MR pancreatography after secretin stimulation. Radiology 2000; 215:358-364.
32. Matos C, Deviere J, Cremer M, et al. Acinar filling during secretin-stimulated MR pancreatography. AJR Am J Roentgenol 1998; 171:165-169.
33. Matos C, Metens T, Deviere J, et al. Pancreatic duct: morphologic and functional evaluation with dynamic MR pancreatography after secretin stimulation. Radiology 1997; 203:435-441.
34. Maldonado A, Gonzalez F, Tamames S, et al. The role of 18F-FDG PET/CT in the evaluation of pancreatic lesions. J Nucl Med 2007; 48(Suppl 2):26P.

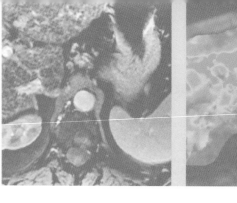
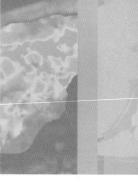

Miscellaneous Pancreatitis

Nisha I. Sainani

AUTOIMMUNE PANCREATITIS

Etiology

Autoimmune pancreatitis (AIP), also known as lympho-plasmacytic sclerosing pancreatitis, is a peculiar form of chronic pancreatitis that has recently gained significant attention. AIP is a heterogeneous, systemic disease characterized by a fibroinflammatory process involving multiple organs, unusual histopathologic and serologic features, an association with other autoimmune disorders, and a propensity to respond to corticosteroid therapy (CST).[1-3] The occurrence of AIP in concordance with other auto-immune disease processes (Table 79-1) has led to the acceptance of its immune-mediated etiology.[3-5] Absence of prior attacks of acute pancreatitis or alcohol abuse is a notable feature of this form of pancreatitis.[6] Although a benign disease, it often mimics pancreatic malignancy clinically and radiologically.[7]

Prevalence and Epidemiology

AIP is more common in elderly males.[8,9] However, the disease does affect a wide age range, with several documented cases in the second and third decades of life.[10] The prevalence of disease in the Western (North America and Europe) and Japanese populations has been studied, and certain differences have been observed.

Clinical Presentation

Clinical presentation of AIP is generally nonspecific with protean manifestations due to pancreatic and extrapancreatic involvement. Symptoms related to pancreatic involvement include vague upper abdominal pain, jaundice, nausea, vomiting, weight loss, back pain, and diabetes mellitus type 2. Some patients may seek medical attention for extrapancreatic manifestations with incidental detection of pancreatic involvement.[2,9,11] Although some patients may present acutely with jaundice, more often the nonspecific or mild symptoms are overlooked, resulting in delay in diagnosis. The disease may relapse a few times or may persist in a milder form for a time period before it is diagnosed. In some patients the diagnosis may be delayed to the stage when changes of chronicity such as atrophy or strictures have set in.[12] More than half of patients show some degree of exocrine and endocrine dysfunction.[9]

Pathophysiology

AIP is a systemic disease with predominant involvement of the pancreas. Other organ systems that may be involved include the biliary tree, liver, kidney, retroperitoneum, bowel, lungs, lymph nodes, and salivary glands.

Pathology

Laboratory

Obstructive jaundice from pancreatic inflammation can result in elevated levels of bilirubin and other biliary enzymes. Serum amylase and lipase values can be marginally abnormal. The pancreatic tumor marker CA 19-9 can be elevated, and this is probably due to cholestasis.[9] The involvement of pancreatic acinar, beta, and alpha cells by the inflammatory process results in exocrine and endocrine dysfunction. The exocrine dysfunction is characterized by reduced volume and amylase content of pancreatic secretions with normal bicarbonate content. This is due to preservation of the basement membrane of pancreatic ducts and also accounts for reversibility of exocrine function with CST. The endocrine abnormality is in the form of reduced insulin secretion from beta cells and glucagon from alpha cells; the beta cells are perturbed by circulatory failure due to inflammation and fibrosis along with reduction in number. The CST can reverse the inflammatory component affecting the beta cells but not the reduction in number, resulting in residual dysfunction.[13-15]

Serology

An elevated serum autoimmune phenomenon such as immunoglobulin level (especially IgG$_4$), is a characteristic feature. Elevated titers of various antibodies such as antinuclear antibodies, rheumatoid factor, anti–carbonic anhydrase antibody, perinuclear antineutrophil cytoplasmic antibody, anti–smooth muscle antibody, and antimitochondrial or antilactoferrin antibody have been variably reported, although none is consistently positive.[3,4,7,9] Serum IgG$_4$ is more sensitive than total IgG for diagnosis of AIP. It is, however, not specific or diagnostic, because elevated levels have also been observed in other forms of acute and chronic pancreatitis, in pancreatic carcinoma, and in individuals without any pancreatic disease (3% to 10%). Also, in the Western population, raised IgG$_4$ levels have been inconsistently observed. A higher IgG$_4$ cutoff value (280 mg/dL, twice the upper limit of normal) is considered highly sensitive and specific (>95%) for distinguishing AIP from pancreatic cancer. Although the positive predictive value of IgG$_4$ is very low (about 36%), owing to the low prevalence of disease as compared with other conditions with raised IgG$_4$, the negative predictive value is very high (99%).[16,17] Whenever elevated, the IgG$_4$ level can be a useful marker to monitor disease activity.[16-19] On the other hand, a high level of CA 19-9 (>100 U/mL) is more suggestive of pancreatic carcinoma. In patients with lower levels of serum IgG$_4$, the combination of clinical picture, other organ involvement, and characteristic imaging features is useful. The diagnosis can be confirmed by obtaining core biopsies of the pancreas.[16]

Gross Pathology

Resection of a pancreas affected by AIP could be difficult owing to smoldering, peripancreatic inflammation and fibrosis causing distortion of surgical planes, making dissection difficult and resulting in higher blood loss and longer operating time.[20] On gross inspection the gland is unremarkable but it is firm to rock hard on palpation. No dominant mass or well-circumscribed nodules are detected.[21,22]

Histopathology

The cardinal features include dense lymphoplasmacytic infiltration in the pancreatic parenchymal lobules with secondary interlobular and intralobular fibrosis. A collar of inflammation is also seen around small and large interlobular ducts. Although the lymphocytes are predominantly T cells, B cells are consistently present. The plasma cells are IgG$_4$ positive.[23] Occasional eosinophils are seen. The inflammatory infiltrate spills into the peripancreatic soft tissue, resulting in a characteristic imaging appearance. The lobular and ductal involvement is often patchy, which sometimes hampers definitive diagnosis on needle biopsy. Acinar loss frequently results, owing primarily to lobular involvement and secondarily to ductal obstruction. Progression of disease results in replacement of dense cellular infiltration with collagen fibrils and fibroblasts/myofibroblasts with lesser lymphoplasmacytic infiltrate. This is seen in chronic cases, particularly with development of focal mass-like swelling on imaging (pseudotumor).[22] The tumorous swellings seen in chronic alcoholic pancreatitis consist of extensive fibrosis with necrosis, abscesses, stones, and reparative granulation tissue, thus distinguishing it from AIP.[24]

Intraductal neutrophilic (granulocytic) infiltration is occasionally observed and has been linked to concurrent presence or future development of ulcerative colitis.[10] Periphlebitis and obliterative phlebitis, sparing the arterioles, is invariably present and useful for establishing the diagnosis. Perineural inflammation, although nonspecific, is frequently encountered.[10,22] Epithelioid cell granulomas especially in a ductocentric location have been reported.[25] Changes associated with chronic alcoholic pancreatitis are typically absent. However, cysts, which probably represent retention cysts due to pancreatic ductal obstruction, and duct stones have been reported.[12,22]

Depending on the preponderance of involvement, histologically, AIP has been substratified into predominant lobular involvement (AIP-PL) (lymphoplasmacytic sclerosing pancreatitis) and predominant ductal involvement (AIP-PD) (idiopathic ductocentric pancreatitis).[10,22] The

TABLE 79-1 Autoimmune Disorders Associated with AIP

Sjögren's syndrome
Idiopathic thrombocytopenic purpura
Rheumatoid arthritis
Systemic lupus erythematosus
Primary sclerosing cholangitis
Primary biliary cirrhosis
Inflammatory bowel disease
Diabetes mellitus

TABLE 79-2 Difference in Two Histologic Subtypes of Autoimmune Pancreatitis

Feature	Predominant Lobular Involvement (AIP-PL)	Predominant Ductal Involvement (AIP-PD)
Gender	Male predominance	—
Age	—	Younger age group
Population predominance	Japanese	Western (North America and Europe)
Inflammation	Predominant lobular and septal	Predominant ductocentric
	Fibroblastic proliferation	Ductocentric granulomas
	Minimal periductal	Minimal or focal lobular
	Higher number of IgG$_4$ + plasma cells	Neutrophilic infiltration more common
Pseudotumors	—	More common
Common extrapancreatic manifestation	Sialadenitis	Inflammatory bowel disease

differences encountered between the two groups are listed in Table 79-2.[22,26,27]

The inflammatory infiltrates invade and compress the walls of the pancreatic duct and common bile duct, resulting in thickening and luminal narrowing. If not treated, the process becomes chronic with progression to fibrosis and stricture formation.[25,28]

The extrapancreatic lesions, like the pancreatic disease, reveal lymphoplasmacytic infiltration, fibrosis, IgG$_4$-positive plasma cells, and obliterative phlebitis. Absence of these features along with low-grade inflammation that is predominantly located beneath the epithelium in primary sclerosing cholangitis can help differentiate it from AIP-associated sclerosing cholangitis.[29] Occasionally, hepatic inflammatory pseudotumors with dense lymphoplasmacytic infiltration, myofibroblastic proliferation, and fibrosis have been reported.[29] A resected gallbladder from a patient with AIP also reveals similar histologic features.[30] Histologically, the renal lesions reveal tubulointerstitial nephritis with lymphoplasmacytic infiltration and fibrosis.[31]

IgG$_4$ Immunohistochemistry

Organs affected by this disease process have a lymphoplasmacytic infiltrate rich in IgG$_4$-positive plasma cells on immunostaining.[11] Tissue infiltration with IgG$_4$-positive plasma cells can be seen even in absence of serum IgG$_4$ elevation. Although higher numbers of pancreatic IgG$_4$-positive plasma cells have been identified in AIP as compared with pancreatic carcinoma and chronic pancreatitis, the existence of this overlap precludes use of immunolabeling as an absolute diagnostic means, particularly when evaluating a biopsy specimen. Absence of IgG$_4$-positive plasma cells weighs against the diagnosis of AIP, whereas presence of large numbers of these cells supports the diagnosis.[2,22]

Immunogeneity

An increased number of HLA class II antigens DR4 and DQ4 (DRB1*0405 and DRB1*0410 alleles) has been associated with AIP. It is speculated that these molecules may present a specific peptide that triggers the autoimmune response. No association has been found with HLA class I antigens.[32]

Imaging

Because of the variegated and heterogeneous renditions of AIP, the diagnosis is currently based on the criteria proposed by the Japan Pancreas Society (Revised proposal, 2006) or the HISORt criteria from the Mayo Clinic.[2,8] These criteria take into consideration the combination of imaging, laboratory, and serologic features, histopathologic findings with extrapancreatic manifestations, associated disorders, and response to corticosteroids.

Radiography

There is no role for radiography in evaluating the pancreatic or extrapancreatic features of AIP.

CT

CT is considered the modality of choice for assessing the varied manifestations of AIP. Focal or, more frequently, diffuse swelling of the pancreas is the most common imaging feature. The classic appearance is that of a diffusely enlarged, sausage-shaped pancreas with sharp borders and absence of normal pancreatic clefts (featureless) with homogeneous attenuation. Moderate heterogeneous and delayed enhancement is often seen. A peripheral, smooth, well-defined rim of hypoattenuation appears as a halo around the pancreatic parenchyma and represents inflammatory exudate (Figs. 79-1 and 79-2).[3] Infrequently, the halo reveals a capsule-like enhancement on the delayed phase of contrast enhancement.[33] Minimal stranding in peripancreatic fat and retraction of the pancreatic tail ("tail cutoff") are commonly seen (see Fig. 79-1).[3] Multifocal enlargement of the pancreas occurring concurrently or spaced in time has been noted.[33,34]

With advanced disease, there may be development of focal mass-like swelling (Fig. 79-3). This has been reported more commonly in Western populations and is known as pseudotumorous pancreatitis or inflammatory pancreatic mass; in Japan it is known as tumor-forming pancreatitis.[26,28] These mass-like swellings are often misdiagnosed as pancreatic carcinomas and are surgically treated.[35] They show homogeneous delayed enhancement on CT.[3]

Segmental or diffuse irregularity and narrowing of the pancreatic duct due to compression from surrounding inflammation, with or without thickening and enhancement, is seen. The distal common bile duct may reveal tapered narrowing owing to compression from adjacent involved pancreatic parenchyma or from involvement of the common bile duct by the disease process itself; the involved duct may also reveal contrast enhancement. Involvement of the common bile duct and resulting biliary obstruction often require biliary drainage (see Fig. 79-2).[1,36]

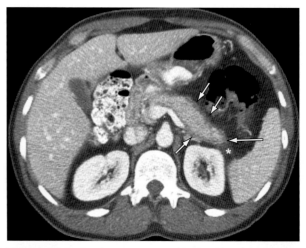

■ **FIGURE 79-1** Autoimmune pancreatitis. On this axial CT image the pancreas is diffusely swollen with loss of lobulations. The pancreatic duct is attenuated (not visualized), and the pancreatic tail is retracted (*long arrow*). A smooth rim of hypoattenuation, a "halo" (*arrows*), is seen around the pancreas. Minimal stranding in seen in the peripancreatic fat (*asterisk*).

The pancreatic swelling, peripancreatic changes, and irregular narrowing of the pancreatic duct usually improve in most of the patients, especially if CST is instituted early in the course of disease. The biliary narrowing also improves with CST, allowing withdrawal of biliary drainage tubes.[37] Ductal stricture develops in the absence of timely institution of CST or with a protracted disease course, which may result in irregular upstream dilatation of the pancreatic duct.[25]

Vascular encasement is conspicuously absent,[33] although mass effect on the vessels and narrowing of peripancreatic veins can be seen. Occasional cysts in relation to the pancreas have been reported; these are known to disappear with or without treatment, without any

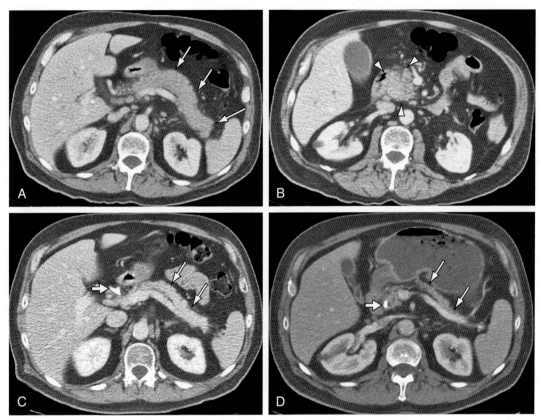

■ **FIGURE 79-2**   Autoimmune pancreatitis. Axial CT images through the pancreas at different time points of disease process in same patient. **A,** The pancreas is diffusely swollen and featureless (sausage-shaped) (*arrows*) with attenuated pancreatic duct (not visualized). **B,** A prominent focal swelling is detected in the pancreatic head (*arrowheads*), with resultant obstruction of the common bile duct requiring biliary drainage. The patient was started on corticosteroid therapy. **C,** CT image 2 months after treatment reveals significant improvement in the diffuse and focal pancreatic swelling (*arrows*). Biliary stent is seen in situ (*thick arrow*). **D,** CT image 5 months after the initial evaluation reveals an atrophic pancreas (*arrows*). A biliary stent is seen in situ (*thick arrow*) and was later removed.

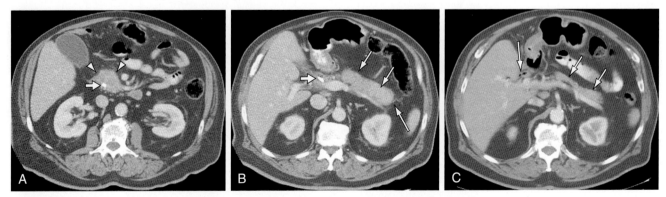

■ **FIGURE 79-3**   Autoimmune pancreatitis. Axial CT images at different time points of disease process. **A,** A focal swelling (*arrowheads*) is seen in the head of pancreas with a biliary stent (*thick arrow*) in situ to relieve the obstruction. **B,** Sausage-shaped enlargement of body and tail of pancreas (*arrows*) with tail cut off (*long arrow*) is also seen. Biliary stent (*thick arrow*) is seen in situ. The focal swelling in the head of pancreas was resected (Whipple's procedure) due to unremitting symptoms and concern for malignancy. Based on histopathologic diagnosis of AIP, the patient was then treated with corticosteroids. **C,** A follow-up CT examination 3 months later reveals near-complete resolution of swelling of body and tail of pancreas (*arrows*). Air is noted in the biliary tree (postoperative finding) (*long thin arrow*).

sequelae.[12] AIP is rarely associated with stone formation, more so in relapsing cases.[38] Pancreatic calcification and ascites are not seen.[1] A long-term, protracted disease course often results in atrophy of the gland (see Fig. 79-2).[37]

The extrapancreatic manifestations associated with AIP are listed in Table 79-3.[31,39,40] Extrapancreatic manifestations can occur simultaneously or can appear before or after detection of pancreatic involvement.[41] Extrapancreatic manifestations may be useful in supporting the diagnosis in equivocal cases.[12]

Sclerosing cholangitis–like involvement of biliary tree, which is a manifestation of AIP, can be differentiated from primary sclerosing cholangitis (a common association with AIP) or cholangiocarcinoma by tissue infiltration with abundant IgG$_4$-positive plasma cells and response to corticosteroids.[11,40]

TABLE 79-3 Extrapancreatic Manifestations of Autoimmune Pancreatitis

Sclerosing cholangitis (68%-88%)
Renal lesions (35%)
Inflammatory bowel disease (17%) (Ulcerative colitis, Crohn's disease)
Sialadenitis (12%-16%)
Retroperitoneal fibrosis (3%-8%)
Chronic thyroiditis
Abdominal, cervical, hilar lymphadenopathy
Interstitial pneumonia
Autoimmune hepatitis
Orbital pseudotumor
Malignant lymphoma

Typically, the renal lesions are parenchymal; however, there can be involvement of the perirenal tissue, renal sinus, and renal pelvis wall. Renal parenchymal lesions are commonly multiple, cortical, and nonenhancing. On imaging, these are represented by either wedge-shaped lesions, ill-defined rounded or nodular lesions, or diffuse patchy lesions, seen on the contrast-enhanced examination (Fig. 79-4A). These lesions may resemble pyelonephritis, vascular insult, lymphoma, renal cell carcinoma, or Wegener's granulomatosis on imaging; associated pancreatic or other extrapancreatic abnormalities should be looked for to appropriately classify these lesions. The soft tissue masses in the renal pelvis associated with AIP can resemble urothelial tumors and lymphomas. The perirenal rim of soft tissue and thickening of renal pelvic wall represent an inflammatory process related to AIP. The renal lesions do not affect the renal function in the early stage; the long-term effects, with or without CST, are not yet clearly known. However, fibrosis in the later stages results in cortical volume loss.[31]

Retroperitoneal fibrosis most commonly appears as a mantle of tissue adjacent to the aorta and other retroperitoneal structures and is morphologically indistinguishable from other causes of retroperitoneal fibrosis (see Fig. 79-4B). If untreated, it can also result in hydronephrosis.[39]

Association of ulcerative colitis with AIP is more frequently observed in the Western population and in a relatively younger age group.[10,26,40,42,43]

Incidence of AIP-associated sialadenitis is higher in the Japanese population.[26] Sialadenitis co-occurring with AIP is negative for anti-SSA and anti-SSB antibodies, shows elevated serum IgG$_4$ levels and IgG$_4$-positive plasma cell

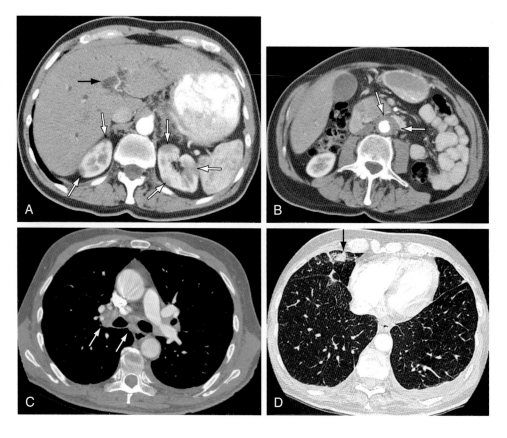

■ **FIGURE 79-4** Autoimmune pancreatitis. Axial CT images revealing extrapancreatic manifestations of AIP in same patient. **A,** Multiple, nonenhancing wedge-shaped and nodular, renal cortical lesions (*arrows*). Note the prominence of the biliary tree (*black arrow*) resulting from involvement of the distal CBD by swelling in the head of pancreas. **B,** A retroperitoneal mantle is seen surrounding the aorta (*arrows*). **C,** Note multiple mediastinal and hilar lymph nodes (*white arrows*). **D,** Parenchymal lesions are seen in the lung (*black arrow*).

infiltration in tissue, and is thus different from the typical Sjögren's syndrome. The involved salivary glands (parotid or submandibular) are enlarged, which can be confirmed by scintigraphy.[39]

Abdominal, cervical, and hilar adenopathy has been reported in association with AIP and tends to respond to CST (see Fig. 79-4C). Pulmonary involvement may result in discrete or diffuse nodules or infiltrates (see Fig. 79-4D).

The wide spectrum of disease manifestations with the prevalence of IgG4-positive plasma cells has justifiably resulted in considering this a systemic IgG4 disease.[11]

MRI

There is no specific indication for MRI in evaluation of AIP. MR cholangiopancreatography (MRCP) can be performed as a noninvasive technique in lieu of endoscopic cholangiopancreatography (ERCP) for evaluation and subsequent follow-up of ductal changes.

The involved pancreas appears hypointense on T1-weighted (T1W) images. The gland may appear hyperintense on T2-weighted (T2W) images when inflammation is predominant; it is hypointense when fibrosis predominates (Fig. 79-5). Delayed parenchymal enhancement is seen after intravenous administration of gadolinium. The "halo" appears hypointense on T1W and T2W images. The seldom-seen, delayed capsule–like enhancement of the halo is better appreciated on T1W fat-suppressed gadolinium-enhanced MR images as compared with CT.[25,33,34]

The renal parenchymal and sinus lesions appear hypointense on T1W and T2W imaging.[31]

ERCP

ERCP has an important role in pretreatment and posttreatment evaluation of ductal changes. Moreover, it is of more value than MRCP because it allows simultaneous biliary drainage in required cases.

The main pancreatic duct reveals focal or diffuse irregularity and narrowing, without upstream dilatation (Fig, 79-6). Segmental involvement of the pancreas with segmental narrowing of the pancreatic duct is more likely to mimic a carcinoma.[44] Narrowing of the distal common bile duct with variable proximal dilatation is often observed (Fig. 79-7).[1,33] On ERCP the features of sclerosing cholangitis associated with AIP are morphologically difficult to distinguish from primary sclerosing cholangitis or even bile duct cancer (Fig. 79-8).[12]

Ultrasonography

Transabdominal ultrasonography of the pancreas is rarely diagnostic of AIP. Moreover, the findings on ultrasonography resemble those of other forms of pancreatitis. The focal or diffusely swollen gland appears hypoechoic. The diffusely altered echotexture of the involved pancreas is better appreciated on endoscopic ultrasonography (EUS), especially when the gland appears normal or

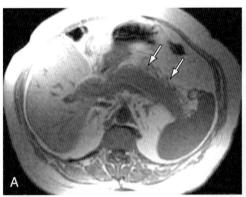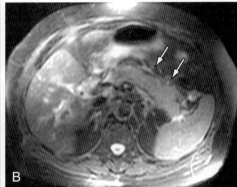

■ **FIGURE 79-5** Autoimmune pancreatitis. **A,** Axial T1W MR image reveals swollen body and tail of the pancreas, which appears hypointense. Stranding in the peripancreatic fat is also seen (*arrows*). **B,** Axial T2W fat-suppressed MR image reveals mildly hyperintense pancreas with peripancreatic stranding (*arrows*).

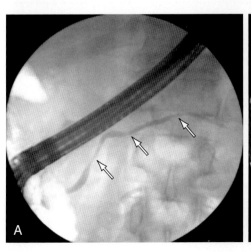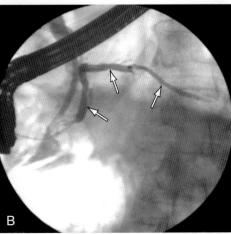

■ **FIGURE 79-6** Autoimmune pancreatitis. **A,** ERCP image reveals irregularity and multisegmental narrowing (*arrows*) of the pancreatic duct. **B,** ERCP performed 2 months after corticosteroid therapy shows improvement of the narrowing and irregularity (*arrows*) with normalization of ductal changes.

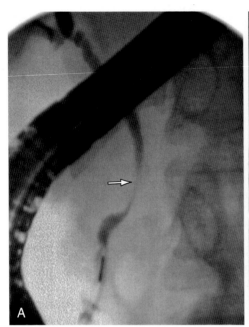
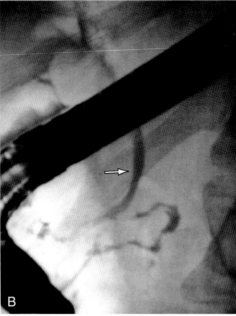

■ **FIGURE 79-7**   Autoimmune pancreatitis. **A,** ERCP reveals a long segment of narrowing of the distal common bile duct (*arrow*) with mild proximal dilatation. **B,** ERCP performed 1 month after corticosteroid therapy shows resolution of common bile duct narrowing (*arrow*).

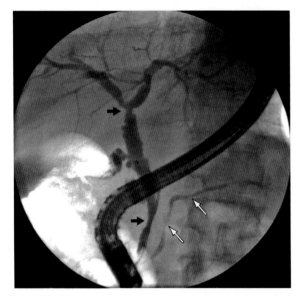

■ **FIGURE 79-8**   Autoimmune pancreatitis. Sclerosing cholangitis. ERCP reveals segments of narrowing in the distal common bile duct and hilar region (*thick arrows*). The pancreatic duct also reveals multiple segments of irregular narrowing (*thin arrows*).

equivocal on CT. This is due to higher sensitivity of EUS and close proximity to the gland.[3] However, the appearance of the focal mass-like swelling may be deceptively similar to that of pancreatic carcinoma. EUS-guided fine-needle aspiration biopsy serves as a relatively less invasive technique to acquire tissue for further evaluation of these focal mass-like swellings (Fig. 79-9). Mural thickening of the distal common bile duct and proximal biliary tree are also clearly visualized with EUS.[7]

Nuclear Medicine

Scintigraphy can confirm enlargement of the salivary glands associated with AIP.[39] Hilar adenopathy in AIP

reveals increased uptake on gallium-67 scintigraphy, which also disappears after CST.[45]

PET/CT

Increased fluorodeoxyglucose (FDG) uptake is seen in the pancreas and other involved organs in the inflammatory phase of the disease. FDG-PET can be useful in evaluating disease activity and discovering other hypermetabolic lesions in the extrapancreatic location. Response to CST is marked by disappearance of the intense uptake and correlates with improvement in the serum IgG$_4$ levels.[46]

Imaging Algorithm

An imaging algorithm is presented in Figure 79-10; see also Table 79-4.

Classic Signs: Autoimmune Pancreatitis

- Diffuse pancreatic swelling: "featureless sausage-shaped pancreas"
- Halo
- Minimal peripancreatic stranding
- Diffuse irregular pancreatic ductal attenuation
- No vascular encasement or invasion in presence of focal mass-like swelling
- Extrapancreatic manifestations
- Resolution with corticosteroid therapy

Differential Diagnosis

AIP should be differentiated from other pancreatic disorders because the morphologic and functional changes of AIP are reversible with CST.[3]

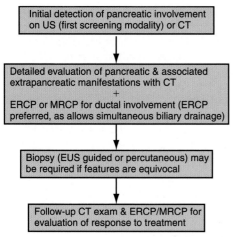

■ **FIGURE 79-10** Imaging algorithm for autoimmune pancreatitis.

The focal form, particularly involving the head and uncinate process of the pancreas, may be difficult to differentiate from pancreatic carcinoma.[3] Focal mass-like swelling associated with AIP enhances like the rest of the pancreas and can thus be differentiated from pancreatic carcinoma, which is generally hypoattenuating in the parenchymal phase. However, this finding alone cannot be relied on for differentiation because hypoattenuating focal AIP lesions and isoattenuating pancreatic carcinomas have been reported.[3,47] Concomitant diffuse changes in the pancreas and ducts, lack of pancreatic duct occlusion or upstream dilatation, absence of substantial parenchymal atrophy, vascular encasement or metastasis, and features of associated autoimmune disorders favor AIP.[3] Adequate imaging criteria to differentiate focal AIP from pancreatic carcinoma have not been established; and thus in suspicious cases, those not responding to

■ **FIGURE 79-9** Autoimmune pancreatitis. **A,** A focal hypoechoic mass-like lesion (inflammatory pseudotumor) is seen in the head of the pancreas (*arrows*) on endoscopic ultrasonography, mimicking a carcinoma. **B,** Endoscopic ultrasound–guided fine-needle aspiration biopsy can be a useful technique to acquire tissue for further evaluation of these lesions. The needle is seen (*arrow*).

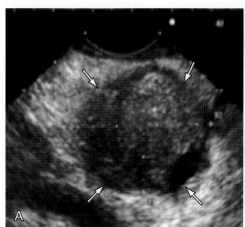
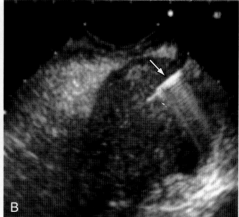

TABLE 79-4 Accuracy, Advantages, Limitations, and Pitfalls of the Modalities Used in Imaging of Autoimmune Pancreatitis

Modality	Accuracy*	Advantages	Limitations	Pitfalls
CT	Imaging modality of choice	Sensitive Detects pancreatic and extrapancreatic lesions Useful for follow-up	Radiation exposure	Ductal changes not distinctly visualized May mimic other forms of pancreatitis or pancreatic carcinoma
MRI		Sensitive MRCP reveals ductal abnormalities better than CT No radiation exposure	Patient cooperation needed High cost Not specific	May mimic other forms of pancreatitis or pancreatic carcinoma
Ultrasonography	First screening modality	No radiation exposure	Not sensitive Not specific Hindrance by bowel gas and obesity Does not give a comprehensive picture of disease process Operator dependent	May mimic other forms of pancreatitis or pancreatic carcinoma
Nuclear medicine		Sensitive Applications in sialadenitis and adenopathy	Not specific Poor spatial resolution No role in evaluation of pancreatic disease process	Mimics other inflammatory or neoplastic processes
PET/CT		Sensitive Detects pancreatic and extrapancreatic hypermetabolic foci	Not specific Radiation exposure High cost	Mimics other inflammatory or neoplastic processes

*No studies evaluating the comparative role of different modalities or accuracy of a modality per se are available because of rarity of this disease process.

corticosteroids, or with persistent intractable symptoms, one has to resort to histopathologic evaluation.[1]

The diffusely enlarged pancreas may morphologically resemble other diffuse disorders such as lymphomas, metastases, or infiltrative processes.

Histopathologic evaluation is the gold standard for confirmation of the diagnosis and excluding the possibility of a carcinoma.[2] Although most often resorted to, pancreatic core biopsies are often nondiagnostic (50% in AIP), owing to patchy involvement of the gland by the disease process and lack of duct or vein in the biopsy specimen.[10] The false-negative rate of core biopsy can be minimized to some extent by performing guided procedures utilizing transabdominal ultrasonography or EUS.[48] EUS-guided fine-needle aspiration biopsy is a relatively less invasive alternative of acquiring the tissue sample and can suggest the diagnosis of AIP in clinically and radiologically suspected cases.[7,12] However, guided fine-needle aspiration cytology has a limited role in detection of malignant cells. The technique of immunostaining for IgG$_4$-positive plasma cells from a biopsy specimen of the pancreas and other involved organs can enhance the diagnostic yield and support the diagnosis of AIP, especially in inexplicable cases or in the event of sole extrapancreatic manifestations.[2] Nonetheless, histopathologic evaluation is an invasive technique that may not be feasible in all patients and also may not be a practical approach.

A constellation of parameters thus may be needed to reliably make a diagnosis. A strong clinical suspicion based on symptoms, serology, laboratory parameters, along with pancreatic and extrapancreatic clinical manifestations can suggest the diagnosis. A response to corticosteroids is an important criterion, not only for the management of the disease but also for gauging the diagnosis.[2]

Treatment

Medical Treatment

CST is now being considered as standard therapy for AIP.[49] The pancreatic, ductal, and extrapancreatic manifestations due to the inflammatory component of the disease process, associated clinical symptoms, and laboratory findings including the endocrine and exocrine dysfunction respond often dramatically to CST. However, because AIP is associated with intense fibrosis, many radiologic changes (ductal changes, retroperitoneal fibrosis) may improve only partially or in some cases remain unchanged after treatment.[50] When the protracted fibrosing process becomes predominant, it results in an unfavorable response and irreversible changes, with lack of restoration of normal structure and function, especially if treatment with CST is delayed.[9,37,51] CST should be used carefully, and the response should be objectively assessed; CST should not be a mere substitute to other investigative parameters.[2] Maintenance CST may be needed for some cases, and this is more likely in patients with extrapancreatic lesions.[26]

For CST, an initial dose of 30 to 40 mg/day for 2 to 4 weeks with careful observation of clinical, laboratory, and imaging findings, followed by gradual reduction of 5 mg/week to a maintenance dose in 2 to 3 months and finally to 2.5 to 5 mg/day after remission, has been recom-

mended. Radiologic response is seen in 2 to 3 weeks. Normalization of radiologic findings can be seen in 4 to 6 weeks. If biliary stenting was done, stent removal is possible within 6 to 8 weeks after starting CST.[50] Although the duration of the maintenance dose is uncertain, therapy can be stopped after 6 to 12 months depending on improvement. Regular clinical and laboratory (including serologic studies every 6 months) follow-up can help detect any recurrence.[41,49] Relapses are seen in 6% to 26% (average, 17%) of cases after tapering of corticosteroids or while on maintenance therapy, and these patients may require a second course with a higher dose or a longer maintenance dose.[37,52] Whether a long-term maintenance dose will prevent relapses is yet to be determined and will have to be balanced with the risk of CST-related adverse effects.

In our experience, atrophy is a late stage of disease; CST has little role to play at this stage, unless there is associated extrapancreatic disease that needs therapy.[51] In fact, atrophy may also be seen after CST, and this is attributed to the acinar loss that is caused by the dynamic disease process.[22] Likewise, strictures and focal mass-like swellings that persist after the course of CST are unlikely to respond to prolonged therapy and need surgical treatment to relieve the symptoms.

Immunomodulatory medications, such as azathioprine or mycophenolate mofetil, have been used for corticosteroid sparing in patients with relapses.[41] Blood sugar needs to be controlled in patients who develop diabetes mellitus.[49]

Although spontaneous resolution of acute presentation of the disease is known to occur, institution of CST is more rational, because it hastens the resolution of clinical and radiologic features and is likely to prevent progression of fibrosis and its consequential complications.[41,51]

CST should be used with caution if the diagnosis is in doubt. Also, if CST does not give a desired response, a re-evaluation with additional diagnostic techniques should be sought to exclude malignancy.[49] This is especially relevant when focal mass-like swellings develop that respond less favorably to CST.

The long-term effect of AIP treated with CST on the pancreatic morphology and pancreatic function is uncertain, and long drawn-out follow-ups would be required to determine this.

Surgical Treatment

Short-term biliary drainage can be performed in patients with biliary obstruction and jaundice.[49] Although in the past surgery was extensively used as a prime approach to treat AIP, improved understanding of the disease process has led to a paradigm shift in the management protocol. Surgical resection is now utilized for focal mass-like swellings or biliary strictures that develop late in the course of the disease, which generally do not respond to CST.

TUMOR LYSIS PANCREATITIS

Tumor lysis syndrome occurs in patients with lymphoproliferative malignancies treated with chemotherapy, radiation therapy, or corticosteroids, although spontaneous occurrence has also been reported.[53,54] Involvement of the pancreas indistinguishable from other causes of acute pancreatitis has been reported to be rarely associated.[55]

What the Referring Physician Needs to Know: Autoimmune Pancreatitis

■ Awareness of the concept of AIP and its diverse manifestations is most important.

■ Imaging findings in combination with the clinical and serologic parameters should alert the clinician to the diagnosis.

■ Imaging is the most important factor in diagnosis because laboratory and histopathologic findings may often be insufficient and nonspecific.

■ Association of other autoimmune diseases provides a potential clue.

■ There is a propensity for AIP to resemble pancreatic carcinoma clinically and radiologically.

■ Recognition of this disease with a preoperative diagnosis is essential because the disease is reversible with timely institution of corticosteroids.

■ Surgery can be avoided.

■ Long-term prognosis appears better than other forms of chronic pancreatitis because morphologic and functional reversal occurs after CST.

EOSINOPHILIC PANCREATITIS

Eosinophilic pancreatitis is most commonly a systemic manifestation of peripheral eosinophilia, elevated serum IgE levels, and/or eosinophilic infiltrates in other organs.[56] On imaging, it may present as diffuse involvement of the pancreas, which histopathologically reveals diffuse, periductal, acinar, and septal eosinophilic infiltrates and eosinophilic phlebitis with arteritis. Focal involvement and pseudocyst formation may also be encountered.[57] This entity may be indistinguishable from other causes of pancreatitis on imaging; clinical and laboratory correlation along with imaging involvement of other organs is necessary for diagnosis.

KEY POINTS: AUTOIMMUNE PANCREATITIS

■ Evolving understanding of the disease process
■ Heterogeneous disorder
■ Association with autoimmune phenomena
■ Serum IgG_4 level
■ Pancreatic and extrapancreatic manifestations
■ Pancreatic carcinoma: main differential diagnosis
■ Response and reversibility with corticosteroids

SUGGESTED READINGS

Chari ST. Current concepts in the treatment of autoimmune pancreatitis. JOP 2007; 8:1-3.

Chari ST, Smyrk TC, Levy MJ, et al. Diagnosis of autoimmune pancreatitis: the Mayo Clinic experience. Clin Gastroenterol Hepatol 2006; 4:1010-1016; quiz 934.

Deshpande V, Mino-Kenudson M, Brugge W, Lauwers GY. Autoimmune pancreatitis: more than just a pancreatic disease? A contemporary review of its pathology. Arch Pathol Lab Med 2005; 129:1148-1154.

Finkelberg DL, Sahani D, Deshpande V, Brugge WR. Autoimmune pancreatitis. N Engl J Med 2006; 355:2670-2676.

Kamisawa T, Okamoto A. Prognosis of autoimmune pancreatitis. J Gastroenterol 2007; 42(Suppl 18):59-62.

Kloppel G, Luttges J, Sipos B, et al. Autoimmune pancreatitis: pathological findings. JOP 2005; 6:97-101.

Kwon S, Kim MH, Choi EK. The diagnostic criteria for autoimmune chronic pancreatitis: it is time to make a consensus. Pancreas 2007; 34:279-286.

Okazaki K, Chiba T. Autoimmune related pancreatitis. Gut 2002; 51: 1-4.

Okazaki K, Kawa S, Kamisawa T, et al. Clinical diagnostic criteria of autoimmune pancreatitis: revised proposal. J Gastroenterol 2006; 41:626-631.

Suda K, Takase M, Fukumura Y, Kashiwagi S. Pathology of autoimmune pancreatitis and tumor-forming pancreatitis. J Gastroenterol 2007; 42(Suppl 18):22-27.

REFERENCES

1. Yang DH, Kim KW, Kim TK, et al. Autoimmune pancreatitis: radiologic findings in 20 patients. Abdom Imaging 2006; 31:94-102.

2. Chari ST, Smyrk TC, Levy MJ, et al. Diagnosis of autoimmune pancreatitis: the Mayo Clinic experience. Clin Gastroenterol Hepatol 2006; 4:1010-1016; quiz 934.

3. Sahani DV, Kalva SP, Farrell J, et al. Autoimmune pancreatitis: imaging features. Radiology 2004; 233:345-352.

4. Okazaki K, Chiba T. Autoimmune related pancreatitis. Gut 2002; 51:1-4.

5. Yoshida K, Toki F, Takeuchi T, et al. Chronic pancreatitis caused by an autoimmune abnormality: proposal of the concept of autoimmune pancreatitis. Dig Dis Sci 1995; 40:1561-1568.

6. Weber SM, Cubukcu-Dimopulo O, Palesty JA, et al. Lymphoplasmacytic sclerosing pancreatitis: inflammatory mimic of pancreatic carcinoma. J Gastrointest Surg 2003; 7:129-137; discussion 137-139.

7. Deshpande V, Mino-Kenudson M, Brugge WR, et al. Endoscopic ultrasound guided fine needle aspiration biopsy of autoimmune pancreatitis: diagnostic criteria and pitfalls. Am J Surg Pathol 2005; 29:1464-1471.

8. Okazaki K, Kawa S, Kamisawa T, et al. Clinical diagnostic criteria of autoimmune pancreatitis: revised proposal. J Gastroenterol 2006; 41:626-631.

9. Kawa S, Hamano H. Clinical features of autoimmune pancreatitis. J Gastroenterol 2007; 42(Suppl 18):9-14.

10. Zamboni G, Luttges J, Capelli P, et al. Histopathological features of diagnostic and clinical relevance in autoimmune pancreatitis: a study on 53 resection specimens and 9 biopsy specimens. Virchows Arch 2004; 445:552-563.

11. Kamisawa T. IgG4-positive plasma cells specifically infiltrate various organs in autoimmune pancreatitis. Pancreas 2004; 29:167-168.

12. Nakazawa T, Ohara H, Sano H, et al. Difficulty in diagnosing autoimmune pancreatitis by imaging findings. Gastrointest Endosc 2007; 65:99-108.

13. Kamisawa T, Egawa N, Inokuma S, et al. Pancreatic endocrine and exocrine function and salivary gland function in autoimmune pancreatitis before and after steroid therapy. Pancreas 2003; 27:235-238.

14. Nishimori I, Tamakoshi A, Kawa S, et al. Influence of steroid therapy on the course of diabetes mellitus in patients with autoimmune pancreatitis: findings from a nationwide survey in Japan. Pancreas 2006; 32:244-248.

15. Ito T, Kawabe K, Arita Y, et al. Evaluation of pancreatic endocrine and exocrine function in patients with autoimmune pancreatitis. Pancreas 2007; 34:254-259.

16. Ghazale A, Chari ST, Smyrk TC, et al. Value of serum IgG4 in the diagnosis of autoimmune pancreatitis and in distinguishing it from pancreatic cancer. Am J Gastroenterol 2007; 102:1646-1653.

17. Hamano H, Kawa S, Horiuchi A, et al. High serum IgG4 concentrations in patients with sclerosing pancreatitis. N Engl J Med 2001; 344:732-738.

18. Pearson RK, Longnecker DS, Chari ST, et al. Controversies in clinical pancreatology: autoimmune pancreatitis: does it exist? Pancreas 2003; 27:1-13.

19. Chen RY, Adams DB. IgG4 levels in non-Japanese patients with autoimmune sclerosing pancreatitis. N Engl J Med 2002; 346:1919.

20. Hardacre JM, Iacobuzio-Donahue CA, Sohn TA, et al. Results of pancreaticoduodenectomy for lymphoplasmacytic sclerosing pancreatitis. Ann Surg 2003; 237:853-858; discussion 858-859.

21. Horiuchi A, Kaneko T, Yamamura N, et al. Autoimmune chronic pancreatitis simulating pancreatic lymphoma. Am J Gastroenterol 1996; 91:2607-2609.

22. Deshpande V, Mino-Kenudson M, Brugge W, Lauwers GY. Autoimmune pancreatitis: more than just a pancreatic disease? A contemporary review of its pathology. Arch Pathol Lab Med 2005; 129:1148-1154.

23. Okazaki K, Uchida K, Matsushita M, Takaoka M. Autoimmune pancreatitis. Intern Med 2005; 44:1215-1223.

24. Takase M, Suda K. Histopathological study on mechanism and background of tumor-forming pancreatitis. Pathol Int 2001; 51:349-354.

25. Kawaguchi K, Koike M, Tsuruta K, et al. Lymphoplasmacytic sclerosing pancreatitis with cholangitis: a variant of primary sclerosing cholangitis extensively involving pancreas. Hum Pathol 1991; 22:387-395.

26. Ohara H, Nakazawa T, Ando T, Joh T. Systemic extrapancreatic lesions associated with autoimmune pancreatitis. J Gastroenterol 2007; 42(Suppl 18):15-21.

27. Deshpande V, Chicano S, Finkelberg D, et al. Autoimmune pancreatitis: a systemic immune complex mediated disease. Am J Surg Pathol 2006; 30:1537-1545.

28. Suda K, Takase M, Fukumura Y, et al. Pathology of autoimmune pancreatitis and tumor-forming pancreatitis. J Gastroenterol 2007; 42(Suppl 18):22-27.

29. Zen Y, Harada K, Sasaki M, et al. IgG4-related sclerosing cholangitis with and without hepatic inflammatory pseudotumor, and sclerosing pancreatitis-associated sclerosing cholangitis: do they belong to a spectrum of sclerosing pancreatitis? Am J Surg Pathol 2004; 28:1193-1203.

30. Abraham SC, Cruz-Correa M, Argani P, et al. Lymphoplasmacytic chronic cholecystitis and biliary tract disease in patients with lymphoplasmacytic sclerosing pancreatitis. Am J Surg Pathol 2003; 27:441-451.

31. Takahashi N, Kawashima A, Fletcher JG, Chari ST. Renal involvement in patients with autoimmune pancreatitis: CT and MR imaging findings. Radiology 2007; 242:791-801.

32. Kawa S, Ota M, Yoshizawa K, et al. HLA DRB10405-DQB10401 haplotype is associated with autoimmune pancreatitis in the Japanese population. Gastroenterology 2002; 122:1264-1269.

33. Irie H, Honda H, Baba S, et al. Autoimmune pancreatitis: CT and MR characteristics. AJR Am J Roentgenol 1998; 170:1323-1327.

34. Mikami K, Itoh H. MR imaging of multifocal autoimmune pancreatitis in the pancreatic head and tail: a case report. Magn Reson Med Sci 2002; 1:54-58.

35. Kamisawa T, Egawa N, Nakajima H, et al. Clinical difficulties in the differentiation of autoimmune pancreatitis and pancreatic carcinoma. Am J Gastroenterol 2003; 98:2694-2699.

36. Kamisawa T, Tu Y, Egawa N, et al. Clinicopathologic study on chronic pancreatitis with diffuse irregular narrowing of the main pancreatic duct. Nippon Shokakibyo Gakkai Zasshi 2001; 98:15-24.

37. Kamisawa T, Okamoto A. Prognosis of autoimmune pancreatitis. J Gastroenterol 2007; 42(Suppl 18):59-62.

38. Takayama M, Hamano H, Ochi Y, et al. Recurrent attacks of autoimmune pancreatitis result in pancreatic stone formation. Am J Gastroenterol 2004; 99:932-937.

39. Kamisawa T, Egawa N, Nakajima H, et al. Extrapancreatic lesions in autoimmune pancreatitis. J Clin Gastroenterol 2005; 39:904-907.

40. Ohara H, Nakazawa T, Sano H, et al. Systemic extrapancreatic lesions associated with autoimmune pancreatitis. Pancreas 2005; 31:232-237.

41. Hirano K, Tada M, Isayama H, et al. Long-term prognosis of autoimmune pancreatitis with and without corticosteroid treatment. Gut 2007; 56:1719-1724.

42. Kamisawa T, Okamoto A, Funata N. Clinicopathological features of autoimmune pancreatitis in relation to elevation of serum IgG4. Pancreas 2005; 31:28-31.

43. Notohara K, Burgart LJ, Yadav D, et al. Idiopathic chronic pancreatitis with periductal lymphoplasmacytic infiltration: clinicopathologic features of 35 cases. Am J Surg Pathol 2003; 27:1119-1127.

44. Horiuchi A, Kawa S, Hamano H, et al. ERCP features in 27 patients with autoimmune pancreatitis. Gastrointest Endosc 2002; 55:494-499.

45. Saegusa H, Momose M, Kawa S, et al. Hilar and pancreatic gallium-67 accumulation is characteristic feature of autoimmune pancreatitis. Pancreas 2003; 27:20-25.

46. Nakajo M, Jinnouchi S, Noguchi M, et al. FDG PET and PET/CT monitoring of autoimmune pancreatitis associated with extrapancreatic autoimmune disease. Clin Nucl Med 2007; 32:282-285.

47. Prokesch RW, Chow LC, Beaulieu CF, et al. Isoattenuating pancreatic adenocarcinoma at multi-detector row CT: secondary signs. Radiology 2002; 224:764-768.

48. Kim KP, Kim MH, Kim JC, et al. Diagnostic criteria for autoimmune chronic pancreatitis revisited. World J Gastroenterol 2006; 12:2487-2496.

49. Ito T, Nishimori I, Inoue N, et al. Treatment for autoimmune pancreatitis: consensus on the treatment for patients with autoimmune pancreatitis in Japan. J Gastroenterol 2007; 42(Suppl 18):50-58.

50. Ghazale A, Chari ST. Optimising corticosteroid treatment for autoimmune pancreatitis. Gut 2007; 56:1650-1652.

51. Chari ST. Current concepts in the treatment of autoimmune pancreatitis. JOP 2007; 8:1-3.

52. Kamisawa T, Yoshiike M, Egawa N, et al. Treating patients with autoimmune pancreatitis: results from a long-term follow-up study. Pancreatology 2005; 5:234-238; discussion 238-240.

53. Veenstra J, Krediet RT, Somers R, Arisz L. Tumour lysis syndrome and acute renal failure in Burkitt's lymphoma: description of 2 cases and a review of the literature on prevention and management. Neth J Med 1994; 45:211-216.

54. Jasek AM, Day HJ. Acute spontaneous tumor lysis syndrome. Am J Hematol 1994; 47:129-131.

55. Spiegel RJ, Magrath IT. Tumor lysis pancreatitis. Med Pediatr Oncol 1979; 7:169-172.

56. Hashimoto F. Transient eosinophilia associated with pancreatitis and pseudocyst formation. Arch Intern Med 1980; 140:1099-1100.

57. Abraham SC, Leach S, Yeo CJ, et al. Eosinophilic pancreatitis and increased eosinophils in the pancreas. Am J Surg Pathol 2003; 27:334-342.

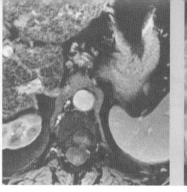
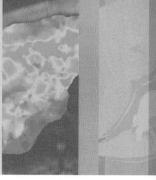

CHAPTER 80

Diffuse Pancreatic Disease

Nisha I. Sainani

Diffuse involvement of pancreas can occur with various inflammatory, infective, infiltrative, or neoplastic disorders. In fact, any pathologic process that involves the pancreas focally can also cause diffuse involvement (Table 80-1).

The more common causes of diffuse pancreatic involvement (viz., pancreatitis) have been discussed in previous chapters. In this chapter the discussion is focused on the infrequent causes and differential features.

GENERAL CONSIDERATIONS

Imaging

Imaging can demonstrate the pattern and extent of pancreatic involvement and other ancillary features, which can suggest and facilitate diagnosis. The imaging features resulting from various causes, however, can be overlapping, although differentiation of these conditions is important from a management perspective.

Radiography

Radiographs can reveal calcification within the pancreas or lymph nodes, which occurs in chronic cases or in lymphomas after treatment. Other than this revelation, there is no clinical significance.

Ultrasonography

Ultrasonography, although being the first screening modality used when a pancreatic pathologic process is suggested, is not sensitive for detection of early or subtle changes. In addition, the evaluation can be hindered by gas in the gastrointestinal tract. Also, in the event of detection of diffuse pancreatic involvement, ultrasonography is not specific.

CT

In most instances, CT is used for diagnosis and further evaluation and is now considered to be a preferred modality.

MRI

MRI offers the advantage of being devoid of ionizing radiation. The sensitivity of MRI for various imaging features is comparable to that of CT, except for detection of calcification, in which CT is superior to MRI. MRI, however, can be particularly advantageous for detection of deposition diseases, which result in changes in signal intensity and evaluation of associated ductal changes.

PET/CT

PET/CT has a role in staging of malignant disorders and evaluation of congenital hyperinsulinism (nesidioblastosis) (see later).

Imaging Algorithm

Figure 80-1 is an imaging algorithm for diffuse pancreatic involvement. The reader also is referred to Table 80-2.

Differential Diagnosis

Because of overlapping imaging features, clinical and laboratory parameters are desirable to elucidate and reinforce the diagnosis. Imaging can guide invasive techniques (biopsy, fine-needle aspiration cytology [FNAC]) in dubious cases, aid in the further substantiation of diagnosis, and thus guide treatment planning. Imaging also plays an important role in screening and post-therapy follow-up to demonstrate resolution, recovery, or recurrence (Table 80-3, Figures 80-2 to 80-5, and Table 80-4).

Treatment

Medical management depends on the underlying disease process involving the pancreas diffusely and is detailed in the discussion of individual diseases presented in this chapter. Surgical management is generally not recommended for diffuse pancreatic disorders, but palliative measures may be required in some cases (see under the discussions of individual diseases).

TABLE 80-1 Diffuse Pancreatic Diseases

Inflammation
Acute pancreatitis
Chronic pancreatitis
  Chronic calcifying pancreatitis
  Chronic obstructive pancreatitis
  Autoimmune pancreatitis

Infiltration
Cystic fibrosis
Fatty replacement of pancreas
Amyloidosis
Hemochromatosis

Infection
Tuberculosis
AIDS

Neoplasm
Lymphoma
Leukemia
Carcinoma
Metastases

Miscellaneous
Congenital hyperinsulinism of infancy
Von Hippel-Lindau disease

What the Referring Physician Needs to Know: General Considerations

■ Imaging features of disorders involving the pancreas diffusely (especially inflammatory, infective, or neoplastic disease) can be overlapping.

■ Clinical and laboratory parameters along with imaging findings are vital for narrowing the differential diagnosis.

■ Histologic diagnosis is crucial before appropriate medical or surgical therapy is instituted.

■ Confirmation of diagnosis can be done by pathologic evaluation of tissue obtained from a pancreatic lesion or other involved organs by image-guided biopsy.

■ Imaging plays an important role in demonstrating the pattern and extent of involvement and helps avoid surgery for diagnostic and therapeutic purposes in medically treatable cases.

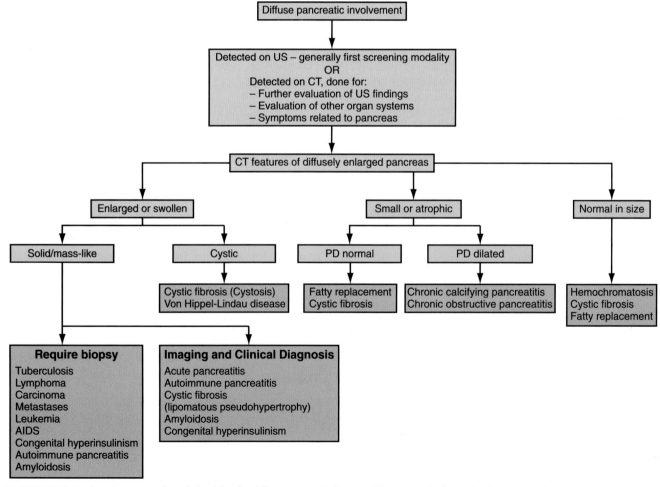

■ **FIGURE 80-1** Imaging pattern–based algorithm for diffuse pancreatic diseases. PD, pancreatic duct; US, ultrasonography.

TABLE 80-2 Accuracy, Limitations, and Pitfalls of the Modalities Used in Imaging for Diffuse Pancreatic Diseases

Modality	Accuracy*/Advantages	Limitations	Pitfalls
General Radiography	Pattern and extent of involvement Can reveal calcifications	Not sensitive Not specific	Overlapping features Cannot identify soft tissue changes
CT	Imaging modality of choice Sensitive Calcification seen Allows comprehensive evaluation Can be used for follow-up	Not always specific Radiation exposure Ductal changes not distinctly visualized	Overlapping features
MRI	Sensitive No radiation Ductal evaluation with MRCP Signal intensity changes in deposition diseases Allows comprehensive evaluation	Not always specific Calcification not seen High cost	Overlapping features
Ultrasonography	First screening modality No radiation Can be utilized as screening tool in familial disorders	Not sensitive Not specific Hindrance by bowel gas and obesity Operator dependent Comprehensive evaluation difficult	Overlapping features
PET/CT	Sensitive Staging of malignant disorders Evaluation of congenital hyperinsulinism	Not specific Radiation exposure High cost	No role in diagnosis due to overlap

*No studies evaluating the comparative role of different modalities or accuracy of a modality per se are available owing to the rarity of these disease processes.

INFILTRATIVE DISORDERS

Cystic Fibrosis

Etiology

Cystic fibrosis (CF) is a multisystem, life-threatening disorder caused by mutation in the cystic fibrosis transmembrane conductance regulator gene (*CFTR*).

Prevalence and Epidemiology

CF is an autosomal recessive disorder that is more prevalent in whites.

Clinical Presentation

Chronic obstructive lung disease and pancreatic insufficiency are the main clinical manifestations of CF. The clinical and imaging changes vary with the severity and duration of disease process in all age groups. Pancreatic involvement can result in endocrine or exocrine dysfunction. Most patients present with exocrine pancreatic insufficiency at or soon after birth. Pancreatic function is, however, preserved in 10% to 15% of patients.[1]

Pathophysiology

The defective transmembrane ion transport in CF leads to accumulation of thick, viscous pancreatic secretions in the pancreatic ducts, leading to ductal ectasia and acinar atrophy. Inflammatory reaction, progressive fatty replacement, fibrosis, and sometimes calcification result.[2] Cyst formation can occur owing to inspissated secretions obstructing the small pancreatic ducts.[3] Extensive fatty replacement, fibrosis, calcification, and atrophy are features of severe long-standing disease.[4]

Imaging

The patterns of pancreatic involvement include (1) partial fibrofatty replacement of pancreas, (2) complete fibrofatty replacement with enlargement of pancreas (lipomatous pseudohypertrophy), (3) pancreatic atrophy without evidence of fatty replacement, (4) diffuse pancreatic fibrosis, and (5) pancreatic cystosis.[1,4] Complete fatty replacement of pancreas is commonly seen, with the fat replacement maintaining the shape of the pancreas. This morphologic finding may be evident in older patients and represents a late stage of the disease, but it also can be seen earlier in the course of the disease with severe involvement.[5]

Radiography

Calcifications that develop with the course of disease may be detectable on radiographs.

Ultrasonography

On ultrasonography, the involved pancreas reveals homogeneously or heterogeneously increased echogenicity (Fig. 80-6A). The pancreas may be normal or small in size, and the typical fine-lobular echo pattern of the pancreas is gradually lost. Pancreatic cystosis is seen as multiple, thin-walled, sonolucent, multiloculated cysts scattered throughout the pancreas with interspersed hyperechoic pancreatic parenchyma (see Fig. 80-6B). Ultrasonography is not sensitive to detect and estimate the extent of pancreatic involvement, and false-negative findings also have been reported.[6]

Text continued on p 811.

TABLE 80-3   Differential Features of Diffuse Pancreatic Diseases

Disease Process	Clinical Data	Specific Laboratory Tests	Radiography	Imaging Ultrasonography	Imaging CT	Imaging MR	ERCP	Imaging Mimics
Acute pancreatitis (Fig. 80-2)	Acute presentation ± history of gallstones and/or alcoholism	Serum lipase & amylase ↑	Small bowel ileus	Enlarged, hypoechoic	Enlarged, hypodense Peripancreatic fat stranding & fluid collection	Enlarged, T1W hypointense, T2W hyperintense	—	Lymphoma
Chronic calcifying pancreatitis (Fig. 80-3)	Chronic presentation History of gallstones, alcohol, ± exocrine & endocrine insufficiency	—	Prevertebral calcification	Small or atrophic, irregular ductal dilatation ± calcification	Small or atrophic, irregular ductal dilatation ± calcification	Small or atrophic, MRCP—PD irregularity, beaded, dilated	PD beaded, irregularly dilated	Pancreatic CA when associated with focal mass-like lesion
Chronic obstructive pancreatitis (Fig. 80-4)	Chronic presentation, history of CA or IPMN	—	—	CA—hypoechoic lesion, small or atrophic pancreas, upstream PD dilatation & irregularity, ± calcification MD IPMN—diffuse PD dilatation	CA—hypoechoic on parenchymal phase of IV contrast, upstream PD dilatation, ± calcification, ± invasion & metastasis MD IPMN—diffuse PD dilatation ± bulging papilla	CA—hypoechoic on parenchymal phase of IV contrast, upstream PD dilatation, ± invasion & metastasis MD IPMN—diffuse PD dilatation ± bulging major papilla	Bulging papilla, PD dilated	Mass-like lesion of chronic pancreatitis
Autoimmune pancreatitis (Fig. 80-5)	Common in males Nonspecific symptoms related to pancreatic involvement	Serum IgG$_4$ ↑	—	Enlarged, hypoechoic	Enlarged, sausage shaped, halo, peripancreatic stranding, PD attenuated or irregular, ± CBD involvement, focal mass-like swelling	T1 hypointense, T2 hyperintense, sausage shaped, halo, peripancreatic stranding, PD attenuated or irregular, ± CBD involvement, focal mass-like swelling	PD attenuated or irregular	Acute pancreatitis, pancreatic CA when associated focal mass-like swelling
Tuberculosis (Fig. 80-13)	Immigrants, immunocompromised HIV patients Constitutional symptoms, symptoms related to pancreas or other organ system involvement	—	Calcification in chronic or treated cases	Enlarged, hypoechoic, heterogeneity due to abscess/ calcification	Enlarged, hypodense, heterogeneity due to abscess/ necrosis, heterogeneous enhancement, peripancreatic edema, peripancreatic, mesenteric, periportal LN, fistulas	Enlarged T1 hypointense T2 hyperintense, heterogeneous enhancement	PD normal, compressed, displaced or stenosed	Carcinoma, lymphoma, AIDS

Disease	Clinical features		Special findings	US	CT	MRI	PD	Differential diagnosis
AIDS (Fig. 80-14)	High-risk behavior, homosexuals, IVDA	—	—	Enlarged, hypoechoic	Enlarged, hypodense, hemorrhagic necrosis with herpes simplex	Enlarged T1 hypointense T2 hyperintense, heterogeneous enhancement	—	Tuberculosis, carcinoma, lymphoma
Lymphoma (Fig. 80-15)	Systemic symptoms, jaundice less common	—	Calcification in treated cases	Enlarged, hypoechoic, mesenteric & retroperitoneal LN	Enlarged, hypodense, peripancreatic infiltration, mild homogeneous enhancement, PD dilation not a feature, mesenteric and retroperitoneal LN extending below renal vein, invasion of other organs, engulfment of vessels Valuable for staging	Enlarged, T1 hypointense, T2 hyperintense, mild homogeneous enhancement, PD dilation not a feature, mesenteric and retroperitoneal LN extending below renal vein, invasion of other organs, engulfment of vessels	PD normal, displaced, narrowed	Tuberculosis, carcinoma, leukemia, AIDS
Leukemia	Systemic symptoms, jaundice not a feature	—	—	Enlarged, hypoechoic, LN, other organ system involvement	Enlarged, hypodense, mild enhancement, LN, other organ system involvement	Enlarged, T1 hypointense, T2 hyperintense, LN, other organ system involvement	—	Lymphoma Carcinoma Tuberculosis AIDS
Carcinoma (Fig. 80-16)	Middle–elderly age Systemic symptoms, painless jaundice	CA 19-9 for follow-up	—	Enlarged, hypoechoic, LN, vascular invasion, metastases	Enlarged, hypodense, heterogeneity due to necrosis/calcification, LN, vascular encasement/invasion, metastases	Enlarged, T1 hypointense, T2 hyperintense, heterogeneity due to necrosis/calcification, LN, vascular encasement/invasion, metastases	Irregularity or narrowing	Lymphoma, tuberculosis, AIDS
Metastases	Known primary illness, occasionally pancreatic metastases —first sign Systemic and local symptoms	—	—	Enlarged, hypoechoic, LN, involvement of other organs	Enlarged, hypodense, occasionally necrosis, LN, involvement of other organs	Enlarged, T1 hypointense, T2 hyperintense, LN, involvement of other organs	Irregularity or narrowing	Lymphoma, carcinoma, tuberculosis

(Continued)

TABLE 80-3 Differential Features of Diffuse Pancreatic Diseases—cont'd

Disease Process	Clinical Data	Specific Laboratory Tests	Imaging					Imaging Mimics
			Radiography	Ultrasonography	CT	MR	ERCP	
Cystic fibrosis (Figs. 80-6 to 80-10)	AR, whites, family history, exocrine & endocrine dysfunction	Sweat chloride test	—	Homogeneously or heterogeneously hyperechoic, multiple hypoechoic cysts	Size—normal or atrophic, hypodense due to fat/fibrosis, ± calcification, low-attenuation cystic lesions without solid component	Fatty T1 & T2 hyperintensity Fibrosis—T1 & T2 hypointensity Cysts—T1 hypointensity, T2 hyperintensity	—	Fatty replacement, VHL
Fatty replacement (Fig. 80-11)	Advanced age, DM, Cushing's, long-term use of corticosteroids, chronic pancreatitis	—	—	Echogenic	Hypodense, prominent lobulations	T1 & T2 hypointense, prominent lobulations	—	Cystic fibrosis
Amyloidosis	Chronic or hematologic illness	—	—	Hypoechoic	Hypodense	T1 hypointense & hyperintense, T2 hyperintense	—	Fatty replacement
Hemochromatosis (Fig. 80-12)	AD, family history, systemic manifestations, endocrine or exocrine pancreatic dysfunction	Serum iron, TIBC, transferrin saturation	—	Normal-appearing pancreas	Hyperdense pancreas and peripancreatic LN	T2 hypointense pancreas and liver	—	—
Hyperinsulinism	Recurrent hypoglycemia in infancy	Insulin and C peptide	—	Enlarged, hypoechoic	Enlarged, hypodense	T1 hypointense, T2 hyperintense	—	—
VHL (Figs. 80-17 and 80-18)	Family history, CNS manifestations, endocrine or exocrine pancreatic dysfunction with severe involvement	Genetic testing	—	Multiple hypoechoic cysts, sometimes solid appearance due to multiple interfaces, ± SCA	Multiple hypodense cysts with thin wall, ± calcification throughout pancreas ± SCA	Multiple cysts, T1 hypointense, T2 hyperintense ± SCA	—	Cystic fibrosis

CA, carcinoma; IPMN, intraductal papillary mucinous neoplasm; PD, pancreatic duct; IVDA, intravenous drug abuse; LN, lymph nodes (lymphadenopathy); AR, autosomal recessive; AD, autosomal dominant; TIBC, total iron-binding capacity; VHL, von Hippel-Lindau disease; SCA, serous cystadenoma; MD, main duct; DM, diabetes mellitus; CBD, common bile duct.
—, Not available or not relevant.

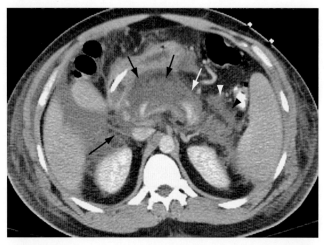

■ **FIGURE 80-2** Acute pancreatitis. Axial CT image reveals a swollen, edematous head and body of pancreas (*arrows*) with peripancreatic fat stranding (*long black arrow at lower left*) and fluid collection (*arrowheads*).

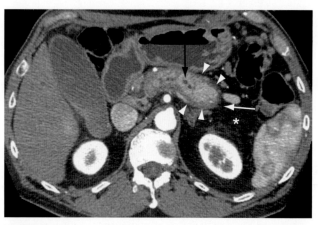

■ **FIGURE 80-5** Autoimmune pancreatitis. Axial CT image reveals a swollen pancreas with a peripancreatic hypodensity (halo) (*arrowheads*), minimal peripancreatic stranding (*asterisk*), irregularity of the pancreatic duct (*vertical black arrow*), and retraction of the pancreatic tail (*long white arrow*).

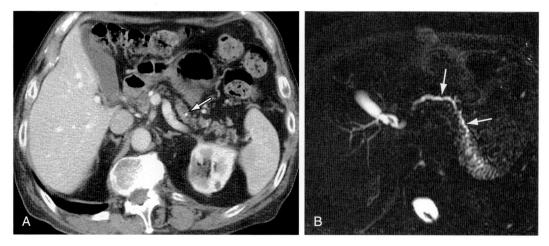

■ **FIGURE 80-3** Chronic calcifying pancreatitis. **A,** Axial CT image shows a small and atrophic pancreas. The pancreatic duct visualized in the region of the body is dilated with an intraductal calcification (*arrow*). **B,** Axial 2D MRCP image in a different patient reveals a beaded irregular pancreatic duct (*arrows*).

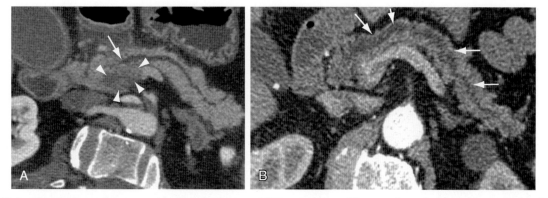

■ **FIGURE 80-4** Chronic obstructive pancreatitis. Curved reformatted CT images in two different patients. **A,** A hypodense mass (carcinoma) (*arrowheads*) is seen in the head and uncinate process of the pancreas with abrupt cutoff of the pancreatic duct (*arrow*) and upstream dilatation. The pancreatic parenchyma reveals mild atrophy. **B,** Diffuse dilatation of the pancreatic duct (*arrows*) with mild parenchymal atrophy without any evident mass lesion in this case of main duct intraductal papillary mucinous neoplasm.

TABLE 80-4 CT Characteristics of Diffuse Pancreatic Diseases

Disease Process	Size	Parenchyma	Peripancreatic Stranding	Necrosis	Calcification	PD	Enhancement	Vascular Invasion	Metastases	Lymphadenopathy	Other Organs	Comments
							CT Features					
Acute pancreatitis	Enlarged	Hypodense	+	±	−	Attenuated	Mild	−	−	−	Ascites, CBD narrowing	Acute presentation
Chronic calcifying pancreatitis	Small or atrophic	Isodense	−	−	+	Beaded, irregular, dilated	Mild-moderate	−	−	±	−	Focal mass may resemble CA
Chronic obstructive pancreatitis	Small or atrophic	Isodense CA: hypodense	−	−	±	Upstream dilatation & irregularity	Mild-moderate CA: lesser than pancreatic parenchyma in parenchymal phase	± with mass lesion	±	±	Biliary	MD IPMN—bulging papilla
Autoimmune pancreatitis	Swollen, later atrophy	Heterogeneous	±	−	−	Attenuated or irregular dilatation	Heterogeneous or homogeneous	−	−	±	Liver, biliary, kidney, lung, retroperitoneum	Halo, elevated IgG$_4$
Tuberculosis	Enlarged	Hypodense, heterogeneity due to abscess/ calcification	±	±	+ in chronic or treated cases	Normal, compressed, displaced or stenosis	Heterogeneous	−	−	±	Multiple organ involvement	Immigrants, immunocompromised, HIV
AIDS	Enlarged	Hypodense	±	Hemorrhagic necrosis with herpes simplex	−	Normal or attenuated	Mild-moderate	−	−	±	Multiple organ involvement	High-risk behavior, IVDA, homosexual
Lymphoma	Enlarged	Hypodense	±	−	+ in treated cases	Normal, displaced or narrowed	Mild	Engulfment	−	±	Multiple organ involvement	Jaundice less common
Leukemia	Enlarged	Hypodense	−	−	−	Normal or narrowed	Mild	−	−	±	Multiple organ involvement	−
Carcinoma	Enlarged	Hypodense	−	±	±	Irregular or narrowed	Heterogeneous	±	±	±	Biliary	Painless jaundice
Metastases	Enlarged	Hypodense	−	±	−	Irregular or narrowed	Heterogeneous, prominent if from a vascular primary lesion	−	+	±	Multiple organ involvement	−
Cystic fibrosis	Enlarged, normal or atrophic	Homogeneous or heterogeneous, multiple hypodense cysts	−	−	±	−	−	−	−	−	−	Positive family history, sweat chloride test
Fatty replacement	Normal or atrophic	Hypodense (fat attenuation)	−	−	−	−	−	−	−	−	−	Advanced age, DM, Cushing's, long-term use of corticosteroids, chronic pancreatitis
Amyloidosis	Enlarged	Hypodense	−	−	−	−	−	−	−	−	−	Chronic or hematologic illness
Hemochromatosis	Normal	Hyperdense	−	−	−	−	−	−	−	± Hyperdense	Liver	Family history, iron panel
Hyperinsulinism	Enlarged	Hypodense	−	−	−	−	Mild-moderate	−	−	−	−	Recurrent hypoglycemia in infancy
VHL	—	Multiple hypodense cysts with thin wall	−	−	±	−	−	−	−	−	Kidney	Positive family history, CNS manifestations

CA, Carcinoma; MD IPMN, main duct intraductal papillary mucinous neoplasm; PD, pancreatic duct; IVDA, intravenous drug abuse; VHL, von Hippel-Lindau disease; SCA, serous cystadenoma; DM, diabetes mellitus; CNS, central nervous system; CBD, common bile duct; IVDA, intravenous drug abuse.

+, Present; ±, may be present or absent; −, absent.

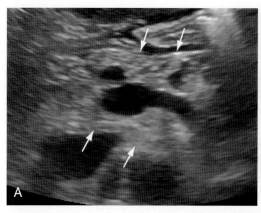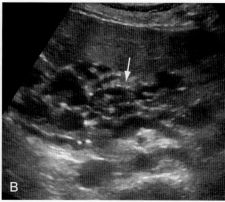

■ **FIGURE 80-6** Cystic fibrosis. Ultrasound images reveal hyperechoic pancreatic parenchyma (*arrows,* **A**) and diffuse cystosis of the pancreas with interspersed echogenic pancreatic parenchyma (*arrow,* **B**).

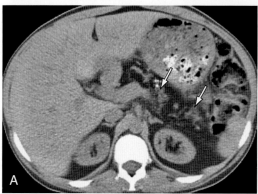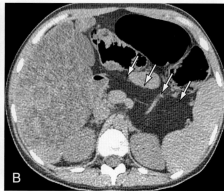

■ **FIGURE 80-7** Cystic fibrosis. Axial CT images demonstrate fatty changes in the pancreas with interspersed residual pancreatic parenchyma (*arrows,* **A**) and complete replacement of pancreas by fat (*arrows,* **B**).

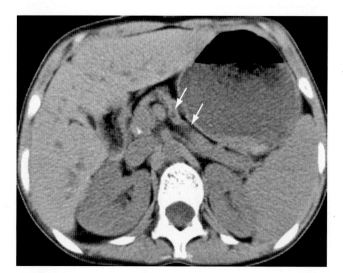

■ **FIGURE 80-8** Cystic fibrosis. Axial CT image reveals atrophy of the pancreas with a few small cystic lesions seen in the proximal body (*arrows*).

CT

Fatty replacement of the pancreas appears as low attenuation (Fig. 80-7). Areas of fibrosis also appear hypodense on CT; the differentiation of these two pathologic processes is possible by measuring the Hounsfield units. Atrophy of the pancreas is indicated by small size (Fig. 80-8). Calcification, when present, is better appreciated on CT.[4] The cystic lesions appear as well-defined low-attenuation structures without any solid portions or excrescences (Fig. 80-9).

MRI

Fatty changes reveal high signal intensity (Fig. 80-10), whereas areas of fibrosis show as low signal intensity on T1- and T2-weighted (T1W, T2W) images. Cysts appear as low signal intensity on T1W images and as high signal intensity on T2W images. Although additional small cysts may be seen on MRI that are not visible on CT and ultrasonography, no additional clinically important information is added to that already obtained.[6]

Classic Signs: Cystic Fibrosis
■ Fatty replacement
■ Cystic changes
■ Calcified foci
■ Fibrosis
■ Atrophy

Differential Diagnosis

Recurrent respiratory tract infections, failure to thrive, exocrine and/or endocrine pancreatic insufficiency, a positive family history, white race, and a positive sweat chloride test are essential for the diagnosis.

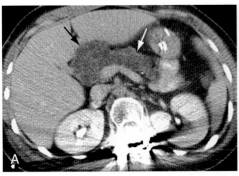 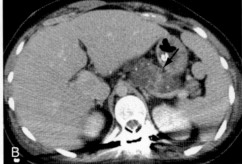

■ **FIGURE 80-9** Cystic fibrosis. Axial CT images reveal diffuse pancreatic cystosis involving the head, neck, body (*black and white arrows,* **A**) and tail of the pancreas (*black arrow,* **B**).

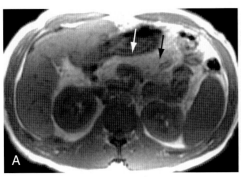 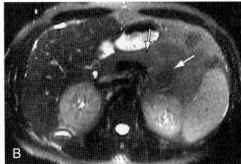

■ **FIGURE 80-10** Cystic fibrosis. Axial T1W (**A**) and T2W fat-suppressed (**B**) MR images reveal near-complete fatty replacement of pancreas (*arrows*), appearing isointense to the retroperitoneal fat.

Treatment

Medical Treatment

Lifelong pancreatic enzyme replacement and insulin therapy are the mainstays of treatment in patients with endocrine or exocrine insufficiency.[7]

Surgical Treatment

End-stage lung disease is treated with bilateral lung transplantation. Immunosuppressive therapy, which is mandatory to prevent transplant rejection, along with exogenous growth hormone administered to these patients and CF per se, is procarcinogenic. These agents can trigger pancreatic malignancies in patients with CF, requiring surgical management.[8,9]

Fatty Replacement (Lipomatosis) of Pancreas

Etiology

Fatty replacement of pancreas is commonly seen with obesity and aging. Other conditions leading to fatty replacement include Cushing's syndrome, adult-onset diabetes mellitus, chronic pancreatitis, hereditary pancreatitis, alcoholic hepatitis, malnutrition, Shwachman-Diamond syndrome, and long-term use of corticosteroids.[4]

Clinical Presentation

Fatty replacement per se does not cause clinical symptoms. The clinical presentation is according to the primary disease process.

What the Referring Physician Needs to Know: Cystic Fibrosis

- Genetic testing can result in early diagnosis and treatment.
- Once the diagnosis is established, CT may be used when complications such as hemorrhage or infection are suspected.
- Asymptomatic patients can be observed with ultrasonography.
- Exocrine pancreatic dysfunction may not become clinically apparent until 98% to 99% of pancreatic parenchyma is damaged.
- Pancreatic insufficiency may lead to an earlier pseudomonal colonization of airways.
- Noninvasive imaging can thus be useful for quantitative evaluation of morphologic changes in the pancreas and monitoring the progress of the disease, before clinical decline becomes apparent.

Pathology

Microscopically, mature adipose tissue and bands of fibrous tissue replace the acini and ducts. The islet cells are preserved and are histologically normal.

Imaging

Ultrasonography

On ultrasonography, the gland appears echogenic.

CT

Fatty replacement can be readily identified on CT performed with or without intravenous administration of a contrast agent, which reveals separation of pancreatic parenchyma with prominence of lobulations interspersed with fat. Fatty replacement can be uniform or may patchily involve a segment or more of pancreas. In the case of patchy involvement, the spared regions can be mistaken as pseudotumors. Associated atrophy of the pancreas may be seen to a variable degree, particularly in elderly individuals (Fig. 80-11). Massive enlargement of the pancreas due to fatty replacement is known as fatty pseudohypertrophy.[10]

MRI

Fatty replacement of the gland appears hyperintense on T1W and T2W imaging.

Classic Signs: Fatty Replacement (Lipomatosis) of Pancreas

- Fatty replacement
- Prominent lobules

Differential Diagnosis

Clinical diagnosis gives an insight to the cause of fatty replacement. In the presence of the clinical diagnosis and imaging findings, no other diagnostic technique is required.

Treatment

No medical treatment is required or available. Fatty replacement is reversible in obesity after weight reduction, in treated Cushing's syndrome, and with discontinuation of corticosteroids.[4]

What the Referring Physician Needs to Know: Fatty Replacement (Lipomatosis) of Pancreas

- Knowledge of this clinical entity helps recognize this condition and avoids mistaking this benign process from other treatable disorders.

Amyloidosis

Etiology

Amyloidosis is a systemic disorder characterized by the extracellular deposition of insoluble fibrillar proteins.

Clinical Presentation

The clinical presentation can be with exocrine or endocrine dysfunction, in addition to the signs and symptoms of associated systemic illness.

Pathology

Pancreas can be involved in primary amyloidosis or, more commonly, as a part of amyloidosis secondary to chronic systemic disease processes.

Imaging

Pancreatic involvement can be focal or diffuse.

Ultrasonography

The diffusely involved gland appears hypoechoic on ultrasonography.[11]

CT

The diffusely involved gland appears hypodense on CT.[11]

MRI

The involved gland appears hypointense or hyperintense on T1W imaging and hyperintense on T2W imaging.[11]

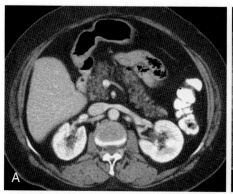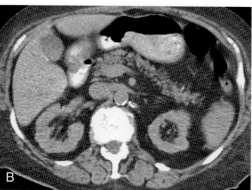

■ **FIGURE 80-11** Fatty replacement of pancreas. **A** and **B**, Axial CT images in two different elderly patients aged 75 and 84 years, respectively, show variable degree of fatty replacement with prominent pancreatic lobulations and mild atrophy.

Differential Diagnosis

Involvement of other organ systems can indicate the diagnosis in secondary amyloidosis. Histopathologic evaluation with Congo red and immunostaining of tissue is required for differentiation from other clinical entities.

Treatment

Medical management involves treatment of the systemic disease process.

What the Referring Physician Needs to Know: Amyloidosis

■ Although amyloidosis is a rare cause of diffuse pancreatic involvement, this disease should be considered when chronic or hematologic illnesses coexist.

Hemochromatosis

Etiology

Hemochromatosis is a disorder resulting from excessive accumulation of iron in several organs.

Prevalence and Epidemiology

Hereditary hemochromatosis is prevalent in people of Northern European descent and is less common in blacks, Hispanics, and Asian-Americans. The disease is five times more common in men, and they usually experience symptoms at an earlier age. Because women lose iron with menstruation and pregnancy, they tend to store less iron than men do. After menopause or a hysterectomy, the risk for women is the same as that for men.

Clinical Presentation

Pancreatic involvement manifests as abdominal pain, in addition to the other systemic manifestations of hemochromatosis owing to involvement of heart, skin, liver, thyroid, joints, and other organ systems.

Pathophysiology

Hemochromatosis can be primary/hereditary or secondary. Hereditary hemochromatosis is an autosomal dominant disorder resulting from excessive absorption of iron; secondary hemochromatosis results from excessive ingestion of iron or from multiple transfusions. Hereditary hemochromatosis is mainly caused by a defect in the *HFE* gene, which helps regulate the amount of iron absorbed from food. The two common mutations involving the *HFE* gene are C282Y and H63D. Juvenile and neonatal hemochromatosis, two additional forms, are caused by a mutation in a gene called hemojuvelin.[12]

Imaging

Radiography

Radiographs have no role in evaluation of pancreatic hemochromatosis. They can assess involvement of the joints when there is skeletal involvement.

Ultrasonography

Ultrasonography is noncontributory in most cases as far as pancreatic involvement is concerned. Liver involvement may be seen as an altered echo pattern or as heterogeneity.

CT

CT characteristically reveals an increased density in the pancreas and adjacent peripancreatic lymph nodes, although no correlation has been found between the amount of increased density and the pancreatic dysfunction or insufficiency.[13] Unopacified vessels may give a spurious impression of low-density masses in the pancreas, but the problem can be resolved by contrast studies.[14]

MRI

Pancreatic involvement is uncommon without cirrhosis. On T2W gradient-recalled-echo MR images, liver and pancreas reveal markedly diminished signal intensity as compared with skeletal muscles (Fig. 80-12). Hypointense

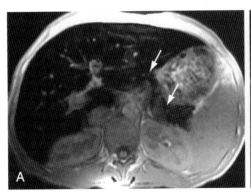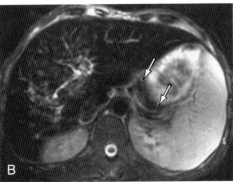

■ **FIGURE 80-12**
Hemochromatosis. Axial T1W (**A**) and T2W fat-suppressed gradient-recalled-echo (**B**) MR images reveal diffusely hypointense pancreas (*arrows*) and liver, as compared with the muscles, due to iron deposition. Spleen is shown as normal signal intensity.

signal can also be seen on spin-echo T2W images, although this sequence is less sensitive. The splenic signal is normal in these patients.[15] Quantification of the liver iron content can be performed using T2W gradient-recalled-echo images. By calculating the ratio of signal intensity of liver to that of fat, mounting iron overload can thus be serially evaluated.[16]

Classic Signs: Hemochromatosis

■ Hyperdense on CT (pancreas and lymph nodes)
■ Hypointense on T2W gradient-recalled-echo MR images

Differential Diagnosis

Systemic involvement of heart, skin, liver, joints, thyroid, and other organ systems supports the imaging diagnosis. Findings of elevated serum iron concentration, total iron-binding capacity, and transferrin saturation values are characteristic. Liver biopsy is done for confirmation of diagnosis.

Treatment

Medical Treatment

Phlebotomy done on a regular basis is effective in removing the excess iron from the body.

Surgical Treatment

No surgical management is recommended for the disease per se. However, patients developing cirrhosis of liver secondary to hemochromatosis are at increased risk of hepatocellular carcinoma, which may require surgical management.

What the Referring Physician Needs to Know: Hemochromatosis

■ Early identification of the disease and appropriate treatment can prevent progression to irreversible pancreatic insufficiency and liver cirrhosis.
■ Genetic testing can be done for early identification of a mutated gene.

INFECTIONS

Tuberculosis

Etiology

Pancreatic tuberculosis is a rare disease entity caused by *Mycobacterium tuberculosis.*

Prevalence and Epidemiology

An increased incidence of tuberculosis is being documented in developed countries owing to immigration, the human immunodeficiency virus (HIV) pandemic with worldwide resurgence of *M. tuberculosis,* and other immunocompromised conditions. Sporadic cases are also noted with propensity to involve malnourished or homeless people or those living in overcrowded situations.[17]

Clinical Presentation

Because of the propensity to involve multiple organ systems, the clinical presentation of tuberculosis varies. Pancreatic involvement can result in moderate intensity, intermittent, or persistent vague upper abdominal pain, obstructive jaundice, portal vein obstruction, acute or chronic pancreatitis, gastrointestinal bleeding, ventral abdominal wall fistula with purulent discharge, and lymphadenopathy. These may be present with or without constitutional signs and symptoms related to tuberculosis or with symptoms of tuberculosis elsewhere in the body (viz., lungs, brain).[18]

Pathophysiology

Within the abdomen, the mesentery, small bowel, peritoneum, liver, and spleen are the common sites of involvement. Tuberculosis of the pancreas usually occurs as a complication of miliary tuberculosis and immunodeficiency; isolated or primary involvement of the pancreas is exceedingly rare. The rarity of occurrence of pancreatic tuberculosis has been attributed to the antibacterial pancreatic factors. The diagnosis is suggested by relevant clinical history or evidence of tuberculosis elsewhere in the body.[17]

Pathology

Lymphatic, hematogenous, and direct extension from adjacent involved organs are the modes theorized to result in pancreatic involvement. The gland may be diffusely involved by the caseating granulomatous process or there may be a combination of granulomas and associated inflammation. Pancreatic tuberculosis can cause biliary obstruction either by compression of the bile duct by lymphadenopathy or by direct involvement of the duct itself.[19] HIV-infected patients also often develop well-formed caseating granulomas because tuberculosis tends to occur before advanced immunocompromise develops.[20]

Imaging

Although focal involvement of pancreas is more common, diffuse involvement has been reported.

Radiography

Plain radiographs of the chest may reveal evidence of pulmonary tuberculosis. Calcification of the granulomatous lesions involving the abdominal organs can occur with treatment and chronicity, which will be evident on abdominal radiographs.[19]

Ultrasonography

The diffusely involved gland appears enlarged and hypoechoic, although heterogeneity due to necrosis, abscess formation, and calcification may be evident, which can be difficult to differentiate from pancreatic carcinoma.[19]

CT

On noncontrast CT, the involved gland appears enlarged and hypodense. Focal areas of necrosis or calcification may result in a heterogeneous appearance (Fig. 80-13). On contrast-enhanced CT, the lesion reveals peripheral enhancement with a nonenhancing central necrotic component. Areas of central enhancement may result in a multiloculated appearance. Peripancreatic edema or collections may be seen. Peripancreatic, mesenteric, or periportal lymphadenopathy is more readily identified on CT. Lymphadenopathy may be homogeneous or may reveal necrotic foci. Fistulas (interbowel loop or enterocutaneous), when present, are also better appreciated on CT.[19]

MRI

On MRI, the involved gland appears hypointense on T1W imaging and hyperintense or heterogeneous on T2W imaging, with heterogeneous enhancement after intravenous contrast agent administration.[21]

PET/CT

Fluorodeoxyglucose (FDG)-PET reveals increased tracer uptake, resulting in a false-positive diagnosis of malignancy.

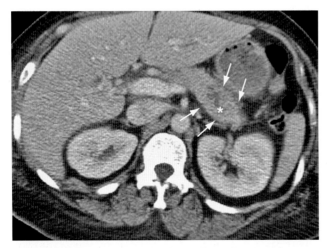

■ **FIGURE 80-13** Tuberculosis. Axial CT image through the pancreas demonstrates diffuse enlargement of the body and tail. The involved pancreas is mildly enhanced peripherally (*arrows*) with a central hypodense nonenhancing area due to necrosis (*asterisk*).

ERCP

Endoscopic retrograde cholangiopancreatography (ERCP) reveals a normal pancreatic duct, or there may be compression, displacement, or stenosis.[22]

Classic Signs: Tuberculosis

- Necrosis and abscess formation
- Peripancreatic, mesenteric, and periportal lymphadenopathy
- Heterogeneous enhancement
- Bowel involvement
- Fistulas

Differential Diagnosis

None of the imaging features are specific, and they may resemble those of other inflammatory or neoplastic lesions of the pancreas. A search for associated radiologic features, such as ileocecal mural thickening or lymphadenopathy in the peripancreatic tissues and mesentery, along with the local and constitutional signs and symptoms, assists in raising the clinical suspicion and confirming the diagnosis.[23]

Histologic diagnosis is crucial before appropriate medical therapy can be instituted. Confirmation of the diagnosis usually requires pathologic evaluation of tissue obtained from a pancreatic lesion or peripancreatic lymph nodes for cytology and culture. This can be procured using CT- or ultrasound-guided percutaneous biopsy or surgical biopsy. The aspirate should be stained for acid-fast bacilli and cultured for *M. tuberculosis*. Image-guided percutaneous aspiration biopsy has a reported sensitivity of less than 50% for pancreatic tuberculosis; surgical biopsy is hence sometimes essential, especially when the image-guided biopsy results are negative in a setting of high clinical and radiologic suspicion.[17]

Acid-fast staining of pathologic material demonstrates organisms in 20% to 40% of cases, and culture is about 77% sensitive. Polymerase chain reaction (PCR) assay has proved useful in identifying *M. tuberculosis* in pathologic material, although the results offer no information regarding drug susceptibility and therefore it is best used as an adjunct to standard culture.[17]

A few investigators have used endoscopic ultrasound-guided fine needle aspiration successfully for definitive histologic and bacteriologic diagnosis of pancreatic tuberculosis. This technique along with PCR shows promise in becoming a minimally invasive technique for improving the diagnostic accuracy for pancreatic tuberculosis.[24]

Treatment

Medical Treatment

Patients with pancreatic tuberculosis typically respond well to conventional antituberculous therapy with rifampin, isoniazid, ethambutol, or pyrazinamide.

Abscesses, particularly large ones, require aspiration to accelerate the response. Prognosis is, however, poor in patients with HIV.[25]

Surgical Treatment

Patients with evidence of biliary obstruction would need either endoscopic or surgical intervention to relieve the obstruction because the ductal narrowing might persist despite treatment with antituberculous therapy.[26] Ultrasonography or CT can be used to observe patients with pancreatic tuberculosis to assess the response to treatment.[27]

What the Referring Treating Physician Needs to Know: Tuberculosis

- Pancreatic tuberculosis can be treated with antituberculous therapy with good results.
- Early diagnosis of pancreatic tuberculosis is important to avoid unnecessary diagnostic or therapeutic procedures.
- Imaging plays an important role for noninvasive and invasive characterization of pancreatic tuberculosis.

Acquired Immunodeficiency Syndrome

Etiology

In patients with AIDS, opportunistic infections (Table 80-5), drug-induced inflammation, or neoplasms may affect the pancreas, in addition to the disorders seen in the general population.

Clinical Presentation

In addition to the constitutional symptoms of AIDS, pancreatic involvement may present as signs and symptoms indistinguishable from other causes of pancreatitis.

Pathology

Multiple organ systems can be involved. The pancreatic involvement may vary from asymptomatic to fulminant pancreatitis and is most commonly a part of a disseminated disease process.

Imaging

The involvement of pancreas in AIDS is more often diffuse (Fig. 80-14). Typically, ultrasonography or CT reveals an enlarged or boggy pancreas with cytomegalovirus infection.[28] Hemorrhagic necrotic lesions are seen with herpes simplex pancreatitis.[29] Medications such as dideoxyinosine, pentamidine, and trimethoprim-sulfamethoxazole used for treating AIDS can result in pancreatitis indistinguishable from other causes.

Ultrasonography and CT

The involved gland is indistinguishable from other forms of pancreatitis.

MRI

The involved gland is hypointense on T1W images and hyperintense on T2W images and indistinguishable from that of other forms of pancreatitis.

Classic Signs: AIDS

- Enlarged boggy pancreas with cytomegalovirus infection
- Hemorrhagic necrosis with herpes simplex infection

Differential Diagnosis

Clinical diagnosis of AIDS is of utmost importance to raise the suspicion of pancreatic involvement by the disease

---

TABLE 80-5 Opportunistic Infections Affecting Pancreas in AIDS

Bacteria
Mycobacterium tuberculosis
Mycobacterium avium-intracellulare complex (MAC)

Fungi
Cryptococcus neoformans
Candida
Histoplasma capsulatum
Aspergillus

Protozoa
Toxoplasma gondii
Pneumocystis jiroveci
Cryptosporidium
Microsporida
Leishmania

Virus
Cytomegalovirus (CMV)
Herpes simplex
Herpes zoster

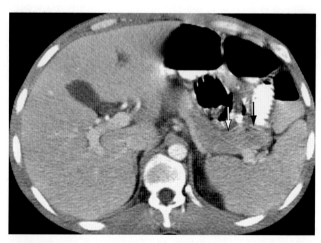

■ **FIGURE 80-14** AIDS. Pancreas is diffusely swollen and hypoechoic (*arrows*) on this axial CT image. *Mycobacterium bovis* was cultured from the pancreatic aspirate.

process. Other organ system involvement should be sought. Histologic evaluation may be necessary for organism-specific diagnosis. Special stains for mycobacteria, fungi, and viral inclusions after biopsy and serologic tests are required for diagnosis.

Treatment

Medical management includes supportive therapy and treatment of the underlying disease process and inciting cause.

What the Treating Physician Needs to Know: AIDS

■ Recognition of AIDS-related pancreatic involvement is important for appropriate management.

NEOPLASMS

Lymphoma

Etiology

Lymphomatous involvement of the pancreas can be primary or secondary.

Prevalence and Epidemiology

Primary pancreatic lymphoma is a rare extranodal manifestation of non-Hodgkin's lymphoma (NHL). NHL commonly involves the pancreas secondarily; only 0.2% to 2% of patients with NHL have primary involvement of the pancreas. A relatively higher incidence (5%) is seen with AIDS-related NHL.[30]

Clinical Presentation

The presenting symptoms of pancreatic lymphoma are usually nonspecific and include abdominal pain, abdominal mass, weight loss, nausea, vomiting, jaundice, and acute pancreatitis.[30] Abdominal pain with a mass without jaundice is a clinical manifestation commonly associated with pancreatic lymphoma and can be valuable in distinguishing these lesions from carcinomas or at least raise the suspicion of an unusual neoplasm.[31]

Pathophysiology

The majority of primary pancreatic lymphomas are the B-cell type, although T-cell types have been reported in the Japanese literature.[32] Most are intermediate- to high-grade NHLs, with diffuse large cell tumors being the predominant histotype.[31] Diagnostic criteria for primary pancreatic involvement include a predominant pancreatic mass with gross involvement of only peripancreatic lymph nodes, no hepatic or splenic involvement, no palpable superficial or mediastinal lymph nodes, and a normal leukocyte count.[33] Secondary involvement of the pancreas occurs by extension of peripancreatic lymphadenopathy to the adjacent gastrointestinal tract.[30,31]

Imaging

The morphologic presentation of pancreatic lymphoma on imaging may be in the form of a localized, well-circumscribed mass or a diffuse enlargement of the pancreas.

Radiography

Calcification can be seen only in treated pancreatic lymphoma on abdominal radiographs.[34]

Ultrasonography

On ultrasonography, the pancreatic involvement, whether focal or diffuse, appears as homogeneously hypoechoic. The involved peripancreatic lymph nodes are isoechoic to the pancreatic lesion. Typically, the peripancreatic vasculature is engulfed by pancreatic lymphoma, the patency of which can be evaluated using color Doppler imaging. On endoscopic ultrasonography, due to high resolution, the wall of the common bile duct appears hyperechoic, contrasting to the adjacent hypoechoic pancreatic parenchyma.[31]

CT

CT by far is the most common imaging modality used for detection and staging of pancreatic lymphoma. The lesions are predominantly homogeneous and hypodense to the musculature, although areas of heterogeneity may sometimes be seen (Fig. 80-15). Infiltration and stranding of peripancreatic fat often may be seen. The lesions reveal poor homogeneous enhancement on intravenous contrast agent administration with occasional heterogeneous enhancement.[31]

The diffuse infiltrating pattern with enlargement and irregular infiltration of the peripancreatic fat may mimic acute pancreatitis on imaging. However, the clinical presentation is never similar to acute pancreatitis and is disproportionate to the extensive pancreatic involvement, even in the presence of abnormal laboratory parameters.

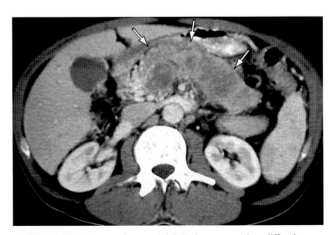

■ **FIGURE 80-15** Lymphoma. Axial CT image reveals a diffusely enlarged pancreas (*arrows*) that is hypodense and has mild heterogeneous enhancement.

Pancreatic ductal dilatation is not marked, despite invasion. Invasion of the retroperitoneum, upper abdominal organs, and gastrointestinal tract and the presence of mesenteric or retroperitoneal lymphadenopathy extending below the renal veins are also signs favoring lymphoma. Calcification and necrosis in an untreated case weighs against lymphoma. The engulfment, rather than stenosis or occlusion of peripancreatic vessels, which characteristically differentiates lymphoma from pancreatic carcinoma, can be appreciated on CT angiography, although stenosis or occlusion of the superior mesenteric, splenic, or portal vein has been seen in a minority of cases.[34]

MRI

On MRI, the diffusely involved gland appears hypointense on T1W imaging and hypointense or hyperintense on T2W imaging, with homogeneous mild to moderate enhancement after intravenous injection of gadolinium. The peripancreatic lymphadenopathy has a similar signal intensity as the pancreas. Ductal involvement can be assessed with magnetic resonance cholangiopancreatography (MRCP), whereas MR angiography can help evaluate peripancreatic vasculature.

ERCP

On ERCP, the Wirsung duct may be normal, displaced, or narrowed in patients with pancreatic lymphoma. This is in contrast to carcinoma, which causes stenosis with moderate to severe upstream dilatation. Although biliary obstruction may be seen, jaundice occurs in less than half the cases of pancreatic lymphoma.

PET/CT

Lymphomas reveal avid FDG uptake. PET/CT has an important role in staging and post-treatment follow-up.

Classic Signs: Lymphoma

- Abdominal pain with mass without jaundice
- Predominantly homogeneous
- Infiltration of peripancreatic fat
- Lack of pancreatic ductal dilatation
- Lack of calcification and necrosis in untreated cases
- Retroperitoneal lymphadenopathy extending below renal veins
- Engulfment rather than stenosis of vessels

Differential Diagnosis

Clinical presentation can be overlapping with other pancreatic neoplasms, but absence of jaundice is an important diagnostic clue to differentiate lymphoma from carcinoma.

Imaging plays an important role in the diagnosis and staging of pancreatic lymphoma. A high degree of suspicion with imaging features favoring lymphoma is needed to differentiate this condition. The treatment and prognosis of lymphoma significantly differ from those of pancreatic carcinoma, which is the main differential disorder. CT- or ultrasound-guided biopsy of a pancreatic mass can be employed to procure tissue for pathologic evaluation, which serves as the gold standard in distinguishing pancreatic lymphoma from carcinoma. Surgery is reserved for cases in which the diagnosis cannot be established by these less invasive methods.[34,35]

Treatment

Medical Treatment

Chemotherapy with the CHOP (cyclophosphamide, hydroxydaunomycin, vincristine [Oncovin], prednisolone) regimen is the treatment of choice; irradiation or immunotherapy drugs (e.g., rituximab) are used as adjuncts to chemotherapy in advanced cases.[31]

Surgical Treatment

Relief of biliary obstruction can be achieved by endoscopic or percutaneous stent insertion or with surgical procedures such as choledochojejunostomy, tumor debulking, or a palliative Whipple procedure, which, however, is no longer performed for this indication.[31]

What the Referring Physician Needs to Know: Lymphoma

- The prognosis of pancreatic lymphoma is much better than the dismal survival rate of pancreatic carcinoma.
- Most pancreatic lymphomas respond well to chemotherapy.
- Imaging diagnosis and staging play a crucial role in management.

Leukemia

Etiology

Leukemia-associated extramedullary disease can occur as lymphoid or myeloid lesions. Extramedullary myeloid lesions are more common and are called granulocytic sarcoma. Granulocytic sarcoma can involve virtually any organ system but has particular predilection for soft tissue, bones, skin, lymph nodes, and periosteum; involvement of the pancreas is extremely rare.[36]

Prevalence and Epidemiology

Pancreatic disease may be seen with preexisting hematologic disease, which suggests the diagnosis, or the pancreas may be the primary site of involvement.[37]

Clinical Presentation

The presentation is similar to that of other pancreatic neoplastic processes. Associated systemic manifestations may be present.

Pathology

In addition to the pancreas, lymph nodes, bones, periosteum, skin, soft tissue, and other organ systems may be involved.

Imaging

Three morphologic patterns of pancreatic leukemia have been described: (1) well or ill-circumscribed focal form, (2) diffuse infiltrative form, and (3) combination of nodular and diffuse infiltrative forms. Leukemic involvement of the pancreas is by and large indistinguishable from that of pancreatic lymphoma on imaging. The diffusely involved gland appears homogeneously hypoechoic or hypodense on CT or ultrasonography, with poor contrast enhancement on CT. As seen in lymphomas, the pancreatic duct is not commensurately dilated. Likewise, the common bile duct may be involved, but jaundice is not a common feature. Lymphadenopathy may or may not be seen with pancreatic leukemia.[37]

Radiography

Radiographic manifestations of skeletal involvement may be a clue to the diagnosis.

Ultrasonography and CT

The involved gland appears hypoechoic on ultrasonography and hypodense on CT.

MRI

The involved gland appears hypointense on T1W images and hyperintense on T2W images.

Classic Sign: Leukemia

■ Overlapping features with lymphoma

Differential Diagnosis

Clinical features and systemic manifestations are a clue to the diagnosis. Associated widespread extramedullary multiple-organ involvement with pathologic evaluation of tissue facilitates the appropriate diagnosis.[37]

Treatment

Pancreatic involvement responds to antileukemic therapy.

What the Referring Physician Needs to Know: Leukemia

■ Because extramedullary involvement of leukemia is known to be highly responsive to systemic antileukemic therapy, consideration of this rare diagnosis in the differential diagnosis is important for management, especially to avoid unnecessary surgery.

Carcinoma

Etiology

Diffuse involvement of the pancreas with a carcinomatous process is rare. The etiology remains the same as for a focal disease process.

Prevalence and Epidemiology

Pancreatic carcinoma appears as a focal mass, most commonly in the head of the pancreas. However, the gland can be diffusely involved in 21% of cases.

Clinical Presentation

Clinical features are similar to those associated with focal involvement of gland (see Chapter 75).

Pathology

Two or more segments (head, neck, body, and tail) or the whole of the pancreas may be involved. The pathologic features are similar to focal involvement of gland (see Chapter 75).

Imaging

Ultrasonography

The diffusely involved gland appears homogeneously hypoechoic, although areas of heterogeneity may be seen due to necrosis and calcification.

CT

On CT, the attenuation values are not significantly different from those of the uninvolved pancreas. Focal areas of hypoattenuation may, however, be seen within, either due to necrosis or due to focal areas of ductal obstruction with dilatation (Fig. 80-16). Focal areas of increased density can be seen due to calcification.[38,39] On intravenous contrast administration, the lesion appears hypodense as compared to enhancing normal pancreatic parenchyma.

Distant metastasis to the liver, peripancreatic and paraaortic lymph nodes, and vascular encasement, when present, can suggest a neoplastic process and facilitate differentiation of pancreatic carcinoma from other lesions. Lymphomas tend to engulf the vessels, in contrast to carcinomas, which encase or infiltrate the vessels (see Fig. 80-15).[39] Diffuse obscuration of posterior pancreatic fat

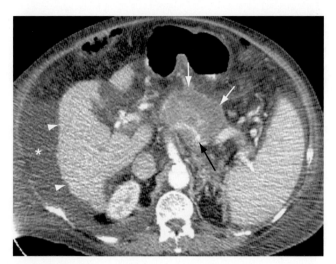

■ **FIGURE 80-16** Carcinoma. Axial CT image reveals a heterogeneously enhancing diffuse mass lesion (*arrows*) encasing the splenic artery (*long arrow*). Also noted is shrunken liver (*arrowheads*) and ascites (*asterisk*) in this patient with cirrhosis.

planes is a finding favoring pancreatitis rather than diffuse carcinoma.[40]

MRI

The diffusely involved gland appears homogeneously or heterogeneously hypointense on T1W images and hyperintense on T2W images. Calcification cannot be appreciated on MRI. The gland reveals heterogeneous enhancement after intravenous administration of gadolinium. MRCP may reveal irregular ductal narrowing.

PET/CT

PET/CT plays an important role in staging and post-treatment follow-up.

Classic Signs: Carcinoma

■ Heterogeneous appearance
■ Necrosis and calcification
■ Irregular ductal dilatation
■ Metastases
■ Lymphadenopathy
■ Vascular encasement

Differential Diagnosis

Clinical features may resemble those of other neoplastic or non-neoplastic processes. However, the presence of jaundice with weight loss with or without abdominal pain and a mass should be viewed with a high level of clinical suspicion, especially in middle-aged and elderly patients.

Histologic confirmation is generally required and can be achieved by image-guided percutaneous biopsy. Several different sites must be sampled from the diffusely enlarged gland to improve diagnostic accuracy and to avoid false-negative findings, which can result from the scattered distribution of tumor cells and associated inflammatory and fibrotic changes.[39]

Treatment

Medical Treatment

Palliative medical management is required.

Surgical Treatment

There are no surgical recommendations for a diffusely involved gland. Palliative procedures for relieving ductal obstruction can be performed.

What the Referring Physician Needs to Know: Carcinoma

■ A diagnosis of pancreatic carcinoma holds a poor prognosis.
■ Imaging features may, however, overlap with other pancreatic neoplastic processes, especially lymphoma, which, however, has a relatively better outcome.
■ Appropriate diagnosis and staging with imaging and histology are mandatory.

Metastases

Etiology

Pancreatic metastases are not as rare as they were once thought to be and must be considered in the differential diagnosis of pancreatic neoplasms.

Prevalence and Epidemiology

The most common primary lesions metastasizing to the pancreas are lung, breast, renal, hepatobiliary, gastrointestinal, and prostate cancers and malignant melanomas and, rarely, osteosarcomas or Ewing's sarcoma.[41] The time interval between diagnoses of primary tumor to development of pancreatic metastases varies from concurrent detection to several years after detection of the primary lesion or even several years after presumed successful treatment of the primary lesion. Occasionally, pancreatic metastasis is the first sign of a malignant disease.[42] The hematogenous route is presumed to be the mode of spread to the pancreas.[43]

Clinical Presentation

The different clinical presentations of pancreatic metastases include abdominal pain, back pain, weight loss, jaundice due to biliary obstruction, gastrointestinal obstruction, upper gastrointestinal bleeding, melena, and acute pancreatitis, or the metastases may be asymptomatic and discovered during a staging CT examination.[44]

Pathology

Metastatic foci in other organs and the primary lesion should be sought. In general, the pathology is similar to that of focal pancreatic metastases (see Chapter 75).

Imaging

On imaging, pancreatic metastases may manifest as a focal lesion, multifocal nodularity, or diffuse enlargement of the gland.[44] On imaging, diffuse pancreatic metastasis is generally morphologically indistinguishable from other diffuse primary neoplasms.[42] Likewise, no distinguishing features of pancreatic metastasis have been found on ERCP.[45] Occasionally, pancreatic metastases can cause severe pancreatitis with necrosis, making it difficult to differentiate it from hemorrhagic necrotizing pancreatitis.[46]

Radiography

Associated skeletal metastases may be seen on radiographs.

Ultrasonography and CT

The appearance is indistinguishable from other pancreatic neoplasms.

MRI

The involved gland appears hypointense on T1W images and hyperintense on T2W images.

PET/CT

Pancreatic metastases reveal increased FDG uptake. PET/CT helps in elucidating the extent of the disease process.

Classic Signs: Metastases

- Overlapping imaging features with other pancreatic neoplasms
- May occasionally mimic the fulminant form of pancreatitis

Differential Diagnosis

Clinical manifestations may support but do not contribute significantly to the diagnosis. Confirmation of the diagnosis with biopsy is mandatory when metastasis is suspected or when the lesions do not reveal any distinguishing features.[43] Although CT-guided biopsy is a common approach, its accuracy (43%) has been found to be less than that of careful analysis of the same CT scan (76%) for diagnosis of cancer.[47] Moreover, doubt remains regarding the safety of biopsy procedures owing to the possibility of malignant cells seeding along the path of the needle. Endoscopic ultrasound–guided biopsy is a relatively lesser invasive and promising technique, found to be as much as 80% sensitive.[48]

Treatment

Medical Treatment

Palliative management is recommended.

Surgical Treatment

No surgical management is available for a diffusely involved gland. Palliative procedures for relieving ductal obstruction can be performed.

What the Referring Physician Needs to Know: Metastases

- Although diffuse involvement of the pancreas by a metastatic process is rare, this diagnosis should be kept in mind, because its presence prevents curative resection.
- The primary site and other metastatic foci need to be elucidated before palliative therapy is done.

MISCELLANEOUS DISORDERS

Congenital Hyperinsulinism of Infancy (Nesidioblastosis)

Etiology

Hyperinsulinism of infancy is a common cause of recurrent hypoglycemia. It results from abnormal hyperfunctioning pancreatic islet tissue and can lead to irreversible brain damage.

Prevalence and Epidemiology

Most cases are sporadic, but familial cases have been reported.

Clinical Presentation

Presentation is within the first year of life in 70% of cases with symptoms of hypoglycemia, including sweating, seizure, pallor, motor abnormalities, and macrosomia.[49]

Pathophysiology

Genetic studies have revealed a number of different mutations in genes encoding the adenosine triphosphate (ATP)–sensitive potassium channels in the cell membrane of beta cells, suggesting that this disorder has a functional basis rather than just representing an increase in the number of beta cells.[50] The severity of symptoms depends on the specific mutations. Histologically, in the diffuse form, the pancreas is studded with abnormally shaped, enlarged beta islet cells, with enlarged and hyperchromatic nuclei and ductuloinsular complexes. On the other hand, in the focal form, the islet cells in the surrounding pancreas are normal.[51]

Imaging

Morphologically, hyperinsulinism of infancy may present as focal (40%) or diffuse (50%). The diffuse form is seen on imaging as a generalized enlargement of the pancreas.[52]

Ultrasonography

The diffusely involved gland appears hypoechoic.

CT

The diffuse enlargement and the homogeneous hypodensity of the gland may resemble the CT appearance of other diffuse disease processes.

MRI

The gland appears hypointense on T1W images and hyperintense on T2W images.

PET/CT

The role of [18F]fluoro-L-DOPA-labeled PET/CT has been evaluated in the preoperative differentiation between focal or diffuse form of hyperinsulinism and has become an important alternate or complementary investigation to pancreatic venous catheterization, which was until now the only method for differential diagnosis between focal and diffuse forms.[53]

Classic Signs: Congenital Hyperinsulinism of Infancy (Nesidioblastosis)

- Homogeneously enlarged gland
- Overlapping imaging features

Differential Diagnosis

The clinical symptoms of hypoglycemia in the appropriate age group should raise the clinical suspicion. Confirmation of the diagnosis with histologic evaluation and now with [18F]fluoro-L-DOPA PET/CT is essential for management planning.

Treatment

Surgical resection of the involved gland is the management of choice. The surgical treatment of diffuse hyperinsulinism involves near-total pancreatectomy with increased risk of diabetes mellitus, whereas focal hyperinsulinism can be treated with partial pancreatectomy.

What the Referring Physician Needs to Know: Congenital Hyperinsulinism of Infancy (Nesidioblastosis)

- In neonates with characteristic clinical findings, the main differentiation is not with other lesions but between focal and diffuse forms.
- Histology, although a gold standard for confirmation of diagnosis, involves an invasive technique.
- [18F]Fluoro-L-DOPA-labeled PET/CT can be utilized to noninvasively distinguish the two forms.

Von Hippel-Lindau Disease

Etiology

Von Hippel-Lindau disease (VHL) is a dominant hereditary multisystem syndrome caused by germline mutations of the *VHL* tumor suppressor gene.[54]

Prevalence and Epidemiology

Pancreatic involvement in VHL varies from 17% to 77%. The pancreas may be the only organ involved in 7.6% of cases.[55,56]

Clinical Presentation

The age at onset of VHL varies and depends on the expression of the disease within the individual or within the family and the intensity with which asymptomatic lesions are sought.[57]

More often, the diagnosis of VHL is due to manifestations of central nervous system (CNS) involvement. Pancreatic involvement rarely results in presenting symptoms. Pancreatic cysts are usually detected incidentally during screening or workup for other abnormalities.[57] However, identification of multiple pancreatic cysts without a prior history of pancreatic inflammation and especially when associated with renal cysts should raise the suspicion and lead to genetic testing for VHL rather than other invasive investigations.[58] Extensive pancreatic involvement can result in exocrine and exocrine dysfunction.

Pathology

VHL is a multisystem disorder involving pancreas, kidneys, adrenals, epididymis, and CNS. The most common pancreatic lesions are single or multiple cysts (90%), the others being nonfunctional neuroendocrine tumors, adenocarcinomas, and serous cystadenomas. Discrete cysts in the pancreas with or without calcified foci are seen early in the course of disease. These gradually increase in number, ultimately replacing the entire pancreatic parenchyma and resulting in pancreatic insufficiency. In severe cases the pancreatic parenchyma may be difficult to distinguish. Solid pancreatic lesions (nonfunctional neuroendocrine tumors or pancreatic adenocarcinomas) are known to be associated with severe cystic disease. The multisystem involvement includes cancers of the central nervous system (retinal and craniospinal hemangioblastomas, endolymphatic sac tumors), pheochromocytomas, benign cysts, and tumors of the pancreas, kidneys, and epididymis. CNS and renal cell carcinomas are major causes of death.[55,56]

Imaging

Ultrasonography

The multiple cystic lesions are seen as well-defined hypoechoic lesions with thin walls. Severe involvement is seen as complete cystic replacement of the pancreas. Serous cystadenomas, when present, appear microcystic and sometimes solid because of the multiple acoustic interfaces caused by innumerable microscopic cysts.

Distinguishing serous cystadenomas from multiple cysts may sometimes be difficult, which is, however, not clinically important unless they cause symptoms.[57]

CT

Multiple cysts appear as thin-walled hypodense structures on CT, with poorly or nonenhancing walls (Fig. 80-17). Diffusely replaced pancreas may be mistaken for a tumor. Calcification is commonly seen throughout the pancreas and is well appreciated on CT. It may be relatively easier to discriminate serous cystadenoma on CT, which appears as focal enlargement of the pancreas and has a microcystic appearance with or without a central scar and calcification.[57,59]

MRI

MRI does not offer any significant additional advantage except for detecting a few more cystic lesions and better characterization (Fig. 80-18).[57]

Classic Signs: Von Hippel-Lindau Disease

- Multiple cysts in pancreas and kidneys
- Solid lesions of pancreas and kidneys

Differential Diagnosis

A correct and early diagnosis of VHL is vital for patient management and the detection of asymptomatic relatives.[58] Screening in families affected by VHL permits timely genetic counseling and early identification of potentially life-threatening sequelae. Screening programs should minimally include evaluation of the eyes, CNS, and abdomen. Accurate, noninvasive imaging of the CNS and abdomen should begin in the early or middle teens.

Abdominal ultrasonography, although an attractive screening tool owing to low cost and the absence of ionizing radiation, is insensitive for isolated pancreatic cysts and small renal and pancreatic tumors. Contrast-enhanced CT of the abdomen is the preferred modality for initial evaluation of pancreatic lesions. Follow-up screening, especially in younger individuals (≤16 years of age) at risk for VHL can be performed using ultrasonography. MRI has a limited role in screening for VHL because of its expense.[60]

Treatment

Solid neoplasms of pancreas and kidney, especially the malignant lesions, need to be surgically treated. Serous cystadenomas may require surgical resection when causing symptoms.

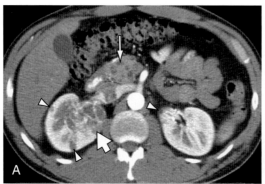
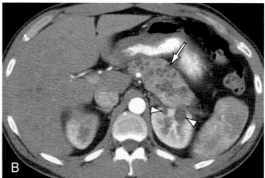

■ **FIGURE 80-17** Von Hippel-Lindau disease. Axial CT images through the head (**A**) and body-tail (**B**) of the pancreas reveal multiple thin-walled cystic lesions in the pancreas (*arrows*) and kidneys (*arrowheads*). In addition is noted a complex cystic lesion in the right kidney (*large arrow,* **A**), which was proven at biopsy to be renal cell carcinoma.

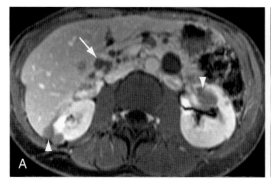
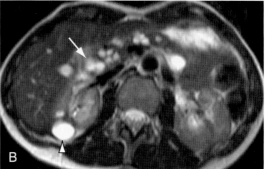

■ **FIGURE 80-18** Von Hippel-Lindau disease. Contrast-enhanced axial T1W (**A**) and T2W fat-suppressed (**B**) gradient-recalled-echo MR images reveal multiple cysts in the pancreas (*arrows*) and kidneys (*arrowheads*).

What the Referring Physician Needs to Know: Von Hippel-Lindau Disease

- Early screening can result in timely recognition of life-threatening manifestations.

KEY POINTS

Cystic Fibrosis

- Autosomal recessive
- Benign, but progressive
- Race and family history
- Sweat chloride test
- Fatty changes, cystosis, fibrosis
- Exocrine/endocrine insufficiency
- Procarcinogenic

Fatty Replacement (Lipomatosis) of Pancreas

- Fatty replacement
- Old age, diabetes mellitus, obesity, Cushing's disease, corticosteroids

Amyloidosis

- Systemic illness
- Secondary involvement
- Primary involvement rare

Hemochromatosis

- Autosomal dominant
- Irreversible changes if not treated
- Race and family history
- Systemic involvement
- Hyperdense pancreas on CT
- Hypointense liver and pancreas on MRI
- Regular phlebotomies

Tuberculosis

- Immunocompromised, HIV patients, immigrants
- Granulomatous disorder
- Caseation, necrosis, abscess
- Lymph nodes with necrosis
- Acid-fast staining
- Polymerase chain assay
- Treatable with antituberculous therapy

AIDS

- Opportunistic infection
- Drug-induced pancreatic involvement
- Disseminated disease

Lymphoma

- Non-Hodgkin's lymphoma
- Secondary involvement common
- Jaundice rare

- Homogeneous
- Lymphadenopathy
- Lack of pancreatic ductal dilatation
- Engulfment of vessels
- PET/CT for staging
- Chemotherapy ± irradiation and immunotherapy
- Prognosis better than that of carcinoma

Leukemia

- Homogeneous appearance
- Pancreatic duct not commensurately dilated
- Jaundice not a common feature
- ± Lymphadenopathy
- Good response to antileukemic therapy

Carcinoma

- Poor prognosis
- Heterogeneous predominantly hypoattenuating
- Necrosis and calcification
- Distant metastases
- Vascular encasement
- Lymphadenopathy
- Lymphoma—main differential disorder
- Palliative management

Metastases

- Rare
- Occasionally first manifestation of metastatic process
- High clinical suspicion
- Overlapping imaging features with other disease processes
- Primary lesion with metastases at other sites

Congenital Hyperinsulinism of Infancy (Nesidioblastosis)

- Neonate
- Hypoglycemia
- Overlapping imaging features
- [18F]Fluoro-L-DOPA-labeled PET/CT
- Surgical resection

Von Hippel-Lindau Disease

- Family history
- Genetic screening
- Multiple cysts in pancreas and kidneys
- Serous cystadenomas of pancreas
- Other organ system involvement
- Regular screening

SUGGESTED READINGS

Beazley RM, Cohn I Jr. Pancreatic cancer. CA Cancer J Clin 1981; 31:346-358.

Choi EK, Byun JH, Lee SJ, et al. Imaging findings of leukemic involvement of the pancreaticobiliary system in adults. AJR Am J Roentgenol 2007; 188:1589-1595.

Falk RH, Comenzo RL, Skinner M. The systemic amyloidoses. N Engl J Med 1997; 337:898-909.

Fishman RS, Bartholomew LG. Severe pancreatic involvement in three generations in von Hippel-Lindau disease. Mayo Clin Proc 1979; 54:329-331.

Katz DS, Hines J, Math KR, et al. Using CT to reveal fat-containing abnormalities of the pancreas. AJR Am J Roentgenol 1999; 172: 393-396.

Knowles KF, Saltman D, Robson HG, Lalonde R. Tuberculous pancreatitis. Tubercle 1990; 71:65-68.

Ladas SD, Vaidakis E, Lariou C, et al. Pancreatic tuberculosis in non-immunocompromised patients: reports of two cases and a literature review. Eur J Gastroenterol Hepatol 1998; 10:973-976.

Merkle EM, Bender GN, Brambs HJ. Imaging findings in pancreatic lymphoma: differential aspects. AJR Am J Roentgenol 2000; 174: 671-675.

Merkle EM, Boaz T, Kolokythas O, et al. Metastases to the pancreas. Br J Radiol 1998; 71:1208-1214.

Miller FH, Gore RM, Nemcek AA Jr, Fitzgerald SW. Pancreaticobiliary manifestations of AIDS. AJR Am J Roentgenol 1996; 166:1269-1274.

Patel S, Bellon EM, Haaga J, Park CH. Fat replacement of the exocrine pancreas. AJR Am J Roentgenol 1980; 135:843-845.

REFERENCES

1. Ferrozzi F, Bova D, Campodonico F, et al. Cystic fibrosis: MR assessment of pancreatic damage. Radiology 1996; 198:875-879.

2. Oppenheimer EH, Esterly JR. Pathology of cystic fibrosis: review of the literature and comparison with 146 autopsied cases. Perspect Pediatr Pathol 1975; 2:241-278.

3. Liu P, Daneman A, Stringer DA, Durie PR. Pancreatic cysts and calcification in cystic fibrosis. Can Assoc Radiol J 1986; 37:279-282.

4. Tham RT, Heyerman HG, Falke TH, et al. Cystic fibrosis: MR imaging of the pancreas. Radiology 1991; 179:183-186.

5. Daneman A, Gaskin K, Martin DJ, Cutz E. Pancreatic changes in cystic fibrosis: CT and sonographic appearances. AJR Am J Roentgenol 1983; 141:653-655.

6. Berrocal T, Pajares MP, Zubillaga AF. Pancreatic cystosis in children and young adults with cystic fibrosis: sonographic, CT, and MRI findings. AJR Am J Roentgenol 2005; 184:1305-1309.

7. Liou TG, Adler FR, Cahill BC, et al. Survival effect of lung transplantation among patients with cystic fibrosis. JAMA 2001; 286:2683-2689.

8. Penn I. De novo malignances in pediatric organ transplant recipients. Pediatr Transplant 1998; 2:56-63.

9. Ibrahim YH, Yee D. Insulin-like growth factor-I and cancer risk. Growth Horm IGF Res 2004; 14:261-269.

10. Matsumoto S, Mori H, Miyake H, et al. Uneven fatty replacement of the pancreas: evaluation with CT. Radiology 1995; 194:453-458.

11. Segovia Garcia C, Quilez Barrenechea JI, Vidales Arechaga L, et al. Pancreatic involvement in primary amyloidosis: radiologic findings. Eur Radiol 2002; 12:774-778.

12. Erdman RA, Vandersall JH. Effect of rumen protein degradability on milk yield of dairy cows in early lactation. J Dairy Sci 1983; 66: 1873-1880.

13. Long JA Jr, Doppman JL, Nienhus AW, Mills SR. Computed tomographic analysis of beta-thalassemic syndromes with hemochromatosis: pathologic findings with clinical and laboratory correlations. J Comput Assist Tomogr 1980; 4:159-165.

14. Haaga JR, Lanzieri CF, Gilkeson RC. The pancreas. In Haaga JR (ed). Computed Tomography and Magnetic Resonance Imaging of the Whole Body, 4th ed. Philadelphia, Elsevier, 2003, pp 1395-1485.

15. Hayes AM, Jaramillo D, Levy HL, Knisely AS. Neonatal hemochromatosis: diagnosis with MR imaging. AJR Am J Roentgenol 1992; 159:623-625.

16. Gandon Y, Guyader D, Heautot JF, et al. Hemochromatosis: diagnosis and quantification of liver iron with gradient-echo MR imaging. Radiology 1994; 193:533-538.

17. Woodfield JC, Windsor JA, Godfrey CC, et al. Diagnosis and management of isolated pancreatic tuberculosis: recent experience and literature review. Aust NZ J Surg 2004; 74:368-371.

18. De Backer AI, Mortele KJ, Bomans P, et al. Tuberculosis of the pancreas: MRI features. AJR Am J Roentgenol 2005; 184:50-54.

19. Schapiro RH, Maher MM, Misdraji J. Case records of the Massachusetts General Hospital. Case 3-2006. A 63-year-old woman with jaundice and a pancreatic mass. N Engl J Med 2006; 354:398-406.

20. Pitchenik AE, Fertel D. Medical management of AIDS patients. Tuberculosis and nontuberculous mycobacterial disease. Med Clin North Am 1992; 76:121-171.

21. De Backer AI, Mortele KJ, Bomans P, et al. Tuberculosis of the pancreas: MRI features. AJR Am J Roentgenol 2005; 184:50-54.

22. Fischer G, Spengler U, Neubrand M, Sauerbruch T. Isolated tuberculosis of the pancreas masquerading as a pancreatic mass. Am J Gastroenterol 1995; 90:2227-2230.

23. Takhtani D, Gupta S, Suman K, et al. Radiology of pancreatic tuberculosis: a report of three cases. Am J Gastroenterol 1996; 91:1832-1834.

24. Itaba S, Yoshinaga S, Nakamura K, et al. Endoscopic ultrasound-guided fine-needle aspiration for the diagnosis of peripancreatic tuberculous lymphadenitis. J Gastroenterol 2007; 42:83-86.

25. Eyer-Silva WA, de Sa CA, Pinto JF, Gameiro CA. Pancreatic tuberculosis as a manifestation of infection with the human immunodeficiency virus. Clin Infect Dis 1993; 16:332.

26. Iwai T, Kida M, Kida Y, et al. Biliary tuberculosis causing cicatricial stenosis after oral anti-tuberculosis therapy. World J Gastroenterol 2006; 12:4914-4917.

27. Teo LL, Venkatesh SK, Ho KY. Clinics in diagnostic imaging. Singapore Med J 2007; 48:687-692; quiz 692.

28. Joe L, Ansher AF, Gordin FM. Severe pancreatitis in an AIDS patient in association with cytomegalovirus infection. South Med J 1989; 82:1444-1445.

29. Drew WL, Buhles W, Erlich KS. Herpesvirus infections (cytomegalovirus, herpes simplex virus, varicella-zoster virus). How to use ganciclovir (DHPG) and acyclovir. Infect Dis Clin North Am 1988; 2:495-509.

30. Saif MW, Khubchandani S, Walczak M. Secondary pancreatic involvement by a diffuse large B-cell lymphoma presenting as acute pancreatitis. World J Gastroenterol 2007; 13:4909-4911.

31. Behrns KE, Sarr MG, Strickler JG. Pancreatic lymphoma: is it a surgical disease? Pancreas 1994; 9:662-667.

32. Nishimura R, Takakuwa T, Hoshida Y, et al. Primary pancreatic lymphoma: clinicopathological analysis of 19 cases from Japan and review of the literature. Oncology 2001; 60:322-329.

33. Dawson IM, Cornes JS, Morson BC. Primary malignant lymphoid tumours of the intestinal tract: report of 37 cases with a study of factors influencing prognosis. Br J Surg 1961; 49:80-89.

34. Prayer L, Schurawitzki H, Mallek R, Mostbeck G. CT in pancreatic involvement of non-Hodgkin lymphoma. Acta Radiol 1992; 33:123-127.

35. Arcari A, Anselmi E, Bernuzzi P, et al. Primary pancreatic lymphoma: a report of five cases. Haematologica 2005; 90:ECR09.

36. Neiman RS, Barcos M, Berard C, et al. Granulocytic sarcoma: a clinicopathologic study of 61 biopsied cases. Cancer 1981; 48: 1426-1437.

37. Matsueda K, Yamamoto H, Doi I. An autopsy case of granulocytic sarcoma of the porta hepatis causing obstructive jaundice. J Gastroenterol 1998; 33:428-433.

38. Kaplan JO, Isikoff MB, Barkin J, Livingstone AS. Necrotic carcinoma of the pancreas: "the pseudo-pseudocyst." J Comput Assist Tomogr 1980; 4:166-167.

39. Wittenberg J, Simeone JF, Ferrucci JT Jr, et al. Non-focal enlargement in pancreatic carcinoma. Radiology 1982; 144:131-135.

40. Mendez G Jr, Isikoff MB, Hill MC. CT of acute pancreatitis: interim assessment. AJR Am J Roentgenol 1980; 135:463-469.

41. Rubin E, Dunham WK, Stanley RJ. Pancreatic metastases in bone sarcomas: CT demonstration. J Comput Assist Tomogr 1985; 9:886-888.

42. Charnsangavej C, Whitley NO. Metastases to the pancreas and peripancreatic lymph nodes from carcinoma of the right side of the colon: CT findings in 12 patients. AJR Am J Roentgenol 1993; 160:49-52.

43. Rumancik WM, Megibow AJ, Bosniak MA, Hilton S. Metastatic disease to the pancreas: evaluation by computed tomography. J Comput Assist Tomogr 1984; 8:829-834.

44. Muranaka T, Teshima K, Honda H, et al. Computed tomography and histologic appearance of pancreatic metastases from distant sources. Acta Radiol 1989; 30:615-619.

45. Swensen T, Osnes M, Serck-Hanssen A. Endoscopic retrograde cholangiopancreatography in primary and secondary tumours of the pancreas. Br J Radiol 1980; 53:760-764.

46. Niccolini DG, Graham JH, Banks PA. Tumor-induced acute pancreatitis. Gastroenterology 1976; 71:142-145.

47. Rodriguez J, Kasberg C, Nipper M, et al. CT-guided needle biopsy of the pancreas: a retrospective analysis of diagnostic accuracy. Am J Gastroenterol 1992; 87:1610-1613.

48. Giovannini M, Seitz JF, Monges G, et al. Fine-needle aspiration cytology guided by endoscopic ultrasonography: results in 141 patients. Endoscopy 1995; 27:171-177.

49. Aynsley-Green A, Hussain K, Hall J, et al. Practical management of hyperinsulinism in infancy. Arch Dis Child Fetal Neonatal Ed 2000; 82:F98-F107.

50. Clayton PT, Eaton S, Aynsley-Green A, et al. Hyperinsulinism in short-chain L-3-hydroxyacyl-CoA dehydrogenase deficiency reveals the importance of beta-oxidation in insulin secretion. J Clin Invest 2001; 108:457-465.

51. Suchi M, MacMullen C, Thornton PS, et al. Histopathology of congenital hyperinsulinism: retrospective study with genotype correlations. Pediatr Dev Pathol 2003; 6:322-333.

52. Fournet JC, Mayaud C, de Lonlay P, et al. Unbalanced expression of 11p15 imprinted genes in focal forms of congenital hyperinsulinism: association with a reduction to homozygosity of a mutation in *ABCC8* or *KCNJ11*. Am J Pathol 2001; 158:2177-2184.

53. Subramaniam RM, Karantanis D, Peller PJ. [18F]Fluoro-L-dopa PET/CT in congenital hyperinsulinism. J Comput Assist Tomogr 2007; 31:770-772.

54. Kim WY, Kaelin WG. Role of *VHL* gene mutation in human cancer. J Clin Oncol 2004; 22:4991-5004.

55. Mohr VH, Vortmeyer AO, Zhuang Z, et al. Histopathology and molecular genetics of multiple cysts and microcystic (serous) adenomas of the pancreas in von Hippel-Lindau patients. Am J Pathol 2000; 157:1615-1621.

56. Hammel PR, Vilgrain V, Terris B, et al. Pancreatic involvement in von Hippel-Lindau disease. The Groupe Francophone d'Étude de la Maladie de von Hippel-Lindau. Gastroenterology 2000; 119:1087-1095.

57. Choyke PL, Glenn GM, Walther MM, et al. von Hippel-Lindau disease: genetic, clinical, and imaging features. Radiology 1995; 194:629-642.

58. Elli L, Buscarini E, Portugalli V, et al. Pancreatic involvement in von Hippel-Lindau disease: report of two cases and review of the literature. Am J Gastroenterol 2006; 101:2655-2658.

59. Bergmann LS, Russell JC, Gladstone A, Devers T. Cystadenomas of the pancreas. Am Surg 1992; 58:65-71.

60. Choyke PL, Filling-Katz MR, Shawker TH, et al. von Hippel-Lindau disease: radiologic screening for visceral manifestations. Radiology 1990; 174:815-820.

Index

Focal xanthogranulomatous cholecystitis, 922-923
Four-dimensional ultrasound
    breast cyst on, 52f
    cholelithiasis on, 52f
    fetal spine on, 52f
    intestinal ascites on, 51f
    limitations of, 53
    opacity mode, 53t
    pregnancy on, 51f
    pros and cons of, 52-53
    rendering methods, 50, 53t
    technical aspects, 49-50
    transducers, 49, 50f
    urinary bladder on, 51f
Fourier transform, 106
Frequency-encoding artifacts, MRI, 115-116, 116t
FSGS. *See* Focal segmental glomerulosclerosis (FSGS).
Functional magnetic resonance cholangiography (fMRC), 929-932, 933t
    biliary leaks in, 934-936
Functional magnetic resonance cholangiopancreatography (fMRC), 787-788
Fungal peritonitis, 1416
Fungal splenic infections, 978-980

G

Gadobenate dimeglumine, 124, 930-931
Gadolinium contrast. *See also* Contrast-enhanced MRI.
    chemical structure of, 118
    liver-specific, 124
    in MRI of liver, 534
    nephrogenic systemic fibrosis and, 109-110
    pregnancy and, 109
Gadolinium-ethoxybenzyl-diethylenetriaminepentaacetic acid, 931
Gallbladder
    adenoma, 919-921
    anatomy, 837-840, 933
    calcified, 8
    carcinoma, 925-927
    congenital anomaly classification, 843t
    ectopic, 844-845, 847
    on endoscopic retrograde cholangiopancreatography, 843t
    imaging
        controversies in, 837
        technical aspects, 833-836
    lymphoma, 909
    malignancy, 909-912
    on MR cholangiopancreatography, 835-836, 843t
    on MRI, 835, 837-840
    pathology, 933-940
    porcelain, 8, 906f, 907
    tumors
        classification of, 876t
        clinical presentation of, 875
        on CT, 877
        differential diagnosis of, 879
        epidemiology of, 875
        etiology of, 875
        imaging algorithm for, 878
        imaging of, 876-878
        medical treatment of, 879
        on MRI, 877-878
        on nuclear medicine, 878
        pathology of, 875-876

Gallbladder *(Continued)*
        pathophysiology of, 875
        on PET, 878, 879f
        prevalence of, 875
        on radiography, 876
        staging of, 876t
        surgical treatment of, 879
        treatment of, 879-880
        on ultrasonography, 878
    on ultrasound, 28, 833-835, 838t, 843t
        cholangiopancreatography *vs.*, 838t
    variants, 842-845, 844f
    varices, 41f
Gallbladder agenesis, 842-844, 846
Gallbladder duplication, 844, 846-847
Gallbladder wall
    normal, 898
    thickened
        diffuse, 898-899
            primary, 899-914
            secondary, 914-917
        focal, 919, 920t
Gamna-Gandy bodies, 993f
Gangrenous cholecystitis, 902-903, 902f
Gantry rotation time, 76t
Gartner's duct cyst, 1385
Gas
    in portal vein, 7-8
    on radiography, 7
        extraluminal, 7-8
        intraluminal, 7, 7f
        in pneumoperitoneum, 7-8, 8f
        in small bowel, 9-10
Gastric adenocarcinoma, 249f
Gastric anatomy and function, 273
Gastric cancer. *See also* Mucosal diseases of stomach, malignant.
    on CT, 223-224
    metastatic lymphadenopathy in, 1032f
    nodal involvement in, 1033-1034
    nodal staging of, 1031t
    on PET, 150-151
    staging, 224t
Gastric distention, 226, 227f
Gastric duplication, 231
Gastric emptying
    delayed, 274-277
        diabetes mellitus and, 275, 275t, 276f
        functional, 275-277, 275t
        mechanical, 275f
    factors affecting, 275
Gastric fold thickening, 219
Gastric function imaging
    accuracy in, 272t
    controversies in, 272
    limitations of, 272t
    normal, 274
    pharmacologic adjuncts in, 271
    pitfalls in, 272t
    pros and cons of, 272
    radiopharmaceuticals in, 271
    technical aspects, 271-272
    technique, 271-272
Gastric hernia, 231-232
Gastric herniation, 232
Gastric leiomyosarcoma, 226
Gastric lymphoma, 224, 249f
Gastric metastases, 226
Gastric mucosal disease
    benign
        clinical presentation of, 240
        on CT, 241, 243t
            diffuse, 243
        differential diagnosis, 243

Gastric mucosal disease *(Continued)*
        epidemiology of, 239-240
        etiology of, 239
        imaging of, 241-243
        in nuclear medicine, 242, 243t
            diffuse, 243
        pathology of, 240-241
        prevalence of, 239-240
        on radiography, 241, 243t
            diffuse, 243
        surgical treatment of, 244
        treatment of, 243-244
    malignant
        clinical presentation of, 246
        on CT, 247, 248f, 250t
        differential diagnosis, 249-250
        epidemiology of, 246
        etiology of, 246
        imaging of, 247-249
        in nuclear medicine, 248
        pathology of, 247
        on PET, 248, 250t
        prevalence of, 246
        on radiography, 247, 248f, 250t
        surgical treatment of, 250
        treatment of, 250
        on ultrasound, 248
Gastric nodes, 1004-1005
Gastric outlet obstruction
    anatomy in, 257
    Brunner's gland hyperplasia and, 256, 257f
    clinical presentation of, 257
    on CT, 258
    differential diagnosis, 259
    epidemiology of, 256-257
    etiology of, 256
    imaging, 258-259
    imaging algorithm, 259
    on MRI, 258
    in nuclear medicine, 259
    pathology of, 257
    on PET, 259
    prevalence of, 256-257
    on radiography, 258
    surgical treatment of, 260
    treatment of, 259-260
    on ultrasound, 258-259
Gastric polyps
    causes of, 240
    on CT, 242
    imaging of, 242
    on radiography, 242
Gastric remnant, 1400f
Gastric ulcer
    in barium study, 217-218, 241f
    causes of, 239
    on CT, 221-222, 241, 242f
    delayed gastric emptying and, 275t
    imaging of, 241-242
    types of, 239
Gastric variants
    acquired, 231-236
    congenital, 231
Gastric varices, 202, 226
Gastric volvulus, 232-234, 262, 264f
Gastrinoma, 735t. *See also* Pancreatic endocrine neoplasms (PENs).
Gastroduodenal artery, 339, 340f-341f
Gastroenteritis
    delayed gastric emptying and, 275t
    eosinophilic, 371-373, 1426-1427
Gastrohepatic ligament, 1397-1398
Gastrohepatic ligament nodes, 1004t, 1005, 1019t

HIV. *See* Human immunodeficiency virus (HIV).
Hollow viscus perforation
  classic signs of, 199b
  clinical presentation of, 195
  on CT, 196f, 197-198, 199f, 199t
  differential diagnosis, 199
  epidemiology of, 195
  etiology of, 195
  imaging algorithm for, 199
  imaging of, 196-199
  pathology of, 196
  pathophysiology of, 195-196
  prevalence of, 195
  on radiography, 196-197, 199t
  surgical treatment of, 200
  treatment of, 200
Horseshoe kidney, 1240
Human immunodeficiency virus (HIV).
  See also Acquired immune deficiency syndrome (AIDS).
  lymphadenopathy in, 1017, 1021
  nephropathy associated with, 1145-1146
Hydrocele, 1359t, 1363-1364
Hydronephrosis
  definition of, 1177
  renal papillary necrosis *vs.*, 1164
Hyperbilirubinemia, 543-544
Hyperinsulinism, 806t-808t, 810t, 822-823
Hyperlipasemia syndrome, 744
Hyperrotation, 442t, 445
Hypertension
  portal, 39-41
  renovascular, 1079-1080, 1150-1154
Hypogastric hernia, 1466t
Hypovascular hepatic metastases, 57t, 574t, 589f

I

Iatrogenic ureteral stricture, 1198-1200
IgA. *See* Immunoglobulin A (IgA).
Ileal carcinoid, 96f
Ileostomy enema, 286
Iliac bone, 1440f
Iliac vessels, 1442f
Iliococcygeus muscle, 1440f
Immunoglobulin A (IgA) disease, 1127, 1132-1133
Impotence. *See* Erectile dysfunction.
Incarcerated inguinal hernia, 1359t
Incisional hernias, 1466t, 1471-1472
Infants
  biliary atresia in, 544-545
  jaundice in, 543-544
  neonatal hepatitis in, 545
  normal hepatobiliary scintigraphy in, 539-540
Infectious colitis
  etiology of, 449
  sites of involvement, 425t
Infectious enteritis
  Crohn's disease *vs.*, 366-367
  on ultrasound, 298t
Infectious small bowel disease, 367-370
Infectious splenic lesions, 970t-971t
Infective lymphadenitis, 1017-1018
Inferior epigastric muscle, 1440f
Inferior epigastric vessels, 1442f
Inferior mesenteric artery, 39, 339, 341f-342f, 445t
Inferior mesenteric nodes, 1004t, 1006-1007
Inferior mesenteric vein, 445t

Inferior vena cava
  anatomy of, 37
  in asplenia, 976
  Doppler ultrasound of, 35t, 38t
Inferior vena cava disorders, 47
Inflammatory bowel disease
  lymphadenitis in, 1018, 1022
  ureteral stricture and, 1204-1205
Inflammatory colonic lesions
  clinical presentation of, 449
  on CT, 452-460
  enhancement patterns in, 450-451
  epidemiology of, 449
  etiology of, 449
  extraintestinal manifestations of, 451
  imaging of, 450-460
  length of involvement in, 450
  location of involvement in, 450
  on MRI, 460
  pathophysiology of, 449-450
  prevalence of, 449
  on radiography, 451-452
  "target" sign in, 452, 454f
  thickening in, 450
  "thumbprinting" sign in, 451, 452f
Inflammatory fibroid polyp, 377
Inflammatory pseudotumor
  mesenteric, 1428-1429
  splenic
    clinical presentation of, 957
    on CT, 957, 957f
    differential diagnosis, 958
    epidemiology of, 957
    etiology of, 957
    imaging of, 957-958
    on MRI, 957
    pathology of, 957
    pathophysiology of, 957
    on PET, 958
    prevalence of, 957
    on radiography, 957
    surgical treatment of, 958
    treatment of, 958
    on ultrasound, 958
  urinary bladder
    on CT, 1220, 1221f
    on MRI, 1221
    pathology of, 1218
    prevalence and epidemiology of, 1217
    treatment of, 1222
Inframesocolic spaces, 1400-1401, 1401f
Infundibulopelvic dysgenesis, 1243
Inguinal canal, 1441-1442
Inguinal hernia, 1466t, 1467-1468
  incarcerated, 1359t, 1368
Inguinal ligament, 1442f
Inguinal nodes, 1004t, 1005f-1006f, 1007, 1012f
Inguinal rings, 1440f
Insulinoma, 735t. *See also* Pancreatic endocrine neoplasms (PENs).
Interfascial spread, 1403-1404
Internal hernia
  on CT, 405, 406f
  imaging of, 405
  pathology of, 401
  on radiography, 405
Internal iliac nodes, 1004t, 1005f-1006f, 1007
Internal inguinal ring, 1440f, 1442f
Internal oblique muscle, 1440f
Interparietal hernia, 1471-1472
Interstitial hernia, 1471-1472
Interventional fluoroscopic procedures, 15

Intestinal atresia
  classic signs of, 403b
  imaging of, 403
  pathophysiology of, 401
  on radiography, 403
Intestinal lymphangiectasia, 371-373
Intestinal malrotation, 235
Intestinal obstruction. *See also* Small bowel obstruction (SBO).
  CT for, 10
  on radiography, 9-10
Intraductal papillary mucinous neoplasms, 757-761
Intrahepatic bile duct tumors
  classification of, 883t
  clinical presentation of, 882
  on CT, 885
  differential diagnosis, 887
  epidemiology of, 882
  etiology of, 882
  imaging algorithm for, 887
  imaging of, 884-887
  medical treatment of, 887-888
  on MRI, 885
  in nuclear medicine, 886
  pathology of, 883-884
  pathophysiology of, 882-883
  on PET, 886
  prevalence of, 882
  on radiography, 884
  staging of, 883t
  surgical treatment of, 888
  treatment of, 887-888
  on ultrasonography, 885-886
Intraoperative cholangiography, 934
Intrapancreatic metastases, 738-740
Intravenous CT contrast media, 93-97, 423
Intravenous pyelography, 1059t, 1244f
Intravenous urography, 1046-1049
Intussusception
  on CT, 329f, 404f, 405
  imaging of, 403-405
  pathophysiology of, 401
  on radiography, 9, 404-405
  on ultrasound, 298, 405
Inverse cecum, 442t, 445-446
Iodine
  as CT contrast agent, 93
  in liver imaging, 517-518
  as fluoroscopic contrast agent, 15f, 16, 18
Iopamidol, 93
Ischemia
  mesenteric, 43, 44t
    imaging of, 347-349
    nonocclusive, 347-349
      on angiography, 348-349
      on CT, 348
      on MRI, 348
  small bowel
    acute
      anatomy in, 339-340
      on angiography, 339t, 344-350, 351f
      clinical presentation of, 338-339
      on CT, 343-344, 345f, 347-349, 350f
      differential diagnosis, 351-352
      epidemiology of, 338
      etiology of, 338
      imaging, 342-350
      on MRI, 339t, 344, 348-349
      pathology of, 340-342
      pathophysiology of, 339-340
      prevalence of, 338
      on radiography, 343
      surgical treatment of, 352

Ischemia *(Continued)*
>treatment of, 352
>on ultrasound, 339t, 344, 347, 349
>chronic
>>on angiography, 356, 357f, 358t
>>clinical presentation of, 354
>>on CT, 355, 358t
>>differential diagnosis, 358
>>epidemiology of, 354
>>etiology of, 354
>>imaging algorithms for, 357
>>imaging of, 354-357
>>on MRI, 355-356
>>pathology of, 354
>>pathophysiology of, 354
>>prevalence of, 354
>>on radiography, 354, 358t
>>treatment of, 358-359
>>on ultrasound, 356, 358t
Ischemic colitis
>in barium enema study, 418
>sites of involvement, 425t
Isolated dextrogastria, 231
Isomolar contrast agents, CT, 87

J

Jejunojejunostomy, 1400f
Junctional parenchymal defect, 1237, 1238f
Juxtaglomerular tumors, 1093-1094

K

Kaposi's sarcoma, 1021
Kidney(s), 1037. *See also Entries at Renal.*
>anatomy, 1045, 1059-1060
>angiography of, 1059t
>ascent anomalies in, 1239
>collecting system, 1045
>computer-aided techniques with, 180
>contrast media and, CT, 88
>on CT, 1046
>>MRI *vs.*, 1068-1069
>>normal anatomy, 1059-1060
>>parameters, 1058t
>>in preoperative planning, 1063-1064
>>pros and cons, 1057-1059
>>technical aspects, 1057
>>in trauma, 1058t, 1065-1066
>horseshoe, 1240
>medullary sponge, 1164, 1246-1247
>on MRI, 1059t
>>morphologic, 1068
>>normal anatomy, 1069-1070
>>pros and cons, 1068-1069
>>solid mass characterization, 1070-1071
>>technical aspects, 1068
>>ultrasound *vs.*, 1068
>multicystic dysplastic, 1241
>in nuclear medicine, 1059t
>>controversies, 1077-1078
>>imaging, 1078-1079
>>pros and cons, 1076-1077
>>technical aspects, 1075-1076
>pancake, 1240
>pelvic, 1239
>on PET, 140, 1059t
>polycystic, 181f
>radiography of, 1046
>response to increase in bulk, 1132f
>response to loss of bulk, 1131f
>trauma to, CT in, 1058t, 1065-1066
>on ultrasound, 1049-1055

Kidney(s) *(Continued)*
>ultrasound of, 28
>>MRI *vs.*, 1068
>vascular anatomy, 1045
>volumetry, 176
Klatskin tumor, 787, 860f-861f, 891
K-space, 106, 106f
KVp. *See* Tube potential (kVp).

L

Lateral conal plane, 1402f
Left inframesocolic space, 1400-1401, 1401f
Left paracolic gutter, 1401f
Left pararectal space, 1401f
Left renal vein abnormalities, 1251
Left supracolic spaces, 1400
Leiomyoma
>female urethral, 1386-1387
>renal, 1092-1093
>small bowel, 375-376
>urinary bladder
>>calcification in, 1219
>>on computed tomography, 1219f
>>on MRI, 1221
>>pathology of, 1218
>>prevalence and epidemiology of, 1217
>>treatment of, 1222
Leiomyosarcoma
>gastric, 226
>urinary bladder, 1230
Lesser sac, 1400, 1401f
Lesser sciatic foramen, 1440f
Lesser space, 1401f
Leukemia
>pancreatic involvement in, 806t-808t, 810t, 819-820
>renal, 1104-1106, 1107t
Leukocyte scintigraphy, 307-309
Leydig cell tumors, 1372. *See also* Testicular cancer.
Lienorenal collateral vessels, 37f
Ligamentum venosum, 1400f
Linea alba, 1440f
Linear sequential array transducer, 21
Linear vascular impressions on renal pelvis, 1239
Linitis plastica, 218-219
Lipoma
>abdominal wall, 1456-1457
>in barium study, 419
>small bowel, 374
Littre hernia, 1471-1472
Liver. *See also Entries at Hepatic.*
>abscess
>>on contrast-enhanced ultrasound, 57t
>>on ultrasound, 514f
>arterial anatomy, 161f, 677
>cirrhosis
>>CT of, 524
>>nonalcoholic
>>>classic signs of, 617b
>>>clinical presentation of, 608-609
>>>on CT, 610f, 611-612, 616f, 617t
>>>differential diagnosis, 618
>>>epidemiology of, 608
>>>etiology of, 607-608
>>>fibrosis in, 611, 614, 616
>>>grading of, 608
>>>hepatic encephalopathy in, 608
>>>hepatorenal syndrome in, 608
>>>hepatorenal syndrome *vs.*, 618
>>>hyperdynamic circulation in, 607-608
>>>imaging algorithm for, 616

Liver *(Continued)*
>>>imaging of, 609-616, 617t
>>>on MRI, 612-615, 616f, 617t
>>>nuclear medicine in, 616
>>>pathology of, 609
>>>prevalence of, 608
>>>on radiography, 609-611
>>>surgical treatment of, 619
>>>treatment of, 618-619
>>>on ultrasound, 615-616, 617t
>>primary biliary
>>>clinical presentation of, 664
>>>on CT, 665-667
>>>differential diagnosis, 670
>>>epidemiology of, 664
>>>etiology of, 663
>>>imaging algorithm for, 668-669
>>>on MRI, 665-667
>>>pathogenesis of, 663
>>>pathology of, 665
>>>prevalence of, 664
>>>treatment of, 671
>>>on ultrasound, 665-667
>computer-aided techniques with, 179
>CT angiography, 161t
>CT of
>>biliary system in, 524-526
>>collimation in, 519
>>contrast delivery in, 519
>>contrast volume in, 519
>>dual-phase, 517
>>iodinated contrast media in, 517-518
>>multidetector protocols for, 520t
>>pitch in, 519
>>postprocessing, 160, 520-521, 523, 523t
>>pros and cons in, 526-527
>>scan delay in, 519
>>technical aspects, 517-526
>>tumors in, 523-524
>>vascular pathologic processes in, 524
>diffuse disease of
>>lymphadenitis in, 1018, 1022
>>ultrasound in, 515
>>ultrasound of, 515
>MDCT angiography protocol for, 675t
>MR angiography protocol for, 675t
>on MRI, 112t
>MRI contrast agents specific to, 123-124
>MRI of
>>contrast-enhanced, 531-533
>>diffusion-weighted, 534-535
>>dynamic contrast-enhanced, 535
>>gadolinium contrast agents in, 534
>>half-Fourier acquisition single-shot turbo spin-echo sequence (HASTE) in, 531
>>indications for, 529, 530t
>>multichannel systems in, 534
>>new developments in, 534-535
>>parallel imaging in, 534
>>pros and cons in, 535
>>protocol, 530t
>>superparamagnetic iron oxide particles in, 534
>>3.0-T considerations in, 534
>>technical aspects in, 529-534
>>technique optimization in, 534-535
>>time-of-flight sequence in, 533-534
>>T1-weighted imaging in, 529-530
>>T2-weighted imaging in, 530-531
>nonalcoholic fatty liver disease
>>clinical presentation of, 596
>>on CT, 597-599, 603t
>>differential diagnosis, 602-603
>>epidemiology of, 595-596
>>etiology of, 595